Mechanical Ventilation

Physiological and Clinical Applications

PILBEAM'S
Mechanical Ventilation

Physiological and Clinical Applications

J.M. Cairo, PhD, RRT, FAARC
Dean of the School of Allied Health Professions
Professor of Cardiopulmonary Science, Physiology, and Anesthesiology
Louisiana State University Health Sciences Center
New Orleans, Louisiana

ELSEVIER

ELSEVIER

3251 Riverport Lane
St. Louis, Missouri 63043

Notices

Knowledge and best practice in this field are constantly changing. As new research and experience broaden our understanding, changes in research methods, professional practices, or medical treatment may become necessary.

Practitioners and researchers must always rely on their own experience and knowledge in evaluating and using any information, methods, compounds, or experiments described herein. In using such information or methods they should be mindful of their own safety and the safety of others, including parties for whom they have a professional responsibility.

With respect to any drug or pharmaceutical products identified, readers are advised to check the most current information provided (i) on procedures featured or (ii) by the manufacturer of each product to be administered, to verify the recommended dose or formula, the method and duration of administration, and contraindications. It is the responsibility of practitioners, relying on their own experience and knowledge of their patients, to make diagnoses, to determine dosages and the best treatment for each individual patient, and to take all appropriate safety precautions.

To the fullest extent of the law, neither the Publisher nor the authors, contributors, or editors, assume any liability for any injury and/or damage to persons or property as a matter of products liability, negligence or otherwise, or from any use or operation of any methods, products, instructions, or ideas contained in the material herein.

Previous editions copyrighted 2012, 2006, and 1998.

Library of Congress Cataloging-in-Publication Data
Cairo, Jimmy M., author.
   Pilbeam's mechanical ventilation : physiological and clinical applications / J.M. Cairo.—Sixth edition.
     p. ; cm.
   Mechanical ventilation
   ISBN 978-0-323-32009-2 (pbk. : alk. paper)
   I. Title.   II. Title: Mechanical ventilation.
   [DNLM: 1. Respiration Disorders—therapy.   2. Respiration, Artificial.   3. Ventilators, Mechanical.
WF 145]
   RC735.I5
   615.8′36—dc23

                                                                    2015016179

Content Strategist: Sonya Seigafuse
Content Development Manager: Billie Sharp
Content Development Specialist: Charlene Ketchum
Publishing Services Manager: Julie Eddy
Project Manager: Sara Alsup
Design Direction: Teresa McBryan
Cover Designer: Ryan Cook
Text Designer: Ryan Cook

Printed in the United States of America

Last digit is the print number: 9   8   7   6   5   4   3   2   1

To Palmer Grace Wade

For reminding us what is truly important in life.

Contributors

Robert M. DiBlasi, RRT-NPS, FAARC
Seattle Children's Hospital
Seattle, Washington

Terry L. Forrette, MHS, RRT, FAARC
Adjunct Associate Professor of Cardiopulmonary Science
LSU Health Sciences Center
New Orleans, Louisiana

Christine Kearney, BS, RRT-NPS
Clinical Supervisor of Respiratory Care
Seattle Children's Hospital
Seattle, Washington

ANCILLARY CONTRIBUTOR

Sandra T. Hinski, MS, RRT-NPS
Faculty, Respiratory Care Division
Gateway Community College
Phoenix, Arizona

REVIEWERS

Allen Barbaro, MS, RRT
Department Chairman, Respiratory Care Education
St. Luke's College
Sioux City, Iowa

Margaret-Ann Carno, PhD, MBA, CPNP, ABSM, FNAP
Assistant Professor of Clinical Nursing and Pediatrics
School of Nursing
University of Rochester
Rochester, New York

J. Kenneth Le Jeune, MS, RRT, CPFT
Program Director, Respiratory Education
University of Arkansas Community College at Hope
Hope, Arkansas

Tim Op't Holt, EdD, RRT, AE-C, FAARC
Professor
University of South Alabama
Mobile, Alabama

Stephen Wehrman, RRT, RPFT, AE-C
Professor
University of Hawaii
Program Director
Kapiolani Community College
Honolulu, Hawaii

Richard Wettstein, MMEd, FAARC
Director of Clinical Education
University of Texas Health Science Center at San Antonio
San Antonio, Texas

Mary-Rose Wiesner, BS, BCP, RRT
Program Director
Department Chair
Mt. San Antonio College
Walnut, California

Acknowledgments

A number of individuals should be recognized for their contributions to this project. I wish to offer my sincere gratitude to Sue Pilbeam for her continued support throughout this project and for her many years of service to the Respiratory Care profession. I also wish to thank Terry Forrette, MHS, RRT, FAARC, for authoring the chapter on Ventilator Graphics; Rob DiBlasi, RRT-NPS, FAARC, and Christine Kearney, BS, RRT-NPS, who authored the chapter on Neonatal and Pediatric Ventilation; Theresa Gramlich, MS, RRT, for her contributions in earlier editions of this text to the chapters on Noninvasive Positive Pressure Ventilation and Long-Term Ventilation; Paul Barraza, RCP, RRT, for his contributions to the content of the chapter on Special Techniques in Ventilatory Support. I also wish to thank Sandra Hinski, MS, RRT-NPS, for authoring the ancillaries that accompany this text, and Amanda Dexter, MS, RRT, and Gary Milne, BS, RRT, for their suggestions related to ventilator graphics. As in previous editions, I want to express my sincere appreciation to all of the Respiratory Therapy educators and students who provided valuable suggestions and comments during the course of writing and editing the sixth edition of *Pilbeam's Mechanical Ventilation*.

I would like to offer special thanks for the guidance provided by the staff of Elsevier throughout this project, particularly Content Development Strategist, Sonya Seigafuse; Content Development Manager, Billie Sharp; Content Development Specialist, Charlene Ketchum; Project Manager, Sara Alsup; and Publishing Services Manager, Julie Eddy. Their dedication to this project has been immensely helpful and I feel fortunate to have had the opportunity to work with such a professional group.

My wife, Rhonda, has provided loving support for me and for all of our family throughout the preparation of this edition. Her gift of unconditional love and encouragement to our family inspires me every day.

The goal of this text is to provide clinicians with a strong physiological foundation for making informed decisions when managing patients receiving mechanical ventilation. The subject matter presented is derived from current evidence-based practices and is written in a manner that allows this text to serve as a resource for both students and for practicing clinicians. As with previous editions of this text, I have relied on numerous conversations with colleagues about how best to ensure that this goal could be achieved.

It is apparent to clinicians who treat critically ill patients that implementing effective interprofessional care plans is required to achieve successful outcomes. Respiratory therapists are recognized as an integral part of effective interprofessional critical care teams. Their expertise in the areas of mechanical ventilation and respiratory care modalities is particularly valuable considering the pace at which technological advances are occurring in critical care medicine. Indeed, ventilatory support is often vital to a patient's well-being, making it an absolute necessity in the education of respiratory therapists. To be successful, students and instructors must have access to clear and well-designed learning resources to acquire and apply the necessary knowledge and skills associated with administering mechanical ventilation to patients. This text and its resources have been designed to meet that need.

Although significant changes have occurred in the practice of critical care medicine since the first edition of *Mechanical Ventilation* was published in 1985, the underlying philosophy of this text has remained the same—to impart the knowledge necessary to safely, appropriately, and compassionately care for patients requiring ventilatory support. The sixth edition of *Pilbeam's Mechanical Ventilation* is written in a concise manner that explains patient-ventilator interactions. Beginning with the most fundamental concepts and expanding to the more advanced topics, the text guides readers through a series of essential concepts and ideas, building upon the information as they work through the text.

The application of mechanical ventilation principles to patient care is one of the most sophisticated respiratory care applications used in critical care medicine, making frequent reviewing helpful, if not necessary. *Pilbeam's Mechanical Ventilation* can be useful to all critical care practitioners, including practicing respiratory therapists, critical care residents and physicians, and critical care nurse practitioners and physician assistants.

ORGANIZATION

This edition, like previous editions, is organized into a logical sequence of chapters and sections that build upon each other as a reader moves through the book. The initial sections focus on core knowledge and skills needed to apply and initiate mechanical ventilation, whereas the middle and final sections cover specifics of mechanical ventilation patient care techniques, including bedside pulmonary diagnostic testing, hemodynamic testing, pharmacology of ventilated patients, a concise discussion of ventilator associated pneumonia, as well as neonatal and pediatric mechanical

ventilatory techniques and long-term applications of mechanical ventilation. The inclusion of some helpful appendixes further assists the reader in the comprehension of complex material and an easy-access Glossary defines key terms covered in the chapters.

FEATURES

The valuable learning aids that accompany this text are designed to, make it an engaging tool for both educators and students. With clearly defined resources in the beginning of each chapter, students can prepare for the material covered in each chapter through the use of Chapter Outlines, Key Terms, and Learning Objectives.

Along with the abundant use of images and information tables, each chapter also contains:

- **Case Studies:** Concise patient vignettes that list pertinent assessment data and pose a critical thinking question to readers to test their understanding of content learned. Answers can be found in Appendix A.
- **Critical Care Concepts:** Short questions to engage the readers in applying their knowledge of difficult concepts.
- **Clinical Scenarios:** More comprehensive patient scenarios covering patient presentation, assessment data, and treatment therapies. These scenarios are intended for classroom or group discussion.
- **Key Points:** Highlights important information as key concepts are discussed.

Each chapter concludes with:

- A bulleted Chapter Summary for ease of reviewing chapter content
- Chapter Review Questions (with answers in Appendix A)
- A comprehensive list of References at the end of each chapter for those students who wish to learn more about specific topics covered in the text

And finally, several appendixes are included to provide additional resources for readers. These include a Review of Abnormal Physiological Processes, which covers mismatching of pulmonary perfusion and ventilation, mechanical dead space, and hypoxia. A special appendix on Graphic Exercises gives students extra practice in understanding the inter-relationship of flow, volume, and pressure in mechanically ventilated patients. Answer Keys to Case Studies and Critical Care Concepts featured throughout the text and the end-of-chapter Review Questions can help the student to track progress in comprehension of the content.

NEW TO THIS EDITION

This edition of *Pilbeam's Mechanical Ventilation* has been carefully updated to reflect the newer equipment and techniques, including current terminology associated with the various ventilator modalities available to ensure it is in step with the current modes of therapy. To emphasize this new information, Case Studies, Clinical Scenarios, and Critical Care Concepts have been added to each chapter. A new updated chapter on Ventilator Graphics has been included in this edition to provide a practical approach to understanding and applying ventilator graphic analysis to the care of mechanically ventilated patients. Robert DiBlasi and Christine Kearney have updated the chapter on Neonatal and Pediatric Mechanical Ventilation (Chapter 22) to include current information related to the goals of newborn and pediatric respiratory support, including noninvasive and adjunctive forms of ventilator support.

LEARNING AIDS

Workbook

The Workbook for *Pilbeam's Mechanical Ventilation* is an easy-to-use guide designed to help the student focus on the most important information presented in the text. The workbook features exercises directly tied to the learning objectives that appear in the beginning of each chapter. Providing the reinforcement and practice that students need, the workbook features exercises such as key term crossword puzzles, critical thinking questions, case studies, waveform analysis, and NBRC-style multiple choice questions.

FOR EDUCATORS

Educators using the Evolve website for *Pilbeam's Mechanical Ventilation* have access to an array of resources designed to work in coordination with the text and aid in teaching this topic. Educators may use the Evolve resources to plan class time and lessons, supplement class lectures, or create and develop student exams. These Evolve resources offer:

- More than 800 NBRC-style multiple choice test questions in ExamView
- A **new** PowerPoint Presentation with more than 650 slides featuring key information and helpful images
- An Image Collection of the figures appearing in the book

Jim Cairo
New Orleans, Louisiana

Contents

Basic Terms and Concepts of Mechanical Ventilation

OUTLINE

PHYSIOLOGICAL TERMS AND CONCEPTS RELATED TO MECHANICAL VENTILATION
Normal Mechanics of Spontaneous Ventilation
Ventilation and Respiration
Gas Flow and Pressure Gradients During Ventilation
Units of Pressure
Definition of Pressures and Gradients in the Lungs
Lung Characteristics
Compliance
Resistance
Time Constants

TYPES OF VENTILATORS AND TERMS USED IN MECHANICAL VENTILATION
Types of Mechanical Ventilation
Negative Pressure Ventilation
Positive Pressure Ventilation
High-Frequency Ventilation
Definition of Pressures in Positive Pressure Ventilation
Baseline Pressure
Peak Pressure
Plateau Pressure
Pressure at the End of Exhalation
Summary

KEY TERMS

- Acinus
- Airway opening pressure
- Airway pressure
- Alveolar distending pressure
- Ascites
- Auto-PEEP
- Bronchopleural fistulas
- Compliance
- Critical opening pressure
- Elastance
- Esophageal pressure
- External respiration
- Extrinsic PEEP
- Functional residual capacity
- Heterogeneous
- High-frequency jet ventilation
- High-frequency oscillatory ventilation
- High-frequency positive pressure ventilation
- Homogeneous
- Internal respiration
- Intrinsic PEEP
- Mask pressure
- Mouth pressure
- Peak airway pressure
- Peak inspiratory pressure
- Peak pressure
- Plateau pressure
- Positive end-expiratory pressure (PEEP)
- Pressure gradient
- Proximal airway pressure
- Resistance
- Respiration
- Static compliance/static effective compliance
- Time constant
- Transairway pressure
- Transpulmonary pressure
- Transrespiratory pressure
- Transthoracic pressure
- Upper airway pressure
- Ventilation

LEARNING OBJECTIVES   *On completion of this chapter, the reader will be able to do the following:*

1. Define *ventilation, external respiration,* and *internal respiration.*
2. Draw a graph showing how intrapleural and alveolar (intrapulmonary) pressures change during spontaneous ventilation and during a positive pressure breath.
3. Define the terms *transpulmonary pressure, transrespiratory pressure, transairway pressure, transthoracic pressure, elastance, compliance,* and *resistance.*
4. Provide the value for intraalveolar pressure throughout inspiration and expiration during normal, quiet breathing.
5. Write the formulas for calculating compliance and resistance.
6. Explain how changes in lung compliance affect the peak pressure measured during inspiration with a mechanical ventilator.
7. Describe the changes in airway conditions that can lead to increased resistance.
8. Calculate the airway resistance given the peak inspiratory pressure, a plateau pressure, and the flow rate.
9. From a figure showing abnormal compliance or airway resistance, determine which lung unit will fill more quickly or with a greater volume.
10. Compare several time constants, and explain how different time constants will affect volume distribution during inspiration.
11. Give the percentage of passive filling (or emptying) for one, two, three, and five time constants.
12. Briefly discuss the principle of operation of negative pressure, positive pressure, and high-frequency mechanical ventilators.
13. Define *peak inspiratory pressure, baseline pressure, positive end-expiratory pressure* (PEEP), and *plateau pressure.*
14. Describe the measurement of plateau pressure.

Physiological Terms and Concepts Related to Mechanical Ventilation

The purpose of this chapter is to review some basic concepts of the physiology of breathing and to provide a brief description of the pressure, volume, and flow events that occur during the respiratory cycle. The effects of changes in lung characteristics (e.g., respiratory compliance and airway resistance) on the mechanics of breathing are also discussed.

NORMAL MECHANICS OF SPONTANEOUS VENTILATION

Ventilation and Respiration

Spontaneous breathing, or *spontaneous ventilation,* is simply the movement of air into and out of the lungs. Spontaneous **ventilation** is accomplished by contraction of the muscles of inspiration, which causes expansion of the thorax, or chest cavity. During a quiet inspiration, the diaphragm descends and enlarges the vertical size of the thoracic cavity while the external intercostal muscles raise the ribs slightly, increasing the circumference of the thorax. Contraction of the diaphragm and external intercostals provides the energy to move air into the lungs and therefore perform the "work" required to inspire, or inhale. During a maximal spontaneous inspiration, the accessory muscles of breathing are also used to increase the volume of the thorax.

Normal quiet exhalation is passive and does not require any work. During a normal quiet exhalation, the inspiratory muscles simply relax, the diaphragm moves upward, and the ribs return to their resting position. The volume of the thoracic cavity decreases and air is forced out of the alveoli. To achieve a maximum expiration (below the end-tidal expiratory level), the accessory muscles of expiration must be used to compress the thorax. Box 1-1 lists the various accessory muscles of breathing.

Respiration involves the exchange of oxygen and carbon dioxide between an organism and its environment. Respiration is typically divided into two components: **external respiration** and **internal respiration.** External respiration involves the exchange of oxygen and carbon dioxide between the alveoli and the pulmonary capillaries. Internal respiration occurs at the cellular level and involves the movement of oxygen from the systemic blood into the cells, where it is used in the oxidation of available substrates (e.g., carbohydrates and lipids) to produce energy. Carbon dioxide, which is a major by-product of aerobic metabolism, is then exchanged between the cells of the body and the systemic capillaries.

Gas Flow and Pressure Gradients During Ventilation

For air to flow through a tube or airway, a **pressure gradient** must exist (i.e., pressure at one end of the tube must be higher than pressure at the other end of the tube). Air will always flow from the high-pressure point to the low-pressure point.

Consider what happens during a normal quiet breath. Lung volumes change as a result of gas flow into and out of the airways caused by changes in the pressure gradient between the airway opening and the alveoli. During a spontaneous inspiration, the pressure in the alveoli becomes less than the pressure at the airway opening (i.e., the mouth and nose) and gas flows into the lungs. Conversely, gas flows out of the lungs during exhalation because the pressure in the alveoli is higher than the pressure at the airway opening. It is important to recognize that when the pressure at the airway opening and the pressure in the alveoli are the same, as occurs at the end of expiration, no gas flow occurs because the pressures across the conductive airways are equal (i.e., there is no pressure gradient).

Units of Pressure

Ventilating pressures are commonly measured in centimeters of water pressure (cm H_2O). These pressures are referenced to atmospheric pressure, which is given a baseline value of zero. In other words, although atmospheric pressure is 760 mm Hg or 1034 cm H_2O (1 mm Hg = 1.36 cm H_2O) at sea level, atmospheric pressure is designated as 0 cm H_2O. For example, when airway pressure increases by +20 cm H_2O during a positive pressure breath, the pressure actually increases from 1034 to 1054 cm H_2O. Other units of measure that are becoming more widely used for gas pressures, such as arterial oxygen pressure (P_aO_2), are the torr (1 Torr = 1 mm Hg) and the kilopascal ([kPa]; 1 kPa = 7.5 mm Hg). The kilopascal is used in the International System of units. (Box 1-2 provides a summary of common units of measurement for pressure.)

Definition of Pressures and Gradients in the Lungs

Airway opening pressure (P_{awo}), is most often called **mouth pressure** (P_M) or **airway pressure** (P_{aw}) (Fig. 1-1). Other terms that are often used to describe the airway opening pressure include **upper-airway pressure, mask pressure,** or **proximal airway pressure.** Unless pressure is applied at the airway opening, P_{awo} is zero or atmospheric pressure.

A similar measurement is the pressure at the body surface (P_{bs}). This is equal to zero (atmospheric pressure) unless the person is placed in a pressurized chamber (e.g., hyperbaric chamber) or a negative pressure ventilator (e.g., iron lung).

BOX 1-1 **Accessory Muscles of Breathing**

Inspiration
Scalene (anterior, medial, and posterior)
Sternocleidomastoids
Pectoralis (major and minor)
Trapezius

Expiration
Rectus abdominus
External oblique
Internal oblique
Transverse abdominal
Serratus (anterior, posterior)
Latissimus dorsi

BOX 1-2 **Pressure Equivalents**

1 mm Hg = 1.36 cm H_2O
1 kPa = 7.5 mm Hg
1 Torr = 1 mm Hg
1 atm = 760 mm Hg = 1034 cm H_2O

Intrapleural pressure (P_{pl}) is the pressure in the potential space between the parietal and visceral pleurae. P_{pl} is normally about −5 cm H_2O at the end of expiration during spontaneous breathing. It is about −10 cm H_2O at the end of inspiration. Because P_{pl} is difficult to measure in a patient, a related measurement is used, the **esophageal pressure** (P_{es}), which is obtained by placing a specially designed balloon in the esophagus; changes in the balloon pressure

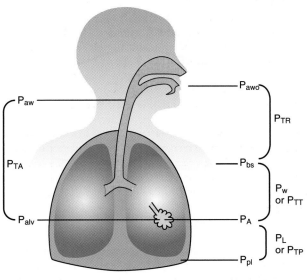

P_{awo} - Mouth or airway opening pressure
P_{alv} - Alveolar pressure
P_{pl} - Intrapleural pressure
P_{bs} - Body surface pressure
P_{aw} - Airway pressure (= P_{awo})

P_L or P_{TP} = Transpulmonary pressure ($P_L = P_{alv} − P_{pl}$)
P_W or P_{TT} = Transthoracic pressure ($P_{alv} − P_{bs}$)
P_{TA} = Transairway pressure ($P_{aw} − P_{alv}$)
P_{TR} = Transrespiratory pressure ($P_{awo} − P_{bs}$)

Fig. 1-1 Various pressures and pressure gradients of the respiratory system. (From Kacmarek RM, Stoller JK, Heuer AJ, editors: Egan's fundamentals of respiratory care, ed 10, St Louis, 2013, Elsevier.)

are used to estimate pressure and pressure changes in the pleural space. (See Chapter 10 for more information about esophageal pressure measurements.)

Another commonly measured pressure is alveolar pressure (P_A or P_{alv}). This pressure is also called *intrapulmonary pressure* or *lung pressure*. Alveolar pressure normally changes as the intrapleural pressure changes. During spontaneous inspiration, P_A is about −1 cm H_2O, and during exhalation it is about +1 cm H_2O.

Four basic pressure gradients are used to describe normal ventilation: transairway pressure, transthoracic pressure, transpulmonary pressure, and transrespiratory pressure (Table 1-1; also see Fig. 1-1).[1]

Transairway Pressure

Transairway pressure (P_{TA}) is the pressure difference between the airway opening and the alveolus: $P_{TA} = P_{aw} − P_{alv}$. It is therefore the pressure gradient required to produce airflow in the conductive airways. It represents the pressure that must be generated to overcome resistance to gas flow in the airways (i.e., airway resistance).

Transthoracic Pressure

Transthoracic pressure (P_W) is the pressure difference between the alveolar space or lung and the body's surface (P_{bs}): $P_W = P_{alv} − P_{bs}$. It represents the pressure required to expand or contract the lungs and the chest wall at the same time. It is sometimes abbreviated to P_{TT}, meaning transthoracic).

Transpulmonary Pressure

Transpulmonary pressure (P_L or P_{TP}), or transalveolar pressure, is the pressure difference between the alveolar space and the pleural space (P_{pl}): $P_L = P_{alv} − P_{pl}$.[2-4] P_L is the pressure required to maintain alveolar inflation and is therefore sometimes called the **alveolar distending pressure**. All modes of ventilation increase P_L during inspiration, either by decreasing P_{pl} (negative pressure ventilators) or increasing P_{alv} by increasing pressure at the upper airway (positive pressure ventilators). The term *transmural pressure* is

TABLE 1-1	**Terms, Abbreviations, and Pressure Gradients for the Respiratory System**	
Abbreviation	**Term**	
C	Compliance	
R	Resistance	
R_{aw}	Airway resistance	
P_M	Pressure at the mouth (same as P_{awo})	
P_{aw}	Airway pressure (usually upper airway)	
P_{awo}	Pressure at the airway opening; mouth pressure; mask pressure	
P_{bs}	Pressure at the body surface	
P_{alv}	Alveolar pressure (also P_A)	
P_{pl}	Intrapleural pressure	
C_{st}	Static compliance	
C_{dyn}	Dynamic compliance	
Pressure Gradients		
Transairway pressure (P_{TA})	Airway pressure − alveolar pressure	$P_{TA} = P_{aw} − P_{alv}$
Transthoracic pressure (P_W)	Alveolar pressure − body surface pressure	P_W (or P_{TT}) = $P_{alv} − P_{bs}$
Transpulmonary pressure (P_L)	Alveolar pressure − pleural pressure (also defined as the *transalveolar pressure*)	P_L (or P_{TP}) = $P_{alv} − P_{pl}$
Transrespiratory pressure (P_{TR})	Airway opening pressure − body surface pressure	$P_{TR} = P_{awo} − P_{bs}$

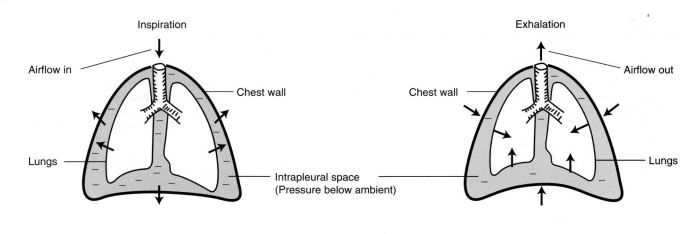

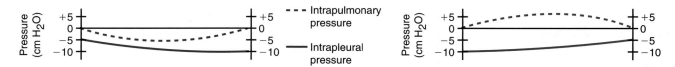

Fig. 1-2 The mechanics of spontaneous ventilation and the resulting pressure waves (approximately normal values). During inspiration, intrapleural pressure (P_{pl}) decreases to −10 cm H_2O. During exhalation, P_{pl} increases from −10 to −5 cm H_2O. (See the text for further description.)

often used to describe pleural pressure minus body surface pressure. (NOTE: An airway pressure measurement called the **plateau pressure** [$P_{plateau}$] is sometimes substituted for P_{alv}. $P_{plateau}$ is measured during a breath-hold maneuver during mechanical ventilation, and the value is read from the ventilator manometer. $P_{plateau}$ is discussed in more detail later in this chapter.)

During negative pressure ventilation, the pressure at the body surface (P_{bs}) becomes negative, and this pressure is transmitted to the pleural space, resulting in an increase in transpulmonary pressure (P_L). During positive pressure ventilation, the P_{bs} remains atmospheric, but the pressures at the upper airways (P_{awo}) and in the conductive airways (airway pressure, or P_{aw}) become positive. Alveolar pressure (P_A) then becomes positive, and transpulmonary pressure (P_L) increases.*

Transrespiratory Pressure

Transrespiratory pressure (P_{TR}) is the pressure difference between the airway opening and the body surface: $P_{TR} = P_{awo} − P_{bs}$. Transrespiratory pressure is used to describe the pressure required to inflate the lungs and airways during positive pressure ventilation. In this situation, the body surface pressure (P_{bs}) is atmospheric and usually is given the value zero; thus P_{awo} becomes the pressure reading on a ventilator gauge (P_{aw}).

Transrespiratory pressure has two components: transthoracic pressure (the pressure required to overcome elastic recoil of the lungs and chest wall) and transairway pressure (the pressure required to overcome airway resistance). Transrespiratory pressure

can therefore be described by the equations $P_{TR} = P_{TT} + P_{TA}$ or $(P_{awo} − P_{bs}) = (P_{alv} − P_{bs}) + (P_{aw} − P_{alv})$.

Consider what happens during a normal, spontaneous inspiration (Fig. 1-2). As the volume of the thoracic space increases, the pressure in the pleural space (intrapleural pressure) becomes more negative in relation to atmospheric pressures. (This is an expected result according to Boyle's law. For a constant temperature, as the volume increases, the pressure decreases.) The intrapleural pressure drops from about −5 cm H_2O at end expiration to about −10 cm H_2O at end inspiration. The negative intrapleural pressure is transmitted to the alveolar space, and the intrapulmonary, or intraalveolar (P_{alv}), pressure becomes more negative relative to atmospheric pressure. The transpulmonary pressure (P_L), or the pressure gradient across the lung, widens (Table 1-2). As a result, the alveoli have a negative pressure during spontaneous inspiration.

The pressure at the mouth or body surface is still atmospheric, creating a pressure gradient between the mouth (zero) and the alveolus of about −3 to −5 cm H_2O. The transairway pressure gradient (P_{TA}) is approximately (0 − [−5]), or 5 cm H_2O. Air flows from the mouth into the alveoli and the alveoli expand. When the volume of gas builds up in the alveoli and the pressure returns to zero, airflow stops. This marks the end of inspiration; no more gas moves into the lungs because the pressure at the mouth and in the alveoli equals zero (i.e., atmospheric pressure) (see Fig. 1-2).

During exhalation the muscles relax and the elastic recoil of the lung tissue results in a decrease in lung volume. The thoracic volume decreases to resting, and the intrapleural pressure returns to about −5 cm H_2O. Notice that the pressure inside the alveolus during exhalation increases and becomes slightly positive (+5 cm H_2O). As a result, pressure is now lower at the mouth than inside the alveoli and the transairway pressure gradient causes air to move out of the lungs. When the pressure in the alveoli and that in the mouth are equal, exhalation ends.

---

*The definition of transpulmonary pressure varies in research articles and textbooks. Some authors define it as the difference between airway pressure and pleural pressure. This definition implies that airway pressure is the pressure applied to the lungs during a breath-hold maneuver, that is, under static (no flow) conditions.

TABLE 1-2   Changes in Transpulmonary Pressure* Under Varying Conditions

Passive Spontaneous Ventilation Pressure	End Expiration	End Inspiration
Intraalveolar (intrapulmonary)	0 cm H_2O	0 cm H_2O
Intrapleural	−5 cm H_2O	−10 cm H_2O
Transpulmonary	$P_L = 0 − (−5) = +5$ cm H_2O	$P_L = 0 − (−10) = 10$ cm H_2O
Negative Pressure Ventilation		
Intraalveolar (intrapulmonary)	0 cm H_2O	0 cm H_2O
Intrapleural	−5 cm H_2O	−10 cm H_2O
Transpulmonary	$P_L = 0 − (−5) = +5$ cm H_2O	$P_L = 0 − (−10) = 10$ cm H_2O
Positive Pressure Ventilation		
Intraalveolar (intrapulmonary)	0 cm H_2O	9-12 cm $H_2O^{\dagger}$
Intrapleural	−5 cm H_2O	2-5 cm $H_2O^{\dagger}$
Transpulmonary	$P_L = 0 − (−5) = +5$ cm H_2O	$P_L = 10 − (2) = +8$ cm $H_2O^{\dagger}$

*$P_L = P_{alv} − P_{pl}$.
†Applied pressure is +15 cm H_2O.

LUNG CHARACTERISTICS

Normally, two types of forces oppose inflation of the lungs: elastic forces and frictional forces. Elastic forces arise from the elastic properties of the lungs and chest wall. Frictional forces are the result of two factors: the resistance of the tissues and organs as they become displaced during breathing and the resistance to gas flow through the airways.

Two parameters are often used to describe the mechanical properties of the respiratory system and the elastic and frictional forces opposing lung inflation: *compliance* and *resistance*.

Compliance

The **compliance** (C) of any structure can be described as the relative ease with which the structure distends. It can be defined as the opposite, or inverse, of **elastance** (e), where *elastance* is the tendency of a structure to return to its original form after being stretched or acted on by an outside force. Thus, C = 1/e or e = 1/C. The following examples illustrate this principle. A balloon that is easy to inflate is said to be very compliant (it demonstrates reduced elasticity), whereas a balloon that is difficult to inflate is considered not very compliant (it has increased elasticity). In a similar way, consider the comparison of a golf ball and a tennis ball. The golf ball is more elastic than the tennis ball because it tends to retain its original form; a considerable amount of force must be applied to the golf ball to compress it. A tennis ball, on the other hand, can be compressed more easily than the golf ball, so it can be described as less elastic and more compliant.

In the clinical setting, compliance measurements are used to describe the elastic forces that oppose lung inflation. More specifically, the compliance of the respiratory system is determined by measuring the change (Δ) of volume (V) that occurs when pressure (P) is applied to the system: C = ΔV/ΔP. Volume typically is measured in liters or milliliters and pressure in centimeters of water pressure. It is important to understand that the compliance of the respiratory system is the sum of the compliances of both the lung parenchyma and the surrounding thoracic structures. In a spontaneously breathing individual, the total respiratory system compliance is about 0.1 L/cm H_2O (100 mL/cm H_2O); however, it can vary considerably, depending on

a person's posture, position, and whether he or she is actively inhaling or exhaling during the measurement. It can range from 0.05 to 0.17 L/cm H_2O (50 to 170 mL/cm H_2O). For intubated and mechanically ventilated patients with normal lungs and a normal chest wall, compliance varies from 40 to 50 mL/cm H_2O in men and 35 to 45 mL/cm H_2O in women to as high as 100 mL/cm H_2O in either gender (Key Point 1-1).

 Key Point **1-1** Normal compliance in spontaneously breathing patients: 0.05 to 0.17 L/cm H_2O or 50 to 170 mL/cm H_2O
Normal compliance in intubated patients: Males: 40 to 50 mL/cm H_2O, up to 100 mL/cm H_2O; Females: 35 to 45 mL/cm H_2O, up to 100 mL/cm H_2O

CRITICAL CARE CONCEPT 1-1

Calculate Pressure
Calculate the amount of pressure needed to attain a tidal volume of 0.5 L (500 mL) for a patient with a normal respiratory system compliance of 0.1 L/cm H_2O.

Changes in the condition of the lungs or chest wall (or both) affect total respiratory system compliance and the pressure required to inflate the lungs. Diseases that reduce the compliance of the lungs or chest wall increase the pressure required to inflate the lungs. Acute respiratory distress syndrome and kyphoscoliosis are examples of pathologic conditions that are associated with reductions in lung compliance and thoracic compliance, respectively. Conversely, emphysema is an example of a pulmonary condition where pulmonary compliance is increased due to a loss of lung elasticity. With emphysema, less pressure is required to inflate the lungs.

Critical Care Concept 1-1 presents an exercise in which students can test their understanding of the compliance equation.

For patients receiving mechanical ventilation, compliance measurements are made during static or no-flow conditions (e.g., this is the airway pressure measured at end inspiration; it is designated as the plateau pressure). As such, these compliance measurements

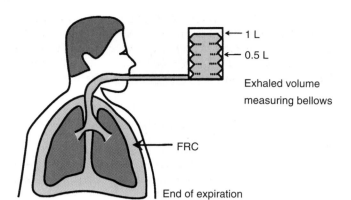

Fig. 1-3 A volume device (bellows) is used to illustrate the measurement of exhaled volume. Ventilators typically use a flow transducer to measure the exhaled tidal volume. The **functional residual capacity** (FRC) is the amount of air that remains in the lungs after a normal exhalation.

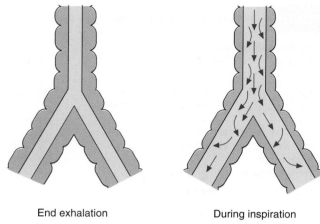

End exhalation   During inspiration

Fig. 1-4 Expansion of the airways during inspiration. (See the text for further explanation.)

BOX **1-3**	**Equation for Calculating Static Compliance**

C_S = (exhaled tidal volume)/(plateau pressure − EEP)
$C_S = V_T/(P_{plateau} − EEP)*$

*EEP is the end-expiratory pressure, which some clinicians call the *baseline pressure;* it is the baseline from which the patient breathes. When PEEP (positive end-expiratory pressure) is administered, it is the EEP value used in this calculation.

---

are referred to as **static compliance** or **static effective compliance.** The tidal volume used in this calculation is determined by measuring the patient's exhaled volume near the patient connector (Fig. 1-3). Box 1-3 shows the formula for calculating static compliance (C_S) for a ventilated patient. Notice that although this calculation technically includes the recoil of the lungs and thorax, thoracic compliance generally does not change significantly in a ventilated patient. (NOTE: It is important to understand that if a patient actively inhales or exhales during measurement of a plateau pressure, the resulting value will be inaccurate. Active breathing can be a particularly difficult issue when patients are tachypneic, such as when a patient is experiencing respiratory distress.)

Resistance

Resistance is a measurement of the frictional forces that must be overcome during breathing. These frictional forces are the result of the anatomical structure of the airways and the tissue viscous resistance offered by the lungs and adjacent tissues and organs.

As the lungs and thorax move during ventilation, the movement and displacement of structures such as the lungs, abdominal organs, rib cage, and diaphragm create resistance to breathing. Tissue viscous resistance remains constant under most circumstances. For example, an obese patient or one with fibrosis has increased tissue resistance, but the tissue resistance usually does not change significantly when these patients are mechanically ventilated. On the other hand, if a patient develops **ascites,** or fluid accumulation in the peritoneal cavity, tissue resistance increases.

The resistance to airflow through the conductive airways (*airway resistance*) depends on the gas viscosity, the gas density, the

length and diameter of the tube, and the flow rate of the gas through the tube, as defined by Poiseuille's law. During mechanical ventilation, viscosity, density, and tube or airway length remain fairly constant. In contrast, the diameter of the airway lumen can change considerably and affect the flow of the gas into and out of the lungs. The diameter of the airway lumen and the flow of gas into the lungs can decrease as a result of bronchospasm, increased secretions, mucosal edema, or kinks in the endotracheal tube. The rate at which gas flows into the lungs can also be controlled on most mechanical ventilators.

At the end of the expiratory cycle, before the ventilator cycles into inspiration, normally no flow of gas occurs; the alveolar and mouth pressures are equal. Because flow is absent, resistance to flow is also absent. When the ventilator cycles on and creates a positive pressure at the mouth, the gas attempts to move into the lower-pressure zones in the alveoli. However, this movement is impeded or even blocked by having to pass through the endotracheal tube and the upper conductive airways. Some molecules are slowed as they collide with the tube and the bronchial walls; in doing this, they exert energy (pressure) against the passages, which causes the airways to expand (Fig. 1-4); as a result, some of the gas molecules (pressure) remain in the airway and do not reach the alveoli. In addition, as the gas molecules flow through the airway and the layers of gas flow over each other, resistance to flow, called *viscous resistance,* occurs.

The relationship of gas flow, pressure, and resistance in the airways is described by the equation for airway resistance, $R_{aw} = P_{TA}/flow$, where R_{aw} is airway resistance and P_{TA} is the pressure difference between the mouth and the alveolus, or the transairway pressure (Key Point 1-2). *Flow* is the gas flow measured during inspiration. Resistance is usually expressed in centimeters of water per liter per second (cm H_2O/[L/s]). In normal, conscious individuals with a gas flow of 0.5 L/s, resistance is about 0.6 to 2.4 cm H_2O/(L/s) (Box 1-4). The actual amount varies over the entire respiratory cycle. The variation occurs because flow during spontaneous ventilation usually is slower at the beginning and end of the cycle and faster in the middle.*

---

*The transairway pressure (P_{TA}) in this equation sometimes is referred to as ∆P, the difference between PIP and $P_{plateau}$. (See the section on defining pressures in positive pressure ventilation.)

Unintubated Patient
0.6 to 2.4 cm $H_2O/(L/s)$ at 0.5 L/s flow

Intubated Patient
Approximately 6 cm $H_2O/(L/s)$ or higher (airway resistance increases as endotracheal tube size decreases)

 Key Point 1-2 $R_{aw} = (PIP - P_{plateau})/flow$ (where PIP is peak inspiratory pressure); or $R_{aw} = P_{TA}/flow$; example

$$R_{aw} = \frac{[40 - 25 \, cm \, H_2O]}{1(L/s)} = 15 \, cm \, H_2O/(L/s)$$

Airway resistance is increased when an artificial airway is inserted. The smaller internal diameter of the tube creates greater resistance to flow (resistance can be increased to 5 to 7 cm $H_2O/[L/s]$). As mentioned, pathologic conditions can also increase airway resistance by decreasing the diameter of the airways. In conscious, unintubated subjects with emphysema and asthma, resistance may range from 13 to 18 cm $H_2O/(L/s)$. Still higher values can occur with other severe types of obstructive disorders.

Several challenges are associated with increased airway resistance. With greater resistance, a greater pressure drop occurs in the conducting airways and less pressure is available to expand the alveoli. As a consequence, a smaller volume of gas is available for gas exchange. The greater resistance also requires that more force must be exerted to maintain adequate gas flow. To achieve this force, spontaneously breathing patients use the accessory muscles of inspiration. This generates more negative intrapleural pressures and a greater pressure gradient between the upper airway and the pleural space to achieve gas flow. The same occurs during mechanical ventilation; more pressure must be generated by the ventilator to try to "blow" the air into the patient's lungs through obstructed airways or through a small endotracheal tube.

Measuring Airway Resistance

Airway resistance pressure is not easily measured; however, the transairway pressure can be calculated: $P_{TA} = PIP - P_{plateau}$. This allows determination of how much pressure is delivered to the airways and how much to alveoli. For example, if the peak pressure during a mechanical breath is 25 cm H_2O and the plateau pressure (pressure at end inspiration using a breath hold) is 20 cm H_2O, the pressure lost to the airways because of airway resistance is 25 cm $H_2O - 20$ cm $H_2O = 5$ cm H_2O. In fact, 5 cm H_2O is about the normal amount of pressure (P_{TA}) lost to airway resistance (R_{aw}) with a proper-sized endotracheal tube in place. In another example, if the peak pressure during a mechanical breath is 40 cm H_2O and the plateau pressure is 25 cm H_2O, the pressure lost to airway resistance is 40 cm $H_2O - 25$ cm $H_2O = 15$ cm H_2O. This value is high and indicates an increase in R_{aw} (see Box 1-4).

Many mechanical ventilators allow the therapist to choose a specific constant flow setting. Monitors are incorporated into the user interface to display peak airway pressures, plateau pressure, and the actual gas flow during inspiration. With this additional information, airway resistance can be calculated. For example, let

us assume that the flow is set at 60 L/min, the PIP is 40 cm H_2O, and the $P_{plateau}$ is 25 cm H_2O. The P_{TA} is therefore 15 cm H_2O. To calculate airway resistance, flow is converted from liters per minute to liters per second (60 L/min = 60 L/60 s = 1 L/s). The values then are substituted into the equation for airway resistance, $R_{aw} = (PIP - P_{plateau})/flow$:

$$R_{aw} = \frac{[40 - 25 \, cm \, H_2O]}{1(L/s)} = 15 \, cm \, H_2O/(L/s)$$

For an intubated patient, this is an example of elevated airway resistance. The elevated R_{aw} may be due to increased secretions, mucosal edema, bronchospasm, or an endotracheal tube that is too small.

Ventilators with microprocessors can provide real-time calculations of airway resistance. It is important to recognize that where pressure and flow are measured can affect the airway resistance values. Measurements taken inside the ventilator may be less accurate than those obtained at the airway opening. For example, if a ventilator measures flow at the exhalation valve and pressure on the inspiratory side of the ventilator, these values incorporate the resistance to flow through the ventilator circuit and not just patient airway resistance. Clinicians must therefore know how the ventilator obtains measurements to fully understand the resistance calculation that is reported.

Case Study 1-1

Determine Static Compliance (C_S) and Airway Resistance (R_{aw})

An intubated, 36-year-old woman diagnosed with pneumonia is being ventilated with a volume of 0.5 L (500 mL). The peak inspiratory pressure is 24 cm H_2O, $P_{plateau}$ is 19 cm H_2O, and baseline pressure is 0. The inspiratory gas flow is constant at 60 L/min (1 L/s).

What are the static compliance and airway resistance? Are these normal values?

Case Study 1-1 provides an exercise to test your understanding of airway resistance and respiratory compliance measurements.

TIME CONSTANTS

Regional differences in compliance and resistance exist throughout the lungs. That is, the compliance and resistance values of a terminal respiratory unit (**acinus**) may be considerably different from those of another unit. Thus the characteristics of the lung are **heterogeneous**, not **homogeneous**. Indeed, some lung units may have normal compliance and resistance characteristics, whereas others may demonstrate pathophysiological changes, such as increased resistance, decreased compliance, or both.

Alterations in C and R_{aw} affect how rapidly lung units fill and empty. Each small unit of the lung can be pictured as a small, inflatable balloon attached to a short drinking straw. The volume the balloon receives in relation to other small units depends on its compliance and resistance, assuming that other factors are equal (e.g., intrapleural pressures and the location of the units relative to different lung zones).

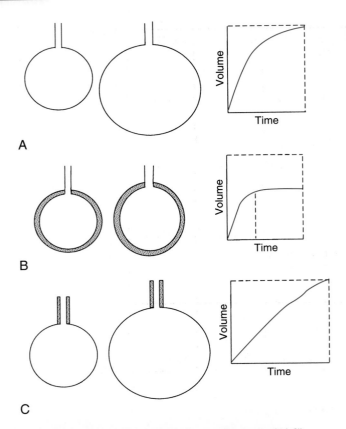

Fig. 1-5 A, Filling of a normal lung unit. **B,** A low-compliance unit, which fills quickly but with less air. **C,** Increased resistance; the unit fills slowly. If inspiration were to end at the same time as in **(A)**, the volume in **(C)** would be lower.

BOX 1-5   Calculation of Time Constant

Time constant = C × R$_{aw}$
Time constant = 0.1 L/cm H$_2$O × 1 cm H$_2$O/(L/s)
Time constant = 0.1 s
    In a patient with a time constant of 0.1 s, 63% of inhalation (or exhalation) occurs in 0.1 s; that is, 63% of the volume is inhaled (or exhaled) in 0.1 s, and 37% of the volume remains to be exchanged.

resistance of 1 cm H$_2$O/(L/s). One time constant equals the amount of time that it takes for 63% of the volume to be inhaled (or exhaled), two time constants represent that amount of time for about 86% of the volume to be inhaled (or exhaled), three time constants equal the time for about 95% to be inhaled (or exhaled), and four time constants is the time required for 98% of the volume to be inhaled (or exhaled) (Fig. 1-6).[2-5] In the example in Box 1-5, with a time constant of 0.1 s, 98% of the volume fills (or empties) the lungs in four time constants, or 0.4 s.

After five time constants, the lung is considered to contain 100% of tidal volume to be inhaled or 100% of tidal volume has been exhaled. In the example in Box 1-5, five time constants would equal 5 × 0.1 s, or 0.5 s. Thus, in half a second, a normal lung unit, as described here, would be fully expanded or deflated to its end-expiratory volume (Key Point 1-3).

Key Point **1-3** Time constants approximate the amount of time required to fill or empty a lung unit.

Calculation of time constants is important when setting the ventilator's inspiratory time and expiratory time. An inspiratory time less than three time constants may result in incomplete delivery of the tidal volume. Prolonging the inspiratory time allows even distribution of ventilation and adequate delivery of tidal volume. Five time constants should be considered for the inspiratory time, particularly in pressure ventilation, to ensure adequate volume delivery (see Chapter 2 for more information on pressure ventilation). It is important to recognize, however, that if the inspiratory time is too long, the respiratory rate may be too low to achieve effective minute ventilation.

An expiratory time of less than three time constants may lead to incomplete emptying of the lungs. This can increase the functional residual capacity and cause trapping of air in the lungs. Some clinicians believe that using the 95% to 98% volume emptying level (three or four time constants) is adequate for exhalation.[3,4] Exact time settings require careful observation of the patient and measurement of end-expiratory pressure to determine which time is better tolerated.

In summary, lung units can be described as fast or slow. **Fast lung units** have short time constants and take less time to fill and empty. Short time constants are associated with normal or low airway resistance and decreased compliance, such as occurs in a patient with interstitial fibrosis. It is important to recognize, however, that these lung units will typically require increased pressure to achieve a normal volume. In contrast, **slow lung units** have long time constants, which require more time to fill and empty compared with a normal or fast lung unit. Slow lung units have

Figure 1-5 provides a series of graphs illustrating the filling of the lung during a quiet breath. A lung unit with normal compliance and airway resistance will fill within a normal length of time and with a normal volume (Fig. 1-5, *A*). If the lung unit has normal resistance but is stiff (low compliance), it will fill rapidly (Fig. 1-5, *B*). For example, when a new toy balloon is first inflated, considerable effort is required to start the inflation (i.e., high pressure is required to overcome the **critical opening pressure** of the balloon to allow it to start filling). When the balloon inflates, it does so very rapidly at first. It also deflates very quickly. Notice, however, that if a given pressure is applied to a stiff lung unit and a normal unit for the same length of time, a much smaller volume will be delivered to the stiff lung unit (compliance equals volume divided by pressure) when compared with the volume delivered to the normal unit.

Now consider a balloon (lung unit) that has normal compliance but the straw (airway) is very narrow (high airway resistance) (Fig. 1-5, *C*). In this case the balloon (lung unit) fills very slowly. The gas takes much longer to flow through the narrow passage and reach the balloon (acinus). If gas flow is applied for the same length of time as in a normal situation, the resulting volume is smaller.

The length of time lung units require to fill and empty can be determined. The product of compliance (C) and resistance (R$_{aw}$) is called a **time constant.** For any value of C and R$_{aw}$, the time constant always equals the length of time (in seconds) required for the lungs to inflate or deflate to a certain amount (percentage) of their volume. Box 1-5 shows the calculation of one time constant for a lung unit with a compliance of 0.1 L/cm H$_2$O and an airway

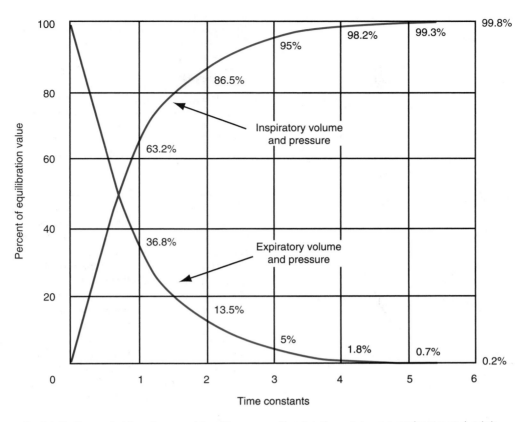

Fig. 1-6 The time constant (compliance × resistance) is a measure of how long the respiratory system takes to passively exhale (deflate) or inhale (inflate). (From Kacmarek RM, Stoller JK, Heuer AJ, editors: Egan's fundamentals of respiratory care, ed 10, St Louis, 2013, Elsevier.)

increased resistance or increased compliance, or both, and are typically found in patients with pulmonary emphysema.

It must be kept in mind that the lung is rarely uniform across ventilating units. Some units fill and empty quickly, whereas others do so more slowly. Clinically, compliance and airway resistance measurements reflect a patient's overall lung function, and clinicians must recognize this fact when using these data to guide treatment decisions.

Types of Ventilators and Terms Used in Mechanical Ventilation

Various types of mechanical ventilators are used clinically. The following section provides a brief description of the terms commonly applied to mechanical ventilation.

TYPES OF MECHANICAL VENTILATION

Three basic methods have been developed to mimic or replace the normal mechanisms of breathing: negative pressure ventilation, positive pressure ventilation, and high-frequency ventilation.

Negative Pressure Ventilation

Negative pressure ventilation (NPV) attempts to mimic the function of the respiratory muscles to allow breathing through normal physiological mechanisms. A good example of negative pressure ventilators is the tank ventilator, or "iron lung." With this device, the patient's head and neck are exposed to ambient pressure while the thorax and the rest of the body are enclosed in an airtight container that is subjected to negative pressure (i.e., pressure less than atmospheric pressure). Negative pressure generated around the thoracic area is transmitted across the chest wall, into the intrapleural space, and finally into the intraalveolar space.

With negative pressure ventilators, as the intrapleural space becomes negative, the space inside the alveoli becomes increasingly negative in relation to the pressure at the airway opening (atmospheric pressure). This pressure gradient results in the movement of air into the lungs. In this way, negative pressure ventilators resemble normal lung mechanics. Expiration occurs when the negative pressure around the chest wall is removed. The normal elastic recoil of the lungs and chest wall causes air to flow out of the lungs passively (Fig. 1-7).

Negative pressure ventilators do provide several advantages. The upper airway can be maintained without the use of an endotracheal tube or tracheostomy. Patients receiving negative pressure ventilation can talk and eat while being ventilated. Negative pressure ventilation has fewer physiological disadvantages in patients with normal cardiovascular function than positive pressure ventilation.[6-9] In hypovolemic patients, however, a normal cardiovascular response is not always present. As a result, patients can have significant pooling of blood in the abdomen and reduced venous return to the heart.[8,9] Additionally, difficulty gaining access to the patient can complicate care activities (e.g., bathing and turning).

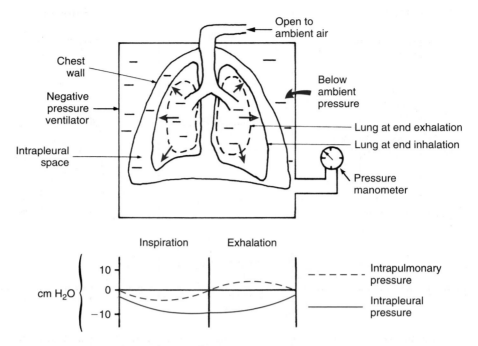

Fig. 1-7 Negative pressure ventilation and the resulting lung mechanics and pressure waves (approximate values). During inspiration, intrapleural pressure drops from about −5 to −10 cm H_2O and alveolar (intrapulmonary) pressure declines from 0 to −5 cm H_2O; as a result, air flows into the lungs. The alveolar pressure returns to zero as the lungs fill. Flow stops when pressure between the mouth and the lungs is equal. During exhalation, intrapleural pressure increases from about −10 to −5 cm H_2O and alveolar (intrapulmonary) pressure increases from 0 to about +5 cm H_2O as the chest wall and lung tissue recoil to their normal resting position; as a result, air flows out of the lungs. The alveolar pressure returns to zero, and flow stops.

The use of negative pressure ventilators declined considerably in the early 1980s, and currently they are rarely used in hospitals. Other methods of creating negative pressure (e.g., chest cuirass, Poncho wrap, and Porta-Lung) have been used in home care to treat patients with chronic respiratory failure associated with neuromuscular diseases (e.g., polio and amyotrophic lateral sclerosis).[9-12] More recently, these devices have been replaced with noninvasive positive pressure ventilators (NIV) that use a mask, a nasal device, or a tracheostomy tube as a patient interface. Chapters 19 and 21 provide additional information on the use of NIV and NPV.

Positive Pressure Ventilation

Positive pressure ventilation (PPV) occurs when a mechanical ventilator is used to deliver air into the patient's lungs by way of an endotracheal tube or positive pressure mask. For example, if the pressure at the mouth or upper airway is +15 cm H_2O and the pressure in the alveolus is zero (end exhalation), the gradient between the mouth and the lung is $P_{TA} = P_{awo} − P_{alv} = 15 − (0)$, = 15 cm H_2O. Thus air will flow into the lung (see Table 1-1).

At any point during inspiration, the inflating pressure at the upper (proximal) airway equals the sum of the pressures required to overcome the resistance of the airways and the elastance of the lung and chest wall. During inspiration the pressure in the alveoli progressively builds and becomes more positive. The resultant positive alveolar pressure is transmitted across the visceral pleura and the intrapleural space may become positive at the end of inspiration (Fig. 1-8).

At the end of inspiration, the ventilator stops delivering positive pressure. Mouth pressure returns to ambient pressure (zero or atmospheric). Alveolar pressure is still positive, which creates a gradient between the alveolus and the mouth, and air flows out of the lungs. See Table 1-2 for a comparison of the changes in airway pressure gradients during passive spontaneous ventilation.

High-Frequency Ventilation

High-frequency ventilation uses above-normal ventilating rates with below-normal ventilating volumes. There are three types of high-frequency ventilation strategies: **high-frequency positive pressure ventilation** (HFPPV), which uses respiratory rates of about 60 to 100 breaths/min; **high-frequency jet ventilation** (HFJV), which uses rates between about 100 and 400 to 600 breaths/min; and **high-frequency oscillatory ventilation** (HFOV), which uses rates into the thousands, up to about 4000 breaths/min. In clinical practice, the various types of high-frequency ventilation are better defined by the type of ventilator used rather than the specific rates of each.

HFPPV can be accomplished with a conventional positive pressure ventilator set at high rates and lower than normal tidal volumes. HFJV involves delivering pressurized jets of gas into the lungs at very high frequencies (i.e., 4 to 11 Hz or cycles per second). HFJV is accomplished using a specially designed endotracheal tube adaptor and a nozzle or an injector; the small-diameter tube creates a high-velocity jet of air that is directed into the lungs. Exhalation is passive. HFOV ventilators use either a small piston or a device similar to a stereo speaker to deliver gas in a "to-and-fro" motion, pushing gas in during inspiration and drawing gas out during exhalation. Ventilation with high-frequency oscillation has been used primarily in infants with respiratory distress and in adults or infants with open air leaks, such as **bronchopleural fistulas.**

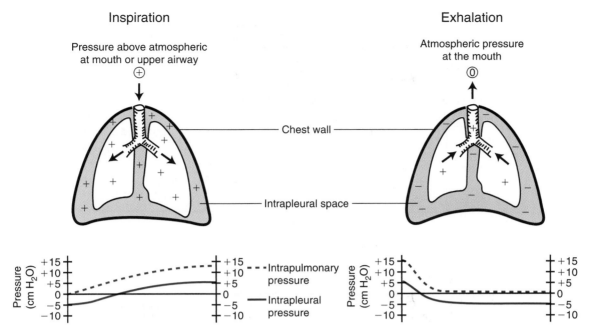

Fig. 1-8 Mechanics and pressure waves associated with positive pressure ventilation. During inspiration, as the upper airway pressure rises to about +15 cm H_2O (not shown), the alveolar (intrapulmonary) pressure is zero; as a result, air flows into the lungs until the alveolar pressure rises to about +9 to +12 cm H_2O. The intrapleural pressure rises from about 5 cm H_2O before inspiration to about +5 cm H_2O at the end of inspiration. Flow stops when the ventilator cycles into exhalation. During exhalation, the upper airway pressure drops to zero as the ventilator stops delivering flow. The alveolar (intrapulmonary) pressure drops from about +9 to +12 cm H_2O to 0 as the chest wall and lung tissue recoil to their normal resting position; as a result, air flows out of the lungs. The intrapleural pressure returns to −5 cm H_2O during exhalation.

Chapters 22 and 23 provide more detail on the unique nature of this mode of ventilation.

DEFINITION OF PRESSURES IN POSITIVE PRESSURE VENTILATION

At any point in a breath cycle during mechanical ventilation, the clinician can check the **manometer,** or pressure gauge, of a ventilator to determine the airway pressure present at that moment. This reading is measured either very close to the mouth (proximal airway pressure) or on the inside of the ventilator, where it closely estimates pressure at the mouth or airway opening. A graph can be drawn that represents each of the points in time during the breath cycle showing pressure as it occurs over time. In the following section, each portion of the graphed pressure or time curve is reviewed. These pressure points provide information about the mode of ventilation and can be used to calculate a variety of parameters to monitor patients receiving mechanical ventilation.

Baseline Pressure

Airway pressures are measured relative to a baseline value. In Fig. 1-9, the baseline pressure is zero (or atmospheric), which indicates that no additional pressure is applied at the airway opening during expiration and before inspiration.

Sometimes the baseline pressure is higher than zero, such as when the ventilator operator selects a higher pressure to be present at the end of exhalation. This is called **positive end-expiratory pressure,** or PEEP (Fig. 1-10). When PEEP is set, the ventilator prevents the patient from exhaling to zero (atmospheric pressure). PEEP therefore increases the volume of gas remaining in the lungs

at the end of a normal exhalation; that is, PEEP increases the functional residual capacity. PEEP applied by the operator is referred to as **extrinsic PEEP.** Auto-PEEP (or intrinsic PEEP), which is a potential side effect of positive pressure ventilation, is air that is accidentally trapped in the lung. **Intrinsic PEEP** usually occurs when a patient does not have enough time to exhale completely before the ventilator delivers another breath.

Peak Pressure

During positive pressure ventilation, the manometer rises progressively to a **peak pressure** (P_{Peak}). This is the highest pressure recorded at the end of inspiration. P_{Peak} is also called **peak inspiratory pressure** (PIP) or **peak airway pressure** (see Fig. 1-9).

The pressures measured during inspiration are the sum of two pressures: the pressure required to force the gas through the resistance of the airways (P_{TA}) and the pressure of the gas volume as it fills the alveoli (P_{alv}).*

Plateau Pressure

Another valuable pressure measurement is the **plateau pressure.** The plateau pressure is measured after a breath has been delivered to the patient and before exhalation begins. Exhalation is prevented by the ventilator for a brief moment (0.5 to 1.5 s). To obtain this measurement, the ventilator operator normally selects a control marked "inflation hold" or "inspiratory pause."

Plateau pressure measurement is similar to holding the breath at the end of inspiration. At the point of breath holding, the

---

*At any point during inspiration, gauge pressure equals $P_{TA} + P_{alv}$. The gauge pressure also will include pressure associated with PEEP.

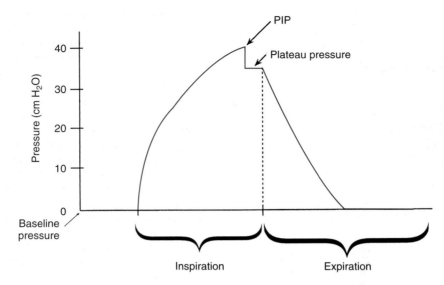

Fig. 1-9 Graph of upper-airway pressures that occur during a positive pressure breath. Pressure rises during inspiration to the peak inspiratory pressure (PIP). With a breath hold, the plateau pressure can be measured. Pressures fall back to baseline during expiration.

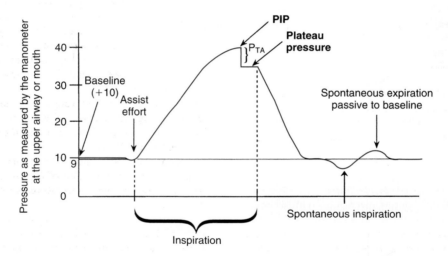

Fig. 1-10 Graph of airway pressures that occur during a mechanical positive pressure breath and a spontaneous breath. Both show an elevated baseline (positive end-expiratory pressure [PEEP] is +10 cm H_2O). To assist a breath, the ventilator drops the pressure below baseline by 1 cm H_2O. The assist effort is set at +9 cm H_2O. *PIP*, Peak inspiratory pressure; P_{TA}, transairway pressure. (See text for further explanation.)

pressures inside the alveoli and mouth are equal (no gas flow). However, the relaxation of the respiratory muscles and the elastic recoil of the lung tissues are exerting force on the inflated lungs. This creates a positive pressure, which can be read on the manometer as a positive pressure. Because it occurs during a breath hold or pause, the manometer reading remains stable and it "plateaus" at a certain value (see Figs. 1-9 through 1-11). Note that the plateau pressure reading will be inaccurate if the patient is actively breathing during the measurement.

Plateau pressure is often used interchangeably with **alveolar pressure** (P_{alv}) and **intrapulmonary pressure.** Although these terms are related, they are not synonymous. The plateau pressure reflects the effect of the elastic recoil on the gas volume inside

the alveoli and any pressure exerted by the volume in the ventilator circuit that is acted upon by the recoil of the plastic circuit.

Pressure at the End of Exhalation

As previously mentioned, air can be trapped in the lungs during mechanical ventilation if not enough time is allowed for exhalation. The most effective way to prevent this complication is to monitor the pressure in the ventilator circuit at the end of exhalation. If no extrinsic PEEP is added and the baseline pressure is greater than zero (i.e., atmospheric pressure), air trapping, or auto-PEEP, is present (this concept is covered in greater detail in Chapter 17).

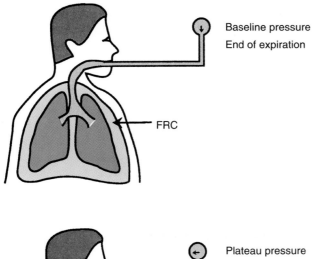

Baseline pressure
End of expiration

FRC

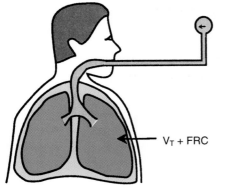

Plateau pressure
End of inspiration
before exhalation
occurs

V_T + FRC

Fig. 1-11 At baseline pressure (end of exhalation), the volume of air remaining in the lungs is the functional residual capacity (FRC). At the end of inspiration, before exhalation starts, the volume of air in the lungs is the tidal volume (V_T) plus the FRC. The pressure measured at this point, with no flow of air, is the *plateau pressure*.

- For air to flow through a tube or airway, a pressure gradient must exist (i.e., pressure at one end of the tube must be higher than pressure at the other end of the tube). Air will always flow from the high-pressure point to the low-pressure point.
- Several terms are used to describe airway opening pressure, including *mouth pressure, upper-airway pressure, mask pressure,* or *proximal airway pressure*. Unless pressure is applied at the airway opening, P_{awo} is zero, or atmospheric pressure.
- Intrapleural pressure is the pressure in the potential space between the parietal and visceral pleurae.
- The plateau pressure, which is sometimes substituted for alveolar pressure, is measured during a breath-hold maneuver during mechanical ventilation, and the value is read from the ventilator manometer.
- Four basic pressure gradients are used to describe normal ventilation: transairway pressure, transthoracic pressure, transpulmonary pressure, and transrespiratory pressure.
- Two types of forces oppose inflation of the lungs: elastic forces and frictional forces.
- Elastic forces arise from the elastance of the lungs and chest wall.
- Frictional forces are the result of two factors: the resistance of the tissues and organs as they become displaced during breathing, and the resistance to gas flow through the airways.
- Compliance and resistance are often used to describe the mechanical properties of the respiratory system. In the clinical setting, compliance measurements are used to describe the elastic forces that oppose lung inflation; airway resistance is a measurement of the frictional forces that must be overcome during breathing.
- The resistance to airflow through the conductive airways *(flow resistance)* depends on the gas viscosity, the gas density, the length and diameter of the tube, and the flow rate of the gas through the tube.
- The product of compliance (C) and resistance (R) is called a *time constant*. For any value of C and R, the time constant approximates the time in seconds required to inflate or deflate the lungs.
- Calculation of time constants is important when setting the ventilator's inspiratory time and expiratory time.
- Three basic methods have been developed to mimic or replace the normal mechanisms of breathing: negative pressure ventilation, positive pressure ventilation, and high-frequency ventilation.

SUMMARY

- Spontaneous ventilation is accomplished by contraction of the muscles of inspiration, which causes expansion of the thorax, or chest cavity. During mechanical ventilation, the mechanical ventilator provides some or all of the energy required to expand the thorax.

REVIEW QUESTIONS *(See Appendix A for answers.)*

1. Using Fig. 1-12, draw a graph and show the changes in the intrapleural and alveolar (intrapulmonary) pressures that occur during spontaneous ventilation and during a positive pressure breath. Compare the two.

2. Convert 5 mm Hg to cm H_2O.

3. Which of the lung units in Fig. 1-13 receives more volume during inspiration? Why? Which has a longer time constant?

4. In Fig. 1-14, which lung unit fills more quickly? Which has the shorter time constant? Which receives the greatest volume?

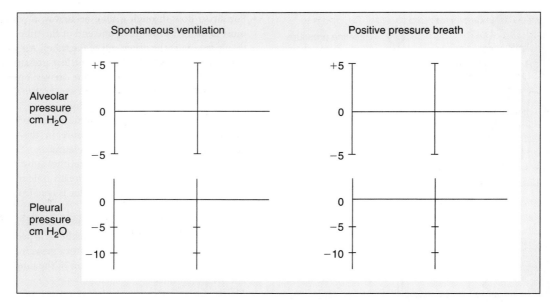

Fig. 1-12 Graphing of alveolar and pleural pressures for spontaneous ventilation and a positive pressure breath.

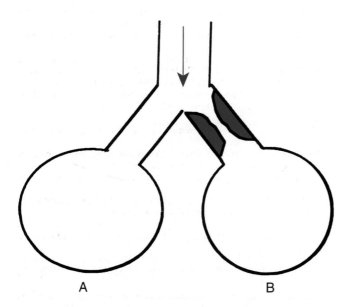

Fig. 1-13 Lung unit **A** is normal. Lung unit **B** shows an obstruction in the airway.

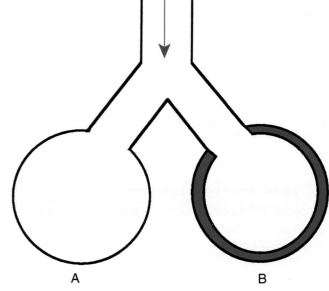

Fig. 1-14 Lung unit **A** is normal. Lung unit **B** shows decreased compliance (see text).

5. This exercise is intended to provide the reader with a greater understanding of time constants. Calculate the following six possible combinations. Then rank the lung units from the slowest filling to the most rapid filling. Because resistance is seldom better than normal, no example is given that is lower than normal for this particular parameter. (Normal values have been simplified to make calculations easier.)
   A. Normal lung unit: $C_S = 0.1$ L/cm H_2O; $R_{aw} = 1$ cm H_2O/(L/s)
   B. Lung unit with reduced compliance and normal airway resistance: $C_S = 0.025$ L/cm H_2O; $R_{aw} = 1$ cm H_2O/(L/s)
   C. Lung unit with normal compliance and increased airway resistance: $C_S = 0.1$ L/cm H_2O; $R_{aw} = 10$ cm H_2O/(L/s)
   D. Lung unit with reduced compliance and increased airway resistance: $C_S = 0.025$ L/cm H_2O; $R_{aw} = 10$ cm H_2O/(L/s)
   E. Lung unit with increased compliance and increased airway resistance: $C_S = 0.15$ L/cm H_2O; $R_{aw} = 10$ cm H_2O/(L/s)
   F. Lung unit with increased compliance and normal airway resistance: $C_S = 0.15$ L/cm H_2O; $R_{aw} = 1$ cm H_2O/(L/s)

6. 1 mm Hg =
   A. 1.63 cm H_2O
   B. 1.30 atm
   C. 1.36 cm H_2O
   D. 1034 cm H_2O

7. The pressure difference between the alveolus (P_{alv}) and the body surface (P_{bs}) is called
   A. Transpulmonary pressure
   B. Transrespiratory pressure
   C. Transairway pressure
   D. Transthoracic pressure

8. Define elastance.
   A. Ability of a structure to stretch
   B. Ability of a structure to return to its natural shape after stretching
   C. Ability of a structure to stretch and remain in that position
   D. None of the above

9. Which of the following formulas is used to calculate compliance?
   A. $\Delta V = C/\Delta P$
   B. $\Delta P = \Delta V/C$
   C. $C = \Delta V/\Delta P$
   D. $C = \Delta P/\Delta V$

10. Another term for airway pressure is
    A. Mouth pressure
    B. Airway opening pressure
    C. Mask pressure
    D. All of the above

11. Intraalveolar pressure (in relation to atmospheric pressure) at the end of inspiration during a normal quiet breath is approximately
    A. -5 cm H_2O
    B. 0 cm H_2O
    C. $+5$ cm H_2O
    D. 10 cm H_2O

12. Which of the following is associated with an increase in airway resistance?
    A. Decreasing the flow rate of gas into the airway
    B. Reducing the density of the gas being inhaled
    C. Increasing the diameter of the endotracheal tube
    D. Reducing the length of the endotracheal tube

13. Which of the following statements is true regarding negative pressure ventilation?
    A. Chest cuirass is often used in the treatment of hypovolemic patients.
    B. Tank respirators are particularly useful in the treatment of burn patients.
    C. The incidence of alveolar barotrauma is higher with these devices compared with positive pressure ventilation.
    D. These ventilators mimic normal breathing mechanics.

14. PEEP is best defined as
    A. Zero baseline during exhalation on a positive pressure ventilator
    B. Positive pressure during inspiration that is set by the person operating the ventilator
    C. Negative pressure during exhalation on a positive pressure ventilator
    D. Positive pressure at the end of exhalation on a mechanical ventilator

15. Which of the following statements is true regarding plateau pressure?
    A. Plateau pressure normally is zero at end inspiration.
    B. Plateau pressure is used as a measure of alveolar pressure.
    C. Plateau pressure is measured at the end of exhalation.
    D. Plateau pressure is a dynamic measurement.

16. One time constant should allow approximately what percentage of a lung unit to fill?
    A. 37%
    B. 100%
    C. 63%
    D. 85%

17. A patient has a PIP of 30 cm H_2O and a $P_{plateau}$ of 20 cm H_2O. Ventilator flow is set at a constant value of 30 L/min. What is the transairway pressure?
    A. 1 cm H_2O
    B. 0.33 cm H_2O
    C. 20 cm H_2O
    D. 10 cm H_2O

References

1. Kacmarek RM, Volsko TA: Mechanical ventilators. In Kacmarek RM, Stoller JK, Heuer AJ, editors: *Egan's fundamentals of respiratory care*, ed 10, St Louis, 2013, Elsevier, pp 1006–1040.
2. Nunn JF: *Applied respiratory physiology*, ed 3, London, 1987, Butterworths.
3. Chatburn RL, Primiano FP, Jr: Mathematical models of respiratory mechanics. In Chatburn RL, Craig KC, editors: *Fundamentals of respiratory care research*, Stamford, Conn., 1988, Appleton & Lange.
4. Chatburn RL, Volsko TA: Mechanical ventilators. In Kacmarek RM, Stoller JK, Heuer AJ, editors: *Egan's fundamentals of respiratory care*, ed 10, St Louis, 2013, Elsevier.
5. Harrison RA: Monitoring respiratory mechanics. *Crit Care Clin* 11(1):151–167, 1995.
6. Marks A, Asher J, Bocles L, et al: A new ventilator assister for patients with respiratory acidosis. *N Engl J Med* 268(2):61–68, 1963.
7. Hill NS: Clinical applications of body ventilators. *Chest* 90:897–905, 1986.
8. Kirby RR, Banner MJ, Downs JB: *Clinical applications of ventilatory support*, ed 2, New York, 1990, Churchill Livingstone.
9. Corrado A, Gorini M: Negative pressure ventilation. In Tobin MJ, editor: *Principles and practice of mechanical ventilation*, ed 3, New York, 2013, McGraw-Hill.
10. Holtackers TR, Loosbrook LM, Gracey DR: The use of the chest cuirass in respiratory failure of neurologic origin. *Respir Care* 27(3):271–275, 1982.
11. Hansra IK, Hill NS: Noninvasive mechanical ventilation. In Albert RK, Spiro SG, Jett JR, editors: *Clinical respiratory medicine*, ed 3, Philadelphia, 2008, Mosby Elsevier.
12. Splaingard ML, Frates RC, Jefferson LS, et al: Home negative pressure ventilation: report of 20 years of experience in patients with neuromuscular disease. *Arch Phys Med Rehabil* 66:239–242, 1983.

How Ventilators Work

OUTLINE

KEY TERMS

- Closed-loop system
- Control system
- Double-circuit ventilator
- Drive mechanism
- External circuit
- Internal pneumatic circuit
- Mandatory minute ventilation
- Open-loop system
- Patient circuit
- Single-circuit ventilator
- User interface

LEARNING OBJECTIVES   *On completion of this chapter, the reader will be able to do the following:*

1. List the basic types of power sources used for mechanical ventilators.
2. Give examples of ventilators that use an electrical and a pneumatic power source.
3. Explain the difference in function between positive and negative pressure ventilators.
4. Distinguish between a closed-loop and an open-loop system.
5. Define *user interface.*
6. Describe a ventilator's internal and external pneumatic circuits.
7. Discuss the difference between a single-circuit and a double-circuit ventilator.
8. Identify the components of an external circuit (patient circuit).
9. Explain the function of an externally mounted exhalation valve.
10. Compare the functions of the three types of volume displacement drive mechanisms.
11. Describe the function of the proportional solenoid valve.

Clinicians caring for critically ill patients receiving ventilatory support must have a basic understanding of the principles of operation of mechanical ventilators. This understanding should focus on patient-ventilator interactions (i.e., how the ventilator interacts with the patient's breathing pattern, and how patient's lung condition can affect the ventilator's performance). Many different types of ventilators are available for adult, pediatric, and neonatal care in hospitals; for patient transport; and for home care. Mastering the complexities of each of these devices may seem overwhelming at times. Fortunately, ventilators have a number of properties in common, which allow them to be described and grouped accordingly.

An excellent way to gain an overview of a particular ventilator is to study how it functions. Part of the problem with this approach, however, is that the terminology used by manufacturers and authors varies considerably. The purpose of this chapter is to address these terminology differences and provide an overview of

ventilator function as it relates to current standards.[1-3] It does not attempt to review all available ventilators. For models not covered in this discussion, the reader should consult other texts and the literature provided by the manufacturer.[3] The description of the "hardware" components of mechanical ventilators presented in this chapter should provide clinicians with a better understanding of the principles of operation of these devices.

HISTORICAL PERSPECTIVE ON VENTILATOR CLASSIFICATION

The earliest commercially available ventilators used in the clinical setting (e.g., the Mörch and the Emerson Post-Op) were developed in the 1950s and 1960s. These devices originally were classified according to a system developed by Mushin and colleagues.[4] Technological advances made during the past 50 years have dramatically changed the way ventilators operate, and these changes

---

> **BOX 2-1**   Components of a Ventilator
>
> 1. Power source or input power (electrical or gas source)
>   a. Electrically powered ventilators
>   b. Pneumatically powered ventilators
> 2. Positive or negative pressure generator
> 3. Control systems and circuits
>   a. Open- and closed-loop systems to control ventilator function
>   b. Control panel (user interface)
>   c. Pneumatic circuit
> 4. Power transmission and conversion system
>   a. Volume displacement, pneumatic designs
>   b. Flow-control valves
> 5. Output (pressure, volume, and flow waveforms)

> **BOX 2-2**   Examples of Electrically Powered Ventilators
>
> Lifecare PLV-102 ventilator (Philips Respironics, Pittsburgh, Pa.)
> Pulmonetics LTV 800, 900, and 1000 ventilators (CareFusion, Minneapolis, Minn.)
> Newport HT50 (Newport Medical Instruments, Costa Mesa, Calif.)

required an updated approach to ventilator classification. The following discussion is based on an updated classification system proposed by Chatburn.[1] Chatburn's approach to classifying ventilators uses engineering and clinical principles to describe ventilator function.[2] Although this classification system provides a good foundation for discussing various aspects of mechanical ventilation, many clinicians still rely on the earlier classification system to describe basic ventilator operation. Both classification systems are referenced when necessary in the following discussion to describe the principles of operation of commonly used mechanical ventilators.

INTERNAL FUNCTION

A ventilator probably can be easily understood if it is pictured as a "black box." It is plugged into an electrical outlet or a high-pressure gas source, and gas comes out the other side. The person who operates the ventilator sets certain knobs or dials on a control panel (**user interface**) to establish the pressure and pattern of gas flow delivered by the machine. Inside the black box, a **control system** interprets the operator's settings and produces and regulates the desired output. In the discussion that follows, specific characteristics of the various components of a typical commercially available mechanical ventilator are discussed. Box 2-1 provides a summary of the major components of a ventilator.

POWER SOURCE OR INPUT POWER

The ventilator's power source provides the energy that enables the machine to perform the work of ventilating the patient. As discussed in Chapter 1, ventilation can be achieved using either positive or negative pressure. The power used by a mechanical ventilator to generate this positive or negative pressure may be provided by an electrical or pneumatic (compressed gas) source.

Electrically Powered Ventilators

Electrically powered ventilators rely entirely on electricity from a standard electrical outlet (110 to 115 V, 60-Hz alternating current [AC] in the United States; higher voltages [220 V, 50 Hz] in other countries), or a rechargeable battery (direct current [DC]) may be used. Battery power is usually used for a short period, such as for transporting a ventilated patient, or in homecare therapy as a backup power source if the home's electricity fails.

An on/off switch controls the main electrical power source. The electricity provides the energy to operate motors, electromagnets, potentiometers, rheostats, and **microprocessors,** which in turn, control the timing mechanisms for inspiration and expiration, gas flow, and alarm systems. Electrical power may also be used to operate devices such as fans, bellows, solenoids, and transducers. All these devices help ensure a controlled pressure and gas flow to the patient. Examples of electrically powered and controlled ventilators are listed in Box 2-2.

Pneumatically Powered Ventilators

Current generation intensive care unit (ICU) ventilators are typically pneumatically powered devices. These machines use one or two 50-psi gas sources and have built-in internal reducing valves so that the operating pressure is lower than the source pressure.

Pneumatically powered ventilators are classified according to the mechanism used to control gas flow. Two types of devices are available: pneumatic ventilators and fluidic ventilators. Pneumatic ventilators use needle valves, Venturi entrainers (injectors), flexible diaphragms, and spring-loaded valves to control flow, volume delivery, and inspiratory and expiratory function (Fig. 2-1). The Bird Mark 7 ventilator, which was originally used for prolonged mechanical ventilation is often cited as an example of a pneumatic ventilator. These devices currently are used primarily to administer intermittent positive pressure breathing (IPPB) treatments. IPPB treatments involve the delivery of aerosolized medications to spontaneously breathing patients with reduced ventilatory function (e.g., chronic obstructive pulmonary disease [COPD] patients).[3]

Fluidic ventilators rely on special principles to control gas flow, specifically the principles of wall attachment and beam deflection. Fig. 2-2 shows the basic components of a fluidic system. An example of a ventilator that uses fluidic control circuits is the Bio-Med MVP-10. (Fluidic circuits are analogous to electronic logic circuits.) Fluidic systems are only occasionally used to ventilate patients in the acute care setting.[3]

Most pneumatically powered ICU ventilators also have an electrical power source incorporated into their design to energize a computer that controls the ventilator functions. Notice that the gas sources, mixtures of air and oxygen, supply the power for ventilator function and allow for a variable fractional inspired oxygen concentration (F_IO_2). The electrical power is required for operation of the computer microprocessor, which controls capacitors, solenoids, and electrical switches that regulate the phasing of inspiration and expiration, and the monitoring of gas flow. The ventilator's preprogrammed ventilator modes are stored in the microprocessor's read-only memory (ROM), which can be updated rapidly by installing new software programs. Random access memory (RAM), which is also incorporated into the ventilator's central processing unit, is used for temporary storage of data,

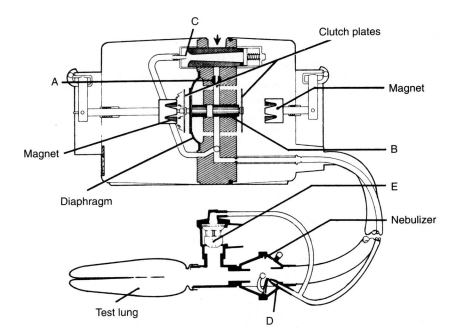

Fig. 2-1 The Bird Mark 7 is an example of a pneumatically powered ventilator. (Courtesy CareFusion, Viasys Corp., San Diego, Calif.)

such as pressure and flow measurements and airway resistance and compliance (Key Point 2-1.)

Case Study 2-1 provides an exercise in selecting a ventilator with a specific power source.

 Key Point **2-1** Pneumatically powered, microprocessor-controlled ventilators rely on pneumatic power (i.e., the 50-psi gas sources) to provide the energy to deliver the breath. Electrical power from an alternating current (AC) wall-socket or from a direct current (DC) battery power source provides the energy for a computer microprocessor that controls the internal function of the machine.

Case Study 2-1

Ventilator Selection
A patient who requires continuous ventilatory support is being transferred from the intensive care unit to a general care patient room. The general care hospital rooms are equipped with piped-in oxygen but not piped-in air. What type of ventilator would you select for this patient?

Positive and Negative Pressure Ventilators

As discussed in Chapter 1, gas flow into the lungs can be accomplished by using two different methods of changing the transrespiratory pressure gradient (pressure at the airway opening minus pressure at the body surface [$P_{awo} - P_{bs}$]). A ventilator can change the transrespiratory pressure gradient by altering either the pressure applied at the airway opening (P_{awo}) or the pressure around the body surface (P_{bs}). With positive pressure ventilators, gas flows into the lung because the ventilator establishes a pressure gradient by generating a positive pressure at the airway opening (Fig. 2-3, *A*). In contrast, a negative pressure ventilator generates a negative

pressure at the body surface that is transmitted to the pleural space and then to the alveoli (Fig. 2-3, *B*).

CONTROL SYSTEMS AND CIRCUITS

The control system (control circuit), or decision-making system that regulates ventilator function internally, can use mechanical or electrical devices, electronics, pneumatics, fluidics, or a combination of these.

Open- and Closed-Loop Systems to Control Ventilator Function

Advances in microprocessor technology have allowed ventilator manufacturers to develop a new generation of ventilators that contain feedback loop systems. Most ventilators that are **not** microprocessor controlled are called **open-loop** systems. The operator sets a control (e.g., tidal volume), and the ventilator delivers that volume to the patient circuit. This is called an **open-loop system** because the ventilator cannot be programmed to respond to changing conditions. If gas leaks out of the patient circuit (and therefore does not reach the patient), the ventilator cannot adjust its function to correct for the leakage. It simply delivers a set volume and does not measure or change it (Fig. 2-4, *A*).

Closed-loop systems are often described as "intelligent" systems because they compare the set control variable to the measured control variable, which in turn allows the ventilator to respond to changes in the patient's condition. For example, some closed-loop systems are programmed to compare the tidal volume setting to the measured tidal volume exhaled by the patient. If the two differ, the control system can alter the volume delivery (Fig. 2-4, *B*).[5-7] **Mandatory minute ventilation** is a good example of a **closed-loop system.** The operator selects a minimum minute ventilation setting that is lower than the patient's spontaneous minute ventilation. The ventilator monitors the patient's spontaneous minute ventilation, and if it falls below the operator's set value, the ventilator increases its output to meet the minimum **set** minute ventilation (Critical Care Concept 2-1).

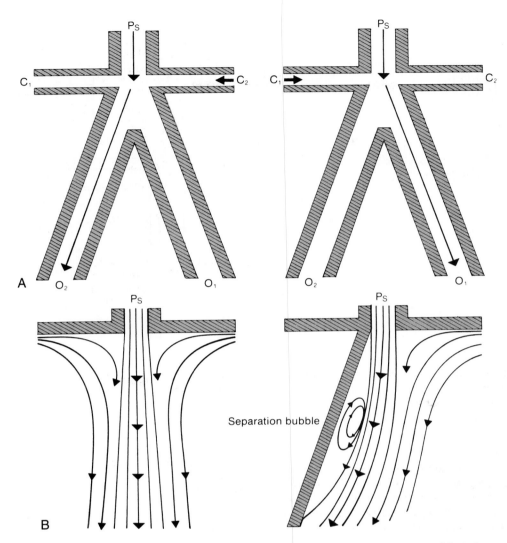

Fig. 2-2 Basic components of fluid logic (fluidic) pneumatic mechanisms. **A,** Example of a flip-flop valve (beam deflection). When a continuous pressure source (P_S at inlet A) enters, wall attachment occurs and the output is established (O_2). A control signal (single gas pulse) from C_1 deflects the beam to outlet O_1. **B,** The wall attachment phenomenon, or *Coanda effect,* is demonstrated. A turbulent jet flow causes a localized drop in lateral pressure and draws in air *(figure on left).* When a wall is adjacent, a low-pressure vortex bubble (separation bubble) is created and bends the jet toward the wall *(figure on right).* (From Dupuis YG: Ventilators: Theory and clinical applications, ed 2, St Louis, 1992, Mosby.)

⬡ CRITICAL CARE CONCEPT 2-1

Open-Loop or Closed-Loop

A ventilator is programmed to monitor S_pO_2. If the S_pO_2 drops below 90% for longer than 30 seconds, the ventilator is programmed to activate an audible alarm that cannot be silenced and a flashing red visual alarm. The ventilator also is programmed to increase the oxygen percentage to 100% until the alarms have been answered and deactivated. Is this a closed-loop or an open-loop system? What are the potential advantages and disadvantages of using this type of system?

Control Panel (User Interface)

The control panel, or *user interface,* is located on the surface of the ventilator and is monitored and set by the ventilator operator. The internal control system reads and uses the operator's settings to control the function of the drive mechanism. The control panel has various knobs or touch pads for setting components, such as tidal volume, rate, inspiratory time, alarms, and F_IO_2 (Fig. 2-5). These controls ultimately regulate four ventilatory variables: flow, volume, pressure, and time. The value for each of these can vary within a wide range, and the manufacturer provides a list of the potential ranges for each variable. For example, tidal volume may range from 200 to 2000 mL on an adult ventilator. The operator also can set alarms to respond to changes in a variety of monitored variables, particularly high and low pressure and low volume. (Alarm settings are discussed in more detail in Chapter 7.)

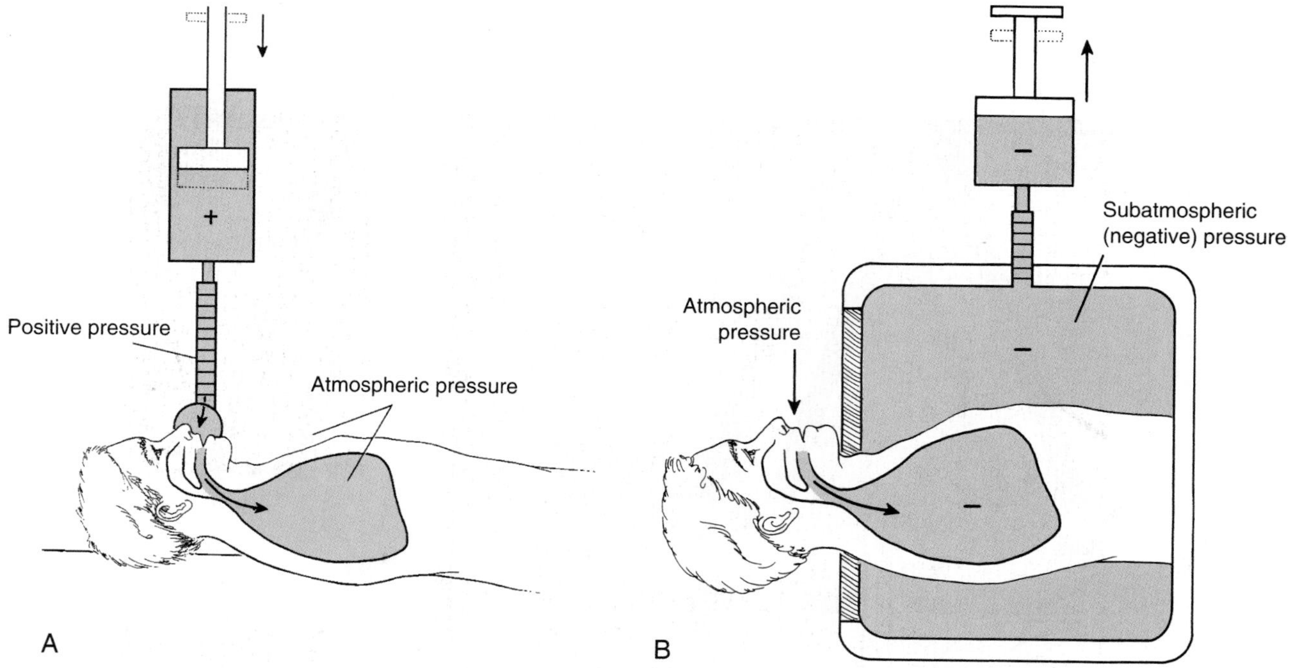

A

B

Fig. 2-3 A, Application of positive pressure at the airway provides a pressure gradient between the mouth and the alveoli; as a result, gas flows into the lungs. **B,** When subatmospheric pressure is applied around the chest wall, pressure drops in the alveoli and air flows into the lungs.

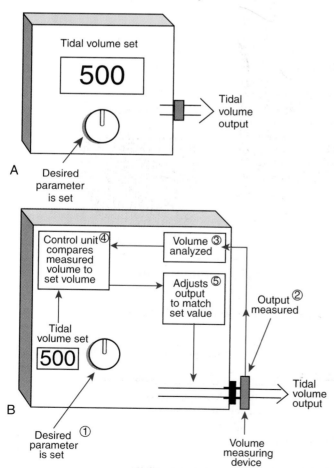

Fig. 2-4 A, Open-loop system. **B,** Closed-loop system using tidal volume as the measured parameter.

Pneumatic Circuit

A pneumatic circuit, or pathway, is a series of tubes that allow gas to flow inside the ventilator and between the ventilator and the patient. The pressure gradient created by the ventilator with its power source generates the flow of gas. This gas flows through the pneumatic circuit en route to the patient. The gas first is directed from the generating source inside the ventilator through the **internal pneumatic circuit** to the ventilator's outside surface. Gas then flows through an **external circuit,** or **patient circuit,** into the patient's lungs. Exhaled gas passes through the expiratory limb of the external circuit and to the atmosphere through an exhalation valve.

Internal Pneumatic Circuit

If the ventilator's internal circuit allows the gas to flow directly from its power source to the patient, the machine is called a **single-circuit ventilator** (Fig. 2-6). The source of the gas may be either externally compressed gas or an internal pressurizing source, such as a compressor. Most ICU ventilators manufactured today are classified as single-circuit ventilators.

Another type of internal pneumatic circuit ventilator is the **double-circuit ventilator.** In these machines, the primary power source generates a gas flow that compresses a mechanism such as a *bellows* or "*bag-in-a-chamber.*" The gas in the bellows or bag then flows to the patient. Figure 2-7 illustrates the principle of operation of a double-circuit ventilator. The Cardiopulmonary Venturi is an example of a double-circuit ventilator currently on the market (Key Point 2-2).

Key Point **2-2** Most commercially available intensive care unit ventilators are single-circuit, microprocessor-controlled, positive pressure ventilators with closed-loop elements of logic in the control system.

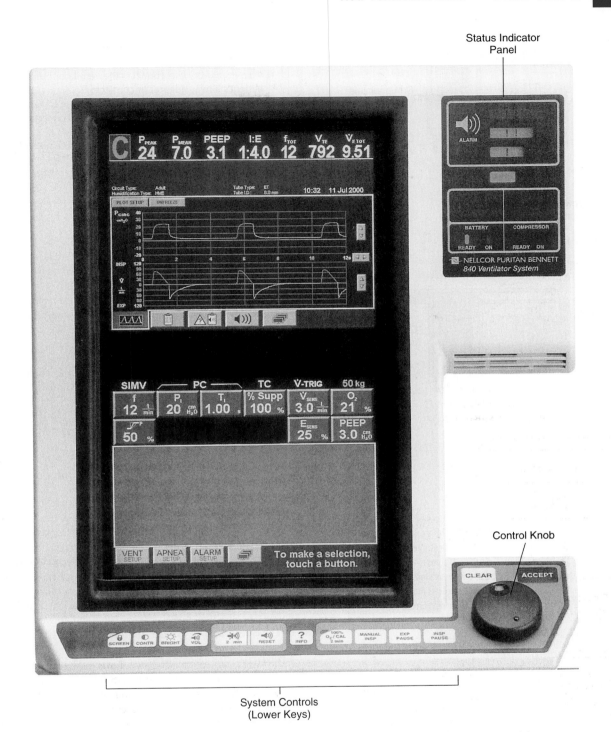

Status Indicator Panel

Control Knob

System Controls
(Lower Keys)

Fig. 2-5 User interface of the Puritan Bennett 840 ventilator. (Courtesy Covidien-Nellcor Puritan Bennett, Boulder, Colo.)

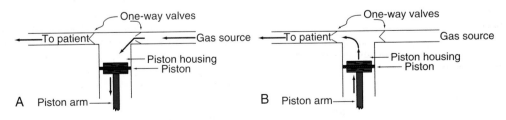

Fig. 2-6 Single-circuit ventilator. **A,** Gases are drawn into the cylinder during the expiratory phase. **B,** During inspiration, the piston moves upward into the cylinder, sending gas directly to the patient circuit.

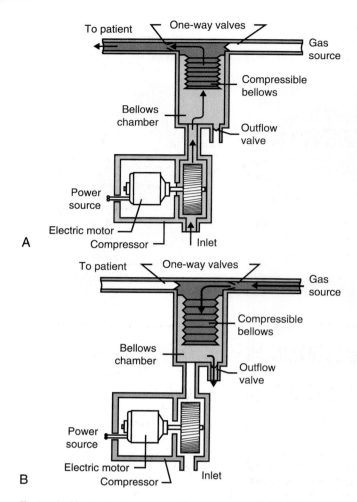

BOX 2-3   **Basic Elements of a Patient Circuit**

1. *Main inspiratory line:* connects the ventilator output to the patient's airway adapter or connector
2. *Adapter:* connects the main inspiratory line to the patient's airway (also called a *patient adapter* or *Y-connector* because of its shape)
3. *Expiratory line:* delivers expired gas from the patient to the exhalation valve
4. *Expiratory valve:* allows the release of exhaled gas from the expiratory line into the room air

Fig. 2-7 Double-circuit ventilator. An electrical compressor produces a high-pressure gas source, which is directed into a chamber that holds a collapsible bellows. The bellows contains the desired gas mixture for the patient. The pressure from the compressor forces the bellows upward, resulting in a positive pressure breath **(A)**. After delivery of the inspiratory breath, the compressor stops directing pressure into the bellows chamber, and exhalation occurs. The bellows drops to its original position and fills with the gas mixture in preparation for the next breath **(B)**.

External Pneumatic Circuit

The external pneumatic circuit, or patient circuit, connects the ventilator to the patient's artificial airway. This circuit must have several basic elements to provide a positive pressure breath (Box 2-3). Figure 2-8 shows examples of two types of patient circuits. During inspiration, the expiratory valve closes so that gas can flow only into the patient's lungs.

In early generation ventilators (e.g., the Bear 3), the exhalation valve is mounted in the main exhalation line of the patient circuit (Fig. 2-8, *A*). With this arrangement, an expiratory valve charge line, which powers the expiratory valve, must also be present. When the ventilator begins inspiratory gas flow through the main inspiratory tube, gas also flows through the charge line, closing the valve (Fig. 2-8, *A*). During exhalation, the flow from the ventilator stops, the charge line depressurizes, and the exhalation valve opens. The patient then is able to exhale passively through the expiratory port. In most current ICU ventilators, the exhalation valve is located inside the ventilator and is not visible (Fig. 2-8, *B*). A

mechanical device, such as a solenoid valve, typically is used to control these internally mounted exhalation valves (see the section on flow valves later in this chapter).

Figure 2-9 illustrates the various components typically included in a patient's circuit to optimize gas delivery and ventilator function. The most common adjuncts are shown in Box 2-4. Additional monitoring devices include graphic display screens, oxygen analyzers, pulse oximeters, capnographs (end-tidal CO_2 monitors), and flow and pressure sensors for monitoring lung compliance and airway resistance (for more detail about monitoring devices, see Chapter 11).

POWER TRANSMISSION AND CONVERSION SYSTEM

A ventilator's power source enables it to perform mechanical or pneumatic operations. The internal hardware that accomplishes the conversion of electrical or pneumatic energy into the mechanical energy required to deliver a breath to the patient is called the *power transmission and conversion system*. It consists of a **drive mechanism** and an output control mechanism.

The drive mechanism is a mechanical device that produces gas flow to the patient. An example of a drive mechanism is a piston powered by an electrical motor. The output control consists of one or more valves that regulate gas flow to the patient. From an engineering perspective, power transmission and conversion systems can be categorized as volume controllers or flow controllers.[2,7]

Compressors (Blowers)

An appreciation of how volume and flow controllers operate requires an understanding of compressors, or blowers. Compressors reduce internal volumes (compression) within the ventilator to generate a positive pressure required to deliver gas to the patient. Compressors may be piston driven, or they may use rotating blades (vanes), moving diaphragms, or bellows. Hospitals use large, piston-type, water-cooled compressors to supply wall gas outlets, which many ventilators use as a power source. Some ventilators (e.g., CareFusion AVEA, Servo-i) have built-in compressors, which can be used to power the ventilator if a wall gas outlet is not available.

Volume Displacement Designs

Volume displacement devices include bellows, pistons, concertina bags, and "bag-in-a-chamber" systems.[7,8] Box 2-5 provides a brief description of the principle of operation for each of these devices, and also examples of ventilators that use these mechanisms.

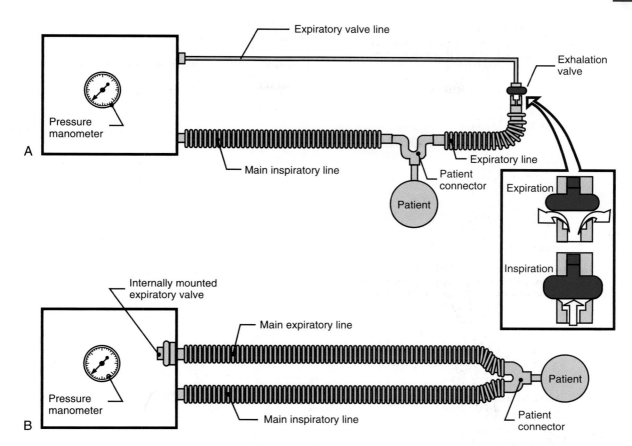

Fig. 2-8 Basic components of a patient circuit that are required for a positive pressure breath. **A,** Ventilator circuit with an externally mounted expiratory valve. The cutaway shows a balloon-type expiratory valve. During inspiration gas fills the balloon and closes a hole in the expiratory valve. Closing of the hole makes the patient circuit a sealed system. During expiration, the balloon deflates, the hole opens, and gas from the patient is exhaled into the room through the hole. **B,** Ventilator circuit with an internally mounted exhalation valve. (From Cairo JM, Pilbeam SP: Mosby's respiratory care equipment, ed 8, St Louis, 2010, Mosby.)

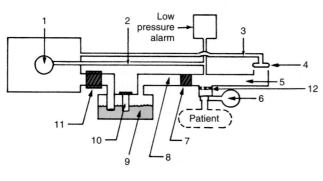

1 — Pressure manometer	5 — Expiratory line	9 — Humidifier
2 — Upper airway pressure monitor line	6 — Expired volume measuring device	10 — Heater and thermostat
3 — Expiratory valve line	7 — Temperature measuring or sensing device	11 — Main flow bacterial filter
4 — Expiratory valve	8 — Main inspiratory line	12 — Oxygen analyzer

Fig. 2-9 A patient circuit with additional components required for optimal functioning during continuous mechanical ventilation.

BOX 2-4   Adjuncts Used with a Patient Circuit

1. A device to warm and humidify inspired air (e.g., heat-moisture exchanger, heated humidifier)
2. A thermometer or sensing device to measure the temperature of inspired air
3. An apnea or low-pressure alarm that indicates leaks or that the patient is not ventilating adequately*
4. A nebulizer line to power a micronebulizer for delivery of aerosolized medications
5. A volume-measuring device to determine the patient's exhaled volume*
6. Bacterial filters to filter gas administered to the patient and exhaled by the patient
7. A pressure gauge to measure pressures in the upper airway*
8. In-line suction catheter

---

*Usually built into the ventilator.

BOX 2-5   **Examples of Volume Displacement Devices**

Spring-Loaded Bellows

In a spring-loaded bellows model, an adjustable spring atop a bellows applies a force per unit area, or pressure (P = Force/Area). Tightening of the spring creates greater force and therefore greater pressure. The bellows contains preblended gas (air and oxygen), which is administered to the patient. The Servo 900C ventilator is an example of a ventilator that uses a spring-loaded bellows (pressure of up to 120 cm H_2O). Although these devices are no longer manufactured, it is worth noting because of their importance in the development of modern mechanical ventilators.

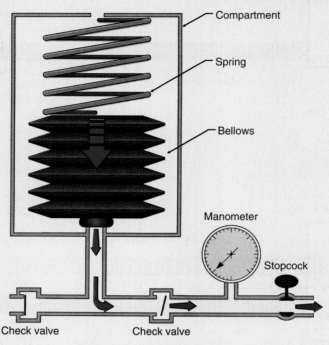

A spring-loaded bellows mechanism.

Linear Drive Piston

In a linear drive device, an electrical motor is connected by a special gearing mechanism to a piston rod or arm. The rod moves the piston forward inside a cylinder housing in a linear fashion at a constant rate. Some high-frequency ventilators use linear or direct drive pistons. Incorporating a rolling seal or using low resistance materials has helped eliminate the friction that occurred with early piston/cylinder designs. The Puritan Bennett 760 ventilator is an example of a linear drive piston device.

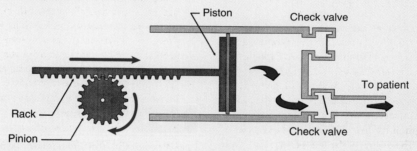

A linear drive piston.

Rotary Drive Piston

This type of drive mechanism is called a *rotary drive*, a *nonlinear drive*, or an *eccentric drive* piston. An electric motor rotates a drive wheel. The resulting flow pattern is slow at the beginning of inspiration, achieves highest speed at midinspiration, and tapers off at endinspiration. This pattern is called a *sine* (sinusoidal) *waveform*. The Puritan Bennett Companion 2801 ventilator, which is used in home care, has this type of piston.

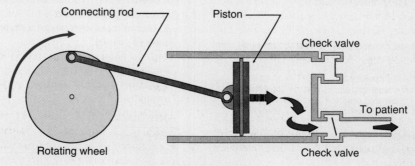

A rotary drive piston.

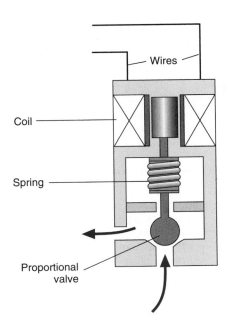

Fig. 2-10 Proportional solenoid valve, a type of flow control valve. In this design, a controllable electrical current flows through the coil, creating a magnetic field. The strength of the magnetic field causes the armature to assume a specified position. With the armature and valve poppet physically connected, this assembly is the only moving part. Coil and armature designs vary, as do strategies for fixing the position of the poppet. (Redrawn from Sanborn WG: Respir Care 38:72, 1993.)

Volume Flow-Control Valves

Current ICU ventilators use flow-control valves to regulate gas flow to the patient. These flow-control valves operate by opening and closing either completely or in small increments. These valves, which are driven by various motor-based mechanisms, have a rapid response time and great flexibility in flow control. Flow-control valves include proportional solenoid valves and digital valves with on/off configurations.

A proportional solenoid valve can be designed with various configurations to modify gas flow. A typical valve incorporates a gate or plunger, a valve seat, an electromagnet, a diaphragm, a spring, and two electrical contacts (Fig. 2-10). An electrical current flows through the electromagnet and creates a magnetic field, which pulls the plunger and opens the valve. The amount of current flowing through the electromagnet influences the strength of the magnetic field; the strength of the field determines the position of the plunger, or *armature*. The design of the plunger can vary from ventilator to ventilator.

Solenoids can be controlled in three ways: by electrical timers or microprocessors, by manual operation, and by pressure. With electrical timers and microprocessors, a current passes to the electromagnet and opens the valve. Manual operation closes a switch, sending a current to the electromagnet and opening the valve. Pressure changes generated by a patient's inspiratory effort can cause a diaphragm to move, closing an electrical contact, and opening or closing the valve.[7,8] Examples of ventilators with this type of valve include the Puritan Bennett 840, the Hamilton Galileo, the Dräger Infinity V500, and the Servo-i.

In the digital on/off valve configuration, several valves operate together. Each valve is either open or closed (Fig. 2-11). A particular valve produces a certain flow by controlling the opening and closing of a specifically sized orifice. The amount of flow varies depending on which valves are open. The Infant Star ventilator used this type of valve configuration.

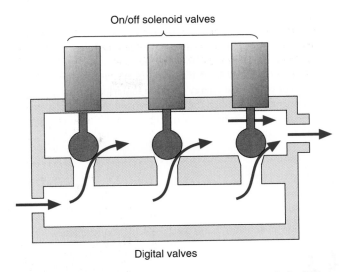

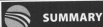

Fig. 2-11 Digital on/off valve, another type of pneumatic flow control valve. With each valve controlling a critical orifice and thus a specified flow, the number of discrete flow steps (including zero) becomes 2^n (where n = number of valves). (Redrawn from Sanborn WG: Respir Care 38:72, 1993.)

SUMMARY

- The major components of a mechanical ventilator include a high-pressure gas source, a control panel (user interface) to establish the pressure and pattern of gas flow delivered by the machine, and a control system that interprets the operator's settings and produces and regulates the desired output.
- Ventilator power sources may operate on electrical or pneumatic (gas) power. Electrically powered ventilators may rely on an AC wall outlet or a direct current DC source, such as a battery. Pneumatically powered ventilators are classified as pneumatic ventilators and fluidic ventilators. Pneumatically powered, microprocessor-controlled ventilators use compressed gas input power to drive inspiration, and use electrical power to control the breath characteristics.
- With positive pressure ventilators, gas flows into the lung because the ventilator establishes a pressure gradient by generating a positive pressure at the airway opening.
- Negative pressure ventilators create a transairway pressure gradient between the airway opening and the alveoli by generating a negative pressure at the body surface. This negative pressure is transmitted to the pleural space and then to the alveoli. The ventilator's control circuit, or decision-making system, uses mechanical or electrical devices, electronics, pneumatics, fluidics, or a combination of these to regulate ventilator function.
- The control panel, or user interface, has various knobs or touch pads for setting components, such as tidal volume, rate, inspiratory time, alarms, and F_IO_2.
- With an open-loop system, the ventilator cannot be programmed to respond to changing conditions. In contrast, a closed-loop system is often described as an "intelligent" system because the ventilator can be programmed to compare the set control variable to the measured control variable.
- The major components of a patient circuit include the main inspiratory line, which connects the ventilator output to the patient's airway adapter or connector; an adapter that connects

the main inspiratory line to the patient's airway; an expiratory line that delivers expired gas from the patient to the exhalation valve; and an expiratory valve that allows the release of exhaled gas from the expiratory line into the room air.

- The internal hardware that accomplishes the conversion of electrical or pneumatic energy required to perform these mechanical operations is called the power transmission and conversion system. It consists of a drive mechanism and the output control mechanism.

- The ventilator's drive mechanism is a mechanical device that produces gas flow to the patient. These are generally classified as volume displacement and flow devices. The output control consists of one or more valves that determine the gas flow to the patient.

- Some ventilators use volume displacement devices, such as bellows, pistons, concertina bags, and "bag-in-a-chamber" systems. Common examples include spring-loaded bellows, linear-drive pistons, and rotary-drive pistons.

REVIEW QUESTIONS *(See Appendix A for answers.)*

1. Name a commercially available ventilator that is entirely pneumatically powered.

2. Name a ventilator that is totally electrically powered.

3. What type of ventilator delivers pressures below ambient pressure on the body surface and mimics the physiology of normal breathing?

4. Explain the operation of an externally mounted exhalation valve.

5. What volume displacement device creates a sine waveform for gas flow?

6. A Dräger Evita Infinity V500 ventilator is set to deliver a minute ventilation of 5 L/min. The patient breathes six times in 1 minute and receives a mandatory breath of 500 mL with each breath. The ventilator detects the difference between the actual and the set minute ventilation and adds four more breaths (500 mL each) to make up the difference. Which of the following best describes this type of ventilator?
   A. Closed loop
   B. Open loop

7. The controls set by the ventilator operator are considered part of the:
   A. Pneumatic drive circuit
   B. Electrical motor
   C. User interface
   D. Pneumatic circuit

8. The gas-conducting tubes that carry gas from the ventilator to the patient are referred to as the:
   A. Internal pneumatic circuit
   B. Control circuit
   C. Control scheme
   D. Patient circuit

9. A ventilator in which the gas that enters the patient's lungs is also the gas that powers the unit is referred to as a:
   A. Direct drive ventilator
   B. Single-circuit ventilator
   C. Double-circuit ventilator
   D. Single-power source ventilator

10. In a spring-loaded bellows volume-delivery device, the amount of pressure is determined by the:
    A. Location of the bellows
    B. Volume setting on the ventilator
    C. Tightness of the spring
    D. Electrical power provided to the spring

11. Which of the following is an example of a flow control valve?
    A. Linear piston
    B. Spring-loaded bellows
    C. Solenoid
    D. Rotary drive piston

12. An electrical current flows through an electromagnet and creates a magnetic field, pulling a plunger and opening a valve. This description best fits which of the following devices?
    A. Proportional solenoid valve
    B. Eccentric valve piston
    C. Digital valve
    D. Linear drive piston

References

1. Chatburn RL: Classification of mechanical ventilators. *Respir Care* 37:1009–1025, 1992.
2. Chatburn RL: Classification of ventilator modes: update and proposal for implementation. *Respir Care* 52:301–323, 2007.
3. Cairo JM: *Mosby's respiratory care equipment*, ed 9, St Louis, 2013, Elsevier.
4. Mushin WW, Rendell-Baker L, Thompson PW, et al: *Automatic ventilation of the lungs*, Philadelphia, 1980, FA Davis.
5. Tehrani FT: Automatic control of mechanical ventilation. Part 1: Theory and history of technology. *J Clin Monit Comput* 22:417–424, 2008.
6. Chatburn RL: Computer control of mechanical ventilation. *Respir Care* 49:507–517, 2007.
7. Sanborn WG: Microprocessor-based mechanical ventilation. *Respir Care* 38:72–109, 1993.
8. Dupuis Y: *Ventilators: Theory and clinical application*, ed 2, St Louis, 1992, Mosby.

How a Breath Is Delivered

OUTLINE

KEY TERMS

- Baseline variable
- Continuous positive airway pressure
- Control variable
- Cycle variable
- Flow cycling
- Flow limited
- Flow triggering
- Limit variable
- Mandatory breath

- Negative end-expiratory pressure
- Patient triggering
- Phase variable
- Plateau pressure
- Positive end-expiratory pressure
- Pressure control
- Pressure cycling
- Pressure limiting
- Pressure support

- Pressure triggering
- Spontaneous breaths
- Time cycled
- Time triggering
- Trigger variable
- Volume cycled
- Volume limiting
- Volume triggering

LEARNING OBJECTIVES *On completion of this chapter, the reader will be able to do the following:*

1. Write the equation of motion, and define each term in the equation.
2. Give two other names for pressure ventilation and volume ventilation.
3. Compare pressure, volume, and flow delivery in volume-controlled breaths and pressure-controlled breaths.
4. Name the two most commonly used patient-trigger variables.
5. Identify the patient-trigger variable that requires the least work of breathing for a patient receiving mechanical ventilation.
6. Explain the effect on the volume delivered and the inspiratory time if a ventilator reaches the set maximum pressure limit during volume ventilation.

7. Recognize the effects of a critical leak (e.g., a patient disconnect) on pressure readings and volume measurements.
8. Define the effects of inflation hold on inspiratory time.
9. Give an example of a current ventilator that provides negative pressure during part of the expiratory phase.
10. Based on the description of a pressure–time curve, identify a clinical situation in which expiratory resistance is increased.
11. Describe two methods of applying continuous pressure to the airways that can be used to improve oxygenation in patients with refractory hypoxemia.

Selecting the most effective mode of ventilation to use once it has been decided that a patient will require mechanical ventilation requires an understanding of how a ventilator works. Answers to several questions can help explain the method by which a ventilator accomplishes delivery of a breath: (1) What is the source of energy used to deliver the breath (i.e., is the energy provided by the ventilator or by the patient)? (2) What factor does the ventilator control to deliver the breath (e.g., pressure, volume, flow, or time)? (3) How are the phases of a breath accomplished (i.e., what begins a breath, how is it delivered, and what ends the breath)? (4) Is the breath mandatory, assisted, or spontaneous? All these

factors determine the mode of ventilation, and each of these concepts is reviewed in this chapter.

BASIC MODEL OF VENTILATION IN THE LUNG DURING INSPIRATION

One approach that can be used to understand the mechanics of breathing during mechanical ventilation involves using a mathematical model that is based on the **equation of motion.** This equation, which is shown in Box 3-1, describes the relationships among pressure, volume, and flow during a spontaneous or mechanical

$$P_{mus} + P_{vent} = P_E + P_R$$

where

Muscle pressure + Ventilator pressure = Elastic recoil pressure + Flow resistance pressure

If one considers that

$$\text{Elastic recoil pressure} = \text{Elastance} \times \text{Volume}$$
$$= \text{Volume/Compliance (V/C), and}$$
$$\text{Flow resistance pressure} = \text{Resistance} \times \text{Flow} = (R_{aw} \times \dot{V})$$

Then the equation can be rewritten as follows:

$$P_{mus} + P_{vent} = V/C + (R_{aw} \times \dot{V})$$

P_{mus} is the pressure generated by the respiratory muscles (*muscle pressure*). If these muscles are inactive, $P_{mus} = 0$ cm H_2O, then the ventilator must provide the pressure required to achieve an inspiration.

P_{vent}, or more specifically, P_{TR}, is the pressure read on the ventilator gauge (manometer) during inspiration with positive pressure ventilation (i.e., the ventilator gauge pressure).

V is the volume delivered, C is respiratory system compliance, V/C is the elastic recoil pressure, R_{aw} is airway resistance, and $\dot{V}$ is the gas flow during inspiration ($R_{aw} \times \dot{V}$ = Flow resistance). It is important to recognize that various combinations of $P_{mus} + P_{vent}$ are used during assisted ventilation.

Because $P_{alv} = V/C$ and $P_{TA} = R_{aw} \times \dot{V}$, substituting in the above equation results in

$$P_{mus} + P_{TR} = P_{alv} + P_{TA}$$

Where P_{alv} is the alveolar pressure and P_{TA} is the transairway pressure (peak pressure minus plateau pressure [PIP − $P_{plateau}$]) (see Chapter 1 for further explanation of abbreviations).

Pressure-Controlled Ventilation
The clinician sets a pressure for delivery to the patient. Pressure-controlled ventilation is also called
- Pressure-targeted ventilation
- Pressure ventilation

Volume-Controlled Ventilation
The clinician sets a volume for delivery to the patient. Volume-controlled ventilation is also called
- Volume-targeted ventilation
- Volume ventilation

breath.[1-4] The equation includes three terms, which were previously defined in Chapter 1, namely, P_{TR}, or transrespiratory pressure; P_E, or elastic recoil pressure; and P_R, or flow resistance pressure. Figure 3-1 provides a graphic representation of each of these pressures.[5]

Notice that energy (i.e., pressure) required to produce motion (i.e., flow) can be achieved by contraction of the respiratory muscles (P_{mus}) during a spontaneous breath, or generated by the ventilator (P_{vent}) during a mechanical breath. In both cases, the total amount of pressure that must be generated to produce the flow of gas into the lungs depends on the physical characteristics of the respiratory system (i.e., elastance or, more specifically, compliance of the lungs and chest wall, plus the amount of airway resistance [R_{aw}] that must be overcome).

If the respiratory muscles are inactive, then the ventilator must perform all of the work required to move air into the lungs. The pressure generated by the ventilator therefore represents the transrespiratory pressure (P_{TR}), that is, the pressure gradient between the airway opening and the body's surface. For example, during positive pressure ventilation, the pressure delivered at the upper airway is positive and the pressure at the body surface is atmospheric (ambient pressure, which is given a value of 0 cm H_2O). Keep in mind that P_{TR} represents the pressure gradient that must be generated to achieve a given flow. (It is important to recognize

that a number of combinations of P_{mus} and P_{vent} can be used to achieve the total force required during assisted ventilation.)

The right side of the equation in Box 3-1 represents the impedance that must be overcome to deliver a breath and can be expressed as the alveolar pressure (P_{alv}) and the transairway pressure (P_{TA}). P_{alv} is produced by the interaction between lung and thoracic compliance and the pressure within the thorax. P_{TA} is produced by resistance to the flow of gases through the conductive airways resistance = P_{TA}/flow).

FACTORS CONTROLLED AND MEASURED DURING INSPIRATION

Delivery of an inspiratory volume is perhaps the single most important function a ventilator accomplishes. Two factors determine the way the inspiratory volume is delivered: the structural design of the ventilator and the ventilator **mode** set by the clinician. The clinician sets the mode by selecting either a predetermined pressure or volume as the target variable (Box 3-2).

The primary variable the ventilator adjusts to achieve inspiration is therefore called the *control variable* (Key Point 3-1).[6] As the equation of motion shows, the ventilator can control four variables: pressure, volume, flow, and time. It is important to recognize that the ventilator can control only one variable at a time. Therefore it must operate as a pressure controller, a volume controller, a flow controller, or a time controller (Box 3-3).

> **Key Point 3-1** The primary variable that the ventilator adjusts to produce inspiration is the **control variable.** The most commonly used control variables are pressure and volume.

Pressure-Controlled Breathing

When the ventilator maintains the pressure waveform in a specific pattern, the breathing is described as *pressure-controlled*. With **pressure-controlled** ventilation, the pressure waveform is unaffected by changes in lung characteristics. The volume and flow waveforms will vary with changes in the compliance and resistance characteristics of the patient's respiratory system.

Volume-Controlled Breathing

When a ventilator maintains the volume waveform in a specific pattern, the delivered breath is *volume-controlled*. During **volume-controlled breathing,** the volume and flow waveforms remain

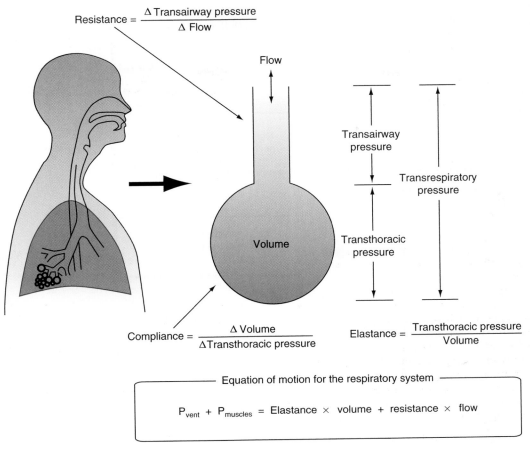

$$Resistance = \frac{\Delta\,Transairway\ pressure}{\Delta\,Flow}$$

Flow

Transairway pressure

Transrespiratory pressure

Volume

Transthoracic pressure

$$Compliance = \frac{\Delta\,Volume}{\Delta\,Transthoracic\ pressure}$$

$$Elastance = \frac{Transthoracic\ pressure}{Volume}$$

Equation of motion for the respiratory system

$$P_{vent} + P_{muscles} = Elastance \times volume + resistance \times flow$$

Fig. 3-1 Equation of motion model. The respiratory system can be visualized as a conductive tube connected to an elastic compartment (balloon). Flow, volume, and pressure are variables and functions of time. Resistance and compliance are constants. Transthoracic pressure is the pressure difference between the alveolar space (P_A), or lung, and the body surface (P_{bs}). (See text for further explanation.) (From Kacmarek RM, Stoller JK, Heuer AJ, editors: Egan's fundamentals of respiratory care, ed 10, St Louis, 2013, Elsevier-Mosby.)

| BOX 3-3 | **Ventilator Control Functions During Inspiration** |

- *Pressure controller:* The ventilator maintains the same pressure waveform at the mouth regardless of changes in lung characteristics.
- *Volume controller:* Ventilator volume delivery and volume waveform remain constant and are not affected by changes in lung characteristics. Volume is measured.*
- *Flow controller:* Ventilator volume delivery and flow waveform remain constant and are not affected by changes in lung characteristics. Flow is measured.*
- *Time controller:* Pressure, volume, and flow curves can change as lung characteristics change. Time remains constant.

*In current intensive care unit ventilators, volume delivery is a product of measured flow and inspiratory time. The ventilator essentially controls the flow delivered to the patient and calculates volume delivery based on the rate of flow and the time allowed for flow. Basically, the same effect is achieved by either controlling the volume delivered or by controlling flow over time.

unchanged, but the pressure waveform varies with changes in lung characteristics.

Flow-Controlled Breathing

When the ventilator controls flow, the flow and therefore volume waveforms remain unchanged, but the pressure waveform changes with alterations in the patient's lung characteristics. Flow can be controlled directly by a device as simple as a flowmeter or by a more complex mechanism, such as a solenoid valve (see Chapter 2).[2] Notice that any breath that has a set flow waveform also has a set volume waveform and vice versa. Thus, when the clinician selects a flow waveform, the volume waveform is automatically established (Flow = Volume change/Time; Volume = Flow × Time). In practical terms, clinicians typically are primarily interested in volume and pressure delivery rather than the contour of the flow waveform.

Time-Controlled Breathing

When both the pressure and the volume waveforms are affected by changes in lung characteristics, the ventilator delivers a breath that is **time-controlled.** Many high-frequency jet ventilators and

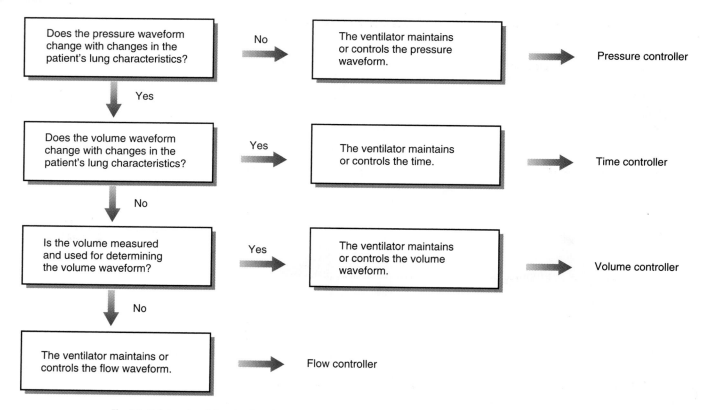

Fig. 3-2 Defining a breath based on how the ventilator maintains the inspiratory waveforms. (Modified from Chatburn RL: Classification of mechanical ventilators, Respir Care 37:1009-1025, 1992.)

oscillators control time (both inspiratory and expiratory); however, distinguishing between inspiration and expiration during high-frequency ventilation can be difficult. Time-controlled ventilation is used less often than pressure- and volume-controlled ventilation.

OVERVIEW OF INSPIRATORY WAVEFORM CONTROL

Figure 3-2 provides an algorithm to identify the various types of breaths that can be delivered by mechanical ventilators. Figure 3-3 shows the waveforms for pressure- and volume-controlled ventilation, and Box 3-4 lists some basic points that can help simplify evaluation of a breath during inspiration.[6]

The airway pressure waveforms shown in Fig. 3-3 illustrate what the clinician would see on the ventilator graphic display as gas is delivered. The ventilator typically measures variables in one of three places: (1) at the upper, or proximal, airway, where the patient is connected to the ventilator; (2) internally, near the point where the main circuit lines connect to the ventilator; or (3) near the exhalation valve.*

Microprocessor-controlled ventilators have the capability of displaying these waveforms as scalar graphs (a variable graphed relative to time) and loops on a screen.[6] Most current generation ventilators, such as the Dräger Infinity V500 and the CareFusion AVEA, have built-in screens. As discussed in Chapter 9, this graphic information is an important tool that can be used for the management of the patient-ventilator interaction.

*Newer ventilators often have a pressure-measuring device on both the inspiratory and expiratory sides of a ventilator circuit.

| BOX **3-4** | **Basic Points for Evaluating a Breath During Inspiration** |

1. Inspiration is commonly described as *pressure-controlled* or *volume-controlled*. Although both *flow-* and *time-controlled* ventilation have been defined, they are not typically used.
2. *Pressure-controlled* inspiration maintains the same pattern of pressure at the mouth regardless of changes in lung condition.
3. *Volume-controlled* inspiration maintains the same pattern of volume at the mouth regardless of changes in lung condition and also maintains the same flow waveform.
4. The pressure, volume, and flow waveforms produced at the mouth usually take one of four shapes:
   a. Rectangular (also called *square* or *constant*)
   b. Exponential (may be increasing [rising] or decreasing [decaying])
   c. Sinusoidal (also called *sine wave*)
   d. Ramp (available as ascending or descending [decelerating] ramp)

PHASES OF A BREATH AND PHASE VARIABLES

The following section describes the phases of a breath and the variable that controls each portion of the breath (i.e., the **phase variable**). As summarized in Box 3-5, the phase variable represents the signal measured by the ventilator that is associated with a specific aspect of the breath. The **trigger variable** begins inspiration. The **limit variable** limits the value of pressure, volume, flow, or time

Pressure-controlled ventilation   **Volume-controlled ventilation**

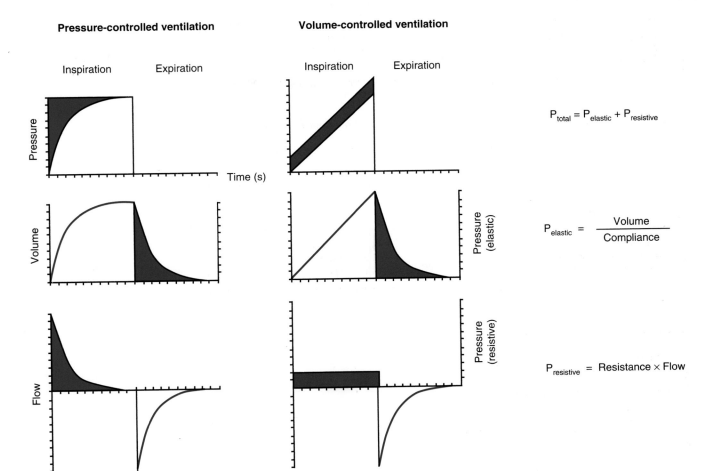

$$P_{total} = P_{elastic} + P_{resistive}$$

$$P_{elastic} = \frac{Volume}{Compliance}$$

$$P_{resistive} = Resistance \times Flow$$

Fig. 3-3 Characteristic waveforms for pressure-controlled ventilation and volume-controlled ventilation. Note that the volume waveform has the same shape as the transthoracic (lung pressure) waveform (i.e., pressure caused by the elastic recoil [compliance] of the lung). The flow waveform has the same shape as the transairway pressure waveform (peak pressure minus plateau pressure [PIP − $P_{plateau}$]) (shaded area of pressure–time waveform). The *shaded areas* represent pressures caused by resistance, and the *open areas* represent pressure caused by elastic recoil. (From Kacmarek RM, Stoller JK, Heuer AJ, editors: Egan's fundamentals of respiratory care, ed 10, St Louis, 2013, Elsevier-Mosby.)

during inspiration. It is important to recognize that the limit variable does not end inspiration. The **cycle variable** ends inspiration. The **baseline variable** establishes the baseline during expiration before inspiration is triggered. Pressure is usually identified as the baseline variable.

Beginning of Inspiration: The Trigger Variable

The mechanism the ventilator uses to begin inspiration is the **triggering mechanism (trigger variable)**. The ventilator can initiate a breath after a set time (**time triggering**), or the patient can trigger the machine (**patient triggering**) based on pressure, flow, or volume changes. Pressure and flow triggering are the most common triggering variables but **volume triggering** and neural triggering from the diaphragm output can be used. Most ventilators also allow the operator to trigger a breath manually (Key Point 3-2).

 Key Point **3-2** The **trigger variable** initiates inspiratory flow from the ventilator.

BOX **3-5**	**Phase Variables**

A *phase variable* begins, sustains, ends, and determines the characteristics of the expiratory portion of each breath. Four phase variables are typically described:
1. The trigger variable begins inspiration.
2. The limit variable limits the pressure, volume, flow, or time during inspiration but it does not end the breath.
3. The cycle variable ends inspiratory phase and begins exhalation.
4. The baseline variable is the end-expiratory baseline (usually pressure) before a breath is triggered.

Time Triggering

With **time triggering**, the ventilator delivers a **mandatory breath** by beginning inspiration after a set time has elapsed. (NOTE: The set time is based on the total cycle time (TCT), which is the sum of inspiratory time (T_I) and expiratory time (T_E), or TCT = T_I + T_E). In other words, the number of mandatory breaths delivered by

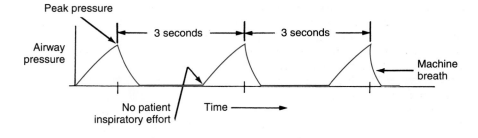

Fig. 3-4 Controlled ventilation pressure curve. Patient effort does not trigger a mechanical breath; rather, inspiration occurs at equal, timed intervals.

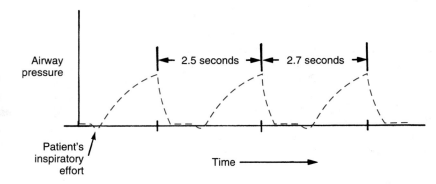

Fig. 3-5 Assist pressure curve. Patient effort (negative pressure deflection from baseline) occurs before each machine breath. Breaths may not occur at equal, timed intervals.

the ventilator is based on the length of the TCT. For example, if the breathing rate is set at 20 breaths per minute, the ventilator triggers inspiration after 3 seconds elapses (60 s/min divided by 20 breaths/min = 3 seconds).

In the past, time-triggered ventilation did not allow a patient to initiate a breath (i.e., the ventilator was "insensitive" to the patient's effort to breathe). Consequently, when the **control mode** setting was selected on early ventilators like the first Emerson Post-Op, the machine automatically controlled the number of breaths delivered to the patient.

Ventilators are no longer used in this manner. Conscious patients are almost never "locked out," and they can take a breath when they need it. The clinician sets up time triggering with the **rate** (or **frequency**) **control**, which may be a knob or a touch pad. Sometimes clinicians may say that a patient "is being controlled" or "is in the control mode" to describe an individual who is apneic *or sedated* or paralyzed and makes no effort to breathe (Fig. 3-4). It should be noted however that the ventilator should be set so that it will be sensitive to the patient's inspiratory effort when the person is no longer apneic or paralyzed.

Patient Triggering

In those cases where a patient attempts to breathe spontaneously during mechanical ventilation, a ventilator must be available to measure the patient's effort to breathe. When the ventilator detects changes in pressure, flow, or volume, a patient-triggered breath occurs. Pressure and flow are common patient-triggering mechanisms (e.g., inspiration begins if a negative airway opening pressure or change in flow is detected). Figure 3-5 illustrates a breath triggered by the patient making an inspiratory effort (i.e., the patient's inspiratory effort can be identified as the pressure deflection below baseline that occurs prior to initiation of the mechanical breath). To enable **patient triggering**, the clinician must specify the sensitivity setting, also called the *patient effort* (or *patient-triggering*) *control*. This setting determines the pressure or flow change that is required to trigger the ventilator. The less pressure or flow change required to trigger a breath, the more sensitive the

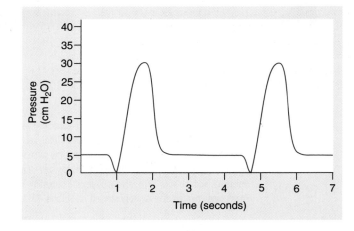

Fig. 3-6 Airway pressure curve during assist ventilation with 5 cm H_2O of positive end-expiratory pressure (baseline), showing a deflection of the pressure curve to 0 cm H_2O before each machine breath is delivered. The machine is not sensitive enough to the patient's effort.

machine is to the patient's effort. For example, the ventilator is more sensitive to patient effort at a setting of −0.5 cm H_2O than at a setting of −1 cm H_2O. Sensing devices usually are located inside the ventilator near the output side of the system; however, in some systems, pressure or flow is measured at the proximal airway.

The sensitivity level for **pressure triggering** usually is set at about −1 cm H_2O. The clinician must set the sensitivity level to fit the patient's needs. If it is set incorrectly, the ventilator may not be sensitive enough to the patient's effort, and the patient will have to work too hard to trigger the breath (Fig. 3-6). If the ventilator is too sensitive, it can **autotrigger** (i.e., the machine triggers a breath without the patient making an effort) (Case Study 3-1).

Flow triggering occurs when the ventilator detects a drop in flow through the patient circuit during exhalation. To enable flow triggering, the clinician must set an appropriate flow that must be sensed by the ventilator to trigger the next breath. As an example, a ventilator has a baseline flow of 6 L/min. This allows 6 L/min of gas to flow through the patient circuit during the last part of exhalation. The sensors measure a flow of 6 L/min leaving the ventilator and 6 L/min returning to the ventilator. If the flow trigger is set at 2 L/min, the ventilator will begin an assisted breath when it detects a drop in flow of 2 L/min from the baseline (i.e., 4 L/min returning to the ventilator [Fig. 3-7]).

When set properly, flow triggering has been shown to require less work of breathing than pressure triggering. Many microprocessor-controlled ventilators (e.g., Servo-i, CareFusion AVEA, Hamilton G5, Covidien PB 840) offer flow triggering as an option.

Volume triggering occurs when the ventilator detects a small drop in volume in the patient circuit during exhalation. The machine interprets this drop in volume as a patient effort and begins inspiration. The Dräger Babylog and the Cardiopulmonary Venturi are volume-triggered ventilators.

As mentioned previously, manual triggering is also available. With manual triggering, the operator can initiate a ventilator breath by pressing a button or touch pad labeled "Manual" breath or "Start" breath. When this control is activated, the ventilator delivers a breath according to the set variables.

It is important to recognize that patient triggering can be quite effective when a patient begins to breathe spontaneously, but occasionally the patient may experience an apneic episode. For this reason, a respiratory rate is set with the rate control to guarantee a minimum number of breaths per minute (Fig. 3-8). Each breath is either patient triggered or time triggered, depending on which occurs first. Although the rate control determines the minimum number of mechanical breaths delivered, the patient

has the option of breathing at a faster rate. Clinicians often refer to this as the *assist-control mode*. (NOTE: The clinician must always make sure the ventilator is sensitive to the patient's efforts [Box 3-6].)

Case Study 3-1

Patient Triggering

Problem 1: A patient is receiving volume-controlled ventilation. Whenever the patient makes an inspiratory effort, the pressure indicator shows a pressure of −5 cm H_2O below baseline before the ventilator triggers into inspiration. What does this indicate?

Problem 2: A patient appears to be in distress while receiving volume-controlled ventilation. The ventilator is cycling rapidly from breath to breath. The actual rate is much faster than the set rate. No discernible deflection of the pressure indicator occurs at the beginning of inspiration. The ventilator panel indicates that every breath is an assisted, or patient-triggered, breath. What does this indicate?

The Limit Variable During Inspiration

Inspiration is timed from the beginning of inspiratory flow to the beginning of expiratory flow. As mentioned previously, the ventilator can determine the waveform for pressure, volume, flow, or time during inspiration. However, it also can **limit** these variables. For example, during volume-controlled ventilation of an apneic patient, the clinician sets a specific volume that the ventilator will deliver.

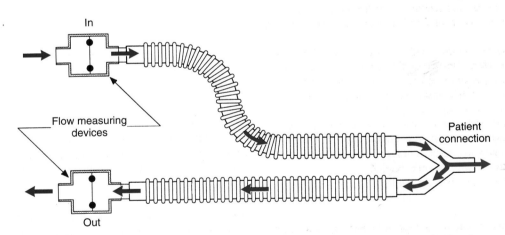

Fig. 3-7 Schematic drawing of the essential features of flow triggering. Triggering occurs when the patient inspires from the circuit and increases the difference between flow from the ventilator (inspiratory side, *in*) and flow back to the exhalation valve (expiratory side, *out*). (From Dupuis Y: Ventilators: theory and clinical application, ed 2, St Louis, 1992, Mosby.)

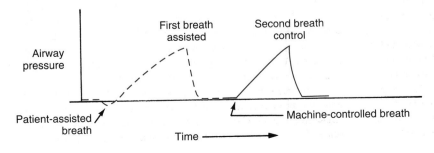

Fig. 3-8 Assist-control pressure curve. A patient-triggered (assisted) breath shows negative deflection of pressure before inspiration, whereas a controlled (time-triggered) breath does not.

In general, the volume delivered cannot exceed that amount; it may be for some reason less than desired, but it cannot be more.

A *limit variable* is the maximum value that a variable (pressure, volume, flow, or time) can attain. It is important to emphasize, however, that reaching the set limit variable **does not** end inspiration. As an example, a ventilator is set to deliver a maximum pressure of 25 cm H_2O, and the inspiratory time is set at 2 seconds. The maximum pressure that can be attained during inspiration is 25 cm H_2O, but inspiration will end only after 2 seconds has passed. Such a breath therefore is described as a *pressure-limited, time-cycled* breath (cycling ends inspiration [see Termination of the Inspiratory Phase: The Cycling Mechanism section]).

Pressure Limiting

As the example mentioned above illustrates, **pressure limiting** allows pressure to rise to a certain value but not exceed it. Figure 3-9 shows an example of the internal pneumatic circuit of a piston ventilator. The ventilator pushes a volume of gas into the ventilator circuit, which causes the pressure in the circuit to rise. To prevent excessive pressure from entering the patient's lungs, the clinician sets a **high** pressure limit control. When the ventilator reaches the high pressure limit, excess pressure is vented through a spring-loaded pressure release, or pop-off, valve (Fig. 3-9). The excess gas pressure is released into the room, just as steam is released by a pressure cooker. In this example, reaching the high pressure limit does not cycle the ventilator and end inspiration.

The pressure–time and volume–time waveforms shown in Fig. 3-10 illustrate how the set pressure and volume curves would appear for a patient with normal lung function and when the patient's lungs are less compliant. Notice that a higher pressure is required to inflate the stiff lungs and the pressure limit would be reached before the end of the breath occurs. Consequently, the volume delivered would be less than desired. In other words, volume delivery is reduced because the pressure limit is reached at Time A even though inspiration does not end until Time B (i.e., the breath is time cycled).

Infant ventilators often pressure limit the inspiratory phase but time cycle inspiration. Other examples of pressure-limiting modes are **pressure support** and **pressure-controlled ventilation.** Remember that when the clinician establishes a set value in pressure-targeted ventilation, the pressure the ventilator delivers to the patient is limited; however, reaching the pressure limit does not end the breath.

Volume Limiting

A volume-limited breath is controlled by an electronically operated valve that measures the flow passing through the ventilator circuit

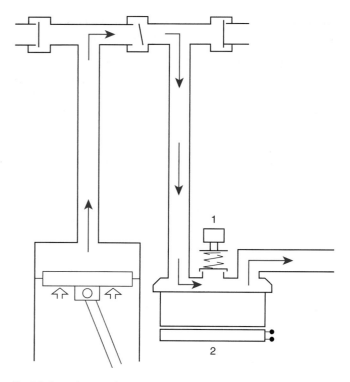

Fig. 3-9 Internal pneumatic circuit on a piston-driven ventilator. 1, Pressure release valve; 2, heated humidifier. (Modified from Dupuis Y: Ventilators: theory and clinical application, ed 2, St Louis, 1992, Mosby.)

during a specific interval. The clinician can set the volume of gas that the ventilator delivers. With volume limiting, the ventilator may include a bag, bellows, or piston cylinder that contains a fixed volume, which establishes the maximum volume of gas that can be delivered. (NOTE: Reaching that volume does not necessarily end inspiration.) A piston-operated ventilator can be used to provide a simple example of **volume limiting.** Volume is limited to the amount of volume contained in the piston cylinder (see Fig. 3-9). The forward movement of the piston rod or arm controls the duration of inspiration (time-cycled breath).

Ventilators can have more than one limiting feature at a time. In the example just provided, the duration of inspiration could not exceed the excursion time of the piston, and the volume delivered could not exceed the volume in the piston cylinder. Therefore a piston-driven ventilator can be simultaneously volume limited and time limited. (NOTE: Current ventilators that are not piston driven [e.g., Servo-i] provide a volume limit option. When special modes are selected, an actively breathing patient can receive more volume if inspiratory demand increases. The advantage of these ventilators is that the volume delivered to the patient during selected modes is adjusted to meet the patient's increased inspiratory needs.)

Flow Limiting

If gas flow from the ventilator to the patient reaches but does not exceed a maximum value before the end of inspiration, the ventilator is **flow limited;** that is, only a certain amount of flow can be provided. For example, the constant forward motion of a linear-drive piston provides a constant rate of gas delivery to the patient over a certain period. The duration of inspiration is determined by the time it takes the piston rod to move forward.

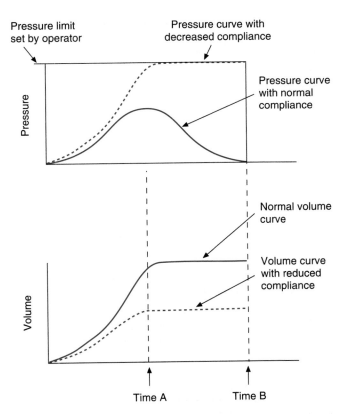

Pressure limit set by operator

Pressure curve with decreased compliance

Pressure curve with normal compliance

Normal volume curve

Volume curve with reduced compliance

Time A   Time B

Fig. 3-10 Waveforms from a volume ventilator that delivers a sine wave pressure curve. The pressure and volume waveforms for normal compliance show pressure peaking at Time A and the normal volume delivered by Time A. Inspiration ends at Time B. With reduced compliance, the pressure rises higher during inspiration. Because excess pressure is vented, the pressure reaches a limit and goes no higher. No more flow enters the patient's lungs. Volume delivery has reached its maximum at Time A, when the pressure starts venting. Inspiration is time cycled at Time B. Note that volume delivery is lower when the lungs are stiffer and the pressure is limited. Some of the volume was vented to the air.

In other ventilators with volume ventilation, setting the flow control also limits the flow to the patient. Even if the patient makes a strong inspiratory effort, the patient will only receive the maximum flow set by the clinician. For example, if the clinician sets a constant flow of 60 L/min, then the maximum flow that the patient can receive is 60 L/min whether or not the patient tries to breathe in at a higher flow. Most current ventilators allow patients to receive increased flow if they have an increased demand because limiting flow is not in the best interest of an actively breathing patient.

Maximum Safety Pressure: Pressure Limiting Versus Pressure Cycling

All ventilators have a feature that allows inspiratory pressure to reach but not exceed a maximum pressure. This maximum safety pressure is used to prevent excessive pressure from damaging a patient's lungs. It is typically set by the operator to a value of 10 cm H_2O above the average peak inspiratory pressure. Manufacturers use various names to describe the maximum pressure control function, such as the *peak/maximum pressure, normal pressure limit, pressure limit, high-pressure limit,* or *upper-pressure limit.*

Most adult ventilators pressure cycle (end inspiration) when the set maximum safety pressure limit is reached, as might occur when

a patient coughs or if there is an obstruction in the ventilator tubing. Some ventilators allow inspiration to continue while excess pressure is vented to the atmosphere through a pressure safety valve. (In newer intensive care unit [ICU] ventilators, a "floating" exhalation valve prevents pressures from abruptly rising as might occur when a patient coughs [Case Study 3-2]).

It is worth mentioning that ventilator manufacturers set an internal maximum safety pressure. By design, the machine cannot exceed that limit, regardless of the value set by the operator. Ventilator manufacturers usually set internal maximum safety pressure at 120 cm H_2O.

Case Study 3-2

Premature Breath Cycling

A patient receiving volume-controlled ventilation suddenly coughs during the inspiratory phase of the ventilator. A high-pressure alarm sounds, and inspiration ends. Although the set tidal volume is 0.8 L, the measured delivered volume for that breath is 0.5 L. What variable ended inspiration in this example?

Termination of the Inspiratory Phase: The Cycling Mechanism (Cycle Variable)

The variable that a ventilator uses to end inspiration is called the *cycling mechanism.* The ventilator measures the cycle variable during inspiration, and uses this information to govern when the ventilator will end gas flow. Only one of four variables can be used at a given time by the ventilator to end inspiration (i.e., volume, time, flow, or pressure).

Volume-Cycled Ventilation

The inspiratory phase of a **volume-cycled** breath is terminated when the set volume has been delivered. In most cases, the volume remains constant even if the patient's lung characteristics change. The pressures required to deliver the set volume and gas flow, however, will vary as the patient's respiratory system compliance and airway resistance change.

In cases where the clinician sets an **inspiratory pause,** inspiration will continue until the pause has ended and expiration begins. (The *inspiratory pause* feature delays opening of the expiratory valve.) In this situation, the breath is volume limited and time cycled. Note that setting an inspiratory pause extends inspiratory time, not inspiratory flow.)

Because most current ICU ventilators do not use volume displacement mechanisms, none of these devices is *technically* classified as *volume cycled.* (NOTE: The Covidien Puritan Bennett 740 and 760 are exceptions[7]; these ventilators use linear-drive pistons and can function as true volume-cycled ventilators.) Ventilators such as the Covidien PB 840, Servo-i, CareFusion AVEA, Hamilton Galileo, and Dräger Evita use sensors that determine the gas flow delivered by the ventilator over a specified period, which is then converted to a volume reading (Volume = Flow/Time). These ventilators are considered volume cycled when the targeted volume is delivered and ends the breath.

Set Volume Versus Actual Delivered Volume

Tubing compressibility. The volume of gas that leaves the ventilator's outlet is not the volume that enters the patient's lungs.

During inspiration, positive pressure builds up in the patient circuit, resulting in expansion of the patient circuit and compression of some of the gas in the circuit (an application of Boyle's law). The compressed gas never reaches the patient's lungs.

In most adult ventilator circuits, about 1 to 3 mL of gas is lost to tubing compressibility for every 1 cm H_2O that is measured by the airway pressure sensor. As a result, a relatively large volume of gas may be compressed in the circuit and never reaches the patient's lungs when high pressures are required to ventilate a patient. Conversely, a patient whose lung compliance is improving can be ventilated at lower pressures; therefore less volume is lost to circuit compressibility.

The actual volume delivered to the patient can be determined by measuring the exhaled volume at the endotracheal tube or tracheostomy tube. If the volume is measured at the exhalation valve, it must be corrected for tubing compliance (i.e., the compressible volume). To determine the delivered volume, the volume compressed in the ventilator circuit must be subtracted from the volume measured at the exhalation valve. Most microprocessor-controlled ICU ventilators (e.g., Covidien PB 840, Servo-i) measure and calculate the lost volume and automatically compensate for volume lost to tubing compressibility by increasing the actual volume delivered. For example, the Covidien PB 840 calculates the circuit compliance/compressibility factor during the establishment of ventilation for a new patient setup. The ventilator measures the peak pressure of a breath delivered to the patient and calculates the estimated volume loss caused by circuit compressibility. Then, for the next breath, it adds the volume calculated to the delivered set volume to correct for this loss. (Determination of the compressible volume is discussed in more detail in Chapter 6.)

System leaks. The volume of gas delivered to the patient may be less than the set volume if a leak in the system occurs. The ventilator may be unable to recognize or compensate for leaks, but the size of the leak can be determined by using an exhaled volume monitor. In cases where a leak exists, the peak inspiratory pressure will be lower than previous peak inspiratory pressures and a low-pressure alarm may be activated. The volume–time graph also can provide information about leaks (see Chapter 9).

Time-Cycled Ventilation

A breath is considered *time cycled* if the inspiratory phase ends when a predetermined time has elapsed. The interval is controlled by a timing mechanism in the ventilator, which is not affected by the patient's respiratory system compliance or airway resistance. At the specified time, the exhalation valve opens (unless an inspiratory pause has been used) and exhaled air is vented through the exhalation valve. If a constant gas flow is used and the interval is fixed, a tidal volume can be predicted:

$$\text{Tidal volume} = \text{Flow (Volume/Time)} \times \text{Inspiratory time}$$

The Servo-i and Dräger Evita XL are examples of time-cycled ventilators. These microprocessor-controlled machines can compare the set volume with the set time and calculate the flow required to deliver that volume in that length of time. Consider the following example. A patient's tidal volume (V_T) is set at 1000 mL and the inspiratory time (T_I) is set at 2 seconds. To accomplish this volume delivery in the time allotted, the ventilator would have to deliver a constant flow waveform at a rate of 30 L/min (30 L/60 s = 0.5 L/s), so that 0.5 L/s × 2 s would provide 1.0 L over the desired 2-second inspiratory time.

With time-cycled, volume-controlled ventilation, an increase in airway resistance or a decrease in compliance does *not* affect the flow pattern or volume delivery as long as the working pressures of the ventilator are adequate. Therefore volume delivery in a fixed period remains the same, although the pressures vary. Appropriate alarms should be set to alert the clinician of any significant changes in airway pressures.

With time-cycled, pressure-controlled ventilation, both volume and flow vary. Volume (and flow) delivery depends on lung compliance and airway resistance, patient effort (if present), the inspiratory time, and the set pressure. Time-cycled, pressure-controlled ventilation is commonly called *pressure-controlled ventilation*. Pressure-controlled ventilation is sometimes used because the inspiratory pressure can be limited, which protects the lungs from injury caused by high pressures. However, the variability of tidal volume delivery can be a concern. Alarm settings must be chosen carefully so that the clinician is alerted to any significant changes in the rate and volume.

Flow-Cycled Ventilation

With flow-cycled ventilation, the ventilator cycles into the expiratory phase once the flow has decreased to a predetermined value during inspiration. Volume, pressure, and time vary according to changes in lung characteristics. **Flow cycling** is the most common cycling mechanism in the pressure support mode (Fig. 3-11). In the Covidien PB 840 ventilator, flow termination occurs when the flow reaches a percentage of the peak inspiratory flow, which is selected by the clinician. In some ventilators, the flow cycle percentage can be adjusted from about 5% to 80%.

 CRITICAL CARE CONCEPT 3-1

Early generation Bennett ventilators (Bennett PR-1 and PR-2) relied on a **Bennett** valve to control gas flow to the patient. The principle of operation of these devices is the valve switches from the inspiratory phase to the expiratory phase when flow to the patient drops to 1 to 3 L/min. This lower flow results when the pressure gradient between the alveoli and the ventilator is small and the pressures are nearly equal. Because equal pressure is nearly achieved, along with the low gas flow, these machines sometimes are called *pressure-cycled ventilators*. However, because the predetermined pressure is never actually reached, these ventilators were in reality examples of *flow-cycled* ventilators. (NOTE: The rate control on these machines allowed them to function as time-cycled ventilators as long as flow and/or pressure limits were not reached first.)

Pressure-Cycled Ventilation

During pressure-cycled ventilation, inspiration ends when a set pressure threshold is reached at the mouth or upper airway. The exhalation valve opens, and expiration begins. The volume delivered to the patient depends on the flow delivered, the duration of inspiration, the patient's lung characteristics, and the set pressure.

A disadvantage of pressure-cycled ventilators (e.g., Bird Mark 7) is that these devices deliver variable and generally lower tidal volumes when reductions in compliance and increases in

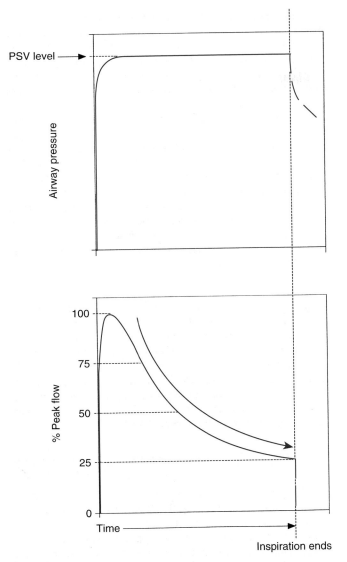

Fig. 3-11 Waveforms from a pressure support breath showing the pressure and flow curves during inspiration. When flow drops to 25% of the peak flow value measured during inspiration, the ventilator flow cycles out of inspiration. (From Dupuis Y: *Ventilators: theory and clinical application,* ed 2, St Louis, 1992, Mosby.)

resistance occur. An advantage of pressure-cycled ventilators is that they limit peak airway pressures, which may reduce the damage that can occur when pressures are excessive. These ventilators are most often used to deliver intermittent positive pressure breathing (IPPB) treatments. These devices have also been used for short-term ventilation of patients with relatively stable lung function, such as postoperative patients. It is important that appropriate alarms are operational to ensure that the patient is being adequately ventilated. Ensuring that the humidification system is adequate is also important. (NOTE: As mentioned previously, **pressure cycling** occurs in volume-controlled breaths when the pressure exceeds the maximum safety high-pressure limit. A high-pressure alarm sounds, and the set tidal volume is not delivered [see Case Study 3-2].)

Inflation Hold (Inspiratory Pause)

Inflation hold is designed to maintain air in the lungs at the end of inspiration, before the exhalation valve opens. During an inflation hold, the inspired volume remains in the patient's lung and the expiratory valve remains closed for a brief period or *pause time*. The pressure reading on the manometer peaks at the end of insufflation and then levels to a plateau (**plateau pressure**). The inflation hold maneuver is sometimes referred to as *inspiratory pause, end-inspiratory pause,* or *inspiratory hold* (Fig. 3-12). As discussed in Chapter 8, the plateau pressure is used to calculate static compliance (Key Point 3-3). The inspiratory pause occasionally is used to increase peripheral distribution of gas and improve oxygenation. Because of the way the pause functions, the normal cycling mechanism no longer ends the breath, resulting in an increase in the inspiratory time and a reduction in the expiratory time.

> **Key Point** **3-3** Calculation of static compliance requires accurate measurement of the plateau pressure. The $P_{plateau}$ value is inaccurate if the patient is actively breathing when the measurement is taken.

Expiratory Phase: The Baseline Variable

During the early development of mechanical ventilation, many clinicians believed that assisting the expiratory phase was just as important as assisting the inspiratory phase. This was accomplished in one of two ways. With the first method, negative pressure was applied with a bellows or an entrainment (Venturi) device positioned at the mouth or upper airway to draw air out of the lungs. This technique was called **negative end-expiratory pressure** (NEEP). Another method involved applying positive pressure to the abdominal area, below the diaphragm. With this latter technique, it was thought that applying pressure below the diaphragm would force the air out of the lungs by pushing the visceral organs against the diaphragm (i.e., similar to the effects of performing a Heimlich maneuver).

Under normal circumstances, expiration during mechanical ventilation occurs passively and depends on the passive recoil of the lung. High-frequency oscillation is an exception to this principle (this type of mechanical ventilation is discussed later in this chapter and in Chapters 22 and 23.)

Definition of Expiration

The *expiratory phase* encompasses the period from the end of inspiration to the beginning of the next breath. During mechanical ventilation, expiration begins when inspiration ends, the expiratory valve opens, and expiratory flow begins. As previously mentioned, opening of the expiratory valve may be delayed if an inflation hold is used to prolong inspiration.

The expiratory phase has received increased attention during the past decade. Clinicians now recognize that air trapping can occur if the expiratory time is too short. Remember that a quiet exhalation normally is a passive event that depends on the elastic recoil of the lungs and thorax and the resistance to airflow offered by the conducting airways. Changes in a patient's respiratory system compliance and airway resistance can alter time constants, which in turn can affect the inspiratory and expiratory times (I:E) required to achieve effective ventilation. If an adequate amount of time is not provided for exhalation, air trapping and hyperinflation can occur, leading to a phenomenon called auto-PEEP or intrinsic PEEP (see the section on Expiratory Hold later in this chapter).

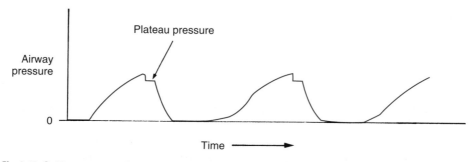

Fig. 3-12 Positive pressure ventilation with an inflation hold, or end-inspiratory pause, leading to a pressure plateau ($P_{plateau}$).

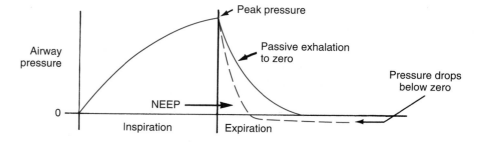

Fig. 3-13 Negative end-expiratory pressure (NEEP). Expiration occurs more rapidly, and the pressure drops below baseline (negative pressure) compared with a normal passive exhalation to zero end-expiratory pressure.

Baseline Pressure

The **baseline variable** is the parameter that generally is controlled during exhalation. Although either volume or flow could serve as a baseline variable, pressure is the most practical choice and is used by all modern ventilators.[7]

The pressure level from which a ventilator breath begins is called the *baseline pressure* (see Figs. 3-5 and 3-6). Baseline pressure can be zero (atmospheric), which is also called *zero end-expiratory pressure* (ZEEP), or it can be positive if the baseline pressure is above zero (*positive end-expiratory pressure* [PEEP]).

Time-Limited Expiration

Current mechanical ventilators (e.g., CareFusion AVEA, Servo-i, Dräger V500, Covidien PB 840) have a mode that allows the clinician to control T_I and expiratory time (T_E). The Dräger Evita was the first ventilator in the United States to provide this mode, which was called *airway pressure release ventilation (APRV)*. During APRV, two time settings are used: Time 1 (T_1) controls the time high pressure is applied, and Time 2 (T_2) controls the *release time*, or the time low pressure is applied. This mode of ventilation limits the expiratory time.

Since the introduction of APRV, other manufacturers of ICU ventilators have chosen to incorporate this mode into their ventilator settings. Interestingly, they use other names for this mode. For example, the Servo-i refers to APRV as Bi-Vent and the Hamilton G5 refers to APRV as Duo-PAP. (APRV is covered in more detail in Chapter 23.)

Continuous Gas Flow During Expiration

Many ICU ventilators provide gas flow through the patient circuit during the latter part of the expiratory phase. When gas flow is provided only during the end of exhalation, resistance to exhalation is minimized. In some ventilators the clinician sets system flow, whereas in others the system flow is automatically set by the ventilator (e.g., Servo-i). This feature provides immediate inspiratory flow to a patient on demand and in most cases also serves as part of the flow-triggering mechanism.

NEEP and Subambient Pressure During Expiration

As mentioned previously, NEEP at one time was used to reduce the airway pressure below ambient pressure during exhalation. The technique was used by physicians who experienced difficulty ventilating newborn infants through narrow endotracheal tubes. Because neonates have high respiratory rates, allowing enough time for exhalation was difficult, and it was proposed that NEEP would facilitate expiration by providing negative pressure at the proximal airway at the end of exhalation (Fig. 3-13).

In addition, NEEP was advocated for adults suffering from shock as a means of increasing venous return to the heart. Unfortunately, the technique presented problems for patients with chronic obstructive airway disease. In these patients, NEEP increased the risk of airway collapse and air trapping and had the potential to increase lung volumes above the resting functional residual capacity (FRC). Because many believed that the benefits were not significant and the hazards were high, the use of NEEP fell into disfavor in the late 1960s and early 1970s. A variety of techniques based on this principle are, however, still used. For example, the Cardiopulmonary Venturi applies a negative pressure to the airway only during the very beginning of the exhalation phase. This facilitates removal of air from the patient circuit and is intended to reduce the resistance to exhalation throughout the circuit at the start of exhalation.[2] Another technique, called *automatic tube compensation*, allows active removal of air (low pressure) during part of exhalation to reduce the expiratory work of breathing associated with an artificial airway (see Chapter 20 for a more detailed discussion of this technique).

High-frequency oscillation (HFO) assists both inspiration and expiration. Oscillators push air into the lungs and pull it back out at extremely high frequencies. These devices function similarly to a speaker system on a stereo. If the mean airway pressure during HFO is set to equal ambient pressure, the airway pressure oscillates

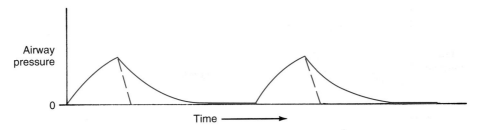

Fig. 3-14 Positive pressure ventilation with expiratory retard *(solid line)* and passive expiration to zero baseline *(dashed line).* Expiratory retard does not necessarily change expiratory time, which also depends on the patient's spontaneous pattern. However, it increases the amount of pressure in the airway during exhalation.

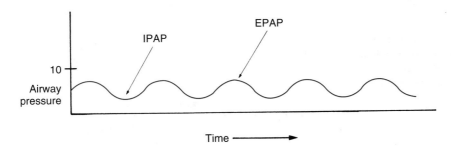

Fig. 3-15 Simplified pressure–time waveform showing continuous positive airway pressure (CPAP). Breathing is spontaneous. Inspiratory positive airway pressure (IPAP) and expiratory positive airway pressure (EPAP) are present. Pressures remain positive and do not return to a zero baseline.

above and below the baseline (i.e., atmospheric pressure). During exhalation, HFO actually creates a negative transrespiratory pressure. HFO is most often used for ventilation of infant lungs, although it has also been used occasionally to treat adult patients with acute respiratory distress syndrome (see Chapters 22 and 23).

Expiratory Hold (End-Expiratory Pause)

Expiratory hold, or end-expiratory pause, is a maneuver transiently performed at the end of exhalation. It is accomplished by first allowing the patient to perform a quiet exhalation. The ventilator then pauses before delivering the next machine breath. During this time, both the expiratory and inspiratory valves are closed. Delivery of the next inspiration is briefly delayed. The purpose of this maneuver is to measure pressure associated with air trapped in the lungs at the end of the expiration (i.e., auto-PEEP).

An accurate reading of end-expiratory pressure is impossible to obtain if a patient is breathing spontaneously. However, measurement of the exact amount of auto-PEEP present is not always necessary; simply detecting its presence may be sufficient. Auto-PEEP can be detected in the flow curve on a ventilator that provides a graphic display of gas flow; it is present if flow does not return to zero when a new mandatory ventilator breath begins (see Chapter 9). (NOTE: A respirometer also can be used if a graphic display is not available. The respirometer is placed in line between the ventilator's Y-connector and the patient's endotracheal tube connector. If the respirometer's needle continues to rotate when the next breath begins, air trapping is present [i.e., the patient is still exhaling when the next mandatory breath occurs].)

Expiratory Retard

Spontaneously breathing individuals with a disease that leads to early airway closure (e.g., emphysema) require a prolonged expiratory phase. Many of these patients can accomplish a prolonged expiration during spontaneous breathing by using a technique called *pursed-lip breathing.* Obviously, a patient cannot use pursed-lip breathing with an endotracheal tube in place. To mimic pursed-lip breathing, earlier ventilators provided an expiratory adjunct called *expiratory retard,* which added a degree of resistance to exhalation (Fig. 3-14). Although theoretically expiratory retard should prevent early airway closure and improve ventilation, this technique is not commonly used in clinical practice. It is important to recognize that ventilator circuits, expiratory valves, and bacterial filters placed on the expiratory side of the patient circuit produce a certain amount of expiratory retard because they cause resistance to flow. This is especially true of expiratory filters, which can accumulate moisture from the patient's exhaled air. The clinician can check for expiratory resistance by observing the pressure manometer and the ventilator pressure–time and flow–time graphics. (Increased resistance is present if pressure and flow return to baseline very slowly during exhalation [see Chapter 9].)

Continuous Positive Airway Pressure (CPAP) and Positive End-Expiratory Pressure (PEEP)

Two methods of applying continuous pressure to the airways have been developed to improve oxygenation in patients with refractory hypoxemia: **continuous positive airway pressure (CPAP)** and PEEP.

CPAP involves the application of pressures above ambient pressure throughout inspiration and expiration to improve oxygenation in a spontaneously breathing patient (Fig. 3-15). It can be applied through a freestanding CPAP system or a ventilator. CPAP has been used for the treatment of a variety of disorders, including postoperative atelectasis and obstructive sleep apnea (see Chapter 13 for more details on the use of CPAP).

Fig. 3-16 Positive end-expiratory pressure (PEEP) during controlled ventilation. No spontaneous breaths are taken between mandatory breaths, and there are no negative deflections of the baseline, which is maintained above zero.

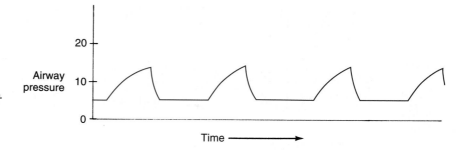

Fig. 3-17 Continuous positive airway pressure (CPAP) or positive end-expiratory pressure (PEEP) with intermittent mandatory breaths (also called intermittent mandatory ventilation [IMV] with PEEP or CPAP). Spontaneous breaths are taken between mandatory breaths, and the baseline is maintained above zero. The mandatory breaths are equidistant and occur regardless of the phase of the patient's spontaneous respiratory cycle.

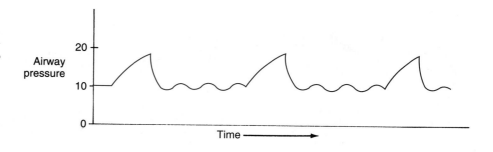

Fig. 3-18 Inspiratory positive airway pressure (IPAP) plus expiratory positive airway pressure (EPAP). IPAP is higher than EPAP when applied to patients. This technique, also called *bilevel positive airway pressure,* or *BiPAP,* is used for noninvasive ventilation in home care.

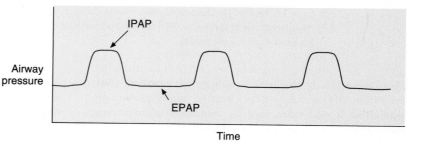

Like CPAP, PEEP involves applying positive pressure to the airway throughout the respiratory cycle. The pressure in the airway therefore remains above ambient even at the end of expiration. According to its purest definition, the term *PEEP* is defined as positive pressure at the end of exhalation during either spontaneous breathing or mechanical ventilation. In practice, however, clinicians commonly use the term to describe the application of continuous positive pressure when a patient is also receiving mandatory breaths from a ventilator (Figs. 3-16 and 3-17). PEEP becomes the baseline variable during mechanical ventilation.

CPAP and PEEP theoretically help prevent early airway closure and alveolar collapse at the end of expiration by increasing (and normalizing) the patient's FRC, which in turn allows for better oxygenation.

Another variation of PEEP and CPAP therapy that is commonly used is bilevel positive airway pressure, or BiPAP. BiPAP is the brand name of a machine manufactured by Philips Respironics (Murrysville, Pa.), which became popular in the 1980s as a home-care device for treating obstructive sleep apnea. The term *BiPAP* has become so commonly used that it is often applied to any device that provides bilevel pressure control (Box 3-7). Figure 3-18 shows a simplified pressure–time waveform generated by a BiPAP machine.

With bilevel positive pressure, the inspiratory positive airway pressure (IPAP) is higher than the expiratory positive airway

| BOX 3-7 | **Other Names for BiPAP** |

Bilevel airway pressure
Bilevel positive pressure
Bilevel positive airway pressure
Bilevel continuous positive airway pressure (CPAP)
Bilevel positive end-expiratory pressure (PEEP)
Bilevel pressure assist
Bilevel pressure support

pressure (EPAP). This form of ventilation is patient triggered, pressure targeted, and flow or time cycled. The application of BiPAP in noninvasive ventilation is discussed in Chapter 19.

TYPES OF BREATHS

Two types of mechanical ventilation breaths can be described: spontaneous breaths and mandatory breaths. **Spontaneous breaths** are initiated by the patient (i.e., patient triggered), and volume delivery is determined by the patient (i.e., patient cycled). With spontaneous breaths, the volume and flow delivered are based on patient demand rather than on a value set by the ventilator operator. During a **mandatory breath,** the ventilator determines the

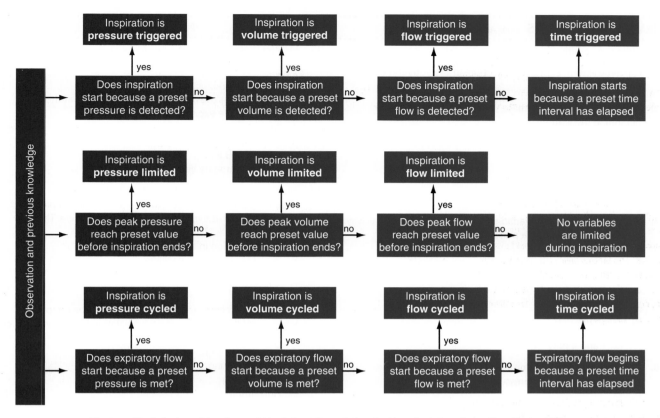

Fig. 3-19 Criteria for determining phase variables during delivery of a breath with mechanical ventilation. (From Kacmarek RM, Stoller JK, Heuer AJ, editors: Egan's fundamentals of respiratory care, ed 10, St Louis, 2013, Elsevier-Mosby.)

BOX 3-8 **Control Variables, Phase Variables, and Types of Breaths**

Control Variables
Control variables are the main variables the ventilator adjusts to produce inspiration. The two primary control variables are pressure and volume.

Phase Variables
Phase variables control the four phases of a breath (i.e., beginning inspiration, inspiration, end inspiration, and expiration). Types of phase variables include
- *Trigger variable* (begins inspiration)
- *Limit variable* (restricts the magnitude of a variable during inspiration)
- *Cycle variable* (ends inspiration)
- *Baseline variable* (the parameter controlled during exhalation)

Types of Breaths
- *Spontaneous breaths:* Breaths are started by the patient (patient triggered), and tidal volume delivery is determined by the patient (patient cycled).
- *Mandatory breaths:* The ventilator determines the start time for breaths (time triggered) or the tidal volume (volume cycled).

start time (time triggering) or tidal volume (or both). In other words, the ventilator triggers and cycles the breath.

Box 3-8 summarizes the main points of control variables, phase variables, and breath types. Figure 3-19 summarizes the criteria for determining the phase variables that are active during the delivery of a breath.[4]

 SUMMARY

- The **equation of motion** provides a mathematical model for describing the relationships among pressure, volume, flow, and time during a spontaneous or mechanical breath.
- The work of breathing can be accomplished by contraction of the respiratory muscles during spontaneous breathing or by the ventilator during a mechanical ventilatory breath.
- Two factors determine the way the inspiratory volume is delivered during mechanical ventilation: the structural design of the ventilator and the ventilator **mode** set by the clinician.
- The primary variable that the ventilator adjusts to produce inspiration is the **control variable.** Although ventilators can be volume, pressure, flow, and time controlled, the two most commonly used control variables are pressure and volume.
- Determining which variable is controlled can be determined by using graphical analysis. The control variable will remain constant regardless of changes in the patient's respiratory characteristics.
- Pressure and flow waveforms delivered by a ventilator are often identified by clinicians as rectangular, exponential, sine wave, and ramp.
- Phase variables are used to describe those variables that (1) begin inspiration, (2) terminate inspiration and cycle the ventilator from inspiration to expiration, (3) can be limited during inspiration, and (4) describe characteristics of the expiratory phase.
- CPAP and PEEP are two methods of applying continuous pressure to the airways to improve oxygenation in patients with refractory hypoxemia.

REVIEW QUESTIONS *(See Appendix A for answers.)*

1. Write the equation of motion.

2. Explain the term *elastic recoil pressure* in the equation of motion.

3. Which of the following phase variables is responsible for beginning inspiration?
   A. Trigger variable
   B. Cycle variable
   C. Limit variable
   D. Baseline variable

4. List two other names for pressure-controlled ventilation.

5. Which of the following variables will remain constant if airway resistance varies during a pressure-controlled breath?
   1. Pressure
   2. Tidal volume
   3. Inspiratory flow
   4. Expiratory time
      A. 1 only
      B. 3 only
      C. 2 and 3 only
      D. 1 and 4 only

6. Compare pressure, volume, and flow delivery in volume-controlled breaths and pressure-controlled breaths.

7. What are the two most common patient-triggering variables?

8. What happens in most ICU ventilators if the pressure alarm is activated?
   1. Inspiration continues, but pressure is limited.
   2. Inspiration ends, and tidal volume is reduced.
   3. An alarm sounds.
   4. Ventilator function does not change.
      A. 1 only
      B. 3 only
      C. 2 and 3 only
      D. 1 and 4 only

9. Flow triggering gained widespread use by clinicians because
   A. The respiratory therapist could set it more easily.
   B. It required less work of breathing for the patient.
   C. It was less expensive to manufacture.
   D. It could be used with any mode of ventilation.

10. A patient is being mechanically ventilated. The tidal volume is set at 600 mL and the rate at 7 breaths/min. The low exhaled volume alarm, set at 500 mL, suddenly is activated. The low-pressure alarm is also activated. The volume monitor shows 0 mL. The peak pressure is 2 cm H_2O. On the volume–time waveform, the expiratory portion of the volume curve plateaus and does not return to zero. The most likely cause of this problem is
    A. Disconnection at the Y-connector
    B. Loss of volume resulting from tubing compressibility
    C. Leakage around the endotracheal tube
    D. Patient coughing

11. Inflation hold increases the inspiratory time.
    A. True
    B. False

12. Which ventilator uses a brief negative pressure at the beginning of the expiratory phase?
    A. Servo-i
    B. Hamilton G5
    C. Covidien PB 840
    D. Cardiopulmonary Venturi

13. On a pressure–time waveform, the curve during the expiratory phase does not return to the baseline rapidly as it normally would. It eventually reaches the baseline. This may be a result of
    A. An obstruction in the expiratory line
    B. PEEP set above zero baseline
    C. NEEP
    D. A leak in the circuit

14. Which of the following can be used to describe the process where inspiratory flow ends and exhalation begins when a set time has elapsed?
    A. Pressure cycling
    B. Time triggering
    C. Time cycling
    D. Flow limiting

15. Which of the following describes the type of ventilation when the pressure–time waveform does not change during inspiration but the volume–time waveform changes when lung characteristics change?
    A. Volume-controlled ventilation
    B. Pressure-controlled ventilation
    C. Time-controlled ventilation
    D. Flow-controlled ventilation

References

1. Mushin WL, Rendell-Baker L, Thompson PW, et al: *Automatic ventilation of the lungs*, ed 2, Oxford, UK, 1969, Blackwell Scientific.
2. Chatburn RL: A new system for understanding mechanical ventilators. *Respir Care* 36:1123–1155, 1991.
3. Chatburn RL: Classification of mechanical ventilators. *Respir Care* 37:1009–1025, 1992.
4. Chatburn RL: Classification of ventilator modes: update and proposal for implementation. *Respir Care* 52:301–323, 2007.
5. Kacmarek RM, Stoller JK, Heuer AJ, editors: *Egan's fundamentals of respiratory care*, ed 10, St Louis, 2013, Elsevier-Mosby.
6. Sanborn WG: Monitoring respiratory mechanics during mechanical ventilation: where do the signals come from? *Respir Care* 50:28–52, 2005.
7. Cairo JM: *Mosby's respiratory care equipment*, ed 9, St Louis, 2014, Elsevier-Mosby.

Establishing the Need for Mechanical Ventilation

OUTLINE

KEY TERMS

- Acute respiratory failure
- Biot respirations
- Cheyne-Stokes respirations
- Functional residual capacity
- Homeostasis
- Permissive hypercapnia
- Residual volume
- Respirometer
- Vital capacity

LEARNING OBJECTIVES *On completion of this chapter, the reader will be able to do the following:*

1. Differentiate between acute respiratory failure (ARF) and respiratory insufficiency.
2. Describe three categories of disorders that may lead to respiratory insufficiency or ARF.
3. Compare normal values for the vital capacity, maximum inspiratory pressure, maximum expiratory pressure (MEP), forced expiratory

volume in 1 second (FEV_1), peak expiratory flow , physiological dead space/tidal volume (V_D/V_T) ratio, alveolar-arterial oxygen pressure difference ($P_{[A-a]}O_2$), and arterial to alveolar partial pressure of oxygen (P_aO_2/P_AO_2) ratio with abnormal values that indicate the need for ventilatory support.

The ability to recognize that a patient requires an artificial airway and mechanical ventilation is an essential skill for clinicians. Although ventilators have been used for more than half a century, surprisingly little evidence and few precise criteria are available to guide clinicians about when to initiate ventilatory support. Originally, mechanical ventilation was instituted because respiratory failure was seen as a "derangement" of gas exchange in the lungs.[1,2] Indeed, clinicians traditionally have relied heavily on arterial blood gas analysis to identify the presence of respiratory failure and the need for ventilatory support.[3] More recently, clinicians have used ventilatory measurements (e.g., respiratory muscle strength) to support their decision to initiate mechanical ventilation. Interestingly, many of these threshold measurements actually reflect criteria that clinicians use to determine when to wean a patient from ventilation.

Decisions made in the acute care setting must be supported by evidence-based criteria. The evidence should clearly demonstrate that a particular intervention is beneficial and is associated with

effective outcomes, such as improved quality of life, reduced length of stay, or a lower mortality rate.[3] This chapter provides information to help clinicians recognize the signs of respiratory distress and respiratory failure. Specific pathologies and methods used to identify the need for an artificial airway and mechanical ventilation are discussed. Noninvasive positive pressure ventilation (NIV), an important alternative to the invasive positive pressure ventilation, is also reviewed. Five patient case studies are presented to demonstrate how clinicians can apply various criteria establishing the need for mechanical ventilation in patients with respiratory failure.

ACUTE RESPIRATORY FAILURE

The primary purpose of ventilation is to maintain **homeostasis.** Mechanical ventilation is indicated when a person cannot achieve an appropriate level of ventilation to maintain adequate gas exchange and acid–base balance. Box 4-1 lists the physiological and clinical objectives of mechanical ventilation.[4]

BOX 4-1 Objectives of Mechanical Ventilation

Physiological Objectives

1. Support or manipulate pulmonary gas exchange:
   - Alveolar ventilation—Achieve eucapnic ventilation or allow **permissive hypercapnia** (NOTE: Permissive hypercapnia sometimes is required in the ventilation of patients with a life-threatening asthma exacerbation, acute lung injury [ALI], or acute respiratory distress syndrome [ARDS] to protect the lung by avoiding high ventilating volumes and pressures.)
   - Alveolar oxygenation—Maintain adequate oxygen delivery ($C_aO_2 \times$ Cardiac output)
2. Increase lung volume:
   - Prevent or treat atelectasis with adequate end-inspiratory lung inflation
   - Restore and maintain an adequate **functional residual capacity** (FRC)
3. Reduce the work of breathing

Clinical Objectives

1. Reverse acute respiratory failure
2. Reverse respiratory distress
3. Reverse hypoxemia
4. Prevent or reverse atelectasis and maintain FRC
5. Reverse respiratory muscle fatigue
6. Permit sedation or paralysis (or both)
7. Reduce systemic or myocardial oxygen consumption
8. Minimize associated complications and reduce mortality

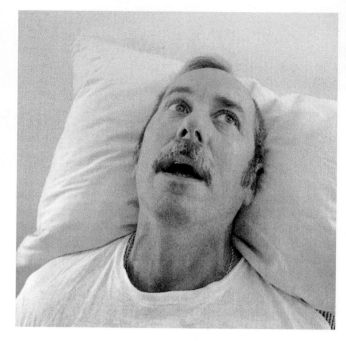

Fig. 4-1 Physical signs of severe respiratory distress. (See text for additional information.)

Recognizing the Patient in Respiratory Distress

Left untreated, acute respiratory failure can lead to coma and eventually death. Early recognition of impending respiratory failure can significantly improve the outcomes for these patients. A number of simple and direct observations can be used to identify impending respiratory failure and guide the selection of an appropriate therapeutic strategy.

The initial assessment of the patient in respiratory distress should focus on several physical findings. First, determine the patient's level of consciousness. Is the patient awake or asleep? If the patient is asleep or unconscious, can the patient be awakened, and if so, to what extent? Second, assess the appearance and texture of the patient's skin? Do the nail beds or lips show evidence of cyanosis? Is the patient pale and diaphoretic (sweating)? Third, evaluate the patient's vital signs (e.g., respiratory rate, heart rate, blood pressure, body temperature, and oxygenation status).

The sudden onset of dyspnea is typically accompanied by physical signs of respiratory distress (Fig. 4-1). For example, patients experiencing respiratory distress appear anxious, with eyes wide open, the forehead furrowed, and the nostrils flared. These patients may be diaphoretic and flushed. They also may try to sit upright or, if seated, lean forward with their elbows resting on a bedside table or their knees. Patients in respiratory or cardiac distress may appear ashen, pale, or cyanotic and be using their accessory muscles of respiration (e.g., the sternocleidomastoid, scalene, and trapezius muscles). In severe respiratory distress, the intercostal spaces and the supraclavicular notch may appear indented (retracted) during active inspiration. The patient may complain of not getting enough air. Paradoxical or abnormal movement of the thorax and abdomen may be noted, and abnormal breath sounds

may be heard on auscultation. Tachycardia, arrhythmias, and hypotension also are common findings.[5] Pulse oximetry is a quick and cost-effective method of assessing arterial oxygen saturation and pulse rate (see Chapter 10). (NOTE: Anemia and reduced cardiac output can compromise oxygen delivery to the tissues. In such cases, reduced pulse pressures and blood flow may prevent the pulse oximeter from accurately estimating the patient's actual arterial oxygen saturation and heart rate.)

It is worth mentioning that in some cases, the signs of respiratory distress are the result of the person experiencing a "panic attack." Simply calming the person and questioning him or her about the distress can usually relieve respiratory distress in this type of patient. (The use of both verbal and nonverbal communication with a patient is vital to effective patient assessment.)

Definition of Respiratory Failure

With **acute respiratory failure** (ARF), respiratory activity is absent or is insufficient to maintain adequate oxygen uptake and carbon dioxide clearance, in spite of initial therapy. Clinically, ARF may be defined as the inability to maintain P_aO_2, P_aCO_2, and pH at acceptable levels. These levels generally are considered to be (1) a P_aO_2 below the predicted normal range for the patient's age under ambient (atmospheric) conditions, (2) a P_aCO_2 greater than 50 mm Hg and rising, and (3) a falling pH of 7.25 and lower.[1-3]

Two forms of ARF have been described: hypoxemic respiratory failure and hypercapnic respiratory failure.[6] Hypoxemic respiratory failure is a result of severe ventilation/perfusion ($\dot{V}/\dot{Q}$) mismatching. It can also occur with diffusion defects, right-to-left shunting, alveolar hypoventilation, aging, and inadequate inspired oxygen. A good working definition of **acute hypoxemic respiratory failure** is acute life-threatening or vital organ–threatening tissue hypoxia.[3] Hypoxemic respiratory failure can be treated with oxygen or in combination with positive end-expiratory pressure (PEEP) or continuous positive airway pressure (CPAP) (see Chapter 13). Mechanical ventilation may also be necessary if

BOX 4-2 Disorders and Agents Associated with Hypoventilation and Possible Respiratory Failure

Central Nervous System Disorders

Reduced Drive to Breathe
- Depressant drugs (barbiturates, tranquilizers, narcotics, general anesthetic agents)
- Brain or brainstem lesions (stroke, trauma to the head or neck, cerebral hemorrhage, tumors, spinal cord injury)
- Hypothyroidism
- Sleep apnea syndrome caused by idiopathic central alveolar hypoventilation

Increased Drive to Breathe
- Increased metabolic rate (increased CO_2 production)
- Metabolic acidosis
- Anxiety associated with dyspnea

Neuromuscular Disorders
- Paralytic disorders (e.g., myasthenia gravis, tetanus, botulism, Guillain-Barré syndrome, poliomyelitis, muscular dystrophy, amyotrophic lateral sclerosis)
- Paralytic drugs (e.g., curare, nerve gas, succinylcholine, insecticides, nondepolarizing neuromuscular blocking agents [See Chapter 15])
- Drugs that affect neuromuscular transmission (e.g., aminoglycoside antibiotics, long-term adrenocorticosteroids, calcium channel blockers)
- Impaired muscle function (e.g., electrolyte imbalances, malnutrition, peripheral nerve disorders, atrophy, fatigue, chronic pulmonary disease with decreasing capacity for diaphragmatic contraction as a result of air trapping)

Disorders That Increase the Work of Breathing
- Pleura-occupying lesions (e.g., pleural effusions, hemothorax, empyema, pneumothorax)
- Chest wall deformities (e.g., flail chest, rib fracture, kyphoscoliosis, obesity)
- Increased airway resistance resulting from increased secretions, mucosal edema, bronchoconstriction, airway inflammation, or foreign body aspiration (e.g., asthma, emphysema, chronic bronchitis, croup, acute epiglottitis, acute bronchitis)
- Lung tissue involvement (e.g., interstitial pulmonary fibrotic diseases, aspiration, ARDS, cardiogenic pulmonary edema, drug-induced pulmonary edema)
- Pulmonary vascular problems (e.g., pulmonary thromboembolism, pulmonary vascular damage)
- Other problems (e.g., increased metabolic rates with accompanying pulmonary problems)
- Postoperative pulmonary complications
- Dynamic hyperinflation (air trapping)

TABLE 4-1 Conditions Seen with Hypoxemia and Hypercapnia

Hypoxemia

	Mild to Moderate	Severe
Respiratory findings	Tachypnea Dyspnea Paleness	Tachypnea Dyspnea Cyanosis
Cardiovascular findings	Tachycardia Mild hypertension Peripheral vasoconstriction	Tachycardia (eventually bradycardia, arrhythmias) Hypertension (eventually hypotension)
Neurologic findings	Restlessness Disorientation Headaches Lethargy	Somnolence Confusion Delirium Blurred vision Tunnel vision Loss of coordination Impaired judgment Slowed reaction time Manic-depressive activity Loss of consciousness Coma

Hypercapnia

	Mild to Moderate	Severe
Respiratory findings	Tachypnea Dyspnea	Tachypnea (eventually bradypnea)
Cardiovascular findings	Tachycardia Hypertension Vasodilation	Tachycardia Hypertension (eventually hypotension)
Neurologic findings	Headaches Drowsiness Dizziness Confusion	Hallucinations Hypomania Convulsions Loss of consciousness (eventually coma)
Signs	Sweating Skin redness	

Recognizing Hypoxemia and Hypercapnia

As shown in Table 4-1, the clinical signs of hypoxemia and hypercapnia closely resemble the signs seen in patients with respiratory distress (see Fig. 4-1 and Key Point 4-1). Tachycardia and tachypnea are early indicators of hypoxia. In some cases of hypoxemic respiratory failure, the patient's condition can be treated successfully by administering enriched oxygen mixtures. However, some hypoxemic conditions, such as severe shunting, are refractory to oxygen therapy (i.e., administering enriched oxygen mixtures does not significantly reduce the level of hypoxemia).

---

hypoxemic respiratory failure occurs along with acute hypercapnic respiratory failure and an increased work of breathing.

Acute hypercapnic respiratory failure, or acute ventilatory failure, occurs when a person cannot achieve adequate ventilation to maintain a normal P_aCO_2. The ventilatory pump consists of the respiratory muscles, thoracic cage, and nerves that are controlled by respiratory centers in the brainstem. Three types of disorders can lead to pump failure (Box 4-2):

- Central nervous system disorders
- Neuromuscular disorders
- Disorders that increase the work of breathing (WOB)

Key Point 4-1 "Tachycardia and tachypnea are nonspecific and mostly subjective signs that may provide only limited help in deciding when to intubate and ventilate a patient."[3]

In patients with hypercapnic respiratory failure, P_aCO_2 levels are elevated with accompanying hypoxemia unless the patient is receiving oxygen therapy. Elevation of P_aCO_2 leads to an increase in cerebral blood flow as a result of dilation of cerebral blood vessels. Severe hypercapnia if left untreated eventually leads to CO_2 narcosis, cerebral depression, coma, and death.

Untreated hypoxemia, hypercapnia, and acidosis can lead to cardiac dysrhythmias, ventricular fibrillation, and even cardiac arrest.[7] The potential for these consequences underscores the importance of recognizing that a patient is in acute or impending respiratory failure and the need to initiate therapy in a timely manner. The elements required to achieve a successful outcome are (1) use of supplemental oxygen therapy, (2) maintenance of a patent airway, and (3) continuous monitoring of oxygenation and ventilatory status with pulse oximetry and arterial blood gas (ABG) analysis.

PATIENT HISTORY AND DIAGNOSIS

The various types of pathologic conditions that increase the risk of a patient developing respiratory failure were mentioned previously (see Box 4-2). The following is a brief discussion of some of these conditions. Several case studies are presented to illustrate the clinical findings associated with respiratory failure.

Central Nervous System Disorders

Central nervous system (CNS) disorders that decrease respiratory drive, such as depression of the respiratory centers induced by drugs or trauma, can lead to significant reductions in minute ventilation ($\dot{V}_E$) and alveolar ventilation ($\dot{V}_A$) and, ultimately, to hypercapnia and hypoxemia. In otherwise normal individuals, an increase in P_aCO_2 greater than 70 mm Hg has a CNS depressant effect, which reduces respiratory drive and ventilation. Hypoxemia, which accompanies this process, normally acts as a respiratory stimulant (through stimulation of the peripheral chemoreceptors) to increase breathing. However, because the CNS already is compromised, the body's response to hypoxemia is diminished.

Other CNS disorders associated with tumors, stroke, or head trauma can alter the normal pattern of breathing. For example, a head injury might result in cerebral hemorrhage and increased intracranial pressure (ICP). If significant bleeding occurs with these types of injuries, abnormal breathing patterns such as **Cheyne-Stokes respirations** or **Biot respirations** may occur. In many cases, cerebral abnormalities can also affect normal reflex responses, such as swallowing. In these cases endotracheal intubation may be required to protect the airway from aspiration or from obstruction by the tongue (Case Study 4-1).

There is considerable debate about whether controlled hyperventilation should be used as a ventilatory technique in patients with a closed head injury. Controlled hyperventilation lowers the P_aCO_2 and increases the pH, resulting in reduced cerebral perfusion and reduced ICP. It is important to understand that this effect is temporary, lasting only about 24 hours, because the body eventually adapts to the change through renal compensatory mechanisms.[8] Although controlled hyperventilation is still used by some clinicians to lower **sudden** increases in ICP, clinicians must keep in mind that the desire to use this technique for patients with traumatic brain injury is not by itself an indication for intubation and mechanical ventilation.[3] Furthermore, patients with traumatic brain injury have a better long-range outcome (3 to 6 months) when controlled hyperventilation is not used.[8]

Case Study 4-1

Stroke Victim

A 58-year-old man is admitted to the emergency department from his home after a suspected stroke (i.e., cerebral vascular accident, or CVA). Vital signs reveal a heart rate of 94 beats/min, respirations of 16 breaths/min, normal temperature, and systemic arterial blood pressure of 165/95 mm Hg. The patient's pupils respond slowly and unequally to light. Breath sounds are diminished in the lung bases. A sound similar to snoring is heard on inspiration. The patient is unconscious and unresponsive to painful stimuli. What is the most appropriate course of action at this time?

Case Study 4-2

Unexplained Acute Respiratory Failure

A stat arterial blood gas evaluation performed on a patient admitted through the emergency department reveals the following: pH = 7.15, P_aCO_2 = 83 mm Hg, P_aO_2 = 34 mm Hg, HCO_3^- = 28 mEq/L on room air. The patient was found unconscious in a nearby park. No other history is available. What is the most appropriate course of action at this time?

Neuromuscular Disorders

Neuromuscular disorders that can lead to respiratory failure usually are the result of one of the following:

- Motor nerve damage
- Problems with transmission of nerve impulses at the neuromuscular junction
- Muscle dysfunction
- Central nervous system disorders
- Drugs that affect neuromuscular function

The onset of respiratory failure can vary considerably depending on the cause of the neuromuscular dysfunction. Drug-induced neuromuscular failure usually has a rapid onset (Case Study 4-2), whereas the onset of respiratory failure in disease states like myasthenia gravis may not occur for days or years, or it might not happen at all. Regardless of the cause, intubation and mechanical ventilation are indicated if respiratory fatigue occurs rapidly in a patient with a neuromuscular disorder and ARF is imminent.[9]

The maximum inspiratory pressure (MIP) and vital capacity (VC) can be used to assess respiratory muscle strength of patients with neuromuscular disorders. These measurements are noninvasive, relatively easy to obtain, and inexpensive. Respiratory therapists can measure MIP and VC every 2 to 4 hours to monitor changes in respiratory status. Commonly cited threshold values are an MIP of −20 to −30 cm H_2O or less (i.e., 0 to −20 cm H_2O) and a VC lower than 10 to 15 mL/kg. Note that although these measures are often used, their effectiveness in improving outcomes has not been established (Table 4-2).[3] (Techniques for measuring MIP and VC are discussed later in this chapter.)

Determination of baseline ABG values, along with periodic measurement of oxygen saturation by pulse oximetry (S_pO_2) is also appropriate when caring for patients with neuromuscular

TABLE 4-2 Indications of Acute Respiratory Failure and the Need for Mechanical Ventilatory Support in Adults		
Criteria	Normal Values	Critical Value
Ventilation*		
pH	7.35-7.45	<7.25
Arterial partial pressure of carbon dioxide (P_aCO_2) (mm Hg)	35-45	>55 and rising
Dead space to tidal volume ratio (V_D/V_T)	0.3-0.4	>0.6
Oxygenation†		
Arterial partial pressure of oxygen (P_aO_2) (mm Hg)	80-100	<70 (on $O_2 \geq 0.6$)
Alveolar-to-arterial oxygen difference $P_{(A-a)}O_2$ (mm Hg)	5-20	>450 (on O_2)
Ratio of arterial to alveolar PO_2 (P_aO_2/P_AO_2)	0.75	<0.15
P_aO_2/F_IO_2	475	<200

F_IO_2, Fraction of inspired oxygen.
*Indicates the need for ventilatory support.
†Indicates the need for oxygen therapy and PEEP/CPAP.

problems. Repeating the ABG analysis may be indicated if the patient's clinical status changes significantly. Furthermore, if the patient's condition progressively worsens, the practitioner should **not** wait until an acute situation develops to intervene (Case Study 4-3). Clinicians generally agree that invasive positive pressure ventilation should be initiated before acute respiratory acidosis develops.[3]

Case Study 4-3

Ventilation in Neuromuscular Disorders

Case 1

A 68-year-old woman with a history of myasthenia gravis has been in the hospital for 12 days. She was admitted because her primary disease had worsened. The patient is unable to perform MIP and slow vital capacity (SVC) maneuvers properly because she cannot seal her lips around the mouthpiece. Her attempts produced these values: MIP = –34 cm H_2O; SVC = 1.2 L. What should the clinician recommend at this time?

Case 2

A 26-year-old man who is recovering from mycoplasma pneumonia complains of tingling sensations and weakening in his hands and feet. He is admitted to the general medicine service for observation. Over several hours the patient becomes unable to move his legs. A respiratory therapist (RT) is called to assess him. What should the RT recommend at this time?

Increased Work of Breathing

An increase in the WOB can lead to respiratory failure secondary to respiratory muscle fatigue. WOB normally accounts for 1% to 4% of total oxygen consumption at rest.[10] In patients experiencing respiratory distress, the WOB can increase to as much as 35% to 40% of total oxygen consumption.[11,12] Increased WOB usually is associated with an increased rate or depth of breathing (or both). More work is required to move the same V_T when the patient has obstructed airways, a restrictive lung disorder, or both (Case Study 4-4). A patient's tolerance to maintain the increased WOB is limited by the eventual fatigue of respiratory muscles. Increased WOB can induce hypoventilation, respiratory insufficiency, and eventually respiratory failure.

An example of a condition that causes increased WOB is severe chest trauma. Flail chest, pneumothorax, and hemothorax can impair the mechanics of breathing and affect the patient's ability to breathe. A reduction in alveolar ventilation leads to $\dot{V}/\dot{Q}$ mismatching; an increased V_D/V_T; and ultimately hypoxemia, hypercapnia, and acidosis. Although the patient's respiratory centers may be intact and responsive to hypercapnia and hypoxemia, his or her ability to maintain the effort to breathe is seriously compromised. Even as the patient initially tries to respond by increasing minute ventilation (i.e., increased respiratory rate and V_T), the P_aO_2 may continue to fall, the P_aCO_2 rises, and the pH decreases despite the patient's compensatory efforts.

In some patients, increased WOB eventually results in rapid, shallow breathing and **paradoxical breathing**.[13] With paradoxical breathing, the abdomen moves out during exhalation and moves in during inhalation while the chest wall moves out during inhalation and moves in during exhalation. This is the reverse of normal breathing, where the chest wall and abdomen move outward together on inspiration and inward on exhalation. This asynchronous motion of the chest and abdomen is an ominous sign in patients with respiratory distress and usually indicates increased WOB and the onset of respiratory muscle fatigue.[3]

At one time physicians commonly used positive pressure to "splint" the chest and "internally stabilize" the chest wall in patients with flail chest. Current evidence suggests that better outcomes are achieved when patients with flail chest are managed without intubation or invasive positive pressure ventilation (IPPV). IPPV is only used for flail chest when it is associated with imminent respiratory failure.

Case Study 4-4

Asthma Case

A 13-year-old girl is seen in the emergency department for an acute exacerbation of asthma. Continuous nebulizer therapy with a β-2 adrenergic bronchodilator is administered. The patient has been given a high dose of corticosteroids and is receiving oxygen. Four hours after admission, she is alert and responsive. Her respiratory rate is 20 breaths/min. Coarse crackles and end-inspiratory wheezes are heard clearly throughout both lung fields. What recommendation for continuous respiratory care should be made for this patient?

PHYSIOLOGICAL MEASUREMENTS IN ACUTE RESPIRATORY FAILURE

Clinicians often use ventilatory mechanics measurements and ABG results to detect respiratory failure. Unfortunately, valid

TABLE 4-3	Normal Adult and Critical Range Values	
Ventilatory Mechanics	**Normal Adult Range**	**Critical Value That May Indicate the Need for Mechanical Ventilation**
Maximum inspiratory pressure (MIP) (cm H_2O)	−100 to −50	−20 to 0
Maximum expiratory pressure (MEP) (cm H_2O)	100	<40
Vital capacity (VC) (mL/kg)	65 to 75	<10 to 15
Tidal volume (V_T) (mL/kg)	5 to 8	<5
Respiratory frequency (f) (breaths/min)	12 to 20	>35
Forced expired volume at 1 second (FEV_1) (mL/kg)	50 to 60	<10
Peak expiratory flow (PEF) (L/min)	350 to 600	75 to 100

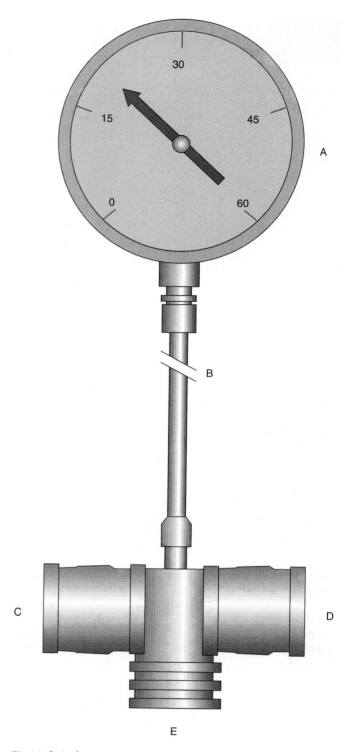

Fig. 4-2 Device for measuring maximum inspiratory pressure. **A,** Pressure gauge. **B,** Connective tubing. **C,** Thumb port, which is occluded during the measurement procedure. **D,** One-way valve connection; the valve allows exhalation into the room but does not allow inhalation. **E,** Connection to the patient's mouth or endotracheal tube. (Modified from Kacmarek RM, Cycyk-Chapman MC, Young-Palazzo PJ, et al: Determination of maximum inspiratory pressure: a clinical study and literature review, Respir Care 34:868-878, 1989.)

predictive threshold values for these measurements have not been substantiated.[3] The absence of guidelines can sometimes make it difficult for a novice clinician to know when to intubate or ventilate a patient in distress.

Table 4-3 lists normal adult values for ventilatory mechanics, as well as the suggested critical range that may indicate a need for mechanical ventilation when considered with other assessment criteria. It is worth mentioning that most of these parameters are probably better used as indications for discontinuing mechanical ventilation, with two exceptions: (1) in patients with neuromuscular disorders, the MIP and the VC may be beneficial in tracking respiratory muscle strength; (2) in patients with reactive airway disease (e.g., asthma and some patients with chronic obstructive pulmonary disease [COPD]), the forced expiratory volume at 1 second (FEV_1) and the peak expiratory flow (PEF) are helpful for quantifying the degree of airway resistance. FEV_1 is more useful to evaluate small airways function than is the PEF.

Bedside Measurements of Ventilatory Mechanics

Abnormal ventilatory mechanics measurements should alert the clinician to the presence of a potentially serious respiratory problem. As previously mentioned, MIP and VC are the bedside measurements most often used to assess respiratory muscle strength in patients with neuromuscular disease. For patients with acute asthma, the PEF is the most frequently used parameter to assess airway resistance. FEV_1 is a better parameter and bedside spirometry is readily available for measuring FEV_1.

Maximum Inspiratory Pressure

The MIP (or P_{Imax}) is the lowest (i.e., most negative) pressure generated during a forceful inspiratory effort against an occluded airway. MIP is also called negative inspiratory force (NIF). At the bedside, MIP usually is measured with a pressure manometer (Fig. 4-2).[14] The device is connected to the patient's airway by means of a mask, mouthpiece, or endotracheal tube adapter. The patient is instructed to inhale forcefully from the device while the respiratory therapist occludes the thumb port of the T-piece connector containing two one-way valves.

Alternative Technique for Measuring Maximum Inspiratory Pressure (MIP)

For accuracy and reproducibility, measurement of the maximum MIP must begin as closely as possible to the residual volume (RV). If the patient cannot perform a maximum exhalation, a one-way valve (see Fig. 4-2) may be used. This valve allows exhalation but prevents inspiration. To perform the technique, the clinician occludes the thumb port and watches the pressure gauge as the patient takes multiple breaths (because the patient cannot inspire air against the occluded valve, this brings lung volume close to the RV as the patient exhales over several breaths). MIP measurement stops when the lowest negative value is reached (this may take up to 20 seconds). Although the one-way valve technique can provide an accurate MIP value, this type of prolonged measurement is extremely uncomfortable for the patient. (Students can gain considerable insight into that discomfort by trying this technique as a laboratory exercise.)

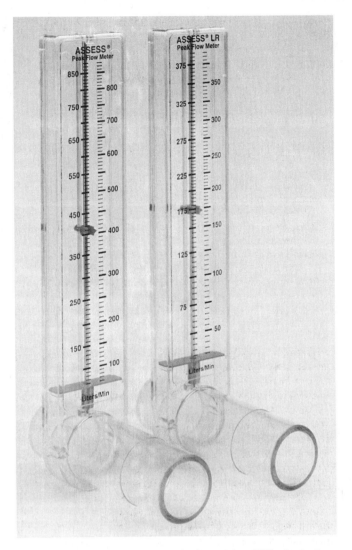

Fig. 4-3 Disposable peak flowmeters. (Used with permission of Philips Respironics, Inc., Murraysville, Pa.)

Values are most accurate and reproducible when MIP is measured from the **residual volume** (RV), that is, after a maximum exhalation.[14-17] At least two measurements should be obtained if possible. Obtaining more than two or three MIP maneuvers from patients in distress may result in erroneous results because the procedure requires significant effort by the patient. MIP normally is −50 to −100 cm H_2O. An MIP of at least −20 cm H_2O is required to generate a V_T large enough to produce a good cough (Box 4-3).[14-18]

Vital Capacity

Vital capacity is the volume of air that can be maximally exhaled following a maximum inspiration. It can provide valuable information about ventilatory function because the patient must be able to take in a large volume of air to produce a cough strong enough to clear the airway. VC is typically 65 to 75 mL/kg of ideal body weight (IBW), but it may be as high as 100 mL/kg IBW. Values less than 10 to 15 mL/kg IBW are considered inadequate to maintain normal ventilation and produce an effective cough.[19] (See Box 6-2 for calculation of IBW.) VC can be measured at the bedside using a pneumotachometer or **respirometer.** Obtaining reliable measurements requires the patient's cooperation, which typically occurs when the patient receives proper instructions from the clinician about how to perform the procedure (Key Point 4-2).

Key Point 4-2 MIP and VC are bedside measurements most often used to assess respiratory muscle strength of patients with neuromuscular disease.

Peak Expiratory Flow and Forced Expiratory Volume in 1 Second

The PEF is a good indicator of airway resistance and a patient's ability to maintain airway patency. Obtaining reliable measurements of PEF is a part of an effective asthma treatment plan for many asthma patients. A peak flowmeter like the one shown in Fig. 4-3 can be used to measure PEF. Acceptable values range from 350 to 600 L/min. Low PEFs most often are seen in patients having an acute asthma episode. Values less than 75 to 100 L/min are cause for alarm and indicate severe airflow obstruction.

The FEV$_1$ is another pulmonary function parameter that can be used to assess airway resistance. FEV$_1$ normally is about 80% of the VC, or about 50 to 60 mL/kg IBW. An FEV$_1$ less than 10 mL/kg IBW is considered extremely low. Although several portable spirometers are available for measuring FEV$_1$ at the bedside, it is **not** an appropriate measurement to perform on a patient who is severely short of breath and in acute respiratory distress.

Respiratory Rate and Minute Ventilation

Two other parameters often mentioned in the assessment of respiratory distress are the respiratory rate (f) and minute ventilation ($\dot{V}_E$). The respiratory rate normally is about 12 to 20 breaths/min in adults. Respiratory rates exceeding 35 breaths/min for extended periods are a sign of inadequate alveolar ventilation or hypoxemia (or both). As mentioned previously, elevated respiratory rates are an indication of an increased WOB, which eventually leads to respiratory muscle fatigue.

Minute ventilation is the product of tidal volume and respiratory rate ($\dot{V}_E = \dot{V}_t \times f_b$). A normal $\dot{V}_E$ is about 5 to 6 L/min, and this value is directly related to the patient's metabolic rate. A $\dot{V}_E$

above 10 L/min is cause for concern. In cases where the patient demonstrates significant pulmonary dysfunction, the $\dot{V}_E$ required to maintain a stable P_aCO_2 may become so high that the patient cannot sustain the required work of breathing. Although V_T and $\dot{V}_E$ can be measured in unintubated patients with respiratory distress, these measurements are seldom obtained.[3]

Failure of Ventilation and Increased Dead Space

Clinicians generally agree that the best single indicator of adequate ventilation is the P_aCO_2 (Key Point 4-3). A P_aCO_2 of greater than 50 to 55 mm Hg with a decreasing pH (less than 7.25) indicates acute hypoventilation or acute hypercapnic respiratory failure.

> **Key Point 4-3** The best single indicator of the adequacy of ventilation is the P_aCO_2.

An elevated P_aCO_2 also suggests that dead space (V_D) is increased relative to V_T. The normal V_D/V_T range is 0.3 to 0.4 at normal tidal volumes. Values greater than 0.6 indicate a critical increase in dead space. For example, in a patient with a V_T of 500 mL and a V_D/V_T of 0.6 mL, for each breath taken, only 40% (200 mL) contacts pulmonary blood flow and contributes to alveolar gas exchange; 60% (300 mL) goes to areas of the pulmonary system that are not in contact with the pulmonary capillary bed. Under these conditions, the patient must increase the rate and depth of breathing (i.e., increase $\dot{V}_E$) to try to achieve adequate gas exchange. Increases in dead space are associated with $\dot{V}/\dot{Q}$ mismatching (i.e., dead space ventilation is defined as ventilation in excess of perfusion). Common causes of increased dead space ventilation include pulmonary thromboemboli, pulmonary vascular injury, and regional hypoperfusion.

In the past, measurement of the V_D/V_T required the collection of expired gases and simultaneous evaluation of arterial CO_2 tensions. This procedure was time consuming and not well tolerated by patients in severe respiratory failure. V_D/V_T can now be estimated by using less cumbersome, noninvasive methods, such as volumetric capnometry (see Chapter 10).

Failure of Oxygenation

P_aO_2 is a good indicator of oxygenation status, assuming that abnormal forms of hemoglobin (e.g., carboxyhemoglobin and methemoglobin) are not present. Normal P_aO_2 is 80 to 100 mm Hg when an individual is breathing room air, but this value varies with age and body position. Monitoring S_pO_2 can also provide an easy, noninvasive means of assessing trends in a patient's oxygenation status (Key Point 4-4).[3] A P_aO_2 less than 70 mm Hg (or S_pO_2 less than 90%) on an oxygen mask ($F_IO_2 \geq 0.6$) indicates refractory hypoxemia or hypoxemic respiratory failure. Additional information about a patient's total oxygen-carrying capacity can be derived from measurements or calculation of his or her arterial oxygen content (C_aO_2) (Box 4-4).

> **Key Point 4-4** P_aO_2 and S_pO_2 are the key indicators of the severity of acute hypoxemic respiratory failure.[3]

As discussed later in this text (see Chapter 13), the $P_{(A-a)}O_2$ can be used to determine the cause of altered oxygenation. The normal range for $P_{(A-a)}O_2$ for patients breathing room air is 5 to 20 mm Hg; the normal range for patients breathing 100% O_2 is 25 to 65 mm Hg.

BOX 4-4 **Calculation of Arterial Oxygen Content**

The arterial oxygen content (C_aO_2) can be calculated with the following equation:

$$C_aO_2 = ([Hb \times 1.34] \times S_aO_2) + (P_aO_2 \times 0.003)$$

where *Hb* is hemoglobin in grams per deciliter of whole blood (g%), S_aO_2 is arterial oxygen saturation, and P_aO_2 is the partial pressure of arterial oxygen in millimeters of mercury (mm Hg).

TABLE 4-4 **Specific Treatments for Arterial Hypoxemia**

Cause	Treatment
Hypoventilation	Increase F_IO_2, increase alveolar ventilation
Low ventilation/ perfusion ratio	Increase F_IO_2, continuous positive airway pressure (CPAP)
Intrapulmonary shunt	Increase F_IO_2, CPAP
Diffusion defect	Increase F_IO_2, steroids (?), diuretics
Low barometric pressure	Descend (to lower altitude)
Low inspired oxygen concentration (<21%)	Increase F_IO_2

From Downs JB: Has oxygen administration delayed appropriate respiratory care? Fallacies regarding oxygen therapy, Respir Care 48:611-620, 2003.

When P_aO_2 is low and $P_{(A-a)}O_2$ is high, hypoxemia is due to one of the other three general causes: shunt, diffusion defects, and $\dot{V}/\dot{Q}$ mismatching (see Appendix B). (NOTE: In these cases P_aCO_2 may even be lower than normal, indicating hyperventilation to compensate for hypoxemia.)

The P_aO_2/P_AO_2 ratio is another approach that can be used to evaluate a patient's oxygenation status. P_aO_2/P_AO_2 normally is about 0.75 to 0.95. This range indicates that 75% to 95% of the oxygen available in the alveoli is diffusing into the pulmonary capillaries. For example, a normal P_aO_2 of 90 mm Hg divided by a normal P_AO_2 on room air (100 mm Hg) gives a ratio of 0.90. A value of 0.15 or less is critical (i.e., only 15% of available oxygen is getting into the artery).

Using a P_aO_2/F_IO_2 ratio eliminates the need to calculate the alveolar PO_2 (P_AO_2). Normal values can be calculated as follows: 90 mm Hg/0.21 = 428 (about 430; range, 350 to 450). A P_aO_2 of 40 mm Hg with an F_IO_2 of 1.0 (40 mm Hg/1.0 = 40) is an example of an extremely severe abnormality (i.e., refractory hypoxemia).[20]

The treatment for hypoxemia is based on its etiology (Table 4-4).[21] For example, when hemoglobin and hematocrit values are low as a result of hemorrhage, the arterial O_2 content is reduced, and a blood transfusion is required to improve oxygen content and transport. In some cases, refractory hypoxemic respiratory failure can be treated with PEEP or CPAP (see Chapter 13). When hypoxemia is accompanied by an increase in WOB or a rising P_aCO_2 and a falling pH, mechanical ventilation is required.[3,22] Mask CPAP and oxygen alone are not considered effective treatments for hypoxemia in patients with acute lung injury (ALI), and intubation is usually required (Key Point 4-5).[23]

| BOX 4-5 | Standard Criteria for Instituting Mechanical Ventilation |

- Apnea or absence of breathing
- Acute ventilatory failure
- Impending ventilatory failure
- Refractory hypoxemic respiratory failure with increased work of breathing or an ineffective breathing pattern

---

Key Point 4-5 No single value for P_aO_2, P_aCO_2, or pH indicates a need for invasive ventilation.[3]

OVERVIEW OF CRITERIA FOR MECHANICAL VENTILATION

The standard criteria for instituting mechanical ventilatory support are listed in Box 4-5. Apnea and impending respiratory failure and arrest are the most obvious indications for invasive ventilation. Current indications for invasive ventilation are shown in Box 4-6.[3]

Reversibility of the underlying disease should always be a consideration. The clinician must consider the patient's medical history, physical assessment, ABG evaluation, lung mechanics measurements, prognosis, and advanced directives (i.e., patient's wishes) when deciding whether to intubate and ventilate a patient's lungs. Thoughtful clinical judgment is essential, as is attention to the goals of therapy for a mechanically ventilated patient[3,4] (Key Point 4-6):

1. Support the pulmonary system so that it can maintain an adequate level of alveolar ventilation
2. Reduce the work of breathing until the cause of respiratory failure can be identified and treated
3. Restore arterial and systemic acid–base balances to levels that are normal **for the patient**
4. Increase oxygen delivery to and oxygenation of body organs and tissues
5. Prevent complications associated with mechanical ventilation

---

Key Point 4-6 Protecting the patient's airway is critical with conditions such as stroke, drug overdose, cerebral damage, and copious or viscous secretions.

POSSIBLE ALTERNATIVES TO INVASIVE VENTILATION

In some cases using a more conservative approach may avoid the need for invasive ventilation. Providing supplemental oxygen through standard oxygen therapy devices or through more specialized respiratory therapy devices (e.g., high flow nasal cannula) may help to relieve hypoxia. For example, high flow nasal cannula therapy allows the delivery of high gas flows through a narrow tube (e.g., nasal or transtracheal cannula) (Fig. 4-4).

Placing the patient in an upright or Fowler position and providing appropriate medications can also be used to avoid the need for mechanical ventilation. However, the clinician must always keep in mind that hypoxemia can arise from a variety of causes, and these

| BOX 4-6 | Indications for Invasive Mechanical Ventilation in Adults with Acute Respiratory Failure |

Invasive mechanical ventilation is indicated in any of the following circumstances:

1. Apnea or impending respiratory arrest
2. Acute exacerbation of chronic obstructive pulmonary disease (COPD)* with dyspnea, tachypnea, and acute respiratory acidosis (hypercapnia and decreased arterial pH) plus at least one of the following:
   - Acute cardiovascular instability
   - Altered mental status or persistent uncooperativeness
   - Inability to protect the lower airway
   - Copious or unusually viscous secretions
   - Abnormalities of the face or upper airway that would prevent effective noninvasive positive pressure ventilation
3. Acute ventilatory insufficiency in cases of neuromuscular disease accompanied by any of the following:
   - Acute respiratory acidosis (hypercapnia and decreased arterial pH)
   - Progressive decline in vital capacity to below 10 to 15 mL/kg
   - Progressive decline in maximum inspiratory pressure to below −20 to −30 cm H_2O
4. Acute hypoxemic respiratory failure with tachypnea, respiratory distress, and persistent hypoxemia despite administration of a high fraction of inspired oxygen (F_IO_2) with high-flow oxygen devices **or** in the presence of any of the following:
   - Acute cardiovascular instability
   - Altered mental status or persistent uncooperativeness
   - Inability to protect the lower airway
5. Need for endotracheal intubation to maintain or protect the airway or to manage secretions, given the following factors:
   - Endotracheal tube (ET) ≤7 mm internal diameter (ID) with minute ventilation >10 L/min
   - ET ≤8 mm ID with minute ventilation >15 L/min

   If any of the conditions listed are not present, emergency intubation and invasive positive pressure ventilation may not be indicated for the following conditions until other therapies have been attempted.
- Dyspnea, acute respiratory distress
- Acute exacerbation of COPD
- Acute severe asthma
- Acute hypoxemic respiratory failure in immunocompromised patients
- Hypoxemia as an isolated finding
- Traumatic brain injury
- Flail chest

Modified from Pierson DJ: Indications for mechanical ventilation in adults with acute respiratory failure, *Respir Care* 47:249-262, 2002.
*Also applies to life-threatening asthma if respiratory acidosis or airflow obstruction has worsened despite aggressive management with bronchodilators and other therapy.

causes should be the focus of therapy. Oxygen therapy, repositioning the patient, and administration of medications such as bronchodilators and mucolytics are palliative measures that usually provide only transient relief of hypoxemia. They do not eliminate the cause.

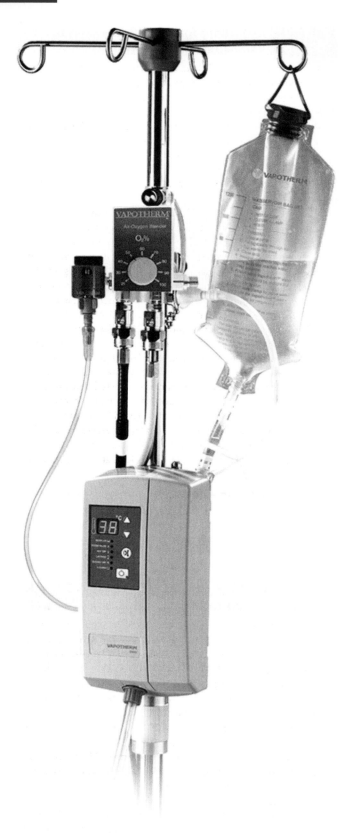

Fig. 4-4 Vapotherm 2000i, a respiratory therapy device that allows very high flows to be administered through a narrow tube such as a nasal or transtracheal cannula. (Courtesy Vapotherm, Stevensville, Md.)

BOX **4-7**	**Indications and Contraindications for Noninvasive Positive Pressure Ventilation (NIV) in Adults**[29,30]

Indications

At least two of the following factors should be present:
- Respiratory rate >25 breaths/min
- Moderate to severe acidosis: pH, 7.25 to 7.30; P_aCO_2, 45 to 60 mm Hg
- Moderate to severe dyspnea with use of accessory muscles and paradoxical breathing pattern

Contraindications

Any of the following factors alone is a contraindication.

Absolute Contraindications
- Respiratory arrest
- Cardiac arrest
- Cardiovascular instability (hypotension, dysrhythmias, acute myocardial infarction)
- Nonrespiratory organ failure (e.g., severe encephalopathy, severe gastrointestinal bleeding or surgery, hemodynamic instability with or without unstable cardiac angina)
- Patent tracheoesophageal fistula
- Inability to protect the airway or high risk of aspiration (or both)
- Uncooperative patient (impaired mental status, hypersomnolence)
- Facial or head surgery or trauma

Relative Contraindications
- Copious or viscous secretions
- Fixed nasopharyngeal abnormalities
- Extreme obesity

Noninvasive Positive Pressure Ventilation

In some patients, noninvasive positive pressure ventilation (NIV) is a viable alternative to invasive positive pressure ventilation and may be a means of avoiding endotracheal intubation.[23] NIV is the treatment of choice for **acute-on-chronic respiratory failure** unless cardiovascular instability is also a factor. The use of NIV for acute-on-chronic respiratory failure has been shown to reduce the need for intubation, reduce complications of ventilation, shorten the hospital stay, and reduce hospital mortality rates.[23-25] It is important to recognize that the patient must meet the criteria for NIV and must not have any of the exclusionary factors (Box 4-7).[21,26-29] Invasive ventilation with intubation is indicated if any of the contraindications for NIV listed in Box 4-7 are present.[27,28]

Although this approach is controversial, NIV may also be beneficial for patients with ARF associated with cardiogenic pulmonary edema.[26] Acute-on-chronic hypercapnic respiratory failure in patients with musculoskeletal problems (e.g., kyphoscoliosis and postpolio syndrome) may be well suited to NIV. NIV also is an alternative to invasive ventilator support for patients with hypercapnic acute exacerbation of COPD and considered a standard of care for these patients (Box 4-8).[29,30] In fact, NIV is an effective method of resting the ventilatory muscles and averting invasive ventilation in this latter group of patients. However, patients with neuromuscular disorders who develop acute respiratory acidosis and evidence of muscle weakness that progressively worsens (decreasing MIP and VC) require prompt intubation to prevent ARF and to protect the airway.[3]

BOX 4-8	**Circumstances in Which Noninvasive Positive Pressure Ventilation Should Be Changed to Invasive Ventilation**

- Respiratory arrest
- Respiratory rate >35 breaths/min
- Severe dyspnea with use of accessory muscles and possibly paradoxical breathing
- Life-threatening hypoxemia: P_aO_2 <40 mm Hg or P_aO_2/F_iO_2 <200
- Severe acidosis (pH <7.25) and hypercapnia (P_aCO_2 >60 mm Hg)
- Hypersomnolence, impaired mental status
- Cardiovascular complications (hypotension, shock, heart failure)
- Failure of noninvasive positive pressure ventilation
- Other circumstances (e.g., metabolic abnormalities, sepsis, pneumonia, pulmonary embolism, barotrauma, massive pleural effusion)

Invasive ventilation also is indicated for patients with severe refractory hypoxemia associated with increased WOB. These patients may suffer adverse events if mask CPAP is used for treatment rather than invasive ventilation.[29,30] Even with appropriately selected patients and skilled clinicians, NIV has been shown to be ineffective in about 25% of cases, and endotracheal intubation is required.[27,28,30] (Chapter 19 discusses many additional important aspects of NIV.)

Intubation Without Ventilation

Some adult patients must be intubated because of an airway obstruction or to protect the airway or facilitate the removal of secretions (Key Point 4-6). If no other indications for ventilatory support are present and if a 7-mm endotracheal tube or larger is used, it is reasonable to conclude that IPPV is not needed. WOB related to the resistance of the endotracheal tube is considered significant only in small tubes (less than 7 mm) and when the minute ventilation is high (over 10 L/min)[3,31] (see Chapter 17 for additional information on the work of breathing through an artificial airway).

Ethical Considerations

Ethical considerations must be part of the decision-making process before initiating mechanical ventilation. First and foremost, does the patient want to be on ventilatory support? If the patient is unable to answer, it is important to determine whether the patient has a designated surrogate. Does the patient have a living will, advance directive, or similar legal document indicating his or her wishes regarding life-support procedures? These significant concerns must be addressed. Invasive ventilation is contraindicated when it is contrary to the patient's advance directives. It might also be considered contraindicated if its use would be medically pointless and futile. If no reasonable chance exists that ventilation would extend a person's quality of life in a meaningful way, it probably is contraindicated.[3]

 Clinical Scenario: Drug Overdose

A 23-year-old woman is taken to the hospital after ingesting an unknown amount of drugs and alcohol. Friends found her unconscious in her apartment. On admission to the emergency department, she is unconscious and unresponsive to verbal commands. Her pulse is 124 beats/min; blood pressure is 85/50 mm Hg. Her respiratory rate is 15 breaths/min, and respirations are shallow. ABG values on room air are as follows: P_aO_2 = 60 mm Hg, P_aCO_2 = 69 mm Hg, and pH = 7.24. Breath sounds reveal bilateral coarse crackles, especially in the bases.

Drugs and alcohol are known to depress the respiratory centers of the brain and also to reduce the normal glottic response. The patient's shallow breathing is most likely caused by the substances ingested. Crackles heard over the right middle lobe may be due to aspiration. Weakening of the normal glottic response causes failure of the glottis to protect the airway, which is important to recognize because drug overdose and alcohol can cause nausea and vomiting.

The ABG values reported indicate ARF. The clinician's first priority is to protect the airway through intubation and provide ventilation to normalize the blood gases. With drug overdose the patient sometimes can be treated pharmacologically, depending on the types of drugs ingested. For example, narcotic overdoses can be treated with naloxone hydrochloride (Narcan), an opioid antagonist. (NOTE: Narcan is used only to reverse the CNS and ventilatory depression caused by a narcotic overdose.) Determining the type and amount of drugs ingested can provide valuable information to guide the immediate treatment of the patient.

Clinical Scenario: Guillain-Barré

A 30-year-old man is admitted to the hospital emergency department complaining of weakness of the limbs, tingling of the hands and feet, and increasing lack of coordination. Two weeks previously he had been treated for a flulike illness. The respiratory care practitioner obtains a baseline ABG evaluation, which is within normal limits. MIP is −70 cm H_2O, and VC is 4.3 L (predicted, 4.8 L).

Over a 36-hour period, VC, MIP, V_T, S_pO_2, and respiratory rate are monitored every 3 to 4 hours. Values progressively decrease to a VC of 2.1 L (44% of predicted [23 mL/kg]) and an MIP of −32 cm H_2O. A repeat ABG evaluation on room air shows the following: P_aO_2 = 70 mm Hg, P_aCO_2 = 48 mm Hg, and pH = 7.34.

The diagnosis of Guillain-Barré syndrome was made based on the patient's history and physical findings. Given the patient's diagnosis and clinical findings, the physician decides to intubate him and begin respiratory support. Guillain-Barré syndrome is a rapidly progressive, ascending, bilateral, flaccid muscle paralysis. Once it begins, it can progress to affect the respiratory muscles and other skeletal muscles.

Often, in neuromuscular disorders, an effective drug therapy is not available to reverse the progression of paralysis. When respiratory mechanics begin to deteriorate, patients are often intubated or provided with invasive respiratory support before the respiratory mechanics reach a critical value. Interestingly, arterial blood gas values and oxygen saturations may often be within normal limits. However, the clinician must remember that it is better to act early than to wait for respiratory arrest.

high minute ventilation (this would indicate an increased V_D/V_T); they do not wait for the P_aCO_2 to exceed 45 mm Hg. Other clinicians use evidence of cardiac failure and a drop in pulse intensity, as well as the presence of dysrhythmias as criteria for intubation and initiating mechanical ventilation. Deterioration in mental status and exhaustion can also be important indicators for intubation and mechanical ventilation.[33]

 ## Clinical Scenario: Asthma

A 15-year-old girl with a life-threatening exacerbation of asthma has been treated in the emergency department over several hours. Administration of oxygen, corticosteroids, heliox, and aerosolized β-2 adrenergic bronchodilators and ipratropium bromide, although appropriate,[32] has not been effective in reducing airway obstruction and WOB. The patient has a respiratory rate of 37 breaths/min and her breathing is labored. Bilateral inspiratory and expiratory wheezes are present in both lungs. PEF is 70 L/min and FEV_1 is 0.75 L. ABG values obtained while the patient is breathing 50% oxygen are as follows: P_aO_2 = 73 mm Hg, P_aCO_2 = 28 mm Hg, HCO_3^- = 19 mEq/L, pH = 7.46. P_aO_2/P_AO_2 is 0.23.

Hyperventilation in moderate or severe attacks of asthma is probably localized to areas of the lung where resistance to flow is lowest. Other areas of the lung are typically underventilated, resulting in shunting and reduced oxygenation. The length of time that a patient can tolerate this amount of work and hypoxemia varies considerably. If the persistent bronchospasm and mucus plugging cannot be alleviated, P_aCO_2 will rise despite a high minute ventilation. In some cases patients may begin to fatigue and may progress to ARF. (A good indication that ARF is imminent is a marked decrease in breath sounds [i.e., **silent chest**].)

Continuous nebulization is started, and after 2 hours of treatment, the patient's ABG values are as follows: P_aO_2 = 75 mm Hg on 80% oxygen, P_aCO_2 = 56 mm Hg, HCO_3^- = 28 mEq/L, pH = 7.31. $\dot{V}_E$ is 18 L/min.

Serious consideration must be given to intubating the patient under mild sedation and initiating mechanical ventilatory support. This decision is often difficult to make for a fully conscious, distressed patient. Even the use of sedation is controversial. Unfortunately, invasive ventilation may be the only alternative. If no intervention is taken, a reduction in previously strong respiratory efforts sometimes occurs. Rates and tidal volumes may start to fall. The patient may become stuporous or uncontrollably agitated, which are often signs of fatigue.

This situation is an example of impending respiratory failure in which aggressive care is required to prevent respiratory failure or possibly cardiopulmonary arrest. NIV may be contraindicated or insufficient for these patients.[33] If NIV is initiated, and the patient's P_aCO_2 rises and a severe acidosis develops during NIV, then a strong argument can be made for intubation and ventilation.[32] Some clinicians start ventilatory support when the P_aCO_2 rises to normal in the presence of

 ## Clinical Scenario: Chronic Restrictive Disorder

An 83-year-old woman with severe kyphoscoliosis is admitted to the hospital from a long-term care facility. She is diagnosed with pneumonia. Evaluation of the patient reveals that she is very weak and pale and has decreased skin turgor (Key Point 4-7). Blood pressure is 110/72 mm Hg, and heart rate is 110 beats/min. Respiratory rate is 28 breaths/min, and breaths are shallow. Breath sounds reveal bilateral crackles scattered throughout both lungs. After 3 days of hospitalization and antibiotic therapy, the patient's condition appears to be progressively worsening. ABG results while the patient receives supplemental oxygen via a nasal cannula (2 L/min) are as follows: P_aO_2 = 58 mm Hg, P_aCO_2 = 68 mm Hg, pH = 7.24. The decision is made to intubate the patient and begin ventilatory support.

The combination of her severe, chronic, restrictive disorder and the unresolved pneumonia have contributed to the deteriorating gas exchange, which indicates ARF and the need for invasive ventilation.[3] No advance directives were available to indicate the patient's wishes regarding invasive ventilation.

 Key Point **4-7** A simple test for dehydration involves gently pinching the skin on the back of the patient's hand. If the skin quickly returns to its normal position, skin turgor is normal. If the skin remains puckered, skin turgor is decreased and the patient probably is dehydrated.

 ## Clinical Scenario: Chronic Obstructive Pulmonary Disease and Congestive Heart Failure

A 78-year-old man with a history of COPD and chronic congestive heart failure (CHF) is admitted to the hospital. He has been admitted to the hospital three times during the past 9 months. The patient has a history of noncompliance with his medications and continues to smoke. He has a long and continued history of alcohol abuse.[25]

The patient is given oxygen therapy via nasal cannula (2 L/min). His respiratory rate is 18 breaths/min. Expirations are prolonged, and he demonstrates pursed-lip breathing and use of his accessory muscles of breathing. The patient is pale and appears anxious. Heart rate and blood pressure are elevated. Auscultation of his chest reveals breath sounds with scattered wheezes and crackles. Sputum is thin and frothy. Current ABG values on an estimated F_IO_2 of 0.28 are as follows: P_aO_2 = 55 mm Hg, P_aCO_2 = 74 mm Hg, HCO_3^- = 34 mEq/L, pH = 7.28.

With an increasing P_aCO_2, moderately severe respiratory acidosis, and an apparently increased WOB, this patient demonstrates all the signs of respiratory distress. Based on the patient's history, the attending physician undoubtedly would have to determine which medications would be appropriate for both the patient's heart failure and his respiratory problems. Blood gas values and respiratory assessment support the need for intervention to improve the patient's ventilation and reduce WOB before his condition becomes more critical.

The presence of acute CHF is one of the exclusionary criteria for NIV in patients with acute-on-chronic COPD. This patient probably needs invasive ventilation. Several measures can be attempted, but they should not preclude intubation if the patient's condition worsens. Two simple measures that can be attempted are continuing oxygen therapy and maintaining the patient in an upright or semi-Fowler position.[23] Determining the patient's wishes is also important. Does he want aggressive support if it becomes necessary? If the patient does not want to be intubated, NIV could be used, particularly considering the alternative if no ventilation is provided.

SUMMARY

- The ability to recognize that a patient needs an artificial airway and ventilation is an essential skill for practitioners.
- Decisions made in the acute care setting must be based on evidence-based criteria that clearly demonstrate that a particular technique is beneficial and is associated with good outcomes, such as improved quality of life, reduced length of stay, or a lower mortality rate.
- ARF is defined as an inability to maintain adequate oxygen uptake and carbon dioxide clearance.
- Two types of ARF are hypoxemic respiratory failure and hypercapnic respiratory failure.
- Hypoxemic respiratory failure can be treated with oxygen or in combination with PEEP or CPAP.
- Acute hypercapnic respiratory failure occurs when a person cannot maintain adequate ventilation to maintain P_aCO_2.
- The primary physiological objectives of mechanical ventilation should include supporting or improving pulmonary gas exchange, increasing lung volume, and reducing the WOB.
- Simple and direct observations can provide valuable information about the cause of respiratory distress and serve as a guide for selecting an appropriate therapeutic strategy.
- Recognizing the clinical signs of hypoxemia and hypercapnia is the first step to the successful treatment of a patient in respiratory distress.
- The onset of respiratory failure can vary considerably depending on the cause of the neuromuscular dysfunction.
- The MIP and VC can be used to assess the respiratory muscle strength of patients with neuromuscular disorders. Determination of baseline ABGs along with periodic measurement of S_pO_2 is also appropriate for the management of these patients.
- WOB normally accounts for 1% to 4% of total oxygen consumption at rest. Increased WOB usually is associated with an increased rate or depth of breathing (or both).
- VC, PEF, respiratory rate, $\dot{V}_E$, and V_D/V_T can provide valuable information about a patient's status and alert the clinician to impending respiratory dysfunction.
- The standard criteria for the initiation of mechanical ventilation include apnea, impending ARF or ARF, and refractory hypoxemia with increased WOB or an ineffective breathing pattern.
- NIV offers a viable alternative to invasive mechanical ventilation in select patients.

REVIEW QUESTIONS (See Appendix A for answers.)

1. Which of the following suggests the presence of respiratory insufficiency and the need for ventilatory support?
   1. MIP of −17 cm H_2O
   2. VC of 2.1 L in a 70-kg man
   3. P_aCO_2 of 81 mm Hg and pH of 7.19
   4. P_aO_2 of 65 mm Hg on room air
      A. 1 and 3 only
      B. 2 and 4 only
      C. 1, 3, and 4 only
      D. 1, 2, 3, and 4

2. Blood gas results on room air from an unconscious patient brought to the emergency department are as follows: pH = 7.23, P_aCO_2 = 81 mm Hg, bicarbonate = 33 mEq/L, P_aO_2 = 43 mm Hg, and S_aO_2 = 71%. With no other data available, which of the following forms of therapy is indicated?
   A. Oxygen with a nonrebreathing mask
   B. CPAP mask
   C. IPPB treatment with albuterol
   D. Mechanical ventilatory support

3. A 30-year-old woman is seen in the emergency department. She demonstrates paralysis of the lower extremities that is progressively worsening. After several hours, during which she was monitored frequently, her VC has decreased to 12 mL/kg and MIP is −30 cm H_2O. The results of blood gas evaluations are not yet available. What type of therapy is most likely needed?
   A. Aerosolized bronchodilator administered with a metered-dose inhaler
   B. Mechanical ventilatory support
   C. Incentive spirometry to improve muscle strength
   D. Narcotic-blocking agent

4. A 28-year-old man with botulism poisoning is beginning to develop progressive paralysis. The respiratory therapist has been monitoring the patient's MIP and VC every 2 hours. The most recent results show that the patient continues to deteriorate: MIP = −27 cm H_2O, VC = 32 mL/kg. Which of the following could be appropriately recommended?
   A. Gastric lavage
   B. Oxygen therapy
   C. Medication to reverse the paralysis
   D. Mechanical ventilatory support

5. A 34-year-old man is taken to the emergency department after a motor vehicle accident. He is unconscious and unresponsive. ABGs obtained while the patient is receiving oxygen via a nonrebreathing mask show the following: P_aO_2 = 47 mm Hg, P_aCO_2 = 93 mm Hg, pH = 7.09, and bicarbonate = 27 mEq/L. Which of the following would the therapist recommend?
   A. Recheck vital signs
   B. Intubate and ventilate
   C. Change to a Venturi mask and coach the patient to breathe
   D. Begin cardiopulmonary resuscitation (CPR)

6. A 68-year-old man with a history of COPD and CO_2 retention is brought to the emergency department by ambulance. He is receiving oxygen through a nasal cannula (2 L/min). He is conscious and cooperative but in distress. He is leaning forward and using accessory muscles to breathe. His vital signs are as follows: heart rate = 100 beats/min, blood pressure = 128/78 mm Hg, temperature = 37.8° C, respiratory rate = 20 breaths/min with prolonged expiration through pursed lips. Breath sounds reveal bilateral crackles and wheezes. Which of the following is most appropriate?
   A. Change to a Venturi mask and coach the patient to breathe
   B. Intubate and ventilate
   C. Change to a nonrebreather mask
   D. Evaluate for NIV

7. A 43-year-old man who weighs 165 lb (75 kg) and has myasthenia gravis is beginning to develop progressive weakness of the muscles. The respiratory care practitioner has been monitoring MIP and VC every 4 hours. The most recent results show that the patient continues to deteriorate despite treatment with anticholinesterase drugs: MIP = −35 cm H_2O, VC = 23 mL/kg. Which of the following would be appropriate to recommend?
   A. Incentive spirometry to improve muscle strength
   B. Oxygen therapy
   C. Mechanical ventilatory support
   D. Administer a neuromuscular blocking agent

8. A 48-year-old woman admitted to the emergency department demonstrates tachypnea, tachycardia, and appears pale. Breath sounds reveal bilateral crackles. ABG results with the patient using a nonrebreathing mask are as follows: P_aO_2 = 45 mm Hg, P_aCO_2 = 32 mm Hg, pH = 7.49, and bicarbonate = 24 mEq/L. Which of the following is the most appropriate initial treatment for this patient?
   A. Increase the flow to the oxygen mask
   B. Begin ventilatory support
   C. Provide CPAP by mask
   D. Administer bronchodilator therapy

9. A 60-year-old man was admitted to the hospital yesterday for a suspected myocardial infarction. Current ABG values on room air are as follows: P_aO_2 = 57 mm Hg, P_aCO_2 = 33 mm Hg, pH = 7.47, and bicarbonate = 25 mEq/L. Which of the following is the most appropriate form of respiratory therapy for this patient?
   A. Oxygen therapy
   B. Noninvasive mechanical ventilation
   C. CO_2/O_2 therapy (5/95)
   D. CPAP by mask

10. Which of the following are goals of mechanical ventilation?
    1. Provide support to the pulmonary system to maintain an adequate level of alveolar ventilation
    2. Reduce the work of breathing until the cause of respiratory failure can be eliminated
    3. Restore arterial blood gas levels to normal
    4. Increase respiratory therapy department revenue
       A. 1 and 2 only
       B. 1 and 3 only
       C. 1, 2, and 3 only
       D. 1, 3, and 4 only

11. A 74-year-old patient with COPD who has acute-on-chronic respiratory failure is supported with NIV. The patient is becoming more confused. Blood gas values are as follows: S_pO_2 = 45 mm Hg, P_aCO_2 = 58 mm Hg, pH = 7.21, and bicarbonate = 23 mEq/L. Which of the following would be appropriate treatment for this patient?
    A. Increase oxygen delivery
    B. Ask the patient if he is comfortable with the mask
    C. Ask the physician for a sedative
    D. Switch to invasive ventilation

12. A 14-year-old boy who previously had been diagnosed with mild persistent asthma has a PEF of 100 L/min. This indicates which of the following?
    A. Increased airway resistance
    B. Heart failure
    C. Increased lung compliance
    D. Inability to take in a deep breath and cough

13. After oxygen is administered, a patient's heart rate changes from 110 beats/min to 85 beats/min. The initial tachycardia was most likely caused by which of the following?
    A. Anxiety
    B. Hypoxemia
    C. Hypercapnia
    D. Pain

14. A 34-year-old patient who was in a motor vehicle crash is admitted to the hospital with crushed chest injuries and a fractured tibia. Two days later the P_aO_2 is 56 mm Hg while he is breathing 80% oxygen, and the respiratory rate is 30 to 34 breaths/min. Based on the history and these findings, which of the following does the patient most likely need?
    A. Invasive ventilation
    B. Noninvasive ventilation
    C. 100% oxygen
    D. CPAP with oxygen

15. Which of the following arterial blood gas parameters is considered the best indicator of a patient's ventilatory status?
    A. pHa
    B. P_aCO_2
    C. P_aO_2
    D. S_aO_2

References

1. Campbell EJM: Respiratory failure. *Br Med J* 1:1451–1460, 1965.
2. Calfee CS, Matthay MA: Recent advances in mechanical ventilation. *Am J Med* 118(6):584–591, 2005.
3. Pierson DJ: Indications for mechanical ventilation in adults with acute respiratory failure. *Respir Care* 47:249–262, 2002.
4. Slutsky AS: ACCP consensus conference: mechanical ventilation. *Chest* 104:1833–1859, 1993.
5. Tobin MJ, editor: *Principles and practice of mechanical ventilation*, ed 3, New York, 2013, McGraw-Hill.
6. Aboussouan LS: Respiratory failure and the need for ventilator support. In Kacmarek RM, Stoller JK, Heuer AJ, editors: *Egan's fundamentals of respiratory care*, ed 10, St Louis, 2013, Elsevier.
7. Pontoppidan H, Geffin B, Lowenstein E: Acute respiratory failure in the adult. Part 2. *N Engl J Med* 287:743–752, 1972.
8. Muizelaar JP, Marmarou A, Ward JD, et al: Adverse effects of prolonged hyperventilation in patients with severe head injury: a randomized clinical trial. *J Neurosurg* 75:731–739, 1991.
9. Provencio JJ, Bleck SP, Connors AF, Jr: Critical care neurology. *Am J Respir Crit Care Med* 164:341–345, 2001.
10. Otis AB: The work of breathing. *Physiol Rev* 34:449–458, 1954.
11. Marini JJ: The role of the inspiratory circuit in the work of breathing during mechanical ventilation. *Respir Care* 32:419–430, 1987.
12. Levison H, Cherniack RM: Ventilatory cost of exercise in chronic obstructive pulmonary disease. *J Appl Physiol* 25:21–27, 1968.
13. Kacmarek RM, Hess D, Stoller JK: *Monitoring in respiratory care*, St Louis, 1993, Mosby.
14. Hess DR, MacIntyre NR: Mechanical ventilation. In Hess DR, MacIntyre NR, Mishoe SC, et al, editors: *Respiratory care: principles and practices*, ed 2, Sudbury, Mass, 2012, Jones and Bartlett, pp 462–500.
15. Marini JJ, Smith TC, Lamb V: Estimation of inspiratory muscle strength in mechanically ventilated patients: the measurement of maximal inspiratory pressure. *J Crit Care* 1:32–38, 1986.
16. Evans JA, Whitelaw WA: The assessment of maximal respiratory mouth pressures in adults. *Respir Care* 54:1348–1359, 2009.
17. Aldrich TK, Prezant DJ: Indications for mechanical ventilation. In Tobin MJ, editor: *Principles and practices of mechanical ventilation*, New York, 1994, McGraw-Hill.
18. Cairo JM: *Mosby's respiratory care equipment*, ed 9, St Louis, 2014, Elsevier.
19. Kacmarek RM, Cheever P, Foley K, et al: Determination of vital capacity in mechanically ventilated patients: a comparison of techniques. *Respir Care* 35:129, (abstract), 1990.
20. Collins SR, Blank RS: Approaches to refractory hypoxemia in acute respiratory distress syndrome: Current understanding, evidence, and debate. *Respir Care* 56:1573–1582, 2011.
21. Downs JB: Has oxygen administration delayed appropriate respiratory care? Fallacies regarding oxygen therapy. *Respir Care* 48:611–620, 2003.
22. Aubier M, Murciano D, Milic-Emili J, et al: Effects of administration of O_2 on ventilation and blood gases in patients with chronic obstructive pulmonary disease during acute respiratory failure. *Am Rev Respir Dis* 122:747–754, 1980.
23. Ritz R: Methods to avoid intubation. *Respir Care* 44:686–701, 1999.
24. Pauwels RA, Buist AW, Calverley PM, et al: Global strategy for the diagnosis, management, and prevention of chronic obstructive pulmonary disease. NHLBI/WHO Global Initiative for Chronic Obstructive Lung Disease (GOLD) Workshop summary. *Am J Respir Crit Care Med* 163:1256–1276, 2001.
25. Wedzicha JA, Donaldson GC: Exacerbations of chronic obstructive pulmonary disease. *Respir Care* 48:1204–1213, 2003.
26. Delclaux C, L'Her E, Alberti C, et al: Treatment of acute hypoxemic nonhypercapnic respiratory insufficiency with continuous positive pressure delivered by face mask: a randomized controlled trial. *J Am Med Assoc* 284:2352–2360, 2000.
27. Kramer N, Meyer TJ, Meharg J, et al: Randomized prospective trial of noninvasive positive pressure ventilation in acute respiratory failure. *Am J Respir Crit Care Med* 151:1799–1806, 1995.
28. Brochard L: Mechanical ventilation: invasive versus noninvasive. *Eur Respir J Suppl* 47:31s–37s, 2003.
29. Hess D: Noninvasive positive pressure ventilation: predictors of success and failure for adult acute care application. *Respir Care* 42:424–431, 1997.
30. Kacmarek RM, Stoller JK, Heuer AJ, editors: *Egan's Fundamentals of respiratory care*, ed 10, St Louis, 2013, Elsevier.
31. Shapiro M, Wilson RK, Casar G, et al: Work of breathing through different-sized endotracheal tubes. *Crit Care Med* 14:1028–1031, 1986.
32. Dhuper S, Maggiore D, Chung V, et al: Profile of near fatal asthma in an inner city hospital. *Chest* 124:1880–1884, 2003.
33. Sydow M: Ventilating the patient with severe asthma: nonconventional therapy. *Minerva Anestesiol* 69:333–337, 2003.

Selecting the Ventilator and the Mode

OUTLINE

KEY TERMS

- Assisted breaths
- Continuous mandatory ventilation
- Control ventilation
- Full ventilatory support
- Mandatory breaths
- Partial ventilatory support
- Patient-ventilator asynchrony
- Spontaneous breaths

LEARNING OBJECTIVES *On completion of this chapter, the reader will be able to do the following:*

1. Select an appropriate mechanical ventilator, breath type, and mode of ventilation based on clinical findings derived from patient assessment data.
2. Describe how continuous positive airway pressure (CPAP) and noninvasive positive pressure ventilation (NIV) are used to deliver noninvasive positive pressure ventilation.
3. Discuss the advantages and disadvantages of volume-controlled and pressure-controlled ventilation.
4. Explain the differences in function among continuous mandatory ventilation, intermittent mandatory ventilation, and spontaneous ventilation.

5. Describe the functions of the *trigger, cycle,* and *limit* variables as they are used in volume-controlled continuous mandatory ventilation, pressure-controlled continuous mandatory ventilation, volume-controlled intermittent mandatory ventilation, pressure-controlled intermittent mandatory ventilation, and pressure support ventilation.
6. Define each of the following terms: *pressure augmentation, pressure-regulated volume control, volume support, mandatory minute ventilation, airway pressure release ventilation, bilevel positive airway pressure,* and *proportional assist ventilation.*

O nce the need for mechanical ventilation has been established, the clinician must select the type of ventilator, the ventilator mode, and the breath type for the patient. This chapter focuses on factors that affect the choice of ventilator, patient interface (i.e., artificial airway or mask), control variable (volume or pressure), breath type, and ventilator mode.

Selecting the appropriate ventilator and mode of ventilation can be challenging even for an experienced clinician. The following questions provide a framework for making the selection process manageable:

- Why does the patient need ventilatory support? (Indication)
- Does the ventilatory problem require a special mechanical ventilation mode? (Pathology)
- What therapeutic goals can be achieved by using a specific ventilator? (Treatment goals)
- Does the patient need to be intubated, or can a mask be used? (Patient interface)
- Will the ventilatory support be provided in the intensive care unit, the patient's home, or an extended care facility? (Location)

- Will ventilatory support be required for a brief period or long term? (Duration)
- How familiar are the staff with the ventilator (or ventilators) under consideration? (Staff training)

If a change is to be made from one type of ventilator to another, the respiratory therapist must know whether the change is being made because a different mode or feature is needed. For example, a patient may have acute respiratory distress syndrome (ARDS) and may need a ventilator that can provide an advanced modality.

If a patient is to be discharged from the hospital to his or her home or to an extended care facility, a ventilator that would be appropriate in that setting should be selected. For example, a patient with amyotrophic lateral sclerosis may be familiar and comfortable with noninvasive ventilation. A patient with postpolio syndrome may be more familiar with a chest cuirass or tank ventilator (negative pressure ventilator [NPV]). (Although NPV is not discussed here, it is important to mention that it is sometimes used in the home-care or alternative-care setting. In rare cases NPV has been used for ventilation of acutely ill infants.[1,2] See Chapter 21 for additional information on NPV.)

This chapter focuses on positive pressure ventilation (PPV). Positive pressure ventilators can function in various types of settings and provide a variety of modes, features, monitors, and alarms.

NONINVASIVE AND INVASIVE POSITIVE PRESSURE VENTILATION: SELECTING THE PATIENT INTERFACE

A patient can be connected to a positive pressure ventilator using either a positive pressure mask or an artificial airway. Face and nasal masks are used to administer NIV. Artificial airways, which include translaryngeal airways (oral or nasal endotracheal tubes [ETs]) and tracheostomy tubes, are required for invasive ventilation. About 75% of patients receiving invasive PPV are intubated (95% with an oral ET and 5% with a nasal ET). Tracheostomy tubes are used in the remaining 25% of patients receiving invasive PPV.[3]

Noninvasive Positive Pressure Ventilation

There are two methods of providing noninvasive positive pressure ventilator support:
- Continuous positive airway pressure (CPAP)
- Noninvasive positive pressure ventilation (NIV)

As previously mentioned, CPAP and NIV are most commonly administered via a face or nasal mask. Ensuring that the mask fits properly will minimize patient discomfort and help prevent air leaks. Mask interfaces are discussed in more detail in Chapter 19.

Continuous Positive Airway Pressure

In hospitalized patients, CPAP has been shown to be an effective method to improve oxygenation. It also is an accepted method used to treat obstructive sleep apnea, especially in the home. In addition, CPAP can be used to assist patients with chronic obstructive pulmonary disease (COPD) who have difficulty breathing. The use of CPAP in COPD patients has received some attention because air trapping can occur in a spontaneously breathing individual with increased airway resistance (R_{aw}). Air trapping in patients with COPD or in patients with acute asthma can lead to an increase in the functional residual capacity (FRC). In the past, CPAP was considered contraindicated in patients with COPD because these patients already had an increased FRC. The concern among some

clinicians was based on the assumption that external CPAP, or positive end-expiratory pressure (PEEP), would further increase the FRC and would not benefit the patient.

Patients with COPD often have difficulty generating the pressure difference between the alveoli and the mouth to begin inspiratory gas flow. The air trapped in the lungs (called *intrinsic PEEP* or *auto-PEEP*) creates a positive alveolar pressure (P_{alv}). If the pressure in the lungs is positive at end exhalation, the pressure must drop below the pressure at the mouth (atmospheric pressure) to start gas flowing into the lungs for inspiration. For example, if auto-PEEP is greater than +5 cm H_2O, the patient must exert an effort of at least −5 cm H_2O to drop the lung pressure below zero. Once alveolar pressure drops below zero, inspiratory gas flow can start.

Externally applied CPAP may reduce the pressure difference between the mouth and the alveoli when flow limitation (increased R_{aw}) is the cause of auto-PEEP. The patient therefore does not have to work as hard to drop the P_{alv} so that inspiratory gas flow enters the lungs. In other words, externally applied CPAP can reduce inspiratory work.[4] Mask CPAP set at 80% to 90% of the measured auto-PEEP (usually about 4 to 10 cm H_2O) reduces diaphragmatic work and dyspnea, improves gas exchange, and does not worsen hyperinflation.[5-7] In many cases, clinicians prefer using noninvasive positive pressure ventilator support in the form of bilevel positive airway pressure (**bilevel PAP**) rather than CPAP for patients with R_{aw}-induced auto-PEEP (Box 5-1). Bilevel PAP also is the method most often used to treat acute-on-chronic respiratory failure (see Chapter 4). An example of an acute-on-chronic respiratory condition is a patient with chronic bronchitis who develops pneumonia (an acute condition).

Noninvasive Positive Pressure Ventilation

Numerous investigators have examined the use of NIV for patients with respiratory failure caused by various neuromuscular disorders, chest wall deformities, COPD, central ventilatory control abnormalities, and acute cardiogenic pulmonary edema (Box 5-2).[8-12] Their findings suggest that NIV can reduce the need for intubation in 60% to 75% of these patients.[9,10,13,14] Two types of ventilators can be used to provide NIV:
- Pressure-triggered, pressure-limited, flow-cycled devices designed specifically for mask ventilation, for example, BiPAP (Philips Respironics, Murrysville, Pa.).[9]
- Critical care ventilators that have a variety of available modes, including NIV in many cases.

Box 5-3 lists some of the advantages and disadvantages of NIV compared with invasive ventilation.[4,11,15] Box 4-7 lists accepted indications and contraindications for NIV. If patients are not excluded by the presence of contraindications, NIV offers the clinician an excellent option for a number of acute and chronic conditions requiring mechanical ventilation.

BOX 5-2	**Disorders Sometimes Managed with Noninvasive Positive Pressure Ventilation**

- Chronic respiratory failure
- Chest wall deformities
- Neuromuscular disorders
- Central alveolar hypoventilation
- Chronic obstructive pulmonary disease (COPD)
- Cystic fibrosis
- Bronchiectasis
- Acute respiratory failure (ARF)
- Acute respiratory distress syndrome (ARDS)
- Pneumonia
- Postoperative complications
- Asthma
- Cardiogenic pulmonary edema
- Heart failure
- Postextubation failure in difficult to wean patients
- Obstructive sleep apnea

From Liesching T, Kwok H, Hill NS: Acute applications of noninvasive positive pressure ventilation, *Chest* 124: 699-713, 2003.

BOX 5-3	**Advantages and Disadvantages of Noninvasive Positive Pressure Ventilation in Acute Respiratory Failure**

Advantages
- Avoids complications associated with artificial airways
- Provides flexibility in initiating and removing mechanical ventilation
- Reduces requirements for heavy sedation
- Preserves airway defense, speech, and swallowing mechanisms
- Reduces need for invasive monitoring

Disadvantages
- Can cause gastric distention, skin pressure lesions, facial pain, dry nose, eye irritation (conjunctivitis), discomfort, claustrophobia, poor sleep, and mask leaks can occur

Invasive Positive Pressure Ventilation

As mentioned previously, a high percentage of patients who need mechanical ventilation require invasive positive pressure ventilation via an artificial airway. Once the appropriate ventilator has been chosen, the clinician must select a mode of ventilation that is most advantageous for the patient's condition.

FULL AND PARTIAL VENTILATORY SUPPORT

The terms *full ventilatory support* (FVS) and *partial ventilatory support* (PVS) describe the extent of mechanical ventilation provided. With FVS the ventilator provides all the energy necessary to maintain effective alveolar ventilation.[15] FVS results in arterial partial pressure of carbon dioxide (P_aCO_2) values less than 45 mm Hg, *or* a P_aCO_2 that is normal for the patient (i.e., eucapnic breathing). FVS is provided when ventilator rates are high (8 breaths/min or more) and tidal volume (V_T) is adequate for the patient. (See Chapter 6 for information on V_T settings and ideal body weight.)[16] FVS is typically provided using a ventilator mode that provides a preset volume or pressure when a breath is delivered. The mode must be set so that the patient receives adequate alveolar ventilation

regardless of whether the person can breathe spontaneously.[15] For example, FVS might include fully controlled and assisted positive pressure ventilation.

Partial ventilatory support is any degree of mechanical ventilation in which set machine rates are lower than 6 breaths/min and the patient participates in the work of breathing (WOB) to help maintain effective alveolar ventilation. A variety of ventilator modes can be used for PVS; however, by definition the patient must actively participate in ventilation to maintain adequate levels of P_aCO_2. PVS modes might include intermittent mandatory ventilation (IMV), pressure support ventilation (PSV), volume support, proportional assist ventilation (PAV), and mandatory minute volume (MMV). All these modes are described later in this chapter.

Strategies for PVS are appropriate when attempts are made to discontinue ventilator support. PVS should be avoided in patients with ventilatory muscle fatigue and when a patient has a high WOB.

When treating patients with acute respiratory failure, the initial goal of mechanical ventilation is to supply all the necessary ventilation (FVS) while the ventilatory muscles are given time to rest.[17,18] Ideally after several hours to several days of FVS, the patient's condition stabilizes and the patient begins to recover. Maintaining complete rest after just a few days on FVS can result in muscle wasting or atrophy; for this reason, some clinicians object to FVS and provide partial support from the very beginning. This is a matter of the clinician's preference and the patient's history. Whether FVS is used or not, the patient assumes part of the WOB within a short time, once other factors have been stabilized, to prevent muscle wasting.

BREATH DELIVERY AND MODES OF VENTILATION

The breath type and pattern of breath delivery during mechanical ventilation constitute the **mode** of ventilation. The mode is determined by the following factors:
- Type of breath (mandatory, spontaneous, assisted)
- Targeted control variable (volume or pressure)
- Timing of breath delivery (continuous mandatory ventilation [CMV], intermittent mandatory ventilation [IMV], or continuous spontaneous ventilation [CSV])

Type of Breath Delivery
Mandatory Breaths

As described in Chapter 3, **mandatory breaths** are breaths for which the ventilator controls the timing, the tidal volume, or the inspiratory pressure. For example, a patient-triggered, volume-targeted, volume-cycled breath is a mandatory breath. The ventilator controls tidal volume delivery.

 Case Study 5-1

What Type of Breath Is It?

1. A patient receives a breath that is patient triggered, volume targeted, and time cycled. What type of breath is it?
2. A patient breathes spontaneously at a baseline pressure of +8 cm H_2O. The pressure stays at +8 cm H_2O during inspiration and exhalation. What type of breath is it?

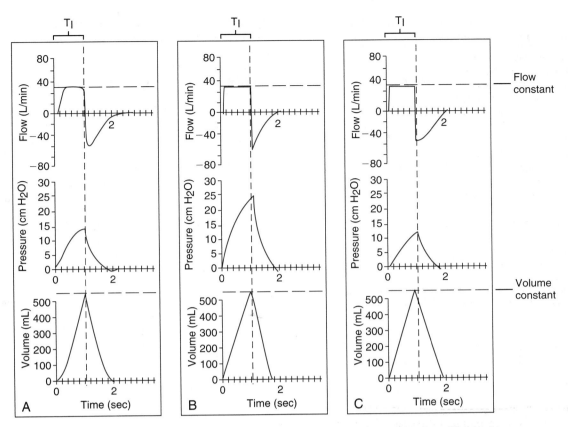

Fig. 5-1 Graphs for constant-flow, volume-targeted ventilation (constant volume) with normal compliance (**A**), reduced compliance (**B**), and increased compliance (**C**). Note that inspiratory flow is above the x-axis and expiratory flow is below the x-axis. (See text for more information.)

Spontaneous Breaths

For **spontaneous breaths**, the patient controls the timing and the tidal volume. The volume or pressure (or both) delivered is not set by the clinician, but rather is based on patient demand and the patient's lung characteristics.

Assisted Breaths

Assisted breaths have characteristics of both mandatory and spontaneous breaths. In an assisted breath, all or part of the breath is generated by the ventilator, which does part of the WOB for the patient. If the airway pressure rises above baseline during inspiration, the breath is assisted.[19] For example, during the pressure support mode the clinician sets the target pressure but the patient initiates the breath (patient triggered). The ventilator delivers the set pressure above baseline pressure to assist the patient's breathing effort. The patient cycles the breath (Case Study 5-1).

Targeting Volume as the Control Variable

By choosing either volume or pressure ventilation, the clinician determines the control variable that will be used to establish gas flow to the patient.[20] Control variables are **independent** variables; in volume control ventilation, for example, the volume selected is constant and independent of what happens to pressure when the patient's lung characteristics (lung compliance and R_{aw}) change or

when the patient's effort changes. The selection of using volume-controlled or pressure-controlled ventilation is based on whether consistency of tidal volume delivery is important or limiting of pressure delivery is important.

The primary advantage of volume control ventilation is that it guarantees a specific volume delivery and volume of expired gas (V_E), regardless of changes in lung compliance and resistance or patient effort.[21] The goal of volume-controlled ventilation is to maintain a certain level of P_aCO_2.

The main disadvantage of volume-controlled ventilation becomes evident when the lung condition worsens. This can cause the peak and alveolar pressures to rise, leading to alveolar over-distention (see Critical Care Concept 5-1 and Fig. 5-1*). Box 5-4 summarizes how changes in lung compliance and airway resistance can affect peak and plateau pressures during volume-controlled ventilation. It is worth noting, however, that these changes are reversible. When the lung condition improves, less pressure is required to deliver the volume, and ventilating pressures decline.

---

*Figures 5-1 and 5-2 introduce ventilator graphics so that the reader can become familiar with this tool. Ventilator graphics are discussed in greater detail in Chapter 9.

| BOX 5-4 | Factors That Affect Pressures During Volume-Controlled Ventilation |

Patient Lung Characteristics
- Reductions in lung or chest wall compliance produce higher peak and plateau pressures; increased compliance produces lower peak and plateau pressures.
- Increased airway resistance produces a higher peak pressure; reductions in airways resistance produce lower peak pressures.

Inspiratory Flow Pattern
- Peak pressure is higher with a constant flow and lower with a decelerating flow pattern. Decelerating flow pattern has a higher mean airway pressure; constant flow generates the lowest mean airway pressure
- High inspiratory gas flow creates a higher peak pressure.

Volume Setting
- High volumes produce higher peak and plateau pressures; low volumes produce lower peak and plateau pressures.

Positive End-Expiratory Pressure (PEEP)
- Increasing PEEP increases the peak and mean pressures.

Auto-PEEP
- Increases in auto-PEEP increase the peak inspiratory pressure.

✿ CRITICAL CARE CONCEPT 5-1

Volume-Controlled Breaths with Changing Lung Characteristics

Use Fig. 5-1 to answer the following questions:
1. What is the approximate inspiratory time? Does it change?
2. What type of flow waveform is used?
3. What is the approximate tidal volume delivery for each breath?
4. What are the peak inspiratory pressures (PIPs) in **A, B,** and **C?**
5. What types of lung or thoracic abnormalities can result in reduced compliance?
6. What would happen to the PIP if compliance remained unchanged but airway resistance increased?

| BOX 5-5 | Factors That Affect Volume Delivery During Pressure-Controlled Ventilation* |

Pressure Setting
- Higher pressure settings produce larger volumes, whereas lower pressure settings produce lower volumes. In other words, increasing the peak inspiratory pressure (PIP) while maintaining a constant end-expiratory pressure (EEP) increases volume delivery (and vice versa).

Pressure Gradient
- Increasing EEP (PEEP + auto-PEEP) while keeping PIP constant reduces the pressure gradient (PIP − EEP) and lowers volume delivery (and vice versa).

Patient Lung Characteristics
- Reduced compliance results in lower volume; increased compliance results in increased volume for a given inspiratory pressure.
- Increased airway resistance (R_{aw}) results in lower volume delivery if active flow is present; reductions in airway resistance results in higher volume delivery if active flow is present.

Inspiratory Time
- When the inspiratory time (T_I) is extended, volume delivery increases. Notice that this is true as long as flow is present during inspiration (i.e., the flow–time curve shows flow above zero when inspiration ends). However, if flow returns to zero before inspiration ends, further increases in T_I can decrease volume delivery if adequate time is not provided for exhalation.

Patient Effort
- Active inspiration by the patient can increase volume delivery.

*See the Review Questions at the end of the chapter for practice problems, which provide examples of how these factors affect volume delivery during pressure ventilation.

Other disadvantages of volume-controlled breaths are related to flow and sensitivity settings. Specifically the delivery of flow is fixed on some ventilators and may not match patient demand. Similarly if the sensitivity level is not set appropriately for the patient, it can make it more difficult for the patient to trigger inspiration. Both situations can lead to **patient-ventilator asynchrony** and patient discomfort.[22,23] The operational controls available for volume ventilation vary depending on the ventilator manufacturers. Operational controls typically include tidal volume, respiratory rate, inspiratory flow, and a flow pattern. With some ventilators, the practitioner can set the tidal volume, respiratory rate, and inspiratory time; the flow pattern is not adjustable. (Chapter 6 reviews guidelines for setting the appropriate volume and rate in volume ventilation.)

Targeting Pressure as the Control Variable

Pressure control ventilation allows the clinician to set pressure as the independent variable; that is, the pressure remains constant, but volume delivery (the dependent variable) changes as lung characteristics change. Volume delivery therefore must be closely monitored (Critical Care Concept 5-2 and Fig. 5-2).

Pressure **control ventilation** has several advantages. First, it allows the clinician to set a maximum pressure, which reduces the risk of overdistention of the lungs by limiting the amount of positive pressure applied to the lung. Second, the ventilator delivers a decelerating flow pattern during pressure control ventilation (Fig. 5-3). It has been suggested that limiting the peak pressure spares more normal areas of the lungs from overinflation.[21] Pressure control ventilation is therefore considered a component of protective strategies for the lung.[16] It also may be more comfortable for patients who can breathe spontaneously. When the patient makes an inspiratory effort, the negative pressure produced at the upper airway causes the ventilator to vary gas flow to match the patient's need. This helps reduce WOB, particularly in patients with ARDS, compared with volume control ventilation.[24] Disadvantages of pressure control ventilation include the following:
- Volume delivery varies as the patient's lung characteristics (i.e., lung compliance and airway resistance) change.
- Clinicians are less familiar with pressure control ventilation (although this is changing).
- V_T and $\dot{V}_E$ decrease when lung characteristics deteriorate (Box 5-5).

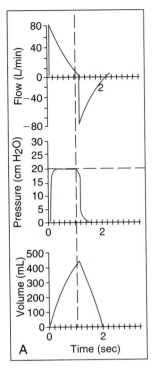
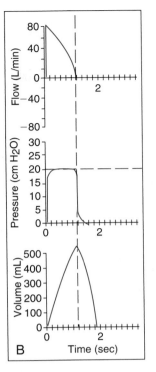
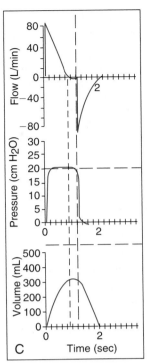

Fig. 5-2 Graphs for pressure-targeted ventilation (constant pressure) with normal compliance (**A**), increased compliance (**B**), and decreased compliance (**C**). (See text for more information.)

CRITICAL CARE CONCEPT 5-2

Pressure-Controlled Breaths with Changing Lung Characteristics

Use Fig. 5-2 to answer the following questions:
1. What type of pressure curve is delivered in **A, B,** and **C?**
2. What type of flow waveform is present during inspiration in **A, B,** and **C?**
3. Compare the flow–time curve during inspiration in **C** with that in **A.** What is the difference between the two?
4. Look at the dotted line in **C** that starts at the flow waveform just when flow drops to zero during inspiration. Look at the volume–time curve **C.** What do you notice about this volume–time curve compared with those in **A** and **B?** Why is it flat at the top?
5. Why is volume delivery higher in **B** than in **A?**

Case Study 5-2

Pressure Control (PC-CMV) or Volume Control Ventilation (VC-CMV)

1. A physician wants to ensure that a patient's P_aCO_2 remains at the person's normal level of 50 mm Hg. Would volume control ventilation or pressure control ventilation best meet this requirement?
2. Ventilating pressure can become very high in patients with acute respiratory distress syndrome. To prevent excessive pressures, what independent variable would be most appropriate, volume or pressure?

Clinical studies comparing pressure control ventilation with volume control ventilation are divided over which method is superior.[21] Pressure control ventilation and volume control ventilation are equally beneficial in patients who are not spontaneously breathing when a targeted flow pattern is used.[21] On the other hand, in spontaneously breathing patients, pressure-controlled ventilation may lower the WOB and improve patient comfort to a greater extent than volume-controlled ventilation, thereby reducing the need for sedatives and neuromuscular blocking agents.[21] Clinician preference and institutional protocol are also important in the selection of pressure control versus volume control ventilation (Case Study 5-2).

Timing of Breath Delivery

Three types of breath delivery timing or sequence are available on current intensive care unit (ICU) ventilators:
1. Continuous mandatory ventilation (CMV)
2. Intermittent mechanical ventilation (IMV)
3. Continuous spontaneous ventilation

With CMV, either time- or patient-triggered breaths are mandatory breaths; the patient is not generating any spontaneous breaths. During IMV, the patient receives a set number of mandatory breaths each minute, but is also allowed to breathe spontaneous breaths between mandatory breaths. Thus the patient breathes spontaneously, and the ventilator intermittently delivers a mandatory breath. In continuous spontaneous ventilation, all breaths are spontaneous and are therefore patient triggered. These spontaneous breaths may be assisted (e.g., pressure support ventilation or PSV), or unassisted (e.g., CPAP). Note that PSV may also refer to PC-CSV.[20]

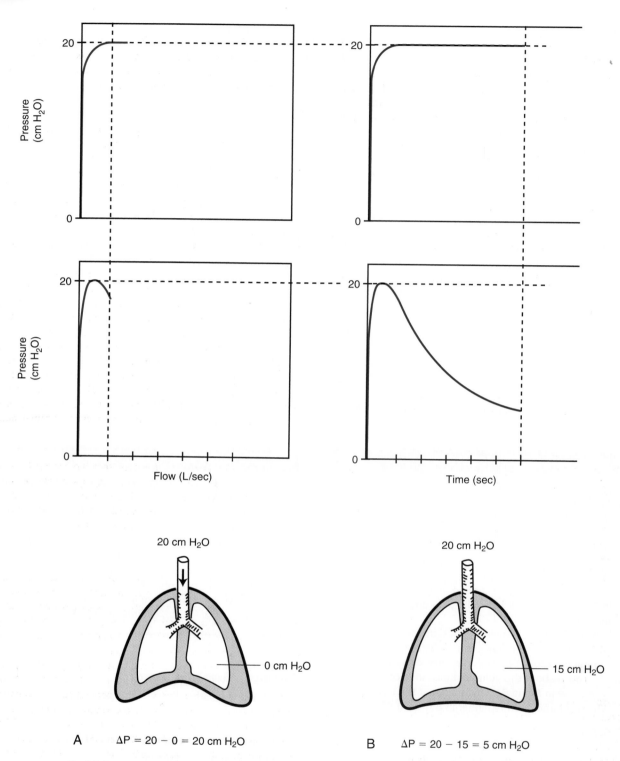

Fig. 5-3 Pressure control ventilation produces a descending waveform. When the ventilator starts gas flow (inspiration), the pressure at the patient's upper airway builds quickly to the set pressure. This produces a pressure (ΔP) gradient between the upper airway and the alveoli (i.e., P_{alv} of 0 cm H_2O or slightly lower). The gradient is highest at the very beginning of inspiration **(A)**; as pressure builds inside the alveolus, the gradient slowly decreases, as does flow **(B)**.

MODES OF VENTILATION

As mentioned previously, the breath type, the targeted control variable, and the timing of breath delivery determine the **mode of ventilation**. Modes of ventilation are often identified using abbreviations (e.g., VC-CMV, PC-IMV, VS, PSV, and MMV). The physicians, therapists, or manufacturers who develop modes of ventilation often create these terms.

The control panel of a ventilator has a dial or touch pad that allows the practitioner to select a particular mode. Unfortunately, considerable variability exists in the way manufacturers name modes; therefore the terminology can be confusing.

This section focuses on describing five basic modes of ventilation (VC-CMV, PC-CMV, VC-IMV, PC-IMV, and CSV), and also briefly introduces several spontaneous modes of ventilation commonly used in the ICU: bilevel positive airway pressure (PAP), dual-control modes, and other closed-loop modes of ventilation (e.g., mandatory minute ventilation [MMV], airway pressure release ventilation [APRV], and proportional assist ventilation [PAV]).

History of Intermittent Positive Pressure Breathing and IPPV: Understanding the Terminology

A positive pressure breath is delivered intermittently during mechanical ventilation. For this reason, in the past this type of ventilation was called *intermittent positive pressure breathing* or *intermittent positive pressure ventilation (IPPV)*. IPPV implied continuous mechanical support of breathing in an apneic patient; every breath was mandatory. In current terminology, the abbreviation *CMV* (which stands for continuous mandatory ventilation) is most often used to describe a mode in which every breath is mandatory. A minimum breathing rate is set, but patients can trigger more breaths if they are able. (NOTE: Another commonly used name for CMV is *assist/control [A/C] ventilation*; this term usually means that a set volume or pressure is delivered with every breath.)

In the early development of mechanical ventilation, small, portable IPPV devices were adapted to deliver aerosolized medications with intermittent positive pressure breaths (IPPB). Consequently, in modern usage, IPPB implies an IPPB aerosol treatment. If correctly adapted, the same equipment (e.g., Bird Mark 7, CareFusion Corp., San Diego, Calif.) also can be used to provide ventilatory support.

Continuous Mandatory Ventilation

With **continuous mandatory ventilation** (CMV), all breaths are mandatory and can be volume or pressure targeted. Breaths can be time triggered or patient triggered. When the breaths are time triggered, the breaths are described as **controlled ventilation** or the *control mode* (see Fig. 3-16). When the breaths are patient triggered during CMV, the breaths are described as **assisted ventilation**. (Key Point 5-1).

> **Key Point 5-1** Historically, clinicians have differentiated between controlled and assisted ventilation by the trigger that is used to initiate a breath. The control mode is time triggered and the patient makes no spontaneous effort, whereas during assisted ventilation, the breath can be either time triggered or patient triggered.

Controlled Ventilation

Controlled (time-triggered) ventilation is appropriate only when a patient cannot make an effort to breathe. Patients who are obtunded because of drugs, cerebral malfunction, spinal cord or phrenic nerve injury, or motor nerve paralysis may be unable to make voluntary efforts; therefore controlled ventilation is appropriate for these patients.

Controlled ventilation may be difficult to use unless the patient is sedated or paralyzed with medications or is deliberately hyperventilated to suppress spontaneous breathing efforts. For example, sedation and paralysis are used if seizure activity or tetanic contractions cannot be prevented. Sedation and sometimes paralysis are recommended during inverse ratio ventilation and with permissive hypercapnia, because these conditions are uncomfortable and not well tolerated by conscious patients.

Deliberate (iatrogenic) hyperventilation occasionally is used to temporarily induce respiratory alkalosis, and thereby reduce intracranial pressure (ICP) in patients with a closed head injury and severely elevated ICP. Iatrogenic hyperventilation also has been used in Reye syndrome and after neurosurgery when ICP is elevated, but as mentioned in Chapter 4, its use is controversial. When iatrogenic hyperventilation is used, it is typically employed for short periods until a more effective strategy can be implemented.

Adequate alarms and monitors must be used to safeguard patients. "Locking out" a patient by making the ventilator totally insensitive to patient effort is rarely advisable.[25] It is important to understand that regardless of the mode selected, sensitivity should be set so that the ventilator responds to even minimal patient effort. (Key Point 5-2).

> **Key Point 5-2** The operator sets the trigger threshold by setting the ventilator's sensitivity. An appropriate sensitivity setting does not require an excessive amount of patient effort to initiate a breath, but it also is not so sensitive that accidental triggering or ventilator self-triggering occurs.

Assisted Ventilation

Assisted ventilation is a term used by many clinicians to describe a time-triggered or patient-triggered CMV mode in which the operator sets a minimum breathing rate, sensitivity level, and type of breath (volume or pressure). Although the patient can trigger breaths at a faster rate than the set mandatory rate, the set volume or pressure is delivered with each breath.

With CMV, every breath (time triggered or patient triggered) is a machine breath. Patient triggering occurs because the ventilator is sensitive to pressure or flow changes that occur as the patient attempts to take a breath. When the ventilator senses a slightly negative pressure (-1 cm H_2O) or a drop in flow (1 to 2 L/min below the expiratory bias flow), the inspiratory cycle begins (see the section on patient triggering in Chapter 3). The clinician must keep in mind that with CMV, a minimum breathing rate is set on the ventilator to guarantee a minimum $\dot{V}_E$.

Several problems can arise with patient-triggered modes. These problems involve the ventilator's sensitivity setting and response time. It is worth noting if the machine is overly sensitive to patient effort, the machine triggers rapidly (autotriggering). This can easily be corrected by adjusting the machine's sensitivity so that it responds to a greater patient effort (-1 to -2 cm H_2O). Conversely if an inspiratory effort shows a pressure reading of -3 to -5 cm H_2O or more below the baseline before an inspiration is initiated,

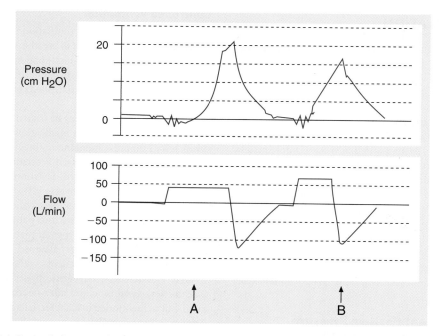

Fig. 5-4 Graphs of volume control continuous mandatory ventilation showing a constant flow waveform. **A,** The curve indicates that the flow, which is set at 50 L/min, is too low for patient demand. Note the concave appearance of the pressure curve; flow begins at one point, but pressure does not rise with the flow curve until much later. This indicates that the machine is not responding to patient effort. **B,** Flow has been increased to 75 L/min. The pressure curve is normal, but sensitivity must also be increased so that the flow and pressure curves begin to rise almost simultaneously. In addition, inspiration time is shortened.

the machine is too insensitive to the patient's effort, and WOB increases.[26] In this case the sensitivity level is set too low and must be increased (see Fig. 3-6).

Historically another common problem that occurs with patient-triggered modes is related to response time. Response time is the time increment between when a patient effort is detected and when flow from the ventilator to the patient begins. Manufacturers of ICU ventilators have made significant strides to improve response times in ventilators used in critical care.

Preventing respiratory alkalosis may be difficult to avoid in some patients on CMV unless respiratory depressants, muscle relaxants, or sedatives are used. The P_aCO_2 may reach the apneic threshold (32 mm Hg) in some patients.[27] It is unknown whether this is due to the mode of ventilation, patient-ventilator asynchrony, or a change in the drive to breathe. Sometimes even switching to intermittent mandatory ventilation (IMV) on similar settings does not significantly change the arterial blood gas value.[28,29]

Volume-Targeted Continuous Mandatory Ventilation

Volume-targeted CMV is often administered using *volume-controlled continuous mandatory ventilation* (VC-CMV). Although VC-CMV was once thought to minimize the WOB during mechanical ventilation, studies have shown that patients receiving this mode of ventilation may actually perform 33% to 50% or more of the work of inspiration.[23,26] This is especially true when inspiration is active and the set gas flow does not match the patient's inspiratory flow demand. Clinically this can be observed by watching the pressure manometer or the pressure–time curve on the graphic display. If the pressure does not rise smoothly and rapidly to peak during inspiration, flow is inadequate. A concave pressure curve

indicates active inspiration. Flow must be increased until the patient's demand is met and the curve assumes a slightly convex shape (Fig. 5-4).

Pressure-Targeted Continuous Mandatory Ventilation

Pressure-targeted CMV is also called *pressure control continuous mandatory ventilation* (PC-CMV) or simply *pressure control ventilation* (PCV). With PC-CMV all breaths are time or patient triggered, pressure targeted, and time cycled. The ventilator provides a constant pressure to the patient during inspiration (Fig. 5-5, *A*). The operator sets the length of inspiration, the pressure level, and the backup rate of ventilation. The V_T delivered by the ventilator is influenced by the compliance and resistance of the patient's lungs, patient effort, and the set pressure.[30] Several studies have shown that the decelerating ramp flow curve associated with PC-CMV (see Fig. 5-5; also see Fig. 5-2) may improve gas distribution and allows the patient to vary inspiratory gas flow during spontaneous breathing efforts.[31-33]

The maximum pressure limit during PC-CMV should be set at about +10 cm H_2O above the target or set pressure, because the set pressure level is not the maximum pressure possible on most ventilators. Active coughing can increase circuit pressure. Reaching the maximum pressure limit usually ends inspiration, as it does in volume ventilation, and prevents excessive system pressures. In some ventilators (e.g., Dräger Evita XL [Dräger Medical Inc, Telford, Pa.] and the Servo-i [Maquet Inc, Wayne, N.J.]) the expiratory valves float. When excessive pressures build in the circuit (e.g., because of coughing), the valves open to release the excess pressure so that the ventilator does not reach the upper pressure limit, which in turn would end inspiration.

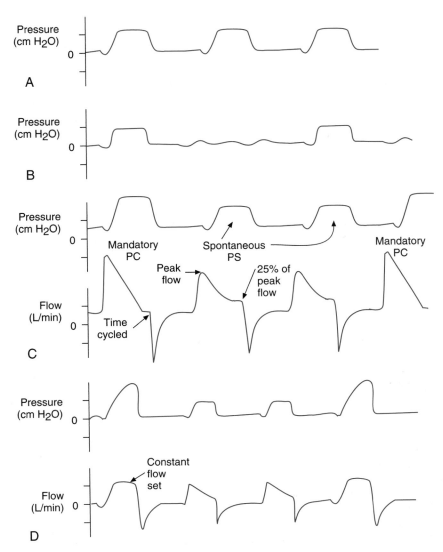

Fig. 5-5 A, Pressure control continuous mandatory ventilation (PC-CMV) mode; breaths are patient triggered. **B,** Pressure control ventilation using the spontaneous intermittent mechanical ventilation (PC-IMV) mode with spontaneous ventilation at zero baseline. **C,** PC-IMV mode in which pressure support (PS) has been added for spontaneous breaths. The *top curve* shows pressure, and the *lower curve* shows flow. Note that peak flow and pressure are higher for mandatory pressure control breaths and that flow returns to zero before end inspiration. In PS breaths, inspiration is flow cycled at 25% of peak flow. **D,** VC-IMV mode with PS added for spontaneous breaths. Compare the upper and lower curves (pressure and flow, respectively) in (**D**) with those in (**C**).

Before 1990, PC-CMV was indicated primarily for patients with ARDS because conventional VC-CMV with PEEP resulted in a high P_{alv} and failed to improve oxygenation.[34-37] Subsequent studies have indicated that PC-CMV with PEEP and VC-CMV with PEEP may be equally effective for ventilating patients with ARDS.[38,39] However, PC-CMV has been shown to reduce the WOB in these patients better than VC-CMV does.[24] Some institutions use PC-CMV for other types of conditions, in which guarding against increasing pressures is more important than guaranteeing a specific tidal volume.

Occasionally the inspiration time T_I is set longer than the expiration time T_E during PC-CMV. Although this approach is the opposite of the process that occurs during normal breathing, it has been shown that a longer T_I provides better oxygenation to some patients by increasing mean airway pressure (P_{aw}). This mode is

referred to as *pressure control inverse ratio ventilation* (PCIRV) because T_I is greater than T_E. Sometimes the goal of PCIRV is to prevent full exhalation, and gas trapping (auto-PEEP) results. PCIRV generally is used only for patients with very stiff lungs, who cannot be ventilated successfully with VC-CMV with PEEP, or PC-CMV with PEEP. PCIRV can be quite uncomfortable for the patient and therefore may require sedation, or in some cases, paralysis.

Intermittent Mandatory Ventilation

Intermittent mandatory ventilation (IMV) involves periodic volume- or pressure-targeted breaths that occur at set intervals (time triggering). During IMV, the patient can breathe spontaneously between mandatory (i.e., machine) breaths at any desired baseline pressure without receiving a mandatory breath.

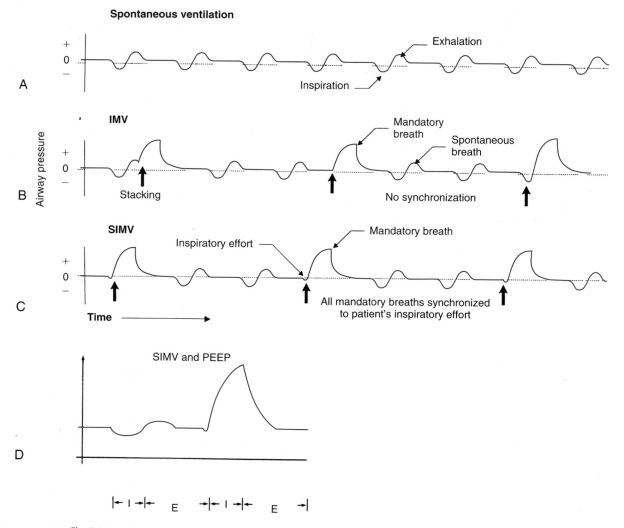

Fig. 5-6 Pressure waveforms showing essential differences in: **A,** spontaneous ventilation; **B,** intermittent mandatory ventilation; **C,** intermittent mandatory ventilation (IMV); **D,** IMV with positive end-expiratory pressure (PEEP). Note that during intermittent mandatory ventilation, mandatory breaths *(vertical arrows)* and spontaneous breaths are not synchronized. (From Dupuis Y: Ventilators: theory and clinical application, ed 2, St Louis, 1992, Mosby.)

The spontaneous baseline pressure between mandatory breaths can be set at ambient (zero gauge) pressures or above ambient pressure if PEEP/CPAP is desired (Fig. 5-6 and Key Point 5-3). During spontaneous breaths, the patient can breathe either from a continuous flow of gas or from a demand valve. Most ventilators can also provide pressure support for spontaneous breaths during the spontaneous breathing period. Critical Care Concept 5-3 provides some historical background about the evolution of IMV.

> **Key Point 5-3** Mandatory breaths are also called *machine breaths.*

The IMV mode is used when the goal is to have the patient breathe spontaneously without receiving a mandatory breath with every effort (i.e., partial ventilatory support). The patient assumes part of the WOB by actively breathing and not receiving complete support from the ventilator. It is thought that one of the main advantages of using IMV is that this mode allows for active participation by the patient in breath delivery, thus preserving a certain amount of respiratory muscle strength. (In fact, the patient's WOB can actually increase with IMV because of a lack of coordination between mandatory and spontaneous breaths. The patient's efforts might not stop just because a mandatory breath is delivered.[40,41] Another potential advantage is that there are fewer cardiovascular side effects because parts of $\dot{V}_E$ occur at lower pressures.[41]

Spontaneous breaths can be supported with PSV if the clinician wants to reduce the WOB for spontaneous breathing. Figure 5-5, *C,* shows the pressure–time curve and the flow–time curve for pressure-targeted IMV with pressure support for spontaneous breaths; these curves should be compared with those for volume-targeted IMV and pressure support in Fig. 5-5, *D.*

IMV has been used to wean patients from mechanical ventilation. As the mandatory rate is lowered, the patient gradually assumes a greater part of the WOB. (NOTE: Many clinicians are moving away from this method of weaning from mechanical ventilation and choosing instead to use spontaneous breathing trials as criteria for discontinuation of mechanical ventilation. [See

CRITICAL CARE CONCEPT 5-3

Successful use of IMV in the 1970s led to the development of a more refined mode of IMV called *synchronized IMV* (SIMV). SIMV operates in the same way as IMV except that mandatory breaths normally are patient or time triggered rather than solely time triggered. Like IMV, the patient can breathe spontaneously through the ventilator circuit between mandatory breaths. At a predetermined interval (i.e., respiratory rate), which is set by the operator, the ventilator waits for the patient's next inspiratory effort. When the ventilator senses this effort, it assists the patient by synchronously delivering a mandatory breath (see Fig. 5-6). The clinician usually sets the volume target or pressure target, a maximum mandatory breath rate, and the sensitivity level. The ventilator then delivers the set volume or pressure breaths, which are patient or time triggered. After delivering the mandatory breath, the ventilator allows the patient to breathe spontaneously without receiving another machine breath until the next mandatory breath is due to occur.

As with IMV, spontaneous breaths that occur during SIMV can be pressure supported. The pressure target for pressure support breaths commonly is set lower than the peak pressure during a mandatory breath. For example, the mandatory breath may generate a peak pressure of 30 cm H_2O, and the pressure support spontaneous breath may be set at 15 cm H_2O. (Pressure support is discussed later in the chapter.)

Originally SIMV was designed to eliminate the problem of *breath stacking*. Breath stacking occurs with IMV when a machine-timed breath accidentally is delivered at the same time the patient spontaneously inhales. Consequently, the patient's lungs receive huge volumes of air, which can cause high pressure in the lungs and result in barotrauma or ruptured lung tissue. Clinicians can prevent this problem by setting an appropriate peak pressure limit. When large volumes reach the pressure limit, they are vented to the atmosphere or the machine ends inspiration. (NOTE: Although a number of current ICU ventilator manufacturers use the term *SIMV* to designate the synchronous nature of coordinating mandatory breaths with spontaneous breaths, the acronym IMV is used in this text because this technology is now considered a built-in feature in all contemporary ICU ventilators.)

Chapter 20 for a more detailed discussion of discontinuation and weaning from mechanical ventilation.]) Table 5-1 presents a comparison of the advantages, risks, and disadvantages of CMV and IMV.[40,42,43]

Spontaneous Modes

The following are the three basic means of providing support for continuous spontaneous breathing (CSV) during mechanical ventilation:

- Spontaneous breathing
- Continuous positive airway pressure (CPAP)
- Pressure support ventilation (PSV)

Spontaneous Breathing

With this mode patients can breathe spontaneously through a ventilator circuit without receiving any mandatory breaths. This is sometimes called a T-piece method because it mimics having the patient's endotracheal tube connected to a Briggs adapter (T-piece) and a humidified oxygen source using large-bore tubing. The advantage of this approach is that the ventilator can be used to monitor the patient's breathing and activate an alarm if an undesirable circumstance arises. The disadvantage is that some ventilator systems require considerable patient effort to open inspiratory valves to receive gas flow, thus increasing WOB. Ventilator manufacturers have attempted to minimize this problem by incorporating rapidly responsive valves into their designs.[44]

A spontaneous breathing trial (SBT) can be used to evaluate a patient's readiness to have ventilation discontinued. During the trial ventilator support is reduced, and the patient is allowed to breathe spontaneously for a brief period (15 to 30 minutes), while the person's vital signs, pulse oximetry, and physical appearance are monitored. A patient who can tolerate the procedure can typically tolerate longer periods of spontaneous breathing and probably is ready to be weaned from ventilation (see Chapter 20).

Continuous Positive Airway Pressure

Ventilators can also provide CPAP for spontaneously breathing patients. In the acute care setting, CPAP may be helpful for improving oxygenation in patients with refractory hypoxemia and a low FRC, which can occur with acute lung injury. As with simple spontaneous breathing, the ventilator can provide a means of monitoring the patient. The advantages and disadvantages of ventilator-provided CPAP are similar to those for spontaneous breathing through a ventilator.

Pressure Support Ventilation

Pressure support ventilation (PSV) is a special form of assisted ventilation.[44-49] The ventilator provides a constant pressure during inspiration once it senses that the patient has made an inspiratory effort (Fig. 5-7). It is important to recognize that the patient must have a consistent, reliable spontaneous respiratory pattern for PSV to be successful. The operator sets the inspiratory pressure, PEEP, flow cycle criteria, and the sensitivity level. The patient establishes the rate, inspiratory flow, and T_I. V_T is determined by the pressure gradient (ΔP = Set pressure – EEP), lung characteristics (lung compliance [C_L] and R_{aw}), and patient effort. PSV is always an assist mode (patient triggered). The flow curve resembles a descending ramp, and the patient can vary the inspiratory flow on demand (see Fig. 5-7). A pressure support breath is patient triggered, pressure limited, and flow cycled. Remember that with flow cycling, the ventilator senses a decrease in flow and determines that inspiration is ending. The decrease in flow corresponds to a decrease in the pressure gradient between the mouth and lungs as the lungs fill (see Fig. 5-3). Sudden pressure changes can pressure cycle a pressure support breath, as can an excessive inspiratory time (which may occur with a leak in the circuit) (Box 5-6). The pressure-cycle and time-cycle capabilities are safety backup features; the manufacturer sets the exact pressure-cycle and time-cycle criteria. (See Fig. 5-8).

Additional settings in pressure support ventilation. With PSV, it is important that the ventilator deliver an appropriate flow at the beginning of inspiration. For example, flow delivery that is set too high can cause a pressure overshoot, and inspiratory flow

TABLE 5-1	Advantages, Risks, and Disadvantages of CMV and IMV	
Mode	**Advantages**	**Risks and Disadvantages**
Volume-targeted or pressure-targeted continuous mandatory ventilation (VC-CMV or PC-CMV)	Set minimum minute ventilation ($\dot{V}_E$) with volume-targeted breaths	Respiratory alkalosis if the number of patient-triggered breaths is high.
		$\dot{V}_E$ may decrease with changes in compliance or airway resistance (R_{aw}) in PC-CMV
	Guaranteed volume or pressure with each breath	High mean airway pressure and related complications
	May synchronize with patient efforts	Patient-ventilator asynchrony if flow or sensitivity is set incorrectly
	Patient may establish rate.	May not be well tolerated in awake patients who are not sedated; high rates can result in auto-PEEP
	Can provide full support in patients who are not breathing spontaneously	Muscle atrophy may result.
Volume-targeted or pressure-targeted synchronized intermittent mandatory ventilation (VC-IMV or PC-IMV)	May lower mean airway pressure compared with CMV	IMV with pressure support ventilation (PSV) may increase mean airway pressure.
	Variable work of breathing for patient may maintain muscle strength and reduce muscle atrophy.	Can significantly increase work of breathing for spontaneous breaths; hypercarbia and muscle fatigue can occur if rate, flow, and sensitivity are set incorrectly
	Can be used for weaning	May increase weaning time
	May reduce alkalosis associated with CMV	Patients may have trouble adjusting to the set mandatory rate; acute hypoventilation can occur with low rates (<6 breaths/min mandatory).
	Full or partial support can be adjusted to meet patient's needs.	Spontaneous work of breathing may increase excessively as set mandatory rate is reduced.
	Sedation and paralysis are not required (unlike with CMV).	Patient-ventilator asynchrony may result if patient actively breathes during a mandatory breath when the set rate is low; rapid, shallow breathing may occur during spontaneous periods.

Data from Hudson LD, Hurlow RS, Craig KC, et al: Does intermittent mandatory ventilation correct respiratory alkalosis in patients receiving assisted mechanical ventilation? Am Rev Respir Dis 132:1071, 1985; Culpepper JA, Rinaldo JE, Rogers RM: Effect of mechanical ventilator mode on tendency towards respiratory alkalosis, Am Rev Respir Dis 132:1075, 1985; Kacmarek RM, McMahon K, Staneck K: Pressure support level required to overcome work of breathing imposed by endotracheal tubes at various peak inspiratory flowrates, Respir Care 33:933, 1988 (abstract).

may end prematurely (i.e., pressure-cycled breath) (see Fig. 5-8). Conversely, a flow set too low may not meet the patient's need, leading to asynchrony.[49] There may also be a natural reflex that is a flow-related inspiratory termination reflex.[50,51] Stimulation of this reflex may shorten inspiration and result in brief, shallow inspiratory efforts. This is especially true for low set pressures in pressure support. The significance of this reflex in clinical practice is not yet known.

Current ICU ventilators allow the operator to adjust the slope of the pressure and flow curves during inspiration (this is sometimes called *sculpturing* or *sloping the breath*). This feature has several names, including rise time, flow acceleration percent, inspiratory rise time, inspiratory rise time percent, and slope adjustment. The term *rise time* refers to the time required for the ventilator to rise to the set pressure at the beginning of inspiration. The clinician can use the ventilator graphics to help establish an appropriate inspiratory flow delivery (Fig. 5-9). If the patient is responsive, the practitioner can ask the person when flow delivery is most comfortable while adjusting this function.

As mentioned previously, inspiratory flow in PSV ends when the ventilator senses that the flow has dropped to a certain level (flow cycling). Current ventilators (e.g., Puritan Bennett 840 [Covidien; Nellcor and Puritan Bennett, Boulder, Colo.] and the Dräger V500 [Dräger Medical, Inc., Telford, Pa.]) have an adjustable flow cycle criterion, which can range from about 5% to about 80% of the measured peak inspiratory flow, depending on the specific ventilator. Manufacturers have given this feature names such as *inspiratory cycle percent*, *inspiratory flow termination*, and *expiratory flow sensitivity*. Patients with increased airway resistance (e.g., COPD) require a shorter T_I or higher flow cycle percentage, whereas patients with parenchymal lung disease (e.g., ARDS) require a longer T_I or lower flow cycle percent.[52,53] Software is available that allows the ventilator to adjust the flow cycle criterion automatically on a breath-to-breath basis, depending

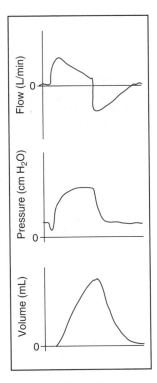

Fig. 5-7 Graph of a pressure support breath. The baseline pressure is above zero; therefore positive end-expiratory pressure (PEEP) has been set. Note the slight negative deflection in the pressure curve before it rises to the set value; this is caused by the patient's inspiratory effort, which triggers the flow from the ventilator. Inspiratory flow is graphed above zero, and expiratory flow is graphed below zero. The flow curve resembles a descending (decelerating) ramp.

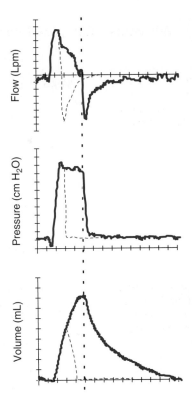

Fig. 5-8 Pressure support ventilation (PSV) graphs with a pressure overshoot at the beginning of inspiration. The *top curve* is flow (L/min), the *middle curve* is pressure (cm H_2O), and the *bottom curve* is volume (mL). The *solid line* of the curves represents PSV without premature termination of inspiration. The *dotted vertical line* through all the curves represents the end of inspiratory flow with normal pressure support breath delivery. The *dashed curve* represents premature cycling caused by pressure overshoot (i.e., a spike at the beginning of the pressure curve). With premature cycling flow ends prematurely; therefore volume delivery is lower than normal. (Courtesy Ted Tabor, RRT, CBET, Paris, France. Redrawn for this text.)

BOX 5-6	**Time-Cycled and Pressure-Cycled Inspiration with Pressure Support Ventilation (PSV) and Volume Support (VS)**

PSV inspiration ends if the inspiratory time (T_I) exceeds a preset value. This most often occurs with a leak in the circuit. For example, a deflated cuff causes a large leak. The flow through the circuit might never drop to the flow cycle criterion required by the ventilator. Therefore inspiratory flow, if not stopped, would continue indefinitely. For this reason, all ventilators that provide pressure support also have a maximum preset inspiratory time. Most ventilators use a fixed value, such as 1.5 to 2 seconds for adult patients and 0.5 seconds for infants, for the maximum inspiratory time. Other ventilators use different maximum time-cycle criteria.

PSV and VS breaths also end if the pressure in the circuit exceeds the preset pressure by a specific margin (the margin is preset by the manufacturer). For adult patients the margin is approximately 2 cm H_2O above the set pressure. For example, if the set pressure is 12 cm H_2O and the patient forcibly tries to exhale or coughs, the circuit pressure might rise to 14 cm H_2O. At this point inspiratory flow delivery ends for the pressure support breath.

The size of the patient (i.e., adult, child, infant) influences the specific time and pressure limits used. It is also important to mention that the specific times and pressure limits are different for every ventilator. The clinician must become familiar with each of these functions for the ventilator used.

PSV is used for three basic functions:
- To reduce work of breathing (WOB) for spontaneously breathing patients breathing through a ventilator circuit.
- To reduce WOB in patients receiving continuous positive airway pressure or spontaneous intermittent mechanical ventilation. This is accomplished by setting the pressure level higher than that required to overcome system resistance.
- To provide full ventilatory support in the assist mode, in which each patient breath is a pressure support (PS) breath. The patient must have a dependable, intact respiratory center and a fairly stable lung condition, because tidal volume can vary when used in this mode. This is sometimes referred to as maximum pressure support (PS_{max}).[17]

PSV can be used with an artificial airway or a mask to provide noninvasive ventilation.

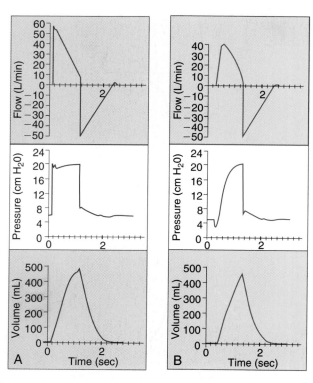

Fig. 5-9 Effect of rise time adjustment during PSV. **A,** Faster rise time. **B,** Slow rise time. (From Hess DR, MacIntyre NR, Mishoe SC, et al: Respiratory care principles and practice, Philadelphia, 2002, Saunders.)

on the lung characteristics and the patients active expiratory efforts.[54,55]

BILEVEL POSITIVE AIRWAY PRESSURE

Bilevel positive airway pressure (bilevel PAP), also called *bilevel pressure assist,* is another form of pressure ventilation often used in NIV. Bilevel intermittent positive airway pressure (bilevel IPAP) is different from classical bilevel PAP and is generally intended for patients with ARDS.[44]

The original BiPAP (Philips Respironics, Murrysville, Pa.), was introduced in the early 1990s. Machines that provide bilevel pressure assist generate a high gas flow through a microprocessor-controlled valve. The operator sets two pressure levels: an inspiratory and an expiratory positive airway pressure. Inspiration is typically patient triggered, but can also be time triggered. It can be flow or time cycled. A full face mask is the most popular technique for starting therapy, but a nasal mask or nasal pillows can also be used. Leakage from the mouth often occurs with the nasal mask and nasal pillows, although chin straps sometimes help eliminate this problem. Some machines require a fixed-leak exhalation port and function best with nasal ventilation, which allows exhalation through the mouth. Most devices now compensate for leaks. Newer designs are even being used with artificial airways (see Chapter 19).

ADDITIONAL MODES OF VENTILATION

Pressure Augmentation

Pressure augmentation (P_{Aug}) is a dual-control mode that provides pressure-limited ventilation with volume delivery targeted for every breath. Another term that is used to describe this mode is *volume-assured pressure support (VAPS).* VAPS is the term used to describe this mode on the Bird 8400st (CareFusion, Viasys Corp, San Diego, Calif.).

With P_{Aug} ventilation, the ventilator begins with a patient-triggered, pressure-targeted breath (e.g., a pressure support breath), but targets the volume preset by the operator and delivers that volume with every breath.[56] A key criterion for P_{Aug} is the ability to initiate breaths. These patients must also have a consistent respiratory frequency or must be able to make consistent attempts at inspiratory triggering. P_{Aug} does not work if the patient has been sedated to the point where the respiratory centers are not active; it is intended for conditions in which the respiratory drive waxes and wanes because of changes in level of alertness or moderate changes in sedation.

When using P_{Aug}, the operator selects a desired volume and minimum rate, a set pressure level above baseline, an inspiratory gas flow, and a sensitivity setting. When the patient triggers a breath, the ventilator delivers the set pressure level and monitors flow and volume. If volume is achieved before the inspiratory gas flow drops to the preset value, the breath cycles into expiration. Cycling occurs when the measured flow drops to 25% to 30% of the patient's peak inspiratory flow. The threshold value depends on the ventilator's flow cycle criterion. If volume is not achieved before flow drops to the set level, the ventilator maintains the flow at the set value until the volume is delivered (volume cycled). If the patient's inspiratory flow demand is high and pressure starts to fall below the set pressure level in this mode, the ventilator provides additional flow to the patient. In this sense, P_{Aug} targets a minimum volume, but the breath is not limited to that volume. Patients can receive more than the set volume if there is a high flow demand.

Pressure-Regulated Volume Control

Pressure-regulated volume control (PRVC) is a volume-targeted, pressure control breath that is available on most ventilators (e.g. Servo-i, CareFusion AVEA, Hamilton-G5, Covidien PB 840, and the Dräger Evita XL). Although PRVC was introduced on the Servo 300 in the 1990s and later has been used to describe this mode on the Servo-i and Servo-s (Maquet, Inc, Wayne, N.J.) and the CareFusion AVEA (CareFusion, Inc., Yorba Linda, Calif.), it subsequently has been given different proprietary names on other ventilators (e.g., *AutoFlow* on the Dräger Evita E-4 [Dräger Medical Inc., Telford, Pa.], and *VC+* on the Covidien PB 840 [Covidien, Puritan Bennett, Boulder, Colo.], *Adaptive Pressure Ventilation* on the Hamilton G5 and C3 ventilators [Hamilton Medical, Bonaduz, Switzerland]).

Pressure-regulated volume control delivers pressure breaths that are patient- or time-triggered, volume-targeted, and time-cycled breaths. During breath delivery, the ventilator measures the tidal volume delivered and compares it to the targeted V_T, which is set by the operator. If the volume delivered is less than the set V_T, the ventilator increases pressure delivery progressively over several breaths until the set and the targeted V_T are about equal (Fig. 5-10). If the measured volume is too high, the pressure is reduced in an attempt to reach the targeted V_T. Generally the ventilator does not allow the pressure to rise higher than 5 cm H_2O below the upper pressure limit setting. For example, if the upper pressure limit is 35 cm H_2O and the ventilator requires more than 30 cm H_2O to deliver a V_T of 500 mL, an alarm activates and the pressure delivery is limited to 30 cm H_2O. The clinician must determine why the higher pressure is required to deliver the set volume

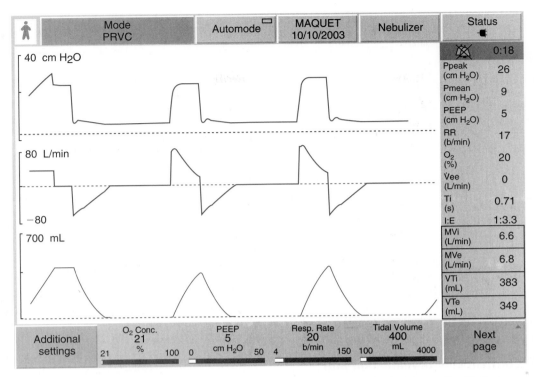

Fig. 5-10 A screen capture of pressure-regulated volume control (PRVC) in an adult patient on the Servo-i ventilator. The first breath (*left*) is a volume-targeted test breath with an inspiratory hold to measure plateau pressure. The second breath is a pressure-targeted breath with a pressure equal to the measured plateau pressure. Set tidal volume is 400 mL. Measured exhaled tidal volume is about 350 mL. Note how the pressure is increased by a few centimeters of H_2O on the third breath for the ventilator to achieve the set tidal volume.

(e.g., the presence of secretions in the airway, bronchospasms, or changes in C_L). The clinician can then choose an appropriate course of action to address the higher pressure required. On the other hand, when a patient's lung condition improves, less pressure is required to achieve the set volume. The ventilator progressively lowers the pressure; however, it does not allow pressure to drop below the set baseline [PEEP].

Volume Support Ventilation

Volume support ventilation (VSV) is very similar to PRVC. It is basically pressure support with a volume target and will have various names depending on the ventilator manufacturer. It is a pressure breath that is patient triggered, volume targeted, and flow cycled. There is no backup rate with VSV; however, there is generally a backup mode in the event that the patient becomes apneic on this purely spontaneous mode. As with PRVC, the ventilator adjusts the pressure, over several breaths, to achieve the set volume. If volume is too low, the pressure is increased. Conversely, the pressure is reduced if the volume is too high. VSV can be used for patients who are ready to be weaned from the ventilator and can breathe spontaneously (Fig. 5-11). Unlike PRVC, it normally is flow cycled when the flow drops to a set percentage of peak flow. It also can be time cycled (if T_I is extended for some reason) or pressure cycled (if the pressure rises too high) (see Box 5-6 and Chapter 6).

Mandatory Minute Ventilation

Mandatory minute ventilation (MMV), also called *minimum minute ventilation* and *augmented minute ventilation*, is used primarily for weaning patients from the ventilator. It allows the operator to set a minimum minute ventilation, which usually is 70% to 90% of a patient's current $\dot{V}_E$. The ventilator provides whatever part of the minute ventilation that the patient is unable to accomplish by increasing the breathing rate or by increasing the preset pressure. The ventilator monitors the patient's spontaneous breathing, and provides additional ventilatory support if the patient does not achieve the set $\dot{V}_E$. If a patient increases the level of his or her spontaneous ventilation, the ventilator reduces its amount of support.

The clinician typically sets high rate and low V_T alarms to monitor significant changes in either of these parameters because either suggests an increased WOB. It is important to monitor these parameters even if the patient can maintain the desired minute ventilation because patients sometimes begin to breathe rapidly and take very shallow breaths. This pattern increases dead space ventilation without effectively increasing alveolar ventilation (Table 5-2). MMV is rarely used in current practice in the United States.

Airway Pressure Release Ventilation

Airway pressure release ventilation (APRV) is designed to provide two levels of CPAP and to allow spontaneous breathing at both levels when spontaneous effort is present.[56-61] Both pressure levels are time triggered and time cycled (Fig. 5-12). Newer ventilators allow for patient triggering and patient cycling. The possible advantage of this modification may be its synchronization with patient breathing.[62-65]

For the initial setup, an optimum high CPAP level is determined much as the optimum PEEP or an ideal P_{aw} is determined

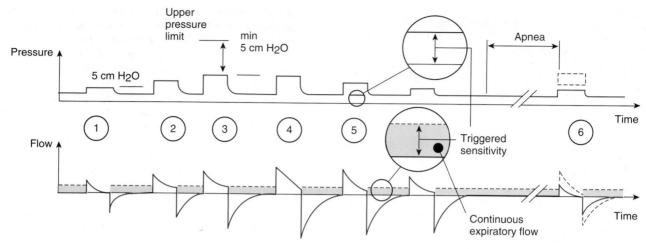

Fig. 5-11 *(1)*, Volume support test breath (5 cm H₂0); *(2)*, pressure is increased slowly until target volume is achieved; *(3)*, maximum available pressure is 5 cm H₂O below upper pressure limit; *(4)*, tidal volume higher than set tidal volume delivered results in lower pressure; *(5)*, patient can trigger breath; *(6)*, if apnea alarm is detected, ventilator switches to pressure-regulated volume. (The 5 cm H₂O test breath and breath delivery pattern are features of the original design; these have been modified in newer models of the Servo 300 and Servo-i.) (Courtesy Maquet, Inc., Wayne, N.J.)

TABLE 5-2	Constant Minute Ventilation with Changing Alveolar Ventilation*			
Tidal Volume (mL)	Dead Space (mL)	Respiratory Rate (breaths/min)	Alveolar Ventilation (L/min)	Minute Ventilation (L/min)
800	150	10	6.5	8
667	150	12	6.2	8
533	150	15	5.75	8
400	150	20	5	8
250	150	32	3.2	8

*If a patient has a constant dead space of 150 mL, minute ventilation remains constant, while alveolar ventilation decreases, rate increases, and tidal volume falls.

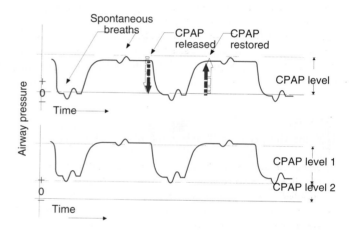

Fig. 5-12 Pressure waveforms for airway pressure release ventilation (APRV) in which alveolar ventilation is enhanced when pressure is released to zero *(upper graph)* and when release pressure is above zero *(lower graph)*. Inspiratory/expiratory ratio for APRV is 2:1. *CPAP,* continuous positive airway pressure. (From Dupuis Y: Ventilators: theory and clinical application, ed 2, St Louis, 1992, Mosby.)

for improving oxygenation (see Chapter 13). The high CPAP level is interrupted intermittently to allow pressures to drop very briefly (for about 1 second or less) to a lower CPAP level. Reducing the CPAP reduces the patient's FRC and allows patient exhalation and ventilation (i.e., exhalation of CO₂). Expiratory flow generally is not permitted to return to baseline (zero); therefore auto-PEEP is intentionally present, which helps maintain an open lung and prevents repeated collapse and reexpansion of alveoli. As soon as the release period is complete, the higher level of CPAP is restored. The optimum duration of the release time is a function of the time constant of the respiratory system.[62] It is worth noting that the pressure curve generated during APRV resembles that of PCIRV if the patient is not breathing spontaneously.

Although originally intended for patients with stiff lungs, APRV has been shown to be as effective as conventional ventilation for ventilating and oxygenating patients with mild pulmonary problems or with normal lung compliance.[61,64-67] Clinical studies have demonstrated that APRV can improve arterial oxygenation, reduce physiological dead space ventilation, and reduce peak airway pressures.[59,60,62,64-67]

Proportional Assist Ventilation

The proportional assist ventilation (PAV) approach is a different approach to mechanical ventilation because pressure, flow, and volume delivery are proportional to the patient's spontaneous effort.[68,69] The amount of pressure the ventilator produces depends on two factors: (1) the amount of inspiratory flow and volume demanded by the patient's effort, and (2) the degree of amplification selected by the clinician (which determines the extent of ventilator response to patient effort). PAV is a positive feedback system.

Basically the ventilator measures airway flow and pressure and compares patient demand with the **gains** (amplification) set by the operator. The amount of flow delivered to the patient is determined from this comparison. As the patient's inspiratory effort increases,

---

| BOX **5-7** | **Determining Proportional Assist** |

$P_{aw} = (f_1 \times volume) + (f_2 \times flow)$
where P_{aw} is the airway pressure; f_1 is the ventilator-supported elastic load (degree of volume assist); and f_2 is the ventilator-supported resistive load (degree of flow assist).

---

the flow from the ventilator increases proportionally. This relationship is described by the equation in Box 5-7.

The clinician sets the gain of the volume amplifier to compensate for the abnormal elastance (f_1) of the patient, and adjusts the gain of the flow amplifier to compensate for the abnormal resistance (f_2) of the patient.[19] The clinician must estimate these values beforehand. Setting the controls and measuring elastance and resistance can be difficult. Indeed, the pressure output from the ventilator can exceed the pressure needed to overcome the respiratory system impedance (C_L and R_{aw}) if the baseline measurements are inaccurate.[70]

Ideally PAV assists the patient's inspiratory effort based on the patient's lung characteristics and the amount of patient effort desired. PAV may prove to be a valuable alternative mode of ventilation. The advantage of PAV is its ability to track changes in patient effort, which can occur rapidly in acute respiratory failure. The disadvantages of PAV are that it provides only for assisted ventilation and cannot compensate for system leaks. Patients experiencing auto-PEEP may also find it more difficult to trigger the ventilator.

 SUMMARY

- Once the need for mechanical ventilation has been established, the clinician must select the type of ventilator, breath type, and ventilator mode appropriate for the patient.
- Mechanical ventilators can function in a wide variety of settings and provide a variety of modes, features, monitors, and alarms.
- The three methods of providing noninvasive ventilatory support include NPV, CPAP, and NIV.
- CPAP has been shown to be an effective method to improve oxygenation in hospitalized patients and as an accepted method to treat obstructive sleep apnea.

- NIV has been successfully used to treat patients with respiratory failure caused by various neuromuscular disorders, chest wall deformities, COPD, central ventilatory control abnormalities, and acute cardiogenic pulmonary edema.
- Invasive positive pressure ventilation can involve full or partial ventilatory support. During full ventilator support, the ventilator provides all of the energy necessary to maintain effective alveolar ventilation. With partial ventilator support, the patient can assume a variable portion of the WOB.
- The breath type and pattern of breath delivery during mechanical ventilation constitute the mode of ventilation. The mode is determined by whether the breath is mandatory, IMV, or spontaneous, the targeted control variable, and the timing of breath delivery.
- The clinician determines the control variable that will be used to establish gas flow to the patient by choosing either volume or pressure ventilation.
- The primary advantage of volume control ventilation is that it guarantees a specific volume delivery and minute ventilation, regardless of changes in lung compliance and resistance or patient effort.
- The main advantage of pressure control ventilation is that it can be used as a lung protective strategy because it reduces the risk of overdistention of the lungs by limiting the amount of positive pressure applied to the lung.
- The goal of IMV is to allow the patient to breathe spontaneously without receiving a mandatory breath with every effort (partial ventilatory support). The primary advantage of IMV is that this mode allows for active participation by the patient in breath delivery thus minimizing the effects of respiratory muscle atrophy.
- Pressure support ventilation can be used with patients who have a dependable, intact respiratory center and a stable lung condition. It is used to reduce WOB in patients receiving CPAP or IMV.
- Volume support, mandatory minute ventilation, airway pressure release ventilation, and proportional assist ventilation provide several alternative methods of ventilating patients.
- Figure 5-13 presents an example of a worksheet the reader can use to evaluate the types of ventilators and their settings. The worksheet also incorporates principles that were discussed in Chapter 4.

Worksheet:
Ventilator, Ventilator Mode, and Breath Delivery

Name _____

Manufacturer _____

Model & No. _____

   I. Power Source: Pneumatic Electric Microprocessor controlled

Other _____

  II. Circuit: Single Double

 III. Drive Mechanism

    Volume displacement design   type _____

    Flow control valve   type _____

    Other _____   type _____

Mode of Ventilation and Breath Description

1. VC-CMV; PC-CMV

    Mandatory breath: volume ventilation or pressure ventilation

    Triggering: time pressure flow

    Limiting: volume pressure flow time

    Cycling: volume pressure flow time

    Inspiratory pause: (time) _____ second(s)

    Other: _____

2. VC-IMV; PC-IMV

    A. Mandatory breaths: volume ventilation or pressure ventilation

      Triggering: time pressure flow

      Limiting: volume pressure flow time

      Cycling: volume pressure flow time

    B. Spontaneous breaths

      Zero baseline

          Auto-PEEP (expiratory pause pressure) = _____ cm H_2O

        Positive baseline

            SET PEEP (positive pressure baseline) = _____ cm H_2O

            Auto-PEEP (expiratory pause pressure) = _____ cm H_2O

            Total end-expiratory pressure = _____ cm H_2O

        PSV

          Set pressure = _____ cm H_2O

          Flow cycling

          or L/min cycling = _____

3. Spontaneous Breathing Through a Ventilator

    A. Zero baseline

      Auto-PEEP (expiratory pause pressure) = _____ cm H_2O

    B. Positive pressure baseline

      SET PEEP (positive pressure baseline) = _____ cm H_2O

      Auto-PEEP (expiratory pause pressure) = _____ cm H_2O

      Total end-expiratory pressure = _____ cm H_2O

    C. PSV set pressure = _____ cm H_2O

      Flow cycling

      or L/min = _____

4. Minimum Mandatory Ventilation

    Volume ventilation   Pressure ventilation   Other

    Set mandatory minute ventilation L/min

    Other settings:

5. APRV

    High CPAP level = _____ cm H_2O

    Low CPAP level = _____ cm H_2O

    Time one = _____ sec

    Time two = _____ sec

Fig. 5-13 Worksheet for reviewing a ventilator's function, mode, and breath delivery.

6. Bilevel PAP

    IPAP = _____ cm H_2O

    EPAP = _____ cm H_2O

    Other settings: _____

7. PAV

    f1 (elastic load) = _____

    f2 (resistive load) = _____

    Volume = _____

    Flow = _____

8. Pressure Ventilation with Volume Guaranteed

    VAPS or pressure augment

    PRVC or _____ VC

    Other _____

    Settings: desired volume _____ pressure (set or limit) _____

        flow (where appropriate) _____ other _____

9. Other: Description

Fig. 5-13, cont'd

REVIEW QUESTIONS *(See Appendix A for answers.)*

1. In which of the following situations would you try NIV?
   A. A patient in whom blood pressure is 65/35, heart rate is 150 beats/min, and respiratory frequency is 34 breaths/min
   B. A patient who nearly drowned who has copious amounts of white, frothy secretions
   C. A patient with COPD and right lower-lobe pneumonia with respiratory acidosis and increased WOB
   D. A 5-year-old child who has aspirated a piece of chicken and is having trouble breathing

2. Which of the following would you use for a trauma victim with crushed chest injuries?
   A. Negative pressure ventilation
   B. Pressure-cycled ventilator
   C. VC-CMV
   D. Noninvasive ventilation

3. A patient with hiccups is ventilated in the VC-CMV mode. Every time he hiccups, he triggers the ventilator. What would you recommend?
   Paralyze the patient and control ventilation
   A. Use PSV
   B. Use PC-CMV
   C. Use VC-IMV

4. A patient with severe tetanus needs ventilatory support. Which of the following modes would you recommend?
   A. Paralyze and sedate the patient; control ventilation using volume control (VC-CMV)
   B. PC-CMV
   C. VC-IMV
   D. PSV with CPAP

5. In which of these four circumstances is it appropriate to select PSV?
   1. As a method of weaning
   2. To overcome the WOB through the endotracheal tube and the circuit
   3. For patients using the IMV mode
   4. For long-term patient support
   A. 1, 2, and 3
   B. 2, 3, and 4
   C. 1, 3, and 4
   D. 1, 2, 3, and 4

6. A patient on PC-CMV has widely fluctuating changes in R_{aw} because of secretions and bronchospasm. The low tidal volume alarm is activated every few hours; the set pressure is 18 cm H_2O. The physician is concerned about consistency in ventilation. What would you recommend?
   A. Increase the set pressure
   B. Sedate the patient
   C. Switch to VC-CMV
   D. Switch to PSV

7. A patient with acute respiratory distress syndrome has a plateau pressure ($P_{plateau}$) of 30 cm H_2O and a peak inspiratory pressure of 39 cm H_2O. V_T is 0.7 on VC-CMV. The decision is made to switch to PC-CMV (PCV) to keep pressures at a safe level. What pressure would you set and why?

8. A patient receiving VC-CMV is actively triggering every breath. The respiratory therapist notices that the patient is using accessory muscles (sternocleidomastoid muscles) during the entire inspiratory phase. The therapist also sees that the pressure–time curve has a negative deflection before inspiration and has a concave appearance during inspiration. What is the apparent problem in this situation?

9. A patient has recovered from a severe pneumonia that required 8 days of PC-CMV ventilation. The patient is now conscious and responsive. She is triggering every breath and has a strong cough. What should the therapist suggest to the physician?

10. A physician is concerned about the high pressures required to perform ventilation for a patient with terminal cancer and severe lung scarring. The lungs are very stiff and fibrous. The physician is also concerned about maintaining a normal CO_2 in this patient. What mode might be appropriate for this patient and why?

References

1. Klonin H, Bowman B, Peters M, et al: Negative pressure ventilation via chest cuirass to decrease ventilator-associated complications in infants with acute respiratory failure: a case series. *Respir Care* 45:486–490, 2000.
2. Kennan SP, Mehta S: Noninvasive ventilation for patients presenting with acute respiratory failure: the randomized controlled trials. *Respir Care* 54:116–124, 2009.
3. Pierson DJ: History and epidemiology of noninvasive ventilation in the acute-care setting. *Respir Care* 54:40–52, 2009.
4. Liesching T, Kwok H, Hill NS: Acute applications of noninvasive positive pressure ventilation. *Chest* 124:699–713, 2003.
5. Hess D: Noninvasive positive pressure ventilation: predictors of success and failure for adult acute care application. *Respir Care* 42:424–431, 1997.
6. Miro AM, Shirvaram U, Hertig E: Continuous positive airway pressure in COPD patients in acute respiratory failure. *Chest* 103:266–268, 1993.
7. Appendini L, Patessio A, Zanaboni S, et al: Physiologic effects of positive end-expiratory pressure and mask pressure support during exacerbations of chronic obstructive pulmonary disease. *Am J Respir Crit Care Med* 149:1069–1076, 1994.
8. Hill NS, Brennan J, Gaspestad E, et al: Noninvasive ventilation in acute respiratory failure. *Crit Care Med* 35:2402–2407, 2007.
9. Hill NS: Where should noninvasive ventilation be delivered? *Respir Care* 54:62–70, 2009.
10. Patrick W, Webster K, Ludwig L, et al: Noninvasive positive-pressure ventilation in acute respiratory distress without prior chronic respiratory failure. *Am J Respir Crit Care Med* 153:1005–1011, 1996.
11. Mehta S, Al-Hashim AH, Keenan SP: Noninvasive ventilation in patients with acute cardiogenic pulmonary edema. *Respir Care* 54:186–195, 2009.
12. Meduri GU, Fox RC, Abou-Shala N, et al: Noninvasive mechanical ventilation via face mask in patients with acute respiratory failure who refused endotracheal intubation. *Crit Care Med* 22:1584–1590, 1996.
13. Ferguson FT, Gilmartin M: CO_2 rebreathing during BiPAP ventilatory assistance. *Am J Respir Crit Care Med* 151:1126–1135, 1995.
14. Meduri GU, Fox RC, Abou-Shala N, et al: Noninvasive face mask mechanical ventilation in patients with acute hypercapnic respiratory failure. *Chest* 100:445–454, 1991.
15. Peruzzi WT: Full and partial ventilatory support: the significance of ventilator mode (editorial). *Respir Care* 35:174, 1990.
16. Respiratory Distress Syndrome Network (ARDS Network): Ventilation with lower tidal volumes as compared with traditional tidal volumes for acute lung injury and the acute respiratory distress syndrome. *N Engl J Med* 342:1301–1308, 2000.
17. MacIntyre NR: Weaning from mechanical ventilatory support: volume-assisting intermittent breaths versus pressure-assisting every breath. *Respir Care* 33:121–125, 1988.
18. MacIntyre NR: Management of obstructive airway disease. In MacIntyre NR, Branson RD, editors: *Mechanical ventilation*, ed 2, Philadelphia, 2009, Saunders-Elsevier, pp 297–305.
19. Chatburn RL: *Fundamentals of mechanical ventilation: a short course in theory and application of mechanical ventilators*, Cleveland Heights, Ohio, 2003, Mandu Press.
20. Chatburn RL: Classification of ventilator modes: update and proposal for implementation. *Respir Care* 52:301–323, 2007.
21. Campbell RS, Davis BR: Pressure-controlled versus volume-controlled ventilation: does it matter? *Respir Care* 47:416–424, 2002.
22. Marini JJ, Rodriguez RM, Lamb V: The inspiratory workload of patient-initiated mechanical ventilation. *Am Rev Respir Dis* 134:902–909, 1986.
23. Marini JJ, Capps JS, Culver BH: The inspiratory work of breathing during assisted mechanical ventilation. *Chest* 87:612–618, 1985.
24. Kallet RH, Campbell AR, Alonso JA, et al: The effects of pressure control versus volume control assisted ventilation on patient work of breathing in acute lung injury and acute respiratory distress syndrome. *Respir Care* 45:1085–1096, 2000.
25. Kirby RR: Modes of mechanical ventilation. In Kacmarek RM, Stoller JK, editors: *Current respiratory care*, Philadelphia, 1988, BC Decker.
26. Marini JJ, Rodriguez RM, Lamb V: Bedside estimation of the inspiratory work of breathing during mechanical ventilation. *Chest* 89:56–63, 1986.
27. Downs JB: Ventilatory patterns and modes of ventilation in acute respiratory failure. *Respir Care* 28:586–591, 1983.
28. Hudson LD, Hurlow RS, Craig KC, et al: Does intermittent mandatory ventilation correct respiratory alkalosis in patients receiving assisted mechanical ventilation? *Am Rev Respir Dis* 132:1071–1074, 1985.
29. Culpepper JA, Rinaldo JE, Rogers RM: Effect of mechanical ventilator mode on tendency towards respiratory alkalosis. *Am Rev Respir Dis* 132:1075–1077, 1985.
30. Kacmarek RM, Hess D: Pressure-controlled inverse-ratio ventilation: panacea or auto-PEEP? (editorial). *Respir Care* 35:945–948, 1990.
31. Kacmarek RM, McMahon K, Staneck K: Pressure support level required to overcome work of breathing imposed by endotracheal tubes at various peak inspiratory flowrates. *Respir Care* 33:933, 1988. (abstract).
32. Banner MJ, Boysen PG, Lampotang S, et al: End-tidal CO_2 affected by inspiratory time and flow waveform: time for a change. *Crit Care Med* 14:374–378, 1986.
33. Al-Saady N, Bennett ED: Decelerating inspiratory flow waveform improves lung mechanics and gas exchange in patients on intermittent positive-pressure ventilation. *Intensive Care Med* 11:68–75, 1985.
34. Hastings D, Sabo J: Pressure-controlled inverse ratio ventilation for adult respiratory distress syndrome. *Respir Care* 33:957, 1988. (abstract).
35. Arnold JS, Summer JL, Tipton RD, et al: Inverse ratio ventilation in hypoxic respiratory failure. *Chest* 96:150S, 1989. (abstract).
36. Greaves TH, Gordon M, Cramolini M, et al: Inverse ratio ventilation in a 5-year-old with severe post-traumatic adult respiratory distress syndrome. *Crit Care Med* 17:588–589, 1989.
37. Marini JJ: Pressure-targeted mechanical ventilation of acute lung injury. *Chest* 105(Suppl):109S–115S, 1994.
38. Lessard MR, Guerot E, Lorino H, et al: Effects of pressure-controlled ventilation with different I:E ratios versus volume-controlled ventilation on respiratory mechanics, gas exchange, and hemodynamics in patients with adult respiratory distress syndrome. *Anesthesiology* 80:983–991, 1994.
39. Muñoz J, Guerrero JE, Escalante JL, et al: Pressure-controlled ventilation versus controlled mechanical ventilation with decelerating inspiratory flow. *Crit Care Med* 21:1143–1148, 1993.
40. Marini JJ, Smith TC, Lamb VJ: External work output and force generation during synchronized intermittent mechanical ventilation: effect of machine assistance on breathing effort. *Am Rev Respir Dis* 138:1169–1179, 1988.
41. Kiiski R, Takala J, Kari A, et al: Effect of tidal volume on gas exchange and oxygen transport in the adult respiratory distress syndrome. *Am Rev Respir Dis* 146:1131–1135, 1992.
42. Mecklenburgh JS, Latto IP, Al-Obaidi TA, et al: Excessive work of breathing during intermittent mandatory ventilation. *Br J Anaesth* 58:1048–1054, 1986.
43. Papdakos PJ, Lachmann B: *Mechanical ventilation: clinical applications and pathophysiology*, Philadelphia, 2007, Saunders-Elsevier.
44. Kuhlen R, Rossaint R: The role of spontaneous breathing during mechanical ventilation. *Respir Care* 47:296–303, 2002.
45. Feeley TW: Mechanical ventilatory support: current techniques and recent advances. *Am Soc Anesthesiology, Refresher Courses* 202:218–219, 1983.
46. Hedley-Whyte J, Pontoppidan H, Morris MJ: The relation of alveolar to tidal ventilation during respiratory failure in man. *Anesthesiology* 27:218–219, 1966.
47. Hess D, Ruppert T, Kemp T: A bench evaluation of pressure-controlled ventilation (PCV). *Respir Care* 34:1045, 1989. (abstract).
48. Kacmarek RM: Point of view: pressure support. *Respir Care* 34:136–138, 1989.

49. Croci M, Pelosi P, Chiumello D, et al: Regulation of pressurization rate reduces inspiratory effort during pressure support ventilation: a bench study. *Respir Care* 41:880–884, 1996.

50. Fernandez R, Mendez M, Younes M: Effect of ventilator flow rate on respiratory timing in normal subjects. *Am J Respir Crit Care Med* 159:710–719, 1999.

51. Manning HL, Molinary EJ, Leiter JC: Effect of inspiratory flow rate on respiratory sensation and pattern of breathing. *Am J Respir Crit Care Med* 151:751–757, 1995.

52. Hess D, Branson R: Ventilators and weaning modes. Part II. *Respir Care Clin N Am* 6:407–435, 2000.

53. Parthasarathy S, Jubran A, Tobin MJ: Cycling of inspiratory and expiratory muscle groups with the ventilator in airflow limitation. *Am J Respir Crit Care Med* 158:1471–1478, 1998.

54. Parthasarathy S, Jubran A, Tobin MJ: Assessment of neural inspiratory time in ventilator-supported patients. *Am J Respir Crit Care Med* 162:546–552, 2000.

55. Yamada Y, Du H-L: Analysis of the mechanisms of expiratory asynchrony in pressure support ventilation: a mathematical approach. *J Appl Physiol* 88:2143–2150, 2000.

56. Amato MB, Barbas CS, Bonassa J, et al: Volume assured pressure support ventilation (VAPSV): a new approach for reducing muscle workload during acute respiratory failure. *Chest* 102:1225–1234, 1992.

57. Putenson C, Rasanen J, Lopez FA, et al: Effect of interfacing between spontaneous breathing and mechanical cycles on the ventilation-perfusion distribution in canine lung injury. *Anesthesiology* 81:921–930, 1994.

58. Putensen C, Muzt NJ, Putensen-Himmer G, et al: Spontaneous breathing during ventilator support improves ventilation-perfusion distribution in patients with respiratory distress syndrome. *Am J Respir Crit Care Med* 159:1241–1248, 1999.

59. Sydow M, Burchardi H, Ephraim E, et al: Long-term effects of two different ventilatory modes on oxygenation in acute lung injury: comparison of airway pressure release ventilation and volume-controlled inverse ratio ventilation. *Am J Respir Crit Care Med* 149:1550–1556, 1994.

60. Frawley PM, Habashi NM: Airway pressure release ventilation: theory and practice. *AACN Clin Issues* 12:234–246, 2001.

61. Neumann P, Golisch W, Strohmeyer A, et al: Influence of different release times on spontaneous breathing pattern during airway pressure release ventilation. *Intensive Care Med* 28:1742–1749, 2002.

62. Davis K, Jr, Johnson DJ, Branson RD, et al: Airway pressure release ventilation. *Arch Surg* 128:1348–1352, 1993.

63. Rouby JJ, Ben Amewr M, Jawish D, et al: Continuous positive airway pressure (CPAP) vs intermittent mandatory pressure release ventilation (IMPRV) in patients with acute respiratory failure. *Intensive Care Med* 18:69–75, 1992.

64. Hering R, Peters D, Zinserling J, et al: Effects of spontaneous breathing during airway pressure release ventilation on renal perfusion and function in patients with acute lung injury. *Intensive Care Med* 29:1426–1433, 2002.

65. Kaplan LJ, Bailey H, Formosa V: Airway pressure release ventilation increases cardiac performance in patients with acute lung injury/acute respiratory distress syndrome. *Crit Care* 5:221–226, 2001.

66. McCunn M, Habashi NM: Airway pressure release ventilation in the acute respiratory distress syndrome following traumatic injury. *Int Anesthesiol Clin* 40:89–102, 2002.

67. Habashi NM: Other approaches to open-lung ventilation: airway pressure release ventilation. *Crit Care Med* 33(Suppl):228–240, 2005.

68. Younes M: Proportional assist ventilation: a new approach to ventilatory support. *Am Rev Respir Dis* 145:114–120, 1992.

69. Younes M, Puddy A, Roberts D, et al: Proportional assist ventilation: results of an initial clinical trial. *Am Rev Respir Dis* 145:121–129, 1992.

70. Branson R: Understanding and implementing advances in ventilator capabilities. *Curr Opin Crit Care* 10:23–32, 2004.

Initial Ventilator Settings

OUTLINE

KEY TERMS

- Compressible volume
- Mechanical dead space
- Overinflation
- System compressibility
- Tubing compliance

LEARNING OBJECTIVES   *On completion of this chapter, the reader will be able to do the following:*

1. Calculate tubing compliance.
2. Determine volume loss caused by tubing compliance.
3. Calculate minute ventilation given a patient's respiratory rate and tidal volume.
4. Calculate total cycle time, inspiratory time, expiratory time, flow in L/sec, and inspiratory-to-expiratory ratios given the necessary patient data.
5. Select an appropriate flow rate and pattern.
6. Calculate initial minute ventilation, tidal volume, and rate for a patient placed on VC-CMV based on the patient's sex, height, and ideal body weight.
7. Identify the source of the problem when an inspiratory pause cannot be measured.
8. Choose an appropriate initial mode of mechanical ventilation, and determine $\dot{V}_E$, tidal volume, respiratory frequency, and positive end-expiratory pressure settings based on the patient's lung
pathology, body temperature, metabolic rate, altitude, and acid-base balance.
9. Evaluate the response in peak inspiratory pressure and plateau pressure when the flow waveform is changed.
10. Recommend the selection and initial settings for the various modes of pressure ventilation, including bilevel positive airway pressure, pressure support ventilation, pressure control ventilation, and Servo-controlled (dual modes) ventilation.
11. Identify a problem in pressure support ventilation from a pressure–time graph.
12. Measure plateau pressure using pressure–time and flow–time waveforms during pressure-controlled mechanical ventilation.
13. List the possible causes for a change in pressure during pressure-regulated volume control.
14. Identify the mode of ventilation based on the trigger, target, and cycle criteria.

The most common reason for instituting mechanical ventilation is to treat respiratory distress in patients who are unable to achieve effective gas exchange.[1] This goal can be accomplished by setting an appropriate tidal volume (V_T) and respiratory rate or frequency (f) to achieve a desired minute ventilation ($\dot{V}_E$). This chapter examines how $\dot{V}_E$ and related variables are set during the initiation of volume ventilation, and then focuses on the settings required to initiate positive pressure ventilation.

DETERMINING INITIAL VENTILATOR SETTINGS DURING VOLUME-CONTROLLED VENTILATION

Initiating volume control ventilation for a patient requires an understanding of the interaction of several key variables, including $\dot{V}_E$ settings (V_T and f), inspiratory gas flow, flow waveform, inspiratory-to-expiratory (I:E) ratio, pressure limit, inflation hold (inspiratory pause), and inspiratory pressure and positive end-expiratory pressure (PEEP).

The design characteristics of mechanical ventilator control panels can vary. For example, many have V_T and rate settings, such as the Puritan Bennett 840 (Covidien, Puritan Bennett, Boulder, Colo.), whereas other ventilators, such as the Servo-i (Maquet Inc, Wayne, N.J.), also allow the operator to set $\dot{V}_E$ and f. Some ventilator manufacturers provide time cycling and have controls for inspiratory time percentage, and still others control total cycle time (TCT).

It is important for clinicians charged with the responsibility of instituting mechanical ventilation to have a fundamental understanding of the various control variables available on intensive care unit (ICU) ventilators. Then regardless of the ventilator involved, they will possess enough information to make an informed decision about how to proceed. The following discussion begins with the basics: $\dot{V}_E$, V_T, and f. A more detailed discussion of initial ventilator setting for patients with specific cardiopulmonary and neuromuscular disorders is provided in Chapter 7.

Initial Settings During Volume-Controlled Ventilation

SETTING MINUTE VENTILATION

The primary goal of volume-controlled, continuous mandatory ventilation (VC-CMV) is to achieve a $\dot{V}_E$ that matches the patient's metabolic needs. A typical healthy person at rest has a total oxygen consumption ($\dot{V}O_2$) of about 250 mL/min, and a carbon dioxide production ($\dot{V}CO_2$) of about 200 mL/min. As the patient's metabolic rate increases, ventilation must change to meet the need for increased oxygen uptake and CO_2 removal (Box 6-1).

Metabolic rate is directly related to body mass and surface area in humans. Measurements of heat production (i.e., direct calorimetry) provide a reliable method to quantify metabolic rate; however, direct calorimetry requires a considerable amount of space and time commitment and is typically reserved for research purposes. Indirect calorimetry, which uses measurements of inspired and expired O_2 and CO_2 to estimate energy expenditure, can be accomplished with significantly less time and effort. Indeed advances in computer technology have made it relatively easy to perform indirect calorimetry in the clinical setting. For example, the Engström Carestation by GE (GE Healthcare, UK) has this technology incorporated into the ventilator's design, making it possible for the clinician to monitor continuously the $\dot{V}O_2$ and $\dot{V}CO_2$ at the bedside. (See Chapter 10 for more information about indirect calorimetry.)

A more commonly used method to estimate metabolic rate and caloric intake involves using equations that were derived from laboratory studies performed in the early part of the twentieth century by scientists like Harris and Benedict. With these equations, metabolic rate is estimated on the basis of an individual's gender and body surface area (BSA).[2] BSA can be calculated using the DuBois BSA formula: $BSA = 0.007184 \times Ht^{0.725} \times W^{0.425}$, where BSA = body surface area in square meters, Ht = body height in centimeters, and W = body weight in kilograms. (It can also be determined using a nomogram like the one shown in Fig. 6-1. Notice that this nomogram is based on the aforementioned DuBois BSA formula.)

As shown in Box 6-1, $\dot{V}_E$ can also be estimated using a patient's BSA. $\dot{V}_E$ is approximately equal to four times the BSA in men and

---

BOX 6-1   Determining Pressure, Tidal Volume, Respiratory Frequency, and Minute Ventilation to Establish Initial Ventilator Settings for Volume and Pressure Ventilation

Volume Control Ventilation

Minute Ventilation ($\dot{V}_E$)
Men $\dot{V}_E = 4 \times$ body surface area (BSA)
Women $\dot{V}_E = 3.5 \times$ BSA

Increase This by
5%/° F above 99° F or 10%/° C above 37° C
20% for metabolic acidosis
50% to 100% if resting energy expenditure is equally increased

Decrease This by
10%/° C between 35° C and 37° C

Tidal Volume (V_T)
Minimum of 6 mL/kg ideal body weight (IBW) (consider sigh or lung recruitment maneuver and high PEEP)*
Maximum of 8 mL/kg IBW (do not use sigh)**
Keep alveolar pressure <30 cm H_2O (assumes thoracic compliance is normal)

Respiratory Frequency (f)
$f = f = \dot{V}_E / V_T$
Respiratory rate typically ranges from 12 to 18 breaths per minute

Pressure Ventilation

Pressure Support Ventilation (PSV)
To overcome system resistance in the spontaneous mode (PSV or continuous positive airway pressure [CPAP]) or in the IMV mode, set pressure at peak inspiratory pressure (PIP) – ($P_{plateau}$), where $P_{plateau}$ is measured in a volume breath or at approximately 5 to 10 cm H_2O. To provide ventilatory support, set pressure to achieve a target V_T as described for VC-CMV.

Pressure Control Ventilation (PC-CMV)
Set pressure to achieve V_T as described for VC-CMV. Set frequency to achieve the same $\dot{V}_E$. $f = \dot{V}_E / V_T$.

Set inspiratory percentage to achieve an inspiratory/expiratory (I:E) ratio of greater than or equal to 1:2.

*For patients being treated for ARDS, lower tidal volumes (e.g., 4 mL/kg) may be necessary to ensure that the $P_{plateau}$ <30 cm H_2O. See Chapter 13 for additional information regarding the use of lung recruitment maneuvers in protective lung strategies used for the treatment of ARDS.
**In patients with neuromuscular disorders or cerebral disorders, a V_T of >10 mL/kg might be required, but $P_{plateau}$ should still be kept below 30 cm H_2O.

---

three and a half times the BSA in women. For example, the estimated $\dot{V}_E$ for an adult male patient with a BSA of 2.1 m^2 would be:

$$\dot{V}_E \text{ for a male} = 4 \times BSA = 4 \times 2.1\,m^2 = 8.4\,L/min$$

Notice that this calculation of $\dot{V}_E$ assumes that the individual is a typical healthy adult. The $\dot{V}_E$ must be adjusted for abnormal conditions, such as the presence of hypothermia or hyperthermia, hypermetabolism, and metabolic acidosis. Lung disorders that increase physiological dead space will also require an increase in $\dot{V}_E$.[2] For example, suppose that the patient already mentioned requires an

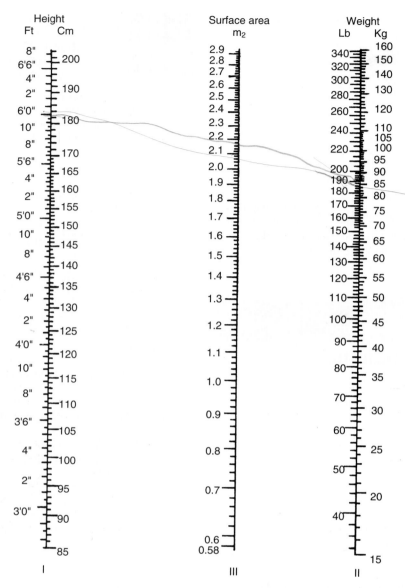

Fig. 6-1 Dubois body surface chart. To determine the body surface area (BSA), locate the height in inches or centimeters on scale I and weight in pounds or kilograms on scale II. Place a straight edge between these two points. Where the straight edge intersects, scale III determines BSA in square meters. (From Boothby WM, Sandiford RB: Nomographic charts for the calculation of the metabolic rate by the gasometry method, Boston Med Surg J 185:337, 1921.)

initial $\dot{V}_E$ of 8.4 L/min but has a temperature of 39° C. $\dot{V}_E$ would have to be increased by 10% for each degree above 37°: a total increase of 20% of 8.4 = 1.68; therefore, the new $\dot{V}_E$ would be 8.4 + 1.68 = 10.08 L/min.

Settings for V_T and f should therefore be derived from the initial calculation of $\dot{V}_E$ (4 × BSA for men and 3.5 × BSA for women) and adjusted if the patient demonstrates a pathologic condition like those mentioned above. V_T can be determined by the method described in the discussion that follows. To determine breathing frequency (f), divide the $\dot{V}_E$ by the V_T ($\dot{V}_E/V_T = f$) (Case Study 6-1).

In many cases, physicians order settings for mechanical ventilation that include volume and rate and do not typically specify $\dot{V}_E$. The respiratory therapist must keep in mind that the ordered rate and volume must reflect the $\dot{V}_E$ needs of the patient.

Case Study 6-1

Minute Ventilation ($\dot{V}_E$) Needs

A physician orders a tidal volume (V_T) of 500 mL and a rate of 12 breaths/min for a 25-year-old woman with a body surface area of 2.0 m². The estimated $\dot{V}_E$ will be: 3.5 × 2.0 = 7.0 L/min. What is the ordered $\dot{V}_E$ compared with the estimated $\dot{V}_E$ needed? If you were the respiratory therapist in this situation, how would you address the discrepancy between the physician's order and the actual $\dot{V}_E$ required?

BOX 6-2 Calculating Ideal Body Weight (IBW) for Women and Men

Women: IBW (lbs) = 105 + 5(H − 60),
where *H* is height in inches.
   For example, the IBW of a 66-inch-tall woman is 105 + 5(66 − 60) = 105 + 5(6) = 135 lb (61.4 kg). (To convert to kilograms, divide by 2.2.)
Men IBW (lbs) = 106 + 6(H − 60).
   For example, the IBW of a 66-inch-tall man is 106 + 6(66 − 60) = 106 + 6(6) = 142 lb (64.5 kg).

 CRITICAL CARE CONCEPT 6-1

Tidal Volume (V_T) and Ideal Body Weight (IBW)
What is the lowest and highest estimated V_T for a 5-foot 6-inch man (IBW = 65 kg)? What would the lowest and highest estimated tidal volume be for a 5-foot 6-inch woman?

 Case Study 6-2

Minute Ventilation ($\dot{V}_E$), Tidal Volume (V_T), and Respiratory Rate
A 6-foot (72-inch)-tall man weighs 190 lb and has a normal metabolic rate, temperature, and acid–base status. What is his body surface area and ideal body weight? What $\dot{V}_E$, V_T, and rate would be appropriate for this patient?

Tidal Volume and Rate

The normal spontaneous V_T for a healthy adult is about 5 to 7 mL/kg with a spontaneous respiratory rate of 12 to 18 breaths/min. $\dot{V}_E$ is about 100 mL/kg of ideal body weight (IBW).[3] Box 6-2 provides formulae that can be used to calculate IBW.[3]

   When determining V_T for ventilated patients, a range of 6 to 8 mL/kg of IBW is typically used for adults, and 4 to 8 mL/kg IBW for infants and children.[4-6] Lower V_T rates (e.g., 4 mL/kg IBW) have been successfully used to ventilate the lungs of adult patients with acute respiratory distress syndrome (ARDS). These lower V_T rates are described as protective strategies that minimize the damaging effects associated with overdistention of the alveoli.[7]

   It is important to understand that an adult's lungs do not get larger as he or she gains weight. For example, a 5-foot 6-inch adult male weighing 100 kg would require the same V_T as a 5-foot 6-inch adult male weighing 65 kg. Remember, however, that a heavier patient would have a higher metabolic rate and thus a higher $\dot{V}_E$. Critical Care Concept 6-1 provides an example of how to estimate tidal volumes based on IBW (Key Point 6-1). (It is interesting to note that the Radford nomogram [Fig. 6-2], which was used in the past by clinicians to estimate the set V_T is based on a V_T range of about 5 to 7 mL/kg IBW.)[8] (See Box 6-3 and Case Study 6-2).

Key Point 6-1 A person's tidal volume increases linearly with body weight up to that person's ideal body weight.

BOX 6-3   Tidal Volume (V_T) Settings

More than 50 years ago, Radford conducted an extensive study to determine normal V_T and rates in human subjects.[8] Radford's findings influenced early recommendations on setting tidal volumes during mechanical ventilation.[9,10] It is worth mentioning that V_Ts derived from Radford's nomogram are low (range, 5 to 7 mL/kg). For example, a 190-lb, 6-foot man breathing at a rate of 10 breaths/min would have a V_T setting of 600 mL (7.4 mL/kg ideal body weight [IBW]) based on Radford's nomogram.

   Early studies in anesthesia, however, showed that using low V_T very rapidly resulted in atelectasis, particularly in the lung bases. An often cited study by Bendixon and colleagues, published in 1964, further demonstrated that a sustained high-pressure inspiration or "sigh" breath could help reverse atelectasis caused by breathing low V_T.[11] Interestingly the actual V_T rates were not reported in this study. The study defined a sigh breath as a sustained high-pressure breath, not just as a single breath with a large V_T.

   Beginning in the 1970s and continuing until the 1990s it was common practice for clinicians to use high V_T settings (e.g., 10 to 15 mL/kg of IBW) for all patients. This practice may have resulted from the fear that using a low V_T would cause atelectasis. Unfortunately, clinicians at that time were unaware of the potential of lung injury and were more concerned with achieving an appropriate V_T and maintaining acceptable arterial carbon dioxide (P_aCO_2) and arterial oxygen (P_aO_2) values. Their focus, while intended for the good of the patient, was nevertheless wrong.

   Preliminary laboratory studies conducted in the 1990s, however, showed that high volumes along with high pressures could cause significant damage to lung tissue (see Chapter 17). In 2000, a landmark multicenter clinical trial conducted involving over 800 patients with acute lung injury and acute respiratory distress syndrome found conclusive evidence that using a V_T setting of 6 mL/kg based on the **predicted** (ideal) body weight (PBW) had a lower mortality rate for this patient population than a V_T of 12 mL/kg PBW.[7] A number of more recent clinical studies conducted to better define the most effective V_T settings to use during mechanical ventilation have corroborated these finding and shown that there are significant benefits associated with using lower a V_T.[3-6]

   Regardless of the method used for selecting the V_T for a patient, it is important for clinicians to be aware of four risks during the setup of V_T:
1. Overdistention of lung tissue
2. Repeated opening and closing (recruitment/derecruitment) of alveoli
3. Atelectasis formation
4. Inadequate V_T setting

An alternative method for calculating initial V_T settings is to use **predicted** values for body weight rather than calculations of IBW. The predicted body weight of male patients can be calculated using the following equation: 50 + 0.91 (centimeters of height − 152.4). For female patients the predicted body weight can be determined using the following equation: 45.5 + 0.91 (centimeters of height × 152.4).[7]

   Recommended tidal volumes for ventilated patients vary depending on the lung pathology. For patients with normal lungs,

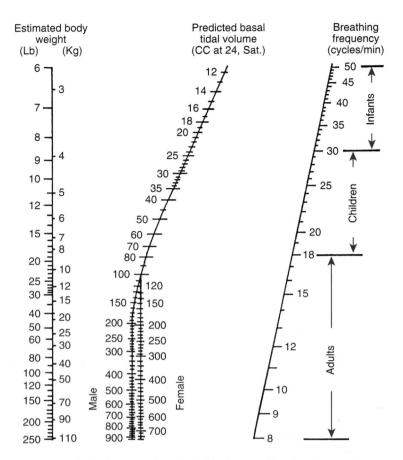

Fig. 6-2 Breathing nomogram (Radford's nomogram) predicted tidal volume V_T and breathing frequency. Corrections to be applied to predict basal (minimum) V_T. Daily activity (patient not in a coma): add 10%; fever: add 5% per ° F above 99° F (rectal) or add 10% per ° C above 37° C (rectal); altitude: add 5% for every 2000 feet above sea level; artificial airway: subtract the volume equal to half the body weight in pounds or subtract 1 mL/kg of body weight; add equipment dead space volume; metabolic acidosis: add 20%. (From Radford EP, Ferris BG Jr, Driete BC: Clinical use of a nomogram to estimate proper ventilation during artificial respirations, N Engl J Med 21:877, 1954.)

such as patients with a drug overdose or patients with the postoperative effects of anesthesia, an initial V_T of 6 to 8 mL/kg and a rate of 10 to 20 breaths/min is generally accepted.[3] In patients with chronic obstructive pulmonary disease (COPD) and asthma, in which airway obstruction and resistance are high, an initial V_T of 6 to 8 mL/kg with a rate of 8 to 12 breaths/min is acceptable.[3,12-14] In patients with chronic or acute restrictive disease, such as pulmonary fibrosis or ARDS, an initial V_T of 4 to 6 mL/kg with a rate of 15 to 25 breaths/min is indicated.[7] As suggested in restrictive disease, lower V_T and higher rates are used. However, high rates may not provide sufficient time for exhalation (short T_E), and air can be trapped in the lungs at the end of exhalation, resulting in intrinsic PEEP (auto-PEEP).[15] The V_T should be adjusted to maintain plateau pressure less than 30 cm H_2O and rates adjusted to minimize auto-PEEP.

A V_T of more than 9 to 10 mL/kg is not recommended because of the risk of high pressures and accompanying overdistention and trauma to the lung, in addition to other complications. Low volume settings (4 to 8 mL/kg) are beneficial in restrictive disease and may help prevent high pressures and alveolar overdistention. It is worth mentioning that using volumes as low as 4 mL/kg may contribute to atelectasis. Using tidal volumes this low may require a recruitment maneuver or sigh breaths to avoid atelectasis. (See

Chapters 7 and 13 for additional information.) Use of lower V_T may be especially important in patients receiving PEEP therapy to avoid high pressures and overdistention[16,17] (Key Point 6-2). Box 6-3 provides some important background on how initial V_T settings were selected for this text.[3,7,9-14] Chapter 13 provides additional information on managing patients with PEEP.

> **Key Point** **6-2** When setting tidal volume (V_T) and rate, the goal is not to focus so much on the exact V_T and rate, but to focus on using settings that do not harm the patient. Maintaining plateau pressure lower than 30 cm H_2O is very important. In some cases it may even be necessary to let P_aCO_2 rise and pH fall outside the patient's normal values to avoid lung injury.[1]

Tubing Compliance

The V_T set on the ventilator control panel represents the amount of gas sent to the ventilator circuit; however, not all of this volume reaches the patient. Some of the gas volume will not be delivered to the patient because of leaks and the effects of tubing compliance.

The **tubing compliance** (C_T), or **system compressibility,** reflects the volume (in milliliters) of gas compressed in the ventilator circuit for every centimeter of water pressure generated by the ventilator during the inspiratory phase: C_T = change in volume divided by change in pressure ($\Delta V/\Delta P$) in mL/cm H_2O.

As pressure builds in the ventilator circuit during inspiration, the circuit expands along with the patient's lungs; therefore, the total volume that goes to the circuit never reaches the patient. As expiration begins, the volume of gas trapped under pressure in the patient circuit flows out the expiratory valve with the air that leaves the patient's lungs. This volume (exhaled volume from the ventilator tubing and the patient's lungs) is often referred to as the *exhaled V_T* .

The volume of gas in the circuit is referred to as the **compressible volume,** or the volume lost as a result of C_T. The compressible volume varies depending on the type of circuit used and is determined for each ventilator system before its use. Calculating compressible volume is especially important in infants, children, or very small patients because of the small V_T they require. A slight change in tidal volume may be insignificant for an adult, but it can be critical for an infant during mechanical ventilation. Thus practitioners routinely use small-bore, rigid circuits with infants because these types of circuits are not very compliant. These ventilator circuits typically have low C_Ts and therefore have low compressible volumes. (NOTE: C_T for a patient's circuit changes slightly as the circuit warms, but this amount is usually not significant.)

Current ICU ventilators (e.g., Hamilton G5 [Hamilton Medical, Switzerland], the Servo-i [Maquet, Inc, Wayne, N.J.], Dräger 500 [Dräger Medical Inc, Telford, Pa.], Puritan Bennett (PB) 980 [Covidien, Mansfield, Mass.], and CareFusion AVEA [CareFusion, Yorba Linda, Calif.]) have the capability of measuring and correcting for C_T. During start-up tests of the system, these ventilators calculate the compressibility of the ventilator circuit. The operator can choose to use this correction or simply ignore it. If correction for C_T is accepted, the ventilator measures the peak pressure during ventilation, calculates the volume lost to the patient circuit, and adds that volume to the set V_T. When the data are displayed on the ventilator, the exhaled V_T measured again corrects for C_T. For example, if the set V_T is 500 mL and the loss of volume is 50 mL, the ventilator actually delivers 550 mL, although it displays 500 mL as V_T inspired and 500 mL of V_T expired. The operator never actually "sees" the correction being made. It is important to recognize that ventilators perform this function in different ways. Therefore, the clinician should understand how this function operates for the ventilator being used.

If a ventilator without this capability is being used, calculation of C_T can be determined during initial setup by doing the following procedure prior to connecting the patient to the ventilator:
1. Confirm there are no leaks in the circuit.
2. Set a low V_T (100 to 200 mL), set PEEP at 0 cm H_2O, and set inspiratory pause at 2 seconds.
3. Place the high-pressure limit on the highest possible setting (e.g., 120 cm H_2O) so the breath does not pressure cycle.
4. Manually trigger the ventilator into inspiration while occluding the Y-connector.
5. Record the static or plateau pressure ($P_{plateau}$).
6. Measure the volume at the exhalation valve using a respirometer.
7. Calculate C_T by dividing measured volume by measured static pressure.

Box 6-4 provides a practice problem for calculating volume lost to C_T.

BOX 6-4   Calculating Volume Lost to Tubing Compliance

A patient's estimated tidal volume (V_T) is 400 mL. Her peak pressure reading during inspiration is 30 cm H_2O and tubing compliance (C_T) is 2.9 mL/cm H_2O. What is the actual V_T delivery to the patient?

Volume lost = 2.9 mL/cm H_2O × 30 cm H_2O = 87 mL; actual volume received by the patient = 400 − 87 mL = 313 mL. To compensate, set V_T is increased to about 487 mL to deliver the 400 mL desired. As mentioned earlier, C_T is very important when V_T settings are very low (<300 mL), such as when setting the V_T for infants and small children.

Mechanical Dead Space Considerations

Another consideration when setting the V_T is the effects of mechanical dead space. **Mechanical dead space** (V_{Dmech}) is defined as the volume of gas that is rebreathed during ventilation. For example, to add flexibility to the patient-ventilator connection, clinicians sometimes add a 6-inch piece of corrugated tubing between the Y-connector and the endotracheal tube connector. When the patient exhales, some of the exhaled gas will occupy the 6 inches of tubing. As the patient inhales during the next breath, the first part of the breath will contain end-expiratory gas from the previous breath, which has a lower oxygen level and a higher carbon dioxide level.

A number of devices can decrease or increase the amount of V_{Dmech} added to the breathing circuit. For example, the use of an endotracheal tube slightly reduces V_{Dmech} by about 1 mL/kg IBW because the tube bypasses the upper airway (mouth and nasal passages). In contrast, the addition of a Y-connector between the ventilator and the patient may add about 75 mL of V_{Dmech}. Interestingly these two factors tend to balance each other. Heat-moisture exchanger (HME) inserted between the endotracheal tube and Y-connector adds V_{Dmech} to the circuit (20 to 90 mL). Fortunately, the low dead space volume associated with these devices (HME of 20 mL) is usually not of clinical significance for adult patients (This is a small dead space volume in relation to an adult V_T and usually does not alter P_aCO_2. However, with a higher-volume HME [90 mL], P_aCO_2 may increase above previous values.)[13]

In the past, respiratory therapists added V_{Dmech} to increase the P_aCO_2 of patients who were hyperventilating and developed a respiratory alkalosis that could not be corrected by other methods. The effectiveness of this practice has been questioned by a number of clinicians.

Relationship of Tidal Volume, Flow, Total Cycle Time, and Inspiratory-to-Expiratory Ratio

Each ventilator has specific settings to select for VC-CMV. For example, the Puritan Bennett 840 allows the operator to set V_T, f, and flow, and the Servo-i allows the operator to set the rate and inspiratory time, or inspiratory-to-expiratory (I:E) ratio.

An understanding of the interrelation of inspiratory flow, inspiratory time (T_I), expiratory time, total cycle time (TCT), and I:E ratio will help the clinician to effectively ventilate a patient regardless of the type of equipment being used. Box 6-5 includes the equations that describe a variety of these interrelations.

Interrelation of Tidal Volume, Flow Rate, Inspiratory Time, Expiratory Time, Total Cycle Time, and Respiratory Rate

I. Total cycle time (TCT) equals inspiratory time (T_I) plus expiratory time:

$$TCT = T_I + T_E$$

II. Respiratory rate (f) equals 1 min (60 seconds) divided by TCT.

$$f = \frac{1\,min}{TCT} = \frac{60\,sec}{TCT\,(sec)} = breaths/min$$

  a. Calculate TCT from f.

$$TCT = 60\,sec/f$$

III. Inspiratory to expiratory ratio equals inspiratory time divided by expiratory time.

$$I:E = T_I/T_E$$

Remember: $TCT = T_I + T_E$ and $TCT - T_I = T_E$

IV. To calculate T_E from f and T_I:

$$f = 60\,sec/TCT \text{ and } TCT = T_I + T_E$$

$$T_E = TCT - T_I$$

V. Reducing the I:E ratio to its simplest form: Divide the numerator and denominator by T_I.

$$I:E = \frac{T_I/T_I}{T_E/T_I}$$

VI. Determine the I:E when inverse ratio ventilation is used: I:E for inverse ventilation equals the division of both the numerator and the denominator by the expiratory time.

$$I:E = \frac{T_I/T_E}{T_E/T_E}$$

VII. Calculate T_I, T_E, and TCT from I:E and f.

$$TCT = T_I + T_E \text{ and } f = 60\,sec/TCT$$

$$f = 60\,sec/(T_I + T_E)$$

$$T_I + T_E = 60\,sec/f$$

VIII. Calculate T_I from V_T and flow ($\dot{V}$)

$$T_I = V_T/\dot{V}$$

IX. Calculate V_T from T_I and $\dot{V}$.

$$V_T = \dot{V} \times T_I$$

X. Calculate $\dot{V}$ from V_T and T_I.

$$\dot{V} = V_T/T_I$$

Fortunately most modern ventilators automatically perform these calculations and display them as measured and calculated values.

Calculating Total Cycle Time and Respiratory Rate

Some ventilators use T_I and T_E or TCT to determine the respiratory rate (or ventilator frequency). To determine these values, calculate the length of the respiratory cycle or the TCT ($TCT = T_I + T_E$) and determine the number of cycles that occur in 1 minute (see Box 6-5, I, II, and IV). For example, if the T_I is 2 seconds and the T_E is 4 seconds, then:

$$TCT = T_I + T_E = 2\,sec + 4\,sec = 6\,sec$$

$$60\,sec/TCT = f$$

$$60\,sec/6\,sec = 10 \text{ breaths in a minute}$$

Calculating Inspiratory-to-Expiratory Ratio

Some ventilators allow the clinician to set either a fixed T_I and rate, or a fixed I:E.* For example, the Servo-i ventilator requires the respiratory therapist to set a T_I. If the rate is set at 10 breaths/min, the TCT is 6 seconds (60 sec/[10 breaths] = 6 sec/breath). If the T_I is set at 2 seconds then the expiratory time is 4 seconds (T_E will be TCT – T_I = 6 sec – 2 sec = 4 sec). The resultant I:E ratio will therefore be 1:2 (T_I/T_E = 2 sec/4 sec = 2:4 or 1:2) (see Box 6-5, I through V).

The I:E ratio is typically expressed so that the T_I is equal to 1. For example, if the I:E ratio is 2:3, then it is expressed as 1:1.5. Dividing the numerator and denominator by T_I reduces the expression to 1:X (see Box 6-5, V).

I:E ratios of 2:1 or 3:1 are called inverse I:E ratios. When I:E ratios are inversed (I greater than E), then T_E takes on the value of 1. For example, if the T_I is 3 seconds and the T_E is 2 seconds, then the I:E ratio is 3:2 or 1.5:1 (see Box 6-5, VI). (NOTE: In previous generation ventilators (e.g., Puritan Bennett 7200 [Covidien, Nellcor and Puritan Bennett, Boulder Colo.]), the digital display of I:E was expressed as 1 : X; thus inverse ratios will appear, for example, as 1:0.5, rather than 2:1.)]

Using inverse ratios can cause significant complications, such as increases in mean airway pressure ($\overline{P}_{aw}$) and physiological dead space, decreases in venous return and cardiac output, and increased air trapping (auto-PEEP). For this reason, I:E ratios are usually set at 1:1.5 to 1:4, so that expiration is longer than inspiration, and the adverse effects of positive pressure are reduced. (NOTE: Inverse I:E ratios have been successfully used in some circumstances, such as to improve oxygenation in patients with ARDS.)

Inspiratory Time, Tidal Volume, and Flow

T_I can be determined if V_T and flow are known and the flow pattern is a constant or square waveform. If V_T is 0.5 L and flow is 2 L/sec, then T_I equals 0.5 L/2 L/sec, or 0.25 seconds. The flow control on adult ventilators is usually calibrated in L/min, so the value for flow needs to be converted to L/sec. For example, a flow of 30 L/min equals 30 L/60s or 0.5 L/sec.[†]

---

*Because ventilation software can be updated frequently, users should check their equipment to determine actual function.

[†]Specifically: (30 L/1 × 1/60 sec) = (30 L/1 min × 1 min/60 sec) = 0.5 L/sec.

gas distribution. Conversely, slower flows may reduce peak pressures, improve gas distribution, and increase $\bar{P}_{aw}$ at the expense of increasing T_I. Unfortunately shorter T_E can lead to air trapping, and using a longer T_I may also cause cardiovascular side effects.[18] In reality actual normal inspiratory times have never been measured, and much of clinical practice involved in setting appropriate T_I requires clinician observation of the patient's response to set values. These may require adjustments.

In general the goal should be to use the shortest T_I possible. Achieving a short T_I is usually not difficult to attain in patients with normal lungs. As a beginning point, flow is normally set to deliver inspiration in about 1 second (range 0.8 to 1.2 seconds).[3,13] An I:E ratio of 1:2 or less (usually about 1:4) is also recommended. This can be achieved with an initial peak flow setting of about 60 L/min (range 40 to 80 L/min). It is important to remember that the flow must be set to meet a patient's inspiratory demand so the spontaneously breathing patient is not trying to breathe in without the ventilator supplying adequate gas flow (see Fig. 5-4).[19]

During VC-CMV where patient-triggered breaths are present, the patient's respiratory rate may actually vary depending on flow and T_I setting. For example, when V_T is constant and the flow setting is increased, T_I will be shorter and the patient may actually begin to increase the rate at which he or she triggers the ventilator. Thus T_I can affect breath frequency when patient triggering is present.[20] The reason this occurs is not known at this time, but clinicians should be aware of this phenomenon.

A long T_I (requiring 3 to 4 time constants) has been shown to improve ventilation in nonhomogeneous lungs like those seen in ARDS.[21] Fast flows (i.e., requiring fewer time constants to fill the lungs) may benefit patients with increased airway resistance (R_{aw}), as in COPD, providing longer T_E, which in turn will reduce or prevent the risk of air trapping (long T_E of 3 to 4 time constants). Tobin has reported that using flow rates up to 100 L/min can improve gas exchange in patients with COPD by providing a longer T_E.[22] Flows that are set too high, however, can result in uneven distribution of inspired air in the lung, and also cause immediate and persistent tachypnea, in addition to increased peak inspiratory pressures[23] (Key Point 6-3).

> **Key Point 6-3** The clinician must carefully adjust the flow and flow pattern to suit the patient's ventilatory needs.

Flow Patterns

Figure 6-3 shows examples of flow patterns available on ICU ventilators. Selecting the most appropriate flow pattern and ventilator

Case Study 6-3

Inspiratory/Expiratory Ratio (I:E) and Flow

You are asked to ventilate a 63-year-old woman who is diagnosed with severe congestive heart failure. She is 5 foot 8 inches tall and weighs 185 lb. She is orally intubated with a 7.5-mm endotracheal tube. Her arterial blood gases on a nonrebreathing mask are pH = 7.18, P_aCO_2 = 83 mm Hg, P_aO_2 = 98 mm Hg, HCO_3^- = 31 mEq/L. What recommendations would you make regarding her initial ventilator settings of V_T, f, I:E, and flow?

CRITICAL CARE CONCEPT 6-2

Inspiratory Flow in a Time-Cycled Ventilator

A time-cycled ventilator is set with the following parameters: V_T = 500 mL (0.5 L), f = 12 breaths/min, and I:E = 1:4. If a constant flow waveform is used, what is the inspiratory gas flow?

Conversely, V_T can be determined when T_I and flow are known and flow is constant: (V_T = flow × T_I). If T_I is 1 second and flow is 0.5 L/sec, V_T = (1 second) × (0.5 L/sec) = 0.5 L (see Box 6-5, VII and VIII).

Flow, Tidal Volume, and Inspiratory Time

Flow can be determined if V_T and T_I are known. For example, if V_T is 500 mL and T_I is 1 second, the flow equals V_T/T_I, which is 500 mL/1 sec, or 0.5 L/($\frac{1}{60}$th of a minute), or 30 L/min (multiply numerator and denominator by 60 to convert to minutes) (see Box 6-5, IX). These examples assume that flow is constant. (See Case Study 6-3 and Critical Care Concept 6-2.)

Inspiratory Flow and Flow Patterns

During VC-CMV, the clinician may have the option to select a variety of ventilator flows and flow patterns. These selections are reviewed in this section.

Rate of Gas Flow

As previously discussed, the flow setting on a mechanical ventilator determines how fast the inspired gas will be delivered to the patient. During controlled mechanical ventilation (CMV), high flows shorten T_I and may result in higher peak pressures and poor

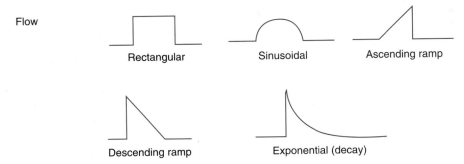

Fig. 6-3 Flow–time waveforms can take on a variety of forms. The most common are rectangular (constant or square) and descending ramp (decelerating ramp).

Tidal Volume (V_T), Rate, Inspiratory Time (T_I), and Flow on the LTV 1000

The Pulmonetics LTV 1000 ventilator has controls for V_T, rate, and a T_I setting. Flow is determined by the set V_T and T_I. (Flow $= V_T/T_I$). Inspiratory flow is a descending ramp during volume-targeted mandatory breaths. The peak flow is determined by the ventilator so that V_T is delivered during the set T_I. Inspiration ends when flow decreases to 50% of peak or 10 L/min, whichever is highest.

Total cycle time (TCT) can be calculated using the following equation: TCT = 60/f. T_E becomes TCT minus T_I (T_E = TCT − T_I). Suppose, for example, that the inspiratory time is set at 1.0 seconds and the rate is set at 12. The TCT will equal 60/12 or 5 seconds. T_E equals 5 seconds − 1 second or 4 seconds and the I:E is therefore 1:4.

TABLE **6-1** **An Example of a Time-Cycled Ventilator***

Flow Waveform	Peak Flow Value (L/min)	Percentage of Set Flow for Constant Flow Pattern
Constant	60	100
Descending ramp	78	133
Sine	94.2	157
Modified sine	78.9	133

*Using V_T = 1000 mL (1.0 L); T_I = 1 second.

rate depends on the patient's lung condition. For example, postoperative patients recovering from anesthesia may have very modest flow demands, whereas a young adult with pneumonia and a strong hypoxemic drive would have a very strong flow demand. The most common flow patterns used clinically are the constant flow and descending (decelerating) flow waveforms.

Constant flow. Clinicians often select the constant flow pattern simply because it is most familiar to them, or it is the only one available on the ventilator in use. Constant flow patterns are also called rectangular and square waveform. For initiating ventilation, a rectangular (constant) flow pattern is acceptable.[13] Generally a constant flow pattern provides the shortest T_I of all the available flow patterns with an equivalent peak flow rate setting.

Descending ramp. The amount of gas flow delivered at the beginning of the breath is probably the major determinant of patient effort and work of breathing. A descending (decelerating) flow waveform has a distinct advantage compared with other waveform patterns. With a descending pattern, flow is greatest at the beginning of inspiration, when patient flow demand is the highest. The descending waveform occurs naturally in pressure ventilation. Box 6-6 shows an example in which the ventilator automatically sets the flow at a descending ramp and calculates the flow rate based on V_T and T_I during VC-CMV.

Ascending ramp. The ascending ramp provides a progressive increase in flow. The ascending ramp is currently not used by most clinicians, and is available only on a few older-generation ventilators. There are no compelling studies that support the use of the ascending flow ramp.[6]

Sine flow. The sine flow pattern produces a tapered flow at the end of inspiratory phase. Although it has been suggested that this type of flow pattern may contribute to a more even distribution of gas in the lungs than the flow of the constant flow ventilator, it is not commonly used clinically and additional clinical studies will be required to verify its efficacy.[24] $\overline{P}_{aw}$ and peak pressures are similar to those seen with the sine and square wave patterns although peak pressures are higher with the sine wave than the square flow when airway resistance is increased, such as in acute asthma.[25]

Comparison of descending ramp and constant flow. Most clinical studies designed to investigate the effects of using various ventilator waveforms have compared the constant waveform with the descending (decelerating) ramp. As one changes from a constant to a descending ramp, peak pressure is lower, and $\overline{P}_{aw}$ is higher.* Studies comparing the descending flow pattern with the constant flow pattern suggest that the descending flow pattern improves the distribution of gas in the lungs, reduces dead space, and increases oxygenation by increasing mean and plateau airway pressures.[3,13,21,25-27] It is important to remember that in situations where plateau pressure ($P_{plateau}$) is critical, changing to a descending ramp to reduce peak pressures may increase the $\overline{P}_{aw}$.

Concerns about high peak inspiratory pressure and mean airway pressure. The clinician must decide whether $\overline{P}_{aw}$ is more important for the patient than are concerns of high peak inspiratory pressure (PIP) when selecting a particular waveform. When R_{aw} and flows are high, peak pressures will be high if an ascending flow pattern is used. Much of this pressure is dissipated in overcoming the R_{aw} and may not reach the alveolar level.[25] Thus high peak pressures do not always increase the risk of damage to lung parenchyma. An example of a patient population in which this can occur involves patients with acute asthma experiencing severe bronchospasm, mucosal edema, and increased secretion production. It is important to recognize, however, there is a risk that some of the high pressures may reach normal lung areas, which could be damaging in this group of patients.[14]

Effects of changing flow pattern in time- vs. volume-cycled ventilators. For time-cycled machines (e.g., Hamilton Galileo G5 [Hamilton Medical, Switzerland], Servo-i, Dräger Evita-4), changing from constant flow to another flow pattern does not change the I:E ratio. However, it does change the peak flow required to deliver the volume in the time provided (T_I). With any ventilator, changing from one waveform to another can vary the peak flow delivery and the distribution of flow. Table 6-1 shows an example of how peak flow varies between four different flow patterns in a time-cycled situation.

In volume-cycled ventilators, changing from a constant flow to a descending flow pattern does not change the peak flow selected. It does, however, change the T_I and I:E ratio (Fig. 6-4). Consequently the clinician may have to change the peak flow setting to accomplish volume delivery at a better I:E ratio. Table 6-2 shows

*T_I will also be longer unless the ventilator is time cycled.

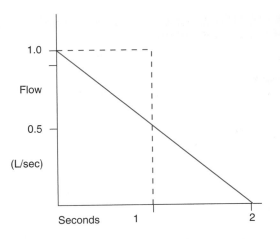

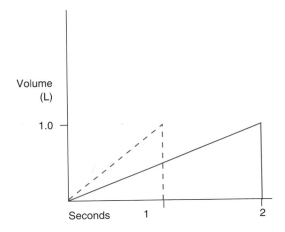

Fig. 6-4 Graphs showing flow and volume delivery in a volume-cycled ventilator with a peak flow set at 1 L/sec (60 L/min). Changing the flow waveform from constant *(dashed line)* to descending ramp *(solid line)* provides the same volume but increases inspiratory time. (Note: Ventilators do not usually allow flow to decrease to zero. It is used here only to simplify the concept.)

TABLE **6-2**	**An Example of a Volume-(Flow–Time) Cycled Ventilator: the Puritan Bennett 840**

Flow Waveform Selected	Determination of Inspiratory Time (T_I Flow Set at 60 L/min)
Constant	$T_I = (V_T)/\text{flow}$
Descending ramp	Begins at 60 L/min; ends at 5 L/min
If flow is set too low or volume too high to be achieved, and the inspiratory-to-expiratory (I:E) ratio becomes greater than 1:1, the ventilator will give a visual warning and a message to "decrease the rate." The alarm becomes audible when the I:E is 3:1 (displayed as "1:0.3").	

V_T is constant. Peak flow does not exceed its set value.

an example of what occurs with the Puritan Bennett 840 ventilator (Covidien, Nellcor and Puritan Bennett, Boulder, Colo.), which cycles based on volume (i.e., flow/time).

With the Maquet Servo-i ventilator, there is no flow waveform selector or peak flow control. During VC-CMV the machine provides a constant (rectangular) waveform. The amount of flow

BOX **6-7**	**Summary of Findings from Flow Waveform Studies**

When initiating mechanical ventilation, most clinicians will choose to start with a descending (decelerating) ramp or a constant (rectangular) waveform for the following reasons:
- The mean airway pressure is higher with descending flow waveforms.
- The peak inspiratory pressure is higher with ascending flow waveforms and lower with descending flow waveforms.
- Descending waveforms improve gas distribution.
- Descending waveforms improve arterial oxygenation.

delivered is based on the V_T selected and the T_I. The flow also varies with patient demand regardless of the method of ventilation. When the patient's inspiratory needs exceed the flow provided and pressure begins to drop by 2 cm H_2O below the measured airway pressure, the ventilator provides additional flow to the patient. Thus volume delivery is not the set value, but rather is influenced by the patient's flow demands. The volume set by the operator becomes the minimum volume. Other more recently released ventilators also provide this feature.

In summary, clinicians must familiarize themselves with how a ventilator functions when selecting peak flow and waveform pattern. When selecting a flow pattern, it is reasonable to assume that there is not one set prescribed pattern or rate of flow that is best for all patients. It is important to match the pattern and rate of gas flow to the patient's needs. Box 6-7 summarizes basic findings in flow waveform studies. The following points can provide some guidance when selecting a flow waveform:
- In patients with normal lung function, flow pattern selection is not a critical issue; descending and constant flow patterns are effective.
- In patients with hypoxemia and low lung compliance (C_L), the descending flow pattern may be beneficial by maintaining low peak pressures and high $\overline{P}_{aw}$, and improving gas distribution.[27,28]
- In patients with high R_{aw}, the descending pattern is more likely to deliver a set V_T at a lower pressure and provide for better distribution of air through the lung than a constant flow.[26-29]

SETTING THE MINUTE VENTILATION: SPECIAL CONSIDERATIONS

Practical considerations for setting a desired $\dot{V}_E$ have been discussed, but a few precautions should be considered before implementing these procedures. An optimum inspiratory flow and flow pattern may exist for every patient. No prescribed formula can be applied to ensure the best possible results for all patients.[29,30] The variability in results related to setting these parameters is influenced by the condition of the patient's lungs and conductive airways and the patient's changing metabolic needs.

Consider a situation where a patient's P_aO_2 falls and his P_aCO_2 rises, while his $\dot{V}_E$ increases. Several reasons could account for this type of situation, including the presence of auto-PEEP, poor ventilation-to-perfusion ($\dot{V}/\dot{Q}$) matching in the nonhomogeneous lung, and changes in venous return. Resolution of this situation may require changing gas flow and/or pattern, V_T, f, or I:E ratio. Using a mode of ventilation that allows some spontaneous breathing may also benefit the patient in this type of situation by allowing the spontaneously breathing patient to have some control over ventilation. There is no "bottom line" and no easy prescription. Management of the patient on mechanical ventilation is both an art and a science requiring the use of sound judgment.

INSPIRATORY PAUSE DURING VOLUME VENTILATION

The inspiratory pause or inflation hold (also called *end-inspiratory pause*) is a maneuver that can be performed by preventing the expiratory valve from opening for a short time at the end of inspiration, when the inspiratory valve is also closed. Most ICU ventilators have an inspiratory pause button or control. As mentioned in Chapter 1, the inspiratory pause maneuver is used to obtain measurements of $P_{plateau}$, which allows estimation of the alveolar pressure (P_{alv}) for the calculation of static compliance (Key Point 6-4).

> **Key Point 6-4** Plateau pressure can only be accurately measured if the patient is not actively breathing so that a stable pressure reading can be obtained.

Inspiratory pauses can also be selected for use with each mandatory breath to improve the distribution of air throughout the lungs regardless of the type of flow pattern used. It is believed that an inspiratory pause provides a longer inspiratory time, which in turn provides optimum ventilation/perfusion ($\dot{V}/\dot{Q}$) matching and reduces dead space to tidal volume ratios (V_D/V_T ratios).[31,32] Note that this maneuver must be used with care, or not at all, in patients with COPD and flow limitation. Inspiratory pause with each breath is not commonly used in clinical practice because it may significantly increase $\overline{P}_{aw}$ and reduce pulmonary blood flow.[33]

Clinical Scenario: Ventilatory Support Postmyocardial Infarction

Following admission to a hospital for myocardial infarction, a 55-year-old man is intubated and placed on ventilatory support. The patient's IBW is 70 kg and BSA is 1.5 m^2. The physician requests the VC-CMV mode. What $\dot{V}_E$, V_T, rate, flow, and flow pattern would be appropriate? A $\dot{V}_E$ of $4 \times 1.5 = 6.0$ L/min is an appropriate starting point. A V_T of 6 mL/kg would equal 420 mL for this patient. A minimum rate setting would be the $\dot{V}_E$ divided by the V_T or 6.0 L/0.42 L = 14.2 or 14 breaths/min. Because no changes in body metabolism such as a fever are evident, we assume these initial settings would be appropriate. No chronic pulmonary disease was mentioned, so we assume a moderate rate setting would be adequate. A flow of 40 L/min or 40 L/60 sec or 0.67 L/sec. using a descending flow pattern would provide sufficient time for exhalation to occur. What is the T_I in this case? Because the V_T is 0.42 L, $T_I = V_T$/flow or $T_I = 0.42$ L/(0.67 L/sec) = 0.63 sec. The TCT is 60 sec/(14 breaths/min) = 4.3 sec/breath. $T_E = TCT - T_I = 4.3$ sec − 0.63 sec = 3.67 sec. T_I is 0.63 seconds and T_E is 3.67 seconds, which is an adequate time for exhalation. Note that this is a fairly short T_I for an adult patient and may need to be increased.

Clinical Scenario: Ventilator Required?

A 45-year-old male receiving VC-CMV ventilation has a V_T of 800 mL and a set rate of 8 breaths/min. The actual total rate is 15 breaths/min because the patient is triggering additional breaths. Flow is set at 40 L/min using a constant flow waveform. Inspiratory pressure actually stays in the negative range (below baseline) during most of inspiration and finally peaks at 60 cm H_2O. The respiratory therapist is unable to obtain a pause pressure to determine $P_{plateau}$ because the patient is actively breathing.

Using the actual rate (15 breaths/min), determine T_I. Total cycle time is 60 sec/(15 breaths/min) = 4 sec/breath. Flow is 40 L/min or 40 L/60 sec = 0.67 L/sec. $T_I = V_T$/flow or 0.8 L/(0.67 L/sec) = 1.19 sec. $T_E = TCT − T_I = 4$ sec − 1.19 sec = 2.81 sec. The I:E ratio is about 1:3, which should be an adequate amount of time for exhalation.

The C_T is 3 mL/cm H_2O and was determined when the ventilator was set up. How much volume is lost to tubing compliance? The peak pressure is 60 cm H_2O, so the lost volume is $C_T \times PIP = 3$ mL/cm $H_2O \times 60$ cm $H_2O = 180$ mL. Of the 800 mL V_T, 180 mL is lost in the circuit and is not delivered to the patient. What is the volume of gas delivered to the patient? 800 mL − 180 = 620 mL is delivered to the patient. How can the respiratory therapist correct for this loss of volume delivery to the patient? The respiratory therapist can either set the ventilator to automatically compensate for C_T, if it has that feature, or manually adjust the set volume. For example, adding about 200 mL to the set volume would help compensate this loss. It is important to remember that making these adjustments will increase the set V_T and also increase the patient's PIP.

In this example, the patient's problem occurs during inspiration. Why does the pressure waveform demonstrate a negative deflection during inspiration? Perhaps the flow is not adequate to meet the patient's demand. The respiratory therapists readjusted the flow to 100 L/min, but this change did not improve the situation, and the therapist reports that occasionally "he seems to trigger two tidal volumes during one inspiratory effort." What would you suggest?

There are several possible solutions. Switching to PC-CMV and adjusting the pressure to achieve the original V_T or even a slightly higher volume might be appropriate. Pressure ventilation modes are more likely to deliver a flow that meets the patient demands because the ventilator can provide all the flow needed to maintain the set pressure. Another option would be to place the patient on continuous positive airway pressure (CPAP) for a trial of spontaneous breathing and see what flow and volume the patient can achieve on his own. (This patient actually achieved a spontaneous volume of 1.2 L.) Other possible solutions are to increase the ventilator rate or V_T to meet patient need or to switch to pressure support ventilation (PSV) and possibly VC-IMV or PC-IMV and use PSV for spontaneous breaths. The original ventilator settings did not provide adequate flow or volume to meet the patient ventilatory demands. (NOTE: With spontaneous V_T this high, one wonders if the patient needs the ventilator.)

TABLE 6-3	Required Setting Selection and Variables During Pressure Ventilation	
Name	**Trigger**	**Cycle**
Pressure support ventilation	Patient	Flow
Pressure control continuous mandatory ventilation	Time/patient	Time
Bilevel positive airway pressure	Time/patient	Flow
Pressure-regulated Volume control	Time/patient	Time
Volume support	Patient	Flow

Determining Initial Ventilator Settings During Pressure Ventilation

As previously defined, pressure-targeted ventilation provides a set pressure to the patient during breath delivery, whereas V_T can vary from breath to breath (see Chapter 5). There are several methods to provide a pressure breath that should be considered. This discussion begins with baseline pressure and then includes PSV, pressure control ventilation, bilevel positive airway pressure, and dual-control modes (pressure-regulated volume control [PRVC] and volume support [VS]). Each of these modes has specific controls that are set by the operator (Table 6-3). Less frequently used pressure-targeted modes, such as pressure control inverse ratio ventilation, are discussed in Chapter 13, and airway pressure release ventilation is reviewed in Chapter 23.

Volume-targeted ventilation has the advantage of guaranteeing volume delivery; however, it has the disadvantage of increasing PIP as C_L decreases or R_{aw} increases. **Overinflation** is also a risk. Pressure-targeted breaths have the advantages of providing flow on demand and potentially limiting pressures to avoid overinflation. With pressure-targeted breath delivery, rapid initial flows may cause frictional forces (shearing) between adjacent alveoli with differing lung inflation characteristics (time constants). In addition, V_T varies as lung characteristics change. There currently are no definitive studies that have demonstrated a clear advantage of one method over the other.[34]

SETTING BASELINE PRESSURE– PHYSIOLOGICAL PEEP

Functional residual capacity (FRC) frequently decreases when a patient is intubated or placed in a supine position.[35,36] In most situations it is appropriate to use minimum levels of PEEP (3 to 5 cm H_2O) to help preserve a patient's normal FRC.* Because only a modest amount of pressure is applied with this minimum level of PEEP, it is not considered a problem in terms of causing complications. In fact, not using a low level of PEEP may result in atelectasis. Use of low levels of PEEP may also be beneficial in patients with COPD who would normally pursed-lip breathe but cannot do so with an artificial airway in place (Box 6-8).

*Sometimes called *compensating PEEP*.

Determining Tidal Volume Delivery in Pressure Ventilation

In any pressure-targeted breath the difference in pressure (ΔP) between baseline (PEEP + auto-PEEP) and PIP determines what is set to establish V_T delivery. Volume delivery will also be affected by the patient's lung characteristics and any patient effort that is present.

There are two ways to set the pressure in pressure-targeted breaths to provide the desired V_T. One way is to deliver a volume-targeted breath to the patient at the desired V_T and measure plateau and baseline pressures. Using the same baseline pressure, the breath can be switched to pressure-targeted breath using a set pressure equal to the $P_{plateau}$. The resulting V_T will be approximately equal to the V_T during the volume breath, as long as inspiratory time is set appropriately. The pressure can then be adjusted as necessary to obtain the desired volume delivery. The V_T is continually monitored.

A second method to initiate pressure ventilation is to start at a low pressure (10 to 15 cm H_2O) and check the V_T before readjusting the pressure to attain the desired volume. (Box 5-5 includes a list of factors that affect volume delivery during pressure-targeted breaths.) Case Study 6-4 offers an exercise to illustrate this concept.

Initial Settings for Pressure Support Ventilation

Usually PSV is started after the patient has been on full ventilatory support and is being changed to partial support to begin the process of discontinuing ventilation. PSV is used to support spontaneous breaths in a patient with an artificial airway when IMV or spontaneous/CPAP modes are used. The pressure is set at a level sufficient to prevent a fatiguing workload on the respiratory muscles.

Some clinicians recommend calculating the level of pressure support based on an estimation of total ventilatory system resistance determined while the patient is receiving VC-CMV. The resistance of the patient and the ventilator circuit during VC-CMV with constant flow can be estimated with the following equation: $R_{aw} = (PIP - P_{plateau})/flow$.[36-39] It is probably easier and just as effective to set the initial PSV level to equal the transairway pressure ($PIP - P_{plateau}$) after establishing these values with VC-CMV. The level of PSV can then be adjusted once it has been initiated to an adequate level. Sometimes simply asking the patient if he or she feels it is easy to breathe and if he or she is getting enough air helps in adjusting initial PSV. (NOTE: Another way to determine whether an adequate amount of pressure support is being provided involves observing the patient's use of the accessory respiratory muscles [e.g., sternocleidomastoid muscle] during inspiration. Increased use of the accessory muscles of inspiration may indicate that the level of PSV is inadequate.)

Case Study 6-4

Tidal Volume (T_v) During Pressure Control Continuous Mandatory Ventilation (PC-CMV)

A patient is set on 12 cm H_2O of pressure during PC-CMV. If the measured V_T is 350 mL and the desired V_T is 550 mL, how would you adjust the pressure to achieve the desired V_T?

| BOX **6-8** | **Factors Affecting Expiratory Gas Flow** |

During normal expiration, gas flow from a lung unit (acinus) is the result of the elastic recoil of the alveolus (+2 cm H_2O) plus the force (pressure) from recoil of the chest wall (+3 cm H_2O) acting on the alveolar gas volume to produce a pressure gradient between the alveoli and the mouth (see Figure below, Part A). Notice that the total pressure (+5 cm H_2O) at the alveolar level is greater than that at the mouth, so the air moves out of the lung.

As the exhaled air moves across the conductive airways, some of the driving pressure is lost to airway resistance, R_{aw} (−1 cm H_2O). In normal lungs, this pressure loss is small because the intrathoracic forces exert pressure both on the alveoli and the conductive airway. In a patient with normal airways, the resilience of the airway combined with the gas pressure in the airway lumen prevents airway collapse in most regions of the lung during most phases of the respiratory cycle. The pressure in the alveolus minus the pressure drop across the airway equals the pressure in the airway lumen (+5 cm H_2O − 1 cm H_2O = +4 cm H_2O intraluminal).*

The pressure gradient changes in patients with weakened airways caused by loss of supportive connective tissue. (Loss of lung elasticity occurs with aging and in patients with pulmonary emphysema.) Part **B** of the figure shows an example of an alveolus with lower than normal lung elastic recoil forces (+1 cm H_2O). The

intrathoracic forces (+3 cm H_2O) will not be affected, but the total force providing gas flow out of the lungs is lower (+4 cm H_2O). When gas flows through an airway where R_{aw} is increased, the pressure drop is greater than in normal airways (−2 cm H_2O). As a result, the intraluminal pressure is lower (+4 cm H_2O − 2 cm H_2O = +2 cm H_2O). Because chest wall elastic recoil pressures are greater than intraluminal pressures in the small airways weakened by loss of elastic recoil forces, these small airways tend to collapse from dynamic compression. Pursed-lip breathing is an effective maneuver that helps prevent airway collapse by resisting expiration, thus raising pressures across the entire length of the airway.

For patients with chronic obstructive pulmonary disease (COPD), it is not possible to pursed-lip breathe with an artificial airway in place and air trapping (auto-positive end-expiratory pressure [auto-PEEP]) is common. Early generation ventilators offered an expiratory retard control, which slowed the rate of exhalation by applying resistance to the expired gas flow. Older expiratory and PEEP valves actually increased resistance to exhalation whether resistance was desired or not. Newer microprocessor ventilators do not provide an expiratory retard option, and resistance through current expiratory valves is very low. Some practitioners consider that using low levels of PEEP (≤5 cm H_2O) offers a means to provide a similar effect.

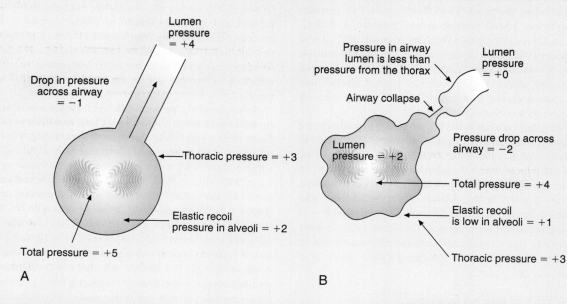

A, Alveolar, thoracic, and airway dynamics during exhalation in a patient with normal lungs (units in centimeters H_2O pressure). **B**, Alveolar, thoracic, and airway dynamics during exhalation in a patient with chronic obstructive pulmonary disease (units in centimeters H_2O pressure).

*The numerical values used here are for the sake of simplicity and are only approximations of actual values.

Appropriate adjustment of PSV level can be done at the bedside. The goal of adjusting PSV is threefold.

1. To help increase V_T (4 to 8 mL/kg)
2. To decrease respiratory rate (to <30 breaths/min)
3. To decrease the WOB associated with breathing through an artificial airway

For patients with lung disease, levels of 8 to 14 cm H_2O are typically used to compensate for additional work associated with breathing through a tube and ventilator system. For patients without lung disease, about 5 cm H_2O should be adequate to compensate for the additional work of breathing.

When patients, particularly infants, are receiving CPAP through a ventilator, it is recommended that pressure support is added if a high level of CPAP (10 cm H_2O) is being used. CPAP by itself may increase WOB, and adding pressure support reduces this workload.[40]

As previously discussed in this chapter, V_T selection varies depending on the patient's lung condition. Low-volume and high-frequency alarms must be set appropriately because a number of factors can change the V_T and $\dot{V}_E$. If a backup ventilation mode is available on the ventilator, it is also appropriate to set the backup ventilation parameters for the patient, particularly if PSV is being used by itself.

When patients with COPD are ventilated with PSV, it may be prudent to use graphic displays of pressure and flow versus time to monitor their status. These patients are known to have active short inspirations. In addition, if the patient begins to exhale actively during flow delivery from the ventilator, the flow may not drop to the necessary cycling value. Consequently the ventilator breath may not end as normally expected, resulting in a sudden rise in the pressure curve at the end of the breath[41] (Fig. 6-5). The breath may actually pressure cycle. The same can occur in other patients when ventilators use a very low flow criterion for ending inspiration. This can also induce expiratory muscle activity.[42] The problem can be avoided by using a ventilator with adjustable flow-cycling characteristics for patients demonstrating expiratory muscle activity. A cycle criteria of 40% of peak flow is an appropriate starting point for a patient with COPD. (NOTE: Using a low-flow cycling value [10%] may be appropriate for patients with restrictive disorders [Case Study 6-5].)

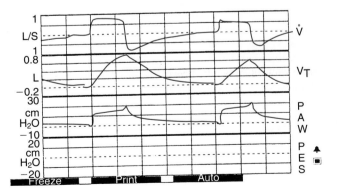

Fig. 6-5 Pressure and flow waveforms depicting a pressure-cycled pressure support ventilation breath delivered by a 7200 series ventilator. Note that the inspiratory flow does not descend to the 5 L/min terminal flow. Pressure rises slightly at the end of inspiration, showing an active exhalation by the patient before the flow cycle criterion is met. V_T, tidal volume. (From Campbell RS, Branson RD: Ventilatory support for the 90s: Pressure support ventilation. Respir Care 38:526-537, 1993.)

Initial Settings for Pressure Control Ventilation

Rate, inspiratory time, and I:E ratio are set in PC-CMV as they are with VC-CMV. The pressure gradient (PIP – PEEP, including auto-PEEP) is adjusted to establish volume delivery based on patient lung characteristics and effort. Initial pressure is set at the $P_{plateau}$ value determined during VC-CMV and must be adjusted as necessary to achieve V_T. If $P_{plateau}$ is not available, the peak pressure from VC-CMV minus 5 cm H_2O (PIP – 5 cm H_2O) can be used as a starting point.[43,44]

If volume readings are not available, an initial pressure of 10 to 15 cm H_2O with simultaneous volume measurement and adjustment is appropriate. The pressure limit must be set, because in some ventilators pressure can be higher than the set pressure control level if the patient actively coughs. Low V_T and high f alarms are also necessary.

An important advantage of PC-CMV is that P_{alv} usually will not exceed the applied pressure. Setting a PIP of less than 30 cm H_2O can therefore help avoid alveolar overinflation. Because it is not possible to measure P_{alv} in all situations, PIP is maintained less than this set pressure. The patient's P_{alv} can be estimated by observing the flow curve. If the flow drops to zero before inspiration ends, then the applied pressure is reaching the alveolar level by the end of inspiration (see Fig. 5-2). If inspiration ends before the flow reaches zero, then P_{alv} is less than applied pressure, but is not measurable. In this case, T_I may need to be adjusted (increased) depending on patient need and V_T delivery.

Normally PC-CMV provides a descending ramp waveform. As with PSV, current generation ventilators (e.g., the CareFusion AVEA) are able to adjust the inspiratory rise time, which is the amount of the T_I required for the ventilator to reach the set pressure at the beginning of inspiration. The practitioner can adjust the rise to meet patient needs as with PSV (see Fig. 5-9). It is advisable to use graphic monitoring to help make adjustments in pressure, T_I, and flow taper. If T_I is too long and the patient starts to actively exhale, a slight rise will occur at the end of the breath on the pressure curve.

Compared with similar settings on VC-CMV, PC-CMV has been shown to improve oxygenation and gas exchange, increase $\bar{P}_{aw}$, and facilitate lung healing. PC-CMV also reduces the PIP, the amount of applied PEEP, V_E, respiratory work, the need for sedation, and the duration of mechanical ventilation.[44-48] Pressure-targeted ventilation is safe and well tolerated as an initial mode of ventilation in patients with acute hypoxemic respiratory failure and may result in greater patient comfort.[43,48]

Initial Settings for Bilevel Positive Airway Pressure Ventilation

Bilevel positive airway pressure (bilevel PAP) can be used for intubated patients or nonintubated patients, although it is most often used as noninvasive positive pressure ventilation (NIV). Initial settings include an inspiratory positive airway pressure (IPAP) of about 5 to 10 cm H_2O. The level of IPAP is increased in increments of 3 to 5 cm H_2O until a rate of 25 breaths/min or lower is achieved and the V_T is 4 to 8 mL/kg or more, depending on the patient's pathology. Expiratory positive airway pressure (EPAP) or PEEP is initiated at 2 to 5 cm H_2O and increased in increments of 3 to 5 cm H_2O. The initial F_IO_2 is set to ensure adequate oxygenation. It is important to recognize that initiating NIV may require a considerable amount of time to achieve patient compliance.

Case Study 6-5

Inspiratory Flow Termination in Pressure Support Ventilation (PSV)

Problem 1

During PSV, a patient's peak flow is 50 L/min. At what flow level will inspiration end if the ventilator has a 25% flow cycle criterion?

Problem 2

A patient on PSV has an endotracheal tube cuff that is not inflated, preventing the ventilator from reaching the flow cycle criterion to end inspiration. What will terminate inspiration?

Problem 3

At the end of inspiration, a patient on PSV actively exhales before the ventilator detects the drop in flow required to cycle the breath. How will this affect the pressure/time waveform of the ventilator?

TABLE 6-4	Names for Pressure-Regulated Volume Control (PRVC) and Volume Support on Different Ventilators
Ventilator Name	**PRVC Name**
Hamilton G5	Adaptive pressure ventilation
CareFusion AVEA	PRVC
Dräger 500	Autoflow
Servo-i	PRVC
Ventilator Name	**VS Name**
Servo-i	VS
Dräger V500	SPN-CPAP/VS
PB 840	VS

For patients with COPD experiencing air trapping (auto-PEEP), EPAP is typically set at 80% to 90% of the level of auto-PEEP, which is usually a range of 3 to 10 cm H_2O. Observing the patient's use of accessory muscles (e.g., sternocleidomastoid muscles) during inspiration can assist in the titration of EPAP when auto-PEEP is present. For patients with hypoxemic respiratory failure, a PEEP/CPAP level greater than 5 cm H_2O is often required. (NOTE: The use of PEEP to help a patient trigger the ventilator is also used in other modes of ventilation besides NIV.) If no improvement is seen after about 2 hours of treatment, this mode of ventilation is probably not benefiting the patient and a more aggressive intervention may be necessary. Additional information on noninvasive ventilation can be found in Chapter 19.

INITIAL SETTINGS FOR PRESSURE VENTILATION MODES WITH VOLUME TARGETING

Pressure ventilation with volume targeting, previously called "dual-control" ventilation, provides the benefits of pressure breaths along with targeting a set volume (see Chapter 5). Pressure-limited, volume-targeted modes are available in two forms, one where volume is targeted for each breath and one where volume is targeted over several breaths. (Additional information on dual-control ventilation is available on the Evolve website.)

Initial Settings of Pressure-Regulated Volume Control (PRVC)

Pressure-regulated volume control (PRVC) is a mode of ventilation that provides closed-loop pressure breaths and targets the pressure to achieve the set volume. PRVC is a pressure-limited, time-cycled mode that uses the set V_T as a feedback control.[49] PRVC was originally available only with the Servo 300 ventilator, but it has now been incorporated into a number of other ventilators. As Table 6-4 shows, the names to describe PRVC vary among manufacturers.

With PRVC, the operator sets a V_T to be delivered that is appropriate for the patient. The baseline pressure and the maximum pressure limit are also set. The ventilator delivers one or more test breaths. For example, in the Servo-i, the test breath is a volume-targeted breath with an inspiratory pause. The test breaths allow the ventilator to calculate static compliance and R_{aw} of the patient and system to determine the pressure required to achieve the set V_T. The first pressure level delivered in PRVC equals the plateau pressure measured during the test breath. The ventilator progressively adjusts the pressure level until the set V_T is achieved. The operator can evaluate volume and pressure graphics to ensure that these parameters are set appropriately (see Fig. 5-10). (NOTE: The exact maximum level of pressure delivery may differ between ventilators, but the ventilator relies on the upper pressure limit to determine how high to go when increasing pressure delivery to deliver the set V_T.)

It is important to set the upper pressure limit for two reasons:
1. It provides the upper limit for the ventilator to use in adjusting the pressure breath. (Pressure will not exceed a fixed amount, usually 5 cm H_2O below the upper pressure limit.)
2. If a patient coughs or forcibly exhales during the inspiratory phase, the ventilator will not permit pressure to exceed the upper pressure limit.

Current-generation ventilators with floating exhalation valves can actually release pressure during a forceful cough. This helps maintain the inspiratory pressure without prematurely ending inspiration as a result of pressure cycling when circuit pressures reach the upper pressure limit.

The following example illustrates how the ventilator adjusts pressure during PRVC. Suppose that the tidal volume is set at 600 mL, the baseline pressure is + 5 cm H_2O of PEEP, and an upper pressure limit of 35 cm H_2O is set. Imagine that the patient begins ventilation with the PRVC mode using a pressure of 20 cm H_2O to achieve the 600-mL volume target. Then suppose the patient suddenly develops a pneumothorax. This would reduce the patient's compliance, thus requiring a higher pressure to deliver the desired V_T of 600 mL. (The ventilator reaches 30 cm H_2O but is unable to deliver the 600 mL.) Circuit pressure is now within 5 cm H_2O of the upper pressure limit and the ventilator's alarm will activate. This will be an audible alarm and perhaps a digital message that might say, "Pressure limited, please evaluate." The clinician must evaluate the patient and determine whether ventilator changes are required (Case Study 6-6).

Initial Settings of Volume Support

Volume support is a purely spontaneous mode (see Fig. 5-11). In addition to setting the ventilator sensitivity, the operator sets the V_T and the upper pressure limit. Again the selection of V_T is based on the same criteria that are used in VC-CMV. The advantage of volume support is that spontaneously breathing patients can establish their own respiratory rate and V_T. (NOTE: In volume support, the set V_T is the minimum V_T. A patient can obtain a higher V_T if desired.) As lung characteristics improve, less pressure is required from the ventilator to deliver the volume, which automatically drops pressure delivery. At the same time, if the patient becomes apneic, volume support modes provide a "safety net," usually as a backup mode that can provide a set rate and volume.

Case Study 6-6

Pressure-Regulated Volume Control (PRVC)
A patient on PRVC has a set volume of 550 mL. The upper pressure limit is set to 30 cm H_2O. Initially, 19 cm H_2O is required to deliver the volume. The pressure is now at 13 cm H_2O. What should the therapist do in this situation?

SUMMARY

- The primary goal of VC-CMV is to achieve a $\dot{V}_E$ that matches the patient's metabolic needs and ensures adequate gas exchange.
- Initiation of VC-CMV requires several considerations, including $\dot{V}_E$ settings (V_T and f), inspiratory gas flow, flow waveform, inspiratory to expiratory (I:E) ratio, pressure limit, inflation hold (inspiratory pause), and inspiratory and expiratory pressure (PEEP).
- Settings for V_T and f should reflect a $\dot{V}_E$ that is derived from the initial calculation based on patient's gender and BSA and pathology.

- Regardless of the method used for selecting the V_T for a patient, it is important for clinicians to be aware of potential risks of causing lung injury, such as overdistention of lung tissue, and atelectasis.
- The tubing compliance, or system compressibility, reflects the volume of gas compressed in the ventilator circuit during the inspiratory phase.
- A number of devices can decrease or increase the amount of V_{Dmech} added to the breathing circuit.
- An understanding of the interrelation between inspiratory flow, inspiratory time (T_I), expiratory time (T_E), TCT, and I:E ratio is necessary for the clinician to effectively ventilate a patient.
- During VC-CMV where patient-triggered breaths are present, the patient's respiratory rate may actually vary, depending on flow and T_I setting.
- A variety of flow patterns are available on most ventilators, including constant flow, descending ramp, ascending ramp, and sine flow patterns. The most common are constant and descending ramp patterns.
- Clinicians must familiarize themselves with how a ventilator functions when selecting peak flow and waveform pattern.
- A constant flow pattern generally provides the shortest T_I of all the available flow patterns with an equivalent peak flow rate setting. Descending flow pattern may improve the distribution of gas in the lungs, reduces dead space, and increases oxygenation by increasing mean and plateau airway pressures.
- PSV is used to support spontaneous breaths in a patient with an artificial airway when the IMV or spontaneous/CPAP modes are used.
- PRVC provides closed-loop pressure breaths and targets the pressure to achieve the set volume.

REVIEW QUESTIONS (See Appendix A for answers.)

1. A respiratory therapist is determining the tubing compliance of a ventilator before use. A volume of 100 mL delivers a pressure of 33 cm H_2O. What is the compliance of the circuit?

2. Following initiation of ventilation using the circuit described in Question 1, the PIP is 15 cm H_2O and the V_T set is 250 mL. About how much volume is actually reaching the patient?

3. A patient being ventilated with a CareFusion AVEA has a set V_T of 700 mL, and f is at 12 breaths/min on the VC-CMV mode. The patient is initiating another 3 breaths/min so that the total f is 15 breaths/min. What is the patient's actual $\dot{V}_E$? Also answer the following questions.
   A. If the flow is set at 30 L/min using a constant flow pattern, what is the flow in L/sec?
   B. What is the TCT based on the set machine f of 12 breaths/min?
   C. What is the TCT based on the actual machine f of 15 breaths/min?
   D. What is the T_I based on the set f, flow, and V_T?
   E. What is the T_E when the f is 12?
   F. What is the T_E when the f is 15?

4. A therapist wants to select a flow waveform and flow setting for a patient with severe asthma. Which of the following is a good initial setting?
   A. Constant flow, 60 L/min
   B. Ascending flow, 80 L/min
   C. Descending flow, 70 L/min
   D. Sine flow, 40 L/min

5. A practitioner sets an inspiratory pause of 0.5 seconds to obtain a $P_{plateau}$ reading and to calculate the patient's static compliance. During the measurement, a stable plateau is not seen on the pressure–time graph. What could be the problem?

6. A post-open heart surgery patient is still intubated and under the effects of anesthesia. He is being transferred from the operating suite to the recovery unit. The surgeon wants to keep ventilating pressures to a minimum and is less concerned about ventilation. The patient's body temperature is 35° C. He is 5 foot 9 inches tall and weighs 210 lb.
   A. What is the patient's BSA?
   B. What is his IBW?
   C. What is an appropriate initial $\dot{V}_E$?
   D. Would you use PC-CMV or VC-CMV, and why?
   E. What V_T would be an appropriate target?
   F. Based on the V_T you selected, what would be an appropriate rate?
   G. What PEEP would you set?

7. A patient with ARDS is to be changed from a CPAP of +10 cm H_2O to VC-CMV. She is 5 foot 4 inches tall and weighs 195 lb. What tidal volume and rate would you set, and why? Would pressure control ventilation be appropriate for this patient?

8. NIV is being initiated on a 54-year-old man with a history of COPD. He has an IBW of 70 kg. The initial settings are IPAP = 8 cm H_2O and PEEP = 3 cm H_2O. The patient's V_T on these settings is 280 mL and f = 27 breaths/min. What change would you recommend?

9. A patient with right lower-lobe pneumonia and a temperature of 100° F must be mechanically ventilated. How should the initial $\dot{V}_E$ be adjusted? (HINT: See Box 6-1.)

10. A physician requested that her patient be switched from PC-CMV to VC-CMV to guarantee volume delivery. Ventilator parameters are VC-CMV + PSV; V_T = 0.6; f = 20 breaths/min, flow = 60 L/min (using constant flow waveform); PSV = 27 cm H_2O; PEEP = +8 cm H_2O; PIP = 56 cm H_2O; and $P_{plateau}$ = 43 cm H_2O. The physician asked the respiratory therapist to find a way to reduce pressures without changing $\dot{V}_E$. What is a possible solution?

11. A ventilator is set with PRVC with a PEEP = +5 cm H_2O, a set V_T of 650 mL, and an upper pressure limit of 30 cm H_2O. Initially the pressure required to deliver the V_T was 20 cm H_2O. After a period of 24 hours, the pressure required to deliver the set V_T increases to 24 cm H_2O. What changes have probably occurred in the patient's lung characteristics?

12. What ventilator mode is patient triggered, pressure targeted, flow cycled, and also targets a set tidal volume?

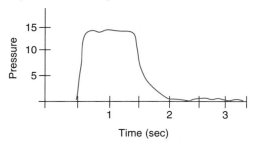

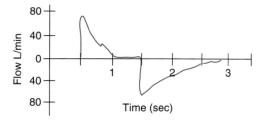

13. The pressure–time and flow–time curves above are viewed during PC-CMV ventilation with an apneic patient. What is the $P_{plateau}$?

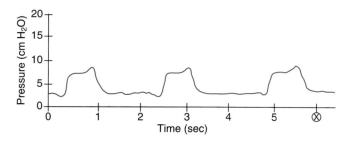

14. The pressure–time curve above is observed during PSV. What is causing the curve to appear like this?
A. Active exhalation
B. No sloping in the presence of increased airway resistance
C. A leak in the circuit
D. Active inhalation

References

1. Laghi F, Tobin MJ: Indications for mechanical ventilation. In Tobin MJ, editor: *Principles and practice of mechanical ventilation*, ed 3, New York, 2013, McGraw-Hill, pp 101–135.
2. Boothby WM, Sandiford RB: Nomographic charts for the calculation of the metabolic rate by the gasometry method. *Boston Med Surg J* 185:337–354, 1921.
3. Slutsky AS, Ranieri M: Ventilator-induced lung injury. *N Engl J Med* 369:2126–2136, 2013.
4. Serpa NA, Cardoso SO, Manetta JA, et al: Association between use of lung-protective ventilation with lower tidal volumes and clinical outcomes among patients without acute respiratory distress syndrome: a meta-analysis. *JAMA* 308:1651–1659, 2012.
5. Spieth PM, Carvalho AR, Pelosi P, et al: Variable tidal volumes improve lung protective ventilation strategies in experimental lung injury. *Am J Respir Crit Care Med* 179:684–693, 2009.
6. Malhostra A: Low tidal volume ventilation in the acute respiratory distress syndrome. *N Engl J Med* 357:1113–1120, 2007.
7. Brower RG, Matthay MA, Morris A, et al: Acute Respiratory Distress Syndrome Network: Ventilation with lower tidal volume as compared with traditional tidal volumes for acute lung injury and the acute respiratory distress syndrome. *N Engl J Med* 342:1301–1308, 2000.
8. Radford EP, Ferris BG, Kriete BC: Clinical use of a nomogram to estimate proper ventilation during artificial respirations. *N Engl J Med* 251:877–884, 1954.
9. Egan DF: *Fundamentals of inhalation therapy*, St Louis, 1969, Mosby.
10. Young J, Crocker R: *Principles and practices of inhalation therapy*, Chicago, 1970, Year Book Medical.
11. Bendixen HH, Bullwinkel B, Hedley-Whyte J, et al: Atelectasis and shunting during spontaneous ventilation in anesthetized patients. *Anesthesiology* 25:297–301, 1964.
12. Hess DR, Branson RD: Mechanical ventilation. In Hess DR, MacIntyre NR, Mishoe SC, et al, editors: *Respiratory care principles and practice*, Philadelphia, 2011, W.B. Saunders, pp 462–500.
13. Campbell RS, Davis K, Richard JC, et al: The effects of passive humidifier dead space on respiratory variables in paralysed and spontaneously breathing patients. *Respir Care* 45:306–312, 2000.
14. Pelosi P, Brusasco C, Gama de Abreu M: Mechanical ventilation during general anesthesia. In Tobin MJ, editor: *Principles and practice of mechanical ventilation*, ed 3, New York, 2013, McGraw-Hill, pp 597–627.
15. Thorevska NY, Manthous CA: Determinants of dynamic hyperinflation in a bench model. *Respir Care* 49:1326–1334, 2004.
16. Quan SF: A ghost from the past: low tidal volume mechanical ventilation revisited (editorial). *Chest* 97:261–262, 1990.
17. Lee PC, Helsmoortel CM, Cohn SM, et al: Are low tidal volumes safe? *Chest* 97:430–434, 1990.
18. Holets SR, Hubmayr RD: Setting the ventilator. In Tobin MJ, editor: *Principles and practice of mechanical ventilation*, ed 3, New York, 2013, McGraw-Hill, pp 101–135.
19. Jubran A: Inspiratory flow rate: more may not be better. *Crit Care Med* 27:670–671, 1999.
20. Laghi F, Karamchandani K, Tobin MJ: Influence of ventilator settings in determining respiratory frequency during mechanical ventilation. *Am J Respir Crit Care Med* 160:1766–1770, 1999.
21. Banner MJ, Boysen PG, Lampotang S, et al: End-tidal CO_2 affected by inspiratory time and flow waveform—time for a change [abstract]. *Crit Care Med* 14:374, 1986.
22. Tobin MJ: Mechanical ventilation. *N Eng J Med* 330:1056–1061, 1994.
23. Tobin MJ: Advances in mechanical ventilation. *N Eng J Med* 344:1986–1996, 2001.
24. Dammann JF, McAslan TC, Maffeo CJ: Optimal flow for mechanical ventilation of the lungs. Part 2: The effect of a sine versus square wave flow pattern with and without an end-inspiratory pause on patients. *Crit Care Med* 6:293–310, 1978.

25. Rau JJ, Shelledy DC: The effect of varying inspiratory flow waveforms on peak and mean airway pressures with a time-cycled volume ventilator: a bench study. *Respir Care* 36:347–356, 1991.

26. Al-Saady N, Bennett ED: Decelerating inspiratory flow waveform improves lung mechanics and gas exchange in patients on intermittent positive-pressure ventilation. *Intensive Care Med* 11:68–75, 1985.

27. Rau JL: Inspiratory flow patterns: the shape of ventilation. *Respir Care* 38:132–140, 1993.

28. Kallet R: The effects of flow patterns on pulmonary gas exchange, lung-thorax mechanics and circulation. *Respir Care* 41:611–624, 1996.

29. Owen-Thomas JB, Ulan OA, Swyer PR: The effect of varying inspiratory gas flow rate on arterial oxygenation during IPPV in the respiratory distress syndrome. *Br J Anaesth* 40:493–502, 1968.

30. Dammann JF, McAslan TC: Optimal flow pattern for mechanical ventilation of the lungs: evaluation with a model lung. *Crit Care Med* 5:128–136, 1977.

31. Marini J, Crooke P, Truwit J: Determinants and limits of pressure-preset ventilation: a mathematical model of pressure control. *J Appl Physiol* 67:1081–1092, 1989.

32. Uttman L, Jonson G: A prolonged postinspiratory pause enhances CO_2 elimination by reducing airway dead space. *Clin Physiol Funct Imaging* 23:252–256, 2003.

33. Kacmarek RM: Initiating and adjusting invasive ventilatory support. In Kacmarek RM, Stoller JK, Heuer AJ, editors: *Egan's fundamentals of respiratory care*, ed 10, St. Louis, 2013, Elsevier, pp 1088–1130.

34. Campbell RS, Davis BR: Pressure controlled versus volume-controlled ventilation: does it matter? *Respir Care* 47:416–424, 2002.

35. Shapiro BA, Cane RD, Harrison RA, et al: Changes in intrapulmonary shunting with administration of 100% oxygen. *Chest* 77:138–141, 1980.

36. Marini JJ: Weaning techniques and protocols. *Respir Care* 40:233–238, 1995.

37. MacIntyre NR: Pressure-limited versus volume-cycled breath delivery strategies, (editorial). *Crit Care Med* 22:4–5, 1994.

38. Hill NS, Brennan J, Garpestad E, et al: Noninvasive ventilation in acute respiratory failure. *Crit Care Med* 35:2402–2407, 2007.

39. Kacmarek RM, McMahon K, Staneck K: Pressure support level required to overcome work of breathing imposed by endotracheal tubes at various peak inspiratory flowrates (abstract). *Respir Care* 33:933, 1988.

40. Heulitt MJ, Holt SJ, Thurman TL, et al: Effects of continuous positive airway pressure/positive end-expiratory pressure and pressure-support ventilation on work of breathing, using an animal model. *Respir Care* 48:689–696, 2003.

41. Branson RD, Campbell RS: Pressure support ventilation, patient-ventilator synchrony and ventilator algorithms (editorial). *Respir Care* 43:1045–1047, 1998.

42. Parthasarathy S, Jubran A, Tobin MJ: Cycling of inspiratory and expiratory muscle groups with the ventilator in airflow limitation. *Am J Respir Crit Care Med* 158:1471–1478, 1998.

43. Böhm S, Lachmann B: Pressure-control ventilation: putting a mode into perspective. *Int J Intensive Care* 3:12–27, 1996.

44. Abraham E, Yoshihara G: Cardiorespiratory effects of pressure controlled inverse ratio ventilation in severe respiratory failure. *Chest* 96:1356–1359, 1989.

45. Lain DC, DiBenedetto R, Morris SL, et al: Pressure control inverse ratio ventilation as a method to reduce peak inspiratory pressure and provide adequate ventilation and oxygenation. *Chest* 95:1081–1088, 1989.

46. Guervitch MJ, Van Dyke J, Young ES, et al: Improved oxygenation and lower peak airway pressure in severe adult respiratory distress syndrome: treatment with inverse ratio ventilation. *Chest* 89:211–213, 1986.

47. Tharratt RS, Allen RP, Albertson TE: Pressure controlled inverse ratio ventilation in severe adult respiratory failure. *Chest* 94:755–762, 1989.

48. Rappaport SH, Shpiner R, Yoshihara G, et al: Randomized, prospective trial of pressure-limited versus volume-controlled ventilation in severe respiratory failure. *Crit Care Med* 22:22–32, 1994.

49. Branson RD, MacIntyre NR: Dual-control modes of mechanical ventilation. *Respir Care* 41:294–305, 1996.

Final Considerations in Ventilator Setup

OUTLINE

KEY TERMS

- Acute severe asthma
- Barotrauma
- Cushing response
- Humidity deficit
- Isothermic saturation boundary
- Pulsus paradoxus
- Relative humidity

LEARNING OBJECTIVES *On completion of this chapter, the reader will be able to do the following:*

1. Recommend fractional inspired oxygen concentration (F_1O_2) settings when initiating mechanical ventilation.
2. Discuss the pros and cons of using the sigh function during mechanical ventilation.
3. Compare the use of sigh with the concept of a recruitment maneuver in acute respiratory distress syndrome.
4. List the actions necessary for final ventilator setup.
5. Explain the concept of using extrinsic positive end-expiratory pressure (PEEP) in patients with airflow obstruction and air trapping who have trouble triggering a breath during mechanical ventilation.

6. Calculate the desired F_1O_2 setting given the current partial pressure of arterial oxygen (P_aO_2) and F_1O_2 values.
7. List the essential capabilities of an adult intensive care unit (ICU) ventilator.
8. Provide initial ventilator settings from the guidelines for patient management for any of the following patient conditions: chronic obstructive pulmonary disease (COPD), acute asthma exacerbation, neuromuscular disorders, closed head injuries, acute respiratory distress syndrome (ARDS), and acute cardiogenic pulmonary edema.

S everal issues must be considered after decisions about the type of ventilator to be used, mode selection, and settings for pressure and volume have been made. These issues include selecting appropriate ventilator settings for the **fractional concentration of inspired oxygen** (F_1O_2), sensitivity, sigh breaths, alarms, and monitors, in addition to concerns regarding humidification of inspired gases. Only after these

issues have been addressed can mechanical ventilation be initiated.

This chapter provides a summary of these issues and also addresses the initial settings for patients with specific pathologic conditions, such as chronic obstructive pulmonary disease (COPD), asthma, neuromuscular diseases, and acute respiratory distress syndrome (ARDS).

Selection of Additional Parameters and Final Ventilator Setup

SELECTION OF FRACTIONAL CONCENTRATION OF INSPIRED OXYGEN

The goal of selecting a specific F_IO_2 for a patient is to achieve a clinically acceptable arterial oxygen tension (e.g., 60 to 100 mm Hg). To accomplish this goal, a baseline arterial blood gas (ABG) should be performed. If the patient's partial pressure of arterial oxygen (P_aO_2) is within the desired range before beginning ventilatory support, the F_IO_2 that the patient is receiving at the time of the baseline ABG can be used when mechanical ventilation is initiated. If the P_aO_2 is not within the desired range, the following equation can be used to estimate F_IO_2:

$$\text{Desired } F_IO_2 = \frac{[P_aO_2(\text{desired}) \times F_IO_2(\text{known})]}{P_aO_2(\text{known})}$$

This relationship is based on the assumption that the patient's cardiopulmonary function will not radically change from the time of the baseline ABG to the time when mechanical ventilation is initiated.[1,2] Some changes will obviously occur because the application of positive pressure ventilation (PPV) can affect a patient's cardiopulmonary status.

If a baseline ABG is not available, it is advisable to select a high initial F_IO_2 setting (≥ 0.50) for patients with presumed severe hypoxemia. This can provide a way of restoring normal oxygenation and replacing tissue oxygen storage when oxygen debt and lactic acid accumulation have occurred. Many practitioners start with an F_IO_2 of 1.0 and then reduce it as quickly as possible. Extended use of 100% O_2 is not recommended because it can quickly result in absorption atelectasis and, in the long term, can lead to oxygen toxicity. It is important to state, however, that 100% oxygen should not be withheld if the patient is seriously ill and requires a high F_IO_2. Indeed, any procedure that places the patient at risk of developing hypoxemia should be performed with the patient breathing 100% O_2. For example, administering 100% O_2 before and after suctioning and also during bronchoscopy is a common practice.

Titrating the F_IO_2 using pulse oximetry and ABG findings can minimize the risk of administering too much oxygen.[3-5] The F_IO_2 can be adjusted after ventilation is started, based initially on the pulse oximetry saturation (S_pO_2).[6] An S_pO_2 greater than 92% ($P_aO_2 \geq 60$ mm Hg) is a common and acceptable goal. Within 10 to 20 minutes of beginning ventilation, an ABG sample should be collected to assess the adequacy of ventilation and oxygenation. Appropriate ventilator changes based on ABG results are reviewed in Chapters 12 and 13.

The equation for obtaining a desired F_IO_2 shown earlier in this section can also be used to adjust the F_IO_2. When an F_IO_2 greater than 0.50 is required to maintain oxygenation, positive end-expiratory pressure (PEEP) may be indicated (see Chapter 13). An F_IO_2 of 0.50 or greater increases the risk of oxygen toxicity and intrapulmonary shunting that occurs with oxygen induced atelectasis.

SENSITIVITY SETTING

Ventilator sensitivity is normally set so that patients can easily flow- or pressure-trigger a breath (see Chapter 3). Flow triggering is set in a range of 1 to 10 L/min below the base flow, depending on the selected ventilator. Pressure sensitivity is commonly set between −1 and −2 cm H_2O.

Many clinicians prefer using flow triggering because it provides a slightly faster response time compared with pressure triggering for two main reasons. First, the exhalation valve does not have to close during flow triggering. With pressure triggering, the exhalation valve must close and the patient's inspiratory effort has to be sufficient to reduce the circuit pressure to the trigger setting. Secondly, during pressure triggering, the circuit pressure has to drop before the inspiratory valve opens and flow goes to the patient.[7] In contrast, with flow triggering, the pressure does not need to drop because the inspiratory valve remains open and the patient receives almost immediate support (Key Point 7-1).

> **Key Point 7-1** Flow triggering has a slightly faster response time compared with pressure triggering.

If auto-PEEP (intrinsic PEEP, or $PEEP_I$) is present, patients often have trouble triggering a breath. Indeed, in cases when auto-PEEP is very high, patients may not be able to trigger a breath at all. It can therefore be particularly difficult when a high level of auto-PEEP is present to adjust the ventilator sensitivity so that it senses a patient's effort. Furthermore, the cause of the problem often goes unsolved unless auto-PEEP is detected and measured (Box 7-1).

When auto-PEEP occurs in mechanically ventilated, spontaneously breathing patients with airflow obstruction (e.g., in COPD), setting the extrinsic PEEP ($PEEP_E$) level to equal about 80% of the patient's auto-PEEP level may improve the ventilator's response (i.e., sensitivity) to the patient's inspiratory efforts. Figure 7-1, A and B, helps illustrate this problem. Imagine that you are trying to sip water through a straw from a glass in which the water level is 10 cm below your mouth. You would have to generate at least −10 cm H_2O to draw the water into your mouth. A similar situation occurs in ventilated patients with air trapping who are trying to trigger a breath. The patient must create a pressure gradient

---

BOX 7-1 Definitions of Positive End-Expiratory Pressure (PEEP)

PEEP = Positive end-expiratory pressure; airway pressure greater than zero at the end of exhalation

  Extrinsic PEEP ($PEEP_E$) = the level of PEEP set by the operator on the ventilator

  Auto-PEEP (Intrinsic PEEP, or $PEEP_I$) = the amount of pressure in the lungs at the end of exhalation when expiration is incomplete (i.e., expiratory flow is still occurring) and no $PEEP_E$ is present ($PEEP_E$ is excluded from this value)

  Intrinsic PEEP can occur in three situations: (1) strong active expiration, often with normal or even with low lung volumes (e.g., Valsalva maneuver); (2) high minute ventilation (>20 L/min), where expiratory time (T_E) is too short to allow exhalation to functional residual capacity; or (3) expiratory flow limitation due to increased airway resistance, as may occur in patients with chronic obstructive pulmonary disease on mechanical ventilation or with small endotracheal tubes or obstructed (clogged) expiratory filters.

  Total PEEP = $PEEP_E$ + auto-PEEP

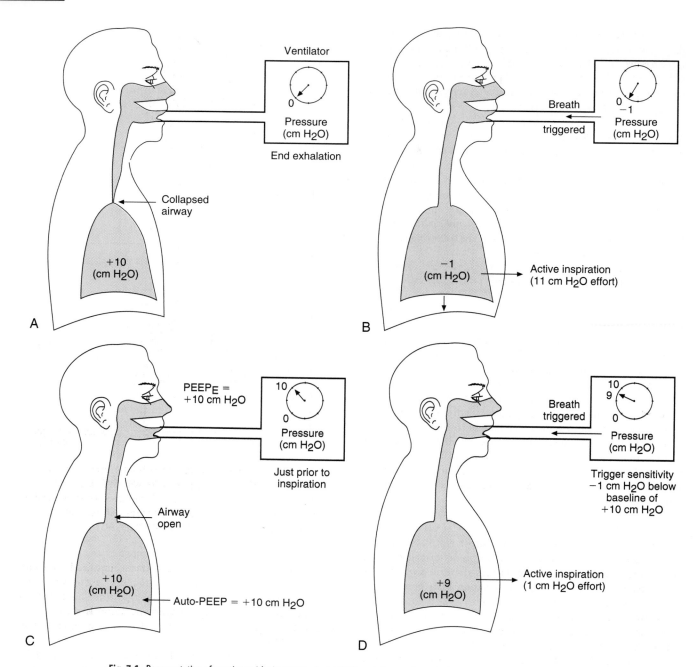

Fig. 7-1 Representation of a patient with air trapping (auto-PEEP) and airway collapse trying to trigger a ventilator breath. **A,** 10 cm H_2O of auto-PEEP at end exhalation. **B,** The patient's alveolar pressure (P_{alv}) must drop to -1 cm H_2O to trigger a ventilator breath. The effort required is the sum of the auto-PEEP level plus the trigger sensitivity setting of the ventilator, $+10$ cm H_2O (auto-PEEP) plus 1 cm H_2O (sensitivity), equals 11 cm H_2O of effort. **C,** Extrinsic PEEP ($PEEP_E$) set to $+10$ cm H_2O helps open airways and, for this example, did not increase peak inspiratory pressure. **D,** Triggering is accomplished with only -1 cm H_2O of effort.

between the alveolus and mouth by decreasing alveolar pressure (P_{alv}) to zero or lower so that mouth pressure (P_M) is greater than P_{alv}. This gradient allows air to flow into the lungs. For example, if $+10$ cm H_2O of auto-PEEP were present, the patient would have to generate an effort equal to -10 cm H_2O to achieve a P_{alv} of zero. Then the patient must generate an additional -1 to -2 cm H_2O to trigger inspiratory flow.

Another approach to solving the straw-sipping problem is to fill the glass with more water, which in turn would bring the water level closer to the mouth. Similarly, the problem that patients with

auto-PEEP have with triggering a breath can be solved by increasing pressure at the mouth (PEEP) until it equals P_{alv} (i.e., the pressure gradient between the mouth and the alveolus is reduced). This reduction is accomplished by applying PEEP with the ventilator (see Fig. 7-1, *C*). PEEP can be added until most of the airways are no longer collapsed, and the patient only has to generate enough pressure to trigger the ventilator based on the sensitivity setting. Note that this technique will not be effective if the auto-PEEP is the result of a high minute ventilation ($\dot{V}_E$) and if there is insufficient expiratory time (T_E).[4]

An easy way to estimate the amount of $PEEP_E$ to add, if auto-PEEP cannot be measured, is to increase $PEEP_E$ until peak inspiratory pressure (PIP) begins to increase. This increase in PIP is an indication that more pressure and volume have been added to the lung. Another technique of estimating the amount of $PEEP_E$ to add is to observe whether activity of the accessory muscles of breathing (e.g., sternocleidomastoids) decreases as $PEEP_E$ is added (Case Study 7-1). Still another technique involves comparing the number of triggered breaths with the number of patient efforts. As the level of set PEEP is increased, the number of triggered breaths should match the patient's efforts. Chapters 13 and 17 provide additional information about the complications associated with auto-PEEP, its causes, and methods to reduce auto-PEEP.

It is important to mention that the type of humidifier system being used also can influence the sensitivity. If the humidifier is located between the patient and the point at which the ventilator detects triggering, the patient has to work harder to trigger a breath. When the trigger device is located proximal to the patient's airway, this is less of a problem.[3]

Humidification

A spontaneously breathing individual's inspired air is typically conditioned down to the fourth or fifth generation of subsegmental bronchi (i.e., the **isothermic saturation boundary**) (Fig. 7-2).[8] Under normal circumstances, conditioning of inspired air occurs as air passes through the nose and upper airway. Because these are bypassed during invasive ventilation, a humidity source must be added to the ventilator circuit.

The humidification system used during mechanical ventilation should provide at least 30 mg H_2O/L of absolute humidity at a temperature range of about 31° to 35° C for all available flows up to a $\dot{V}_E$ of 20 to 30 L/min.[9,10] Some clinicians prefer a delivered temperature range of 35° to 37° C.[5]

Heated Humidifiers

Humidity can be provided by a variety of heated humidification systems. Devices in this category include the following types of humidifiers: passover, vapor phase, wick, and active heat and moisture exchanger.[10-12] Refilling heated humidifiers is best accomplished by using closed-feed system. With a closed-feed system, the water level in the reservoir is either maintained manually by adding water from a bag through a fill port or by a float-feed system that maintains a relatively constant water level. (Notice that another advantage of the closed-feed system is that the water temperature can be better regulated.) Both types avoid the need to open the ventilator circuit to refill the device and thus reduce the risk of potential contamination.

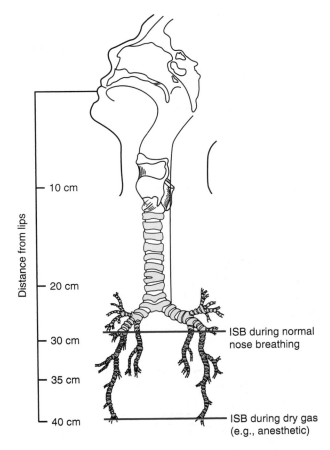

Fig. 7-2 Position of the isothermic saturation boundary (ISB) during normal nose breathing and during inhalation of dry gases (during intubation). (Redrawn from Branson RD, Campbell RS, Johannigman JA, et al: Comparison of conventional heated humidification with a new active hygroscopic heat and moisture exchanger in mechanically ventilated patients, Respir Care 44:912-917, 1999.)

Heated humidifiers typically include a servo-controlled heater with a temperature probe that is placed close to the patient airway. These devices are typically equipped with a temperature display and a temperature alarm. The high-temperature alarm is set at 37° to 38° C so that inspired gas does not exceed 37° C. A minimum alarm setting of 30° C is appropriate.[8,9,13]

Whenever the temperature in the patient circuit is less than the temperature of the gas leaving the humidifier, condensate accumulates in the circuit. Notice that condensate accumulation (rain-out) will increase as the room temperature becomes cooler.[14,15] (Using heated wire circuits on the inspiratory and expiratory lines of the circuit can significantly reduce the amount of rain-out.)

It is important to understand that if the temperature of the gas in the patient circuit is higher than the humidifier, the **relative humidity** in the circuit decreases (Critical Care Concept 7-1).[8] (This can occur when using heated wire circuits.) Anytime a deficit exists between the amount of humidity provided and the amount needed by the patient, drying of secretions can occur. Assessing whether a **humidity deficit** is present can be easily determined by examining the patient's secretions. For example, thick secretions that are difficult to suction or the presence of bronchial casts and mucous plugs are signs of drying of the airways.

Without a heated wire circuit, the humidifier may need to be heated to as much as 50° C for the gas temperature to come near

 Case Study 7-1

Auto-PEEP and Triggering

A 60-year-old man with COPD is receiving pressure-supported ventilation (PSV). He appears to be having difficulty triggering ventilator breaths. Auto-PEEP is measured at +8 cm H_2O and no $PEEP_E$ is being used. Sensitivity is set at −1 cm H_2O. How much of an effort (in cm H_2O) must the patient generate to trigger a breath?

to body temperature (37° C) by the time it reaches the patient's upper airway. As the highly saturated and warm gas passes through the ventilator circuit, ambient air surrounding the circuit tubing cools this gas and condensate forms in the circuit. Placing water traps at gravity-dependent parts of the circuit to catch excessive rain-out can help alleviate this problem. Water traps should be emptied regularly in a manner that protects the practitioner from any aerosolized spray that may be produced when the trap is opened. Some traps have spring-loaded caps that seal the circuit when they are unscrewed. Others have suction ports from which excess water can be suctioned. Traps that remain sealed during emptying help avoid interruption in ventilation during the process (Key Point 7-2). Maintaining a seal prevents breaking the circuit and thus reduces the risk of introducing contaminants.

CRITICAL CARE CONCEPT 7-1

Changes in Relative Humidity
Gas leaves a heated humidifier at a temperature of 34° C and 100% relative humidity. The absolute humidity is 37 mg/L. The gas enters a heated wire circuit that is heated to 37° C at the proximal airway. What is the absolute humidity of the gas that is 100% saturated at normal body temperature? What is the **humidity deficit** (i.e., the difference between what is provided by the humidifier and the amount of humidity required by the patient)? What happens to the relative humidity of the gas as it leaves the humidifier and enters the circuit?

Key Point 7-2 Condensate in the circuit tubing can potentially be a source of accidental lavage when the patient is turned. This water should be directed away from the patient and never allowed to enter the patient's airway.

Heat-Moisture Exchangers

Heat-moisture exchangers (HMEs), or artificial noses, can also be used for humidification in patients receiving mechanical ventilation. However, there are some circumstances when HMEs should **not** be used (Box 7-2).[9,13,16] HMEs can provide 10 to 14 mg/L of water at tidal volumes (V_T) of 500 to 1000 mL. More efficient hygroscopic heat and moisture exchangers (HHME) can provide 22 to 34 mg/L at similar volumes.[8] Because a net heat and water loss occurs when HMEs are used for extended periods, the patient should be assessed for signs of drying secretions.

Most HMEs have a resistance to flow of between 2.5 and 3.5 cm H_2O/L/min.[8] During extended use, HMEs can accumulate moisture and secretions, resulting in an increased resistance to flow. This increased resistance can cause gas trapping (i.e., auto-PEEP) and increase expiratory work of breathing (WOB). If more than four HMEs are used during a 24-hour period because of secretion buildup, it is probably advisable to change to a heated humidifier that provides 100% RH at 31° to 35° C.[17]

It is also important to recognize that HMEs add mechanical dead space (V_{Dmech}) to the ventilator circuit. The dead space for most HMEs ranges from about 50 to 100 mL. This is an important

---

BOX 7-2 | Contraindications for Heat-Moisture Exchangers

1. The presence of thick, copious, or bloody secretions. These secretions can accumulate on the heat-moisture exchanger (HME) and increase both inspiratory and expiratory resistance.
2. The patient's exhaled tidal volume (V_T) is less than 70% of inhaled V_T (e.g., in bronchopleural fistulas or when endotracheal tube cuffs are absent).
3. Body temperatures below 32° C (hypothermia).
4. Spontaneous high minute ventilation ($\dot{V}_E$) is greater than 10 L/min.
5. An aerosolized medication must be given.
6. Very small V_T must be delivered (lung protective ventilation); in which case the HME may significantly increase mechanical dead space (V_{Dmech}) and compromise CO_2 clearance. Notice that large V_T delivery may compromise the ability of the HME to humidify inspired gases.

---

consideration when HMEs are used on patients with low V_T, such as infants, children, and adult patients with V_T of 400 mL or less (Key Point 7-3).

Key Point 7-3 Passive humidifiers (heat-moisture exchangers [HMEs]) placed at the endotracheal tube should not be used simultaneously with heated humidifiers. Water produced by the heated humidifier can occlude the filter and significantly reduce airflow to the patient.[8]

Heat-moisture exchangers should be taken out of line during delivery of an aerosolized medication. It should be kept in mind, however, that circuit disconnection increases the risk of circuit contamination. An alternative approach is to use a meter dose inhaler (MDI) with an MDI adapter placed between the HME and the endotracheal tube (ET). If a spacer is used with the MDI on the inspiratory line, the HME must still be removed. Another solution is to use a circuit adapter that does not require the HME to be removed during aerosol treatments (Fig. 7-3).

Although some manufacturers recommend changing HMEs every 24 hours, replacement may be required only every 2 to 3 days if the HME is not partially obstructed with secretions.[3,8,18] Clinicians have reported using HMEs for up to 5 days without difficulties.[19] However, if secretions appear thick after two consecutive suctioning procedures, the HME should be removed and the patient switched to a heated humidification system.[8] For critically ill patients requiring more than 5 days of ventilation, it is probably better to use a heated humidification system that will optimize humidification and help prevent secretion retention. Long-term use (>7 days) of HMEs for the critically ill patient can increase the rate of ET occlusion. On the other hand, patients in long-term care facilities with tracheostomy tubes in place can use artificial noses for more extended periods of time without difficulty, as long as secretions do not present a problem.[19]

ALARMS

Audible and visible alarm systems are designed to alert the clinician of potential dangers related to the patient-ventilator

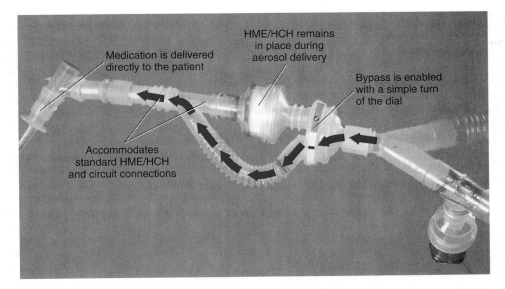

Medication is delivered directly to the patient

HME/HCH remains in place during aerosol delivery

Bypass is enabled with a simple turn of the dial

Accommodates standard HME/HCH and circuit connections

Fig. 7-3 The CircuVent ventilator circuit adapter. Aerosol delivery can be accomplished with a heat-moisture exchanger (HME) in line without breaking (disconnecting) the circuit. The practitioner turns the dial to redirect flow during medication delivery. (From DHD Healthcare, Wampsville, N.Y.)

interaction. This section reviews the most commonly used ventilator alarms and how they are set by most clinicians.[20,21] Box 7-3 shows the various levels of alarms and gives some examples of what causes them to become activated.

Low-pressure alarms are usually set about 5 to 10 cm H_2O below PIP. These alarms are useful for detecting patient disconnections and leaks in the system. High-pressure alarms are set about 10 cm H_2O above PIP. High-pressure alarms can be activated when the patient coughs, if secretions increase, compliance drops, or there are kinks in the ET or circuit tubing. Low PEEP/continuous positive airway pressure (CPAP) alarms are usually set about 2 to 5 cm H_2O below the PEEP level. Activation of these latter alarms usually indicates the presence of a leak in the patient-ventilator circuit.

Apnea alarms are used to monitor mandatory or spontaneous breaths. An apnea period of 20 seconds is the highest accepted maximum. In some situations, apnea alarms are set so the patient will not miss two consecutive machine breaths (apnea time > total cycle time [TCT] and < [TCT × 2]). Apnea settings provide full ventilatory support for the patient if apnea occurs and should be set appropriately (e.g., V_T 6 to 8 mL/kg ideal body weight [IBW], rate 10 to 20 breaths/min with a high percentage of oxygen [80% to 100%]).

Most ventilators also have an alarm or indicator that alerts the operator when the inspiratory time (T_I) is more than half the set TCT. Some ventilators, such as the Servo-i (Maquet Inc. Wayne, N.J.), will automatically end inspiration if the T_E is so short that the patient does not have time to exhale. The shortest possible T_E is 20% of any cycle time unless the patient is receiving bilevel PAP (bilevel positive airway pressure), and can be activated or inactivated.

Low-source gas alarms alert the operator that the available high-pressure gas source is not functioning. This alarm is critical for microprocessor ventilators that rely on high-pressure gas to function, particularly for ventilators that do not have a built-in compressor (Key Point 7-4).

BOX 7-3 **Levels of Alarm and Example Events During Mechanical Ventilation**

Level 1: Immediately Life-Threatening
Example events:
- Electrical power failure
- No gas delivery to patient
- Exhalation valve failure
- Excessive gas delivery to patient
- Timing failure

Level 2: Potentially Life-Threatening
Example events:
- Circuit leak
- Circuit partially obstructed
- Heater/humidifier malfunction
- Inspiratory-to-expiratory (I:E) ratio inappropriate
- Inappropriate oxygen level (gas/blender failure)
- Autocycling
- Inappropriate PEEP/CPAP level (too low/too high)

Level 3: Not Life-Threatening but a Potential Source of Patient Harm
Example events:
- Changes in lung characteristics (compliance/resistance)
- High respiratory rates
- Auto-PEEP
- Changes in ventilatory drive (e.g., central nervous system [CNS] or muscle function)

Sources: Hess D: Noninvasive monitoring in respiratory care—present, past and future: an overview, *Respir Care* 35:482-499, 1990; MacIntyre NR, Day S: Essentials for ventilator-alarm systems, *Respir Care* 37:1108-1112, 1992.

Key Point **7-4** Low-source gas alarms cannot be silenced if gas is critical to ventilator operation.

An intensive care unit (ICU) patient receiving mechanical ventilatory support is on an air-filled mattress, and there is a fan in his room to help cool him. He has a pleural drainage system with suction in place.

A nurse at the ICU station hears the ECG monitor alarm, which shows a pattern of asystole. She goes to the patient's bedside, begins cardiopulmonary resuscitation, and a normal sinus rhythm is quickly restored.

The nurse notes that the patient had been disconnected from the ventilator and attributed the life-threatening event to this occurrence. The nurse also notes that when the ventilator alarm was sounding, it could barely be heard. When confronted with the nurse's concerns about alarm failure, the respiratory therapist notices that the alarm's volume adjustment is on the lowest setting and resets it to a higher volume.

This scenario occurs all too frequently in the clinical setting and represents a critical medical error that can be avoided. What would you suggest to prevent a recurrence of this situation?

| BOX 7-5 | History of Sighs and Mechanical Ventilation |

Bendixen and colleagues demonstrated that anesthetized and intubated surgical patients developed increased intrapulmonary shunting, decreased P_aO_2 values, and reduced compliance following mechanical ventilation. They attributed these findings to microatelectasis from constant low tidal volumes.[22] When patients were given periodic deep breaths (sighs), these changes were reversed. Unfortunately, the effectiveness of periodic hyperinflation (sighing) continues to be debated because subsequent studies did not entirely support Bendixen's findings.[23-29] The decrease in lung compliance (C_L) and in P_aO_2 values seen in surgical patients may actually be due to a loss of functional residual capacity in the supine position and to the effects of anesthetics, muscle relaxants, and similar medications on diaphragm and intercostal muscles function. It has been suggested that this decrease in C_L and P_aO_2 can often be improved by the addition of low levels of PEEP.[29,30]

Most ventilators also include alarms for low V_T, low and high $\dot{V}_E$, low and high respiratory rates (f), and low and high oxygen F_IO_2. Alarms should not be set so sensitively that they are constantly being triggered. The following suggestions can be used as a guide:

- Low exhaled V_T: 10% to 15% below set V_T.
- Low exhaled minute volume: 10% to 15% below average minute volume.
- F_IO_2: 5% above and below set oxygen percentage.

Other alarms are available for detecting low battery levels, if the ventilator is inoperative, ventilator circuit malfunction, exhalation valve leaks, and inappropriately set parameters. For example, a set parameter (e.g., V_T) may be outside the range of the ventilator.

Unfortunately, because there are so many alarms and warning indicators on ICU equipment, many clinicians can become desensitized to audible alarms causing the clinicians to respond slowly, or not at all to these alerts.

Action During Ventilator Alarm Situations

When a ventilator malfunctions during use, the clinician must first ensure that the patient is being ventilated. When in doubt, the practitioner should disconnect the patient from the ventilator, start manual ventilation using a manual resuscitation bag, silence the alarms, and call for help. If the practitioner cannot immediately correct the problem, it may be necessary to replace the ventilator (Box 7-4). The operating manuals provided with ventilators usually have troubleshooting sections to solve most problems and can be consulted when time permits. If a ventilator problem cannot be resolved by the in-house biomedical technician support team, it will be necessary to call the local maintenance representative for the company.

PERIODIC HYPERINFLATION OR SIGHING

A *sigh* is a deep breath that occurs regularly as part of a normal breathing pattern. It is used occasionally during mechanical ventilation and related maneuvers (e.g., deep breaths or sighs are used before and after suctioning a patient) (Box 7-5).[22-30]

The sigh or deep breath was a popular idea that was introduced during the 1960s. Ventilators developed in the 1970s and 1980s incorporated sigh breaths into their designs, although traditional sigh breaths had not been shown to be clinically beneficial. These ventilators were capable of providing one or more deep breaths at periodic timed intervals (i.e., three or four times per hour or once every 10 minutes), depending on the ventilator. Because a normal sigh in a spontaneously breathing, nonintubated person occurs about every 6 minutes, ventilator manufacturers designed their machines to deliver sighs at a similar frequency.[28] Sigh volumes were set at one and a half to two times the regular low V_T setting.[28] (Interestingly, low V_T settings [e.g., 5 to 7 mL/kg IBW] were popular at the time.)

Other investigators found that large V_T (10 to 15 mL/kg) in anesthetized patients reduced atelectasis.[31,32] As already discussed, using these higher volumes for patients with acute respiratory failure can cause alveolar overdistention and increase the risk of ventilator-induced lung injury. Mechanical ventilator sigh breaths are therefore **not** recommended in the presence of plateau pressures greater than 30 cm H_2O.

Mild hypoxemia sometimes occurs in patients receiving pressure-supported ventilation (PSV) with low volumes (4 to 6 mL/kg). Studies of the use of sigh breaths in these patients may be worth examining.[29] However, sigh breaths are not indicated for these patients and may be harmful to spontaneously breathing patients receiving CPAP for the treatment of hypoxemia.[33]

With the advent of low V_T strategy in patients with ARDS, another ventilator strategy called *lung recruitment* has been successfully used in selected patients.[34,35] The recruitment maneuver is not unlike sigh breaths. The recruitment maneuver, which is used to expand collapsed areas of the lung, involves using a sustained high pressure of 35 to 45 cm H_2O for 40 to 60 seconds.[35-37] Interestingly, the sigh breaths used by Bendixen and colleagues in 1963,[22] more than 50 years ago, were as follows:

- One breath at 20 cm H_2O for 10 seconds
- A second breath at 30 cm H_2O for 15 seconds
- A third breath at 40 cm H_2O for 15 seconds

These sustained high-pressure maneuvers are not unlike the recruitment maneuvers that are used in the management of patients with ARDS (Key Point 7-5).

Key Point 7-5 When low tidal volumes are used, such as in patients with ARDS, a recruitment maneuver may be an effective method to avoid atelectasis.

Sighs or deep breaths may be appropriate in the following situations:
- Before and after suctioning
- Before and after bronchoscopy
- During an extubation procedure
- During chest physiotherapy
- During low V_T ventilation
- As a recruitment maneuver in some patients with ARDS

FINAL CONSIDERATIONS IN VENTILATOR EQUIPMENT SETUP

Before initiating mechanical ventilation, the respiratory therapist should perform a final check of the equipment to be used. This check should include the following steps:

1. Check ventilator and circuit function to ensure they are operating correctly and no significant leaks are present.
2. Fill the humidifier with sterile water, and set the humidifier temperature so that the final gas temperature at the airway will be approximately 31° to 35° C, or place an HME in line.
3. Place a temperature monitoring device near the patient connector when heated humidification is used.
4. Check the F_IO_2, set V_T (or inspiratory pressure) and f.
5. Adjust the alarms.
6. Ensure that the patient is connected to an electrocardiographic monitor.
7. Have an emergency airway tray available in case the patient's airway is removed or damaged.
8. Check that suctioning equipment is available and functioning.
9. Select a volume-monitoring device and an oxygen analyzer if one is not available with the ventilator.
10. Ensure that a manual resuscitation bag is available and easily accessible.

Once the decision has been made to connect the patient to a ventilator, several steps should be taken, including the following:
- Preparing the patient
- Establishing an airway interface
- Manually ventilating the patient
- Ensuring that the patient's cardiovascular status is stable
- Meeting ventilation needs
- Treating the cause of respiratory failure

Preparing the Patient

Mental preparation of a patient who will require mechanical ventilation is an obvious part of preoperative planning for patients that will likely need short-term postoperative ventilatory support. It is an important part of patient preparation because it can significantly reduce the patient's anxiety and discomfort.

Before initiating mechanical ventilation, conscious patients must be prepared for what to expect once they are connected to the ventilator. The clinician should give a brief explanation about how the ventilator works and why it is being used. The patient must also be informed that the use of an artificial airway will inhibit verbal communication.

Unconscious patients should be informed about their situation as soon as they regain consciousness. This is crucial because these patients will be unable to speak and may be completely unaware of what has occurred. Often the explanation will need to be repeated because sedatives and similar agents can alter a patient's mental status.

Establishing an Interface

For noninvasive ventilation, a face or nasal mask is snugly fitted (see Chapter 19). During invasive ventilation, the three most commonly used artificial airways are orotracheal, nasotracheal, and tracheostomy tubes. Orotracheal tubes are used for emergencies and are generally kept in place for several days. Nasotracheal tubes provide better patient comfort but may require more insertion time. Nasotracheal tubes usually have smaller diameters than orotracheal tubes and are associated with increased incidence of sinus infections. Tracheostomy tubes must be inserted surgically, but these tubes can be used for extended periods. They also allow for easier pulmonary hygiene and are apparently most comfortable for the patient, even allowing the patient to talk in some cases.

Manual Ventilation

Before initiating mechanical ventilation, the patient's ventilatory requirements can be supported by using a manual resuscitation bag. These devices are easy to operate and allow the clinician to monitor closely the patient's breathing efforts and changes in airway resistance (R_{aw}) or lung compliance (C_L).

Cardiovascular Stabilization

The combined stress of acute or impending respiratory failure and endotracheal intubation can reveal undiagnosed cardiovascular complications, which may already be present. For example, patients with existing or borderline myocardial ischemia may develop cardiac dysrhythmias. The effects of any of the pharmacologic agents used during intubation (e.g., topical anesthetics, sedatives, narcotics, and muscle-paralyzing agents) can lead to hypotension and relative hypovolemia, resulting in reduced venous return and cardiac output. Appropriate cardiovascular support is therefore essential to a successful outcome.

Ventilator Needs

After the patient's cardiovascular status is stabilized and primary ventilatory needs are being met, the clinician can then select the appropriate mechanical ventilator mode and appropriate ventilator settings. (See Chapter 6.)

Treating the Cause of Respiratory Failure

Once a life-threatening situation no longer exists, attention can be turned to treating the initial problems that caused the patient to require ventilation. Mechanical ventilation is not curative; the underlying problem must be resolved regardless of whether it is the result of central nervous system or neuromuscular problems or increased WOB caused by trauma, ARDS, or COPD with complications. It makes little sense to be overly aggressive with palliative methods if the underlying pathology is irreversible.

Selecting the Appropriate Ventilator

Specific ventilator selection depends not only on theoretical but also practical considerations. The ventilators available at an institution and the familiarity of personnel with this equipment usually determine ventilator choice. Detailed descriptions of many available ventilators and their features are available from other sources.[38]

The selected ventilator should offer a variety of modes of ventilation, including volume or pressure continuous mandatory ventilation (VC- or PC-CMV), volume or pressure intermittent mandatory ventilation (VC- or PC-IMV), and spontaneous CPAP/PSV.

Adult ventilators are typically capable of delivering V_T in the range of 100 to 2000 mL and respiratory rate from 1 to 60 breaths/min. Pressures from 0 to 100 cm H_2O are adequate, and the driving pressure must be high enough to maintain the gas flow pattern throughout inspiration regardless of how high peak pressures may rise. PEEP/CPAP should be in the range of 0 to 30 cm H_2O. Flow rates should range from 10 to 180 L/min. Constant flow or descending flow patterns probably have more clinical benefit than others and should be included.[37] An inspiratory-to-expiratory (I:E) ratio display may be useful in the management of patients that are difficult to oxygenate.

Response time, patient circuits, exhalation valves, PEEP, and demand valves should be designed to reduce WOB and patient resistance to inspiration and expiration. Two important ventilatory adjuncts are inflation hold and expiratory pause. Inflation hold is used to measure $P_{plateau}$, which is used to calculate static compliance. Expiratory pause is used for auto-PEEP measurements.

The mechanical ventilator should be able to deliver F_IO_2 values from 21% to 100% in increments of 1% to 2%. Alarms should include apnea, pressure limit, power failure, gas source, and low- and high-pressure alarms. If available, high f, low V_T, and high and low $\dot{V}_E$ alarms are particularly important for monitoring pressure-targeted ventilation and spontaneous modes such as PC-CMV, PC-IMV, CPAP, and PSV.

It is important to recognize that these are the fundamental features of adult ventilators, not a description of an ideal ventilator. In fact, most microprocessor ventilators may be equipped with additional modes and features.

EVALUATION OF VENTILATOR PERFORMANCE

The cost of purchasing a particular ventilator and the specific needs of the patients served by the institution should be considered before purchasing a new ventilator; specifically, whether these patients will require short-term or long-term ventilation. The needs of the medical staff should also warrant consideration. For example, the amount of in-service training that will be required to ensure that the respiratory therapy staff is proficient in the use of the equipment should be part of the selection process.

A performance evaluation, or bench test, must be conducted on every ventilator brand before purchase and certainly before patient connection. Forms for conducting these tests are available from the Joint Commission and the American National Standards Institute. A bench test requires the use of a lung analog, which can simulate alterations in respiratory system function. Instruments for measuring volume, pressure, flow, and time are also needed. Bench tests examine ventilator performance during changes in compliance and resistance and leak conditions, and check general features,

parameter ranges, and alarm systems. These tests must also account for various simulated conditions, such as very low and very high $\dot{V}_E$ values, air trapping (auto-PEEP), function during added nebulization, and CPAP function.

Once purchased, ventilators must be checked regularly with maintenance, testing, and calibration programs. Records must be maintained for each ventilator, as well as documentation of personnel training for ventilator use.

Initial Ventilator Settings for Specific Patient Situations

The following cases offer the reader some guidance for making initial ventilator settings. The study questions at the end of the chapter provide additional practice in this area.

A number of published reviews along with several other textbooks provide information about currently accepted practices for managing various pulmonary disorders requiring mechanical ventilation.[3-5,40-43] The settings recommended in the following cases reflect the standard of practice suggested by these sources.

CHRONIC OBSTRUCTIVE PULMONARY DISEASE

Patients with COPD have increased R_{aw} and may also have increased C_L, which, when combined, cause significant expiratory obstruction, lengthen the time constant, and lead to air trapping. When patients with COPD require mechanical ventilation, it is often because their chronic disease has been coupled with another problem, such as a respiratory infection, leading to an **acute-on-chronic** respiratory failure.

Mechanical ventilation in COPD is associated with increased morbidity because of air trapping, nosocomial infections, barotrauma and volutrauma, cardiac problems, aspiration, and difficulty weaning. The goals of mechanical ventilation are to maximize patient-ventilator synchrony, reduce WOB and patient anxiety, and avoid the complications associated with mechanical ventilation, such as ventilator-associated pneumonia (VAP) and ventilator-induced lung injury.

Guidelines for Patients with Chronic Obstructive Pulmonary Disease

Basic guidelines for mechanically ventilating patients with COPD have been established.[3-5,40-44] These guidelines include the following:

- If possible, use noninvasive ventilation to avoid problems associated with artificial airways. Bilevel positive airway pressure (bilevel PAP) is ideal for patients with chronic pulmonary disorders (see Chapter 19).
- If intubation is necessary, an orotracheal intubation is recommended.
- The clinician can select a ventilator mode that he or she feels is most familiar. It has been noted, however, that VC- or PC-CMV may unload the work of the respiratory muscles more than IMV.[44] Using patient-triggered CMV in an alert patient with COPD may increase the risk of hyperinflation and elevated lung pressures. This mode should be monitored carefully.[44]
- Adjust the peak inspiratory flow to meet the patient's demand in VC-CMV using the descending flow pattern: flow >60 L/min.
- In patients with COPD and asthma, where airway obstruction and resistance are high, an initial V_T of 6 to 8 mL/kg with a rate of 8 to 16 breaths/min, and T_I 0.6 to 1.2 seconds is acceptable.

- PEEP 5 cm H_2O or lower, or about 50% of auto-PEEP, should be used initially.
- Monitor for and minimize dynamic hyperinflation (auto-PEEP) by setting the lowest possible $\dot{V}_E$ that produces acceptable gas exchange, targeting the patient's baseline P_aCO_2 and pH.
- Provide the longest expiratory time (T_E) possible. This may include decreasing T_I, increasing T_E, reducing f or V_T, and accepting hypercapnia (P_aCO_2 higher than the patient's normal). (NOTE: Patients with COPD are usually ventilated in their normal P_aCO_2 range (e.g., P_aCO_2 = 50 to 60 mm Hg; pH 7.3 to 7.4.)
- If the patient is initiating inspiration once ventilation has started and auto-PEEP is present, set PEEP near 80% of the auto-PEEP level, but do not exceed it (3 to 5 cm H_2O is often adequate). If PIP begins to rise because PEEP is increased, the safe PEEP level has probably been exceeded and will result in lung overinflation.
- $P_{plateau}$ should be monitored and maintained below 30 cm H_2O to avoid alveolar overdistention and, consequently, lung injury. Accurate measurement of $P_{plateau}$ may require sedation and paralysis. The decision to medicate patients is generally based on physician preference and institutional policy.
- Maintain P_aO_2 at 55 to 75 mm Hg or near the patient's normal P_aO_2, with F_IO_2 less than 0.5, unless the patient's condition worsens and he or she requires more oxygen.

Pressure control ventilation (PC-CMV) may be ideal for this group of patients for several reasons. PC-CMV provides flow on demand to meet the patient's needs. T_I can be set along with a backup rate, but patient triggering is still permitted. PC-CMV has a distinct advantage over PSV for this patient population because inspiration during PSV can be too long or too short, depending on the patient's active breathing patterns. This can result in increased WOB and poor patient-ventilator synchrony. Auto-PEEP can be a lethal complication. Current ventilators that allow an adjustable expiratory flow cycle may allow for the use of PSV in COPD.

Volume-assured pressure support (VAPS) or volume support (Servo-i) can also provide pressure ventilation with a set targeted volume delivery (see Chapter 6). Although these modes are also well suited for patients with COPD, clinicians must be familiar with their use.

An important part of patient care is providing adequate hydration and pharmacologic therapy (i.e., bronchodilators and corticosteroids) to reverse airflow limitation. Secretions must be mobilized and removed, and if infections are present, appropriate antibiotic medication must be administered. The primary problem necessitating ventilation must be corrected to ensure that weaning will be successful. Because many of these patients are malnourished, an evaluation of their nutritional needs must be part of any follow-up program.

⊘ Clinical Scenario: Chronic Obstructive Pulmonary Disease

A 65-year-old man with a history of COPD is brought to the emergency department complaining of severe shortness of breath. Below is the information obtained from the patient assessment. The S_pO_2 of 75% obtained while he was breathing room air is very low. Because pulse oximetry may be inaccurate in this range, an ABG was obtained. A 28% air-entrainment mask was placed on the patient.

Initial Patient Assessment on Admission: History of COPD

The patient is a retired salesman and lives at home with his wife. He has a 40-pack-per-year history of cigarette smoking.

Mental Status

Alert and oriented but shows signs of fatigue
Speaks in halting sentences and appears to be catching his breath between efforts to talk

Physical Appearance

- Tall and thin
- Barrel chest
- Pale skin
- Pitting edema of the ankles
- Prolonged expiration through pursed lips with labored breathing
- Sitting in a chair, leaning forward with his arms on the chair arms
- Active use of the sternocleidomastoid muscles

Vital Signs

f = 35 to 40 breaths/min
Heart rate = 135 beats/min
Blood pressure = 185/110 mm Hg
Temperature = 98.6° F

Breath Sounds

Bilateral wheezes, crackles in the bases, hyperresonance to percussion bilaterally

Cough

Weak, producing a moderate amount of thick, yellow secretions

S_pO_2

75% on room air

Chest Radiograph

Increased bilateral radiolucency, flattened diaphragm, widened rib spaces; scattered infiltrates in both bases

The patient is given an aerosol treatment with albuterol by small-volume nebulizer followed by an aerosolized mucolytic. He does not tolerate the treatment well and is unable to take a deep breath or to perform a breath-hold maneuver. His dyspnea persists. ABGs on an F_IO_2 of 0.28 are pH = 7.24; P_aCO_2 = 97 mm Hg; P_aO_2 = 38 mm Hg; and HCO_3^- = 41 mEq/L.

The ABGs indicate chronic CO_2 retention (elevated HCO_3^-) that has now progressed to an acute-on-chronic phase (elevated P_aCO_2 and low pH). His level of hypoxemia is also severe. The infiltrates in the lower lung fields and the production of thick yellow sputum suggest the presence of a respiratory infection, but the absence of an elevated temperature is confusing. (NOTE: Elderly patients, particularly those with chronic health problems, do not always develop a fever. If patients take aspirin or nonsteroidal or steroidal antiinflammatory medications, an elevated temperature might be masked.) A sputum specimen is sent to the laboratory for culture and sensitivity testing.

Based on the assessment, a decision is made to begin mechanical ventilatory support. The patient is 5 ft 10 in tall and weighs 148 lb. What are his body surface area (BSA) and IBW? What initial settings for $\dot{V}_E$, f, T_I, and flow would be appropriate? Would you use pressure or volume ventilation? The box below answers these questions and provides the initial settings selected in this case.

Initial Ventilator Settings—COPD Patient

BSA = 1.85 m²
IBW = 106 + 6(10) = 166 lb (75.5 kg)
Initial $\dot{V}_E$ = 4 × 1.85 = 7.4 L/min
Because of concern for air trapping, consider a lower set $\dot{V}_E$
Attempt to synchronize the ventilator with the patient
Noninvasive ventilation is appropriate

A Respironics BiPAP ventilator is selected. With this ventilator, a low level of CPAP/PEEP (2 cm H_2O) is maintained in the airway even when the expiratory positive airway pressure (EPAP) control is minimal.

Rate is set at 8 breaths/min; TCT = 60/8 = 7.5 seconds; and T_I = 13% of TCT

I:E ratio = 1:6.5; T_I = 1.0 seconds; and T_E = 6.5 seconds
Inspiratory positive airway pressure (IPAP) = 10 cm H_2O initially and is titrated to obtain an exhaled V_T of 600 mL (0.6 L)
Final IPAP is 14 cm H_2O
EPAP = set at 4 cm H_2O

Spontaneous/timed setting is selected, providing a backup rate, at which point time-triggered breaths are modified pressure-controlled (PC) breaths; spontaneous breaths are pressure-supported (PS) breaths.

Oxygen is titrated to ≥90% oxygen saturation measured by pulse oximetry (S_pO_2).

The patient is transferred to the ICU and the settings are maintained for 2 hours. It becomes increasingly difficult for the patient to clear secretions, and he continues to try to remove the mask. He eventually consents to intubation and is intubated using a size 8-Fr orotracheal ET. The physician asks the respiratory therapist to maintain similar settings but wants to use Dräger Evita Infinity V500 in the VC-CMV mode. The box below shows the selected ventilator settings.

VC-CMV Settings—Patient with COPD

- Pressure required during inspiration was 14 cm H_2O
- PEEP at 4 cm H_2O, as previously present
- Set rate at 8 breaths/min
- V_T (set) of 600 mL (0.6 L) to match previous setting
- Flow at 80 L/min to start
- Flow waveform is constant (the current recommended setting for this mode)
- F_iO_2 at 0.3 to 0.5, since exact setting is unknown; titrate to achieve S_pO_2 of ≥ 90%

The following information is noted after assessment:
- The patient triggers every breath but at a rate >8 breaths/min. TCT is about 2.5 seconds.
- T_I is about 1 second and T_E is about 1.5 seconds.
- Expiratory flow does not return to zero before the next breath indicating the presence of auto-PEEP.[45]
- During inspiration, following an initial high flow, flow drops to 80 L/min and stays there until V_T is delivered.

This flow may not be adequate to keep T_I short.
Possible solutions to minimize air trapping might include:
- Switching to PC-CMV with a short T_I.
- Setting a lower V_T.

- Checking the patient's airway to be sure it is clear of secretions and possibly administering a bronchodilator.
- Increasing inspiratory flow.

Appropriate adjustments are made, and the patient is successfully managed using PC-CMV. The respiratory infection is resolved 5 days later. Secretion clearance is improved. Occasional scattered crackles are heard on auscultation, but otherwise breath sounds have cleared. Infiltrates are no longer present on chest radiographs. Weaning should now be considered for this patient.

ASTHMA

Patients presenting an exacerbation of **acute severe asthma** that requires mechanical ventilation are among the most difficult to manage. Increased R_{aw} from bronchospasm, increased secretions, and mucosal edema increase the incidence of air trapping. Trapped air can cause uneven hyperexpansion of various lung units, which can rupture or compress other areas of the lungs, leading to pneumothorax, pneumomediastinum, subcutaneous emphysema, and other forms of barotrauma.

During an asthma exacerbation, the patient struggles to breathe while trying to move air against increasing loads. The result is dramatic changes in intrapleural pressures (P_{pl}) during inspiration and expiration that not only affect gas distribution in the lungs but also alter cardiac function, resulting in **pulsus paradoxus.** Progressive hypoxemia further enhances the patient's drive to breathe and compounds anxiety. Even aggressive treatment with bronchodilators and steroids might not be enough to reverse the course of an acute asthma exacerbation.

Box 7-6 lists indications for mechanical ventilation for this group of patients. The primary goal during mechanical ventilation of these patients is to focus on reversing the high R_{aw} while avoiding or reducing air trapping. If the patient has anxiety and the drive to breathe produces patient-ventilator asynchrony during mechanical ventilation, then sedation and possibly paralysis may be

---

BOX 7-6 **Indications for Mechanical Ventilation in Acute Exacerbation of Asthma**

1. Exhaustion (e.g., respiratory rate progressively decreases and level of consciousness is altered), with developing metabolic acidosis, and decreasing pH in the presence of a normal or rising carbon dioxide pressure (P_aCO_2).
2. If audible, bilateral wheezes become distant as air trapping increases (e.g., breath sounds absent, chest hyperresonant to percussion or fixed on palpation).
3. Severe hypoxemia while receiving oxygen (e.g., inability to oxygenate with supplemental oxygen).
4. Chest radiograph with depression of the hemidiaphragms and increased radiolucency, suggestive of air trapping.
5. Altered mental status, confusion, or decreased level of consciousness.
6. Life-threatening dysrhythmias.
7. P_aCO_2 rises while pH declines (e.g., ≥40 mm Hg; pH ≤7.25 [progressive respiratory acidosis superimposed on a metabolic acidosis]).
8. Cardiac or respiratory arrest.

required. (NOTE: The use of certain paralytics may result in a neuropathy that can produce prolonged paralysis, which can hinder weaning from ventilatory support. Indeed, prolonged paralysis can have long-term effects, such as reducing a patient's ability to ambulate for several weeks or months. [This can be a particularly serious complication in patients with renal insufficiency or hepatic disease, particularly when paralytic agents and corticosteroids are used in combination for extended periods of time.])

Guidelines for Patients with Asthma

The following guidelines provide suggestions for mechanically ventilating patients with asthma.[3-5,41-43,45-50]

- VC- or PC-CMV are acceptable modes immediately following intubation. It is easier to control airway pressure with PC-CMV.
- Maintain peak and plateau pressures at minimal levels. PIP may be high due to the high R_{aw} and the use of high inspiratory gas flows. Alveolar (plateau) pressures must still be maintained at <30 cm H_2O despite the high PIP.
- Ensure that the patient's oxygenation status is adequate by using an F_IO_2 as needed to achieve a P_aO_2 from 60 to 100 mm Hg (usually $F_IO_2 \geq 0.5$). Monitor hemodynamic status to ensure cardiac output is stable.
- Permissive hypercapnia (P_aCO_2 45 to 80 mm Hg) is acceptable as long as pH is acceptable (i.e., ≥ 7.2). (NOTE: Trishydroxymethyl-aminomethane [THAM] or bicarbonate is administered by some physicians to keep pH greater than 7.2. The preference between these agents varies among physicians.)
- If the ventilator settings cannot accommodate the patient's needs, the use of sedatives and paralytics may be necessary. The use of sedation and paralysis may permit resting of fatigued respiratory muscles, particularly during the first 24 hours.[46]
- When patients are spontaneously breathing and having trouble triggering breaths, setting the $PEEP_E$ at about 80% of intrinsic PEEP may allow for easier triggering of ventilator breaths. (NOTE: $PEEP_E$ is indicated in only a few situations because these patients already have an increased functional residual capacity.) In some cases, applied PEEP may recruit lung units that are collapsed (even in the presence of auto-PEEP) and may also assist with expired gas flows.[51] In other cases it may worsen the patient's condition. If PIP increases with the application of $PEEP_E$, decrease the level of $PEEP_E$.
- Reduce the incidence of air trapping by providing long expiratory times:
- f = <8 breaths/min; V_T = 6 to 8 mL/kg; $T_I \leq 1$ sec; inspiratory gas flow = 80 to 100 L/min descending flow waveform.[51]
- The occurrence of **barotrauma** in the form of pneumothorax, for example, is not uncommon in these patients. Regular assessment of breath sounds and diagnostic chest percussion, along with chest radiographs, can help guide therapy to avoid this potential problem.

Clinical Scenario: Patient with Asthma

A 13-year-old girl with a history of severe persistent asthma is brought to the emergency room at 2:30 AM. Wheezing is audible without the use of a stethoscope. Auscultation of the chest confirms that the wheezing is bilateral. The patient has used her albuterol MDI 10 times (20 puffs) in the past 4 hours. Current peak expiratory flow rate (PEFR) is 150 L/

min. A chest radiograph shows increased radiolucency and depressed hemidiaphragms. ABGs on a 2 L/min nasal cannula are: pH = 7.43; P_aCO_2 = 25 mm Hg; P_aO_2 = 43 mm Hg; HCO_3^- = 17 mEq/L. Her S_pO_2 is 73%. She is started on bronchodilators (albuterol and Atrovent) via continuous aerosol and intravenous corticosteroids (Solu-Medrol).

The patient's condition does not improve over the next 5 hours, in spite of therapy. Her breath sounds are more distant and there is hyperresonance to percussion of the chest wall. She is cyanotic and anxious and her breaths are labored. On a 4 L/min O_2 nasal cannula, ABGs are: pH = 7.25; P_aCO_2 = 59 mm Hg; P_aO_2 = 53 mm Hg; HCO_3^- = 25 mEq/L. S_pO_2 is 79%. PEFR is 120 L/min and f is 16 breaths/min (down from 30 breaths/min on admission). Blood pressure (BP) is 160/100 and heart rate (HR) is 175 beats/min. She is transferred to the ICU, and the decision is made to intubate her and begin mechanical ventilatory support. To calculate initial settings, see below.

Initial Ventilator Settings—Patient with Acute Asthma

Based on this patient's history and size (5 ft 3 in [63 in], 108 lbs [49 kg])
- IBW = 105 + 5(3) = 120 lb (54.5 kg)
- BSA = 1.5 m²
- Initial $\dot{V}_E$ = 1.50 × 3.5 = 5.25 L/min
- Targeted V_T (6 to 8 mL/kg); 327 to 435 mL
- f = $\dot{V}_E/V_T$ = (5.25 L/min)/0.435 L = 12 breaths/min.

NEUROMUSCULAR DISORDERS

It is not unusual for patients with neuromuscular disorders to require ventilatory support. Examples of disorders that are included in this category are myasthenia gravis, amyotrophic lateral sclerosis, muscular dystrophy, postpolio syndrome, Guillain-Barré syndrome, tetanus, cervical spinal cord injury, and botulism. Patients with ventilatory failure because of a neuromuscular disorder usually have a normal ventilatory drive and normal or near-normal lung function. Most of the neuromuscular disorders cited cause respiratory muscle weakness, which can limit these patients' abilities to cough and clear secretions. As a result, they tend to develop atelectasis and pneumonia. If the glottic response is weak, they also may have an increased risk of aspiration. Mechanical ventilation is most often required if progressive respiratory muscle weakness will eventually lead to respiratory failure.

Patients with neuromuscular problems can be effectively ventilated with either positive or negative pressure ventilation. In the hospital environment, PPV is most often selected and can be either noninvasive or invasive. Negative pressure ventilation (NPV) is rarely used.

The patients most often seen in hospitals are those with a rapid onset of their disease that requires admission (e.g., Guillain-Barré syndrome and myasthenia gravis). Because these patients often have normal lung function, they are at low risk for barotrauma and are most comfortable when ventilated with higher V_T values (i.e., 6 to 8 mL/kg) and high inspiratory flow rates greater than 60 L/min using a constant flow or descending flow pattern when VC-CMV is used. (NOTE: Some clinicians prefer starting with a lower V_T and adjusting the volume as needed.) Patients with spinal cord injuries resulting in quadriplegia require full ventilatory support. Patients with myasthenia gravis usually require only partial support until their own breathing capacity returns.

Guidelines for Patients with Neuromuscular Disorders

The following guidelines are recommended for mechanically ventilating patients with neuromuscular disorders[3-5,41-43]:

- Full or partial support
- Negative or positive pressure ventilation
- Noninvasive or invasive ventilation
- Assist/control mode (CMV)
- Volume control ventilation
- V_T (6 to 8 mL/kg) while maintaining the $P_{Plateau}$ at less than 30 cm H_2O
- f = 8 to 16 breaths/min
- Inspiratory flow rates ≥60 L/min to meet patient need (T_I about 1 second to start)
- Flow waveform: constant or descending flow pattern
- PEEP = 5 cm H_2O may be needed to relieve dyspnea
- $F_IO_2 = 0.21$

⊘ Clinical Scenario: Neuromuscular Disorder

A 5-ft 2-in, 115-lb, 67-year-old woman with a history of myasthenia gravis was brought to her physician's office by her daughter. She complained of progressive muscle weakness. Physical examination revealed that she demonstrated drooping eyelids and difficulty talking and swallowing. She was unable to walk more than a step or two. She was transferred to the hospital, where she was given edrophonium (Tensilon), which improved her muscle function for 10 to 15 minutes. On admission, her vital signs were unremarkable. Her maximum inspiratory pressure (MIP) was −35 cm H_2O, and her vital capacity (VC) was 1.8 L (predicted was 3.3 L). Her S_pO_2 on room air was 96%.

Anticholinesterase therapy was administered, and MIP and VC were monitored every 8 hours. The nursing staff reported that the patient was having trouble swallowing when she ate and they feared that she would aspirate. MIP and VC values progressively declined. After being hospitalized for 24 hours, her MIP was −25 cm H_2O and VC was 1.0 L. ABGs on room air were as follows: pH = 7.36; P_aCO_2 = 48 mm Hg; P_aO_2 = 62 mm Hg; HCO_3^- = 27 mEq/L. The section below provides a summary of the therapeutic intervention used for this patient. Could noninvasive positive pressure ventilation (NIV) be used in this situation?

Initial Ventilator Settings with Neuromuscular Disorder (Myasthenia Gravis)

The patient was intubated because of increased risk of aspiration. (Invasive mechanical ventilation was initiated rather than NIV because her ability to swallow was compromised and she showed signs of acute respiratory failure despite anticholinesterase therapy.)

Patient is 5 ft 2 in tall and weighs 115 lbs, so:

- IBW = 105 + 5(2) = 115 lb (52 kg)
- BSA is 1.5 m^2
- Estimated $\dot{V}_E$ is 3.5 × 1.5 = 5.25 L

- V_T = 420 mL (8 mL/kg); (VC-CMV)
- Rate = 13 breaths/min
- Flow = 60 L/min using a constant waveform
- PEEP = 2 cm H_2O and F_IO_2 = 0.21
- Calculate T_I and T_E
- $T_I = V_T$/flow (L/sec) = 0.420 L/(1 L/sec) = 0.42 sec
- TCT = 60 sec/12 = 5.0 sec
- T_E = 6.0 − 0.42 = 5.58 sec
- PIP = 20 cm H_2O
- $P_{plateau}$ = 12 cm H_2O
- What is the transairway pressure? 20 − 12 = 8 cm H_2O
- What is the patient's C_L and is it normal?
- $C_L = V_T/(P_{plateau} − PEEP)$ = 0.420/(12 − 3) = 0.046 L/cm H_2O or 46 mL/cm H_2O
- C_L is normal

Ventilatory support was maintained for a total of 10 days with one occurrence of a respiratory infection that responded to antibiotic therapy. She was successfully weaned and extubated on the 10th day.

CLOSED HEAD INJURY

Closed head injury is an injury to the brain in which the skull remains intact. It is most commonly caused by trauma to the head from falls, automobile accidents, and blows to the head. Because the skull is a closed container, bruising the brain tissue can result in swelling (edema) and increased intracranial pressures (ICP). Similar effects may occur following surgery (postcraniotomy), medical accidents (i.e., cerebral vascular accident [stroke], and postresuscitation hypoxemia.)[3,37,41,42]

The cranial vault contains the brain, blood, and cerebral spinal fluid (CSF). Assessment of cerebral blood flow is important because the brain relies on steady blood flow to provide oxygen. Maintaining sufficient cerebral blood flow requires an adequate cerebral perfusion pressure (CPP). CPP is defined by the equation: CPP = mean arterial pressure (MAP) − ICP. Normal values for MAP are 90 to 95 mm Hg and ICP less than 10 mm Hg. Normal CPP is 80 to 85 mm Hg. Values of CPP lower than 60 mm Hg indicate poor cerebral perfusion.

Clinically, it is important to keep ICP low and MAP in the normal range to maintain CPP in brain-injured patients. Several techniques can be used to accomplish this goal. Mannitol infusion can be used to increase osmotic pressures and reduce ICP in acute situations; diuretics can reduce fluid volume (may reduce MAP, which may reduce CPP); and barbiturates can be used to reduce cerebral oxygen demand and lower ICP when conventional therapy fails. Patients should be maintained with their heads in a neutral position and the head of the bed elevated by 30 degrees.

Iatrogenic hyperventilation, or the deliberate lowering of P_aCO_2, is sometimes used to reduce ICP, but its effectiveness remains controversial. The theory is that acute reductions in P_aCO_2 are believed to result in cerebral vasoconstriction, reducing cerebral blood volume and ICP. Note that a decreasing CO_2 is associated with an increase in pH. The effect of CO_2 and pH change on ICP is most pronounced when it is acute and loses its effect as the pH of the CSF becomes normalized. Therefore, P_aCO_2 should be normalized as soon as possible, depending on ICP response. It is important to mention that not all physicians advocate the use of this technique. Furthermore, if an increased ICP is not present, iatrogenic hyperventilation is not indicated (current standards

BOX 7-7 Indications for Mechanical Ventilation in Patients with Head Injuries

Assisted Ventilation
1. Respiratory depression associated with injury. It may be manifested as Cheyne-Stokes respiration, central neurogenic hyperventilation, or apnea.
2. Additional injuries to the chest, abdomen, back, or neck.
3. Use of medications that depress respiration.
4. Neurogenic pulmonary edema (an acute respiratory distress syndrome [ARDS]-like pattern that can occur following head trauma).
5. Impending or actual cardiac arrest.
6. Upper airway compromise (e.g., presence of stridor or loss of airway clearance mechanisms).
7. Aspiration at the time of loss of consciousness.

Airway Management (Intubation)
1. Head injury (particularly with Glasgow Coma Score* of ≤8).
2. Face, jaw, neck injuries with bleeding.

Oxygen Delivery
1. Head injury.
2. Pulmonary contusion, edema, or both.

*See Box 7-8.

BOX 7-8 Glasgow Coma Score*

Verbal Response:
1 = None
2 = Incomprehensible sounds
3 = Inappropriate words
4 = Confused
5 = Oriented

Eye Opening:
1 = None
2 = To pain
3 = To speech
4 = Spontaneously

Motor Response:
1 = None
2 = Abnormal extension to pain
3 = Abnormal flexion to pain
4 = Withdraws from pain
5 = Localizes pain
6 = Follows commands

*The Glasgow Coma Score evaluates a patient's verbal, eye, and motor responses. Scores range from 3 to 15.

suggest that the P_aCO_2 should be maintained between 35 and 40 mm Hg). When a high ICP is present, iatrogenic hyperventilation can be used for a short time. Box 7-7 lists the indications for mechanical ventilation in patients with head injury.[3] Box 7-8 provides information on the Glasgow Coma Score mentioned in Box 7-7.

Guidelines for Patients with a Closed Head Injury

The following guidelines are recommended for mechanically ventilating patients with closed head injuries[3-5,41-43]:

- Following head injury, protect the airway because patients with altered levels of consciousness may be unable to do so. There is a high risk for vomiting and aspiration. Orotracheal intubation is often required.
- PC-CMV and PEEP can actually increase ICP. These patients often have normal lungs, so high P_{alv} can be transmitted to the blood vessels, thus affecting venous return from the head. Monitoring for elevated ICP can help to evaluate this effect.
- Monitor for increased ICP and hypoxemia so that a rapid increase in ventilation and oxygenation can be instituted if needed or if recommended by institutional policy.
- When there is acute uncontrolled increased ICP, maintain P_aCO_2 from 25 to 30 mm Hg or titrate the ICP if it is being monitored.
- If iatrogenic hyperventilation is used, this should only be temporary, with P_aCO_2 gradually returning to normal levels in 24 to 48 hours, allowing acid–base balance to restore itself. Sudden increases in P_aCO_2 could trigger increases in cerebral blood flow and ICP. A normal response to acute increases in ICP is hypertension with bradycardia, which is called the *Cushing response.*[3]
- Ventilator settings include the following:
  - Provide full ventilatory support to start.
  - Either PC- or VC-CMV can be used.

- Maintain V_T from 6 to 8 mL/kg IBW while maintaining $P_{plateau}$ at less than 30 cm H_2O.
- An f of 15 to 20 breaths/min to provide normal acid–base status, as long as auto-PEEP is avoided.
- $F_IO_2 = 1.0$ initially and titrate as needed to keep P_aO_2 from 70 to 100 mm Hg to avoid hypoxemia.
- High inspiratory flow (>60 L/min) to keep T_I short, about 1 second (avoid auto-PEEP) using a descending ramp pattern or constant flow pattern.
- PEEP = 0 to 5 cm H_2O, as long as ICP is being measured and is 10 mm Hg or less. Because PEEP can increase ICP, it is used only if necessary to avoid severe hypoxemia.
- Suctioning and chest physiotherapy can dramatically increase ICP but maintaining a clear airway is also essential. Consequently, bronchial hygiene therapy must be done with extreme caution.
- Monitor for complications of pulmonary infections and pulmonary emboli.

Clinical Scenario: Acute Head Injury

A 23-year-old man is admitted to the emergency department after hitting his head against a tree in a skiing accident. He is unconscious on admission. There are no fractures to his head, neck, thorax, or limbs, but some bruising is present on his arms and legs. On admission his vital signs are blood pressure = 150/90 mm Hg; heart rate = 110 beats/min and regular; f = 12 breaths/min; and temperature = 35.6° C. Breath sounds are equal and clear bilaterally. He withdraws from painful stimuli but is otherwise unresponsive. His pupils respond equally to light.

The decision is made to intubate the young man to protect his airway. A computed tomogram (CT) of the head reveals an intracranial hemorrhage. Following neurosurgery, the patient is transferred to the ICU; an ICP monitor is in place, along with an arterial line and a pulmonary artery catheter. He is receiving phenobarbital (a barbiturate) and midazolam (a short-acting benzodiazepine). The patient is 6 ft 4 in (76 in) and weighs 225 lb (102 kg). ICP is 15 mm Hg, and hemodynamic data are within normal limits. The following box provides suggestions for his initial ventilator setting.

Suggesting Initial Ventilator Settings—Patient with Head Injury

- Patient's IBW: $106 + 6(16) = 202$ lb (92 kg)
- Patient's BSA: 2.32 m^2
- Settings: $V_T = 552$ to 736 mL (range of 6 to 8 mL/kg IBW)
- Normal $\dot{V}_E = 4 \times 2.32 = 9.28$ L/min
- Lung condition assumed to be normal at this time

Possible Initial Settings

VC-CMV, $V_T = 0.6$ L; $f = 15$ breaths/min; flow = 60 L/min using descending ramp

$F_IO_2 = 1.0$; PEEP = 3 cm H_2O

After 30 minutes on the initial settings, ABGs are pH = 7.43; $P_aCO_2 = 36$ mm Hg; $P_aO_2 = 450$ mm Hg; and HCO$_3^-$ = 24 mEq/L. ICP = 18 mm Hg. F_IO_2 is reduced to 0.5, and the patient is maintained on these settings until reevaluation in 2 hours. Additional changes should be directed toward reducing ICP.

ACUTE RESPIRATORY DISTRESS SYNDROME

Acute respiratory distress syndrome (ARDS) is recognized as one of the most complex pulmonary disorders to manage. Mortality rates have been reported to range from 30% to 70%.[34-39] Box 7-9 lists the diagnostic criteria for ARDS, and Box 7-10 lists some precipitating factors leading to this disorder. The characteristic pathophysiological findings associated with ARDS include hypoxemia, increased pulmonary vascular permeability, bilateral radiographic opacities, venous admixture, increased lung weight, and decreased lung compliance. ARDS has been described as having two phases: an early phase (first 7 to 10 days), which is characterized by increased vascular permeability, lung water, and lung protein; and a later phase (after 10 days), which is accompanied by extensive lung fibrosis.[52-54] Management of ARDS inevitably includes mechanical ventilatory support.[55]

Guidelines for Patients with Acute Respiratory Distress Syndrome

For patients with ARDS, a V_T of 6 to 8 mL/kg with a respiratory rate of 15 to 25 breaths/min is indicated. Use of lower than normal tidal volumes ($V_T = 4$ to 6 mL/kg) may be necessary to maintain the $P_{plateau}$ <30 cm H_2O. This protective lung strategy has been shown to reduce the risk of ventilator-induced lung injury and improve outcomes for ARDS patients. As discussed in earlier chapters, it is important to remember that the use of high respiratory rates and low V_T may not provide sufficient time for exhalation and ultimately lead to air being trapped in the lungs during exhalation (auto-PEEP).

The following guidelines are suggested for ventilating patients with ARDS[3-5,34-36,43,52-55]:

BOX 7-9 Diagnostic Criteria for Acute Respiratory Distress Syndrome[39]

- History of precipitating condition (see Box 7-10) that occurs within 1 week of a known clinical insult
- Diffuse bilateral alveolar infiltrates on chest radiograph (or computed tomography scan) not fully explained by effusions, lobar/lung collapse, or nodules
- Pulmonary edema that is not fully explained by cardiac failure or fluid overload. Objective assessment to verify if no risk factor is present
- Reduced lung compliance (C_L) (<40 mL/cm H_2O)
- Refractory hypoxemia (reduced partial pressure of arterial oxygen [P_aO_2]/fractional inspired oxygen concentration [F_IO_2])

• Mild	≤200 mm Hg P_aO_2/F_IO_2 ≤ 300 mm Hg with 5 cm H_2O PEEP
• Moderate	<100 mm Hg ≤ 200 mm Hg with 5 cm H_2O PEEP
• Severe	≤100 mm Hg with 5 cm H_2O PEEP

BOX 7-10 Examples of Conditions Associated with Development of Acute Respiratory Distress Syndrome

- Sepsis
- Aspiration of gastric contents
- Thoracic and nonthoracic trauma
- Heroin or other drug overdose
- Massive blood transfusions
- Fat emboli
- Smoke inhalation or chemically induced lung injury
- Pulmonary vasculitis
- Burns
- Pancreatitis
- Near-drowning
- Interstitial viral pneumonitis
- Disseminated intravascular coagulation
- Oxygen toxicity
- Prolonged cardiopulmonary bypass

- Choose a mode capable of supporting oxygenation and ventilation, such as PC- or VC-CMV.
- Maintain S_aO_2 at 88% to 90% or greater. Start at 100% oxygen. To support oxygenation, use PEEP$_E$ at a level that prevents alveolar collapse but minimizes overdistention to prevent lung damage. PEEP$_E$ may allow reduction of F_IO_2 to safe levels.
- When oxygenation is inadequate, sedate, paralyze, and change patient position. Cardiac output and hemoglobin levels should be optimized. High PEEP$_E$ levels greater than 15 cm H_2O may be required in ARDS.
- Keep $P_{plateau}$ below 30 cm H_2O by lowering V_T to 4 to 6 mL/kg, if necessary. Allow P_aCO_2 to rise above normal (permissive hypercapnia) if necessary, unless there is a risk of increased ICP or contraindications exist that demand a normal P_aCO_2 or pH. Rapid rises in P_aCO_2 should be avoided.

There is no evidence to date that PC-CMV is superior to VC-CMV, or vice versa. The selection of one mode over the other may depend on clinician comfort levels. If VC-CMV is selected, the clinician should use the descending flow waveform to help ensure early delivery of V_T and provide a higher mean airway pressure ($\bar{P}_{aw}$) than a constant flow pattern, which may benefit oxygenation and minimizes the difference between PIP and $P_{plateau}$.

During the acute phase of the disease, patients typically require high levels of ventilatory support, although full support is usually not necessary. These levels can be attained with either CMV or IMV + PSV. Adequate ventilation can generally be provided with V_T in the range of 4 to 6 mL/kg while $P_{plateau}$ is maintained at below 30 cm H_2O with rates of 15 to 25 breaths/min. Use flow greater than 60 L/min for volume-controlled ventilation. During pressure-controlled ventilation, use a T_I that is long enough to enhance oxygenation but short enough to allow adequate T_E to avoid auto-PEEP (e.g., T_I <1 second). Because time constants are short for many lung units (decreased compliance), this is usually not difficult even for I:E ratios of 1:1.5 or higher (e.g., 1:1 or 2:1).

$PEEP_E$ is required for the management of ARDS to prevent the opening and closing of alveoli during each breath. This opening and closing can cause lung injury from the shear stress (frictional forces) between alveoli that have different time constants and may also result in surfactant being "milked" from the alveoli (Fig. 7-4).[54,55] During the early phase of ARDS, it is important to keep $PEEP_E$ high enough at least to exceed the inflection point on a slow or static pressure–volume curve (see Chapter 13).[56] It is generally accepted by clinicians that the deflation limb of a slow pressure–volume loop best approximates the end-expiratory pressure range required to prevent alveolar collapse.[57] Maintaining $PEEP_E$ above this pressure range helps to prevent opening and closing of small airways and alveoli (i.e., this is often referred to as the *open lung approach* to ventilator management).[55-59] Even if a ventilator does not have a graphics package, this curve can be graphed by hand.

$PEEP_E$ may also be beneficial in later stages of ARDS to maintain oxygenation and reduce the F_IO_2 levels (<0.5). More information about the management of ARDS is presented in Chapter 13.

Acceptable endpoints for the management of ARDS based on ABGs are P_aCO_2 = 40 to 80 mm Hg; pH = 7.20 to 7.40; P_aO_2 = 60 to 100 mm Hg. Note that these values may vary between institutions. Some physicians prefer to use THAM or sodium bicarbonate when pH drops below 7.20.[42,59]

 Clinical Scenario: Patient with ARDS

A 60-year-old man sustained multiple lacerations from a motor vehicle crash. Admission to the emergency department for evaluation revealed a fractured left femur, a deep laceration of the right arm, an open pneumothorax on the right side of the chest, and abdominal bruising. There was evidence of injury to the head or neck. The patient was taken to surgery for repair of internal injuries; a chest tube with pleural drainage was inserted for the pneumothorax.

The patient developed a fever of 39.5° C and severe refractory hypoxemia 4 days after surgery. A chest radiograph showed resolution of the pneumothorax and the presence of bilateral fluffy infiltrates. ABGs on a nonrebreathing mask at the time were pH = 7.29; P_aCO_2 = 51 mm Hg; P_aO_2 = 76 mm Hg; HCO_3^- = 24.8 mEq/L. Vital signs were blood pressure = 148/90 mm Hg; heart rate = 152 beats/min; f = 40 to 42 breaths/min and labored. The patient was restless and anxious. Mask CPAP was initiated with F_IO_2 = 1.0 and greater than 10 cm H_2O. The face mask was not well tolerated. The patient, who was 6 ft 2 in (72 in) and weighed 258 lb (117 kg), was sedated, paralyzed, orally intubated, and placed on ventilatory support (Case Study 7-2). (NOTE: The progress of this patient is continued in Chapter 13.)

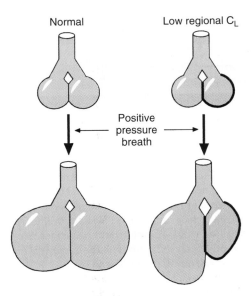

Fig. 7-4 The volume from a positive pressure breath distributes homogeneously throughout the lung with normal lung compliance (C_L) (left panel). In a lung with low regional C_L, the volume from a positive pressure breath distributes preferentially to the regions with more normal C_L (right panel). Thus, a tidal volume (V_T) of normal size in a lung with regions of low C_L can overdistend the healthier regions. This may create shear stress (frictional forces) between adjacent lung units. (Redrawn from MacIntyre NR: Minimizing alveolar stretch injury during mechanical ventilation, Respir Care 41:318-326, 1996.)

Normal | Low regional C_L

Positive pressure breath

Case Study 7-2

Key Questions for ARDS Patient

1. What were the indications for ventilation of this patient?
2. What clinical information suggests that this patient may have developed ARDS?
3. What would be appropriate initial ventilator settings for this patient?

ACUTE CARDIOGENIC PULMONARY EDEMA AND CONGESTIVE HEART FAILURE

Cardiovascular disease is the most common cause of death in the United States (Centers for Disease Control and Prevention). It is not surprising that many patients with cardiovascular problems seek medical help both in emergency departments and urgent care centers. These problems can take the form of shortness of breath with or without accompanying chest pain.

Patients with congestive heart failure (CHF) can rapidly develop acute pulmonary edema. Box 7-11 lists the most common causes of cardiogenic pulmonary edema.

| BOX **7-11** | **Common Causes of Acute Pulmonary Edema** |

- Acute myocardial infarction
- Hypertension
- Rapid heart rates with inadequate filling time
- Valvular heart disease
- Fluid overload

| BOX **7-12** | **Potential Effects of PEEP in Left Ventricular Dysfunction** |

1. Increased mean airway pressure ($\bar{P}_{aw}$) and intrathoracic pressure lead to reduced venous return, which can reduce preload to a failing heart, improving its function.
2. Increased functional residual capacity from PEEP leads to increased pulmonary vascular resistance and increased afterload to the right heart, and decreased left heart filling. Increased right heart pressures with the increased afterload may shift the interventricular septum to the left. This does not seem to alter right ventricular contractility until values for pulmonary artery pressure are critical.
3. With the left shift of the interventricular septum, the left ventricular volume is reduced. This may reduce the load it must pump. However, it may also affect the compliance of the left ventricle and either increase or decrease left heart function (the response varies).
4. The mechanical compression of the heart and aorta by the pleural pressure surrounding them can also alter ventricular function. The vascular pressure in the heart and thoracic aorta is transiently increased relative to the extrathoracic aorta (i.e., left ventricular afterload decreases). This response is not always consistent, and cardiac tamponade from PEEP can negatively alter myocardial compliance as well.
5. If ventilator modes increase work of breathing, this increases oxygen demand and can lead to increased myocardial ischemia and a reduction in left ventricular compliance.

Much of the treatment of acute heart failure is based on medical management. For example, diuretics are given to reduce vascular fluid load, positive inotropic agents are given to improve cardiac contractility, and vasodilators can improve myocardial oxygenation and reduce preload and afterload. Many patients can be successfully managed with drug therapy and do not require mechanical ventilatory support. However, mechanical ventilation may be indicated when severe heart failure leads to increased myocardial work, increased WOB, and hypoxemia. In patients with left ventricular failure the use of positive pressure, particularly PEEP (see 1 through 4 in Box 7-12), can effectively reduce the size of the heart and therefore reduce venous return and reduce preload to left ventricles.[3,37] Reducing the size of an overdistended left ventricle can improve the left ventricular length–tension relationship and allow for an increase in stroke volume. PEEP increases intrathoracic pressures and reduces venous return, and thus reduces preload to the heart.

Guidelines for Patients with Congestive Heart Failure

The following guidelines are recommended for mechanically ventilating patients with acute cardiogenic pulmonary edema and CHF[3-5,41-43]:

- Select a mode of ventilation that reduces WOB. This may be as simple as noninvasive mask CPAP. NIV by mask CPAP may improve oxygenation, reduce P_aCO_2, reduce the WOB, and reduce myocardial work. NIV in patients with CHF may allow sufficient time for pharmacologic treatment to become effective.
- When life-threatening hypoxemia occurs with severe CHF, PEEP or PPV may have beneficial effects on myocardial function and improve oxygenation.
- Careful evaluation of the effects of PPV on hemodynamics is essential. This may include the use of a pulmonary artery catheter in severe cases, particularly if $PEEP_E$ greater than 10 to 15 cm H_2O is used. However, the use of pulmonary catheters carries a risk of increased mortality and morbidity and is controversial (see Chapter 11 for more details about hemodynamic monitoring).
- The use of VC- or PC-CMV is recommended to minimize spontaneous breathing, which may divert increased blood flow and oxygen consumption to the respiratory muscles.
- V_T range is moderate from 6 to 8 mL/kg; set f from 10 or more breaths/min and peak flows 60 L/min or greater using either descending or constant waveforms. T_I range is 1 to 1.5 seconds.
- Set a PEEP of 5 to 10 cm H_2O to support the cardiac function.
- Start F_IO_2 at 1.0 and titrate quickly with S_pO_2 to maintain S_pO_2 greater than 90% to 92%.
- Monitor S_pO_2, ABGs, urine output, electrolytes, and systemic hemodynamic status.

⊘ Clinical Scenario: Patient with Congestive Heart Failure

A 63-year-old man who is complaining of severe shortness of breath is brought by ambulance to the emergency department. He is 5 ft 11 in (71 in) and weighs 175 lb (79.5 kg). His vital signs are blood pressure = 175/115 mm Hg; heart rate = 140 beats/min and the rhythm is irregular; f = 22 to 24 breaths/min; and he has a normal temperature. His lips are cyanotic, his neck veins are distended, and both of his ankles show evidence of pitting edema. Breath sounds reveal bilateral basilar crackles and wheezes. He has a productive cough with small amounts of pink, frothy secretions. He is very anxious and refuses to lie down on the gurney, saying, "I get too short of breath when I lie down."

A chest radiograph shows cardiomegaly and dense, fluffy opacities in the lower lung fields. The electrocardiogram reveals atrial fibrillation with a ventricular rate of 138 to 140 beats/min and occasional premature ventricular contractions. The respiratory therapist places a pulse oximeter sensor on the patient's left index finger and notices that the patient's hand is cold. The respiratory therapist is unable to obtain an accurate pulse oximeter reading (Case Study 7-3). After placing the sensor on the right index finger and rubbing the hand to warm it, an S_pO_2 reading of 87% is obtained.

The patient is started on a nasal cannula at 2 L/min and given intravenous furosemide, dobutamine, and digitalis. ABGs obtained 1 hour later are pH = 7.16; P_aCO_2 = 79 mm Hg; P_aO_2 = 33 mm Hg; HCO_3^- = 28 mEq/L on 2 L/min by nasal cannula. The patient's urine output was 580 mL in the past hour, and he remained cyanotic. The 2 L/min nasal cannula was not adequate. He is slow to respond to verbal commands. The following information provides an alternative therapeutic approach utilizing NIV.

Alternative Solution to Patient Treatment—CHF

Noninvasive ventilation is started for this patient using a full face mask and bilevel PAP with IPAP at 9 cm H_2O, EPAP at 3 cm H_2O, and F_IO_2 of approximately 0.5. The patient's spontaneous respiratory rate on these settings is 25 breaths/min, and the S_pO_2 is now 88%.

To reduce f and S_pO_2, the IPAP and EPAP are increased. After several adjustments, the final values for adequate ventilation are IPAP = 15 cm H_2O; EPAP = 5 cm H_2O; approximate F_IO_2 = 0.6; f = 16 breaths/min; and V_T = 760 mL. S_pO_2 = 95%.

The patient's condition improves with treatment. Urine output is 850 mL over a 2-hour period. Breath sounds reveal a moderate amount of crackles in the lung bases. The patient's color improves and he is alert, responsive, and cooperative. The pressure support levels are gradually reduced. The patient is alternately tested with a 50% oxygen mask and returned to the noninvasive ventilator until he is stable on the 50% mask. ABGs on an F_IO_2 = 0.5 are pH = 7.38; P_aCO_2 = 45 mm Hg; P_aO_2 = 73 mm Hg; HCO_3^- = 26 mEq/L. The patient is monitored over the next 24 hours, stabilized on medication, and discharged into the care of his wife.

Although NIV was successful in this individual, it is important to recognize that it is not always successful. Some patients with decompensated heart failure will temporarily improve with NIV but then worsen and may even go into cardiac arrest. Some clinicians prefer to intubate and provide invasive ventilation rather than NIV in this patient population because invasive ventilation provides more controlled conditions.

 Case Study 7-3

Troubleshooting: The Pulse Oximeter
Why was the therapist unable to get an initial reading from the pulse oximeter? What would you suggest to alleviate this situation?

 SUMMARY

- Numerous issues must be considered before connecting a patient to a mechanical ventilator. These include selecting appropriate ventilator settings for F_IO_2, sensitivity, sigh breaths, alarms, and monitors, as well as concerns regarding humidification of inspired gases.
- Once the patient is connected to the ventilator, the clinician should perform a careful assessment of the patient's response to these initial parameters.
- Titrating the F_IO_2 using pulse oximetry and ABG findings can minimize the risk of administering too much oxygen.
- Ventilator sensitivity is normally set so that patients can easily flow- or pressure-trigger a breath.
- It can be particularly difficult to adjust the ventilator sensitivity so that it senses a patient's effort when auto-PEEP is present.
- Humidity can be provided by a variety of humidification systems. Devices in this category include the following types of humidifiers: passover, vapor phase, wick, and active heat and moisture exchangers.
- Audible and visible alarm systems are designed to alert the operator of potential dangers related to the patient-ventilator interaction.
- Initial ventilator setting should be based on the patient's condition. Table 7-1 provides a summary of initial ventilator settings for patients commonly encountered in the clinical setting.
- Mechanical breaths of V_T 6 to 8 mL/kg IBW are usually effective but lower V_Ts may be required for patients with ARDS to maintain $P_{Plateau}$ <30 cm H_2O. Low levels of PEEP (3 to 5 cm H_2O) can reduce atelectasis formation.

TABLE 7-1	Initial Ventilator Settings Based on Pulmonary Disorder*							
Lung Disease	Mode	V_T (mL/kg IBW)	Rate (breaths/min)	Flow (L/min)	Flow Waveform	T_I (sec)	PEEP (cm H_2O)	F_IO_2
Normal lungs	VC- or PC-CMV	6-8	10-15	60	Descending or constant	1	≤5	≤0.5
COPD[†]	VC- or PC-CMV	6-8	8-12	>60 (80-100)	Descending or constant	0.6-1.2	≥5 or 50% of intrinsic PEEP	<0.5
Neuromuscular disorder	VC-CMV	6-8	8-12	≥60	Descending or constant	1	5	0.21
Asthma	VC- or PC-CMV	6-8	10-14	60-70	Descending	≤1	Only to offset intrinsic PEEP and improve triggering	≥0.5
Closed head injury	PC- or VC-CMV	6-8	15-20	60	Descending or constant	1	0-5 with caution Only in severe hypoxemia	1.0
ARDS	PC- or VC-CMV	4-8	12-35	≥60	Descending or constant	1	5 to >15	1.0
CHF	VC- or PC-CMV	6-8	≥10	≥60	Descending or constant	1-1.5	5-10	1.0

Sources: Meade MO, Herridge MS: An evidence-based approach to acute respiratory distress syndrome, Respir Care 46:1368-1376, 2001; Slutsky AS, Ranieri M: Ventilator-induced lung injury, N Engl J Med 369:2126-236, 2013.
ARDS, Acute respiratory distress syndrome; *CHF*, congestive heart failure; *CMV*, continuous mandatory ventilation; *F_IO_2*, fractional inspired oxygen concentration; *IBW*, ideal body weight; *PC*, pressure control; *PEEP*, positive end-expiratory pressure; *V_C*, volume control; *V_T*, tidal volume.
*For all disorders it is very important that the plateau pressure be maintained lower than 30 cm H_2O.
[†]An initial attempt at bilevel PAP should be tried using NIV with IPAP = 10 to 12 cm H_2O and EPAP = 2 to 3 cm H_2O before intubation is considered. An exception would be a critical emergency with these patients.

REVIEW QUESTIONS *(See Appendix A for answers.)*

1. A male patient has a BSA of 1.5 m², is 5 ft 8 in, and weighs 175 lb. The patient has a history of lung damage resulting from old tuberculosis scars. He demonstrates a restricted breathing pattern. What ventilator settings would you select for this patient?

   $\dot{V}_E$: _____

   V_T: _____

   f: _____

2. A patient with COPD is being ventilated with a Puritan Bennett 840 ventilator. Ventilator parameters are as follows: VC-CMV: flow = 40 L/min with descending ramp flow waveform; V_T = 0.65; F_IO_2 = 0.3. **At 2:00** PM, total f = 10 breaths/min, PIP = 28 cm H_2O, there are no assisted breaths, and the pressure–time curve is normal. **At 4:00** PM, total f = 20 breaths/min, PIP = 37 cm H_2O, the patient is actively assisting and using accessory muscles to breathe, and the pressure–time graphic shows a concave appearance.

   What do you think has caused the changes in the patient's condition? What would you do to correct this situation?

3. An 83-year-old man with COPD is being treated in the emergency department. His wife, who brought him in, states, "He's been so short of breath and pale and I'm worried." Oxygen by a 28% air-entrainment mask is begun. The patient is given an aerosol treatment with albuterol. Despite continued therapy, the patient does not improve and continues to use accessory muscles to breathe. He is diaphoretic and pale and his temperature is 102° F. The decision is made to begin noninvasive ventilation. A BiPAP unit is set up with initial pressures of inspiratory positive airway pressure (IPAP) = 6 cm H_2O and expiratory positive airway pressure (EPAP) = 2 cm H_2O. These were then adjusted based on pulse oximetry and patient f. With an IPAP to EPAP ratio of 12 cm H_2O to 4 cm H_2O and a measured F_IO_2 of 0.3, the patient has a rate of 25 breaths/min and S_pO_2 of 87%. Vital signs, S_pO_2, and respiratory rate remain fairly stable.

   Two hours later, the patient's respiratory rate has increased to 35 breaths/min. ABGs reveal pH = 7.21; P_aCO_2 = 105 mm Hg; P_aO_2 = 47 mm Hg; HCO_3^- = 40 mEq/L. Repeated adjustments of the IPAP:EPAP ratio fail to improve the patient's condition; the decision is made to intubate him and provide him with volume-targeted ventilation. The patient is 5 ft 8 in and weighs 148 lbs (IBW = 70 kg). BSA = 1.78 m². The VC-IMV mode is selected.

   What initial V_T, $\dot{V}_E$, and f would you select?

   After initiating ventilation the following values are noted: PIP = 33 cm H_2O; $P_{plateau}$ = 25 cm H_2O; transairway pressure (P_{TA}) = 33 − 25 = 8 cm H_2O. The patient is spontaneously breathing an additional 10 breaths/min with a V_T of 200 mL. The decision is made to add pressure support for the spontaneous breaths to overcome the WOB imposed by the artificial airway.

   What is an estimated resistance on this patient, assuming a constant flow of 80 L/min is used for calculation? Where would you set pressure support?

4. A 50-year-old patient is receiving VC-CMV following surgery for a bowel resection. He is in the recovery room. The patient has an IBW of 80 kg and a BSA of 1.8 m². This patient's lungs are normal. What initial settings would be appropriate?

References

1. Mithoefer JC, Holford FD, Keighley JFH: The effect of oxygen administration on mixed venous oxygenation in chronic obstructive pulmonary disease. *Chest* 66:122–132, 1974.
2. Mithoefer JC, Keighley JF: Karetzkey MS: Response of the arterial PO_2 to oxygenation administration in chronic pulmonary disease. *Ann Intern Med* 74:328–335, 1971.
3. Hess DR, Kacmarek RM: *Essentials of mechanical ventilation*, ed 2, New York, 2002, McGraw-Hill.
4. Hess DR, MacIntyre NR: Mechanical ventilation. In Hess DR, MacIntyre NR, Mishoe SC, editors: *Respiratory care principles and practices*, Sudbury, Mass., 2011, Jones and Bartlet Learning, pp 462–500.
5. Kacmarek RM: Initiating and adjusting invasive ventilatory support. In Kacmarek RM, Stoller JK, Heuer AJ, editors: *Egan's fundamentals of respiratory care*, ed 9, St Louis, 2013, Mosby, pp 1088–1130.
6. Jubran A, Tobin MJ: Reliability of pulse oximetry in titrating supplemental oxygen therapy in ventilator-dependent patients. *Chest* 97:1420–1425, 1990.
7. Branson RD: Understanding and implementing advances in ventilator capabilities. *Curr Opin Crit Care* 10:23–32, 2004.
8. Branson RD: Humidification for patients with artificial airways. *Respir Care* 44:630–641, 1999.
9. AARC clinical practice guideline: Humidification during mechanical ventilation, American Association for Respiratory Care. *Respir Care* 37:887–890, 1992.
10. Branson RD, Campbell RS: Humidification in the intensive care unit. *Respir Care Clin N Am* 4:305–320, 1998.
11. Branson RD, Campbell RS, Johannigman JA, et al: Comparison of conventional heated humidification with a new active hygroscopic heat and moisture exchanger in mechanically ventilated patients. *Respir Care* 44:912–917, 1999.
12. Cairo JM: *Mosby's respiratory care equipment*, ed 9, St Louis, 2014, Elsevier.
13. Shelly MP: Inspired gas conditioning. *Respir Care* 37:1070–1080, 1992.
14. Chatburn RL: Physiologic and methodologic issues regarding humidity therapy (editorial). *J Pediatr* 114:416–420, 1989.
15. Chatburn RL: Principles and practice of neonatal and pediatric mechanical ventilation. *Respir Care* 36:569–595, 1991.
16. Hess D: Prolonged use of heat and moisture exchangers: why do we keep changing things? *Crit Care Med* 28:1667–1668, 2000.
17. Branson RD, Davis K, Campbell RS, et al: Humidification in the intensive care unit. Prospective study of a new protocol utilizing heated humidification and a hygroscopic condenser humidifier. *Chest* 104:1800–1805, 1993.
18. Davis K, Evans SL, Campbell RS, et al: Prolonged use of heat and moisture exchangers does not affect device efficiency or frequency rate of nosocomial pneumonia. *Crit Care Med* 28:1412–1418, 2000.
19. Collard HR, Saint S, Matthay MA: Prevention of ventilator-associated pneumonia: an evidence-based systematic review. *Ann Intern Med* 138:494–501, 2003.
20. Hess D: Noninvasive monitoring in respiratory care—present, past and future: an overview. *Respir Care* 35:482–499, 1990.
21. MacIntyre NR, Day S: Essentials for ventilator-alarm systems. *Respir Care* 37:1108–1112, 1992.
22. Bendixen HH, Hedley-White J, Laver MB: Impaired oxygenation in surgical patients during general anesthesia with controlled ventilation: a concept of atelectasis. *N Engl J Med* 269:991–996, 1963.
23. Brochard L: Pressure-limited ventilation. *Respir Care* 41:447–455, 1996.
24. Laver MB, Morgan J, Bendixen NH, et al: Lung volume, compliance, and arterial oxygen tensions during controlled ventilation. *J Appl Physiol* 19:725–733, 1964.
25. Housley E, Louzada N, Becklake MR: To sigh or not to sigh. *Am Rev Respir Dis* 101:611–614, 1970.
26. Bergman NA: Concerning sweet dreams, health and quiet breathing (editorial). *Anesthesiology* 32:297–298, 1970.
27. Levine M, Gilbert R, Auchincloss JH, Jr: A comparison of the effects of sighs, large tidal volumes, and positive end expiratory pressure in assisted ventilation. *Scand J Respir Dis* 53:101–108, 1972.
28. Colgan FJ, Marocco PP: Cardiorespiratory effects of constant and intermittent positive-pressure breathing. *Anesthesiology* 36:444–448, 1970.
29. Branson RD, Campbell RS: Sighs: wasted breath or breath of fresh air? *Respir Care* 37:462, 1992.
30. Dammann JF, McAslan TC: PEEP: its use in young patients with apparently normal lungs. *Crit Care Med* 7:14–19, 1979.
31. Sykes MK, Young WE, Robinson BE: Oxygenation during anesthesia with controlled ventilation. *Br J Anaesth* 33:314–325, 1965.
32. Visick WD, Fairley HB, Hickey RE: The effects of tidal volume and end-expiratory pressures on pulmonary gas exchange during anesthesia. *Anesthesiology* 19:285–290, 1973.
33. Bruce RD, et al: Does a sigh breath improve oxygenation in the intubated patient receiving CPAP? *Respir Care* 37:1409–1413, 1992.
34. Acute Respiratory Distress Syndrome Network: Ventilation with lower tidal volume as compared with traditional tidal volumes for acute lung injury and the acute respiratory distress syndrome. *N Engl J Med* 342:1301–1308, 2000.
35. Amato MB, Barbas CSV, Medeiros DM, et al: Effect of a protective-ventilation strategy on mortality in the acute respiratory distress syndrome. *N Engl J Med* 338:347–354, 1998.
36. Zambon M, Vincent JL: Mortality rates for patients with acute lung injury/ARDS have decreased over time. *Chest* 133(5):1120–1127, 2008.
37. Tobin MJ, editor: *Principles and practices of mechanical ventilation*, ed 3, New York, 2014, McGraw-Hill.
38. Forrette TR: Mechanical ventilators: general-use devices. In Cairo JM, editor: *Mosby's respiratory care equipment*, ed 9, St Louis, 2014, Elsevier-Mosby, pp 421–460.
39. ARDS Definition Task Force, Ranieri VM, Rubenfeld GD, et al: Acute respiratory distress syndrome: the Berlin Definition. *JAMA* 307:2526–2533, 2012.
40. Slutsky AS, Ranieri M: Ventilator-induced lung injury. *N Engl J Med* 369:2126–2136, 2013.
41. Slutsky AS: Ventilator-induced lung injury: from barotrauma to biotrauma. *Respir Care* 50:646–659, 2005.
42. Slutsky AS: Consensus conference on mechanical ventilation. Northbrook, Ill, Jan 27-30, 1994. *Intensive Care Med* 20:64–79, 1994.
43. MacIntyre NR, Branson RD: *Mechanical ventilation*, ed 2, Philadelphia, 2008, W.B. Saunders.
44. Sethi JM, Siegel MD: Mechanical ventilation in chronic obstructive lung disease. *Clin Chest Med* 21:799–818, 2000.
45. Dhand R: Ventilator graphics and respiratory mechanics in the patient with obstructive lung disease. *Respir Care* 50:246–261, 2005.
46. Georgopoulos D, Kondili E, Prinianakis G: How to set the ventilator in asthma. *Monaldi Arch Chest Dis* 55:74–83, 2000.
47. Rowe BH, Edmonds ML, Spooner CH, et al: Evidence-based treatments for acute asthma. *Respir Care* 46:1380–1390, 2001.
48. Tuxen DV, Lane S: The effects of ventilatory pattern on hyperinflation, airway pressures, and circulation in mechanical ventilation of patients with severe airflow obstruction. *Am Rev Respir Dis* 136:872–879, 1987.
49. Menchon MN, Palacios IE, Alapont MI: Ventilation in special situations. Mechanical ventilation in status asthmaticus. *An Pediatr (Barc)* 59:352–362, 2003.
50. Rodrigo GJ, Rodrigo C, Hall JB: Acute asthma in adults: a review. *Chest* 125:1080–1102, 2004.
51. Leatherman JW: Mechanical ventilation for severe asthma. In Tobin MJ, editor: *Mechanical ventilation: principles and applications*, ed 3, New York, 2013, Elsevier, pp 727–739.
52. Bernard GR, Artigas A, Brigham KL, et al: The American-European Consensus Conference on ARDS: definitions, mechanisms, relevant outcomes, and clinical trial coordination. *Am J Respir Crit Care Med* 149:819–824, 1994.
53. MacNaughton PD, Evans TW: Management of adult respiratory distress syndrome. *Lancet* 339:469, 1992.
54. MacIntyre NR: Minimizing alveolar stretch injury during mechanical ventilation. *Respir Care* 41:318–326, 1996.
55. Meade MO, Herridge MS: An evidence-based approach to acute respiratory distress syndrome. *Respir Care* 46:1368–1376, 2001.
56. Gattinoni L, Pelosi P, Crotti S, et al: Pressure-volume curve of total respiratory system in acute respiratory failure. *Am Rev Respir Dis* 136:730–736, 1987.
57. Harris RS: Pressure-volume curves of the respiratory system. *Respir Care* 50:78–98, 2005.
58. Marini JJ, Gattinoni L: Ventilatory management of acute respiratory distress syndrome: a consensus of two. *Crit Care Med* 32:250–255, 2004.
59. Marini JJ: Mechanical ventilation in Acute Respiratory Distress Syndrome. In Tobin MJ, editor: *Mechanical ventilation: principles and applications*, ed 3, New York, 2013, McGraw-Hill, pp 699–726.

Initial Patient Assessment

OUTLINE

KEY TERMS

- Ascites
- Inflection point
- Operational verification procedure
- Patient-ventilator system check
- Upper inflection point
- Ventilator flow sheet

LEARNING OBJECTIVES *On completion of this chapter, the reader will be able to do the following:*

1. Understand the importance of performing an operational verification procedure.
2. State the recommended times when an oxygen analyzer is used to measure the fractional inspired oxygen concentration (F_IO_2) during mechanical ventilation.
3. Identify various pathophysiological conditions that alter a patient's transairway pressure, peak pressure, and plateau pressure.
4. Use pressure–time and flow–time curves obtained during pressure-controlled continuous mandatory ventilation (PC-CMV) to determine the plateau pressure.
5. Identify a system leak from a volume–time curve.
6. Use physical examination and radiographic data to determine whether pneumonia, acute respiratory distress syndrome (ARDS), flail chest, pneumothorax, asthma, pleural effusion, or emphysema is present.
7. Determine whether a lung compliance problem or an airway resistance problem is present, using the ventilator flow sheet and time, volume, peak inspiratory pressure (PIP), and plateau pressure data.
8. Evaluate a static pressure–volume curve for static compliance and dynamic compliance to determine changes in compliance or resistance.
9. Estimate a patient's alveolar ventilation based on ideal body weight, tidal volume, and respiratory rate.
10. Detect a cuff leak by listening to breath sounds.
11. Recognize inappropriate endotracheal tube cuff pressures and an inappropriate tube size, and recommend measures to correct these problems.
12. Evaluate flow sheet information about a patient on pressure control ventilation and recommend methods for determining whether compliance and airway resistance have changed.
13. Explain the technique for measuring endotracheal tube cuff pressure using a manometer, syringe, and three-way stopcock.
14. Describe two methods that can be used to remedy a cut pilot tube (pilot balloon line) without changing the endotracheal tube.

Assessing a patient's skin color, respiratory rate, breathing pattern, use of accessory muscles, chest movement, and breath sounds, along with estimates of work of breathing (WOB), and evaluation of their level of consciousness can provide valuable information about a patient's physiological status. These observations, along with information derived from ventilator displays and hemodynamic monitoring, are among the first assessments the clinician records for a patient who is undergoing mechanical ventilation.[1]

This chapter reviews assessment and documentation of patient-ventilator interactions after a patient has been placed on a mechanical ventilator. The first step in this process involves verification of the physician's orders for initiating mechanical ventilator support (Box 8-1). Once the physician's orders have been verified, the respiratory therapist ensures that the designated ventilator has passed an **operational verification procedure** (OVP). The OVP process is typically described in the respiratory therapy department's policies and procedures manual.

It is important that the respiratory therapy department maintains records showing the OVP history for each ventilator. In addition, a label or form should be attached to each ventilator showing when the OVP was performed, by whom, and whether the ventilator passed the multiple-part test. Newer microprocessor-controlled ventilators are designed to perform a series of automated self-tests once the operator initiates the self-test process. This self-test record may be part of the OVP.

The equipment evaluation process should also involve checking the integrity of the ventilator circuit and humidifier system, and ensuring that related equipment has been correctly attached and tested to ensure that the system is free of leaks (Box 8-2).

DOCUMENTATION OF THE PATIENT-VENTILATOR SYSTEM

In addition to documentation of the OVP, patient information and ventilator settings should be documented regularly when a patient is receiving ventilatory support. These data can be recorded on a computer software program with specific entry fields or kept as a paper record. Regardless of the form it takes, the document often is called a *ventilator flow sheet.*

The frequency of patient-ventilator system checks depends on the institution's policy. They generally are performed every 1 to 4 hours.[3] In addition to this schedule, patient-ventilator system checks are performed:

- Before an arterial blood gas (ABG) sample is drawn
- When the physician has entered new orders
- Before hemodynamic data or bedside pulmonary function data are measured
- After a ventilator change has been made
- If an acute change occurs in the patient's condition (such changes should be documented as soon as possible after the event)
- After a patient returns from testing (e.g., x-ray or magnetic resonance imaging [MRI])
- Whenever the ventilator's performance is questionable

It is important to recognize that **patient-ventilator system checks** represent a documented evaluation of the ventilator's function and the patient's response to ventilatory support. Several points regarding patient-ventilator system checks should be emphasized:

- Data relevant to the patient-ventilator system check are recorded on the appropriate hospital form and are part of the patient's medical record.
- The patient-ventilator system check includes observations of ventilator settings at the time of the check.
- The record should include the physician's order for mechanical ventilator settings.
- The patient-ventilator system check includes a brief narrative of the clinical observations of the patient's response to mechanical ventilation at the time of the check.

Figure 8-1 shows a typical ventilator flow sheet used to record patient-ventilator system check data. The top of the form contains basic patient information, including the patient's name and

---

BOX 8-1   **Physician's Orders for Mechanical Ventilation**

The orders written by the physician for mechanical ventilation settings vary between institutions. In some cases the physician's orders may be very specific, with little flexibility for respiratory therapist involvement. More commonly the physician orders simply request a particular protocol for mechanical ventilation, which is then followed by the respiratory therapist, nurse, and other staff members involved with the care of the patient.[2]

The orders or protocol should include at least one (and preferably both) of the following:

- Desired range for the arterial carbon dioxide partial pressure (P_aCO_2) or end-tidal carbon dioxide partial pressure ($P_{ET}CO_2$), and/or for the arterial oxygen partial pressure (P_aO_2), arterial oxygen saturation (S_aO_2), oxygen saturation as measured by pulse oximetry (S_pO_2), or transcutaneous oxygen partial pressure ($P_{tc}O_2$).
- Ventilator variables to be initiated or manipulated to achieve the desired arterial blood gases (e.g., mode, tidal volume [V_T], respiratory rate [f], set pressure, and fractional inspired oxygen [F_IO_2]) while protecting the lung.

BOX 8-2   **Simple Verification of Ventilator Operation**

A simple ventilator check should be performed:
- Before connecting a patient to a ventilator for the first time.
- Before reconnecting the patient to a ventilator if the circuit has been changed or disassembled for any reason.

The operational verification procedure should also include checking the system for leaks before the patient is connected to the ventilator. To check for leaks, the operator should:
- Set the tidal volume (V_T) at 500 mL, the gas flow low (e.g., 20 L/min), the maximum pressure limit high (e.g., 100 to 120 cm H_2O), and an inspiratory pause of 1 to 2 seconds.
- Occlude the Y-connector, cycle the ventilator, and observe the airway pressure rise and pause on the pressure manometer; if no leak is present, the circuit will hold the pressure steady.
- Change the ventilator settings to those appropriate for the patient before connecting the patient to the ventilator.
- Newer microprocessor-controlled ventilators automatically perform a test to check for leaks in the patient-ventilator circuit. This test can be performed at any time, but the patient must be disconnected from the ventilator to perform the test.

Patient Name _____   Medical Record Number_____   Date of Birth _____   Age _____

Physician _____   Diagnosis _____   Vent. Start Date _____   Vent Day_____

Height _____   Weight _____   IBW ____   BSA____   ET size_____   Position (teeth/lips/nose) _____

Original Physician Order _____;   Circuit Change Due Date _____

	Date	___	___	___
	Time			
	Therapist Initials			
	MODE*			
V	Auto-Wean Mode (on/off)			
O	$V_T$set/$V_T$exh			
L	V_T spont			
U	Machine rate/Total rate			
M	I:E ratio (or Set T_I%)(or T_{HI}/T_{LO})			
E	Minute Ventilation			
	Increase $V_D$mech (mL)			
P	Ppeak/Pplateau			
R	Compliance (V_T/PIP-PEEPtot)			
E	Raw [(PIP-Pplat)/flow(L/sec)]			
S	IPAP/EPAP (P_{HI}/P_{LO})			
S	Mean Airway Pressure			
U	Set Pressure (PCV or PS)			
R	Set PEEP/CPAP			
E	Auto-PEEP			
	Sensitivity (P or Flow setting)			
M	F_IO_2 (set/analyzed)			
I	Flow rate			
S	Flow waveform			
C	Insp. Rise Setting			
	Inspir Flow cycle			
	Automatic Tube Comp. Set (yes/no)			
	Air Temperature			
A	Apnea Parameters Set (yes/no)			
L	Press. Limit (high/low)			
A	Low V_T			
R	V_E (high/low)			
M	High Rate			
	Low PEEP			
A	Suctioned (yes/no)			
I	Secretion color			

Fig. 8-1 Example of a ventilator flow sheet.

R	Secretion consistency			
W	Secretion Amt. (small/mod./lg)			
A	ET Repositioned/Taped (yes/no)			
Y	Cuff (Press/Vol.)/Tube position			
	MLT or MOV			
	Aerosol Therapy (MDI or Neb)			
	Medication/Dose			
	pH/$PaCO_2$			
A	$P_{ET}CO_2$			
B	PaO_2			
G	SpO_2			
	Hb			
	HCO_3^-			
	B.E.			
	PaO_2/F_IO_2 or PaO_2/P_AO_2			
	$CaO_2/CaO_2-C\bar{v}O_2$			
H	Pulse			
E	Blood Pressure			
M	CVP			
O	PAP (sys/dys)			
	PAWP			
	C.O./C.I. (C.O./BSA)			
	SVR			
	PVR			
S	Spontaneous rate			
P	Spontaneous V_T			
O	RSBI [f/V_T (breaths/min/L)]			
N	MIP (NIF)			
T	VC			
	Time of SBT			
	COMMENTS			
M	*VC-CMV (A/C), PC-CMV (PCV),			
O	VC-SIMV; PC-SIMV			
D	VC-SIMV+PS; PC-SIMV+PSV			
E	PRVC; APRV			
S	Spontaneous, PSV, VS, CPAP			
	BiLevel PAP			

Fig. 8-1, cont'd

anthropometric data (e.g., age, weight, height, ideal body weight [IBW], body surface area [BSA]), the medical record identification number, the patient's diagnosis, the name of the attending physician along with the physician's orders, date of intubation, the ventilator start date, and the ventilator day (number of days on the ventilator).

The form will typically include spaces for entering current information about the patient and measurements of ventilator parameters. These may include the following:

- Date
- Time
- Mode of ventilation

- Minute ventilation ($\dot{V}_E$)
- Respiratory rate (f)
- Tidal volume (V_T)
- Peak inspiratory pressure (PIP)
- Plateau pressure ($P_{plateau}$)
- Static compliance (C_s)
- Airway resistance (R_{aw})
- Fractional inspired oxygen (F_IO_2)
- Temperatures of inspired gases
- Inspiratory-to-expiratory (I : E) ratio
- Continuous positive airway pressure (CPAP) or positive end-expiratory pressure (PEEP)
- Inspiratory and end-expiratory positive airway pressures (IPAP/EPAP)
- Arterial blood gases (ABGs)
- Alveolar-to-arterial partial pressure of oxygen ($P_{(A-a)}O_2$) or ratio of arterial oxygen partial pressure to fractional inspired oxygen (P_aO_2/F_IO_2)
- Vital capacity (VC)
- Maximum inspiratory pressure (MIP)
- Vital signs
- Alarm settings

Volumes, pressures, temperature, vital signs, and F_IO_2 are measured during each patient-ventilator system check. Most intensive care unit (ICU) ventilators have oxygen analyzers that provide continuous monitoring of F_IO_2. In cases where continuous F_IO_2 measurements are not available on a particular ventilator, intermittent measurements of F_IO_2 are usually sufficient for adult patients. F_IO_2 should be continuously monitored, however, for infants receiving mechanical ventilation. Alarms should be regularly checked to ensure that they have been set appropriately. ABGs, shunt fraction, $P_{(A-a)}O_2$, and P_aO_2/F_IO_2 should be determined when the patient's condition or the ventilator settings change significantly.

Despite the importance of regular, accurate documentation, many respiratory therapy departments do not follow specific guidelines for patient-ventilator system checks or a similar model.[2-4] Case Study 8-1 provides a clinical scenario illustrating the important of maintaining accurate patient-ventilator records.[5]

 Case Study 8-1

The Importance of Documentation

A 38-year-old woman is intubated for respiratory failure secondary to severe pneumonia. After 24 hours her status improves. The endotracheal tube is kept in place to allow suctioning, because she has large amounts of secretions. On the third day after intubation, her respiratory status declines. She has a cardiac arrest and is resuscitated but suffers brain injury as a result. She dies several weeks later.

The family hires an attorney. At issue is the fact that in the medical record, the respiratory therapist's notes with the ventilator flow sheet indicate that the patient had been suctioned about every 2 hours for large amounts of thick, yellow secretions. However, during the 8 hours before the arrest, nowhere did the notes state that the patient had been suctioned. The therapist states that he had suctioned the patient but had not recorded it in the chart. Was the therapist negligent and did his actions lead to the wrongful death of the patient?

The following clinical laboratory tests may be included in the initial evaluation of the patient:
- Complete blood count (CBC)
- Blood chemistries (glucose, sodium, potassium, chloride, carbon dioxide [CO_2], blood urea nitrogen, creatinine, phosphate, magnesium)
- Prothrombin time, partial thromboplastin time, international normalized ratio (PT/PTT/INR) and platelet count
- Blood, sputum, and urine cultures

THE FIRST 30 MINUTES

Immediately after the patient is connected to a mechanical ventilator, the clinician should perform auscultation of the patient's chest to confirm adequate volume delivery and proper placement of the endotracheal tube (ET). The patient's vital signs are checked, making particular note of heart rate and blood pressure, because ventilation may affect these parameters (Key Point 8-1). The alarms (e.g., apnea, low pressure, low V_T, and high pressure limit) are activated.[6] An arterial blood sample is obtained about 15 minutes after mechanical ventilation is initiated for evaluation of the effectiveness of ventilation and oxygenation.[3,7] If not already done, a chest radiograph is obtained to confirm proper placement of the ET. Box 8-3 lists other clinical laboratory tests a physician might order to assess the patient's status when mechanical ventilation is initiated.[3]

Once the patient assessment shows the individual is stable, the respiratory therapist then performs the first ventilator check.

Key Point **8-1** Positive pressure ventilation can reduce venous return to the heart, cardiac output, and blood pressure. (See Chapter 16 for more information on the cardiovascular effects of mechanical ventilation.)

Mode

The mode of ventilation is recorded in the appropriate space on the ventilator flow sheet. It may be recorded as follows:
- Volume-controlled continuous mandatory ventilation (VC-CMV)
- Pressure-controlled continuous mandatory ventilation (PC-CMV)
- Intermittent mandatory ventilation (IMV), using either volume-controlled ventilation (VC-IMV) or pressure-controlled ventilation (PC-IMV), with or without pressure support ventilation (PSV)
- Pressure-regulated volume control (PRVC)*
- Airway pressure release ventilation (APRV)
- PSV, volume support (VS), CPAP, unsupported spontaneous ventilation (these are spontaneous modes)
- Bilevel positive airway pressure (bilevel PAP; noninvasive positive pressure ventilation [NIV])

---

*Other names associated with this mode include *AutoFlow* (Dräger V500) and *VC+* (Puritan Bennett 840 ventilators).

Sensitivity

If a patient-triggered mode is used (i.e., inspiration is initiated by patient effort), the pressure or flow required to trigger the ventilation should be checked; no more than −1 or −2 cm H_2O should be required. If the ventilator is flow triggered, the sensitivity should be set so that the ventilator will trigger at a flow change of 2 to 3 L/min. The ventilator should be checked for autotriggering, and the patient's ability to trigger a breath should be assessed. Adjustments are made as needed.

As discussed previously, when auto-PEEP is present, the patient has more difficulty triggering breaths. The presence of auto-PEEP should be suspected if the patient is using his accessory muscles of inspiration or demonstrates labored breathing. Ventilator graphics that show failure of the expiratory flow to return to zero before the next breath also is an indicator of auto-PEEP (see Chapter 9).[8]

If auto-PEEP is present, a number of strategies can be used to reduce its effects, including increasing the flow (reducing the inspiratory time [T_I]), reducing V_T, or reducing the rate [i.e., reducing $\dot{V}_E$]), suctioning the patient, or changing modes to allow for more spontaneous breaths. It is important to recognize that it may not always be possible to eliminate auto-PEEP, particularly in patients with increased flow resistance and airway closure. The addition of extrinsic PEEP ($PEEP_E$) in these cases may make triggering easier (see Fig. 7-1). $PEEP_E$ is increased progressively during VC-CMV until the patient's use of accessory muscles diminishes or until PIP and $P_{plateau}$ begin to rise. (Additional information about treatment of auto-PEEP can be found in Chapter 17.)

Tidal Volume, Rate, and Minute Ventilation

V_T, f, and $\dot{V}_E$ are typically displayed digitally on the front panel of the ventilator in the data display window. Most ventilators display the set V_T (V_{Tset}) and the exhaled V_T (V_{Texh}). Newer microprocessor-controlled ventilators provide excellent, reliable flow and pressure

monitoring. If this information is not available, V_T can be measured using a handheld bedside pulmonary function device or other volume-measuring device (e.g., respirometer) and a watch or clock with a sweep second hand. Although this technique generally is used only with older ventilators, it can also be used to verify digital readouts if a question arises about the machine's reliability (Fig. 8-2 and Box 8-4).

BOX 8-4 | **Respirometer Technique for Measuring Tidal Volume (V_T) and Minute Ventilation (V_E)**

Modern microprocessor-controlled ventilators provide digital displays for the clinician to monitor a patient's tidal volume and minute ventilation. Before the introduction of these devices, clinicians typically relied on handheld respirometers to measure these variables. The procedure for measuring V_T and $\dot{V}_E$ with a respirometer is relatively easy to accomplish.

- The respirometer is connected directly to the patient's endotracheal tube and to the Y-connector of the ventilator circuit (see Fig. 8-2). This allows easy measurement of the V_T that does not have to be corrected for compressible volume from the ventilator circuit. (NOTE: In cases where the V_T was measured at the expiratory port, the compressible volume [volume lost to C_T] must be subtracted from the V_T reading on the respirometer.)
- Gas exhaled from the lungs is measured for 1 minute and the f is simultaneously counted. $\dot{V}_E$ can be calculated ($\dot{V}_E = V_T \times f$) or measured directly. If the patient is on intermittent mandatory ventilation (IMV), the total $\dot{V}_E$ is measured. Mandatory V_T and f can be measured separately, and mandatory $\dot{V}_E$ can be subtracted from the total $\dot{V}_E$ to determine a patient's spontaneous $\dot{V}_E$.

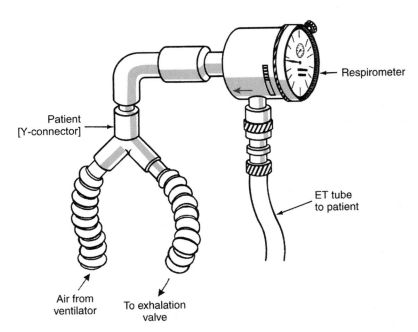

Fig. 8-2 Measurement of tidal volume (V_T) at the endotracheal tube (ET). The respirometer is attached to the ET so that the patient's actual exhaled air can be measured. The respirometer can also be attached at the exhalation valve, but those readings would include compressible volume from the ventilator circuit in addition to volume from the patient's lungs.

Correcting Tubing Compliance

Accurate reporting of volumes requires correction for volume loss within the patient circuit due to the effects of tubing compliance (also called *compressible volume*). As discussed in Chapter 6, tubing compliance (C_T) for most ventilator circuits ranges from about 1.5 to 2.5 mL/cm H_2O.[9]

Most microprocessor-controlled ventilators (e.g., Puritan Bennett 840 [Covidien-Nellcor and Puritan Bennett, Boulder, Colo.] Servo-i [Maquet Inc, Wayne, N.J.]) do not require calculation of tubing compliance because these machines automatically compensate for this factor. As discussed previously, ventilators that perform this function typically increase the delivered volume so that the set volume is the amount provided to the patient (i.e., the digital readout indicates the V_T actually delivered to the patient's airway). With older ventilators, the operator can set the value for the circuit's C_T and the ventilator will add volume to the set V_T to compensate for volume loss due to tubing compliance.

Alveolar Ventilation

Monitoring of alveolar ventilation ($\dot{V}_A$) has declined in popularity in recent years because many acute care facilities do not include this variable on the ventilator flow sheet. Unfortunately, its importance often is overlooked when using low V_T strategies. In-line heat and moisture exchangers (HMEs), closed suction systems, and other circuit adapters and equipment can add mechanical dead space (V_{Dmech}) to the ventilator circuit and affect the V_D/V_T. Knowledge of the effect of dead space on alveolar volume delivery can be particularly important in infants, children, and smaller adults with ARDS.

Two factors must be considered in determining alveolar ventilation:
1. Anatomic dead space
2. Mechanical dead space

Dead Space

Normal anatomic dead space (V_{Danat}) is about 1 mL/lb IBW.* Bypassing the upper airway with an artificial airway reduces V_{Danat} by about one half. Using a Y-connector, additional flex tubing between the Y-connector and the ET, or a HME adds mechanical dead space.

Added Mechanical Dead Space

Because HMEs or other adapters attached to the ET (Fig. 8-3) add to mechanical dead space (V_{Dmech}), the volume of these devices, along with the V_{Danat}, must be subtracted from the V_T to determine actual alveolar ventilation (Box 8-5). For example, if a 150-lb adult has a V_T of 500 mL and the added V_{Dmech} is 100 mL, the alveolar ventilation for each breath would be:

$$V_T - V_{Dmech} - V_{Danat} = 500 \text{ mL} - 100 \text{ mL} - 150 \text{ mL} = 250 \text{ mL (Key Point 8-2)}$$

> **◖ Key Point 8-2** The volume of mechanical dead space can be easily measured for any device added to a ventilator circuit. The device is simply filled with water and then emptied into a graduated container; the volume measured is the volume of mechanical dead space for the device. (A piece of equipment [i.e., tubing] similar to that being placed on the patient should be used for this type of measurement.)

*Physiological dead space is reviewed in Appendix B.

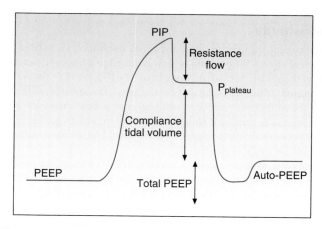

Fig. 8-3 Airway pressure waveform during volume control ventilation. An end-inspiratory breath hold and an end-expiratory breath hold are applied to measure the plateau pleasure and the auto-PEEP, respectively. Note the difference between the peak inspiratory pressure (PIP) and the plateau pressure ($P_{plateau}$); this is the transairway pressure (P_{TA}), which is produced by the interaction of the set flow and airway resistance. The V_T is the product of the pressure difference between $P_{plateau}$ and total PEEP (set PEEP and auto-PEEP) and lung compliance. (From Hess DR, MacIntyre NR, Mishoe SC, et al: Respiratory care principles and practice, Philadelphia, 2002, WB Saunders.)

BOX 8-5 **Added Mechanical Dead Space**

Some patient situations require the addition of a small amount of mechanical dead space. For example, in Fig. 7-3 a small circuit has been added at the Y-connector to allow for intermittent use of a metered-dose inhaler (MDI) without removing the heat and heat-moisture exchanger (HME) or disconnecting the circuit.

Excessive turbulence at the upper airway and Y-connector sometimes can produce a pressure spike at the beginning of a breath during pressure-targeted ventilation. This has been noted with CareFusion (Pulmonetics) LTV-1000 ventilator (CareFusion, Yorba Linda, Calif.) in a clinical situation.[10] Auto-triggering occasionally occurs in this same ventilator. These two phenomena can be prevented in most cases by adding about 2 inches of corrugated tubing between the Y-connector and the endotracheal tube (or between the HME and the endotracheal tube) but must be accounted for as additional V_{Dmech}.

Final Alveolar Ventilation

During VC-CMV (A/C), $\dot{V}_A$ is calculated by multiplying the number of breaths counted for 1 minute by the corrected V_T: $\dot{V}_A = (V_T - V_{Danat} - \text{Added } V_{Dmech}) \times f$. When a patient is on VC-IMV, the mandatory rate and volume delivery must be calculated separately from the patient's spontaneous rate and volume; these values then are added to determine the total minute ventilation (Box 8-6).

MONITORING AIRWAY PRESSURES

All positive pressure ventilators have a pressure monitor or display that continuously shows the upper airway pressure. The pressure monitor is probably most accurate when it shows pressures measured very near the patient's upper airway because this eliminates the effects of the humidifying device and the breathing circuit on

---

BOX 8-6 Calculation of Alveolar Ventilation in VC-IMV

Calculations are made using the following data:
- Intermittent mandatory ventilation (IMV) rate = 5 breaths/min
- Tidal volume (V_T) = 600 mL
- Anatomic dead space (V_{Danat}) = 100 mL
- Added mechanical dead space (V_{Dmech}) = 50 mL
- Mandatory alveolar ventilation per minute ($\dot{V}_A$) = 5 × [600 − 100 − 50] = 2250 mL or 2.25 L/min
- Patient spontaneous rate = 10 breaths/min
- Spontaneous V_T = 350 mL
- Spontaneous alveolar ventilation = 10 × [350 − 100 − 50] = 2000 mL or 2 L
- Total alveolar ventilation = 2.25 + 2 = 4.25 L/min

---

the measurement. Proximal pressure measurements are obtained by connecting the monitor tubing (usually a small-diameter plastic tube) to the Y-connector of the patient circuit. If the tubing is not visible on the circuit, pressures are detected through the main patient circuit and not at the upper airway. Although these values are not measured at the proximal airway, ICU ventilators are generally very accurate and clinically useful[1] (Key Point 8-3).

> **Key Point** 8-3 Proximal pressure and flow monitor lines must be free of moisture and secretions to provide accurate readings.

Pressure monitoring allows the clinician to assess pressure delivery to the upper airway. It ensures that a minimal pressure is maintained (low-pressure limit) and that high-pressure limits are not exceeded during mechanical ventilation. Intermittent readings of PIP, $P_{plateau}$, set pressure (for pressure-targeted modes such as PC-CMV and pressure support [PS]), transairway pressure (P_{TA} = PIP − $P_{plateau}$), mean airway pressure $\overline{P}_{aw}$, and end-expiratory pressure (EEP) can provide valuable information about the patient's condition.

Peak Inspiratory Pressure

PIP (or P_{peak}), which is the highest pressure observed during inspiration, can be used to calculate dynamic compliance (C_D; also called *dynamic characteristic*). A fairly constant V_T with an increasing P_{peak} may indicate a reduction in lung compliance (C_L) or an increase in airway resistance (R_{aw}). Conversely, a declining PIP may indicate a leak or may be a sign of improvement in compliance or resistance.

Plateau Pressure

A $P_{plateau}$ reading can be obtained by using the ventilator's inspiratory pause control or by setting a pause time of about 0.5 to 1.5 seconds. Remember that the static pressure is read when no gas flow is occurring. Traditionally, $P_{plateau}$ was determined by occluding the ventilator's expiratory port at the end of inspiration and reading the pressure registered on the ventilator's pressure manometer. After PIP is reached, the manometer needle or pressure indicator shows a drop of a few centimeters from peak and then briefly remains in a plateau (static) position before dropping to zero (see Fig. 8-3). It is important to remember that $P_{plateau}$ cannot be measured accurately if the patient makes active respiratory efforts, has a high f, or resists extending T_I; therefore measurement of $P_{plateau}$ is difficult, if not impossible, to obtain in spontaneously breathing individuals.

$P_{plateau}$ most often is used to calculate C_S, which reflects the elastic recoil of the alveoli and thoracic cage against the volume of air in the patient's lungs. Current practice strongly recommends keeping $P_{plateau}$ below 30 cm H_2O (Key Point 8-4). Notice that during either pressure or volume ventilation, if a condition of no gas flow occurs near the end of inspiration (i.e., the flow–time waveform graphic shows a reading of zero), the corresponding pressure on the pressure–time curve is an indicator of $P_{plateau}$ (Fig. 8-4 and Key Point 8-5).

> **Key Point** 8-4 Current practice strongly recommends keeping $P_{plateau}$ below 30 cm H_2O to avoid ventilator-induced lung injury.

> **Key Point** 8-5 Remember flow occurs because of a pressure difference between two points. If the pressure is the same at any two points within a tube or conductive airway, no flow will occur between those points.

Set Pressure

During PC-CMV, PC-IMV, and PSV the operator sets a target pressure to be delivered to the patient. As shown in Fig. 8-1, many institutions include a separate space on the flow sheet for entering the target pressure.

Transairway Pressure: PIP Minus $P_{plateau}$

The difference between the PIP and $P_{plateau}$ readings (PIP − $P_{plateau}$) is the transairway pressure (P_{TA}). P_{TA} is the amount of pressure required to overcome R_{aw} ($R_{aw} = P_{TA}$/Flow). Notice that P_{TA} includes the resistance of the ET. A higher than expected difference between PIP and $P_{plateau}$ suggests an increased R_{aw}. R_{aw} most often increases when the patient's airway requires suctioning, the patient is biting the tube or it is kinked, or the patient has mucosal edema, or bronchospasms (or both). It may also increase if the HME is partially occluded by accumulation of moisture or secretions.

Mean Airway Pressure

Many of the newer microprocessor-controlled ventilators automatically calculate and display $\overline{P}_{aw}$. $\overline{P}_{aw}$ is affected by PIP, EEP, the duty cycle (T_I/Total cycle time [TCT]) and f. Inspiratory flow patterns and modes also can influence $\overline{P}_{aw}$. Monitoring $\overline{P}_{aw}$ can be useful when examining the benefits and side effects of positive pressure ventilation (PPV), because it closely parallels the mean alveolar pressure. As discussed later in Chapter 13, the mean airway pressure influences tissue oxygenation and affects both lung volumes and cardiac output. (See Chapter 13 for additional information for the calculation of mean airway pressure.)

End-Expiratory Pressure

End-expiratory pressure (EEP) is the lowest pressure measured during the expiratory phase of a breath. The EEP is above atmospheric pressure when $PEEP_E$ or CPAP is administered. EEP is also elevated when auto-PEEP occurs.

An expiratory pause maneuver can be used to measure auto-PEEP, and most ventilators have a control for this purpose. The expiratory pause typically lasts 0.5 to 1.5 seconds, but some

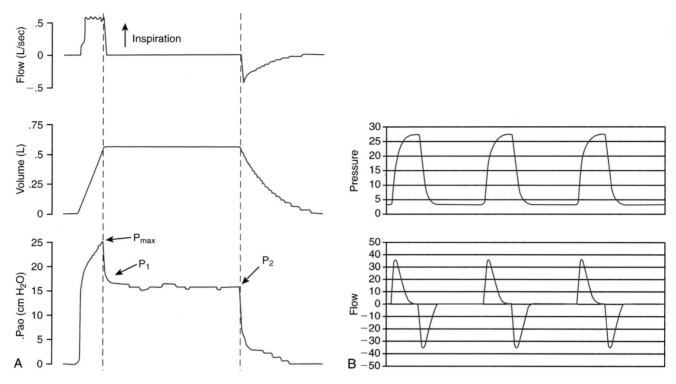

Fig. 8-4 A, VC-CMV with an inspiratory pause set. *Top curve,* Flow–time curve. *Middle curve,* Volume–time curve. *Bottom curve,* Pressure–time curve. After PIP, P_{max} is reached, the pressure drops to a plateau (begins at P_1 and ends at P_2). At the same time, inspiratory flow delivery ends and the flow drops to zero. The exhalation valve does not open until the end of the pause time. Expiratory flow does not occur until then. **B,** PC-CMV in which flow drops to zero during inspiration before the exhalation valve opens. The pressure measured during the no-flow period is an indicator of $P_{plateau}$. (NOTE: For a plateau to be visible in PC-CMV, T_1 must be long enough to allow ventilator pressure and lung pressure to equilibrate. If no pressure difference exists, no flow occurs.) (**A** from Pelosip P, Cereda M, Foti G, et al: Am J Respir Crit Care Med, 152:531-537, 1995. **B** from MacIntyre NR, Branson RD: Mechanical ventilation, ed 2, Philadelphia, 2009, Saunders/Elsevier.)

ventilators allow a pause of up to 15 to 20 seconds. As with the $P_{plateau}$ measurement, the EEP reading is accurate only if the patient is **not** actively breathing.

Sometimes the total PEEP ($PEEP_{TOT}$), which is the sum of the $PEEP_E$ and auto-PEEP, is recorded on the flow sheet. It is important to understand that $PEEP_{TOT}$ must be subtracted from $P_{plateau}$ to calculate C_S and from PIP to calculate C_D (Key Point 8-6).

> **Key Point 8-6** $PEEP_{TOT}$ must be subtracted from $P_{plateau}$ to calculate C_S, and from PIP to calculate C_D.

An airway pressure slightly greater than zero can occur at the upper airway during exhalation if a constant gas flow is moving through the circuit. This constant flow is referred to as *bias flow* or *base flow*. It is used to help the ventilator detect flow changes during exhalation and to allow flow triggering (see Chapter 3).

In most modern ventilators, bias flow occurs only at the end of exhalation; consequently no resistance to flow exists at the beginning of exhalation. (Microprocessor-controlled ventilators include software that corrects for bias flow, which does not appear in the graphics for the pressure–time and flow–time curves.) For example, the CareFusion Pulmonetics LTV 1000 ventilator (CareFusion, San Diego, Calif.) has a constant bias flow of gas during exhalation of 10 L/min. Note that a flow of 10 L/min is the current base flow for the LTV 1000. The manufacturer may change this value in the future. The presence of bias flow usually is not clinically significant and does not cause increased resistance to exhalation except in small infants, in whom it can increase WOB.

Pressure Limit

Audible and visual alarms are activated if PIP exceeds a set limit (this setting usually is about 10 cm H_2O above PIP). Activation of the high-pressure limit alarm ends inspiration. Some newer ventilators have an alarm delay that allows the limit to be exceeded for two or three breaths before the audible portion of the alarm is activated. It is worth noting, however, that in those instances when the pressure limit is exceeded, the breath ends, and flow to the patient stops for that breath.

Although high-pressure alarms frequently are activated when the patient coughs, activation of the alarm may indicate an increase in R_{aw} or a decrease in C_L. As mentioned earlier, increases in R_{aw} may signal that the patient's airway needs suctioning, that bronchospasm is occurring, or that the patient is biting the tube. Decreased C_L is associated with a number of conditions, such as pulmonary edema, pneumonia, pleural effusion, and pneumothorax.

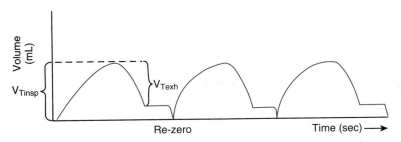

Fig. 8-5 Volume–time waveform during VC-CMV. Note that inspired tidal volume (V_{Tinsp}) is greater than expired V_T (V_{Texh}). All the volume measures are the same; therefore the leak is constant. Note that the software program for this waveform causes the line to drop to baseline before another breath is delivered.

| BOX **8-7** | **False Pressure Readings or Alarm Failure** |

False pressure readings can occur if the tubing leading to the pressure indicator (whether digital or an analog manometer) is twisted or plugged with water or secretions. This is especially true for ventilators with plastic monitoring tubes that attach close to the Y-connector (proximal pressure lines), such as the Hamilton G5 (Hamilton Medical, Bonaduz, Switzerland) and the CareFusion (Pulmonetics) LTV series. These monitoring lines not only measure pressure, but they may also detect flow, which in some cases is used to trigger the ventilator.

Manufacturers typically use air purging to maintain the patency of these monitoring lines. They also recommend that the connection tubes are mounted above the endotracheal connection to prevent the entry of water and secretions. Regardless of the setup, respiratory therapists should be vigilant about checking this type of monitoring system.

Low-Pressure Alarm

Audible and visual alarms alert the clinician when PIP falls below a designated level (this setting usually is 5 to 10 cm H_2O below PIP). These alarms indicate that the pressure has fallen significantly and usually are associated with a leak in the patient-ventilator circuit. The most common cause of a leak is patient disconnection from the ventilator, which typically can easily be seen and quickly corrected. If a leak in the patient-ventilator circuit is not obvious, the patient must be manually ventilated with a resuscitation bag until the respiratory therapist can identify the cause of the leak (Box 8-7 and Case Study 8-2).

Checking the Circuit: Checking for Leaks

Evaluation of the integrity of the ventilator circuit is part of a standard ventilator check. It includes checking for leaks, disconnected tubing, and other circuit problems.

A leak can be identified in a number of ways. The simplest way is to note whether the peak pressure and the exhaled volume are lower than previous measurements. The volume–time waveform also can be checked; if it resembles an igloo, the inspired V_T is greater than the expired V_T (Fig. 8-5).

 Case Study 8-2

Circuit Disconnect

The cardiac monitor on a mechanically ventilated patient suddenly activates. The patient demonstrates sinus tachycardia. The nurse and respiratory therapist check the patient but do not immediately find the cause of the tachycardia.

The nurse pulls back the bedding sheet covering the patient's upper chest and discovers that the patient is disconnected from the ventilator. What probably prevented the ventilator's low-pressure alarm from activating?

To find a leak, the practitioner first should check the patient's airway by listening over the trachea with a stethoscope to determine whether the ET or tracheostomy tube cuff is adequately inflated. (If the cuff is not adequately inflated, abnormal breathing sounds will be heard as air leaks around the ET.) The clinician should then check for leaks in the ventilator circuit, starting at the point where the patient circuit attaches to the ventilator outlet and working toward the exhalation valve. Before beginning the test, it is prudent to hyperventilate and hyperoxygenate the patient. The patient is then disconnected from the ventilator and his or her lungs manually ventilated with a resuscitation bag by another therapist or a nurse (Key Point 8-7).[2]

Key Point 8-7 Disconnecting a patient from the ventilator can result in hypoventilation, hypoxemia, bradycardia, and/or hypotension. Before disconnecting the patient, it is prudent to hyperventilate and hyperoxygenate to reduce the risk of these complications.[2]

The procedure for identifying the origin of a leak is fairly straightforward. First, the Y-connector is occluded, and the ventilator is cycled. If the high-pressure limit is not reached, a significant leak is present. Second, the main inspiratory tubing on the distal side of the humidifier (the side farthest from the ventilator) is pinched closed. If the PIP alarm sounds, no leak exists in the humidifier system between the respiratory therapist's hand and the ventilator. If the alarm does not sound, the leak is in the humidifier assembly or at the point where the circuit attaches to the ventilator or to the humidifier. Third, the large-bore expiratory line is pinched shut, and the ventilator is cycled manually. If the PIP limit alarm fails to activate, the leak is located near the Y-connector. This technique works well for large leaks, but may not be as useful for identifying smaller leaks.

Leaks most often occur around the humidifier, through humidifier water-feed lines, at water traps, or anywhere tubing connections join. Other possible sources are closed suction catheters, in-line thermometers, and end-tidal carbon dioxide (CO_2) monitors. A normal leak may be present around the ET if the minimum leak technique (MLT) is used to inflate the cuff

---

BOX 8-8 **Minimum Leak and Minimum Occlusion Techniques for Cuff Inflation**

Two techniques are commonly used to inflate tube cuffs:
1. Minimum occlusion technique (MOT)

The cuff is inflated during positive pressure ventilation until no leak is heard at end inspiration. The leak is detected by listening with a stethoscope over the suprasternal notch or lateral neck. With the MOT, just enough measured volume is injected into the cuff to stop all leakage around the cuff resulting in the lowest cuff pressure needed to create a seal. The required volume is then recorded. (NOTE: Increasing the volume to slightly above that needed to occlude the airway can significantly increase cuff pressure.)
2. Minimum leak technique (MLT).

The cuff is inflated during positive pressure ventilation until a leak is no longer heard on inspiration. A small amount of air is removed from the cuff so that the leak can just be heard at end inspiration. Some clinicians prefer MOT because of concerns about aspiration with MLT.

Although MLT can provide low cuff pressures in some situations, it cannot do so if the cycling pressure necessary to achieve tidal volume (V_T) delivery is too high. This occurs in patients with low lung compliance (C_L) or high airway resistance (R_{aw}), in which case a significant amount of volume may be lost. A solution may be simply to increase the set volume on the ventilator to compensate for the volume loss.

During VC-CMV, the amount of the leak that occurs with MLT changes as the peak inspiratory pressure (PIP) changes. If MLT is used when PIP is high and PIP gradually decreases, cuff volume eventually becomes higher than necessary. The leak actually may be eliminated and MLT would have to be performed again. Conversely, if MLT is used at low PIP, the leak becomes too great if P_{peak} increases (see Case Study 8-3).

 Case Study 8-3

Cuff Inflation Techniques

The minimum leak technique (MLT) has been used to establish cuff inflation with a cuff pressure of 20 mm Hg. At this same time (13:00), the respiratory therapist records a ventilator peak inspiratory pressure (PIP) of 28 cm H_2O, a set volume of 520 mL, and a measured exhaled volume of 500 mL. At 21:00 the PIP is 23 cm H_2O and the exhaled volume is 520 mL. What might account for an increase in volume while the pressure is decreasing?

VITAL SIGNS, BLOOD PRESSURE, AND PHYSICAL EXAMINATION OF THE CHEST

Observing and recording a patient's vital signs (i.e., systemic arterial blood pressure [BP], heart rate [HR], temperature [T], f, oxygen saturation measured by pulse oximetry [S_pO_2], and physical appearance) can help staff members evaluate possible changes in the patient's overall condition. In mechanically ventilated patients, f, HR, and S_pO_2 are monitored continuously. Temperature and arterial BP may also be monitored continuously, but more often they are measured intermittently. It is important for the clinician to remember that alarms are activated only by critical changes. Moderate changes in vital signs during hourly or bihourly checks should alert the practitioner to the possibility of hypoxemia, impending cardiovascular collapse (decreased or increased BP and HR), or infection (elevated temperature).

Heart Rate

An electrocardiogram (ECG) is a noninvasive means of continuously monitoring HR and heart rhythm. All hospitalized patients receiving ventilatory support must be continuously monitored with a three-lead ECG. The ECG provides minimum and maximum HR alarms (audible and visual), and therefore can alert the ICU staff if significant bradycardia or tachycardia occurs.

The ECG leads generally are placed on the chest, one near each clavicle, and one near the fourth intercostal space at the left midaxillary line. It is important to place the leads so that a clearly discernible QRS complex can be displayed on the monitor (a standard lead II configuration is typically used for monitoring ICU patients).

The ECG monitor is viewed or scanned by a computer for changes in HR and rhythm. Activation of an audible alarm alerts personnel when a potentially dangerous event has occurred. Activation of an HR alarm may simply indicate that the ECG electrodes have become disconnected from the patient, or it may signal a more critical event (e.g., the patient has become disconnected from the ventilator, and is experiencing severe hypoxemia or hypercapnia, or both). Other factors that can affect HR include pathologic changes in the myocardium (e.g., infarction, hypoxia, and drug reaction), anxiety, pain, and stress. An initial 12-lead ECG should be obtained when mechanical ventilation is initiated in patients older than 21 years with acute respiratory failure.[3]

Temperature

A patient's temperature can be measured orally (by mouth), aurally (by ear), or by an axillary technique (from the armpit). Core temperature measurements typically are obtained using rectal, esophageal, or pulmonary artery temperatures. A number of factors can

---

(Box 8-8[11,12] and Case Study 8-3). The leak associated with the MLT usually is insignificant, and very little volume is lost with adult patients. A chest tube may be another source of leaks. A pleural drainage system is a likely source if a leak is detected with the volume–time waveform, but cannot be found in the circuit.

A system leak can prevent flow cycling during PSV. For example, during PSV with the Servo-i ventilator, inspiration is adjusted to end when the flow falls below 5% of the peak inspiratory flow. If a leak in the system allows flow out of the circuit at more than 5% of the peak flow rate, the ventilator continues inspiratory gas flow to the patient. Most microprocessor-controlled ventilators have a backup cycling time of 1.5 to 3 seconds to end inspiration, if flow does not drop the set amount.

It is critical that no leaks exist in the ventilating system when expired gas is collected, as is done for measurement of the dead space–to–tidal volume ratio (V_D/V_T), oxygen consumption per minute ($\dot{V}O_2$), and carbon dioxide production per minute ($\dot{V}CO_2$) (see Chapter 10). In these situations the cuff must be sufficiently inflated to occlude the airway completely. Once the measurements have been obtained, the cuff is reinflated using MLT or reinflated to the previous low pressure.

affect body temperature.[13] For example, hyperthermia can be caused by infection, tissue necrosis, late-stage carcinoma, Hodgkin disease, leukemia, and metabolic abnormalities, such as hyperthyroidism. Low-grade fever can be a result of accidental or surgical trauma, atelectasis, fistulas, hematomas, or foreign bodies.

Hypothermia can result from metabolic diseases (e.g., hypothyroidism), central nervous system disorders, drugs (e.g., phenothiazines, tricyclic antidepressants, and benzodiazepines), and other substances (e.g., alcohol, heroin, carbon monoxide).[13]

Systemic Arterial Blood Pressure

A patient's BP should be checked intermittently with a stethoscope and sphygmomanometer or an automatic BP cuff. It also can be measured continuously with invasive intravascular arterial catheters. Invasive arterial pressure monitoring is typically used after open heart surgery and for critically ill patients requiring continuous, direct measurements of BP (see Chapter 11).

Arterial catheters usually are placed in a peripheral vessel, such as the radial artery, where collateral circulation exists. A modified Allen test (Box 8-9) should be performed whenever a radial artery catheter is placed.

Central Venous Pressure

Indwelling venous catheters placed in the superior vena cava or right atrium can be used to monitor central venous pressure (CVP), myocardial function, and fluid status in critically ill patients (see Chapter 11). CVP measurements reflect right arterial pressure

---

BOX 8-9   The Modified Allen Test

The modified Allen test for collateral circulation is performed by holding a patient's hand with the palm up, occluding the radial and ulnar arteries, and having the patient open and close the hand. The hand is opened to make sure it is drained of blood (blanched), and the pressure over the ulnar artery is then released. The palm flushes with blood in 15 seconds or less if collateral circulation to the hand through the ulnar artery is present. The process is repeated with the radial artery to demonstrate perfusion in this vessel. Note that the modified Allen test results are not always reliable and the results must be interpreted with caution.

---

and right ventricular end-diastolic pressure, and therefore can provide valuable information about venous return and right heart function.

Because CVP is elevated during a positive pressure breath, it is measured at the end of expiration when intrapleural pressure returns to normal or its lowest value during the respiratory cycle.

Pulmonary Artery Pressure

The pulmonary artery pressure can be monitored continuously with a balloon-tip, flow-directed, pulmonary artery (PA) catheter that is connected to a monitor by a transducer. PA catheters are typically used to monitor the hemodynamic status of critically ill patients with severe cardiopulmonary complications and problems with fluid management (see Chapter 11).

Physical Examination of the Chest

Ideally physical examination of a patient should be performed at least once every shift. This examination should include inspection, palpation, percussion, and auscultation of the chest. The results are recorded on the chart and compared with previous findings. Abnormal findings or significant changes must be evaluated and treated promptly.

Different conditions can produce a variety of physical findings (e.g., hyperresonance occurs on chest percussion of a patient with severe asthma and air trapping). Additionally, breath sounds and chest excursion are diminished, accessory muscle use is increased, and high-pitched wheezes are present. For patients with pneumonia, the chest is dull to percussion, breath sounds are decreased, and crackles (rales) occur late in inspiration over the affected area. With pleural effusion, the affected area produces a dull percussion note, breath sounds are absent, and a pleural friction rub may be audible on auscultation. Patients with a large pneumothorax show a shift in their tracheal position away from the affected side. Chest percussion in these patients is hyperresonant over the affected area, and breath sounds are absent. Table 8-1 presents a list of the physical changes associated with various pulmonary disorders.

Auscultation of the chest that reveals low-pitched breath sounds with a rattle-like quality (rhonchi) may indicate secretions in the larger airways and the need for suctioning. The presence of wheezes often suggests the need for bronchodilator therapy, although wheezes can also occur when secretions are retained in the small airways and with some cardiac conditions. Absence of breath

---

TABLE 8-1   Physical and Radiologic Findings in Common Pulmonary Disorders

Diagnosis	Auscultation	Percussion	Tracheal Excursion	Chest Wall Movement	Chest Radiograph
Asthma	High-pitched wheezing	Hyperresonant R and L	WNL	↓ R and L	↑ Radiolucency
Pneumonia (R)	Late inspiratory crackles	Dull (R)	WNL; if massive, L-shift	↓ R	Infiltrates (R)
Pleural effusion (R)	Friction rub, just above fluid level	Dull (R)	L-shift	↓ R	Blunting of costophrenic angle (R)
Pneumothorax (R)	Decreased or absent on R	Hyperresonant (R)	L-shift	↓ R	Lack of vascular markings (R); mediastinal shift (L)
Emphysema	Diminished; vary; early expiratory crackles	Hyperresonant	WNL	↓ R and L	↑ Radiolucency; widened rib spaces; flattened diaphragm

L, Left; *R,* right; *WNL,* within normal limits; ↓, decrease; ↑, increase.

sounds may indicate a pneumothorax, complete airway obstruction, complete lung collapse, improper placement of the ET, or a pleural effusion. Evaluation of both the physical and ventilatory findings (e.g., increased PIP and chest radiographs results) can confirm the presence of abnormal findings and point to appropriate treatments.

Patient assessment should also include evaluation of respiratory muscle use. Increased use of the accessory muscles of inspiration or *paradoxical breathing* (retraction of the abdomen during inspiration and protrusion during exhalation) indicates an increased WOB and the potential for respiratory muscle fatigue.[13]

Abdominal distention suggests several problems, including postoperative intestinal accumulation of gas, air swallowing, bleeding, or **ascites** (fluid in the abdominal space). Regardless of the cause, abdominal distention can impair ventilation by applying upward pressure on the diaphragm, creating restrictive breathing difficulties. The cause must be determined and the problem should be corrected if possible (Case Study 8-4).

 Case Study 8-4

Patient Assessment Cases

Problem 1

Physical examination of a patient on mechanical ventilation reveals bilateral low-pitched lung sounds and normal resonance to percussion. The patient has a temperature of 39° C. Heart rate is 122 beats/min and blood pressure is 135/85 mm Hg. What is the possible cause of this patient's abnormal breath sounds? What therapeutic procedure is indicated?

Problem 2

On chest auscultation, the practitioner hears no breath sounds on the left, but distant breath sounds on the right. The percussion note on the left is hyperresonant, and the note on the right has normal resonance. The trachea is deviated to the right. In the past hour cardiac output has dropped from 6 L/min to 4.5 L/min. What is the most likely problem?

Problem 3

A female patient has been intubated for 4 hours and is receiving 100% oxygen. Auscultation of the patient's chest reveals normal breath sounds on the right, but no breath sounds on the left. The percussion note is normal on the right, and dull on the left. The oral endotracheal tube indicates a 26-cm marking at the teeth. What is the most likely problem?

MANAGEMENT OF ENDOTRACHEAL TUBE AND TRACHEOSTOMY TUBE CUFFS

During the initial assessment of a ventilated patient, the respiratory therapist evaluates endotracheal and tracheostomy tube position, in addition to cuff integrity and pressures. The following section reviews the procedures for measuring cuff pressures and for dealing with inappropriate cuff pressures and cuff leaks.

Cuff Pressure Measurement

The endotracheal or tracheostomy cuff pressure is typically checked during the initial evaluation of the patient and once every 8 to 12

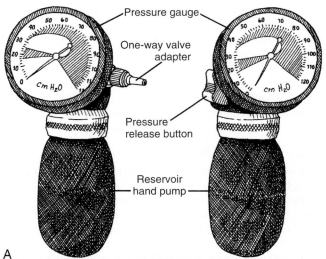

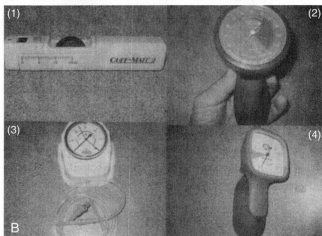

Fig. 8-6 A, Posey Cuffalator device used to measure cuff pressures. **B,** Four types of cuff inflator devices: *(1),* DHD CuffMate; *(2),* Posey Cuffalator; *(3),* SIMS-Portex Cuff Pressure Indicator; *(4),* Rüsch Endotest. (**A** from Sills JR: Comprehensive respiratory therapist exam review, entry and advanced level, ed 5, St Louis, 2010, Mosby. **B** Redrawn from Blanch PB: Laboratory evaluation of 4 brands of endotracheal tube cuff inflator, Respir Care 49:166-173, 2004.)

hours to ensure that cuff pressures do not exceed 20 to 25 mm Hg (27 to 34 cm H_2O). It is generally accepted that maintaining the cuff pressure below 34 cm H_2O (25 mm Hg) reduces the risk of tracheal damage associated with overinflated tube cuffs. Although the pressure transmitted to the tracheal wall generally is lower than the pressure in the cuff, some clinicians contend that using a low cuff pressure reduces the risk of tracheal damage and necrosis associated with tube cuffs.[12,14] Tracheal damage and necrosis can occur if the cuff pressure transmitted to the trachea is greater than the perfusion pressure. This is particularly important in hypotensive patients, where even an ET and tracheostomy cuff pressure of only 34 cm H_2O (25 mm Hg) can exceed the perfusion pressure to the trachea, resulting in significant tracheal damage.

Cuff pressure measuring devices are a convenient means of monitoring cuff pressure and for adding or removing air from the cuff. These devices have either an analog (gauge) or a digital readout. A small volume of air is lost when the cuff pilot balloon is connected to the device, because these devices use very short connecting tubes (Fig. 8-6, *A*). The pressure may be shown in centimeters of water (cm H_2O) or millimeters of mercury (mm Hg) depending on the device (Fig. 8-6, *B*).[15] Unfortunately, these devices are often inaccurate, and clinicians may find it advisable to use an alternative method for measuring cuff inflation pressures (Box 8-10).[15]

ET and tracheostomy cuff pressures can also be measured using a mercury column manometer, like those used to measure BP. A three-way or four-way stopcock between the cuff pilot balloon and the manometer should be used to pressurize the manometer before the cuff pressure is measured. If this is not done, a significant amount of the cuff volume or pressure will be lost in the connecting tube. Air is injected into the manometer with a syringe to pressurize it. The amount of pressure added must equal previous pressure readings or must be approximately 20 to 25 mm Hg (27 to 34 cm H_2O). The cuff and manometer can be pressurized simultaneously if the cuff is being inflated or was deflated before measurement (Fig. 8-7).

A five-step protocol was developed to minimize the risk of tracheal necrosis associated with cuff overinflation[16]:

1. The minimal leak technique (MLT) should be used whenever possible.
2. A reasonable MLT should be established, one in which only 50 to 100 mL of V_T is lost during inspiration. For example, in VC-CMV with a 600 mL V_T setting and delivery, the exhaled V_T is 500 to 550 mL.
3. A high-volume/low-pressure cuff should not require more than 5 mL for inflation. If it does, the tube probably is too small.
4. If a minimal leak cannot be maintained with a cuff volume of less than 5 mL, the practitioner should make sure that the cuff pressure is less than 25 mm Hg and that the cuff-to-tracheal diameter ratio checked on chest radiograph is 1:1.5 or less.

BOX 8-10	Improving the Accuracy of Cuff Pressures Measured with a Cuff Inflation Device

1. Place a stopcock into the pilot valve of the endotracheal tube (ET).
2. Set the stopcock to the closed-in-all-directions position.
3. Attach a cuff inflator and a syringe to the two open ports of the stopcock. (NOTE: The Cuffalator and the Endotest have their own bulbs, which can be used in place of a syringe.)
4. Turn the stopcock to the syringe or bulb to prepressurize the cuff inflator. (NOTE: If the device has a built-in inflator bulb, the stopcock can remain in the closed-in-all-directions position.)
5. Pressurize the cuff to 27 cm H_2O (20 mm Hg) using the syringe or bulb.
6. Once the cuff has been pressurized, rotate the position of the stopcock to connect the cuff inflator to the ET cuff.
7. If the cuff pressure is not approximately 27 cm H_2O (20 mm Hg), it will rise or fall, depending on the difference. The range should be 27 to 34 cm H_2O (20 to 25 mm Hg) or less.

Modified from Blanch PB: Laboratory evaluation of 4 brands of endotracheal tube cuff inflator, *Respir Care* 49:166-173, 2004.

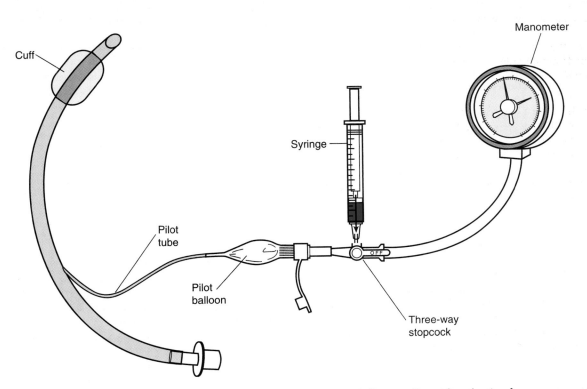

Fig. 8-7 A syringe, manometer, and three-way stopcock can be used to measure cuff pressure. (See text for explanation of procedure.)

5. If steps 1 through 4 cannot be achieved, the patient should be followed up for tracheal stenosis for at least 1 year after discharge.

High Cuff Pressure

The most common cause of an excessively high cuff pressure is simply an overinflated tube cuff. Occasionally cuff pressures are high because a low-volume/high-pressure cuff is used. However, most cuffs currently used are the high-volume/low-pressure type unless a specialty tube is used.

Sometimes a higher-than-acceptable cuff pressure is required to maintain a minimum occlusion, and none of the problems previously mentioned are present. There are two reasons why this may occur. First, the cuff and artificial airway may have moved up (cephalad) in the patient's airway and become lodged in the larynx or pharynx. The markings at the lips or teeth may indicate the depth of the tube in the airway. In this situation, the tube should be moved farther into the airway. Second, the ET may be too small for the patient; in this situation, a very large volume is required to seal the tube in the trachea. This is a particularly difficult problem because the clinician may be reluctant to change to a larger tube. However, if the ET will be needed for several days, changing it is the wise course. This can be done using a tube changer (Fig. 8-8). The tube changer is inserted into the current ET, which is removed while the changer is left in place. A larger ET is inserted over the tube changer and into the trachea, and the tube changer is then withdrawn.

On rare occasions a high cuff pressure may be required to maintain either a minimum leak or minimum occlusion because the patient's trachea is dilated at the level of the cuff (Fig. 8-9). Occasionally, the cuff can be repositioned but a dilated trachea suggests that the cuff has been in place and overinflated for quite some time, resulting in the tracheal injury (see Case Study 8-3).

Nonexistent or Low Cuff Pressure

If the cuff pressure is very low or nonexistent, the respiratory therapist should first check that the cuff has been properly inflated and is in the appropriate position in the airway. If the pressure is still low (or absent) or continues to drop after inflation and positioning,

the most common cause is a leak in the ET cuff or pilot system. Fig. 8-10 presents an algorithm for determining the cause of a cuff leak and loss of pressure.[17,18]

The location of the leak must be determined. First, the cuff is inflated to an appropriate pressure, and the pilot tube is clamped. The clinician then listens for an air leak in the upper airway. For example, if a leak is present during a positive pressure breath, air can be heard over the neck area or may even be escaping from the patient's mouth. If the cuff continues to lose pressure with the pilot tube clamped, the leak probably is in the cuff itself. As a temporary solution, cuff inflation can be maintained with a continuous low flow of gas to the pilot line until the ET can be changed.[19]

If the leak is not in the cuff, it may be in the pilot balloon or the valve. To detect these types of leaks, the cuff is inflated and a

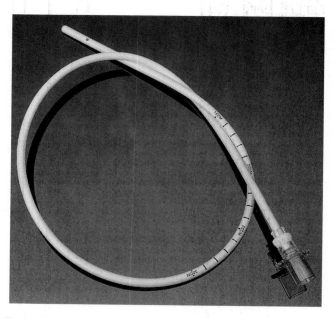

Fig. 8-8 Endotracheal tube changer (see text for further information). (From Cairo JM: Mosby's respiratory care equipment, ed 9, St Louis, 2014, Elsevier.)

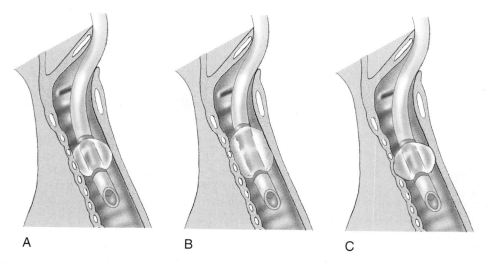

Fig. 8-9 A, Low-volume/high-pressure cuff. **B,** High-volume/low-pressure cuff. **C,** Tracheal dilation adjacent to the cuff. (Modified from Hess DR, MacIntyre NR, Mishoe SC, et al: Respiratory care principles and practice, Philadelphia, 2002, W.B. Saunders.)

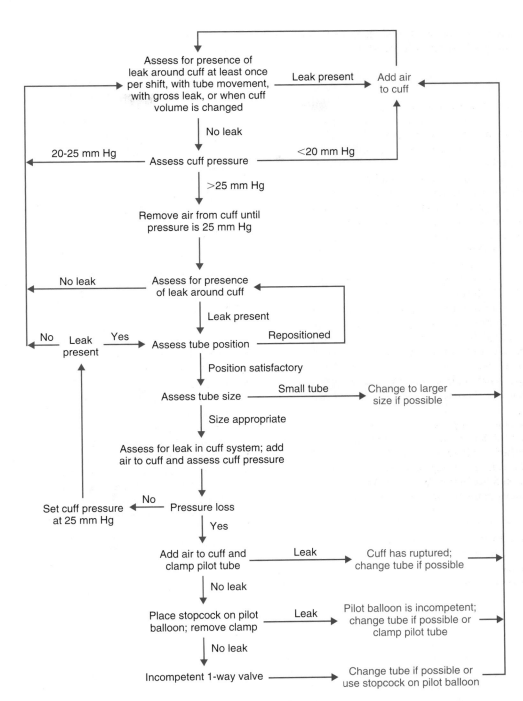

Fig. 8-10 Algorithm for resolution of a cuff leak in an artificial airway. (Modified from Hess DR: Managing the artificial airway, Respir Care 44:759-772, 1999.)

stopcock is attached to the pilot balloon. The stopcock is turned to the off position. If the leak is still present, it is located in the pilot balloon. This problem can be solved temporarily by clamping the pilot line. If the stopcock on the pilot balloon resolves the leak, the valve is not working. Simply leaving the stopcock on the pilot balloon temporarily solves this problem. The tube should be changed if possible.

A 2-year study of massive airway leaks produced an important finding: a large number of ETs that were removed for apparent defects or damage were actually flawless. Tube malposition was the most likely explanation for these results. Careful investigation of a leaking airway should precede any decision to change the tube to solve the problem.[20]

Cut in the Pilot Tube

An accidental cut in the pilot tube is a common occurrence. This often happens when clinicians change the tape that secures the tube. This problem can be remedied by positioning a three-way stopcock between a blunt-tipped needle inserted into the cut pilot tube and a syringe (Fig. 8-11). Some manufacturers specifically

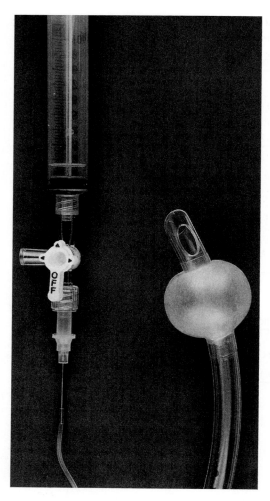

Fig. 8-11 A cut pilot tube can be repaired temporarily by inserting a cutoff 19-gauge needle with a stopcock into the pilot tubing. This system can also be used to repair a failed pilot balloon/valve assembly by cutting the pilot tube and inserting the needle.

design blunt-tipped needle devices with pilot balloons. The blunt-tipped needle can be inserted into the cut pilot tube and the cuff of the ET can be inflated (Fig. 8-12).

Tube and Mouth Care

About once every shift (approximately 8 to 12 hours) the ET must be repositioned in the mouth and retaped if needed. Repositioning the ET helps prevent pressure injuries to the gums, mouth, lips, or nose that can occur as a result of the constant pressure of the tube. Oral hygiene also should be performed routinely. Although oral hygiene often is the responsibility of the patient's nursing staff, the process of retaping and repositioning the tube is a two-person procedure. One practitioner holds the tube in place, while the other person secures the tube with surgical tape.

MONITORING COMPLIANCE AND AIRWAY RESISTANCE

Static Compliance

Normal C_S is approximately 70 to 100 mL/cm H_2O ($C_S = V_T/[P_{plateau} - EEP]$). When C_S is less than 25 mL/cm H_2O, WOB is very high. The accuracy of the C_S calculation depends on the accuracy of the actual delivered V_T and $P_{plateau}$ measurements.

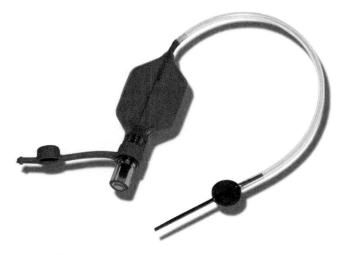

Fig. 8-12 Pilot tube repair kit. (Courtesy Instrumentation Industries, Inc., Bethel Park, Pa.)

Chest wall recoil and the elastic recoil of the patient circuit remain fairly constant in most patients. Therefore a change in C_S readings over time usually is considered a result of change in the patient's alveolar elastic recoil.

In cases where chest wall compliance does change, C_S readings can be used to identify the presence of a significant problem. For example, air trapping, pulmonary edema, atelectasis, consolidation, pneumonia, pneumothorax, hemothorax, and pleural effusion will cause a decrease in C_S. Reductions in chest wall compliance also can occur with flail chest, changes in chest wall muscle tension, pneumomediastinum, and abdominal distention (e.g., peritonitis, ascites, herniation, or abdominal bleeding). Note that clinicians can also detect many of these conditions by evaluating breath sounds and percussion notes, palpating the chest and abdominal wall, obtaining a chest radiograph, and studying laboratory data.

Regardless of the method that is used to determine that an abnormal condition exists, appropriate medical intervention must be initiated and the problem corrected. Reduced C_S implies that ventilation is less effective. In PC-CMV, pressure remains constant, while the delivered V_T decreases. In VC-CMV, PIP and $P_{plateau}$ increase, while the delivered V_T remains fairly constant (Table 8-2, A and B). In PC-CMV, pressure must be increased when compliance decreases to maintain V_T delivery. Reduced C_S can result in a decreased P_aO_2 and an increased arterial carbon dioxide partial pressure (P_aCO_2); therefore determining the cause of the condition and treating it are important.

Dynamic Characteristic (Dynamic Compliance)

The **dynamic characteristic** (C_D), often called *dynamic compliance* or *dynamic effective compliance,* is the volume delivered by the ventilator divided by (PIP − EEP): C_D = Volume/PIP − EEP).[21] C_D is measured during airflow; therefore it is influenced by the patient's lung and chest wall elastic recoil and by airway resistance, the ET, and the ventilator circuit. Because C_D includes both compliance and resistance components, it is more accurately described as an impedance measurement; however, most practitioners still refer to it as dynamic compliance.

The C_D decreases whenever C_S decreases or R_{aw} increases. Lung problems can easily be differentiated from airway problems simply by monitoring changes in PIP, $P_{plateau}$, and the difference between

| TABLE 8-2 | Simplified Examples of Changes in Delivered Tidal Volume (V_T) and Peak Inspiratory Pressure (PIP) and Pressure Plateau ($P_{plateau}$) Reflecting Changes in Dynamic Compliance (C_D) |

A. DECREASING C_D DURING PC-CMV

Time	PIP	V_T	C_D*
01:00	25	500	20
02:00	25	400	16
03:00	25	300	12

Constant pressures with decreasing volume.

B. DECREASING C_D DURING VC-CMV

Time	PIP	V_T	C_D
01:00	25	500	20
02:00	30	500	17
03:00	35	500	14

Constant volume with increasing pressures.

C. DECREASING C_S AND C_D DURING VC-CMV WITH CONSTANT R_{AW}

Time	PIP	C_D	$P_{plateau}$	C_S*	P_{TA}	Volume†
01:00	25	20	20	25	5	500
02:00	30	17	25	20	5	500
03:00	35	14	30	17	5	500

Increasing PIP and $P_{plateau}$. Volume and pressure lost to the airways are constant. The lung is less compliant.

D. DECREASED C_D, CONSTANT C_S DURING VC-CMV WITH INCREASED R_{AW}

Time	PIP	C_D	$P_{plateau}$	C_S	P_{TA}	Volume
01:00	25	20	20	25	5	500
02:00	30	17	20	25	10	500
03:00	35	14	20	25	15	500

Increasing PIP with constant volumes and $P_{plateau}$. R_{aw} is increased (P_{TA} = PIP − $P_{plateau}$).

E. IMPROVING C_D AND C_S DURING VC-CMV

Time	PIP	C_D	$P_{plateau}$	C_S	P_{TA}	Volume
01:00	25	20	23	22	2	500
02:00	23	22	21	24	2	500
03:00	20	25	18	28	2	500

PIP and $P_{plateau}$ are decreasing; delivered volume and P_{TA} are constant; the lungs are more compliant.

F. COMPLIANCE MEASUREMENTS WITH PEEP DURING VC-CMV

Time	PIP	C_D	$P_{plateau}$	C_S	P_{TA}	PEEP	Volume
01:00	30	20	28	22	2	+5	500
02:00	35	20	33	22	2	+10	500
03:00	40	18	37	20	3	+12	500

The addition of increasing PEEP results in increasing PIP and $P_{plateau}$. Delivered V_T and P_{TA} remain constant.

C_D, Dynamic compliance (C_D = Volume/[PIP − EEP]); C_S, static compliance (C_S = Volume/[$P_{plateau}$ − EEP]); *EEP*, end-expiratory pressure; *PEEP*, positive end-expiratory pressure; *PIP*, peak inspiratory pressure (cm H_2O); *PC-CMV*, pressure-controlled, continuous mandatory ventilation; $P_{plateau}$, plateau pressure (cm H_2O); P_{TA}, transairway pressure (cm H_2O); R_{aw}, airway resistance; *VC-CMV*, volume-controlled, continuous mandatory ventilation; V_T, tidal volume (mL).
*Volume is shown in mL throughout the table.
†Compliance is shown in mL/cm H_2O throughout the table.

them (P_{TA}). If PIP and $P_{plateau}$ both are increasing with the same volume delivery and the P_{TA} is fairly constant, C_S is decreasing (see Table 8-2, *B* and *C*). If PIP increases along with P_{TA}, R_{aw} is increasing (see Table 8-2, *D*). Calculation of C_D and C_S confirms these findings.

With VC-CMV, volume delivery remains nearly constant regardless of changes in C_D; however, delivery pressures may become dangerously high. In PC-CMV, a decrease in C_D will result in a reduction in the delivered V_T. Pressure must therefore be increased to maintain the delivered V_T. During VC-CMV, a decreasing PIP with a constant delivered V_T may signal improvement in compliance or R_{aw} (see Table 8-2, *E*). Because a drop in pressure might also indicate a leak, the delivered V_T must be checked. Remember that when extrinsic PEEP ($PEEP_E$) and/or auto-PEEP is present, it must be subtracted from $P_{plateau}$ and PIP readings to calculate C_S and C_D (see Table 8-2, *F*).

During PC-CMV, increased V_T delivery with the same pressure indicates an improvement in compliance or a decrease in R_{aw} (or both) (Case Study 8-5).

Airway Resistance

Total resistance is the sum of R_{aw} and tissue resistance, although tissue resistance remains relatively constant in most cases. Tissue resistance can increase in conditions, such as ascites and pleural effusion. R_{aw} normally ranges from 0.6 to 2.4 cm H_2O/L/sec, and can be estimated for ventilated patients by measuring P_{TA}, and using the inspiratory flow and a constant flow waveform. Although this is not an accurate flow measurement, it can be used over time to indicate relative changes in R_{aw}. For example, if PIP is 35 cm H_2O; $P_{plateau}$ is 34 cm H_2O; and flow is 30 L/min (0.5 L/sec), Raw is calculated as follows:

$$R_{aw} = P_{TA}/Flow\,(L/sec)$$
$$R_{aw} = (PIP - P_{plateau})/Flow$$
$$R_{aw} = (35 - 34\,cm\,H_2O)/(0.5\,L/sec)$$
$$R_{aw} = 2\,cm\,H_2O/L/sec$$

Many microprocessor-controlled ventilators utilize software programs that can calculate and display compliance and resistance values. Some of the values are taken from measurements of pressure, expired flow, and volume.

Case Study 8-5

Exercises
Problem 1

While checking the ventilation parameters during VC-CMV, you notice the following changes in positive inspiratory pressure (PIP) and plateau pressure ($P_{plateau}$):

Time	Volume (L)	PIP (cm H_2O)	$P_{plateau}$ (cm H_2O)
01:00	0.7	23	15
03:00	0.7	28	16
05:00	0.7	35	17

What is the likely cause of the problem? How would you assess the patient to determine the appropriate treatment?

Problem 2

During PC-CMV, the following changes are noted:

Time	Volume (L)	Set Pressure (cm H_2O)
01:00	0.65	20
03:00	0.60	20
05:00	0.55	20

What is the likely cause of the problem? How would you assess the patient to determine treatment?

Treatment for increased R_{aw} must be directed at the specific cause of the increase. For example, suctioning the airway, clearing an obstruction, or giving a bronchodilator treatment may correct the problem.

Bedside Measurement of Pressure–Volume Curves

The pressure–volume relationships for C_D and C_S can be plotted by ventilating the lung at different volumes and recording the PIP and $P_{plateau}$.[22,23] Bone and colleagues first described a bedside measurement technique for drawing static pressure–volume (P-V) curves nearly 40 years ago.[20,22,23] Plotting of P-V curves, which was done

BOX 8-11 Technique for Obtaining Pressure–Volume Curves

1. The patient normally is placed in the supine position, or the head of the bed is slightly elevated and the patient is relaxed. The person cannot be spontaneously breathing because the $P_{plateau}$ measurements will be inaccurate. (Use of sedation may be necessary.) Explain the procedure to the patient if appropriate.
2. Inflate the airway cuff to eliminate leaks; check the system for leaks and remove all of them.
3. Select the inspiratory pause control for each volume measurement.
4. Select a series of tidal volume (V_T, such as 6, 8, 10, 12, and 14 mL/kg or 250, 500, 750, 1000, and 1250 mL. Do not let $P_{plateau}$ become excessively high.)*
5. For each volume setting, record the peak inspiratory pressure (PIP), $P_{plateau}$, end-expiratory pressure (EEP), and V_T. (Subtract EEP from PIP and $P_{plateau}$ before recording.)
6. Closely monitor the patient's hemodynamic status during the procedure.
7. Allow return to normal settings for several breaths between each test volume setting.
8. Remove the inspiratory pause.
9. Return cuff pressures to minimum leak or initial pressure or volume.
10. Perform a complete patient-ventilator system check.
11. Plot the data (see Fig. 8-14).

*If pressure rises rapidly and markedly, discontinue study to prevent lung injury.

by hand in the 1970s and 1980s,[21,22] is still a valuable tool (Fig. 8-13).[24] Box 8-11 explains the procedure for obtaining static P-V curves.

Current ICU ventilators with graphic displays can automatically generate P-V loops and save a reference loop to make comparisons over time. Daily evaluation of the pressure–volume relationship (either static or dynamic) is recommended to track progression of lung and airway changes. (Chapters 10 and 13 contain additional information on P-V curves.)

Figure 8-13 shows changes in the curves that can be associated with patients demonstrating sudden hypoxemia caused by airway problems, lung parenchymal problems, and pulmonary emboli.[22-24] Conditions that affect the airway shift the dynamic curve to the right and flatten it. If neither curve changes position but the patient develops hypoxemia, pulmonary embolus should be suspected. Table 8-3 correlates P-V curve data with clinical findings to aid evaluation of the patient's pulmonary condition.

Figures 9-19 and 9-20 present examples of C_D curves or P-V loops graphed by newer ventilators such as the Hamilton Galileo (Hamilton Medical, Bonaduz, Switzerland), CareFusion Avea (CareFusion Corp, San Diego, Calif.), Puritan Bennett 840 (Covidien-Nellcor and Puritan Bennett, Boulder, Colo.), Dräger Evita XL (Dräger Medical, Inc, Telford, Pa.), and Servo-i (Maquet Inc, Wayne, N.J.) (Key Point 8-8).

Key Point **8-8** Dynamic P-V loops reflect changes in compliance during gas flow. Static P-V loops represent changes in compliance when no gas flow is present.

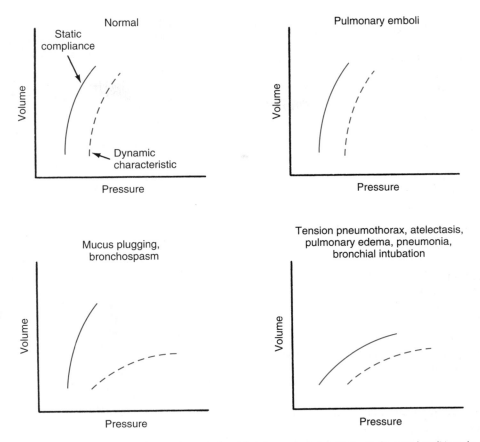

Fig. 8-13 Pressure—volume curves reflecting changes in C$_S$ and C$_D$ during mechanical ventilation. Under normal conditions, the C$_S$ and C$_D$ curves are similar. Because pulmonary emboli do not affect resistance or compliance, neither curve changes with this condition. With mucus plugging or bronchospasm, airway resistance increases, the C$_D$ curve shifts to the right and flattens (more pressure is required), and the C$_S$ curve remains unchanged. With conditions that reduce C$_L$, both curves shift to the right and flatten. (From Bone RC: Monitoring ventilatory mechanics in acute respiratory failure, Respir Care 28:597-603, 1983.)

| TABLE 8-3 | Correlation of Pressure–Volume Curve Data and Clinical Findings to Evaluate Pulmonary Condition | | | | | |

Diagnosis	C$_S$	C$_D$	Chest Radiograph	P$_a$O$_2$	PAOP	Treatment
Pulmonary edema (cardiogenic)	↓	↓	↑ Vascular markings; possible heart size	↓	↑	Diuretics, digitalis, morphine, oxygen
ARDS	↓	↓	Diffuse infiltrate	↓	Normal	PEEP and supportive care
Pneumonia	↓	↓	Consolidation in affected area	↓	Normal	Antibiotics and supportive care
Atelectasis	↓	↓	Collapse of affected area	↓	Normal	Treat cause and give supportive care
Pneumothorax	↓	↓	No vascular markings in affected area	↓	Normal	Chest tube; chest drainage if severe
Bronchospasm	No change	↓	Possible hyperinflation	↓	Normal	Bronchodilator therapy

ARDS, Acute respiratory distress syndrome; *C$_D$,* dynamic compliance; *C$_S$,* static compliance; *P$_a$O$_2$,* arterial oxygen partial pressure; *PAOP,* pulmonary artery occlusion pressure; *PEEP,* positive end-expiratory pressure; ↓, decreased; ↑, increased.

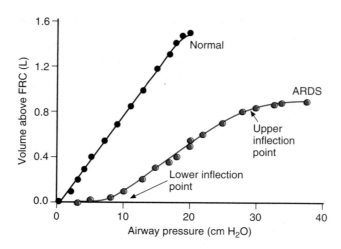

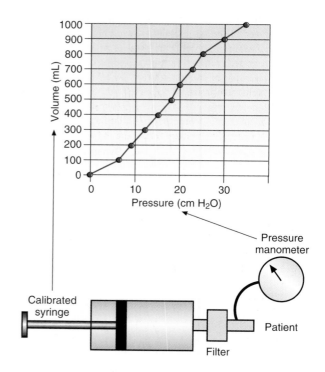

Fig. 8-14 Pressure–volume curves for normal lungs and the lungs of patients with ARDS. Note the lower and upper inflection points on the pressure–volume curve for ARDS. *FRC,* Functional residual capacity. (From Hess DR, MacIntyre NR, Mishoe SC, et al: Respiratory care principles and practice, Philadelphia, 2002, W.B. Saunders.)

Fig. 8-15 Super syringe technique used to measure the P-V curve and an example of a P-V curve produced with this technique. (From Hess DR, MacIntyre NR, Mishoe SC, et al: Respiratory care principles and practice, Philadelphia, 2002, W.B. Saunders.)

Some ventilators, such as the Hamilton G5, can graph a slow dynamic P-V loop using very slow flows and preset PEEP levels. A software program manages the maneuver and draws the resulting graph. Slow P-V loops may have value for establishing inflection points on the curve (see Chapter 13).

Figure 8-14 shows a static P-V curve for a patient with normal lungs and one for a patient with ARDS. The curve for the patient with ARDS has a sigmoid shape (S shape). The lower inflection point marks a significant change in the slope of the curve and may indicate the pressure at which large numbers of alveoli are recruited. The **upper inflection point** indicates a point at which large numbers of alveoli are becoming overinflated. Attempts should be made to ventilate the patient somewhere between these two points.

The value of static P-V curves has been shown to be a useful in patients with ARDS.[24-27] During the procedure, the patient is typically heavily sedated, and short-acting paralytic agents may be required. Lung inflation can be accomplished with the ventilator if it has the appropriate software. Alternatively, lung inflation can be accomplished with a super syringe (i.e., a 1 to 3 L syringe). With the syringe technique, a graduated, super syringe is attached to the ET (Fig. 8-15). Precise volumes of gas (e.g., 100 to 200 mL) are pushed into the lung and held for 2 seconds or long enough to allow measurement of $P_{plateau}$. The pressure is measured after the administration of each volume, and the P-V curve is then plotted manually. It is important to obtain measurements during the slow deflation of the lungs. The **inflection point,** which occurs during deflation (also sometimes called the *deflection point*), represents collapse of a significant number of lung units following full inflation (recruitment) of the lungs. It is worth mentioning that obtaining PV measurements using the syringe technique is generally well tolerated by patients; however, the procedure can cause significant changes in the patient's hemodynamic and oxygenation status. It is therefore prudent to closely monitor the patient during the procedure.[28]

Setting PEEP above the lower inflection point on the deflation part of the loop may help prevent inflated alveoli from collapsing and reexpanding with each breath. Setting the V_T low enough so that PIP remains below the upper inflection point may reduce the risk of ventilator-induced lung injury. Assessment of the clinical data and analysis of the P-V curve can help the clinician both establish the cause of a change in the patient's condition and determine the appropriate treatment (see Chapter 13).

COMMENT SECTION OF THE VENTILATOR FLOW SHEET

The patient-ventilator system check sheet includes a section for comments. The respiratory therapist can use this section to comment on any of the following:

- Patient assessment (e.g., breath sounds, chest wall movement, percussion note, presence of cyanosis, cutaneous perfusion, and level of consciousness)
- Changes in ventilator settings
- Changes in the physician's orders
- Description of any equipment problems

Some medical centers use a separate patient assessment sheet in which subjective findings, objective findings, the assessment, and the treatment plan (SOAP notes) can be summarized.

 SUMMARY

- Before connecting a patient to a mechanical ventilator, the respiratory therapist should verify that the designated ventilator has passed an operational verification procedure (OVP).
- The initial assessment of a patient receiving mechanical ventilation should include evaluation of the patient's physical appearance, vital signs, ABGs, S_pO_2, and ventilator settings (e.g., f, sensitivity, F_IO_2, volumes, and pressures).

- The ventilator flow sheet is a necessary and valuable record of measured and observed patient and ventilator clinical values.
- Volumes, pressures, temperature, vital signs, and F_IO_2 are measured during each patient-ventilator system check.
- Initial assessment of the position of the ET and cuff pressure measurements establishes that the ET is positioned properly and that the cuff pressures have been set correctly.
- Calculation of V_D/V_T, compliance and resistance, and evaluation of P-V curves/loops help determine the baseline condition of the lung mechanics, and can serve as a means to monitor changes.
- Evaluation of the integrity of the ventilator circuit is part of a standard ventilator check. It includes checking for leaks, disconnected tubing, and other circuit problems.
- Visual and auditory alarms are essential components of the patient-ventilator system.

REVIEW QUESTIONS *(See Appendix A for answers.)*

1. Before a ventilator is used, an operational verification check is performed. A simple variation of this procedure is also performed under which of the following circumstances?
   A. Before a blood gas sample is obtained
   B. When the physician's order specifies a change in ventilator settings
   C. Before a patient is reconnected to a ventilator after the ventilator circuit has been changed or disassembled for any reason
   D. Before the patient's hemodynamic status is monitored

2. When should the F_IO_2 be measured with an oxygen analyzer?
   1. At least every 24 hours
   2. Continuously with infants
   3. During suctioning procedures
   4. When static P-V loops are determined
      A. 1 and 2 only
      B. 2 and 3 only
      C. 1 and 4 only
      D. 1, 2, 3, and 4

3. A patient has a P_{TA} of 5 cm H_2O. Three hours later a high-pressure alarm activates. The patient's P_{TA} is now 14 cm H_2O. What is the most likely cause of this change?
   A. Pneumothorax
   B. Deflated ET cuff
   C. Water in the circuit
   D. Secretions in the airway

4. A 36-year-old man with ARDS is ventilated with a V_T of 400 mL. The patient's IBW is 176 lb (80 kg). The HME has a volume of 50 mL. What is an approximate alveolar volume for one breath for this patient?
   A. 350 mL
   B. 260 mL
   C. 270 mL
   D. 190 mL

5. The figure below shows pressure–time and flow–time curves obtained during PC-CMV. What is the $P_{plateau}$?

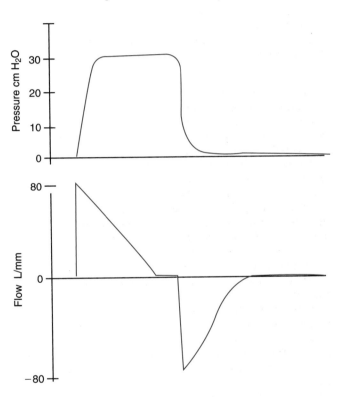

   A. It cannot be determined from this graph
   B. 30 cm H_2O
   C. 30 cm H_2O – Set PEEP
   D. 25 cm H_2O

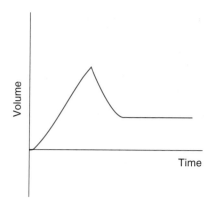

6. Which of the following problems is illustrated in the above figure?
   A. A leak in the patient-ventilator system
   B. Water in the inspiratory line
   C. A set inspiratory pause
   D. Active exhalation

7. A physical examination of the chest is performed on a mechanically ventilated patient. Breath sounds and percussion are normal except over the right middle lobe, where late inspiratory crackles are heard. This area is dull to percussion. A bedside chest radiograph reveals infiltrates in the right middle lobe. Based on these findings alone, which of the following is the most likely problem?
   A. Pneumothorax in the right hemithorax
   B. Congestive heart failure
   C. Right middle lobe pneumonia
   D. Asthma affecting the right side only

8. The following values are obtained from a patient's ventilator flow sheet:

Time	Volume (mL)	PIP (cm H_2O)	$P_{plateau}$ (cm H_2O)
01:00	850	36	33
02:00	850	39	32
03:00	850	43	33

   Which of the following statements about these conditions is correct?
   A. C_L is improving
   B. C_D has not changed
   C. R_{aw} is improving
   D. R_{aw} is getting worse

9. A static P-V curve for C_S and C_D reveals a widening gap between the two curves. What does this probably represent?

10. A patient has an IBW of 150 lb, a V_T of 0.55 L, and an f of 8 breaths/min. What is the estimated alveolar ventilation?

11. While listening with a stethoscope over the trachea during VC-CMV, the respiratory therapist hears a slight leak at the end of inspiration on an orally intubated patient. What change should the therapist make?
   A. Increase cuff pressure until no sound is heard
   B. Check cuff pressure and delivered volume
   C. Check cuff volume
   D. Recommend changing the artificial airway

12. A 215-lb, 6-foot 4-inch-tall man has a size 7 oral ET in place. Cuff pressure is 35 mm Hg. The set V_T is 600 mL (0.6 L), and the delivered V_T is 500 mL (0.5 L). The patient is likely to need

mechanical ventilation for at least a week. What would you recommend?
   A. Increase the set V_T
   B. Reduce the cuff pressure to 20 mm Hg
   C. Change the ET to a size 8
   D. Make no changes at this time

13. The following data were obtained for a patient on PC-CMV:

Time	Set Pressure (cm H_2O)	V_T (mL)
21:00	20	550
23:00	20	575
01:00	20	620

   What do you think is causing the change in V_T and what should the respiratory therapist evaluate?

14. A high-volume/low-pressure cuff has a pressure of 15 mm Hg as measured with a BP manometer technique. The respiratory therapist does not hear a leak when listening over the tracheal area with a stethoscope. What should the respiratory therapist do?
   A. Reevaluate the cuff pressure because this technique is not trustworthy
   B. Increase the cuff pressure to 20 to 25 mm Hg
   C. Maintain the current pressure because this will augment tracheal perfusion
   D. Be concerned about high cuff pressures damaging the airway

15. While changing the tape on the ET, the respiratory therapist accidentally cuts the pilot balloon line. This problem can be corrected by:
   A. Using a stopcock, blunt-tipped needle, and syringe to reinflate the cuff and keep it inflated
   B. Changing the ET
   C. Clamping the pilot line with a hemostat
   D. Increasing the flow on the ventilator

References

1. Campbell RS: Managing the patient-ventilator system: system checks and circuit changes. *Respir Care* 39:227–236, 1994.
2. Kacmarek RM, Stoller JK, Heuer AH, editors: *Egan's fundamentals of respiratory care*, ed 10, St Louis, 2012, Elsevier.
3. Task Force on Guidelines, Society of Critical Care Medicine: Guidelines for standards of care for patients with acute respiratory failure on mechanical ventilatory support. *Crit Care Med* 19:275–278, 1991.
4. Akhtar SR, Weaver J, Pierson DJ, et al: Practice variation in respiratory therapy documentation during mechanical ventilation. *Chest* 124:2275–2282, 2003.
5. Gialanella KM: *Documentation, advance for nurses—Florida*, King of Prussia, Pa., 2004, Motion Publ.
6. Greenwald I, Rosonoke S: Mechanical ventilation: understanding respiratory physiology and the basics of ventilator management. *JEMS* 28:74–86, 2003.
7. Sasse SA, Jaffe MB, Chen PA, et al: Arterial oxygenation time after an F_IO_2 increase in mechanically ventilated patients. *Am J Respir Crit Care Med* 152:148–152, 1995.
8. Blanch L, Bernabé F, Lucangelo U: Measurement of air-trapping, intrinsic positive end-expiratory pressure, and dynamic hyperinflation in mechanically ventilated patients. *Respir Care* 50:110–123, 2005.
9. Hess D, McCurdy S, Simmons M: Compression volume in adult ventilator circuits: a comparison of five disposable circuits and a nondisposable circuit. *Respir Care* 36:1113–1118, 1991.
10. Abramson NS, Wald KS, Grenvik ANA, et al: Adverse occurrences in intensive care units. *JAMA* 244:1582–1584, 1980.
11. Shilling AM, Durbin CG: Airway management devices and advanced cardiac life support. In Cairo JM, editor: *Mosby's respiratory care equipment*, ed 9, St Louis, 2014, Elsevier, pp 113–157.

12. Branson RD, Gomaa D, Rodriquez D: Management of the artificial airway. *Respir Care* 59:974–990, 2014.
13. Hall JL: *Guyton and Hall textbook of physiology*, ed 12, Philadelphia, 2010, Saunders.
14. Bernhard WN, Cottrell JE, Sivakumaran C, et al: Adjustment of intra-cuff pressure to prevent aspiration. *Anesthesiology* 50:363–366, 1979.
15. Blanch PB: Laboratory evaluation of 4 brands of endotracheal tube cuff inflator. *Respir Care* 49:166–173, 2004.
16. Neff TA, Clifford D: A new monitoring tool: the ratio of the tracheostomy tube cuff diameter to the tracheal air column diameter (C/T ratio). *Respir Care* 28:1287–1290, 1983.
17. Davies JD, May RA, Bortner PL: Airway management. In Hess DR, MacIntyre NR, Mishoe SC, editors: *Respiratory care principles and practices*, ed 2, Sudbury, Mass., 2012, Jones and Bartlett Learning, pp 376–418.
18. Hess DR: Managing the artificial airway. *Respir Care* 44:759–772, 1999.
19. Tinkoff G, Bakow ED, Smith RW: A continuous flow apparatus for temporary inflation of damaged endotracheal tube cuffs. *Respir Care* 31:423–426, 1990.
20. Kearl RA, Hooper RG: Massive airway leaks: an analysis of the role of endotracheal tubes. *Crit Care Med* 21:518–521, 1993.
21. Fleming WH, Bowen JC, Petty C: The use of pulmonary compliance as a guide to respiratory therapy. *Surg Gynecol Obstet* 134:291–292, 1972.
22. Bone RC: Diagnosis of causes for acute respiratory distress by pressure-volume curves. *Chest* 70:740–746, 1976.
23. Bone RC: Pressure-volume measurements in detection of bronchospasm and mucous plugging in acute respiratory failure. *Respir Care* 21:620–626, 1976.
24. Bigatello LM, Davignon KR, Stelfox HG: Respiratory mechanics and ventilator waveforms in the patient with acute lung injury. *Respir Care* 50:235–245, 2005.
25. Jamil SM, Spragg RG: Acute lung injury: Acute respiratory distress syndrome. In Papadakos PK, Lachmann B, editors: *Mechanical ventilation: clinical applications and pathophysiology*, Philadelphia, 2008, Saunders-Elsevier, pp 28–41.
26. Harris RS, Hess DR, Venegas JG: An objective analysis of the pressure-volume curve in the acute respiratory distress syndrome. *Am J Respir Crit Care Med* 161:432–439, 2000.
27. Amato MB, Barbas CSV, Medeiros DM, et al: Effect of a protective ventilation strategy on mortality in the acute respiratory distress syndrome. *N Engl J Med* 338:347–354, 1998.
28. Lee WL, Stewart TE, MacDonald R, et al: Safety of pressure-volume curve measurement in acute lung injury and ARDS using a syringe technique. *Chest* 121:16595–16601, 2002.

CHAPTER 9

Ventilator Graphics

TERRY L. FORRETTE, MHS, RRT, FAARC

OUTLINE

Relationship of Flow, Pressure, Volume, and Time
A Closer Look at Scalars, Curves, and Loops
Scalars
Comparison of Pressure-Controlled Ventilation and
Volume-Controlled Ventilation
Determining the Mode of Ventilation
Components of the Pressure–Volume Loop
Components of the Flow–Volume Loop
Summary: Normal Scalars, Loops, and Curves
Using Graphics to Monitor Pulmonary Mechanics

Assessing Patient-Ventilator Asynchrony
Advanced Applications
Auto-PEEP and Air Trapping
Titrating PEEP
APRV Settings
Integrated Ventilator and Esophageal Graphics
Assessing Overdistension During Pressure-Controlled Ventilation
Inspiratory Rise Time Control: Sloping or Ramping
Flow Cycling During Pressure Support Ventilation
Summary

KEY TERMS

- Asynchrony
- Hysteresis
- Scalar

LEARNING OBJECTIVES *On completion of this chapter, the reader will be able to do the following:*

1. Identify ventilator variables (e.g., the target variable and trigger variable) and ventilator parameters and their values (e.g., peak inspiratory pressure and plateau pressure) using pressure, flow, and volume scalars generated using various modes of mechanical ventilation.
2. Identify ventilator variables and ventilator parameters and their values from flow–volume and pressure–volume loops.
3. Use ventilator scalars and loops to detect changes in lung compliance and airway resistance, inappropriate sensitivity settings, inadequate inspiratory flow, auto-positive end-expiratory pressure (auto-PEEP), leaks in the ventilator circuit, active exhalation during pressure support ventilation, and an inspiratory pressure overshoot during pressure support ventilation.

4. Describe how changes in airway resistance and lung compliance affect scalars and loops during volume-targeted and pressure-targeted ventilation when airway resistance increases and lung compliances decreases.
5. Recognize periods of patient-ventilator asynchrony using scalars and loops.
6. Determine the presence of auto-PEEP using ventilator graphics.
7. Explain the phases of ventilation during airway pressure release ventilation (APRV) using pressure and flow scalars.
8. Describe the relationship between airway and esophageal pressure changes using ventilator graphics.

Modern mechanical ventilators (e.g., Dräger v500 [Dräger Medical Inc., Telford, Pa.], CareFusion AVEA [CareFusion, Viasys Corp, San Diego, Calif.], Maquet Servo-i [Maquet Inc. Wayne, N.J.], Puritan Bennett 840 [Covidien-Nellcor and Puritan Bennett, Boulder, Colo.], and Hamilton G5 [Hamilton Medical, Bonzduz, Switzerland]) incorporate graphic displays into their ventilator interfaces to provide instantaneous displays of pressure, flow and volume. These graphic displays allow clinicians to obtain real-time measurements of the patient-ventilator interaction, which can provide insight into a patient's mechanics of breathing. As such, ventilator graphics offer valuable information for clinicians making adjustments to ventilator settings.[3,4]

Becoming proficient in the use of ventilator graphics typically requires dedicated time and practice. Once this skill is mastered, however, it can greatly enhance a clinician's ability to assess patient-ventilator interactions and improve patient care. Indeed, ventilator graphics can alert the clinician to abnormalities even before clinical signs are obvious, and provide a graphic record of the pathophysiologic changes that can lead to patient-ventilator **asynchrony** and respiratory distress.

Proprietary software programs offered by the ventilator manufacturers allow for flow, pressure, and volume measurements to be displayed as different types of waveforms. The term *scalar* is used to specify the flow, pressure, and volume waveforms that are graphed relative to time (i.e., pressure, flow, and volume scalars).[5]

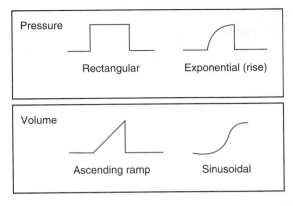

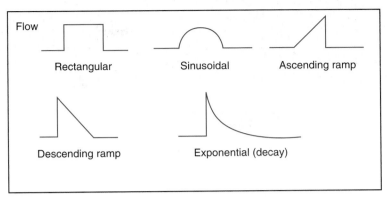

Fig. 9-1 Examples of waveforms for pressure, volume, and flow. Pressure waveforms usually are the rectangular or rising exponential *(similar to an ascending ramp)* type. Volume waveforms usually are the ascending ramp or sinusoidal type. Flow waveforms can take various forms; the rectangular, ramp *(ascending or descending)*, sinusoidal, and decaying exponential waveforms are seen most often.

BOX **9-1**	**Six Basic Curves (Waveforms)**

Rectangular (often called the square wave or constant waveform)
Descending ramp (also called a decelerating ramp)
Ascending ramp (also called an accelerating ramp)
Sinusoidal (often called the sine wave; only one-half or part of this wave is present)
Rising exponential
Decaying exponential

Basically, six shapes (waveforms) are produced with scalars during mechanical ventilation (Fig. 9-1 and Box 9-1).[5-7] The term *loop* is used to describe a graph of two variables plotted on the *x* and *y* coordinates, such as pressure–volume and flow–volume loops (these are discussed later in the chapter).

RELATIONSHIP OF FLOW, PRESSURE, VOLUME, AND TIME

Flow, pressure, volume, and time must be determined to produce the various waveforms and loops. The following principles explain the basic interrelationship of volume, pressure, flow, and time as they are used to create a waveform display:

1. The flow of gas into the lungs depends on the difference between the pressure from the power source (the ventilator) and the pressure inside the lungs. The greater the pressure gradient, the higher the flow of gas, and the faster the lungs fill. Flow is measured as a volume change per unit of time, where time is the inspiratory time (Flow = V/T_I).
2. The amount of pressure (ΔP) required to inflate the lungs depends on the patient's lung compliance and airway resistance. If the lungs are very compliant and easy to inflate, relatively low pressures are required. If the lungs are very stiff (low compliance), considerably higher pressures are required to inflate them ($\Delta P = \Delta V/C_L$). For airway resistance, the most important factor affecting the degree of resistance is the diameter of the airways (or more specifically the radius according to Poiseuille's law). Airway resistance decreases as the diameter of the airway increases, resulting in an increased flow. Conversely airway resistance increases as the diameter of the airway is reduced causing a decreased flow (Key Point 9-1). Note that the ventilator's microprocessor can calculate both compliance and resistance using the measured data.
3. The volume (V) delivered depends on the amount of flow and the inspiratory time (T_I) (V = Flow $\times$ T_I).

> **Key Point** **9-1** The amount of pressure (ΔP) required to inflate the lungs depends on the patient's lung compliance and airway resistance.

A CLOSER LOOK AT SCALARS, CURVES, AND LOOPS

Scalars

Figure 9-2 shows a typical set of scalars for volume-controlled continuous mandatory ventilation (VC-CMV). Note the directional arrows indicating the movement of flow into the lungs and the corresponding rise in airway pressure and resulting delivered volume. Also, notice that flow rises to its peak value and remains constant throughout inspiration.

Figure 9-3 presents a closer look at a flow scalar. At point *A*, the inspiratory valve opens allowing gas flow into the lungs. Keep in mind that this is also the point where expiration ends. Flow rises quickly to point *B*, which is the peak inspiratory flow set on the control panel of the ventilator. What is the inspiratory flow setting in this example? At point *C*, inspiratory flow delivery stops. Has an inspiratory pause been set on the ventilator? What is the length of T_I? What is the flow during the pause period?

In this example, as the expiratory valve opens at point *D*, gas leaves the patient and the ventilator circuit and passes through the ventilator's expiratory valve. Flow during exhalation is graphed below the baseline, as specified by the software program. Look at the expiratory flow curve. What is the peak expiratory flow rate (PEFR)?*

Continue to follow the expiratory flow curve. Note that at point *E*, expiratory flow ends; however, the total expiratory time (TE)

---

*PEFR is 80 L/min. (Even though the graph indicates minus [−] 80 L/min, the value is read without the minus sign.)

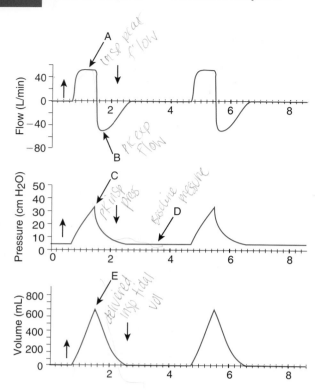

Fig. 9-2 Time-triggered, constant flow, volume-targeted ventilation (VC-CMV). **A,** Peak inspiratory flow; **B,** peak expiratory flow; **C,** peak inspiratory pressure; **D,** baseline pressure; **E,** delivered inspiratory tidal volume. (Modified from Hess DR, MacIntyre NR, Mishoe SC, et al: Respiratory care principles and practice, Philadelphia 2002, WB Saunders.)

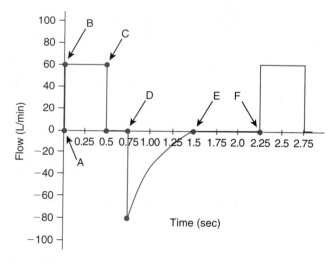

Fig. 9-3 Flow–time graph showing inspiration and expiration during volume ventilation with a constant flow. (See text for explanation.)

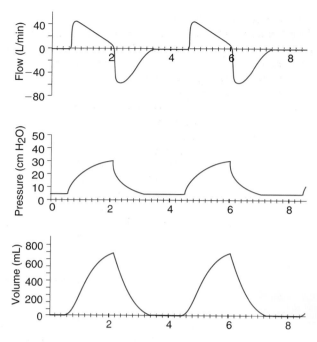

Fig. 9-4 Time-triggered, descending-flow, volume-targeted ventilation (VC-CMV). (Modified from Hess DR, MacIntyre NR, Mishoe SC, et al: Respiratory care principles and practice, Philadelphia 2002, Saunders.)

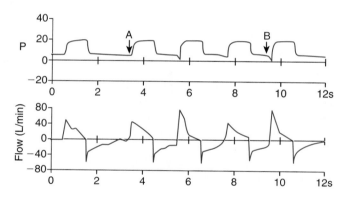

Fig. 9-5 Pressure and flow scalars for time-triggered **(A)** and patient-triggered **(B)** breaths.

lasts from point *D* to point *F,* and the TE continues until the next inspiration begins (point *F*). How long is TE? How much of TE is represented by a period of no gas flow?*

Figure 9-4 shows a VC-CMV breath but notice that the flow pattern has been set to decelerating pattern. Can you explain why

this would not be representative of a pressure-controlled continuous mandatory ventilation (PC-CMV) breath? (Hint, look at the contour of the pressure scalar.)

Scalars can also be used to identify how a ventilator breath is initiated (i.e., time- or patient-triggered). In Fig. 9-5 arrow *A* indicates a time-triggered breath and arrow *B* shows a patient-triggered breath. Notice that for breath B there is a slight drop in baseline pressure indicating a patient effort. Can you determine if this is a PC or VC breath? (Hint: Look at the flow scalar.) Additional information about PC versus VC breaths is presented in the following section on the comparison of pressure-controlled ventilation and volume-controlled ventilation.

As described in Chapter 5, intermittent mandatory ventilation (IMV) is a mode of ventilation that allows spontaneous breaths interspersed with mandatory breaths. Figure 9-6 shows an example

---

*T_E = 1.5 seconds. 1.5 to 2.25 seconds (0.75-second total) is the interval during exhalation when no more gas leaves the patient.

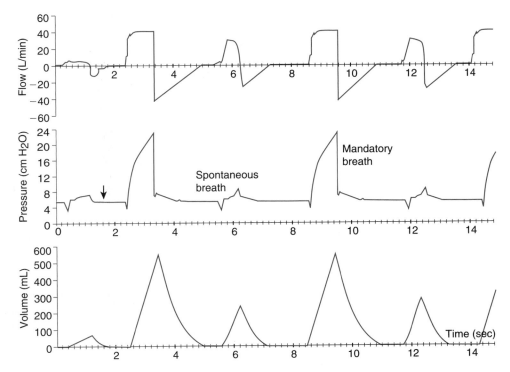

Fig 9-6 Volume-controlled intermittent mandatory ventilation (VC-IMV) plus continuous positive airway pressure/positive end-expiratory pressure (CPAP)/PEEP. (See text for explanation.) (From Hess DR, MacIntyre NR, Mishoe SC, et al: Respiratory care principles and practice, Philadelphia 2002, WB Saunders.)

of a VC-IMV breath. Notice the minimal rise in pressure and tidal volume for each spontaneous breath and the contour difference in flow, pressure, and volume between the mandatory and spontaneous breaths. The elevated baseline pressure (see *arrow* on the pressure scalar) indicates that the patient is receiving PEEP.

During PC-CMV, the flow and pressure patterns differ from those of VC-CMV breaths. As shown in Fig. 9-7, the flow pattern for PC-CMV is decelerating with a constant *(square)* pressure pattern. PC-CMV breaths always generate a decelerating flow pattern whereas the flow pattern for VC-CMV can be changed from square to decelerating. Notice also the change in peak flow that occurs with changes in patient demand during PC-CMV *(dashed line)*.

Mandatory pressure-targeted breaths can also be delivered with PC-IMV as shown in Fig. 9-8. Compare the difference in the flow and pressure scalars for the mandatory breaths and spontaneous breaths in this graphic to those in Fig. 9-6. The spontaneous breaths have a flow and pressure pattern typically associated with a pressure-targeted breath and are representative of a pressure support (PS) breath.

Comparison of Pressure-Controlled Ventilation and Volume-Controlled Ventilation

When pressure and volume breaths are compared, the pressure and flow curves demonstrate the most distinct differences. Volume-controlled ventilation with constant flow produces a rectangular flow curve, which can be changed by selecting a different flow waveform.

During pressure-controlled ventilation the flow waveform is a descending curve that varies with both lung characteristics and

patient flow demand; it therefore is referred to as a *continuously variable decelerating waveform* (Key Point 9-2).

During volume-controlled ventilation, the pressure scalar resembles an ascending ramp, or a *rising exponential curve*. During pressure-controlled ventilation, it is rectangular, assuming T_I is long enough. (See section on monitoring pulmonary mechanics for additional information.)

> **Key Point 9-2** Volume-controlled ventilation with constant flow produces a rectangular flow curve, which can be changed by selecting a different flow waveform. During pressure-controlled ventilation the flow waveform is a descending curve that varies with both lung characteristics and patient flow demand.

Determining the Mode of Ventilation

Scalars can also be used to identify the mode of ventilation being used. By carefully examining the pressure and flow scalars, it is possible to determine whether mandatory, spontaneous, or IMV is being used. Figure 9-9 illustrates the flow, pressure, and volume scalars for mandatory and spontaneous breaths during IMV. Figure 9-10 also demonstrates flow, pressure, and volume scalars during IMV; however, careful examination of the spontaneous breaths shows that the spontaneous breaths are not being pressure supported. (Case Study 9-1 provides an example illustrating how ventilator graphic can be used to identify the mode of ventilation being used.)

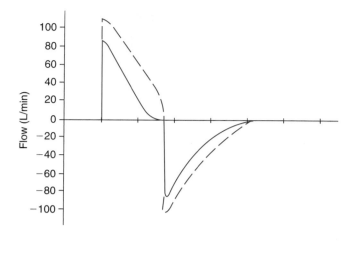

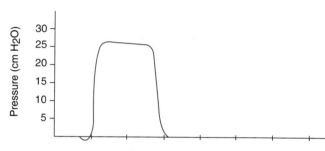

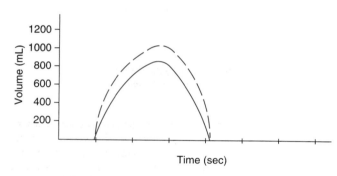

Time (sec)

Fig. 9-7 Flow, pressure and volume. Scalars seen during pressure-controlled continuous mandatory ventilation (PC-CMV).

 Case Study 9-1

A patient is switched from PC-CMV to PC-IMV to promote respiratory muscle activity. Initially the patient does not exhibit a spontaneous breathing frequency but spontaneous efforts are subsequently noted on ventilator graphics (See Figure 9-11). Notice that the two different breath types can be easily distinguishable by analyzing the pressure and flow scalars.

Components of the Pressure–Volume Loop

Pressure–volume (P-V) loops can be used to monitor changes in lung compliance (C = ΔV/ΔP) and airway resistance. Figure 9-12 shows a typical P-V loop generated during a positive pressure

breath. This breath is time-triggered by the ventilator rather than patient-triggered. It is important to recognize that the P-V loop is drawn in a counterclockwise direction when a ventilator breath is delivered. Notice also that the inspiratory and expiratory curves are not perfect arcs. The maximum pressure shown on the x axis is the peak inspiratory pressure (PIP), and the maximum volume reached on the y axis is the tidal volume (V_T).

Figure 9-13 provides additional information regarding pressure gradients that can be determined using a P-V loop. The *solid line* of the loop in Fig. 9-13 represents pressure at the airway opening (P_awo) during a V_T. The *dashed line* represents the static P-V line, which reflects the alveolar pressure (P_alv) under no-flow conditions. The transairway pressure (P_TA), or flow-resistive pressure, is the difference between the P_alv and P_awo. P_TA is represented by a *double-headed arrow* in this figure. See if you can determine the values for PIP, V_T, P_TA, and peak P_alv for the P-V loop shown in Fig. 9-13.

Spontaneous Breaths and Pressure–Volume Loops

The clinician can learn to distinguish mandatory breaths from spontaneous breaths by observing the way the P-V loop is generated during breath delivery. When a patient makes a spontaneous inspiration, the P-V loop tracks in a clockwise fashion (see Fig. 9-14). This is the reverse of a positive pressure breath, which creates a counterclockwise tracing (as shown in Fig. 9-12).

Now look at Fig. 9-15, which shows the P-V loop for a patient-triggered mandatory breath. When the patient breathes in spontaneously, the curve moves to the left *(clockwise)*, reflecting the patient's effort. As the positive pressure from the ventilator is triggered, the curve crosses to the right and is traced in a counterclockwise fashion, which indicates that the machine is doing the work.

Components of the Flow–Volume Loop

Figure 9-16 illustrates a typical flow–volume (F-V) loop recorded during a positive pressure breath. Inspiratory flow appears above the baseline and expiratory flow is below the baseline. (NOTE: This is the reverse of the way F-V loops are usually reported for spirometry obtained during a standard laboratory pulmonary function test.) PEFR is the highest value on the expiratory flow curve. What is the PEFR in Fig. 9-16? What type of flow waveform is the ventilator delivering? What is the set inspiratory flow?*

Summary: Normal Scalars, Loops, and Curves

As you can see in the previous discussion, with the diagnostic use of scalars, P-V, and F-V loops, several key points should be reiterated:

- Scalars can be used to identify the phases and characteristics of mechanical ventilatory breaths including PIP, PEEP, peak flow, expiratory flow, and patient-triggered and time-triggered breaths.
- The contour of the flow pattern identifies the type of preset flow for volume-controlled breaths and when viewed with the pressure pattern, volume-controlled breaths can be differentiated from pressure-controlled breaths.
- In addition to identifying the breath type, scalars are useful in identifying the mode of ventilation.
- P-V curves can be an effective method to monitor pulmonary compliance and airways resistance.

*PERF is approximately 70 LPM, flow pattern is square, and inspiratory flow is approximately 55 LPM.

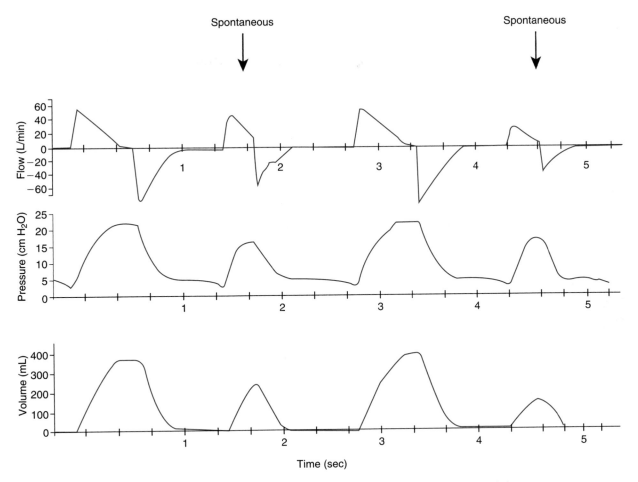

Fig. 9-8 Pressure, flow, and volume scalars for pressure-controlled intermittent mandatory ventilation (PC-IMV) plus pressure support and continuous positive airway pressure (CPAP). Arrows indicate spontaneous breaths. (See text for further information.)

- F-V loops can be a useful way to show the PEFR and inspiratory flow.

USING GRAPHICS TO MONITOR PULMONARY MECHANICS

Most intensive care unit (ICU) ventilators have the capability of measuring and displaying digital calculations of pulmonary compliance and airways resistance. Figure 9-17 illustrates the flow, pressure, and volume scalars obtained during an inspiratory pause with a patient on VC-CMV.

Look first at the inspiratory portion of the pressure–time curve. Notice that the baseline pressure is 5 cm H_2O, indicating that 5 cm H_2O of PEEP is being used. (It is important to recognize that although the baseline pressure is positive, the flow and volume curves start from a zero baseline and end at a zero baseline.) Now observe the flow scalar during the inspiratory pause. Compare the flow and volume scalars at the same moment in time. Notice that when no flow occurs, there is no volume delivery. The volume curve also looks as if it has a pause, or plateau (Key Point 9-3).

Key Point **9-3** When flow drops to zero at the end of inspiration, an inspiratory pause is present. When flow is zero, the pressure gradient between the ventilator and the patient's lungs is the same.

P-V loops can also be used to assess changes in pulmonary mechanics. In Fig. 9-18, line *AB* (peak P_{alv}) represents the pressure–volume relationship of the normal lung under static *(no-flow)* conditions, that is, it is the P_{alv} during static conditions. *C* represents the elastic component of the lungs and chest wall (Fig. 9-18). Triangle *ABE* represents the amount of mechanical work required to overcome the elastic resistance of the lungs and chest wall. For a given amount of pressure applied to the lungs, a certain volume results. When flow is present, the direct *(straight-line)* relationship no longer exists; rather, as seen in previous P-V loops, the line curves during inspiration and expiration.

A certain amount of pressure is required during inhalation (see curve *ACB* in Fig. 9-18) and exhalation (curve *BDA*) to overcome the resistance of the airways and the tissues. These curves represent the nonelastic *(frictional)* forces opposing ventilation. Force *(pressure)* is applied to the lung by the action of the ventilator, but a slight lag time elapses before the volume actually increases. The area between curves *ACB (the inspiratory curve)* and *ADB (the expiratory curve)* is the result of **hysteresis** (Box 9-2). For any given lung volume, the elastic recoil in the lungs is less during exhalation than during inhalation.

The total mechanical work of breathing (WOB) is the sum of triangle *ABE* and curve *ACB*. Recall from physics that work equals force times distance. (In respiratory physiology, force is expressed as pressure and distance is expressed as volume.) In the lungs this

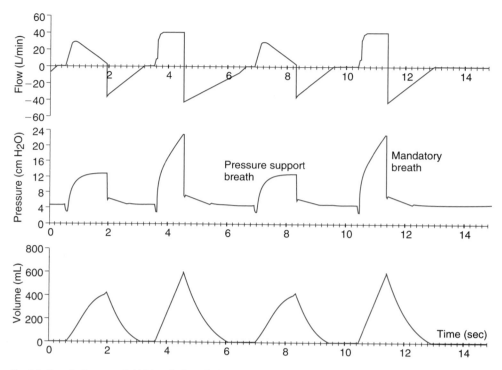

Fig. 9-9 Flow *(top),* pressure *(middle),* and volume *(bottom)* scalars during volume-controlled intermittent mandatory ventilation (VC-IMV) with pressure support ventilation PSV and continuous positive airway pressure (CPAP). (From Hess DR, MacIntyre NR, Mishoe SC, et al: Respiratory care principles and practice, Philadelphia, 2002, WB Saunders.)

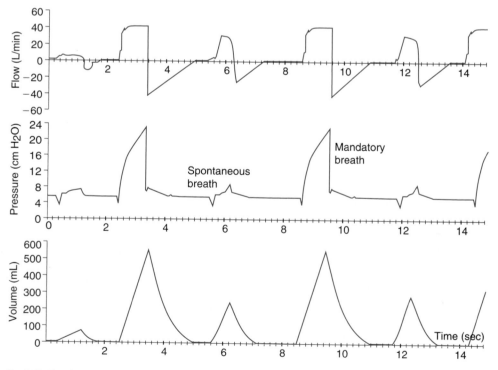

Fig. 9-10 Flow *(top),* pressure *(middle),* and volume *(bottom)* scalars during volume-controlled intermittent mandatory ventilation (VC-IMV) plus continuous positive airway pressure/positive end-expiratory pressure (CPAP/PEEP). (See text for explanation.) (From Hess DR, MacIntyre NR, Mishoe SC, et al: Respiratory care principles and practice, Philadelphia, 2002, WB Saunders.)

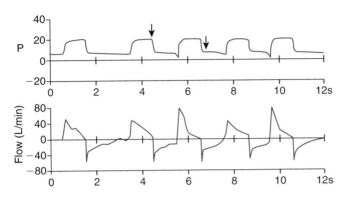

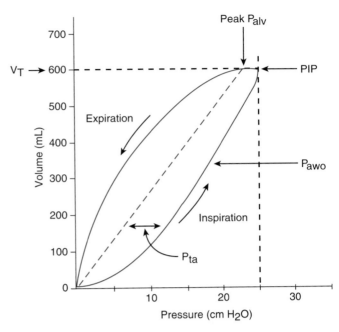

Fig. 9-11 Ventilator graphic of a patient receiving pressure-controlled continuous mandatory ventilation (PC-CMV). The arrows point to patient-triggered breaths, while the other breaths shown are time-triggered. Notice also the difference in the flow scalar for the patient-triggered breaths. In pressure-controlled breaths flow and tidal volume (V_T) are dependent on patient effort.

Fig. 9-13 P-V loop showing the peak inspiratory pressure (PIP), pressure at the airway opening (P_{awo}), alveolar pressure (P_{alv}), and transairway pressure (P_{TA}). (See text for additional information.)

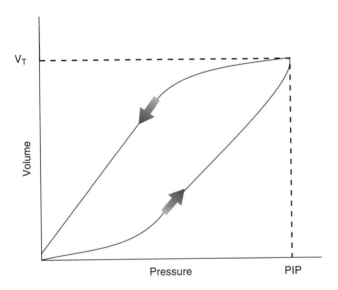

Fig. 9-12 Typical pressure–volume loop for a positive pressure breath. The loop represents the pressure and volume measured at the upper airway opening (P_{awo}). The highest point for tidal volume (V_T [*vertical axis*]) and peak inspiratory pressure (PIP [*horizontal axis*]) represents the dynamic compliance for that pressure–volume relationship.

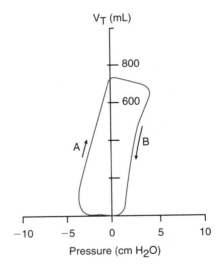

Fig. 9-14 Pressure–volume loop recorded during a spontaneous, unsupported breath. No continuous positive airway pressure (CPAP) or pressure support ventilation (PSV) is delivered. *Arrow A* indicates inspiration, and *arrow B* indicates expiration. (Modified from Puritan Bennett: Waveforms: the graphical presentation of ventilator data, Form AA-1594 [2/91], Pleasanton, Calif., Puritan Bennett Tyco, 1991.)

> **BOX 9-2   Hysteresis**
>
> *Hysteresis* can be thought of as a lagging of one of two associated phenomena; that is, two associated phenomena fail to coincide or occur simultaneously. An example of hysteresis is the difference between the inspiratory and expiratory curves in a pressure–volume loop for the lungs as shown in Fig. 9-13.

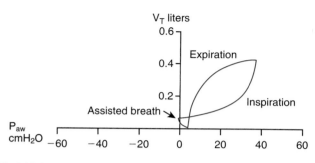

Fig. 9-15 Pressure–volume loop for a patient-triggered breath during pressure-controlled continuous mandatory ventilation (PC-CMV). Notice that part of the curve moves to the left of the y axis, reflecting a drop in pressure during inspiration **(pressure value becomes negative)**; the curve traces to the right of the y axis as the ventilator delivers a positive pressure breath **(pressure value becomes positive).**

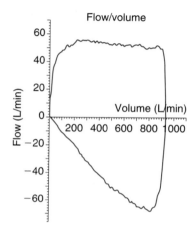

Fig. 9-16 Normal F-V loop during volume-controlled ventilation. The inspiratory curve is on the top, and the expiratory curve is on the bottom. Note the linear change in expiratory flow from peak to end expiration. Also, the end-expiratory flow is zero. (From Kacmarek RM, Hess D, Stoller JK: Monitoring in respiratory care, St Louis, 1993, Mosby.)

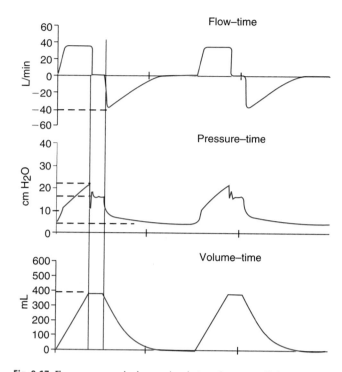

Fig. 9-17 Flow, pressure, and volume scalars during volume-controlled continuous mandatory ventilation (VC-CMV) with constant flow and an inspiratory pause. (See text for explanation.)

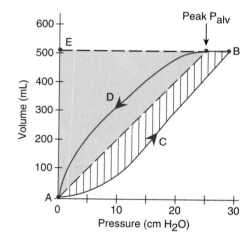

Fig. 9-18 P-V loop for a normal lung. Line *AB* represents compliance or the pressure–volume relation of the lung under static **(no flow)** conditions. Curve *ACB* is inspiration. Curve *BDA* is expiration. Blue shaded area *ABE* denotes work to overcome the elastic resistance of the lungs alone. Cross-hatched area *ACB* represents work performed to overcome nonelastic air flow resistance during inspiration. Area *ABD* represents airflow resistance during exhalation. The sum of the latter two areas represents the resistive work of breathing in one breath. Note that work is not performed during a normal exhalation. P_A, Alveolar pressure. (Modified from Dupuis Y: Ventilators: theory and clinical application, ed 2, St Louis, 1992, Mosby.)

translates to WOB, which approximately equals the pressure required to ventilate the lungs times the volume the lungs accumulate (WOB = P × V). The inspiratory work resulting from airway resistance (R_{aw}) and partly from tissue resistance is curve *ACB*. The expiratory work is represented by curve *ADB*. Chapter 10 provides more information on the monitoring of WOB; it also reviews the pressure–time product and the use of transdiaphragmatic pressure monitoring as a technique for estimating WOB.[25]

During positive pressure ventilation for less compliant (stiffer) lungs, greater pressure is required to achieve a given volume. The P-V loop therefore tends to flatten (Fig. 9-19).[1] Examples of lung conditions demonstrating reduced compliance include fibrotic diseases of the lung and conditions that flood the alveoli with fluids (e.g., pulmonary edema, pneumonia, and acute respiratory distress syndrome [ARDS]). Reduced compliance also is seen in conditions in which the alveoli are deflated (e.g., atelectasis). It is important to understand that as compliance decreases, airway pressure increases, but volume delivery remains constant during volume-targeted ventilation.

When compared to volume-targeted ventilation, lung volume decreases, while pressure remains at the preset level during a pressure-targeted breath as compliance changes (Fig. 9-20).

Pressure–volume curves can also reflect changes in airways resistance. Notice in the P-V curve in Fig. 9-18, the dashed line

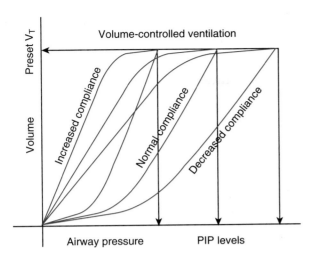

Fig. 9-19 Changes in the P-V loop during volume-targeted ventilation as lung compliance changes. Volume delivery remains constant, but peak inspiratory pressure (PIP) changes. (From Dhand R: Ventilator graphics and respiratory mechanics in the patient with obstructive lung disease, Respir Care 50:246-261, 2005.)

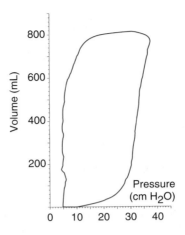

Fig. 9-21 Airway P-V loop recorded in a patient with chronic obstructive pulmonary disease (COPD) during controlled ventilation. Note the increased nonelastic inspiratory and expiratory work *(widening of the loop)* and the shift of the dynamic compliance curve *(P-V loop)* upward and to the left. (From Kacmarek RM, Hess D, Stoller JK: Monitoring in respiratory care, St Louis, 1993, Mosby.)

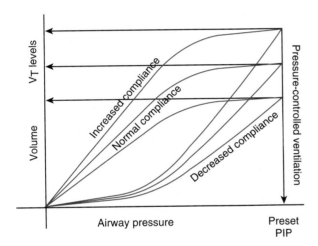

Fig. 9-20 P-V loops during pressure ventilation. As compliance changes, volume delivery changes, but pressure delivery remains constant. (From Dhand R: Ventilator graphics and respiratory mechanics in the patient with obstructive lung disease, Respir Care 50:246-261, 2005.)

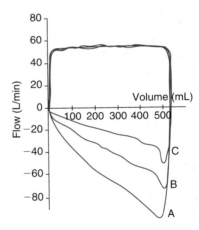

Fig. 9-22 F-V loops showing volume-targeted breaths with a constant flow but changing airway resistance *(compliance constant)*. Loop *A* shows a normal R_{aw}. Loops *B* and *C* represent progressively increasing R_{aw}. Note the drop in expiratory flow and peak expiratory flow rate (PEFR) as airway resistance increases.

dividing the curve into an inspiratory and expiratory component. The width of each component reflects the resistive forces during the respective phase of ventilation. Now compare the width of the P-V curve shown in Fig. 9-21 to that of a P-V curve with normal resistance (see Fig. 9-18). Note how the width of the curve increases, while the compliance *(slope of the isoflow line)* remains normal.

Flow–volume loops are routinely used in a pulmonary function laboratory to assess changes in airways resistance. Figure 9-22 illustrates one of the most valuable uses of the F-V loop, evaluating R_{aw}. Loop *A* in Fig. 9-22 reflects normal R_{aw} during volume ventilation with a constant flow and a normal compliance. Loops *B* and *C* show the effects of increasing R_{aw}. The inspiratory F-V curve is not significantly affected because the ventilator is set to deliver a constant flow (50 L/min) and volume (about 530 mL). However, PEFR progressively decreases as R_{aw} increases.

A reduction in PEFR is most often associated with airway obstruction (e.g., secretions and bronchospasm). Figure 9-23 shows examples of F-V curves that would be obtained in patients with increased airway resistance, such as in a patient with chronic obstructive pulmonary disease (COPD). Note the scooped-out appearance of the expiratory curve.

The F-V loops are helpful for evaluating a patient's response to bronchodilator therapy. Figure 9-24 shows two flow–volume loops that reflect a patient's response to an aerosol treatment with a β-adrenergic agent (e.g., albuterol). Note the improvement in expiratory flow. In the inner loop, a high expiratory flow can be seen at the start of expiration; this spike in flow is an artifact that reflects the release of gas trapped in the patient circuit during inspiration. The clinician can confirm this finding clinically by noting whether the corrugated tubing of the patient circuit "exhales" at the start of expiration.

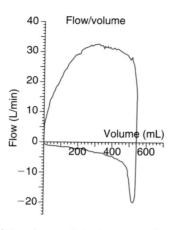

Fig. 9-23 F-V loop during volume ventilation in a patient with chronic obstructive pulmonary disease (COPD). Note the diminished peak expiratory flow and the scooped-out *(concave)* shape of the expiratory F-V curve. (NOTE: The flow scale is 0 to 30 L/min during inspiration and 0 to −20 L/min during exhalation.) The clinician must make sure to check the scale when reading graphs. Inspiration *(top)* and expiration *(bottom)*. (From Kacmarek RM, Hess D, Stoller JK: Monitoring in respiratory care, St Louis, 1993, Mosby.)

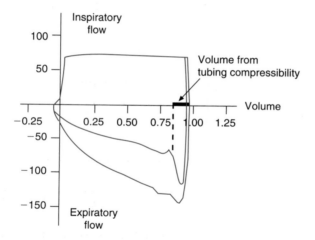

Fig. 9-24 Two F-V loops produced during volume ventilation *(constant flow waveform)*. The inner loop indicates increased airway resistance. The outer loop represents the patient's response to bronchodilator therapy. Note the improvement in expiratory flow. (NOTE: The high expiratory flow spike in the lower right corner of the inner loop results from gas decompression of the patient circuit. The initial expiratory flow spike is an artifact and represents release of the volume of gas trapped in the patient circuit at the beginning of the breath.) (Redrawn from Nilsestuen JO, Hargett K: Managing the patient-ventilator system using graphic analysis: an overview and introduction to Graphics Corner, Respir Care 41:1105-1122, 1996.)

ASSESSING PATIENT-VENTILATOR ASYNCHRONY

Patient-ventilator asynchrony has been identified as one of the major issues in the management of ventilated patients. As discussed in Chapter 17, asynchrony can be simply defined as a mismatching between the patient's ventilatory drive and the response of the ventilator (Key Point 9-4). One type of asynchrony may occur at the onset of breath when the ventilator either delivers a premature breath or fails to recognize a patient effort.

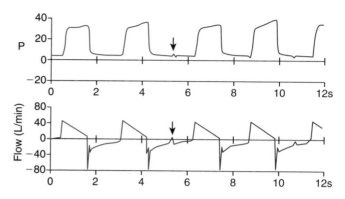

Fig. 9-25 Ventilator graphic demonstrating trigger asynchrony. Notice that the arrows point to a change in baseline pressure and flow without a response from the ventilator. This situation is often seen if the ventilator's sensitivity is set to low.

These situations are often referred to as trigger asynchrony (Fig. 9-25).

> **Key Point** **9-4** Asynchrony occurs when the neural ventilatory demands of the patient are not recognized by the ventilation.

Trigger asynchrony can also be assessed using a P-V loop. Figure 9-26, *A* shows how the patient's inspiratory effort results in a considerable reduction in pressure below the PEEP level creating the characteristic "fish tail" appearance. In Fig. 9-26, *B* trigger sensitivity has been adjusted resulting in an improved trigger synchrony.

In Fig. 9-27, the arrows are pointing at a premature initiating of a breath independent of time or patient effort. This is often referred to as "autotriggering" and may be caused by too sensitive a trigger setting or a leak in the patient-ventilator circuit. A convenient method to differentiate an inappropriately set trigger sensitivity resulting in autotriggering from a leak is to observe the P-V and F-V tracings as shown in Fig. 9-28, *A* and *B*.

Asynchrony can also occur when inspiratory flow from the ventilator does not match the patient's demands (i.e., flow asynchrony), or when the patient wants inspiration to end but the ventilator fails to cycle to exhalation (i.e., cycle asynchrony). Flow asynchrony can occur when the set flow rate, as in volume control ventilation, is insufficient to meet the patient's inspiratory demands. Notice the deflection *(arrows)* in the pressure scalar mid-way through inspiration, which creates an M-shaped pressure pattern associated with flow asynchrony (Fig. 9-29, *A*). Remedies for flow asynchrony may include increasing the set flow in volume-targeted ventilation, changing to a pressure-targeted breath, switching to hybrid breath type such as volume control plus (VC+), pressure-regulated volume control (PRVC), or autoflow (AF). Figure 9-29, *B* illustrates the flow scalar changes that occur when the patient was switched to VC+. Notice how the delivered flow rate changes between the first and second breath in response to patient demand and flow asynchrony is avoided (see Fig. 9-29, *B*).

Failure to cycle or termination asynchrony often results in an inappropriate set inspiratory time during a mandatory breath or an incorrect flow termination level on a spontaneous breath. Figure 9-30 is an example of cycle asynchrony. The arrow points to rise in PIP at the end of inspiration created by the patient actively exhaling to end inspiration.

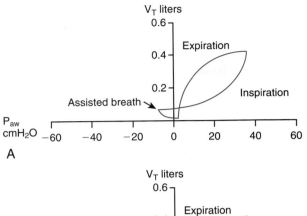

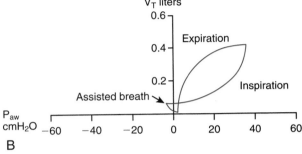

Fig. 9-26 Pressure–volume loops illustrating trigger asynchrony. (A) Deflection below the set level of PEEP indicating increased patient effort to trigger a breath (B) Trigger sensitivity has been adjusted resulting a minimal effort to initiate the breath.

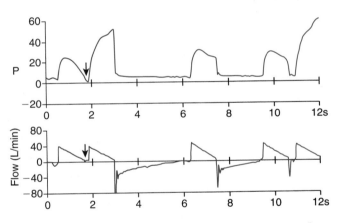

Fig. 9-27 Pressure and flow scalars showing the effects of "autotriggering."

ADVANCED APPLICATIONS

Auto-PEEP and Air Trapping

Auto-PEEP, sometime referred to as intrinsic PEEP or airtrapping, occurs when the patient does not complete exhalation prior to the onset of the next breath. Chapter 17 discussed the causes, occurrence, and remedy in detail. Figure 9-31 indicates pressure and flow scalars for a patient demonstrating auto-PEEP.

AutoPEEP initially can be observed on a P-V curve (Fig. 9-32, A) and F-V loop (Fig. 9-32, B). The characteristic finding is the appearance of an incomplete exhalation with the expiratory portion

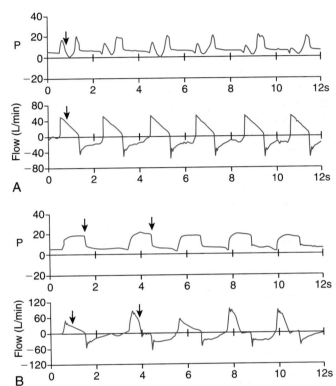

Fig. 9-29 **A,** Pressure and flow scalars demonstrating flow asynchrony. **B,** After the patient was switched to volume control plus (VC+) the contour of the pressure pattern becomes stable *(first breath)*. Notice how the delivered flow rate changes between the first and second breath in response to patient demand and flow asynchrony is avoided.

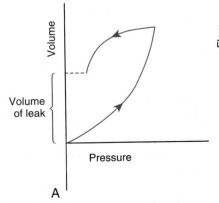

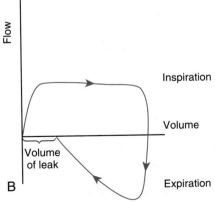

Fig. 9-28 Pressure–volume loop **(A)** and flow–volume loop **(B)** indicating an air leak.

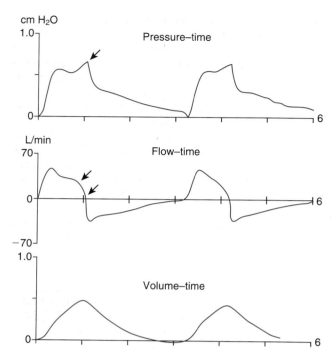

Fig. 9-30 Pressure, flow, and volume scalars illustrating a patient receiving 5 cm H_2O of pressure support. The patient's neural timing precedes the end of the mechanical inflation and results in a pressure spike *(large arrow)* on the pressure waveform. Note the rapid decline in the inspiratory flow waveform at the end of inspiration *(double arrows)* as a result of the patient's active exhalation. (From Nilsestuen JO, Hargett KD: Using ventilator graphics to identify patient-ventilator asynchrony, Respir Care 50:202-234, 2005.)

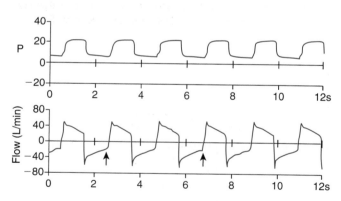

Fig. 9-31 Pressure and flow scalars demonstrating auto-PEEP. The arrows on the flow scalar show how flow does not return to baseline prior to the beginning of the next breath.

of the loop not returning to baseline *(arrow)*. It is interesting to note that an air leak would look similar to auto-PEEP.

Titrating PEEP

There are several methods that can be used to correctly set PEEP including observing changes in P-V loops as PEEP levels are changed. As previously discussed, the slope of the isoflow line reflects lung-thorax compliance (Key Point 9-4 and Fig. 9-20). As shown in Fig. 9-33, the slope of loop *A* is less than loop *B*, indicating that *B* represents a more compliant lung-thorax unit. Careful

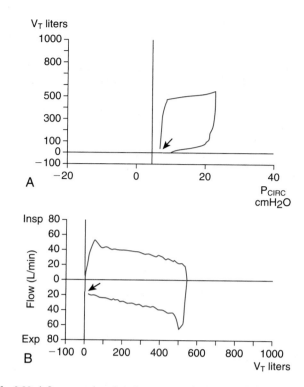

Fig. 9-32 A. Pressure–volume loop demonstrating the presence of auto-PEEP. B. Flow–volume loop demonstrating the presence of auto-PEEP. Notice that the expiratory portion of the P-V loop and the F-V loop does not return to baseline.

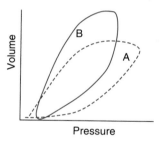

Fig. 9-33 Pressure–volume loops showing the effects of increasing levels of applied PEEP on lung-thorax compliance.

examination of these two curves shows that the curve *B* has a higher baseline (PEEP) level than curve *A* demonstrating that the application of a higher PEEP level results in improved compliance.

APRV Settings

Airway pressure release ventilation (APRV) is often used as lung recruitment mode of ventilation. One of the unique features of this mode is the inversing of high-pressure time to that of low pressure. Graphics can be useful in determining the setting of high pressure and low pressure times to create a period of static flow (see Chapter 23). Additionally this mode, by design, is often configured to generate auto-PEEP (Fig. 9-34).

Upper and lower inflection points can be used to determine the high and low PEEP settings in APRV. Figure 9-35 provides an example of how the upper and lower inflections points affect the pressure scalar and P-V loop for during APRV.

Integrated Ventilator and Esophageal Graphics

Several ventilators provide an auxiliary pressure monitoring port that can be connected to an esophageal catheter. Esophageal pressure measurements may be employed to determine transpulmonary pressure (P_{TP}), which then can be used to set plateau and PEEP pressures. Additionally, esophageal manometry is often used in conjunction with scalars to further identify patient-ventilator asynchrony as shown in Fig. 9-36.

Assessing Overdistension During Pressure-Controlled Ventilation

Determining the appropriate amount of pressure to use with PC-CMV or PC-IMV can often be a challenging procedure. Although tidal volume delivery should be a primary criterion when

setting the rise in pressure above baseline (PC+PEEP), often a secondary criterion can be used to avoid overdistension of the lung. Figure 9-37 illustrates how ventilator graphics can be used to set ventilation parameters. Just as graphics can be used to set baseline pressures, they also can aid in determining the appropriate pressure level when a pressure-controlled breath is delivered. Notice in Fig. 9-37 how at the end of inspiration the P-V loop flattens out creating a pressure overshoot sometimes referred to as a "bird beak." Compare the tidal volume delivery at 15 cm H_2O of pressure to that of 18, and notice that there is very little difference between the two pressure levels. When ventilating a premature infant, keeping the peak pressures at a minimum is critical. In this case the PC level could be dropped to 15 with little effect on tidal volume delivery.

Figure 9-38 was obtained from an adult patient receiving PC-CMV. Again notice the pressure overshoot creating a "bird

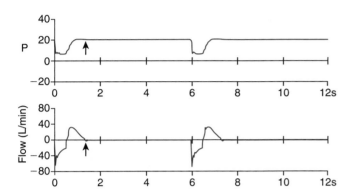

Fig. 9-34 Pressure and flow scalars for a patient receiving airway pressure release ventilation (APRV). Note the extended high-pressure time, short low-pressure period, and resulting auto-PEEP. The arrows are pointed to the period of constant pressure with zero flow. This period is believed to promote recruitment of low compliant alveolar units.

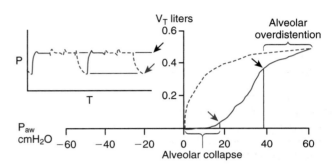

Fig. 9-35 Ventilator graphics illustrating how the upper and lower inflections points for an airway pressure release ventilation (APRV) breath would appear for a pressure scalar and a P-V loop (Settings for APRV are often established by institutional protocol or through waveform analysis. See Chapter 23 for a detailed discussion on APRV).

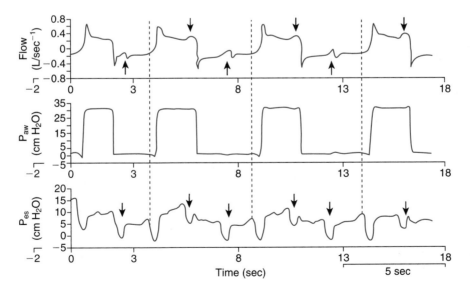

Fig. 9-36 Flow, air pressure (P_{aw}), and esophageal pressure (P_{es}) in a patient with chronic obstructive pulmonary disease (COPD) during PSV. *Dotted lines* indicate the beginning of an inspiratory effort that triggers ventilator gas flow. *Black arrows* in the P_{es} curve indicate patient efforts that did not trigger ventilatory flow. Note the time delay between the beginning of the effort and ventilator triggering. Ineffective efforts occur during both mechanical inspiration and expiration. During inspiration, the *flow scalar* can be used to identify ineffective patient efforts and a rise in the inspiratory flow. During expiration, ineffective efforts are identified by *open arrows* showing a small convex shape in the flow curve. Note how no apparent change occurs in P_{aw}. (From Kondili E, Prinianakis G, Georgopoulos D: New concepts in respiratory function. Br J Anaesthesiol 91:106-119, 2003.)

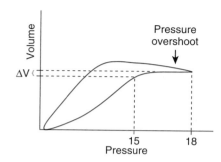

Fig. 9-37 Pressure–volume loop showing the effects of overdistension of the lung during pressure-controlled intermittent mandatory ventilation (PC-IMV).

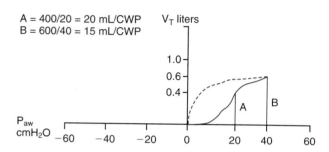

Fig. 9-38 Pressure–volume loop showing the effects of overdistension of the lung during pressure-controlled intermittent mandatory ventilation (PC-IMV). Point *A* indicates the pressure at which tidal volume delivery is optimized in terms of pressure. Point *B* represents the peak inspiratory pressure.

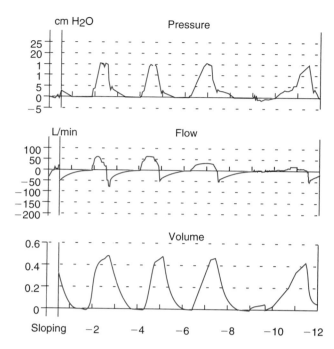

Fig. 9-39 Changes in the gas delivery system produced by adjusting the pressure slope, or rise time function, during pressure-targeted ventilation. (See text for additional information.) (Redrawn from Nilsestuen JO, Hargett K: Managing the patient-ventilator system using graphic analysis: an overview and introduction to Graphics Corner, Respir Care 41:1105-1122, 1996.)

beak" appearance on the P-V loop. Point *B* represents the peak inspiratory pressure and Point *A* indicates the pressure at which tidal volume delivery is optimized in terms of pressure. Note the difference in lung compliance between the two pressure levels indicating that pulmonary mechanics would be optimized at 20 cm H_2O of ventilating pressure.

Inspiratory Rise Time Control: Sloping or Ramping

A pressure breath produces a high flow at the beginning of inspiration. With small diameter ETs (i.e., increased R_{aw}), the high flow through the narrow opening creates turbulence. As a result, a pressure overshoot can occur at the beginning of the pressure curve before the pressure adjusts to the set value.

If the flow and pressure delivery are tapered at the start of inspiration, the waveform can be adjusted to reduce this overshoot. Most current acute care ventilators have a function that can taper the flow during pressure ventilation. When tapering is used, the pressure curve may no longer be constant but may be tapered at the beginning of the breath.

Inspiratory flow delivery during PC-CMV can therefore be adjusted with an inspiratory rise time control, also called a *slope control* (Fig. 9-39).

Flow Cycling During Pressure Support Ventilation

The normal flow-cycling mechanism of pressure support ventilation (PSV) was discussed in Chapters 3 and 5. Flow cycling occurs when the ventilator detects a decreasing flow, which represents the end of inspiration. The ventilator's software determines the point at which flow cycling occurs; in most ventilators this point is a percentage of the peak flow measured during inspiration.

Unfortunately, no single flow cycle percentage is ideal for all patients. Patients with COPD or increased R_{aw} have a slower flow rate drop-off during inspiration with pressure ventilation than do patients with normal R_{aw}. Because flow does not drop normally, patients with COPD are more comfortable with a higher flow cycle percentage (e.g., 40%). The clinician can determine the appropriate cycling criterion by evaluating the P-T curve during PVS. If an active rise in pressure occurs at end inspiration, the flow cycle percentage may be increased to reduce the amount of expiratory work the patient must perform.

The graphics in Fig. 9-40 show two flow cycle percentages. What is the peak flow in *A*? What is the flow value where inspiratory flow ends? What is the approximate flow cycle percentage?* What is the peak flow in *B*? What is the flow value where inspiratory flow ends? What is the approximate flow cycle percentage in *B*?[†]

 Case Study 9-2

A patient receiving PC-CMV demonstrates auto-PEEP on several breaths on the flow scalar (see *arrow* in Fig. 9-41, *A*). The therapist recommends a change in the inspiratory time setting to increase expiratory time. After 5 minutes on the new settings the following flow scalar was seen (see Fig. 9-41, *B*). Note that the expiratory flow now reaches the zero (*see arrow*) prior to the onset of the next breath.

---

*The peak flow is about 30 L/min, and the cycle occurs at about 5 L/min. The percentage cycle is 5/30 or 17%.

[†]In B, the peak flow is about 35 L/min, and the cycle occurs at about 20 L/min. The percentage cycle in B is 20/35 or 57%.

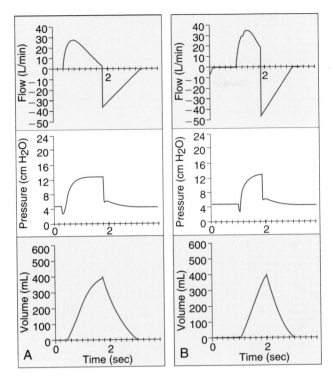

Fig. 9-40 Effect of changes in termination flow during PSV. **A,** A low percentage flow cycle is set so that inspiratory time (T$_I$) is longer. **B,** A higher percentage flow cycle is set so that T$_I$ is shorter. (See text for additional explanation.) (From Hess DR, MacIntyre NR, Mishoe SC, et al: Respiratory care principles and practice, Philadelphia, 2002, WB Saunders.)

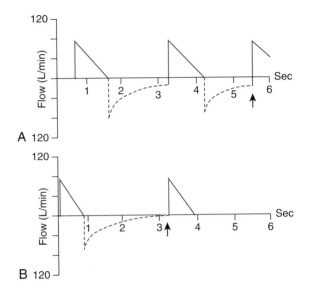

Fig. 9-41 Flow scalars for a patient showing the presence of auto-PEEP during pressure-controlled continuous mandatory ventilation (PC-CMV). See text for more details.

![SUMMARY]

- Modern microprocessor ventilators provide graphic waveforms, including flow, volume, and pressure scalars, and pressure–volume and flow–volume loops.
- Ventilator graphics can be used to monitor ventilator function, to evaluate a patient's response to the ventilator, and to help the clinician adjust ventilator settings.
- It is important to comprehend how the ventilator measures, computes, and displays various parameters. Clinicians also must study actual ventilator graphics to fully understand the usefulness of this application.
- The scalars most often displayed on the ventilator screen are P$_{awo}$, flow, and V.

- Pressure and flow scalars can provide an effective tool for identifying the PIP, PEFR, and the presence of leaks in the patient circuit and auto-PEEP during VC-CMV.
- The flow waveform during volume-targeted ventilation may be set as rectangular or descending, whereas it is by default a descending waveform in pressure-targeted ventilation.
- The pressure waveform varies with changes in static lung compliance C$_S$ and R$_{aw}$ during volume-targeted ventilation. During pressure-targeted ventilation, changes in C$_S$ and R$_{aw}$ will affect the flow and volume waveforms.
- As lung characteristics deteriorate, the pressure delivered to a patient during PVS remains constant but the delivered volume may decrease.
- Pressure–volume loops can alert the clinician to changes in a patient's lung compliance, airway resistance, and work of breathing.
- Pressure and flow scalars are useful to detect patient-ventilator asynchrony.
- Flow–volume loops allow the clinician to evaluate a patient's response to bronchodilator therapy during mechanical ventilation. These loops can also be used to detect leaks and auto-PEEP.

REVIEW QUESTIONS *(See Appendix A for answers.)*

1. Refer to the scalars for pressure, flow, and volume in pressure support ventilation (PSV) in the figure below to answer the following questions.
   A. What caused the pressure spike indicated by arrow *A* on the pressure–time waveform?
   B. What ventilator parameter might be adjusted to eliminate this problem?
   C. What caused the flow waveform during exhalation indicated by arrow *B?*
   D. What parameters might be adjusted on the ventilator to eliminate this problem?
   E. What pulmonary change is suggested by the exhalation volume waveform indicated by arrow *C?*
   F. Is the flow cycle percentage set at a high or low percentage of peak flow?
   G. Is there any indication of inadequate inspiratory flow?

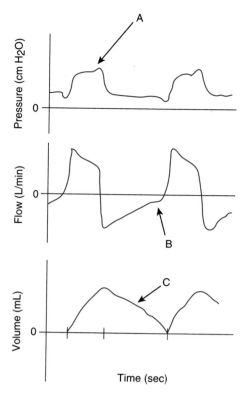

Pressure, flow, and volume scalars for PSV (see Review Question 1).

2. Use the scalars for a specific mode of ventilation in the figure below, *A*, to answer the following questions.
A. What target variable is illustrated?
B. What is the set pressure?

C. What is the delivered V_T?
D. What is the $P_{plateau}$?
E. What problem is indicated by the volume–time curve?

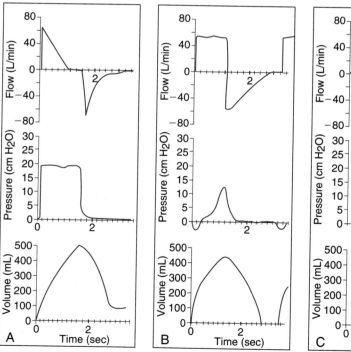
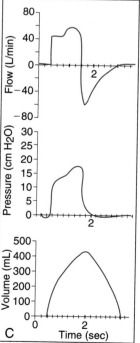

Flow, pressure, and volume scalars for three different ventilation situations (see Review Questions 2 through 4).

3. The scalars in the figure in Question 1, *B,* are for a different mode of ventilation from that in the figure in Question 2, *A.* Use the scalars in part *B* to answer the following questions.
  A. What is the target variable illustrated and how do you determine the mode?
  B. What is the total cycle time?
  C. Is the breath patient-triggered or time-triggered?
  D. What problem is indicated by the pressure scalar?

4. Answer the following questions with regard to the scalars for VC-CMV shown in the figure in Question 2, *C.*
  A. What is the set flow?
  B. Why is the flow delivery variable during inspiration?
  C. What causes the change in flow delivery and how does this affect volume delivery?

5. Answer the following questions using the figure below.
  A. What is the PIP?
  B. What is the approximate delivered V_T?
  C. Has a PEEP been set?
  D. What is the compliance?
  E. What is the approximate P_{TA} during inspiration as indicated by the double-headed arrow? Is this normal?
  F. From the appearance of this P-V loop, what do you think is the patient's primary problem?

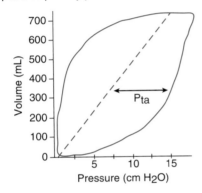

P-V loop (see Review Question 5).

6. Answer the following questions using the figure below.
  A. What is the target variable in this figure?
  B. What is the flow setting and flow waveform?
  C. What is the V_T delivery?
  D. What causes the artifact indicated by arrow *A?*
  E. What does arrow *B* indicate?
  F. What might be the cause of this patient's pulmonary problem?

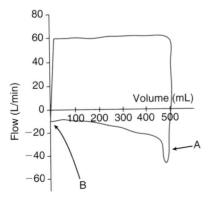

F-V loop (see Review Question 6).

7. A ventilator is set for volume-targeted ventilation, constant flow, and control mode. What will happen to the PIP, $P_{plateau}$, T_I, and V_T if lung compliance (C_L) decreases? (Assume that the pressure limit is not reached.)

8. A ventilator is set for pressure-targeted ventilation, patient triggering, and time cycling. What will happen to the set pressure, T_I, and V_T if C_L increases? (Assume that the pressure limit is not reached.)

9. A patient receiving pressure ventilation has a C_L of 15 mL/cm H_2O (0.015 L/cm H_2O). The pressure is set at 35 cm H_2O. The ventilator is time cycled at 2 seconds. Flow drops to zero before the end of inspiration.
  A. What will the P_{alv} be?
  B. What is an estimated volume delivery?
  C. C_L changes to 30 mL/cm H_2O with improvement in the patient's lung condition. What will happen to the flow and volume delivery?
  D. How would you change volume delivery to return it to its previous value?

10. What type of asynchrony is show in the figures below?

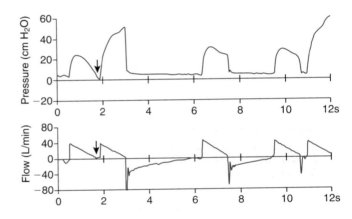

  A. Flow asynchrony
  B. Trigger asynchrony
  C. Termination asynchrony
  D. Cycle asynchrony

11. What would be your suggestion to resolve the problem shown in Question 10?
  A. Increase PEEP
  B. Reduce inspiratory time
  C. Adjust trigger sensitivity
  D. Use a variable flow breath type.

References

1. Benditt JO: Esophageal and gastric pressure measurements. *Respir Care* 50:68–75, 2005.
2. Branson RD: Enhanced capabilities of current ICU ventilators: do they really benefit patients? *Respir Care* 36:362–376, 1991.
3. Branson R: Understanding and implementing advances in ventilator capabilities. *Curr Opin Crit Care* 10:23–32, 2004.
4. Brochard L, LeNouche, F: Pressure support ventilation. In Tobin MJ, editor: *Principles and practices of mechanical ventilation,* ed 2, New York, 2006, McGraw-Hill.
5. Cairo JM: *Mosby's respiratory care equipment,* ed 9, St Louis, 2014, Elsevier.
6. Chatburn RL: Classification of mechanical ventilators. *Respir Care* 37:1009–1025, 1992.
7. Chatburn RL: A new system for understanding mechanical ventilators. *Respir Care* 36:1123–1155, 1991.

8. Croci M, Pelosi P, Chiumello D, et al: Regulation of pressurization rate reduces inspiratory effort during pressure support ventilation: a bench study. *Respir Care* 41:880–884, 1996.

9. Dhand R: Ventilator graphics and respiratory mechanics in the patient with obstructive lung disease. *Respir Care* 50:246–261, 2005.

10. Du HL, Ohtsuji M, Shigeta M, et al: Expiratory asynchrony in proportional assist. *Am J Respir Crit Care Med* 165:972–977, 2002.

11. Durbin CG: Applied respiratory physiology: use of ventilator waveforms and mechanics in the management of critically ill patients. *Respir Care* 50:287–293, 2005.

12. Harris RS, Hess DR, Venegas JG: An objective analysis of the pressure-volume curve in the acute respiratory distress syndrome. *Am J Respir Crit Care Med* 161:432–439, 2000.

13. Hess DR: Mechanical ventilation strategies: what's new and what's worth keeping? *Respir Care* 47:1007–1017, 2002.

14. Hess DR, Branson RD: Mechanical ventilation. In Hess DR, MacIntyre NR, Mishoe SC, et al, editors: *Respiratory care principles and practice*, ed 2, Sudbury, Mass., 2012, Jones and Bartlett.

15. Kacmarek RM, Hess D, Stoller JK: *Monitoring in respiratory care*, St Louis, 1993, Mosby, 1993.

16. Kondili E, Prinianakis G, Georgopoulos D: New concepts in respiratory function. *Br J Anaesthesiol* 91:106–119, 2003.

17. Lucangelo U, Bernabé F, Blanch L: Respiratory mechanics derived from signals in the ventilator circuit. *Respir Care* 50:55–65, 2005.

18. Nilsestuen JO, Hargett K: Managing the patient-ventilator system using graphic analysis: an overview and introduction to Graphics Corner. *Respir Care* 41:1105–1122, 1996.

19. Nilsestuen JO, Hargett KD: Using ventilator graphics to identify patient-ventilator asynchrony. *Respir Care* 50:202–234, 2005.

20. Rodriguez PO, Bonelli I, Setten M, et al: Transpulmonary Pressure and Gas Exchange During Decremental PEEP Titration in Pulmonary ARDS Patients. *Respir Care* 58(5):754–763, 2013.

21. Sanborn WG: Monitoring respiratory mechanics during mechanical ventilation: where do the signals come from? *Respir Care* 50:28–52, 2005.

22. Sassoon CSH, Mahutte CK: What you need to know about the ventilator in weaning. *Respir Care* 40:249–256, 1995.

23. Waugh JB, Deshpande VM, Brown MK, et al: *Rapid interpretation of ventilator waveforms*, ed 2, Upper Saddle River, NJ, 2007, Prentice Hall.

24. Yamada Y, Du HL: Effects of different pressure support termination on patient-ventilator synchrony. *Respir Care* 43:1048–1057, 1998.

25. Henning RJ, Shubin H, Weil MH: The measurement of the work of breathing for the clinical assessment of ventilator dependence. *Crit Care Med* 5:264, 1977.

Assessment of Respiratory Function

KEY TERMS

- Capnography
- Fractional hemoglobin saturation
- Functional hemoglobin saturation
- Indirect calorimetry
- Pulse oximetry
- Qualitative
- Quantitative
- Transcutaneous monitoring

LEARNING OBJECTIVES *On completion of this chapter, the reader will be able to do the following:*

1. Describe the principle of operation of the pulse oximeter.
2. Identify physiological and technical factors that can influence the accuracy of pulse oximetry readings.
3. Describe how various clinical conditions can affect CO-oximetry, oxygen saturation (S_aO_2) and pulse oximetry, oxyhemoglobin saturation (S_pO_2).
4. Discuss the normal components of a capnogram.
5. Give examples of pathophysiological conditions that can alter the contour of the capnogram.
6. Discuss how arterial-to-end-tidal partial pressure of carbon dioxide ($P_{(a-et)}CO_2$) is affected by changes in ventilation-perfusion relationships.
7. Discuss how volumetric CO_2 tracings can be used to assess gas exchange during mechanical ventilation.
8. Describe how exhaled nitric oxide measurements can be used in the management of patients with asthma.
9. Explain the theory of operation of transcutaneous PO_2 and PCO_2 monitors and list the clinical data that should be recorded when making transcutaneous measurements.
10. Provide the respiratory quotient (RQ) value associated with substrate utilization patterns in normal, healthy subjects.
11. Discuss some clinical applications of metabolic monitoring in critically ill patients.
12. Briefly describe devices that are used to measure airway pressures, volumes, and flows during mechanical ventilation.
13. Calculate mean airway pressure, dynamic compliance, static compliance, and airway resistance.
14. Identify pathologic conditions that alter lung compliance and airway resistance and measurements of the work of breathing.
15. Define the pressure–time product, and discuss its application in the management of mechanically ventilated patients.

Procedures and devices, such as pulse oximetry, capnography (capnometry), transcutaneous monitoring of blood gases, exhaled nitric oxide (NO), indirect calorimetry, and bedside lung function testing have made it possible for respiratory therapists to monitor respiratory function noninvasively in mechanically ventilated patients. When it is used appropriately, noninvasive monitoring can provide valuable information for clinicians managing patients receiving ventilatory support. However, if it is used indiscriminately, it can be distracting and confusing for the clinician and economically costly for the patient.

Noninvasive Measurements of Blood Gases

PULSE OXIMETRY

Hypoxemic events in mechanically ventilated patients are most often associated with apnea, airway obstruction, equipment failure or disconnection, and incorrect gas flow settings. Visual recognition of hypoxemia by physical examination is often unreliable because of intraobserver variability, differences in patients' skin pigmentation, and interference by ambient lighting.[1,2] Laboratory measurement of arterial blood gases (ABGs) remains the gold standard for measuring the level of hypoxemia (see Evolve website for a review of ABGs); however, this procedure is performed intermittently and may fail to detect transient hypoxic episodes.

Pulse oximetry provides continuous, noninvasive measurements of arterial oxygen saturation.[3] A sensor is placed over a digit, an earlobe, the forehead, or the bridge of the nose; this sensor measures the absorption of selected wavelengths of light beamed through the tissue (Fig. 10-1). For example, oxyhemoglobin can be differentiated from deoxygenated hemoglobin by shining two wavelengths of light (660 and 940 nm) through the sampling site.

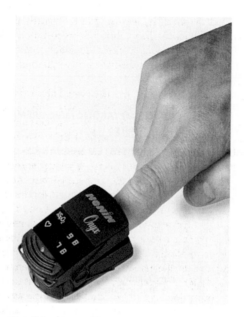

Fig. 10-1 Pulse oximeter. (Courtesy Nonin Medical, Plymouth, Minn.)

As Fig. 10-2 illustrates, at a wavelength of 660 nm (red light), deoxygenated hemoglobin absorbs more light than oxyhemoglobin. Conversely, oxyhemoglobin absorbs more light at 940 nm (infrared light [IR]) than does deoxygenated hemoglobin.

Pulse rate is determined by relating cyclical changes in light transmission through the sampling site with blood volume changes that occur during ventricular systole and diastole. That is, as local (e.g., finger, toe, or earlobe) blood volume increases during ventricular systole, light absorbency increases and transmitted light decreases. In contrast, as blood volume decreases during diastole, absorbency decreases, and transmitted light increases. Figure 10-3 illustrates the pulsatile or alternating current (AC) and nonpulsatile or direct current (DC) components of a typical pulse oximetry signal.

The percentage of oxyhemoglobin present can be determined by first calculating the ratio of absorbencies for pulsatile and nonpulsatile flow, at the two specified wavelengths, or

$$Red/Infrared = Pulsatile_{660\,nm}/Nonpulsatile_{660\,nm}$$
$$\div Pulsatile_{940\,nm}/Nonpulsatile_{940\,nm}$$

This ratio is then applied to an algorithm that relates ratios of these two absorbencies to oxyhemoglobin saturation.[4]

Physiological and Technical Concerns

Pulse oximeters generally are accurate for oxygen saturations greater than 80%.[5,6] Pulse oximeter saturations less than 80% should be confirmed with laboratory analysis of ABGs, including CO-oximetry.[7,8] A number of physiological and technical factors can influence the accuracy of pulse oximetry measurements, including low perfusion states, the presence of dysfunctional hemoglobins and dyes, variations in patients' skin pigmentation, and ambient light interference. The following is a summary of various factors that can influence pulse oximetry readings. A more detailed discussion of each of these factors can be found in the references listed at the end of this chapter.

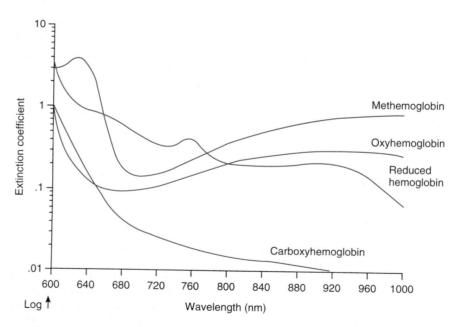

Fig. 10-2 Absorption characteristics of four types of hemoglobin: reduced hemoglobin, oxyhemoglobin, carboxyhemoglobin, and methemoglobin.

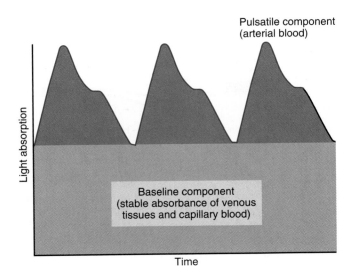

Fig. 10-3 Output signal generated by pulse oximeter illustrating pulsatile and nonpulsatile components. Saturation is based on the ratio of light absorption during pulsatile and baseline phases. (From Kacmarek RM, Stoller JK, Heurer AJ, editors: Egan's fundamentals of respiratory care, ed 10, St Louis, 2013, Elsevier.)

Low Perfusion States

It should be apparent that the accuracy of a pulse oximeter reading is dependent on the identification of an arterial pulse. In cases where perfusion is low, such as hypovolemia, the pulse oximeter may not be able to accurately identify a pulsatile signal, resulting in either an intermittent or absent S_pO_2 reading. Other situations that may contribute to this problem include administering peripheral vasoconstrictors, hypothermia, and heart–lung bypass (i.e., extracorporeal membrane oxygenation).[9] Although some oximeters are better than others in dealing with low perfusion states, compensation for the weak signal associated with low perfusion states is limited. The reason for this limitation is that a low perfusion state produces a low signal-to-noise ratio and, thus, a signal that can potentially be altered by motion artifacts.

The Masimo Signal Extraction Technology (SET) (Masimo Corp, Irvine, Calif.) pulse oximeter is a relatively new processing system that uses special algorithms to minimize interference from motion artifacts. Conventional pulse oximetry assumes that arterial blood accounts for the pulsations or AC component of the pulse oximetry signal, while venous blood produces a nonpulsatile or DC component of the signal. During patient motion, the venous blood may also contribute to the pulsatile signal and cause the pulse oximeter to underestimate the S_pO_2 because it cannot distinguish between the arterial and venous blood. Masimo SET signal processing identifies the venous blood signal, isolates it, and using adaptive filters, cancels the noise and extracts the arterial signal. When tested on healthy individuals simulating various motion artifacts, the Masimo SET oximeter exhibited a much lower error rate compared with conventional pulse oximeters. Studies with critically ill patients also demonstrated fewer false alarms of hypoxemia when compared to conventional pulse oximeters.[10]

Dysfunctional Hemoglobins and Dyes

Adult blood typically contains four types of hemoglobin: reduced or deoxygenated hemoglobin (HHb), oxyhemoglobin (O_2Hb), carboxyhemoglobin (COHb), and methemoglobin (MetHb). Two terms that are often used when describing oxyhemoglobin

saturation are fractional and functional saturations. **Fractional hemoglobin saturation** is calculated by dividing the amount of oxyhemoglobin measured by the sum of concentrations of all four types of hemoglobin present, or

$$Fractional\ O_2Hb = O_2Hb/[HHb + O_2Hb + COHb + MetHb]$$

Functional hemoglobin saturation is calculated by dividing the oxyhemoglobin concentration by the concentration of hemoglobin capable of carrying oxygen, or

$$Functional\ O_2Hb = O_2Hb/[HHb + O_2Hb]$$

Laboratory CO-oximeters measure all four types of hemoglobin by using separate wavelengths of light to identify each species, whereas pulse oximeters use only two wavelengths to quantify the amount of O_2Hb and HHb present. Laboratory CO-oximeters are therefore capable of reporting fractional oxyhemoglobin saturations, and pulse oximeters are typically described as evaluating functional hemoglobin saturations.

This description of a pulse oximeter capability may be somewhat misleading because, as Fig. 10-2 shows, O_2Hb and COHb have similar absorption coefficients for red light (660 nm), whereas COHb is relatively transparent to infrared light (940 nm). Additionally, MetHb and HHb have the same absorption coefficients for red light; however, MetHb demonstrates a greater absorbency for infrared light (940 nm) than does oxyhemoglobin. Accordingly, the presence of significant levels of COHb, as occurs in carbon monoxide poisoning, will lead to an overestimation of S_pO_2 (Key Point 10-1).[8] Methemoglobinemia, a potential complication of administering nitric oxide, benzocaine (topical anesthetic), and dapsone (an antibiotic used to treat malaria and *Pneumocystis carinii*), can cause erroneous S_pO_2 values because MetHb absorbs both red and IR light.[6,11] If enough MetHb is present to dominate all pulsatile absorption, the pulse oximeter will measure a red-to-IR ratio of 1:1, corresponding to an S_pO_2 of about 85%. Consequently, the pulse oximeter reading will overestimate or underestimate the **true oxyhemoglobin** saturation, depending on whether the actual S_aO_2 is less than or greater than 85%.[9,11]

> **Key Point 10-1** Abnormal hemoglobin, such as carboxyhemoglobin (smoke exposure), produces an erroneously high S_pO_2. If abnormal hemoglobin levels are suspected, a CO-oximeter should be used to evaluate the oxygen saturation.

It is well documented that intravascular dyes can adversely affect S_pO_2 values by absorbing a portion of the incident light emitted by the pulse oximeter diodes. Scheller and colleagues[12] demonstrated that injection of methylene blue and indigo carmine into human volunteers caused a false drop in S_pO_2, whereas indocyanine green had little effect on pulse oximeter values.

Nail Polish

Nail polish (particularly blue and black nail polish) can affect S_pO_2 readings. It has been suggested that nail polish causes light to be shunted around the finger periphery (called *optical shunting*).[13,14] The transmitted light never comes in contact with the vascular bed; consequently, S_pO_2 values can be erroneously high or low, depending on whether this light takes on a pulsatile character. Placing the device over the lateral aspects of the digit rather than over the nail can largely alleviate this problem.

Skin Pigmentation

Theoretically, skin pigmentation should have no effect on pulse oximeter readings. In practice, however, S_pO_2 readings are typically higher for patients with dark skin pigmentation. For example, an S_pO_2 of 95% in an African American patient may actually represent an S_aO_2 of only 92%.[15-17] Many clinicians, therefore, use higher threshold values (i.e., S_pO_2 >92%) for initiating oxygen therapy in African American patients. Although using higher target S_pO_2 values does not lead to untreated hypoxemia in most of these patients, some will have arterial oxygen pressure (P_aO_2) values as high as 200 mm Hg when therapy is based on measured S_pO_2.

Bilirubin, a breakdown product of heme metabolism, is the pigment responsible for the yellow discoloration seen in jaundiced patients. Although an elevated bilirubin level (>20 mg/dL) has been shown to affect O_2Hb values recorded with CO-oximetry, pulse oximetry measurements do not appear to be affected by hyperbilirubinemia.[18,19]

Ambient Light

Direct sunlight and external light sources (e.g., fluorescent lights, heat lamps, fiberoptic light sources, and surgical lamps) have been shown to affect S_pO_2 readings adversely.[20-22] Most commercially available pulse oximeters attempt to compensate for this interference by continually cycling the transmitted red and IR light on and off at a rate of about 480 cycles per second.

Clinical Applications

The usefulness of pulse oximetry as an early warning system for detecting hypoxemia in patients with unstable oxygenation status is well recognized. Pulse oximetry is an excellent trending device in critically ill patients, providing a continuous display of oxygen saturation. However, changes in S_pO_2 may not represent an equivalent change in actual S_aO_2.[23,24] This discrepancy is particularly evident when pulse oximetry is used in the neonatal intensive care unit (ICU). Although it is generally used to trend oxygen saturations in neonates, pulse oximetry is not used as a basis for prescribing oxygen therapy in neonates; most neonatologists prefer to base oxygen therapy decisions on P_aO_2 rather than oxygen saturation.[25,26]

A review of the relationship between S_aO_2 and P_aO_2 (i.e., the oxyhemoglobin dissociation curve) is helpful before the use of pulse oximetry to detect hypoxemia is discussed. S_aO_2 varies with the P_aO_2 in a sigmoidal or S-shaped manner. (See Fig. 10-4 for the oxyhemoglobin dissociation curve for arterial blood.) For oxygen saturations greater than 90% saturation, P_aO_2 may rise considerably without much change in S_aO_2. When saturation is less than 80%, the PO_2 values fall rapidly. Although an S_aO_2 of 97% is considered normal, maintaining an oxyhemoglobin saturation of at least 90% is considered acceptable for adult patients. As a result, many algorithms for oxygen therapy typically use 90% or slightly higher as an indication for increasing the fractional inspired oxygen concentration (F_IO_2). (As mentioned, because dark skin pigmentation can lead to erroneously high S_pO_2, many clinicians use a threshold of 94% to 95% for these patients as an indication for adjusting the F_IO_2.) In the case of hyperoxygenation, pulse oximeters can provide limited information about P_aO_2 values because of the flat portion of the oxyhemoglobin dissociation curve above 90%.

Several criteria should be met to ensure that pulse oximetry values are meaningful. Box 10-1 contains a summary of the American Association for Respiratory Care (AARC) clinical practice

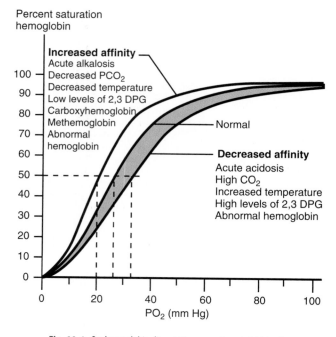

Fig. 10-4 Oxyhemoglobin dissociation curve for arterial blood.

guidelines for pulse oximetry. These guidelines provide valuable information, which practitioners should use to determine whether S_pO_2 values are valid.

Advances in light-emitting diode (LED) technology have led to simplification of pulse oximeter transmitters and sensors, making them easy to use and available at a relatively low cost. Pulse oximetry probes are available in neonatal, pediatric, and adult sizes. The response time of the pulse oximeter (i.e., the time required for the pulse oximeter to detect a change in central oxygenation level [left-heart PO_2]) depends on the location of the probe. The lag time is shortest for probes placed on the earlobe; on the finger, the lag time is longer by 12 seconds or more than for the earlobe; and probes placed on the toe have the longest lag time.

As mentioned earlier, pulse oximetry routinely is used to monitor the oxygenation status of critically ill patients continuously with unstable oxygenation status and to monitor oxygen saturation during surgery and bronchoscopy. Pulse oximetry can be particularly useful in the ICU for titrating F_IO_2 and positive end-expiratory pressure (PEEP) in mechanically ventilated patients and for monitoring the oxygenation status of patients undergoing chest physical therapy and suctioning.[22]

Although pulse oximetry can be effective when prescribing oxygen therapy in hospitalized patients, it may not be as useful in prescribing oxygen therapy for homecare patients. Carlin and colleagues[25] demonstrated that the use of pulse oximetry only can disqualify a significant number of patients applying for reimbursement for oxygen therapy. Under the guidelines of the Centers for Medicare and Medicaid Services (CMS), a patient must demonstrate a P_aO_2 of 55 Torr or lower or a saturation of 88% or lower to qualify for oxygen therapy.[24] It is important to recognize that any of the aforementioned physiological or technical problems can significantly affect S_pO_2 measurements. To resolve this problem, invasive ABG analyses should be done in chronically ill patients to establish the need for oxygen therapy. Case Study 10-1 involves pulse oximetry.

Summary of the American Association for Respiratory Care (AARC) Clinical Practice Guideline for Pulse Oximetry

Indications

Based on current evidence, pulse oximetry is useful for:

1. Monitoring arterial oxyhemoglobin saturation
2. Quantifying the arterial oxyhemoglobin saturation response to therapeutic intervention
3. Monitoring arterial oxyhemoglobin saturation during bronchoscopy

Contraindications

Pulse oximetry may not be appropriate in situations where measurements of pH, P_aCO_2, and total hemoglobin are required. The presence of abnormal hemoglobins may be a relative contraindication.

Limitations

A number of factors, agents, and situations can affect readings and limit precision and performance of pulse oximetry. These include the following:

1. Motion artifacts
2. Abnormal hemoglobins (particularly carboxyhemoglobin and methemoglobin)
3. Intravascular dyes
4. Exposure of the measuring sensor to ambient light sources
5. Low perfusion states
6. Skin pigmentation
7. Nail polish
8. Low oxyhemoglobin saturations (i.e., below 83%)

Monitoring

The following information should be recorded during pulse oximetry:

1. Probe type and site of measurement, date and time of measurement, patient position, activity level
2. F_IO_2 and mode of supplemental oxygen delivery
3. Arterial blood gas measurements and CO-oximetry results that may have been made simultaneously
4. Clinical appearance of the patient (presence of cyanosis, skin temperature)
5. Agreement between pulse oximeter heart rate and heart rate determined by palpation or electrocardiographic recordings

(Source: AARC Clinical Practice Guideline: Pulse oximetry, *Respir Care* 37: 891-897, 1992.)

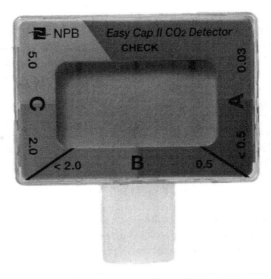

Fig. 10-5   Example of a chemical capnometer. (EasycapII, Nellcor-Puritan-Bennett, a subsidiary of Covidien, Irvine, Calif.)

CAPNOGRAPHY (CAPNOMETRY)

Capnography is the measurement of carbon dioxide concentrations in respired gases. Although the terms *capnography* and *capnometry* often are thought to be synonymous, capnography describes the continuous display of carbon dioxide concentrations as a graphic waveform called a *capnogram;* capnometry involves the display of exhaled CO_2 numerically without a waveform.[27]

Technical Considerations

Both chemical and spectroscopic methods can be used to perform capnometry. Chemical devices that rely on a disposable colorimetric detector provide **qualitative** estimates of exhaled CO_2. Spectroscopic devices (e.g., IR, Raman, acoustic, and mass spectroscopy) provide **quantitative** data on the concentration of expired CO_2. Because chemical and IR analyzers are most often used for mechanically ventilated patients in the critical care setting, the following discussion will focus on these devices.

Chemical Methods

Chemical capnometers are handheld devices composed of specially treated filter paper in a plastic casing that can be attached to the patient's endotracheal tube (ET) (Fig. 10-5). The amount of CO_2 present in the patient's inspired and exhaled gas can be estimated by noting the color changes in the filter paper. Each device uses a characteristic series of colors to indicate the approximate CO_2 concentrations. For example, the Portex CO_2 Clip device, which is manufactured by Smiths Medical Canada (St Paul, Minn.), appears blue when 0 to less than 1% CO_2 is in the respired gas, green when the exhaled gas contains 1% to 2%, green-yellow to indicate a CO_2 concentration of 2% to 5%, and yellow for CO_2 concentrations over 5.0%.

Chemical capnometers are particularly useful in emergency situations in assessing airway placement. It is important to understand that changes in the color of the filter paper are the result of a chemical reaction that affects the pH of the filter paper. (Note that if acidic liquids like regurgitated gastric contents contact the filter paper, an irreversible color change will occur and render the device unusable.[28]) Proper placement of an ET can be determined

Case Study 10-1

Causes of Cyanosis

You are preparing a patient for bronchoscopy. As you are administering an aerosol treatment with benzocaine, you note that the patient appears to be cyanotic but does not demonstrate any signs of distress. Pulse oximetry readings indicate that the S_pO_2 is 85%. You immediately obtain arterial blood gases that demonstrate a pH of 7.36, PCO_2 of 42 Torr, and PO_2 of 80 Torr. Explain the cause of the cyanosis. What diagnostic test would confirm this explanation?

because the color of the paper will change continually as inhaled and exhaled CO_2 levels vary while the patient breathes into and out of the device. In some cases, ET placement in the trachea rather than the stomach may be difficult to determine because the patient's gastric PCO_2 may be elevated after receiving mouth-to-mouth breathing or if the patient has recently ingested a carbonated beverage.

Infrared Spectroscopy

Infrared spectroscopy is based on the principle that molecules containing more than one element absorb infrared light in a characteristic manner.[29] CO_2 absorbs IR radiation maximally at 4.26 μm. The concentration of CO_2 in a gas sample can be estimated because its concentration is directly related to the amount of IR light absorbed.[30] The presence of other gases (e.g., water [H_2O] and nitrous oxide [N_2O]) can adversely affect the accuracy of CO_2 measurements by causing a phenomenon called *pressure broadening*. This phenomenon occurs because the peak absorbance of IR radiation by CO_2 lies between the peak absorbencies of H_2O and N_2O. The presence of these gases increases the absorption of infrared radiation and results in erroneously high CO_2 readings. **Pressure broadening** can be minimized by removing water vapor from the gas sample before it is analyzed and by using electronic filters to subtract the IR absorption by gases other than CO_2.[21]

Figure 10-6 is a schematic of a double beam, positive-filter capnograph. The gas is drawn into a cuvette inside the sample chamber. IR radiation is beamed through the cuvette and through a reference chamber containing CO_2-free gas. The CO_2 in the sample chamber absorbs some of the radiation, reducing the amount of radiation that reaches the detector. The difference between the radiation transmitted through the sample cell and the radiation transmitted through the reference is converted into an electrical signal, which is amplified and displayed. The displayed value can be displayed in millimeters of mercury (mm Hg) representing the partial pressure, or as percent CO_2 (% CO_2).

In clinical practice, IR analyzers are typically classified according to the method of sampling of respired gases. Figure 10-7 illustrates two methods: sidestream sampling devices and mainstream sampling devices. In sidestream sampling devices, gas from the airway is extracted through a narrow plastic tube to the measuring chamber, which is located in a separate console. In mainstream devices, the sampling chamber attaches directly to the ET and analysis is performed at the airway.

Sidestream sampling devices show a slight delay between sampling and reporting times because of the time required to transport the sample from the airway to the measuring chamber. The plastic tube that transports the sample of gas to the analyzer is prone to

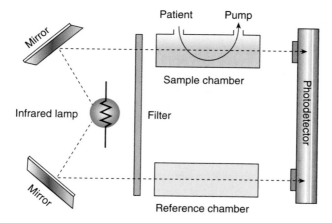

Fig. 10-6 Schematic diagram of a double beam positive, infrared capnograph. (From: Kacmarek RL, Stoller JK, Heurer AJ, editors: Egan's fundamentals of respiratory care, ed 9, St Louis, 2009, Mosby Elsevier.)

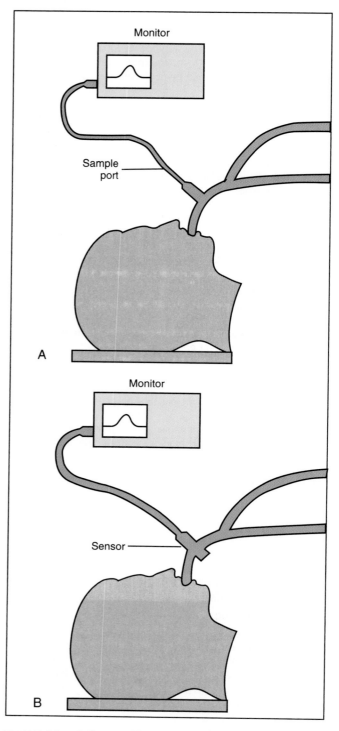

Fig. 10-7 Schematic illustrating **(A)** sidestream and **(B)** mainstream capnographs. (From Cairo J: Mosby's respiratory care equipment, ed 9, St Louis, 2014, Elsevier.)

plugging with water and secretions, which interferes with the delivery of gas to the analyzer. Contamination with ambient air, caused by leaks in the sample line, is also a concern.

In mainstream sampling devices the analyzer is attached directly to the ET; therefore no delay occurs between sampling and reporting times. However, this type of device adds a small amount of dead space to the airway. The analyzer must be properly supported because the added weight it places on the artificial airway increases the possibility of dislodgement or complete extubation. Also, because the analyzer is attached directly to the airway, it is handled often and subject to damage from mishandling (e.g., dropping).

Physiological Considerations

Inspired air contains essentially no carbon dioxide ($\approx 0.3\% \, CO_2$). Expired air normally contains about 4.5% to 5.5% CO_2, which is primarily the product of cellular metabolism. Figure 10-8 illustrates a capnogram for a healthy, resting adult breathing room air. The waveform, which displays the fractional concentration of expired CO_2 (F_ECO_2) versus time, is divided into four phases. In phase 1, the initial gas exhaled is from the conducting airways, which contain low levels of CO_2 from inspired air. During phase 2, alveolar gas containing CO_2 mixes with gas exhaled from the anatomic airways, and the CO_2 concentration rises. In phase 3, the curve plateaus as alveolar gas is exhaled (this phase is often referred to as the *alveolar plateau*). The concentration of CO_2 at the end of the alveolar phase (just before inspiration begins) is referred to as the *end-tidal* PCO_2, or $P_{et}CO_2$. In phase 4 (inspiration), the concentration falls to zero.

The $P_{et}CO_2$ is dependent on the alveolar PCO_2 (P_ACO_2), which is ultimately influenced by CO_2 production ($\dot{V}CO_2$) and the effectiveness of ventilation (i.e., matching of ventilation to perfusion).

The production of CO_2 is primarily determined by the metabolic rate. Fever, sepsis, hyperthyroidism, and seizures increase metabolic rate and $\dot{V}CO_2$. Hypothermia, starvation, and sedation reduce metabolic rate and $\dot{V}CO_2$.

The relationship between ventilation and perfusion of the lung and gas exchange (i.e., P_ACO_2) can be expressed using $\dot{V}/\dot{Q}$ relationships.[31] Figure 10-9 shows three $\dot{V}/\dot{Q}$ relationships that can potentially affect the level of alveolar PCO_2. In Fig. 10-9, *A*, ventilation and perfusion are equally matched. The partial pressure of arterial CO_2 (P_aCO_2) and P_ACO_2 are nearly equal. The $P_{et}CO_2$ is normally about 4 to 6 mm Hg lower than the P_aCO_2. In Fig. 10-9, *B*, ventilation decreases relative to perfusion (low $\dot{V}/\dot{Q}$). The P_ACO_2 eventually equilibrates with the mixed venous PCO_2 ($P_{\bar{v}}CO_2$). Clinical situations in which this type of $\dot{V}/\dot{Q}$ relationship can exist throughout the lung (leading to higher than normal $P_{et}CO_2$ values)

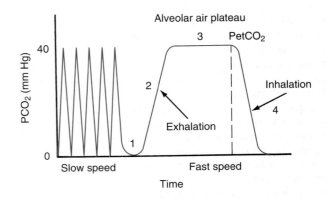

Fig. 10-8 Capnogram from a normal, healthy, resting subject breathing room air.

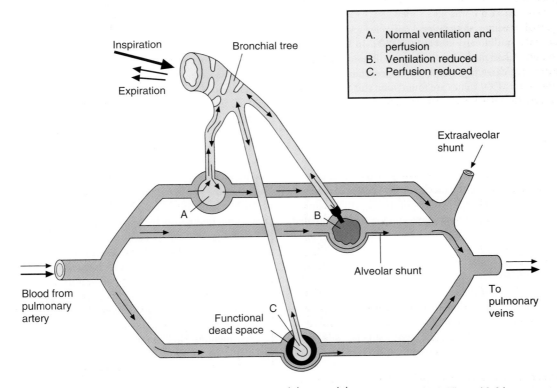

Fig. 10-9 Ventilation-perfusion relationships: **A**, Normal. **B**, Low $\dot{V}/\dot{Q}$. **C**, High $\dot{V}/\dot{Q}$. (Source: Despopoulos A, Silbernagl S: Color atlas of physiology, ed 4, New York, 1991, Thieme Medical Publishers.)

BOX 10-2	Summary of AARC Clinical Practice Guideline for Capnography/Capnometry During Mechanical Ventilation

Indications

Based on current evidence, capnography is useful for the following:

1. Monitoring the severity of pulmonary disease and evaluating the response to therapy, especially therapy intended to improve V_D/V_T and ventilation/perfusion $\dot{V}/\dot{Q}$ relationships. It may also provide valuable information about therapy directed at improving coronary blood flow.
2. Used as an adjunct to verify that tracheal rather than esophageal intubation has taken place.
3. Graphic evaluation of the integrity of the patient-ventilatory interface.
4. Monitoring the adequacy of pulmonary and coronary blood flow.
5. Screening patients for pulmonary embolism.
6. Detection of CO_2 rebreathing and the waning effects of neuromuscular blockade.
7. Monitoring CO_2 elimination.
8. Optimization of mechanical ventilation.

Contraindications/Complications

There are no absolute contraindications to capnography in mechanically ventilated adult patients. Mainstream devices increase the amount of dead space added to the ventilator circuit. The sampling rate of respired gases when using sidestream analyzers may be high enough to cause autotriggering when flow triggering of mechanical breaths is used. The effect is inversely proportional to the size of the patient. The gas-sampling rate can also diminish delivered tidal volume in neonates and small patients while using volume-targeted or volume-controlled ventilation.

Monitoring

During capnography, the following should be recorded:

1. Ventilatory variables, including tidal volume, respiratory rate, positive end-expiratory pressure, inspiratory/expiratory ratios, peak airway pressures, concentrations of respiratory gases.
2. Hemodynamic variables, including systemic and pulmonary pressures, cardiac output, shunt, and $\dot{V}/\dot{Q}$ imbalances.

Limitations

Although capnography can provide valuable information about the efficiency of ventilation, as well as systemic, pulmonary, and coronary perfusion, P_aCO_2 should be routinely determined by standard arterial blood gas analysis. Leaks in the ventilator circuit or leaks around the tracheal tube can lead to inaccurate measurements of expired CO_2. The reliability of the contour of the capnogram can also be affected by the stability of the minute volume, tidal volume, cardiac output, and CO_2 body stores. High breathing frequencies may exceed the response capabilities of the capnograph and therefore affect the integrity of the capnogram recorded. Low cardiac output may cause a false-negative result when attempting to verify the endotracheal tube (ET) position in the trachea. Positioning the ET in the pharynx, as well as the presence of antacids and carbonated beverage in the stomach, can lead to false-positive results when assessing ET placement.

(Source: AARC Clinical Practice Guideline: Capnography/capnometry during mechanical ventilation, 2011, *Respir Care* 56(4): 503-509, 2011.)

---

include respiratory center depression, muscular paralysis, and chronic obstructive pulmonary disease (COPD). In Fig. 10-9, *C*, ventilation is higher than perfusion (high $\dot{V}/\dot{Q}$). Physiological dead space ventilation increases, and the P_aCO_2 approaches inspired air (0 Torr). Decreased $P_{et}CO_2$ values are found with this type of $\dot{V}/\dot{Q}$ relationship in patients with pulmonary embolism, excessive PEEP (extrinsic or intrinsic), and any disorder marked by pulmonary hypoperfusion.

Clinical Applications

Capnography has been shown to be a useful measurement in both spontaneously breathing and mechanically ventilated patients. Box 10-2 summarizes the key points of the AARC's clinical practice guideline for using capnography/capnometry in ventilated patients.[27] The following section discusses some of the most common uses of capnography.

Capnograph Contours

Changes in the contour of the capnogram can be used to detect increases in dead space ventilation, hyperventilation and hypoventilation, apnea or periodic breathing, inadequate neuromuscular blockade in pharmacologically paralyzed patients, and CO_2 rebreathing. They can also be used to monitor the effectiveness of gas exchange during cardiopulmonary resuscitation (CPR) and to detect accidental esophageal intubation.

Phase 3 (i.e., alveolar plateau) becomes indistinguishable from airway obstruction (i.e., increased physiological dead space) as occurs in COPD (Fig. 10-10, *A*). Hyperventilation is characterized by a reduction in P_aCO_2 and, therefore, $P_{et}CO_2$ (Fig. 10-10, *B*). Conversely, hypoventilation is associated with elevated P_aCO_2 and $P_{et}CO_2$ (see Fig. 10-10, *B*). Figure 10-10, *C*, is a capnogram of a patient with Cheyne-Stokes breathing. During bradypnea, phase 4 will occasionally show cardiac oscillations resulting from the motion of the beating heart transferred to the conducting airways (Fig. 10-10, *D*). Failure of the capnogram to return to baseline is an indicator of rebreathing of exhaled gas (Fig. 10-10, *E*). Figure 10-10, *F*, shows a capnogram for a paralyzed patient, demonstrating the characteristic "curare cleft" during phase 3. This is a positive sign that the paralyzed patient is receiving insufficient neuromuscular blockade; however, other factors can contribute to this capnographic finding, such as patient-ventilator asynchrony.

Capnography can be used to detect pulmonary blood flow cessation, such as occurs with pulmonary embolism or during cardiac arrest. A number of investigators have advocated the use of capnography as an adjunct to CPR. Laboratory studies suggest that the capnogram can be used as an indication of the progress and success of the event. These studies demonstrated that $P_{et}CO_2$ increases as $\dot{V}/\dot{Q}$ is restored to normal.

As mentioned, capnography can also be used to detect accidental esophageal intubation. The gastric PCO_2 generally is equal to room air; therefore failure to detect the characteristic changes in CO_2 concentration during ventilation possibly indicates esophageal intubation. However, low perfusion of the lungs is associated with low $P_{et}CO_2$ and should not be confused with esophageal

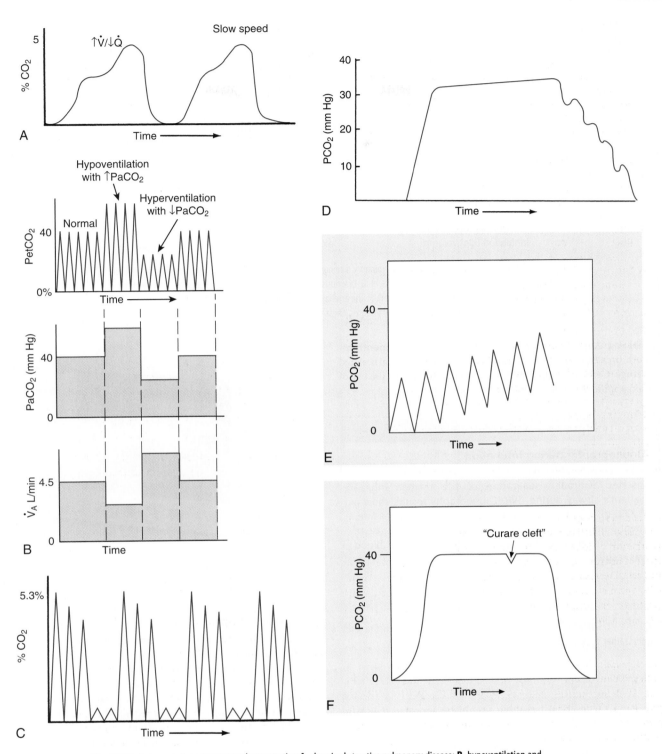

Fig. 10-10 Representative capnograms demonstrating **A,** chronic obstructive pulmonary disease; **B,** hypoventilation and hyperventilation; **C,** Cheyne-Stokes breathing; **D,** cardiac oscillations; **E,** rebreathing exhaled air; **F,** "curare cleft." P_aCO_2, Arterial carbon dioxide pressure; PCO_2, partial pressure of carbon dioxide.

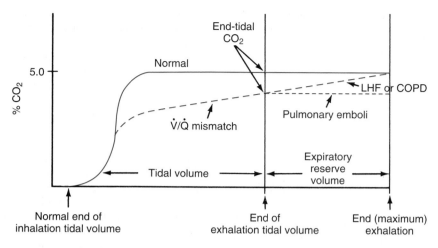

Fig. 10-11 $P_{(a\text{-}et)}CO_2$ for a normal and a forced expiratory capnogram. (Sources: Darin J: Capnography, Curr Rev Respir Ther 3:146-150, 1981; Erickson L, Wollmer P, Olsson CG, et al: Diagnosis of pulmonary embolism based upon alveolar dead space analysis, Chest 96:357-362, 1989; Hatle CJ, Rokseth R: The arterial to end expiratory carbon dioxide tension gradient in pulmonary embolism and other cardiopulmonary diseases, Chest 66:352-357, 1974.)

intubation. Also, the gastric PCO_2 may be elevated after mouth-to-mouth breathing or if the patient recently ingested a carbonated beverage. Case Study 10-2 gives an example situation of the use of capnographic data (Key Point 10-2).

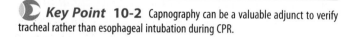

Case Study 10-2

Capnography During Intubation

After considerable difficulty, an endotracheal tube is inserted without visualization of the trachea into a patient's airway during CPR. Capnography results show a $P_{et}CO_2$ of 3 Torr; a standard arterial blood gas measurement demonstrates a P_aCO_2 of 75 Torr. Explain the cause of this discrepancy in the capnography and arterial blood gas results.

 Key Point 10-2 Capnography can be a valuable adjunct to verify tracheal rather than esophageal intubation during CPR.

Arterial to Maximum End-Expiratory PCO₂ Difference

The $P_{(a\text{-}et)}CO_2$ for tidal breathing should be approximately 4 to 6 mm Hg. It is elevated in patients with COPD, left-sided heart failure, and pulmonary embolism caused by an increase in physiological dead space.[31] Another technique that can be used to further evaluate the severity of the disease is to compare arterial PCO_2 measurements with maximum expired PCO_2 measurements (the arterial to maximum expiratory PCO_2 gradient). With this technique, the expired PCO_2 recorded at the end of a maximum exhalation is compared with the P_aCO_2. The difference normally is minimal. Patients with COPD and left-sided heart failure do not show an arterial to maximum expired PCO_2 difference, whereas patients with pulmonary embolism do show an increased gradient. Figure 10-11 shows the capnographic appearance of these differences.

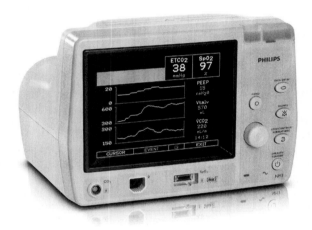

Fig. 10-12 A NICO₂ capnometer. (Courtesy Respironics, Inc, Murrysville, Pa.)

Volumetric Capnometry

In addition to end-tidal CO_2 monitoring, another application that has been available for about a decade is volumetric capnometry. End-tidal CO_2 monitoring focuses on exhaled CO_2 plotted over time, whereas volumetric capnometry focuses on exhaled CO_2 plotted relative to exhaled volume. The Respironics NICO₂ is an example of a capnometer that can provide this type of monitoring (Fig. 10-12) (The NICO₂ monitor [Philips Respironics, Inc., Murrysville, Pa.] can also be used to estimate cardiac output noninvasively; see Chapter 11.)

Description of the Single-Breath CO₂ Curve

The single-breath CO_2 graph (SBCO₂) is produced by the integration of airway flow and CO_2 concentration; it is presented on a breath-to-breath basis. As shown in Fig. 10-13, the graph can provide information on anatomic dead space, alveolar dead space (when P_aCO_2 is known), and CO_2 elimination (VCO₂) for each breath. If a horizontal line is drawn at the top of the curve, representing $\%CO_2$ in arterial blood, three distinct regions of the curve are established.

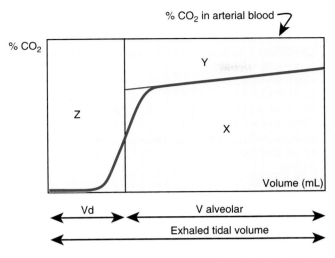

Fig. 10-13 Graph of exhaled volume (x axis) versus % CO_2 (y axis). A horizontal line drawn at the top of the curve represents the % CO_2 in arterial blood. Three distinct regions are illustrated: Area X represents actual CO_2 exhaled in one breath; area Y is the amount of CO_2 not eliminated because of alveolar dead space; and area Z is the amount of CO_2 not eliminated because of anatomic dead space. Vanatomic, Alveolar volume; Vd, dead space volume. (Redrawn from material from Respironics, Murryvillle, PA.)

Area X represents the actual amount of CO_2 exhaled in the breath, assuming that no exhaled air is rebreathed. In other words, the area under the $SBCO_2$ curve is the volume of CO_2 in a single breath. Adding all the single breaths in a minute gives the $\dot{V}CO_2$, the same results that would occur if exhaled gas were collected using a Douglas bag. Thus, the CO_2 monitor can provide information about the volume of CO_2 in one breath (VCO_2) and the volume of CO_2 produced in one minute ($\dot{V}CO_2$).

Area Y represents the amount of CO_2 that is not eliminated because of alveolar dead space (i.e., ventilated alveoli that are poorly perfused or receive no perfusion at all). *Area Z* represents the amount of CO_2 that was not eliminated because of the anatomic dead space.

The relationship of the areas (with the added arterial blood line) provides some important parameters for analysis. The ratios of the areas created in the $SBCO_2$ curve are the same as the relationship seen in the Enghoff modified Bohr equation:

$$[P_aCO_2 - P_{\bar{E}}CO_2]/P_aCO_2 = (Y+Z)/(X+Y+Z),$$

where P_aCO_2 is arterial partial pressure for carbon dioxide, and $P_{\bar{E}}CO_2$ is mixed expired partial pressure for CO_2. (XYZ were defined previously.) Four major factors influence the amount of CO_2 exhaled: CO_2 production, perfusion of the lungs, diffusion, and ventilation.

Altering the production of CO_2 or any one of the factors involved in transport of CO_2 without compensation will result in changes in P_aCO_2 and the volume of CO_2 eliminated through the lungs.[32,33]

As previously mentioned, conditions that can alter the volume of CO_2 produced are related to changes in metabolic rate. For example, $\dot{V}CO_2$ increases in patients with sepsis, fever, severe burns to the body, trauma, and with increases in work of breathing (i.e., the respiratory muscles produce additional CO_2). If metabolic rate increases and ventilation does not increase, P_aCO_2 rises, and therefore the amount of CO_2 exhaled during the $SBCO_2$ maneuver increases.

Reductions in perfusion to the lungs, as occurs with pulmonary emboli, can lead to changes in the contour of the $SBCO_2$ curve. As perfusion to the lung decreases, the phase 2 portion of the curve shifts to the right, showing increased dead space in the system (i.e., less CO_2 exhaled). In this situation, physiological dead space increased. In addition, the area under the curve contains less CO_2; therefore, less $\dot{V}CO_2$ per breath is eliminated due to the fact that less CO_2 is being delivered to the alveoli. (It is important to recognize that overall CO_2 production is not reduced.)

Application of PEEP can also alter the contour of the volumetric $SBCO_2$ curve. As PEEP is increased from zero to 15 cm H_2O, the phase 2 portion of the curve shifts to the right because of expanding airways (increasing PEEP keeps the airways open) and reduced perfusion. The addition of PEEP can cause compression of the pulmonary capillaries and a drop in perfusion to the lungs, reducing effective perfusion to the ventilated alveoli. This change represents an increase in alveolar dead space. The slope of phase 2 decreases as well; this is a result of lower CO_2 concentration occurring at an identical volume point on the x-axis, causing a rise in P_aCO_2.

Case Study 10-3 provides an example of how volumetric capnography can be used clinically.

Case Study 10-3

Exercise
Dead Space Ventilation

A 35-year-old 60-kg man is admitted to the ICU following a motor vehicle accident in which he sustained multiple rib fractures. He is receiving volume-targeted mechanical ventilation and is being monitored with pulse oximetry and volumetric capnography. You are asked to increase his PEEP level from +5 cm H_2O to +10 cm H_2O. After making the change, you notice that his S_pO_2 decreases from 93% to 90%. His $SBCO_2$ curve has shifted to the right and the $P_{et}CO_2$ decreased from 30 mm Hg to 25 mm Hg. Briefly describe why these changes may have occurred.

Single-Breath CO_2 Loop of Inspiration and Exhalation

When the $SBCO_2$ graph includes both inspiration and exhalation, a loop is produced (Fig. 10-14). The net volume of CO_2 exhaled in one breath is the area between the exhaled and inhaled CO_2 of this loop. The net CO_2 in one breath is the difference between the amount of CO_2 inhaled (which is typically negligible) and the amount of CO_2 exhaled.

Trending CO_2 Production and Alveolar Minute Ventilation Over Time

As mentioned, the $NICO_2$ monitor can trend data over time. The display for this purpose reports the CO_2 produced each minute ($\dot{V}CO_2$) rather than $SBCO_2$ curves (Fig. 10-15). Trended data can be used to monitor a variety of clinical procedures. For example, during a recruitment maneuver in a patient with acute respiratory distress syndrome, trended CO_2 data will reveal a transient rise in CO_2 when previously closed alveoli are reopened. This tool can also be used in weaning patients from the ventilator. For example, if the patient's respiratory rate increases during a spontaneous breathing trial (SBT), monitoring CO_2 can help determine whether the

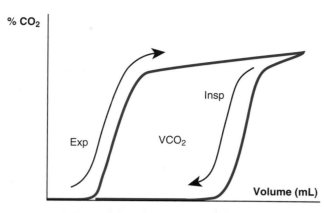

Fig. 10-14 A single-breath CO_2 curve ($SBCO_2$) recorded during inspiration and expiration. (Courtesy Ted Tabor, RRT, Paris, France.)

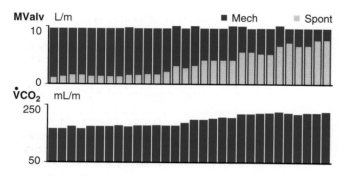

Fig. 10-15 An example of a $\dot{V}CO_2$ trended over time *(bottom bar graph)* compared with corresponding $\dot{V}_E$ *(top bar graph; L/min)*. During the successful weaning trial illustrated in these graphs, mandatory breaths are reduced *(gray area, top graph)*, and the patient's spontaneous breath rate increases *(dark bars in $\dot{V}_E$, top graph)*. At the same time a progressive rise occurs in $\dot{V}CO_2$ as the expected work of the respiratory muscles increases. (Courtesy Philips Respironics, Inc., Murrysville, Pa.)

patient's metabolic rate is increasing (and thus working the respiratory muscles) or whether a change in dead space affects the patient's ability to wean.

Trending of CO_2 can also be useful for noting the time lag that can occur in CO_2 removal as a result of CO_2 stores (CO_2 bound in the cells or through bicarbonate or bound in the blood). Large stores result in the long time lags, and small stores result in short time lags. For example, if the alveolar ventilation increases, P_aCO_2 decreases and the stores of CO_2 also begin to decline; however, this second part requires time to happen and can be identified by the trending of CO_2. In this situation, if $\dot{V}_E$ increases, $SBCO_2$ increases and P_aCO_2 initially declines. After a slight delay, because the production of CO_2 remains constant, the P_aCO_2 remains low and the monitored exhaled $\dot{V}CO_2$ returns to baseline, indicating that a balance has returned. Plotting $SBCO_2$ curve trends over time using a trending graph is the best way to monitor these types of changes.

EXHALED NITRIC OXIDE MONITORING

Nitric oxide (NO) has potent dilatory effects on the pulmonary vessels and airways. It has also been shown to facilitate coordinated beating of ciliated epithelial cells. The synthesis of NO by the body is mediated through a series of enzymes that are referred to as NO

BOX 10-3	Factors Affecting Levels of Exhaled Nitric Oxide (NO)

Conditions Associated with Reductions of Exhaled NO
Systemic hypertension
Pulmonary hypertension
Cystic fibrosis
Sickle cell anemia
Ciliary dyskinesis
Conditions Associated with Elevated Levels of Exhaled NO
Asthma
Bronchiectasis
Airway viral infections
Alveolitis
Allergic rhinitis
Pulmonary sarcoidosis
Chronic bronchitis
Systemic sclerosis
Pneumonia

(Courtesy Aerocrine, Solna, Sweden.)

synthases (NOS), which exist in constitutive and inducible forms. The constitutive form is associated with endothelial and neural cells; the inducible NOS is particularly seen in epithelial cells. Although both forms of NOS are present in the airways, the expression of the inducible NOS appears to correlate with the level of NO found in exhaled air.

The most common method used to quantify the level of exhaled NO is chemiluminescence, which occurs when NO reacts with ozone. Exhaled NO (eNO) can be detected in exhaled gas in the range of 7.8 to 41.1 parts per billion (ppb). Note that the concentration of NO can vary with the flow of exhaled air because it is continually formed in the airways. The range of eNO is also affected by the presence of pathologic conditions, as well as the patient's gender, atopic status, smoking habits, and use of medications.[33] Box 10-3 provides a list of factors that have been shown to affect the levels of eNO.

Exhaled NO is currently used as a marker for airway inflammation associated with asthma.[32] Several studies have shown a positive correlation between the eNO and disease severity.[33] Monitoring the level of eNO can also be used to monitor the effectiveness of inhaled corticosteroid in the treatment of asthmatic patients.

TRANSCUTANEOUS MONITORING

Transcutaneous monitoring is another noninvasive method that can be used to indirectly assess a patient's oxygenation (P_aO_2) and ventilation (P_aCO_2) status. Unlike pulse oximetry and capnography, which rely on spectrophotometric analysis, transcutaneous monitoring uses modified blood gas electrodes to measure the oxygen and carbon dioxide tensions at the skin surface (Box 10-4).[34,35]

Transcutaneous PO_2

Devices used to monitor the transcutaneous partial pressure of oxygen ($P_{tc}O_2$) consist of a servo-controlled, heated (Clark) polarographic electrode connected to a central processing unit (Fig. 10-16, *A*).[36-38] The electrode housing, which is covered with a Teflon

BOX **10-4** Summary of AARC Clinical Practice Guideline for Transcutaneous Blood Gas Monitoring

Setting

1. Monitoring mechanically ventilated patients (e.g., conventional modes of ventilation, high-frequency ventilation, and noninvasive ventilation.
2. Bronchoscopies and procedures requiring sedation or patient-controlled analgesia.
3. Sleep studies.
4. Pulmonary function testing (e.g., stress testing, bronchoprovocation).
5. Trending HCO_3^- in patients with diabetic ketoacidosis.
6. Apnea testing.
7. Patient transport.
8. Evaluation of tissue perfusion.
9. Evaluation of hyperventilation during phonation of patients with vocal cord disorders.
10. Titrating long-term oxygen therapy.

Indications

1. Monitoring the adequacy of arterial oxygenation and/or ventilation.
2. The need to quantify the response to diagnostic and therapeutic interventions (e.g., administering enriched oxygen mixtures, application of PEEP).
3. Transcutaneous oxygen index ($P_{tc}O_2/F_IO_2$) can be used as a marker of hypoperfusion and mortality.
4. Tissue perfusion status and revascularization in wound care (e.g., during hyperbaric oxygen therapy) and peripheral vascular disease.
5. Monitoring response to therapy in patients with diabetic ketoacidosis, as $P_{tc}CO_2$ correlates with serum HCO_3^- levels.

Contraindications/Complications

Transcutaneous monitoring may be relatively contraindicated in patients with poor skin integrity and/or adhesive allergy. Complications may include thermal injury at the sensor site resulting in erythema, blisters, burns, and skin tears. Misinterpretation of data may lead to inappropriate treatment of a patient.

Monitoring

The following should be recorded when monitoring transcutaneous measurements:

1. Clinical appearance of the patient, including subjective assessment of perfusion, pallor, and skin temperature
2. Date and time of the measurement
3. Patient position
4. Respiratory rate
5. Physical activity level
6. F_IO_2 and the type of oxygen delivery device if supplemental oxygen is being administered
7. Mode of ventilator support (i.e., ventilator or CPAP settings)
8. Electrode placement site, electrode temperature, and time of placement
9. Results of simultaneous measurements of P_aO_2, P_aCO_2, and pH

Limitations

Technical and clinical factors may affect the reliability of transcutaneous readings and therefore limit the application of transcutaneous monitoring. Improper calibration, trapped air bubbles, and damaged membranes can affect the accuracy of the measurements of $P_{tc}O_2$ and $P_{tc}CO_2$. The presence of hyperoxemia (P_aO_2 > 100 mm Hg) or a hypoperfused state (e.g., shock) can increase the difference between $P_{tc}O_2$ and P_aO_2.

(Source: AARC Clinical Practice Guideline: transcutaneous monitoring of carbon dioxide and oxygen: 2012, *Respir Care* 57(11):1955-1962, 2012.)

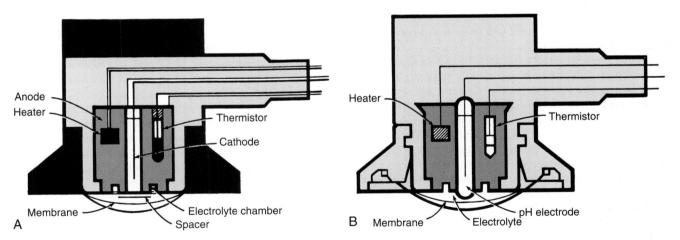

Fig. 10-16 Transcutaneous electrodes. **A,** Transcutaneous partial pressure of oxygen ($P_{tc}O_2$). **B,** Transcutaneous partial pressure of carbon dioxide ($P_{tc}CO_2$). (From Deshpande VM, Pilbeam SP, Dixon RJ: A comprehensive review in respiratory care, East Warwick, CT, 1988, Appleton & Lange.)

membrane, attaches to the skin surface with a double-sided adhesive ring. The electrode is heated to 42° to 45° C to produce capillary vasodilation below the surface of the electrode. Note that heating improves diffusion of gases across the skin because it increases local blood flow at the site of the electrode, as well as altering the structure of the stratum corneum. The stratum corneum has been described as a mixture of fibrinous tissue within a lipid and protein matrix. It has been suggested that heating the skin to temperatures greater than 41° C melts the lipid layer, thus enhancing gas diffusion through the skin.

Although correlation of $P_{tc}O_2$ and P_aO_2 ($P_{tc}O_2/P_aO_2$ index) has been shown to be good for neonates, it is often unreliable for critically ill adult patients.[39] A decrease in peripheral perfusion caused by reductions in cardiac output or by increases in peripheral (cutaneous) resistance can significantly affect the accuracy of $P_{tc}O_2$ measurements.[40,41] Data indicate that when the cardiac index is greater than 2.2 L/min/m², the $P_{tc}O_2/P_aO_2$ index is 0.5, whereas for a cardiac index less than 1.5 L/min/m², it is only 0.1.[42] Therefore hypoperfusion of the cutaneous circulation caused by pathologic states (e.g., septic shock, hemorrhage, or heart failure) or by increased vascular resistance (e.g., hypothermia or pharmacologic intervention) can produce erroneous data. Because the $P_{tc}O_2$ is influenced by blood flow to the tissues, as well as by oxygen utilization by the tissues, changes in this value may be used as an early indicator of vascular compromise or shock.

Transcutaneous PCO₂

Measurement in the transcutaneous CO_2 partial pressure ($P_{tc}CO_2$) was introduced into clinical practice in the late 1970s after the successful use of $P_{tc}O_2$ monitors in neonatal ICU patients was demonstrated. Standard devices use a modified Stowe–Severinghaus blood gas electrode, which is composed of pH-sensitive glass with an Ag/AgCl electrode (Fig. 10-16, *B*). As with the $P_{tc}O_2$ electrode, the $P_{tc}CO_2$ electrode is heated to 42° to 45° C. $P_{tc}CO_2$ values are slightly higher than P_aCO_2, primarily because of the higher metabolic rate at the site of the electrode caused by heating the skin. Most commercial instruments incorporate correction factors into their system's software to remove this discrepancy between $P_{tc}CO_2$ and P_aCO_2.

Technical Considerations

Some simple rules apply when using transcutaneous monitors. These relate to care, placement, and calibration of the electrodes. Establishing a set routine for these three tasks will help to ensure accurate and useful measurements[41]:

1. The transcutaneous monitor manufacturer should have validated transcutaneous monitor, electrodes, calibration gases, and supplies, using accepted quality control procedures and clinical reliability studies.
2. Transcutaneous electrodes are bathed by an electrolyte solution (see Fig. 10-16). This solution can easily evaporate because of the heat applied to the electrode. The electrolyte and the sensor's membrane should be changed weekly or whenever the respiratory care practitioner notices a signal drift during calibration. Because silver can become deposited on the cathode, periodic cleaning of the electrode is suggested, using the manufacturer's recommendations.
3. Before placing an electrode on the patient's skin, the site should be cleansed using an alcohol swab. In cases where hair may be present, the site should be shaved to ensure good contact between the electrode and the skin. Before applying the electrode to the skin, a drop of electrolyte gel or deionized water should be placed on the electrode's surface to enhance gas diffusion between the skin and the electrode.
4. $P_{tc}O_2$ monitors are calibrated using a two-point calibration in which room air (PO_2 of about 150 mm Hg) serves as the high PO_2 of the calibration and an electronic zeroing of the system serves as the low PO_2 of the calibration.
5. $P_{tc}CO_2$ monitors are also calibrated with a two-point calibration procedure. In this calibration, a 5% CO_2 calibration gas and a 10% CO_2 calibration gas are used for low and high calibration

points, respectively. Electrodes should be calibrated before their initial use on a patient. Manufacturers typically suggest that the electrode should be recalibrated each time it is repositioned.

6. Reports of $P_{tc}O_2$ and $P_{tc}CO_2$ readings should include notation of the date and time of the measurement, the patient's activity level and body position, and the site of electrode placement, along with the electrode temperature. The inspired oxygen concentration and the type of equipment used to deliver supplemental oxygen should always be included. The clinical appearance of the patient, including assessment of peripheral perfusion (i.e., pallor, skin temperature), is important data to note. In cases where invasive ABG measurements are available, these data are recorded for comparison with $P_{tc}O_2$ and $P_{tc}CO_2$ readings.

Burns are probably the most common problem that clinicians encounter during transcutaneous monitoring. Burns can occur because the site of measurement must be heated to 42° to 45° C. Repositioning the sensor every 4 to 6 hours can help to avoid this problem.[41] When transcutaneous monitoring is used with neonates, the sensor should be repositioned more often (e.g., every 2 hours).

A problem can occur with $P_{tc}O_2$ and $P_{tc}CO_2$ readings if the electrode is applied improperly. A leak-proof seal must be maintained at the skin surface for the readings to be meaningful. A leak allows room air to contact the sensor and results in higher than actual $P_{tc}O_2$ and lower than actual $P_{tc}CO_2$ readings even though the patient's clinical condition has not changed.

When combined O_2/CO_2 electrodes are used, hydroxyl (OH^-) ions produced at the PO_2 cathode may interfere with $P_{tc}CO_2$ readings. This problem has been reduced by stoichiometric consumption of OH^- by an anodized anode.[24]

Indirect Calorimetry and Metabolic Measurements

OVERVIEW OF INDIRECT CALORIMETRY

Indirect calorimetry allows the clinician to estimate energy expenditure from measurements of oxygen consumption ($\dot{V}O_2$) and carbon dioxide production ($\dot{V}CO_2$).[43] This technique is based on the theory that all the energy that a person uses is derived from the oxidation of carbohydrates, fats, and proteins and that the ratio of carbon dioxide produced to oxygen consumed (i.e., the respiratory quotient or $\dot{V}CO_2/\dot{V}O_2$) is characteristic for the fuel being burned (Box 10-5).[44] Although the use of metabolic measurements varies considerably, many clinicians are becoming comfortable with this emerging technology and recognize that metabolic measurements can provide valuable information for designing nutritional support regimens.

Technical Considerations

The most commonly used devices for indirect calorimetry are open-circuit gas exchange monitors (Fig. 10-17). They are often referred to as *metabolic monitors* or *metabolic carts*. A typical **metabolic monitor** includes analyzers for measuring the concentration of inspired and expired gases, as well as a sensor for measuring the volume and/or flow of respired gases. The O_2 analyzer is a rapid responding polarographic or zirconium oxide oxygen analyzer. The CO_2 analyzer is a nondispersive, infrared analyzer. Volume and flow measurements can be obtained using pneumotachometers,

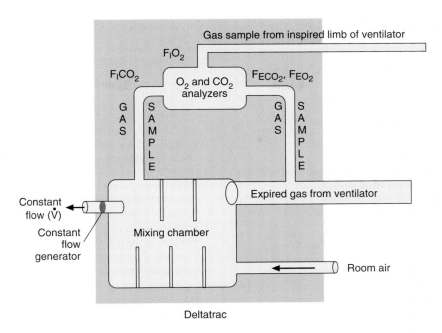

Fig. 10-17 Major components of a metabolic monitoring system. (Source: Weissman CM, Sadar A, Kemper MA: In vivo evaluation of a compact metabolic measurement instrument, J Parenter Enteral Nutr 14:216-221, 1990. Redrawn from Levine RL, Fromm RE: Critical care monitoring, St Louis, 1995, Mosby.)

BOX **10-5**	Variations in Respiratory Quotient (RQ)

Substrate	RQ
Carbohydrate oxidation	1.0
Fat oxidation	0.7
Protein oxidation	0.8
Lipogenesis	>1.0

turbine flow meters, or ultrasonic vortex flow meters. Barometric pressure and expired gas temperatures are monitored with temperature-sensitive, solid-state (integrated circuit) transducers.

Obtaining Indirect Calorimetry Measurements

A spontaneously breathing patient who is breathing room air can be connected to the system by having the patient breathe through a mouthpiece or a mask that is attached to a nonrebreathing valve. Specially designed canopies and hoods can also be used for spontaneously breathing patients who are not receiving ventilatory support.

Patients with ETs or tracheostomy tubes who are being mechanically ventilated can be connected to the system by placing the nonrebreathing valve directly onto the airway opening and directing the expired gases into the system. It is important to inflate the cuffs of ETs and tracheostomy tubes when measuring inspired and expired gases. Failure to inflate the cuff will result in loss of expired air around the tube (system leak) and erroneous measurements of $\dot{V}O_2$ and $\dot{V}CO_2$. For patients receiving a continuous flow of gas during ventilatory support, such as occurs when an external flow from a flow meter is used to power a small volume nebulizer inline, an isolation valve must be used to ensure that only the patient's exhaled gases are delivered to the system.[45-47]

$\dot{V}O_2$ and $\dot{V}CO_2$ are calculated by comparing the fractional concentrations of O_2 and CO_2 of inspired and expired air. For patients breathing room air, the F_IO_2 can be assumed to be 0.209 and the F_ICO_2, 0.03. For patients receiving enriched oxygen mixtures, the F_IO_2 must be measured by the system.[46,47] Fluctuations in F_IO_2 can be caused by air leaks in the patient-ventilator-metabolic monitor system and also by varying gas volumes and pressure demands, such as occur during intermittent mandatory ventilation (IMV). Unstable air–oxygen blending systems within the ventilator circuit may also contribute to unstable F_IO_2 values (this problem can be prevented with the use of an external air–oxygen blender). Clinical studies have shown that some systems may not provide accurate and reproducible $\dot{V}O_2$ measurements for patient breathing F_IO_2 values greater than 0.5.[46] Box 10-6 provides a summary of the AARC Clinical Practice Guideline for using indirect calorimetry during mechanical ventilation.

Clinical Applications of Metabolic Measurements

Indirect calorimetry can provide information on energy expenditure (EE) and the pattern of substrate utilization. EE represents an individual's caloric expenditure calculated from measured $\dot{V}O_2$ and $\dot{V}CO_2$ values. EE can be calculated with the deWeir equation shown in Box 10-7. Note that the urinary nitrogen (UN) is determined separately by the clinical laboratory using a 24-hour urine sample. The UN is one of the end products of protein metabolism; therefore the number of grams of nitrogen excreted in the urine is directly related to the amount of protein used by the individual. If nitrogen excretion data are not available, EE can be calculated using the modified deWeir equation. In this latter equation, it is assumed that protein represents 12% to 15% of the total energy expenditure.

Energy expenditure can be expressed in kilocalories per day (kcal/day) or relative to the individual's body surface area

BOX 10-6	Summary of AARC Clinical Practice Guideline for Metabolic Measurement Using Indirect Calorimetry During Mechanical Ventilation

Indications

1. Metabolic measurements may be indicated in patients with known nutritional deficits and derangements. Multiple nutritional risk and stress factors that may skew predictions made using the Harris-Benedict equation (e.g., neurologic trauma, COPD, acute pancreatitis, multiple trauma, severe sepsis, extreme obesity, severe hypermetabolic or hypometabolic patients).
2. To measure O_2 cost of breathing in patients who fail attempts at liberation from mechanical ventilation.
3. To measure $\dot{V}O_2$ and cardiac output by the Fick equation for patients requiring hemodynamic monitoring.

Contraindications/Complications

1. Manipulation of the ventilator circuit for connection of measurement lines may cause leaks that may lower alveolar ventilation and result in hypoxemia, bradycardia, or other adverse connections.
2. Inappropriate calibration or system setup may result in erroneous results leading to incorrect patient management.
3. Isolation valves may increase circuit resistance and cause increased work of breathing and/or dynamic hyperinflation (auto-PEEP).

4. Inspiratory reserves may cause a reduction in alveolar ventilation due to increased compressible volume of the breathing circuit.

Inaccurate measurements of REE and RQ during open circuit measurements may be caused by:

1. Instability of F_IO_2 within a breath or breath to breath due to changes in the source gas pressure and ventilator blender characteristics.
2. $F_IO_2 > 0.60$.
3. Inability to separate inspired and expired gases due to bias flow and flow-triggering systems, IMV systems, or specific ventilator characteristics.
4. Presence of anesthetic gases or gases other than O_2, CO_2, and nitrogen in the patient-ventilator circuit.
5. Presence of water vapor resulting in sensor malfunction.
6. Inadequate length of the measurement.

Assessment of Test Quality and Outcome

1. RQ is consistent with the patient's nutritional intake.
2. RQ at rest is in the normal physiological range (0.67 to 1.3).
3. Variability of $\dot{V}O_2$ and $\dot{V}CO_2$ measurements should be within a physiological range (0.7 to 1.0).

(Source: AARC Clinical Practice Guideline: Metabolic measurement using indirect calorimetry during mechanical ventilation—2004 revision and update, *Respir Care* 49(9):1073-1079, 2004.)

BOX 10-7	Formulas Used During Indirect Calorimetry

Harris-Benedict Equations*

Men: Energy expenditure (EE) = 66.5 + (13.75 × weight) + (5.003 × height) − (6.775 × age)

Women: EE = 655.1 + (9.563 × weight) + (1.85 × height) − (4.676 × age)

where weight is measured in pounds, height is measured in inches, and age is determined in years.

Energy Expenditure†

deWeir equation: EE = [3.941 ($\dot{V}O_2$) + 1.106 ($\dot{V}CO_2$)] × 1.44 − [2.17 UN]

Modified deWeir equations: EE = [3.9 ($\dot{V}O_2$) + 1.1 ($\dot{V}CO_2$)] × 1.44

Substrate Utilization‡

Carbohydrates: dS = 4.115 $\dot{V}CO_2$ − 2.909 $\dot{V}O_2$ − 2.539 UN

Fats: dF = 1.689 ($\dot{V}O_2$ − $\dot{V}CO_2$) − 1.943 UN

Proteins: dP = 6.25 UN

---

dS, dF, and *dP* represent grams of carbohydrate, fat, and protein, respectively, for a fasting individual.

*Harris JA, Benedict FG, eds: Standard basal metabolism constants for physiologists and clinicians: a biometric study of basal metabolism in man, Philadelphia, 1991 Lippincott Williams & Wilkins.

†Weir JB: A new method for calculating metabolic rate with special reference to protein metabolism, *J Physiol* 109:1-9, 1949.

‡Burszein S, Saphar S, Singer P, et al: A mathematical analysis of indirect calorimetry measurement in acutely ill patients, *Am J Clin Nutr* 50:227-230, 1980.

(kcal/h/m²). A normal, healthy adult uses about 1500 to 3000 kcal/day or about 30 to 40 kcal/h/m².[48]

Another method used to express the level of energy metabolism is to compare the measured EE to predicted EE, which is based on the individual's age, weight, and height. (The Harris-Benedict equations shown in Box 10-7 are examples of reference equations used in clinical practice.) If the measured EE is greater than 120% of the predicted EE, a hypermetabolic state exists. Conversely, when the measured EE is less than 80% of the predicted EE, a hypometabolic state exists.

Numerous factors can influence the metabolic rate, including the type and rate of nutrition that is ingested; the time of day the measurement is made; the patient's level of physical activity; and whether he or she is recovering from infection, surgery, or trauma.[49] The presence of chronic gastrointestinal, hepatic, renal, endocrine, cardiovascular, and pulmonary diseases can also influence the metabolic rate.[50] Box 10-8 lists several conditions that are associated with hypermetabolic and hypometabolic states.

Prolonged starvation is associated with a decreased metabolic rate. Feeding raises metabolic rate through a mechanism referred to as *specific dynamic action*. It is thought that specific dynamic action is related to the digestion and absorption of food. EE can show diurnal variation; it usually is lowest on awakening in the morning and increases 10% to 15% by late afternoon.[50,51] This increase in energy expenditure may be related to hormonal changes that occur during the day.

Sleep is associated with a reduction in metabolic rate, whereas even the slightest exertion is associated with increases in metabolic rate. Changes in body temperature, as occur with bacterial and viral infections, can profoundly affect the metabolic rate. For example, an increase in body temperature of 1°C will cause 10%

Examples of Hypermetabolic and Hypometabolic States

Hypermetabolic States
Pancreatitis
Hyperthyroidism
Pregnancy
Drugs (e.g., stimulants)
Hyperthermia (fever)
Seizures
Burns

Hypometabolic States
Starvation
Hypothyroidism
Anesthesia
Sedation
Hypothermia
Coma

increase in metabolic rate. Burns, long-bone fractures, and surgery can increase the metabolic rate by as much as 200%.[50]

The substrate utilization pattern is the proportion of carbohydrates, fats, and proteins that contribute to the total energy metabolism. The percentage of the total energy that a substrate contributes can be derived from measurements of the RQ (the ratio of $\dot{V}CO_2$ to $\dot{V}O_2$). The RQ levels for the various foods are known; when pure fat is burned, the RQ equals 0.7. The RQ for pure carbohydrate is 1.0, and the RQ for protein is approximately 0.8. RQ levels greater than 1.0 are associated with lipogenesis (fat synthesis) and hyperventilation. RQ levels less than 0.7 are associated with ketosis.

A healthy adult consuming a typical American diet derives 45% to 50% of his or her calories from carbohydrates, 35% to 40% from lipids, and 10% to 15% from proteins. The resultant RQ will range from 0.80 to 0.85. Note that proteins normally contribute only minor amounts to energy metabolism. The percentage of protein used represents the normal turnover rate for replenishing structural and functional proteins in the body. Proteins may contribute significantly to EE in cases of starvation. For this reason, a nonprotein RQ is usually reported to indicate the contribution to RQ made by carbohydrates and lipids.

The types of substrates ingested and the ability of the individual to use various foods determine substrate utilization. For example, feeding large amounts of glucose will raise the RQ to about 1.0, suggesting that carbohydrates are providing most of the EE. Prolonged starvation will lower the RQ to about 0.7, indicating that the individual is relying almost completely on fats for energy. Many systemic diseases will adversely affect an individual's ability to use various substrates. For example, several studies have shown that patients with severe sepsis demonstrate RQ levels of approximately 0.7 because of reliance on lipid metabolism for energy and their inability to use carbohydrates.

Monitoring of substrate utilization patterns also can assist the clinician who is trying to wean patients with limited ventilatory reserve from mechanical ventilation (Key Point 10-3). It has been demonstrated that feeding these patients diets containing a high percentage of carbohydrates will raise their $\dot{V}CO_2$ to a greater extent than their $\dot{V}O_2$ (RQ approaches 1.0).[52,53] The added CO_2 load placed on these patients (remember they have limited ventilatory reserve) is greater than their own ventilatory capacity, and they fail to wean. Switching their diet to one that has a higher fat/carbohydrate ratio lowers their $\dot{V}CO_2/\dot{V}O_2$ ratio (RQ levels approach 0.7) and reduces the CO_2 load to the lungs. It is reasonable to suggest that this change would enhance the potential for a successful weaning outcome. See Critical Care Concept 10-1 for a discussion of the advantages of using indirect calorimetry in the management of critically ill patients.

 Key Point **10-3** The types of substrates ingested and the ability of an individual to use various foods influence substrate utilization.

CRITICAL CARE CONCEPT 10-1

Indirect Calorimetry
Prediction equations used by clinicians to determine energy needs for hospitalized patients are derived from studies of healthy subjects. Clinicians generally agree that using standard prediction equations to estimate energy needs for critically ill patients provides values that compare poorly with measured values, such as those reported from indirect calorimetry. The energy needs of these patients tend to be quite diverse and can lead to over- or undernutrition. Although stress factors can be added to the calculation of predicted caloric intake, these factors may be misleading, particularly in those patients demonstrating multisystem problems.

Assessment of Respiratory System Mechanics

The assessment of respiratory system mechanics for patients receiving ventilatory support begins with measurements of pressure, volume, and flow events. Once these measurements have been made, the clinician can calculate derived values for respiratory system compliance, airway resistance, and the work of breathing.[54] Chapter 1 discusses the physiological concepts required for an understanding of respiratory mechanics in mechanically ventilated patients. The following is a brief description of the devices and techniques that are used to measure airway pressures, volumes, and flows.

MEASUREMENTS

Airway Pressure Measurements

Mechanical ventilators have traditionally allowed for measurements of airway pressures by incorporating an aneroid manometer into the ventilator circuit. With this arrangement, the manometer records pressure changes within the ventilator, which includes contributions from ventilator resistance. Measuring airway pressure near the airway opening can minimize the effects associated with ventilator resistance. Thus, in the current generation of adult and neonatal ventilators, airway pressure is measured using electromechanical transducers (e.g., piezoelectric, variable capacitance, strain gauge) that connect to pressure sampling ports that are located near the airway opening (i.e., measurements can be made on the inspiratory limb of the ventilator circuit, the expiratory side of the circuit, or directly at the ET).

An alternative method of recording airway pressures during mechanical ventilation is to use a strain gauge pressure transducer

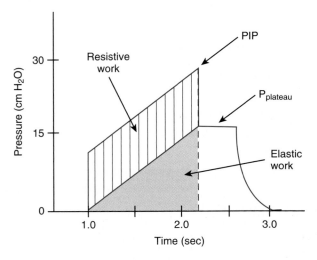

Fig. 10-18 Airway pressure tracing for a patient on mechanical ventilation. *PIP,* Peak inspiratory pressure; *P_plateau,* plateau pressure.

that is normally used for measuring systemic and pulmonary arterial pressures. These transducers can be adapted for respiratory pressure measurements because respiratory pressures are similar in magnitude to those found in the systemic or pulmonary arterial vasculature.[24,55] There are several points to remember when using these types of pressure transducers. Hemodynamic pressures are recorded in millimeters of mercury (mm Hg) and respiratory pressures are recorded in centimeters of water (cm H_2O); to convert from millimeters of mercury to centimeters of H_2O, the mm Hg value is multiplied by 1.36. Second, the transducer needs not be filled with fluid for making airway pressure measurements. Third, the same transducer should not be used to obtain both airway pressure and hemodynamic measurements, to avoid the possibility of introducing an air embolus into the circulation.

The most common airway pressure measurements are **peak inspiratory pressure** (PIP) and **static,** or **plateau, pressure** ($P_{plateau}$) (Fig. 10-18). As discussed in Chapter 1, PIP is the maximum pressure generated during inspiration. During volume-targeted ventilation, PIP is determined by the tidal volume, peak flow, and inspiratory flow. It is also influenced by the resistance and compliance of the patient's lungs and chest wall and by ET resistance and the compliance of the ventilator circuit. During pressure-targeted ventilation, the target pressure set on the ventilator determines the PIP. Patient-triggering efforts can increase or decrease the PIP, depending on the patient-ventilator synchrony.[55]

$P_{plateau}$ is the amount of pressure that is required to maintain the tidal volume within the patient's lungs during a period of no gas flow. As such, $P_{plateau}$ reflects that alveolar pressure (P_{alv}), and it is ultimately influenced by the tidal volume, the lung and thorax compliance, circuit elastance, and the total measured PEEP (including applied and auto-PEEP) (Key Point 10-4).

⚡ Key Point 10-4 $P_{plateau}$ reflects alveolar pressure, and it is ultimately influenced by the tidal volume, the lung and thorax compliance, circuit elastance, and the total measured PEEP.

$P_{plateau}$ can be measured by occluding the expiratory valve at the end of a tidal inspiration. Many current ICU ventilators have an

inspiratory pause control incorporated into the ventilator system that closes the inspiratory and expiratory valves at the end of inspiration so that $P_{plateau}$ measurement can be obtained. As illustrated in Fig. 10-18, $P_{plateau}$ measurements require the establishment of a period of zero flow for 1 to 2 seconds to allow pressure equilibration to occur across the airway. This delay in pressure equilibration and establishment of the $P_{plateau}$ is the result of redistribution of the tidal volume and stress relaxation. True $P_{plateau}$ measurements can be obtained only during a passive inspiration, and failure to establish a stable $P_{plateau}$ can result from patient breathing activity or a leak in the ventilator circuit.[55,56]

Flow Measurements

Gas flow during mechanical ventilation can be monitored with a number of different types of flow meters, including vortex ultrasonic flow meters, variable orifice pneumotachometers, thermal flow meters, and turbine flow meters. With these devices, volume changes can be calculated by integrating the flow signal relative to time.[57,58]

Vortex ultrasonic flow meters and variable orifice pneumotachometers use resistive elements to create a pressure drop that is proportional to the flow of gas through them.[57] Vortex ultrasonic flow meters use struts to create a partial obstruction to gas flow. As gases flow past these struts, whirlpools or vortices are produced. The frequency at which these whirlpools are produced is related to the flow of gas through the struts. These devices are not affected by the viscosity, density, or temperature of the gas being measured. They are unidirectional devices and therefore cannot be used to measure inspiratory and expiratory flow simultaneously.[57] The Servo-i (Maquet, Bridgewater, N.J.) uses ultrasonic transducer technology to measure expiratory gas flow. Rather than struts, two ultrasonic transducers that alternate function are used. One acts as the transmitting device and the other the receiver (Fig. 10-19). The ultrasonic waves detect the expiratory gas flow characteristics as the patient's exhaled air moves through the expiratory cassette and provide a measure of exhaled tidal volumes and flows.

Variable orifice pneumotachometers are disposable, bidirectional flow measuring devices that use a variable area, flexible obstruction for measuring flow as a function of the pressure differential generated by the obstruction. They contain minimal dead space (about 10 mL), and they can measure flow from 0.02 to 3.0 L/sec.[59] Although the flow-pressure characteristics of these devices are nonlinear, nonlinearity is typically compensated electronically. Variable orifice pneumotachometers are used in the Bicore CP-100 pulmonary monitor, the Novametrics Ventrak monitoring system, and the Hamilton Galileo ventilator (Fig. 10-20).

Thermal flow meters ("hot wire" anemometers) use sensors that are temperature-sensitive, resistive elements (e.g., thermistor beads or heated wires). These devices operate on the principle that as gas passes over the thermistor bead or the heated wire, the sensor cools and its resistance changes in proportion to the gas flow. Note that the amount of cooling depends on the viscosity and the thermal conductivity of the gas measured. With thermistor beads, cooling increases resistance, whereas with a heated platinum wire, cooling decreases resistance. The wire is typically heated above 37° C and protected by a low-resistance screen to prevent moisture accumulation and debris impaction on the wire. The gas flow can be calculated because the amount of power needed to maintain the temperature of the heating element above the temperature (e.g., 37° C) is related to the log of the velocity of gas flow, and therefore must be linearized. Thermal flow meters are unidirectional devices

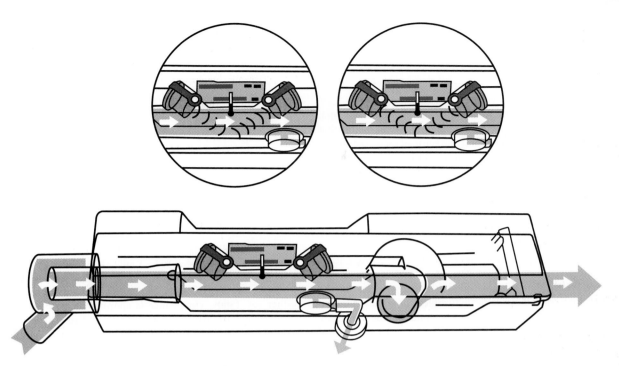

Fig. 10-19 Ultrasonic flow transducers within the Servo-i expiratory cassette. (Courtesy Maquet, Inc, Wayne, N.J.)

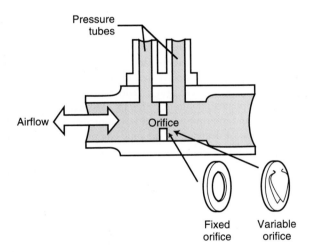

Fig. 10-20 A pneumotachograph illustrating a fixed orifice and a variable orifice (contains a moveable flap). (Redrawn from Sullivan WJ, Peters GM, Enright PL: Pneumotachographs: theory and clinical application, Respir Care 29:736-749, 1984.)

and cannot be used for measuring bidirectional flows during breathing. It is important to recognize that the density and viscosity of the gas being measured can affect the accuracy and precision of the flow measurement. Correction factors for various gases can be applied through computer software.[4] Thermal anemometers are available with the Covidien PB 840 ventilator and Dräger Oxylog 3000 ventilators.

Turbine flow meters use a rotating vane that is placed in the path of gas flow. As gas flows through the device, the vane turns at a rate that is dependent on the flow rate of the gas. Gas flow therefore can be measured by counting the number of times the vane turns. This can be done mechanically by linking the vane to a needle attached to a calibrated display. The rate of gas flow can be measured electronically using a light beam that is interrupted each time the vane turns. Rotating vane devices are portable and easy to use; however, they are slow to respond to flow changes resulting from inertia and as such are inaccurate for measuring bidirectional flows. As discussed in Chapter 8 (Figure 8-2), portable turbine flow meters can be used during patient-ventilator checks when a flow meter has not been incorporated into the ventilator's design.

Clinical Applications

Respiratory systems mechanics data can provide valuable information for the clinician caring for a mechanically ventilated patient. These data are generally divided into **measured** and **derived variables.** Measured variables include airway pressures, volumes, and airflow. Derived variables, which are calculated from measured values, include respiratory system compliance, airway resistance, and work of breathing. The following is a brief description of how pathophysiological events and conditions can affect respiratory system mechanics.

Measured Variables

As mentioned previously, PIP reflects the total force that must be applied to overcome elastic and frictional forces offered by patient-ventilator systems, and $P_{plateau}$ represents that portion of the total pressure required to overcome only elastic forces. Increases in the elastance of the respiratory system (i.e., decreases in compliance of the lung and/or chest wall) will increase both peak and plateau pressures. Increases in respiratory system compliance will lower both PIP and $P_{plateau}$. Increases in airway resistance increase PIP without concomitant increases in $P_{plateau}$. Decreases in airway resistance (R_{aw}) will lower PIP but not affect $P_{plateau}$. It is important to recognize that changes in inspiratory flow or tidal volume should not be made when monitoring R_{aw} by this method. Also, the addition of PEEP (i.e., applied and auto-PEEP) will affect both PIP and $P_{plateau}$ and should be taken into account (see the discussion on R_{aw} later in this chapter) (Key Point 10-5).

> **Key Point** 10-5 Addition of PEEP (applied and auto-PEEP) affects both PIP and $P_{plateau}$ and should be taken into account when assessing changes in R_{aw}.

Sudden increases in PIP should alert the clinician to a potential problem like bronchospasm or mucus plugging. Other factors that should be checked when determining the cause of increased airway resistance include partially blocked heat and moisture exchanger (HME), incorrect ET size, water in ventilator tubing, and malfunctioning expiratory valves. Increases in PIP can also be associated with barotrauma or ventilator-induced lung injury; if these conditions are suspected, $P_{plateau}$ should be monitored because alveolar overdistension and rupture are associated with high P_{alv}, which in turn results in a higher $P_{plateau}$.

Airflow monitoring can also alert the clinician to significant changes in the resistance or compliance (or both) of the patient's respiratory system. For example, high-frequency ripples on the inspiratory flow tracing can indicate turbulent flow caused by the presence of secretions in the airway or water in the ventilator circuit.[54,59] Expiratory flow limitations should be suspected if the decay in expiratory flow is linear rather than exponential (see Chapter 9). Flow measurements can also be used to detect the presence of auto-PEEP because flow will still be present at the end exhalation. This approach to detecting auto-PEEP is more of a qualitative assessment and does not provide an accurate measurement of the level of auto-PEEP (see Fig. 9-7).

Derived Variables

Mean airway pressure. The mean airway pressure ($\overline{P}_{aw}$) represents the average pressure recorded during the respiratory cycle. It is influenced by peak inspiratory pressure, PEEP, inspiratory time (T_I), and total cycle time (TCT). It can be calculated using the following equation:

$$\overline{P}_{aw} = \frac{1}{2}[(PIP - PEEP) \times (T_I/TCT)] + PEEP$$

$\overline{P}_{aw}$ can also be obtained by integrating the area under the pressure–time curve. In most ICU ventilators, microprocessors incorporated into their electronic circuitry perform this calculation and provide a continuous display of $\overline{P}_{aw}$. Oxygenation status can be significantly improved by increases in $\overline{P}_{aw}$, and the application of PEEP has the greatest effect. However, excessive increases in $\overline{P}_{aw}$ can also adversely affect cardiac performance and lead to significant reductions in cardiac output (see Chapter 11).

Dynamic and static compliances. Compliance can be simply defined as the lung volume achieved for a given amount of applied pressure.[60] Two types of compliance calculations can be used to describe this pressure–volume relationship: dynamic compliance and static compliance. Dynamic compliance takes into account the total impedance to volume changes (i.e., flow resistive and elastic characteristics of the patient-ventilator interface); static compliance is only influenced by the elastic characteristics of the lung-thorax unit.

Dynamic compliance is calculated by dividing the tidal volume by the PIP minus the PEEP, or

$$\text{Dynamic compliance} = \text{Exhaled } V_T/(PIP - P_{plateau})$$

For mechanically ventilated patients, the compliance of the ventilator circuit (C_T)* must be included in the calculation, so the formula is more accurately stated as:

$$\text{Dynamic compliance} = V_T - [(PIP - PEEP) \times C_T]/(PIP - PEEP)$$

Static compliance is calculated by dividing the delivered tidal volume by the $P_{plateau}$ minus the total PEEP (i.e., applied PEEP plus auto-PEEP):

$$\text{Static compliance} = \text{adjusted } V_T/(P_{plateau} - PEEP)$$

As with dynamic compliance, the compliance of the ventilator circuit must be included in the calculation. The resultant formula is therefore

$$\text{Static compliance} = V_T - [(P_{plateau} - PEEP) \times C_T]/(P_{plateau} - PEEP)$$

Static compliance in healthy adult subjects is approximately 100 mL/cm H_2O; it is lower in adult patients receiving positive pressure ventilation. It ranges from 40 to 50 mL/cm H_2O (men) or 35 to 45 mL/cm H_2O (women) to as high as 100 mL/cm H_2O in either sex. (Static compliance is approximately 40 to 50 mL/cm H_2O in pediatric patients and 10 to 20 mL/cm H_2O in neonates.) Pathophysiological conditions, such as pulmonary interstitial fibrosis, pleural effusion, hyperinflation, consolidation, respiratory distress syndrome, and pulmonary vascular engorgement, are associated with decreases in lung compliance. Conditions such as kyphoscoliosis and myasthenia gravis are also associated with increased chest wall elastic recoil and decreases in chest wall compliance.

Serial measurements of dynamic and static compliance provide considerably more information than single measurements can provide. For example, congestive heart failure will lead to pulmonary vascular engorgement and a reduction in both static and dynamic compliance. Diuretics therapy reduces the level of engorgement and improves static and dynamic compliance. Bronchospasm causes a decrease in dynamic compliance but does not always affect static compliance (static compliance may decrease if air trapping occurs). If bronchodilator therapy resolves the bronchospasm, dynamic compliance returns to normal.

Airway resistance. Airway resistance (R_{aw}) is the opposition to airflow from nonelastic forces of the lung. R_{aw} for the respiratory system in a ventilated patient is about 5 to 7 cm H_2O/L/sec. As mentioned in Chapter 1, R_{aw} is calculated by dividing the difference between PIP and $P_{plateau}$ by the airflow (constant flow with volume ventilation), or

$$R_{aw} = (PIP - P_{plateau})/\dot{V} \text{ (L/sec)}$$

Airway resistance is primarily determined by the diameter of the airway. A twofold decrease in airway diameter will result in a 16-fold increase in airway resistance (Poiseuille's law).† Retention of secretions, peribronchiolar edema, bronchoconstriction, or dynamic compression of the airways results in increased airway resistance. Bronchodilation results in reduced R_{aw}.

---

*Ventilator tubing compliance varies depending on the type and diameter of tubing used. It is typically 2 to 3 mL/cm H_2O.
†Poiseuille's law describes the factors that affect laminar flow through a smooth tube with a constant diameter. $\Delta P = \dot{V} \times [(8\eta l)/(\pi r^4)]$, where ΔP = driving pressure (dynes/cm^2), η = coefficient of viscosity of the gas, l = tube length (cm), $\dot{V}$ = gas flow (mL/sec), r = radius of tube (cm) (π and 8 are constants).

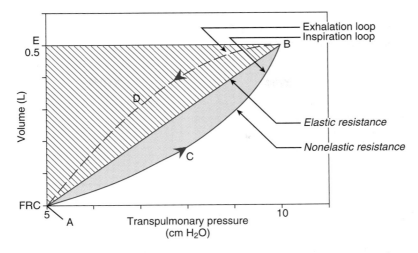

Fig. 10-21 Pressure/volume changes that occur in a patient receiving controlled ventilation with a constant flow ventilator.

Work of breathing. The normal work of breathing (WOB) is related to the energy required to take in a breath. WOB normally is associated with nonelastic forces from gas moving through the airway and inertial forces to move structures in the thorax. **Intrinsic** work is a result of work done to overcome these normal elastic and resistive forces and work to overcome a disorder or disease process affecting normal workloads in the lungs and thorax. For example, abnormal (increased) intrinsic work occurs in chronic bronchitis, in which the resistance to gas flow through the conductive airways increases. In fibrotic diseases of the lung, compliance is reduced and alveolar movement is restricted. This reduced movement impedes the ability of the lungs to expand, thus increasing intrinsic work.

Extrinsic work is work imposed (WOBi) by systems that are added to the patient. Common examples are the ET, trigger sensitivity, demand valve systems, the humidifying device, and the patient circuit.[61] Expiratory work is increased by the resistance offered by the exhalation valve or PEEP valve.

Work of breathing defined. In physics, work (W) is defined as the product of force (F) acting on a mass to move it through a distance (d), or $W = F \times d$. In fluid systems, such as the respiratory system, we say that work is performed when an applied force or pressure causes a volume to displace, as in inspiration and expiration. The WOB is the integral of the product of pressure and volume ($W = \int PV$). That is, work is the amount of pressure that must be generated to result in the movement of a certain volume of gas. Work is reported in kilogram-meters (kg·m) or joules (J; 0.1 kg·m = 1 J). In healthy individuals, the WOB is about 0.5 J/L, which represents only 2% to 5% of the total $\dot{V}O_2$ or 0.35 to 1.0 mL/L of ventilation. Oxygen consumption by the respiratory muscles may be as high as 35% to 40% of total $\dot{V}O_2$ in patients with COPD. WOB is sometimes described by the amount of oxygen consumed by the working respiration muscles, although this is difficult to measure.[61,62] WOB can also be defined as the pressure–time product when intrapleural pressure is monitored.

Graphic representation of WOB. The WOB can now be monitored through the use of graphic displays and calculated data provided by newer microprocessor-controlled ventilators and by special monitoring devices (esophageal pressure monitors). Note

that the accuracy of the calculation still needs to be studied. The amount of work expended during a respiratory cycle can be estimated by multiplying the pressure changes associated with a given volume change, or $W = P \times V$. Alternatively, WOB can be calculated as $W = (PIP - 0.5 \times P_{plateau})/100 \times V_T$ to estimate WOB during constant flow passive inflation of the lungs.[63] A pressure–volume curve can be used to make this estimate.[63] Figure 10-21 illustrates the pressure and volume changes that occur in a patient receiving controlled mechanical ventilation (CMV) with a constant flow with the ventilator doing the resistive and elastic work of breathing.[64] Contrast this to Fig. 10-22, which shows WOB required during continuous positive airway pressure (CPAP). In this figure, WOB is the integral of airway pressure and V_T; the greater the area of the loop, the greater the WOB. Loop A is an example of a free-standing CPAP system. Spontaneous breaths occur clockwise—inspiration to expiration. Loop B is CPAP through a ventilator demand valve system and shows an increased WOBi. The area to the left of the vertical lines (baseline pressure of 5 cm H_2O) is the WOBi during inspiration. The area to the right of the line represents WOBi during expiration.

Figure 10-23 shows the components of a spontaneous breath and a ventilator breath. It distinguishes those parts of the breath that the patient must do and those parts that the ventilator provides.[64]

Figure 10-24 compares the components of a normal spontaneous breath with a spontaneous breath with high impedance to breathing (ET in place), and with a mandatory controlled breath.[65] Curve A represents breathing through an ET by a patient with high impedance (increased R_{aw} or decreased compliance, or both). This occurs during T-tube trials for ventilator liberation or during spontaneous breathing through a continuous flow system. Curve B represents the work done by the ventilator during a volume-controlled breath. The ventilator is doing all the work of breathing. A spontaneous breath under normal conditions is represented by curve C.

Some have suggested that measuring the work of breathing in this way may underestimate the total amount of work that a patient expends during assisted ventilation.[66] Measurements of transdiaphragmatic pressures and pressure–time products may provide accurate estimates of the work of breathing and the metabolic cost of breathing in mechanically ventilated patients.[67]

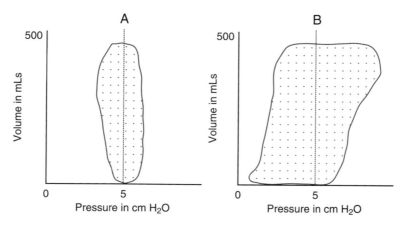

Fig. 10-22 Work of breathing (WOB) during continuous positive airway pressure (CPAP). WOB in this figure is the integral of airway pressure and tidal volume. *Loop A* is an example of a freestanding CPAP system. Spontaneous breaths occur clockwise, inspiration to expiration. *Loop B* is CPAP through a ventilator demand valve system. (Sources: Hirsch C, Kacmarek RM, Stankek K: Work of breathing during CPAP and PSV imposed by the new generation mechanical ventilators: a lung model study, Respir Care 36:815-828, 1991; Kacmarek RM: The role of pressure support ventilation in reducing the work of breathing, Respir Care 33:99-120, 1988; Kirby RR, Banner MJ, Downs JB: Clinical applications of ventilatory support, New York, 1990, Churchill-Livingstone.)

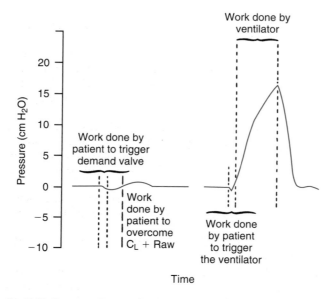

Fig. 10-23 Pressure requirements for a spontaneous *(left)* and an assisted breath *(right)*. The imposed work of breathing (WOBi) can occur during triggering of the breath. In the spontaneous breath, the patient performs work to overcome elastic and resistive forces, while in the assisted breath, the ventilator provides the work. C_L, Lung compliance. (From Branson RD: Enhanced capabilities of current ICU ventilators: do they really benefit patients? Respir Care 36:362-376, 1991.)

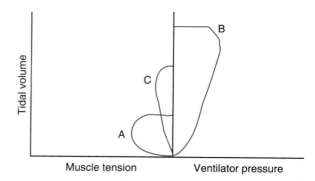

Fig. 10-24 Pressure–volume loops under various conditions. **A,** Patient breathing through an endotracheal tube with high impedance (increased resistance and/or decreased compliance). **B,** Patient receiving a controlled volume breath. **C,** Spontaneous breath under normal circumstances. (Sources: Kacmarek RM: The role of pressure support ventilation in reducing the work of breathing, Respir Care 33:99-120, 1988; MacIntyre NR: Weaning from mechanical ventilatory support: volume-assisting intermittent breaths versus pressure-assisting every breath, Respir Care 33:121-125, 1988.)

Pressure–time product. Measurement of the maximum inspiratory pressure (MIP) and the maximum expiratory pressure (MEP) provides nonspecific information about the strength of the respiratory muscles. It is possible to obtain more specific information about the contributions of diaphragmatic contractions on breathing by measuring transdiaphragmatic pressure and the pressure–time product.[68,69] **Transdiaphragmatic pressure** is a measure of the forcefulness of diaphragmatic contractions. The **pressure–time**

product, which is an assessment of transdiaphragmatic pressure during the inspiratory portion of the breathing cycle, is one method of estimating the contributions of the diaphragm during inspiration. It is probably a better indication of a patient's effort to breathe than measurement of work derived from pressure–volume curves.

Figure 10-25, *A,* shows the positioning of the two balloon-tipped catheters used to measure transdiaphragmatic pressures and thus the pressure–time product. The catheters are inserted through the nose; one is positioned in the stomach (below the diaphragm), and the other is positioned in the lower third of the esophagus (above the diaphragm). Gastric (P_{GA}) and esophageal (P_{es}) pressures are measured during the respiratory cycle. The electronic difference between these two pressures is referred to as the *transdiaphragmatic pressure.* When the transdiaphragmatic

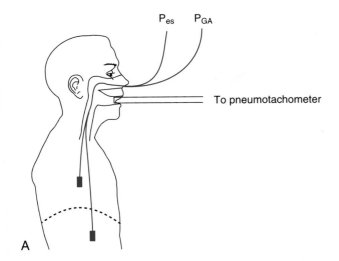

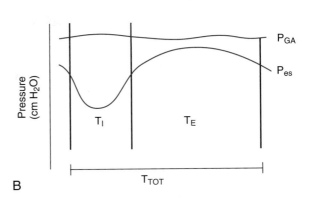

Fig. 10-25 A, Apparatus for measuring transdiaphragmatic pressures and the pressure–time product. **B,** Pressure–time curve for a spontaneous breath. The waveforms illustrate pleural pressure changes during a breath. A variety of waveforms can be displayed with the current respiratory mechanics software. P_{es}, Esophageal pressure; P_{GA}, gastric pressure; T_E, expiratory time; T_I, inspiratory time; T_{TOT}, total time.

pressure is plotted over time, it provides a pressure–time curve that can be used to estimate the activity of the diaphragm (Fig. 10-25, *B*). Thus, diaphragmatic activity during inspiration can be estimated by integrating the area within the curve during inspiration; the resultant value is called the *pressure–time product.* Increases in the pressure–time product indicate a greater force of contraction by the diaphragm. Conversely, decreases in the pressure–time product are associated with less muscular force.[69-71]

Although some clinicians consider the pressure–time product a useful measurement for determining the effectiveness of diaphragm function during weaning from mechanical ventilation, its use is limited in the clinical setting.[69,70]

Occlusion pressure measurements. The **occlusion pressure** ($P_{0.1s}$ or P_{100}) is the airway pressure measured after occluding the airway during the first 100 msec of a patient's spontaneous inspiration. Clinical data suggest that $P_{0.1}$ provides a useful index of ventilatory drive and may be used as a predictor of weaning success (i.e., elevated $P_{0.1}$ is associated with weaning failure). For ventilator-dependent patients, the $P_{0.1}$ has also been shown to correlate with the work of breathing during pressure support ventilation.[17] (See Chapter 20 for additional information on $P_{0.1}$.)

SUMMARY

- Noninvasive monitoring has become common practice in the care of mechanically ventilated patients.
- Pulse oximeters, capnographs, and transcutaneous monitors have greatly improved the respiratory care practitioner's ability to monitor changes in patients' ABG levels.
- The presence of abnormal hemoglobin, such as carboxyhemoglobin (smoke inhalation), produces an erroneously high S_pO_2 and CO-oximetry should be performed to determine the true oxygen saturation.

- Exhaled NO measurements can be used to assess the severity of a patient's asthma exacerbation.
- Transcutaneous O_2 and CO_2 measurements provide a noninvasive method of assessing oxygenation and ventilation status.
- Indirect calorimetry provides new insights about the nutritional status of spontaneously breathing and mechanically ventilated patients.
- Several factors can influence the metabolic rate, including the type and rate of food ingested, the time of day the measurements are made, the patient's level of physical activity, and whether the person is recovering from surgery or an acute or chronic illness.
- The substrate utilization pattern is the proportion of carbohydrates, fats, and proteins that contribute to the total energy expenditure.
- Bedside mechanics testing is an invaluable resource for optimizing mechanical ventilatory support.
- Current ICU mechanical ventilators incorporate microprocessors that can provide breath-by-breath and summative reports of pressure and flow events along with calculations of airways resistance, respiratory compliance, and work of breathing.
- Dynamic compliance takes into account flow resistive and elastic characteristics of the patient-ventilator interface, whereas static compliance is influenced only by elastic characteristics of the lung-thorax unit.
- Airway resistance is primarily determined by the diameter of the airway.
- The work of breathing is influenced by intrinsic and extrinsic factors. Intrinsic factors include the elastic and resistive forces that must be overcome during inspiration and expiration. Extrinsic factors are related to the work imposed by systems that are added to the patient, such as endotracheal tubes, demand valve systems, the humidifying devices, and exhalation valve or PEEP valve.
- The pressure–time product uses transdiaphragmatic pressure measurements to estimate the contributions of the diaphragm during inspiration.

REVIEW QUESTIONS (See Appendix A for answers.)

1. Draw and label the normal components of the capnogram.

2. What is the pressure–time product? How can this variable be used in the management of mechanically ventilated patients?

3. Which of the following conditions will adversely affect pulse oximeter readings?
   1. Hypovolemia
   2. Methemoglobinemia
   3. Anemia
   4. Hyperbilirubinemia
      A. 1 and 2
      B. 1 and 3
      C. 1, 2, and 3
      D. 2, 3, and 4

4. Which of the following actions is indicated when there is disparity between S_pO_2, S_aO_2, and the clinical presentation of a patient?
   A. Moving the probe to an alternative site to check for S_pO_2
   B. Replacing the pulse oximeter probe
   C. Measuring arterial oxygen saturation by CO-oximetry
   D. Disregarding the S_aO_2

5. Which of these parameters is measured to obtain a functional hemoglobin saturation?
   1. O_2Hb
   2. HHb
   3. COHb
   4. MetHb
      A. 1 and 2
      B. 1 and 3
      C. 2 and 3
      D. 3 and 4

6. An indistinct phase 3 on a patient's capnogram is most often associated with:
   A. Rebreathing exhaled gas
   B. Anemia
   C. Chronic obstructive pulmonary disease
   D. Cheyne-Stokes breathing

7. In the clinical setting, the $P_{(a-et)}CO_2$ is normally:
   A. −2 to −5 mm Hg
   B. 1 to 3 mm Hg
   C. 4 to 6 mm Hg
   D. 10 to 15 mm Hg

8. Which of the following data should be recorded when making transcutaneous measurements?
   1. Date and time of the measurement
   2. Clinical appearance of the patient
   3. Site of electrode placement on the patient
   4. Type of oxygen delivery device and the F_IO_2
      A. 1 only
      B. 2 and 4 only
      C. 1 and 3 only
      D. 1, 2, 3, and 4

9. Which of the following conditions could lead to an elevated RQ (>1.0)?
   A. Hyperventilation
   B. Starvation
   C. Diabetes mellitus
   D. Sepsis

10. Which of the following conditions is associated with hypermetabolism?
    A. Starvation
    B. Hypothyroidism
    C. Pregnancy
    D. Anesthesia

11. The following data were obtained from a mechanically ventilated patient: V_T = 600 mL, PIP = 30 cm H_2O, P_{Plat} = 20 cm H_2O. What is this patient's static compliance?
    A. 20 mL/cm H_2O
    B. 25 mL/cm H_2O
    C. 30 mL/cm H_2O
    D. 60 mL/cm H_2O

12. Which of the following conditions will cause a decrease in static and dynamic compliance?
    1. Bronchospasm
    2. Congestive heart failure
    3. Partial occlusion of the endotracheal tube
    4. Atelectasis
       A. 1 and 2
       B. 1 and 4
       C. 2 and 3
       D. 2 and 4

13. What is associated with an increase in the work of breathing in mechanically ventilated patients?
    A. Bronchodilation
    B. Decreased spontaneous breathing frequency
    C. Switching from controlled mechanical ventilation to assisted ventilation
    D. Using a larger endotracheal tube

14. Phase 3 of an $SBCO_2$ curve represents which of the following?
    A. Dead space
    B. Alveolar dead space
    C. A mixture of airway and alveolar gas
    D. Alveolar gas

15. The PEEP is increased on a patient receiving mechanical ventilation. The $SBCO_2$ curve shows a simultaneous shift to the right and an increase in the area of zone Y. This would indicate which of the following?
    A. Lung recruitment and emptying of previously collapsed alveoli
    B. Increased alveolar dead space from reduced pulmonary perfusion
    C. Decreased P_aCO_2 from improvement in oxygenation
    D. Increase in rebreathed volume

16. Which of the following will affect the level of exhaled NO in exhaled gas?
    1. Presence of a pathologic condition
    2. Smoking habits
    3. Atopic status
    4. Patient's gender
       A. 1 and 3 only
       B. 2 and 4 only
       C. 1, 2, and 4 only
       D. 1, 2, 3, and 4

References

1. Malley WJ: *Clinical blood gases: Assessment and intervention*, ed 2, St Louis, 2005, Elsevier-Saunders.
2. Comroe JH, Botelho SH: The unreliability of cyanosis in recognition of arterial anoxemia. *Am J Med Sci* 214:1–6, 1947.
3. Severinghaus JW, Astrup PB: History of blood gas analysis. VI. Oximetry. *J Clin Monit* 2:270–288, 1986.
4. Cairo JM: *Mosby's respiratory care equipment*, ed 9, St Louis, 2014, Elsevier.
5. Hannhart B, Habberer JP, Saunier C, et al: Accuracy and precision of fourteen pulse oximeters. *Eur Respir J* 4:115–119, 1991.
6. Kacmarek RM, Stoller JK, Heuer AJ: *Egan's fundamentals of respiratory care*, ed 10, St Louis, 2013, Elsevier.
7. Kelleher JF: Pulse oximetry. *J Clin Monit* 5:37–62, 1989.
8. Tremper KK, Barker SJ: Pulse oximetry. *Anesthesiology* 70:98–108, 1989.
9. Jubran A: Pulse oximetry. *Crit Care* 3:R11–R17, 1999.
10. Dumas C, Wahr JA, Tremper KK: Clinical evaluation of a prototype motion artifact resistant pulse oximeter in the recovery room. *Anesth Analg* 83:269–272, 1996.
11. Trillo RA, Aukburg S: Dapsone-induced methemoglobinemia and pulse oximetry. *Anesthesiology* 77:594–596, 1992.
12. Scheller MS, Unger RJ, Kelner MJ: Effects of intravenously administered dyes on pulse oximetry readings. *Anesthesiology* 65:550–552, 1986.
13. Coté CJ, Goldstein EA, Fushsman WH, et al: The effect of nail polish on pulse oximetry. *Anesth Analg* 67:683–686, 1988.
14. Rubin AS: Nail polish color can affect pulse oximeter saturation. *Anesthesiology* 68:825, 1988.
15. Emery JR: Skin pigmentation as an influence on the accuracy of pulse oximetry. *J Perinatol* 7:329–330, 1987.
16. Ries AL, Prewitt LM, Johnson JJ: Skin color and ear oximetry. *Chest* 96:287–290, 1989.
17. Jubran A: Advances in respiratory monitoring during mechanical ventilation. *Chest* 116:1416–1425, 1999.
18. Chelluri L, Snyder JV, Bird JR: Accuracy of pulse oximetry with hyperbilirubinemia. *Respir Care* 36:1383–1386, 1991.
19. Veyckemans F, Baele P, Guillaume JE, et al: Hyperbilirubinemia does not interfere with hemoglobin saturation measured by pulse oximetry. *Anesthesiology* 70:118–122, 1989.
20. Amar D, Neidswski J, Wald A, et al: Fluorescent light interferes with pulse oximetry. *J Clin Monit* 5:135–136, 1989.
21. Jubran A, Tobin MJ: Monitoring during mechanical ventilation. In Tobin MJ, editor: *Principles and practice of mechanical ventilation*, ed 3, New York, 2013, McGraw-Hill, pp 1139–1165.
22. Fluck RR, Schroeder C, Frani G, et al: Does ambient light affect the accuracy of pulse oximetry? *Respir Care* 48:677–680, 2003.
23. Perkins GD, McAuley DF, Giles S, et al: Do changes in pulse oximeter saturation predict equivalent changes in arterial oxygen saturation? *Crit Care* 7:R67–R71, 2003.
24. Kacmarek RM, Hess D, Stoller JK: *Monitoring in respiratory care*, St Louis, 2003, Mosby.
25. Carlin BW, Claussen JL, Ries AL: The use of cutaneous oximetry in the prescription of long-term oxygen therapy. *Chest* 94:239–241, 1988.
26. Baeckert P, Bucher HU, Fallenstein F, et al: Is pulse oximetry reliable in detecting hypoxemia in the neonate? *Adv Exp Med Biol* 220:165–169, 1987.
27. AARC Clinical Practice Guideline: Capnography/capnometry during mechanical ventilation, 2011. *Respir Care* 56:503–509, 2011.
28. Gravenstein JS, Paulus DA, Hayes TJ: *Gas monitoring in clinical practice*, ed 2, Newton, Mass., 1995, Butterworth-Heinemann.
29. Gravenstein JS, Jaffe MB, Paulus DA: *Capnography*, Cambridge, UK, 2011, Cambridge University Press.
30. Hess D: Capnometry and capnography: technical aspects, physiologic aspects, and clinical applications. *Respir Care* 35:557–573, 1990.
31. West JB: *Ventilation/blood flow and gas exchange*, ed 5, New York, 1990, Blackwell.
32. Ludviksdottir D, Janson C, Hogman M, et al: Exhaled nitric oxide and its relationship to airway responsiveness and atopy in asthma. BHR Study Group. *Respir Med* 93:552–556, 1999.
33. Franklin PJ, Stick SM, LeSouef PN, et al: measuring exhaled nitric oxide levels in adults: the importance of atopy and airway responsiveness. *Chest* 126:1540–1545, 2004.
34. Huch A, Huch R, Arner B, et al: Continuous transcutaneous oxygen tension measurement with a heated electrode. *Scand J Clin Lab Med* 31:269–275, 1973.
35. Huch R, Huch A, Albani M, et al: Transcutaneous PO_2 monitoring in routine management of infants and children with cardiorespiratory problems. *Pediatrics* 57:681–690, 1976.
36. Lubbers DW: Theory and development of transcutaneous oxygen pressure measurement. *Int Anesthesiol Clin* 25:31–65, 1987.
37. Severinghaus JS, Bradley FA: Electrodes for blood PO_2 and PCO_2 determination. *J Appl Physiol* 13:515–520, 1958.
38. Severinghaus JS, Stafford M, Bradley FA: Transcutaneous PO_2 electrode design, calibration, and temperature gradient problems. *Acta Anaesthesiol Scand* 68(Suppl):118–122, 1978.
39. Reed RL, Maier RV, Del Londicho M, et al: Correlation of hemodynamic variables with transcutaneous PO_2 measurements in critically ill patients. *J Trauma* 25:1045–1053, 1985.
40. Lubbers DW: Theoretical basis of transcutaneous blood gas measurements. *Crit Care Med* 9:721–733, 1981.
41. AARC Clinical Practice Guideline: Transcutaneous monitoring of carbon dioxide and oxygen 2012. *Respir Care* 57:1955–1962, 2012.
42. Wahr JA, Tremper KK: Noninvasive oxygen monitoring techniques. *Crit Care Clin* 11:199–217, 1995.
43. AARC Clinical Practice Guideline: Metabolic measurement using indirect calorimetry during mechanical ventilation—2004 revision and update. *Respir Care* 39:1170–1175, 2004.
44. Ferrannini E: The theoretical basis of indirect calorimetry: a review. *Metabolism* 37:287–301, 1987.
45. Head CA, Grossman GD, Jordan JC, et al: A valve system for the accurate measurement of energy expenditure in mechanically ventilated patients. *Respir Care* 30:969–973, 1985.
46. Browning JA, Linberg SE, Turney SZ, et al: The effects of a fluctuating F_1O_2 on metabolic measurements in mechanically ventilated patients. *Crit Care Med* 10:82–85, 1982.
47. Ultman JS, Bursztein S: Analysis of error in determination of respiratory gas exchange at varying FIO_2. *J Appl Physiol* 50:210–216, 1981.
48. Consolazio CF, Johnson RE, Pecora IJ: *Physiological measurements of metabolic function in man*, New York, 1963, McGraw-Hill.
49. Aschoff P, Pohl J: Rhythm variations in energy metabolism. *Fed Proc* 29:1541–1542, 1970.
50. Weissman C, Kemper M: Metabolic measurements in the critically ill. *Crit Care Clin* 11:169–197, 1995.
51. Vermeij C, Feenstra BWA, Van Lanchot JB, et al: Day to day variability of energy expenditure in critically ill surgical patients. *Crit Care Med* 17:623–626, 1989.
52. Askanazi J, Carpentier YA, Elwyn D, et al: Influence of total parenteral nutrition on fuel utilization in injury and sepsis. *Ann Surg* 191:40–46, 1980.
53. Askanazi J, Rosenbaum SH, Hyman AL, et al: Respiratory changes induced by large glucose loads of total parenteral nutrition. *JAMA* 243:1444–1447, 1980.
54. Marini JJ: Lung mechanics determination at the bedside: instrumentation and clinical application. *Respir Care* 35:669–696, 1990.
55. Kacmarek RM, Hess DR: Airway pressure, flow, and volume waveforms and lung mechanics during mechanical ventilation. In Kacmarek RM, Hess DR, Stoller JK, editors: *Monitoring in respiratory care*, St Louis, 1993, Mosby, pp 497–544.
56. Nilsestuen JO, Hargett KD: Using ventilator graphics to identify patient-ventilator asynchrony. *Respir Care* 50:202–234, 2005.
57. East TD: What makes noninvasive monitoring tick? A review of basic engineering principles. *Respir Care* 35:500–519, 1990.
58. Sanborn WG: Monitoring respiratory mechanics during mechanical ventilation: where do the signals come from? *Respir Care* 50:28–52, 2005.
59. Osborne JJ, Wilson RM: Monitoring mechanical properties of the lung. In Spence AA, editor: *Respiratory monitoring in the intensive care clinic*, New York, 1982, Churchill-Livingstone.
60. Levitzky MG: *Pulmonary physiology*, ed 8, New York, 2013, McGraw-Hill.
61. Branson RD, Davis K: Work of breathing by five ventilators used for long-term support: the effects of PEEP and simulated patient demand. *Respir Care* 40:1270–1278, 1995.
62. Marini JJ: The role of the inspiratory circuit in the work of breathing during mechanical ventilation. *Respir Care* 32:419–430, 1987.
63. Hess DR, Kacmarek RM: *Essentials of mechanical ventilation*, ed 2, New York, 2002, McGraw-Hill.

64. Branson RD: Enhanced capabilities of current ICU ventilators: do they really benefit patients? *Respir Care* 36:362–376, 1991.

65. MacIntyre NR: Weaning from mechanical ventilatory support: volume-assisting intermittent breaths versus pressure-assisting every breath. *Respir Care* 33:121–125, 1988.

66. Marini JJ, Capps J, Culver B: The inspiratory work of breathing during assisted mechanical ventilation. *Chest* 87:612–618, 1985.

67. Henning RJ, Shubin H, Weil MH: The measurement of the work of breathing for the clinical assessment of ventilator dependence. *Crit Care Med* 5:264–268, 1977.

68. Benditt JO: Esophageal and gastric pressure measurements. *Respir Care* 50:68–75, 2005.

69. Bellemare F, Grassino A: Effect of pressure and timing of contraction on human diaphragm fatigue. *J Appl Physiol* 53:1190–1195, 1982.

70. Field S, Sanci S, Grassino A: Respiratory muscle oxygen consumption estimated by the diaphragm pressure-time index. *J Appl Physiol* 57:44–51, 1984.

71. Sassoon CSH, Light RW, Lodia R, et al: Pressure-time product during continuous positive airway pressure, pressure support ventilation, and T-piece during weaning from mechanical ventilation. *Am Rev Respir Dis* 143:469–475, 1991.

Hemodynamic Monitoring

OUTLINE

KEY TERMS

- Afterload
- Balloon-tipped, flow-directed catheter
- Bradycardia
- Cardiac index
- Cardiac work
- Central venous lines
- Contractility
- Diastole
- dP/dT
- Ejection fraction
- Fick principle
- French size
- Incisura
- Physiological shunt
- Preload
- Pulmonary artery catheter
- Pulmonary vascular resistance
- Pulse pressure
- Retrograde
- Stroke index
- Stroke work
- Swan-Ganz catheter
- Systemic vascular resistance
- Tachycardia

LEARNING OBJECTIVES   *On completion of this chapter, the reader will be able to do the following:*

1. Discuss how changes in heart rate, preload, contractility, and afterload can alter cardiac function and cardiac output.
2. Identify indicators of left ventricular preload, contractility, and afterload.
3. Name the major components of a hemodynamic monitoring system.
4. Explain the proper technique for insertion and maintenance of a systemic arterial line, and list the most common complications that can occur with this type of monitoring system.
5. Describe the procedures for insertion and placement of a central venous line, and list the potential complications associated with these devices.
6. Interpret the waveforms generated during the insertion of a pulmonary artery catheter.
7. Calculate arterial and venous oxygen content, cardiac output, cardiac index, stroke index, cardiac cycle time, left ventricular stroke work index, right ventricular stroke work index, and pulmonary and systemic vascular resistance.

8. List normal values for measured and derived hemodynamic variables.
9. Describe the most common complications associated with pulmonary artery catheterization, and discuss strategies that can be used to minimize these complications.
10. Compare the effects of spontaneous and mechanical ventilation breathing on hemodynamic values.
11. Define the following terms: *incisura, pulse pressure, stroke index, stroke work, systemic vascular resistance, pulmonary vascular resistance, ejection fraction.*
12. Explain how measurements of pulmonary artery occlusion pressure can be used to evaluate left ventricular function.
13. Differentiate between cardiogenic and noncardiogenic pulmonary edema using hemodynamic parameters.
14. From a patient case, describe how hemodynamic monitoring can be used in the diagnosis and treatment of selected cases of critically ill patients.

The primary indication for hemodynamic monitoring is the management of critically ill patients who demonstrate evidence of compromised cardiovascular function. As such, hemodynamic monitoring can be used for the diagnosis and treatment of life-threatening conditions, such as shock, heart failure, pulmonary hypertension, complicated myocardial infarction, post–cardiac surgery, acute respiratory distress syndrome (ARDS), chest trauma, severe burn injury, and severe dehydration.

Invasive hemodynamic monitoring requires the insertion of arterial and intracardiac catheters. Measurements typically include systemic arterial pressure, central venous pressure, pulmonary artery (PA) pressures, as well as arterial and mixed venous blood gases and cardiac output. Once obtained, these measurements can be used to calculate a series of derived variables, including oxygen delivery, cardiac index (CI), stroke index, vascular resistance, and cardiac work, which in turn can be used to better define abnormalities in cardiopulmonary function and ultimately guide therapeutic interventions.

The efficacy and potential risks of hemodynamic monitoring have been the subject of considerable debate. Although the frequency of using invasive techniques has significantly decreased with the introduction of noninvasive technology (e.g., pulse oximetry, cardiac ultrasound), most agree that the benefits outweigh the risks in critically ill patients who require continuous invasive hemodynamic monitoring. A consensus statement released in 2000 by the National Heart, Lung, and Blood Institute and the U.S. Food and Drug Administration suggested that more randomized clinical studies should be performed to better determine which patients would benefit most from hemodynamic monitoring.[1] Furthermore, it was agreed that all clinicians involved in hemodynamic monitoring should have a working knowledge of cardiovascular physiology and the technical problems most often encountered with this type of monitoring. This chapter presents information that will help clinicians avoid many of the technical problems associated with hemodynamic monitoring. It also provides a concise description of the measurements and derived variables that are most often used and explains how they can be applied to patient treatment.

REVIEW OF CARDIOVASCULAR PRINCIPLES

It is important to understand the sequence of mechanical events occurring during the cardiac cycle to appreciate fully the various factors that influence hemodynamic measurements. Figure 11-1 is a Wiggers diagram that illustrates the pressure and volume events that occur in the right atrium, left ventricle, and aorta during a single heartbeat. A more detailed description of these events can be found in the references listed at the end of this chapter.[2,3]

Factors Influencing Cardiac Output

The outputs of the right and left ventricle are ultimately influenced by four main factors: heart rate, preload, contractility, and afterload. An individual's heart rate, which is simply the number of times the heart beats per minute, can vary considerably, depending on the patient's age and body habitus, core temperature, level of activity, and even psychological state. Indeed, heart rates can range from 50 to 200 beats per minute in a normal healthy adult.

The **preload,** which is typically defined as the filling pressure of the ventricle at the end of ventricular **diastole,** is estimated by measuring the end-diastolic pressures (EDP). The amount of blood present in the ventricle at the end of ventricular diastole depends on the level of venous return and the compliance of the ventricle. Ultimately preload reflects the length of the ventricular muscle fibers and thus the ability of these fibers to generate the necessary tension in the next ventricular contraction. This is a basic principle of cardiovascular physiology (sometimes called the Frank-Starling mechanism or length–tension relationship). This principle states in most basic terms that the heart pumps what it receives. This relationship holds until one reaches relatively high ventricular volumes, when the muscle fibers are overstretched and unable to generate the necessary tension to elicit a contraction that will adequately eject the required stroke volume. The end result at these higher ventricular volumes is ventricular dilation and failure.

The right ventricular end-diastolic pressure (RVEDP) is typically used as an indicator of the right ventricular preload, and the left ventricular end-diastolic pressure (LVEDP) is used to estimate the left ventricular preload. Because both of these intracardiac pressures are difficult to measure in the critical care setting, clinicians rely on measurements of right atrial (RAP) or central venous pressure (CVP) and pulmonary artery occlusion pressure (PAOP, which for practical purposes is equivalent to pulmonary capillary wedge pressure, or PCWP) to estimate the RVEDP and LVEDP, respectively. It is important to understand that CVP and PAOP can accurately reflect the RVEDP and LVEDP only when the former measurements are made at the end of ventricular diastole and if there is no evidence of valve dysfunction because they are registering **retrograde*** pressures in the right and left atria.

Contractility, which is related to the force that the ventricle generates during each cardiac cycle, can be estimated using the **ejection fraction,** which is calculated as the ratio of the stroke volume to the ventricular end-diastolic volume. For example, a 154-lb (70-kg) adult male typically has a stroke volume of about 70 mL and an end-diastolic volume of about 140 mL. His ejection fraction would be equal to 0.5 (70 mL/140 mL). Alternatively, contractility can be estimated by calculating the slope of ventricular pressure time interval during the initial period of contraction. This change in pressure relative to time (**dP/dT**) is thought to be a practical way of estimating the force of ventricular muscle contraction.

Afterload is usually defined as the impedance that the left and right ventricles must overcome to eject blood into the great vessels. Clinically, this impedance is better expressed as systemic and pulmonary vascular resistances. The **systemic vascular resistance (SVR)** is used to describe the afterload that the left ventricle must overcome to eject blood into the systemic circulation. The **pulmonary vascular resistance (PVR)** reflects the afterload that the right ventricle must overcome to eject blood into the pulmonary circulation. Increases in afterload are generally associated with reductions in cardiac output, whereas decreases in afterload are associated with increases in cardiac output. For example, systemic hypertension and pulmonary hypertension lead to increases in SVR and PVR, respectively. In both cases, the cardiac output will be reduced. Administering a systemic vasodilator (e.g., nitroprusside) or a pulmonary vasodilator (e.g., tolazoline) will reduce the SVR and PVR, respectively, and result in an increase in cardiac output.

---

*Retrograde means moving in the opposite direction. In this case, the catheter is measuring pressures downstream from the catheter tip. Measurements made at the end of diastole will occur when the atrioventricular valves are open. Any type of valve dysfunction that alters the path between the atria and the ventricles will therefore lead to erroneous measurements.

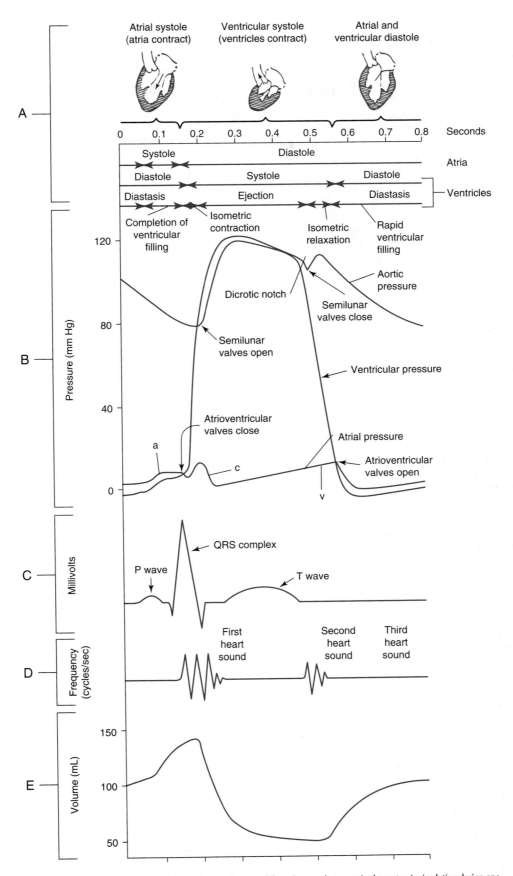

Fig. 11-1 Wiggers diagram illustrating the pressure, volume, and flow changes that occur in the systemic circulation during one cardiac cycle. **A,** Timing of cardiac events; **B,** simultaneous pressures created in the aorta, left ventricle, and left atrium during the cardiac cycle; **C,** electrical activity during the cardiac cycle; **D,** heart sounds corresponding to the cardiac cycle; **E,** ventricular blood volume during the cardiac cycle. (See text for additional information.) (From Moffett DF, Moffett SB, Schauf CL: Human physiology: foundations and frontiers, ed 2, St Louis, 1993, Mosby.)

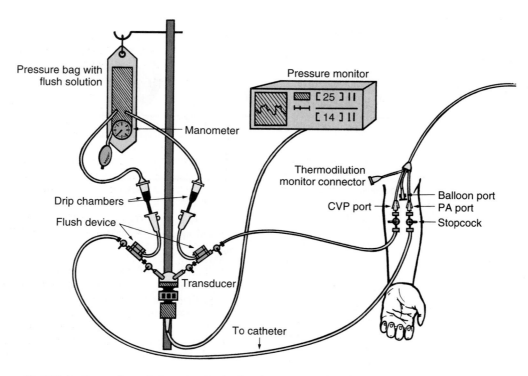

Fig. 11-2 Invasive vascular monitoring system showing the catheter connected from the vessel to a transducer and pressurized intravenous bag containing heparinized saline. The transducer is connected to an amplifier and recording device and monitor. (The transducer pictured is an older model used here for easier visualization.)

OBTAINING HEMODYNAMIC MEASUREMENTS

Clinicians who perform hemodynamic monitoring must understand the physical and technical factors that can influence intravascular measurements and thus determine the likelihood of obtaining meaningful data. The following sections first describe how hemodynamic measurements are obtained and then discuss how various pathophysiological events can alter pressure, volume, and flow tracings.

Hemodynamic Monitoring Systems

Hemodynamic monitoring systems consist of equipment that detects small physiological signal (vascular pressure) changes and converts them to electrical impulses, which can then be amplified and recorded on a computer monitor or strip chart recorder. As shown in the invasive vascular monitoring system in Fig. 11-2, a catheter is inserted into a peripheral artery, a central vein, or pulmonary artery. The catheter transmits pressure changes within the vessel or cardiac chamber through a hollow, plastic tubing filled with a heparinized solution of saline to a transducer, which converts these fluid pressure changes to a digital signal for display.

A strain gauge pressure transducer (Fig. 11-3) uses an electrical circuit known as a *Wheatstone bridge*.[3] The operating principle for this type of device is fairly straightforward. Fluid enters the dome portion of the transducer by way of the fluid-filled plastic line (see Figs. 11-2 and 11-3). A diaphragm separates the fluid-filled compartment from the electronic portion of the transducer. Pressure transmitted to the fluid-filled dome portion of the transducer causes movement of the diaphragm, which alters the length of the

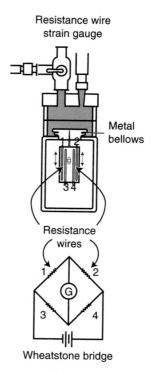

Fig. 11-3 Strain gauge pressure transducer incorporating a Wheatstone bridge. (From Cairo JM: Respiratory care equipment, ed 9. St Louis, 2014, Elsevier-Mosby.)

wires of the Wheatstone bridge. Changes in the length of the wires result in changes in resistance to the current flow through the Wheatstone bridge (i.e., an increase in the length of the wires results in an increased electrical resistance; decrease in length results in a decrease in resistance to electron flow). Thus the pressure changes are directly proportional to the change in current flow through the circuit and inversely proportional to the resistance offered by the circuit.

Fluid Pressures

Fluid can exert pressure while it is in motion (hydrodynamic pressure) or while at a standstill (hydrostatic pressure). These pressures play integral roles when using hemodynamic monitoring systems. Two factors affect fluid-filled systems:

1. A dynamic pressure element
2. Static pressure head

The dynamic pressure element is pressure applied to fluid inside a system by fluid outside a system. It has to do with catheter position in relation to the flow of the blood within the vessel. For example, for an arterial line placed in a radial artery to accurately measure pressures that are the direct result of the work of the left heart, it must be placed with the end of the catheter facing the source of blood flow ("looking" upstream toward the left ventricle). A PA catheter, which measures pressures within a vessel (e.g., pulmonary capillaries) or left heart chamber, must be placed so that the tip of the catheter is facing downstream of the flow of blood (i.e., right ventricle) to estimate blood pressures filling the left side of the heart.

Static pressure head refers to the pressure placed on the transducer as related to the tip of the catheter. To measure pressure accurately, the transducer must be at the same height or level as the catheter tip. If the catheter tip is higher than the transducer, the monitor will read higher than the actual pressure as a result of the fluid "pushing" downstream (because of gravity) from the catheter tip to the transducer. If the catheter tip is placed below the level of the transducer, the fluid will flow away from the transducer toward the catheter tip and produce a reading lower than the actual pressure. The degree of error is about 1.86 mm Hg for each centimeter of distance from the reference point (e.g., if the transducer is 5 cm above the reference point, then the corrected measurement should be 9.3 mm Hg [5 × 1.86 = 9.3]). This adjustment can be avoided by positioning the transducer at the level of the midthoracic line of the patient—the **epistatic** line—to measure CVP accurately. This is about 5 cm behind the sternal angle (the angle of Louis). Once the epistatic line has been determined, it is important to zero-balance the transducer to this reference point. Zero-balancing the transducer references the transducer to atmospheric pressure, which is usually read as 0 mmHg.

Systemic Artery Catheterization

Direct measurement of the systemic arterial pressure requires the insertion of a catheter into a peripheral artery, such as the radial, brachial, or femoral arteries. Note that the radial artery is the most commonly used site because of easy accessibility and because of collateral circulation to the hand from the ulnar artery. Either a percutaneous technique or a surgical cut-down technique can be used to insert the catheter. The percutaneous approach is most often used in the critical care setting; the surgical cut-down procedure is used when the percutaneous technique is unsuccessful.[4,5] Box 11-1 summarizes the recommended technique for inserting and maintaining a systemic arterial line (Key Point 11-1).

BOX 11-1 **Insertion and Maintenance of Arterial Catheters**

- Aseptically assemble, flush, and test tubing and catheter.
- Perform a modified Allen test to ensure ulnar artery refill time of 5 to 10 seconds.
- Prepare and drape the area of insertion (sterile technique is necessary).
- If necessary, infiltrate the skin around the insertion site with a local anesthetic (e.g., lidocaine).
- Percutaneously insert the catheter at approximately 30-degree angle. (If pulse is weak or otherwise inaccessible, surgical cut-down may be necessary.)
- Advance the catheter into the artery while holding the needle secure.
- Remove the needle and secure the catheter.
- Attach tubing for drip solution and observe monitor for proper waveform.
- Frequently monitor:
  - Insertion site for signs of infection
  - Extremity distal to insertion site for adequate circulation
- Catheter should be removed if:
  - There is clot formation as evidenced by difficulty with blood sampling or a persistently dampened waveform
  - Extremity distal to insertion site becomes ischemic
  - Insertion site becomes infected

Key Point **11-1** The Modified Allen test must be performed before a radial artery catheter is inserted.

After the catheter has been positioned in the artery, a surgical dressing is applied and the catheter is secured with tape or sutured to the skin. Maintenance of the arterial line requires the use of a continuous pressurized flush mechanism to irrigate the catheter with a heparinized solution at a low flow (e.g., 2 to 3 mL/h).[5] The irrigating solution of 0.9% sodium chloride (NaCl) containing 1 to 2 units of heparin per milliliter of normal saline (i.e., 100 to 200 units of heparin/dL). Commercially available arterial line sets also have a rapid flush mechanism for quickly clearing the catheter. Prolonged or frequent flushing of the arterial line should be avoided because this can lead to the inadvertent administration of large amounts of flush volume to the patient. This latter point is a particularly important issue for neonatal and pediatric patients who weigh less than 44 lb (20 kg).

Daily inspection of the insertion site for signs of infection, ischemia, and bleeding is essential to avoid serious complications. Certain factors can increase the risk of infections in patients with arterial lines:

- Insertion of the arterial line by surgical cut-down
- Prolonged cannulation (>4 days)
- Altered host defense

Distal ischemia should be suspected when pallor distal to the insertion site occurs, particularly if it is accompanied by pain and paresthesia in the affected limb. The most common cause of decreased perfusion is thrombus formation, which occludes the catheter tip. Other risk factors for acute distal ischemia include hypotension, severe peripheral vascular disease, and the use of vasopressor drugs.[4,5]

Fever in any patient with an intravascular line should alert the clinician to infectious complications. The catheter is removed if there is evidence of local infection or the presence of distal ischemia. Difficulty withdrawing blood or persistence of damped tracings should also alert the clinician to possible complications, such as the presence of air bubbles in the line or occlusion of the catheterized artery.

Bleeding can occur if the line becomes disconnected or is improperly handled. Hemorrhage is a distinct possibility if the line is left open; therefore the clinician should stabilize the catheterized site by taping the patient's arm to a board and placing it above the bed linen for easy observation. Another common problem encountered with the insertion of arterial lines is hematoma formation, which can occur if bleeding occurs under the skin during or immediately after the catheterization procedure. Hematoma typically occurs more often when the catheter is placed through a large-gauge needle.

Central Venous Lines

Catheters placed in the vena cava or right atria are generally called *central venous lines.* Although these lines are most often used to administer fluids, drugs, and nutritional solutions, they can also be used to monitor right heart pressures. During ventricular systole or atrial diastole, when the tricuspid valve is closed, the pressure measured in the right atrium or vena cava reflects the RAP. At the end of ventricular diastole and atrial systole, when the tricuspid valve is open, the pressure measured in the right atrium reflects the right ventricular pressure (RVP). Thus, the CVP measured at the end of ventricular diastole can be used to monitor intravenous (IV) fluid administration and to estimate the filling pressure or the preload of the right ventricle (i.e., RVEDP).

CVP catheters are usually inserted percutaneously into a large central vein, such as the internal jugular, or peripherally through the medial basilic or lateral cephalic vein.[6] Pressure measurements are usually performed during exhalation and when the patient is supine. The transducer is zeroed at the level of the right atrium. A normal value for CVP is 2 to 6 mm Hg.

The most common problems encountered with insertion of CVP catheters are pneumothorax, hemothorax, and vessel damage. Other potential complications include infection, thrombosis, and bleeding. Placement of the catheter usually is confirmed using radiography.

Pulmonary Artery Catheterization

Bedside catheterization of the right heart and pulmonary artery (PA) became possible when Swan and colleagues[7] introduced a **balloon-tipped, flow-directed catheter** in the early 1970s.[8] The balloon-tipped, flow-directed catheter (also referred to as the *Swan-Ganz catheter* or *pulmonary artery catheter*) (Fig. 11-4) is a multiple-lumen catheter constructed of radiopaque polyvinyl-chloride. The standard adult catheter is 110 cm in length and is available in 7 or 8 **French (Fr) sizes.** Remember that the *French* size divided by π or 3.14 equals the external diameter of the catheter in millimeters. Pediatric catheters are 60 cm in length and available in 4 or 5 Fr sizes. Both adult and pediatric catheters are marked at 10-cm increments. As with systemic arterial catheters, a pressurized flush solution must be run through the catheter at a rate of 1 to 5 mL/h (except when making pressure measurements) to prevent clot formation within the catheter's lumen.

Dual-lumen catheters have one lumen that connects to a balloon located near the tip of the catheter and a second lumen that runs the length of the catheter terminating at a port at the distal end of the catheter. Triple-lumen catheters have an additional proximal port that terminates approximately 30 cm from the tip of the catheter, or at the level of the right atrium. This third lumen can be used to measure right atrial pressures or for administrating intravenous medications.

Thermodilution catheters incorporate a fourth lumen, which contains electrical wires that connect to a thermistor located approximately $1\frac{1}{2}$ inches (3 cm) from the tip of the catheter. When measuring cardiac output using the thermodilution technique, a bolus of saline or 5% dextrose (cold or room temperature) is injected through the catheter's third lumen, which is positioned at the level of the right atrium. The cardiac output is calculated by

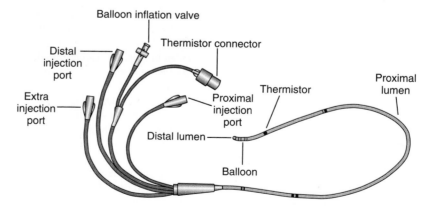

Fig. 11-4 Balloon-tipped, flow-directed right-sided heart catheter showing many of the features that are typically available on pulmonary artery (PA) catheters. Distal lumen opens into the PA. Fiberoptic filaments used for mixed venous oxygen saturation ($S\overline{V}O_2$) monitoring and the balloon are also located at the tip. The thermistor bead is located 1.5 inches from the tip and is connected by a wire through the catheter to the connector for the thermodilution cardiac output computer. The proximal lumen located 30 cm back from the tip opens into the right atrium. Catheters are available for ventricular, atrial, or atrioventricular sequential pacing using either pacemaker bands positioned on the catheter or pacing leads, which are passed through the lumen. Ventricular bands or lumens are located 20 cm from the tip; atrial, 30 cm from the tip.

integrating the change in temperature that is sensed by the thermistor near the tip of the catheter as the injected saline (or dextrose) solution mixes with the patient's pulmonary blood flow.

Pacing catheters with bands for atrial, ventricular, and atrioventricular (AV) cardiac pacing are also available. The bands, which are located approximately 20 cm from the tip of the catheter, have external leads that connect to a pacemaker.

As with CVP catheters, PA catheters can be inserted using a percutaneous approach or via surgical cut-down technique. The subclavian, internal jugular, external jugular, femoral, or antecubital veins are usually used for percutaneous insertion; surgical cut-down is often necessary when the subclavian or antecubital veins are used. The clinician must consider a number of potential complications when choosing an insertion site, including pneumothorax, arterial lacerations, venous thrombosis or phlebitis, and air embolism (Table 11-1).

TABLE **11-1**	**Insertion Sites of the Pulmonary Artery Catheter and Associated Problems**
Site	**Associated Problems**
Internal jugular	Pneumothorax, hemothorax
Subclavian	Severe thrombocytopenia (difficult-to-control bleeding), pneumothorax (more frequently than with internal jugular), hemothorax
Antecubital	Phlebitis; catheter tip may migrate with movement of the arm; difficult site for catheter advancement
Femoral	Phlebitis; catheter tip may migrate with movement of the leg

Positioning the catheter can be accomplished by fluoroscopy or by monitoring the pressure tracings generated as the catheter is slowly advanced into the right side of the heart and pulmonary artery. Fluoroscopy typically is reserved for the catheterization laboratory, whereas continuous pressure monitoring with electrocardiography is routinely used in the critical care setting.

Figure 11-5 shows a series of tracings obtained during PA catheter placement.[8,9] The catheter is introduced into the peripheral vein and slowly advanced until it enters the intrathoracic vessels (i.e., superior or inferior vena cava). When the catheter enters into the intrathoracic vessels, venous pulse waveforms with characteristic respiratory fluctuations are recorded. If these respiratory fluctuations are absent, the results obtained will be erroneous. Loss of these respiratory fluctuations may indicate that the stopcock is closed between the catheter and the pressure transducer. It can also occur if the catheter is kinked or a blood clot or air is present in the tubing. Once the catheter enters the intrathoracic vessels, the balloon is inflated with air so that it can be flow-directed by the blood through the right atrium and right ventricle into the pulmonary artery. (NOTE: It is important to fully inflate the balloon to avoid endocardial or pulmonary artery damage or induce ventricular arrhythmias.) Pediatric (4 to 5 Fr) catheters have a balloon volume of 0.8 mL; the balloon volume for adult (7 to 8 Fr) catheters is 1.5 mL. The catheter is slowly advanced until it wedges in a small pulmonary artery.

As shown in Fig. 11-5, the wedged position can be easily identified because the pulmonary artery occlusion pressure (PAOP) is characteristically lower than or equal to the pulmonary artery diastolic pressure. An overdamped tracing (i.e., loss of a distinctive PAOP waveform) usually indicates a mechanical problem, such as the presence of an air bubble in the catheter tubing, or the protrusion of the balloon over the tip of the catheter. The mean PAOP may exceed the PA diastolic pressure in patients with mitral

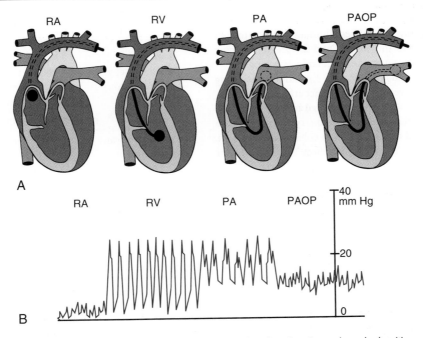

Fig. 11-5 The waveforms seen during the advancement of the catheter from the right atrium to the wedged position. **A,** Position of the pulmonary artery catheter in the heart. **B,** Corresponding waveforms seen on a pressure–time tracing as the catheter is advanced from the right atrium to the wedged position. *PA,* pulmonary artery; *PAOP,* pulmonary artery occlusion pressure; *RA,* right atrial pressure; *RV,* right ventricle. (From Adams AB: Monitoring the patient in the intensive care unit, In Kacmarek RM, Stoller JS, Heuer AJ, editors: Egan's fundamentals of respiratory care, ed 10, St Louis, 2013, Elsevier-Mosby.)

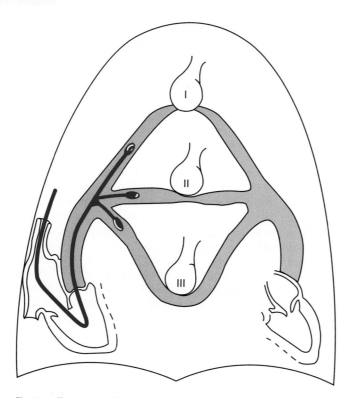

Fig. 11-6 The position of the pulmonary artery catheter tip in relation to West's zone of the lung. For the PAOP to be a valid estimate of left heart pressures, a continuous column of blood needs to be present between the catheter tip and the left atrium. In zones I and II, the pulmonary vessels may be partially or completely compressed by adjacent pulmonary alveolar pressures. (See text for additional information).

stenosis or mitral regurgitation.[10] The PAOP can be identified by another means; when the catheter occludes a small pulmonary artery, a continuous column of blood equilibrates between the left atrium and the distal port of the catheter and the pressure tracing will register a left atrial waveform (i.e., a, c, and v waves).

The catheter must be wedged in a zone 3 position in the lung to reflect the pulmonary venous pressure accurately.[11] As illustrated in Fig. 11-6, if the catheter is positioned in zone 1 or zone 2, the alveolar pressure will exceed the pulmonary venous pressure and cause the vessels distal to the balloon to collapse (Table 11-2). The intravascular pressure reading will reflect the intraalveolar pressure rather than the pressure transmitted from the left atrium. This problem is accentuated by the application of positive end-expiratory pressure (PEEP) during mechanical ventilation (i.e., the alveolar pressure rises) or by hemorrhage when the pulmonary venous pressure is reduced. We will discuss this problem in more detail later in this chapter (Key Point 11-2).

Key Point 11-2 The PA catheter must be wedged in a zone 3 position in the lung to reflect the pulmonary venous pressure accurately.

Table 11-3 lists the most common complications associated with right heart catheterization using a balloon-tipped, flow-directed catheter. Ventricular arrhythmias are fairly common during catheter insertion and often are self-limiting. Electrolyte disturbances, hypoxemia, and acidosis increase the risk of developing ventricular

TABLE 11-2   **West's Zones of the Lung**

Lung Zone	Pressure Relationships	Explanation
Zone 1	$P_{alv} > P_a > P_v$	Basically functions as alveolar dead space—ventilation in excess of perfusion
Zone 2	$P_a > P_{alv} > P_v$	Blood flow is due to the pressure difference between pulmonary artery and alveolar pressures
Zone 3	$P_a > P_v > P_{alv}$	Blood flow is due to arteriovenous pressure differences

P_a, Arterial pressure; P_{alv}, alveolar pressure; $P_{\bar{v}}$, venous pressure.

TABLE 11-3   **Complications Associated with Pulmonary Artery Catheterization**

Complications	Causes
Cardiac Arrhythmias	Heart valve or endocardium irritation by the catheter
Premature ventricular contraction (PVC)	
Premature atrial contraction (PAC)	
Ventricular tachycardia	
Ventricular fibrillation	
Atrial flutter	
Atrial fibrillation	
INSERTION PROCEDURE OR INSERTION SITE	
Infection	Nonsterile technique or irritation of the wound
Pneumothorax	Air entering pleural space during insertion
Air embolism	Air entering vessel during insertion
Access vessel thrombosis	Irritation of vessel by catheter or nonsterile insertion technique or phlebitis
PULMONARY CIRCULATION	
Pulmonary artery rupture or perforation	Overinflation of balloon
Pulmonary infarction	Overinflation of balloon, prolonged wedging, clots formed in or near the catheter, or catheter advancement into a smaller artery
PULMONARY ARTERY CATHETER	
Balloon rupture—air embolism	Loss of balloon elasticity or overinflation
Catheter knotting	Excessive catheter movement
Dampened waveform	Air in line, clot in the system, kinks in line, catheter tip against vessel wall, overwedging, or blood on the transducer
Catheter whip or fling	High cardiac output or abnormal vessel diameter.

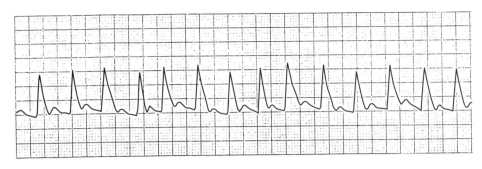

Fig. 11-7 A typical arterial pressure tracing.

BOX 11-2 Risk Factors for Catheter-Associated Pulmonary Artery Rupture

- Age >60 years
- Pulmonary hypertension
- Improper balloon inflation
- Improper catheter positioning
- Cardiopulmonary bypass surgery
- Anticoagulation therapy

TABLE 11-4 Normal Blood Pressures and Heart Rates in Children

Age	Blood Pressure Average for Males (girls 5% lower)	HEART RATE Average	Range
Neonate	75/50	140	100-190
1-6 months	80/50	145	110-190
6-12 months	90/65	140	110-180
1-2 years	95/65	125	100-160
2-6 years	100/60	100	65-130
6-12 years	110/60	80	55-110
12-16 years	110/65	75	55-100

Data from Rubenstein JS, Hageman JR: Monitoring of critically ill infants and children, Crit Care Clin 4:621-639, 1988.

ectopy. Careful monitoring of the patient's electrocardiogram (ECG) during catheter placement can alert the clinician of the development of arrhythmias and reduce chances of provoking a potentially lethal complication such as ventricular tachycardia and fibrillation.

Box 11-2 lists the risk factors most often associated with PA infarction and rupture.[12,13] PA infarction and rupture can be minimized by preventing thrombus development, which is accomplished by instilling a continuous flushed solution containing heparin. Pulmonary infarction and rupture can also be reduced by ensuring that the catheter balloon is deflated after wedge pressure measurements are made. Furthermore, it is important that the balloon is inflated for only 15 to 30 seconds when measuring the PAOP, particularly in patients with pulmonary hypertension. Balloon rupture is most often associated with prolonged duration of catheterization because the balloon will typically lose its elasticity with exposure to blood.

INTERPRETATION OF HEMODYNAMIC PROFILES

As mentioned previously, accurate interpretation of hemodynamic data requires a working knowledge of cardiovascular physiology. The hemodynamic profile ultimately focuses on those factors that influence cardiac output, namely, heart rate, preload, contractility, and afterload.

The information in this section provides an overview of basic measurements and derived variables used in a standard hemodynamic profile. A list of excellent references related to the use of hemodynamic monitoring in critical care can be found at the end of this chapter for more detailed information about this area of clinical physiology.

Heart Rate

The resting heart rate of a healthy adult is typically 60 to 100 beats/min. The heart rates for neonates and infants are considerably

higher. Although the resting heart rates for toddlers and adolescents are higher than for adult subjects, the difference is minimal by the end of the first decade of life.[14] Table 11-4 compares the mean and normal range for heart rate at various stages of life.[14]

Bradycardia (heart rates <60 beats/min) is associated with increases in parasympathetic tone or decreases in sympathetic tone. **Tachycardia** (heart rates >100 beats/min) is associated with increases in sympathetic tone or decreases in parasympathetic tone.

The typical adult can maintain an adequate cardiac output at heart rates of 40 to 50 beats/min as long as stroke volume increases proportionally. (Well-trained athletes are good examples of this concept.) Cardiac output will increase with heart rates up to about 200 to 220 beats/min, assuming that the patient responds normally to sympathoadrenal stimulation.[15] Heart rates above 220 beats/min cause a decrease in cardiac output because diastolic filling time is reduced (i.e., decreased ventricular filling from reduced venous return).

Systemic Arterial Pressure

Figure 11-7 illustrates a typical systemic arterial pressure tracing. Normal systemic arterial pressure (systolic/diastolic pressures) for adult subjects range from 90 to 140 mm Hg/60 to 90 mm Hg with a normal mean arterial pressure (MAP) of 70 to 100 mm Hg.*

*The MAP can be calculated in two ways. MAP = diastolic pressure + ⅓ (pulse pressure). Alternatively, MAP can be calculated as (systolic pressure + 2[diastolic pressure])/3.

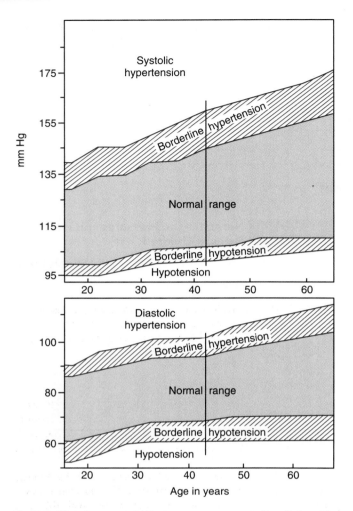

Fig. 11-8 Effect of age on arterial blood pressure measurements. (From Rushmer RF: Cardiovascular dynamics, ed 4, Philadelphia, 1976, W.B. Saunders.)

Figure 11-8 shows the effect of age on systolic and diastolic pressure in adult subjects.[16] It is generally accepted that systemic hypertension exists when the systolic arterial pressure is greater than 140 mm Hg and the diastolic pressure is greater than 90 mm Hg. Systemic hypotension is associated with systolic pressures less than 100 mm Hg and diastolic pressures less than 60 mm Hg. It is important to recognize that systemic arterial pressures in children, particularly very young children, are significantly different from adult subjects (Table 11-4).[14]

Although it may not be apparent, the systemic arterial pressure waveform will change in shape and magnitude, depending on the site of the measurement and the age of the patient. For example, systolic pressure increases as the site of measurement moves away from the heart. This effect is more obvious in young patients than in older patients. Diastolic pressure, on the other hand, is affected by vascular tone. An increase in diastolic pressure is associated with vasoconstriction, whereas a decrease in diastolic pressure is associated with vasodilation.

Changes in vascular tone can also cause the **incisura** to shift on the downslope of the arterial pressure tracing.[16,17] Vasodilation will cause it to shift closer to the baseline. The dicrotic notch also becomes less distinct as the site of measurement is moved farther

from the heart. Indeed, it may not be present in arterial pressure tracing obtained from the femoral artery.

Pulse pressure, which is the difference between the systolic and diastolic pressures, is influenced primarily by the stroke volume and the arterial compliance. A wide pulse pressure is associated with an increased stroke volume and a decreased arterial compliance; a narrow pulse pressure is associated with a decreased stroke volume and an increased arterial compliance.

Right Atrial and Pulmonary Artery Pressures

Proper positioning of the balloon flotation catheter allows for continuous monitoring of RAP and PA pressure, and intermittent measurements of the PAOP. The RAP can be continuously monitored through the proximal lumen of a PA catheter or through a CVP line. PA pressures can be monitored continuously through the distal lumen of a PA catheter. Left atrial and ventricular pressures can be measured intermittently during PAOP determinations. PAOP determinations represent retrograde pressure measurements that are obtained by inflating the balloon of the pulmonary artery catheter until it occludes a small pulmonary artery and wedges to block blood flow past the catheter tip. As mentioned previously, PAOP measured at the end of ventricular diastole reflects LVEDP because the mitral valve is open and the pressure in the left ventricle is transmitted backwards into the pulmonary circulation to the catheter tip.

Direct measurements of right ventricular pressures are usually only obtained during insertion of the catheter. Identification of the right ventricular pressure waveform during continuous monitoring indicates that the catheter has slipped into the right ventricle. It should be repositioned by reinflating the balloon and allowing the blood flow to carry the catheter back into the pulmonary artery. The balloon should be deflated after the catheter is repositioned in the PA. As mentioned, the balloon should be inflated for short periods of time when measuring PAOP.

Atrial Pressures

The RAP and left atrial pressure (LAP) are reported as mean values rather than as systolic and diastolic values. The RAP (more specifically CVP) normally ranges from 2 to 6 mm Hg; the LAP, as estimated from PAOP, ranges from 5 to 12 mm Hg. CVP and PAOP measurements commonly are used to determine overall fluid balance. A low CVP or PAOP suggests hypovolemia, whereas elevations of either of these pressures indicates hypervolemia or ventricular failure (Key Point 11-3).

Key Point 11-3 It is important to remember that CVP and PAOP reflect right and left ventricular pressures and volumes, respectively, only when the measurements are made at the end of ventricular diastole. Also tricuspid and mitral valve disease (e.g., stenosis or regurgitation) can alter the retrograde transmission of pressure from the right ventricle to the right atrium (CVP) or from the left ventricle to the left atrium and ultimately the pulmonary circulation (PAOP).

The PAOP also plays an important role in assessment of pulmonary hydrostatic pressure in the formation of pulmonary edema. PAOP can help distinguish cardiogenic pulmonary edema (increased pulmonary capillary hydrostatic pressure) from noncardiogenic pulmonary edema (normal pulmonary capillary hydrostatic pressure) as occurs in ARDS. For example, the finding of bilateral infiltrates

| BOX 11-3 | Causes of Abnormal Right Atrial and Pulmonary Artery Occlusion Pressure (PAOP) Values and Patterns |

Abnormal Values

Elevated Right Atrial Pressure (RAP)
Volume overload
Right ventricular (RV) failure
Tricuspid stenosis or regurgitation
Cardiac tamponade
Constrictive pericarditis
Chronic left ventricular (LV) failure

Elevated Pulmonary Artery Occlusion Pressure (PAOP)
Volume overload
Left ventricle failure
Mitral stenosis or regurgitation
Cardiac tamponade
Constrictive pericarditis
High PEEP

Low RAP or PAOP
Hypovolemia

Abnormal Patterns

Large a Waves
Tricuspid/mitral stenosis
Decreased ventricular compliance
Compliance
Loss of atrioventricular synchrony
Third-degree block
Any other electrical dissociation

Absent a Waves
Atrial fibrillation
Atrial flutter
Junctional rhythms
Paced rhythms
Ventricular rhythms

Modified from Daily EK: Hemodynamic waveform analysis, *J Cardiovasc Nurs* 15:6-22, 2001, p. 11.

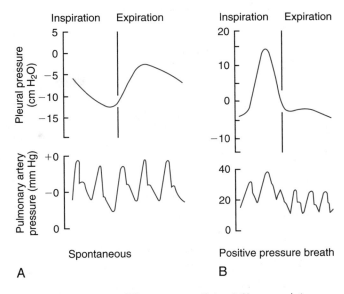

Fig. 11-9 Pulmonary artery (PA) response to ventilation. **A,** PA response during ventilation. The PA pressure falls during inspiration and rises during expiration. **B,** PA pressure response during mechanical ventilation. Notice that the PA pressure rises during inspiration and falls during expiration.

on chest radiographs coupled with a PAOP greater than 25 mm Hg suggests the presence of cardiogenic pulmonary edema resulting from left-sided heart failure.[18,19] This is in contrast to a finding of bilateral infiltrates on chest radiography with a normal PAOP, which would indicate the presence of noncardiogenic pulmonary edema resulting from damage to the alveolar-capillary membrane and suggests the presence of ARDS.

Box 11-3 lists several other conditions that can adversely affect RAP and PAOP values and waveforms.[17,18] Some conditions affect the magnitude of the RAP and LAP, whereas other pathophysiological events alter the contour of these atrial waveforms.

Pulmonary Artery Pressure

The PA pressure waveform resembles the systemic arterial waveform previously discussed. However, the PA systolic and diastolic pressures are considerably lower than the systemic pressures (e.g., the PA systolic pressure for a healthy adult is 15 to 35 mm Hg and the PA diastolic pressure is 5 to 15 mm Hg). As does the systemic arterial pressure tracing, the PA pressure tracing shows a rapid rise to peak pressure during systole followed by a gradual tapering to the dicrotic notch (which in this case represents closure of the pulmonic valve) and eventual descent to the end-diastolic level.

The baseline of the PA pressure tracing shows characteristic respiratory fluctuations arising from changes in the intrathoracic pressure (Fig. 11-9).[17] With spontaneous breathing, the intrapleural pressure decreases during inspiration, causing the PA wave pattern to descend. Conversely, with spontaneous expiration, intrapleural pressure increases and the wave rises. With positive pressure breathing, the curve rises as intrapleural pressures become positive

and falls during the expiratory phase.[19] The intrapleural pressure is the same for spontaneous (negative pressure) and positive pressure breathing at the end of expiration as long as PEEP is not used. For this reason, PA pressure, by convention, is measured at end expiration.

The mode of mechanical ventilation used can also significantly affect measured hemodynamic parameters.[19,20] It has been shown that the lower mean inspiratory pressures present with IMV and PSV minimize the hemodynamic effects of positive intrathoracic pressure and help maintain right heart preload and cardiac output.[20] Pressure-controlled ventilation has about the same effect on hemodynamic values as does volume-controlled ventilation. However, pressure control inverse ratio ventilation (PC-IRV) decreases CI and thus oxygen delivery (DO$_2$).[21-23]

Use of PEEP, either applied or inadvertent (e.g., auto-PEEP), at levels greater than 15 cm H$_2$O, can produce erroneously elevated pressure readings. The pressures in the thoracic circulation will rise when using PEEP therapy because of compression of the vessels by the increased lung volumes (increased functional residual capacity (FRC). PAOP, which reflects preload of the left side of the heart, is a valuable parameter to monitor when performing an optimum PEEP study. If PAOP increases significantly during the study, it could indicate overinflation of the alveoli. Actual blood flow through the vessels might not be affected because the transmural pressure (the pressure difference between inside and outside a vessel) may not have actually decreased.

It is recommended that a patient not be taken off the ventilator, nor should PEEP be discontinued to measure PAOP, if it is desirable to assess cardiac filling during mechanical ventilation.[20] If the patient requires high levels of ventilatory support or PEEP or both, discontinuing this support for the time it would take to measure PAOP accurately could produce hypoxemia and hypoventilation, from which the patient would recover very slowly.

Some practitioners calculate an airway pressure transmission ratio (APTR) and correct the PAOP obtained during ventilation by

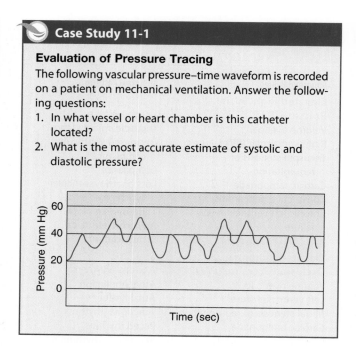

Fig. 11-10 Tracings illustrating both airway pressures and hemodynamic waveforms used to identify end expiration. (Redrawn from Ahrens TS, Taylor LA: Hemodynamic waveform analysis, Philadelphia, 1992, W.B. Saunders. Used with permission.)

this ratio. APTR is calculated by measuring the airway pressure change during a breath and the respiratory variation in PAOP. This procedure is performed with the catheter in the wedge position and evaluated over several breaths. Change in pressure (ΔP) equals the plateau pressure ($P_{plateau}$) − EEP (end-expiratory pressure). The respiratory-induced change in PAOP is the maximum mean PAOP minus the minimum mean PAOP (during a ventilator breath).[20] The transmission ratio is the PAOP divided by the change in airway pressure. The resulting "true" PAOP is:

$$PAOP = EEP \times (1 - PT_{PAOP} \times PAOP)$$

where PT_{PAOP} is the PAOP pressure transmission ratio.[20]

It may not be appropriate to correct PAOP relative to the PEEP level because the practitioner does not know what effect lung zones and lung compliance actually have on PAOP. It may be prudent to trend the patient data rather than to try to obtain an absolute value. It is interesting to note that right atrial pressure (i.e., CVP) may be a more accurate indicator of LV end-diastolic volume than estimating APTR when a total PEEP of 10 cm H_2O or greater is present.[20]

Figure 11-10 shows both airway pressures and pulmonary artery pressure during positive pressure breathing. Figure 11-11 shows the effect of varying levels of PEEP on PA pressure measurements.

Pathologic conditions and pharmacologic interventions can significantly affect PA pressure. Pulmonary hypertension, pulmonary embolus, and congestive heart failure are associated with increased PVR, which in turn leads to increased PA systolic pressure. In contrast, inhaled nitric oxide, which selectively dilates the pulmonary vasculature, decreases PVR and PA systolic pressure (Case Study 11-1).

Case Study 11-1

Evaluation of Pressure Tracing

The following vascular pressure–time waveform is recorded on a patient on mechanical ventilation. Answer the following questions:

1. In what vessel or heart chamber is this catheter located?
2. What is the most accurate estimate of systolic and diastolic pressure?

Cardiac Output

Cardiac output ($\dot{Q}$) is the volume of blood that is pumped by the heart per minute, and it is usually expressed in liters per minute (L/min) or milliliters per minute (mL/min). Cardiac output normally ranges from 4 to 8 L/min. It can be calculated by multiplying the heart rate by the stroke volume (SV). The SV is the volume of blood pumped by the heart per beat; it can be expressed in liters per beat (L/beat) or milliliters per beat (mL/beat). In many cases, the cardiac output and the SV may be reported relative to the person's body surface area (BSA), which can be easily obtained using a Dubois chart like the one found in Fig. 6-1. This indexing technique allows the clinician to compare an individual's cardiac output or stroke output with that of normal healthy individuals of the same weight and height (BSA is calculated using these two anthropometric values).

Cardiac index (CI) is calculated by dividing the cardiac output by the BSA, or

$$CI = Cardiac\ Output/BSA\ or\ CI = \dot{Q}/BSA$$

Similarly, **stroke index** (SI) is calculated by dividing SV by body surface area, or

$$SI = SV/BSA$$

A normal CI for an adult is about 2.5 to 4.0 L/min/m². The stroke index normally ranges from 35 to 55 mL/beat/m² (Case Study 11-2).

Decreases in either heart rate or SV can cause reductions in cardiac output. Decreases in the effective ventricular rate are usually associated with the following:

- A decrease in sympathetic tone as occurs with the use of β-adrenergic blockade or
- An increase in parasympathetic tone and
- The presence of various types of bradyarrhythmias

Decreases in SV are associated with reduced preload or contractility of the heart or with an abnormally high afterload. Note that

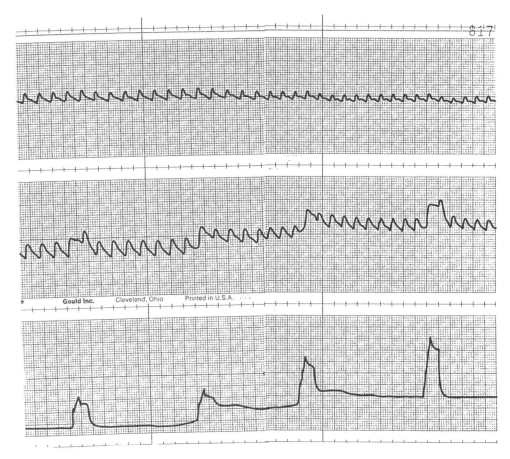

Fig. 11-11 Effects of varying levels of positive end-expiratory pressure (PEEP) on hemodynamic measurements. As PEEP is raised from 5 to 10 to 15 cm H_2O *(bottom panel)*, you can see the corresponding rise in pulmonary artery pressure *(middle panel)* and fall in systemic arterial pressure *(top panel)*. (Courtesy Jon Nilsestuen, PhD, RRT, University of Texas at Galveston.)

tachyarrythmias associated with very high heart rates can lead to decreases in ventricular filling, which can ultimately result in reductions in cardiac output.

In contrast, increases in cardiac output are associated with increases in heart rate or SV. Increases in heart rate associated with either an increase in sympathetic tone or a decrease in parasympathetic tone will lead to an increased cardiac output. Increases in SV are associated with increases in preload and contractility and with reductions in afterload.

Case Study 11-2

Cardiac Index and Stroke Index
A patient has a BSA = 1.7 m², a heart rate of 110 beats/min, and $\dot{Q}$ of 3 L/min. Calculate C.I. and S.I. How do this patient's values compare with normal values?

Fick Principle and Cardiac Output Measurements

Most experts agree that the gold standard for determining cardiac output involves direct measurements of oxygen consumption and arterial and mixed venous oxygen contents. Once these measurements are made, cardiac output can be calculated using the **Fick principle**,

$$\dot{Q} = \dot{V}O_2/[(C_aO_2 - C\overline{v}O_2) \times 10]$$

where $\dot{Q}$ is cardiac output, $\dot{V}O_2$ is oxygen consumption, C_aO_2 is the oxygen content of arterial blood, and $C\overline{v}O_2$ is the oxygen content of mixed venous blood.

Oxygen consumption ($\dot{V}O_2$) can be derived from measurements of the fractional concentration of inspired and expired oxygen and minute ventilation. If these measurements are not available, many clinicians use an oxygen consumption of 3.5 mL/kg/min as an estimate of the person's $\dot{V}O_2$. For example, a 154-lb (70-kg) individual would have a $\dot{V}O_2$ of about 250 mL/min in the calculation of cardiac output. As you might expect, this practice may lead to erroneous results, particularly in critically ill patients.

Calculation of oxygen content requires the measurement of oxygen partial pressures and saturations for oxygen of arterial and mixed venous blood. Arterial samples can be obtained from a peripheral artery; mixed venous blood samples can only be obtained during right heart catheterization by withdrawing blood from the PA (i.e., the distal port of the PA catheter). The oxygen saturation of arterial blood (S_aO_2) is normally about 98%, and the arterial oxygen content (C_aO_2) of a normal healthy individual is approximately 20 vol% (200 mL/L of whole blood). The mixed venous oxygen saturation ($S\overline{v}O_2$) is normally about 75%, and the mixed venous oxygen content ($C\overline{v}O_2$) is about 15 vol% (150 mL/L of whole blood). Critical Care Concept 11-1 provides a sample calculation of cardiac output using the Fick principle.

CRITICAL CARE CONCEPT 11-1

Fick Principle

A 70-kg man receiving volume-targeted mechanical ventilation at an F_iO_2 of 0.35 has an oxygen consumption of 300 mL/min, a C_aO_2 of 18 vol%, and a $C\overline{v}O_2$ of 13 vol%. What is his cardiac output ($\dot{Q}$)?

See Appendix A for the answer.

Indirect Fick Method

A variation on this method of determining cardiac output is the indirect Fick method, which involves the collection and analysis of exhaled gas in place of arterial and mixed venous blood gas samples. With the indirect Fick method of calculating $\dot{Q}$, carbon dioxide production ($\dot{V}CO_2$) is used in place of $\dot{V}O_2$. Arterial and mixed venous oxygen difference is replaced with arterial CO_2 content and mixed venous CO_2 content, respectively. $\dot{V}CO_2$ is obtained from continuous measurements of the fractional expired CO_2 (F_ECO_2) and minute ventilation ($\dot{V}_E$). The arterial CO_2 content is calculated from measurements of the partial pressure of mixed expired CO_2 ($P_{\overline{E}}CO_2$), which are obtained while the patient intermittently rebreathes a fixed volume (at 10- to 15-second intervals). Cardiac output therefore is calculated as

$$\dot{Q} = \dot{V}CO_2/(P\overline{v}CO_2 - P_{ET}CO_2)$$

The application of CO_2 monitoring to estimate cardiac output is currently available with the NICO system (Philips Respironics, The Netherlands; see Fig. 10-12 and Fig. 11-12).

Mixed Venous Oxygen Saturation

If the $\dot{V}O_2$ and cardiac output remain constant, then the difference between the arterial oxygen content and the mixed venous oxygen

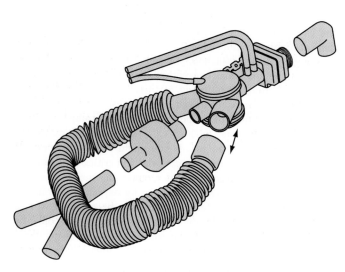

Fig. 11-12 The rebreathing circuit used by the Respironics NICO Capnometer to estimate cardiac output using measurements of rebreathed CO_2. (Courtesy Philips Respironics, The Netherlands.)

content also remain constant. Mixed venous oxygen values decline when arterial oxygenation is decreased. They also decrease when cardiac output is reduced. With a reduced cardiac output, more time is available for the extraction of oxygen from blood delivered to the tissues. Reductions in $S\overline{v}O_2$ are also associated with increases in metabolic rate in patients with limited cardiac output. Mixed venous oxygen values can be higher than normal in patients with histotoxic hypoxia (e.g., cyanide poisoning) and in situations where intrapulmonary shunting occurs, (i.e., ventilation/perfusion mismatching).

With recent advances in fiberoptic reflectance oximetry, continuous recordings of $S\overline{v}O_2$ can be obtained.[23] Reflectance oximetry technology has been incorporated into specialized balloon-flotation catheters that are used for right heart catheterization. Although the potential for this type of monitoring is promising, more studies are required to delineate more clearly the indications for its use in critical care (Case Study 11-3).

Case Study 11-3

Application of the Fick Principle

A patient has a constant $\dot{V}O_2$ of 350 mL/min. At 13:00 hours C_aO_2 is 20 vol% and $C\overline{v}O_2$ is 14 vol%. At 15:00 hours C_aO_2 is 20 vol% and $C\overline{v}O_2$ is 12 vol%. What is one possible cause in the drop in $C\overline{v}O_2$?

Calculate the cardiac output for both times.

Oxygen Delivery

Oxygen delivery (DO_2) is the product of cardiac output and arterial oxygen content. It represents the total amount of oxygen that is carried in the blood to the tissues each minute. Under normal circumstances, DO_2 is approximately 1000 mL/min or about 550 to 650 mL/min/m^2 (Key Point 11-4).[24]

DO_2 is increased in situations where cardiac output or arterial oxygen content is elevated. A reduced DO_2 indicates a decrease in cardiac output or arterial oxygen content.[24] For example, DO_2 is increased in hyperdynamic states (increased cardiac output) such as septic shock. Conversely, DO_2 is decreased following hemorrhage where there is a decrease in arterial oxygen content.

Key Point 11-4 DO_2 represents the total amount of oxygen that is carried in the blood to the tissues each minute.

Shunt Fraction

A *shunt* is defined as that portion of the cardiac output that does not participate in gas exchange with alveolar air (i.e., *perfusion without ventilation*). Shunts are usually identified as anatomical shunts, intrapulmonary shunts, and physiological shunts, with the latter being the sum of anatomical and intrapulmonary shunts.

Normal anatomical shunts exist because venous blood that would ideally return to the right side of the heart (deoxygenated blood) drains into vessels served by the left side of the heart (oxygenated blood). This venous admixture includes deoxygenated blood from bronchial veins, pleural veins, and thebesian veins, and it typically only represents about 2% to 3% of the normal cardiac output. Abnormal anatomic shunts can occur when blood is allowed to bypass the pulmonary circulation and enter directly into the left atrium or left ventricle, as occurs with atrial and ventricular septal wall defects.

Intrapulmonary shunts occur when blood passes through pulmonary capillaries that are not ventilated. Shunt-like states can exist in either poorly ventilated alveolar units that are well perfused or in alveolar-capillary units where oxygen diffusion is impaired. Intrapulmonary shunts can be caused by disorders such as atelectasis, pulmonary edema, pneumonia, pneumothorax, complete airway obstruction, consolidation of the lung, ARDS, and on rare occasions by arterial-to-venous fistulas.

The total shunt fraction or, more specifically, **physiological shunt** can be determined by the following classic shunt equation:

$$\dot{Q}_S/\dot{Q}_T = (C_cO_2 - C_aO_2)/(C_cO_2 - C\bar{v}O_2)$$

where $\dot{Q}_S$ is the shunted portion of the cardiac output, $\dot{Q}_T$ is total cardiac output, C_cO_2 is the content of oxygen of the pulmonary end-capillary following oxygenation of the blood, C_aO_2 is the arterial O_2 content, and $C\bar{v}O_2$ is the mixed venous oxygen content (i.e., pulmonary capillary blood before oxygenation). C_cO_2 is calculated based on the assumption that pulmonary end-capillary PO_2 is the same as P_AO_2. Mixed venous blood can be obtained from a PA catheter. As discussed later in this text, calculation of shunt fraction can be useful in the differential diagnosis of hypoxemia.

Vascular Resistance

As mentioned earlier, the vascular resistance represents the impedance or opposition to blood flow offered by the systemic and pulmonary vascular beds, and it influences the force that the ventricular muscle must generate during cardiac contractions. Although SVR and PVR have been reported historically as dyne × sec × cm^{-5}, recent publications have tended to use the units of mm Hg/L/min. In this text, we use the units of dyne × sec × cm^{-5} for the sake of continuity.

Taking a simple way to approach the calculation of SVR or PVR (R in the following equation), ΔP represents the pressure gradient across the vascular bed and $\dot{Q}$ is the blood flow through the vascular bed, or

$$R = \Delta P/\dot{Q}$$

Thus, SVR can be calculated as follows:

$$SVR = ([MAP - MRAP]/SBF) \times 80$$

where MAP is the mean aortic or arterial blood pressure, expressed in millimeters of mercury (mm Hg), MRAP is the mean right atrial pressure (in mm Hg), and SBF is the systemic blood flow or cardiac output (in L/min). Multiplying the equation by 80 is routinely used by clinicians to convert the units of mm Hg/L/min to dyne × sec × cm^{-5}. Note that CVP may be substituted for MRAP. When CVP is used, the formula can be written as

$$SVR = ([MAP - CVP]/\dot{Q}) \times 80$$

Similarly, PVR can be calculated as

$$PVR = ([MPAP - MLAP]/PBF) \times 80$$

where MPAP is the mean pulmonary artery pressure, MLAP is the mean left atrial pressure (both measured in mm Hg), and PBF is the pulmonary blood flow or cardiac output (C.O.) (in L/min). In the critical care setting, the PAOP may be used instead of MLAP, and the formula becomes

$$PVR = ([MPAP - PAOP]/C.O.) \times 80$$

The normal SVR ranges from 900 to 1500 dyne × sec × cm^{-5}, and the PVR ranges from 100 to 250 dyne × sec × cm^{-5}. The two most important factors that influence vascular resistance are the caliber of the blood vessels and the viscosity of the blood. The SVR is therefore increased in left ventricular failure and hypovolemia arising from vasoconstriction caused by stimulation of the baroreceptor reflex.[16]

The SVR may also be increased if blood viscosity increases, as occurs in polycythemia. SVR decreases during systemic vasodilation, such as occurs with moderate hypoxemia or following the administration of systemic vasodilators such as nitroglycerin or hydralazine.[20]

The PVR increases during periods of alveolar hypoxia or in cases where high intraalveolar pressures are generated, such as during positive pressure ventilation. A low cardiac output can increase PVR by causing derecruitment of pulmonary vessels. PVR is reduced by the administration of pulmonary vasodilator drugs like tolazoline and prostacyclin.[25]

Ejection Fraction

The ejection fraction (EF) is a derived variable that provides an estimate of ventricular contractility. It is calculated by dividing the stroke volume by the end-diastolic volume. The EF shows a positive correlation with CI in most cases, and it is a valuable measurement in the prognosis of heart failure.[26] Note that the correlation between EF and CI may be inaccurate in cases of mitral regurgitation. EF values of 0.5 to 0.7 are considered normal for healthy adults. EF values lower than 0.30 are associated with compromised cardiovascular function and imminent heart failure.

Cardiac Work

In physics work is defined as the product of a force acting on an object to move it a certain distance. In calculations of **cardiac work,** or more specifically **stroke work,** the pressure generated by the heart during a ventricular contraction is used to quantify the amount of force developed; the SV represents the distance portion of the equation. The amount of work performed by each ventricle during the cardiac cycle by applying the following formulas:

$$LVSW = ([MAP \times SV] \times 0.0136)$$

$$RVSW = ([MPAP \times SV] \times 0.0136)$$

where LVSW and RVSW are left ventricular stroke work and right ventricular stroke work, respectively; MAP is the mean arterial pressure; MPAP is the mean pulmonary artery pressure; SV represents stroke volume; and 0.00136 is a factor to convert millimeters of mercury (mm Hg)-milliliters (mL) to gram-meters (g-m). In most clinical situations, stroke work measurements are indexed to BSA. Therefore, the left ventricular stroke work index (LVSWI) and right ventricular stroke work index (RVSWI) are calculated as follows:

$$LVSWI = LSW/BSA$$

$$RVSWI = RSW/BSA$$

LSWI normally ranges from 40 to 60 g-m/m^2 (0.4 to 0.6 kg-m/m^2), and RSWI ranges are normally between 7 and 12 g-m/m^2 (0.07 to 0.12 kg-m/m^2).* Conditions that increase the stroke volume

---

*Alternative methods for calculation of LVSW and RVSW are LVSW = SV × (BPsys − PAOP) × 0.0136; RVSW = SV (PAsys − CVP) × 0.0136, where BPsys is systolic blood pressure (systemic) and PAsys is pulmonary artery systolic pressure.

and/or mean pressure generated by the ventricles will increase the amount of work that the ventricle must perform (Case Study 11-4).

CLINICAL APPLICATIONS

Case Studies 11-5 through 11-7 present clinical cases to demonstrate the application of the concepts reviewed in this chapter. Tables 11-5 and 11-6 may assist the reader in solving the problems presented in these Case Studies.

 Case Study 11-4

Stroke Work

A patient has a mean arterial pressure of 80 mm Hg and a stroke volume of 60 mL/beat. He is given a cardiac stimulant and MAP increases to 100 mm Hg and SV to 70 mL/beat. His BSA is 1.5 m². Calculate his left ventricular stroke work index before and after delivery of the medication.

 Case Study 11-5

Hemodynamic Monitoring: After Open-Heart Surgery

A 59-year-old, 154-lb (70-kg) man is being ventilated with a Puritan Bennett 840 ventilator following open-heart surgery for a triple coronary bypass. Vital signs are stable, with a heart rate of 100 beats/min, a temperature of 37.5° C, and a blood pressure of 130/70. Breath sounds are normal. The tidal volume is 550 mL on VC-IMV, with no spontaneous breaths. The respiratory rate is 12 breaths/min. The F_IO_2 is 0.4. The PEEP is set at 5 cm H_2O. Peak airway pressures are 30 cm H_2O and his pulmonary compliance is 22 mL/cm H_2O. The following data were obtained immediately following surgery:

- Hemoglobin = 13 g%
- Systemic arterial pressure = 135/70 mm Hg
- Pulmonary arterial pressure = 25/10 mm Hg
- Pulmonary artery wedge pressure = 12 mm Hg
- CVP = 2 mm Hg

- pH_a = 7.42; P_aCO_2 = 36 mm Hg; P_aO_2 = 60 mm Hg; S_aO_2 = 90%
- $pH\bar{v}$ = 7.35; $P\bar{v}CO_2$ = 45 mm Hg; $P\bar{v}O_2$ = 40 mm Hg; $S\bar{v}O_2$ = 75%
- P_ECO_2 = 24 mm Hg; $\dot{V}O_2$ = 250 mL/min; $\dot{V}CO_2$ = 200 mL/min

The surgeon asks you to increase the PEEP to 10 cm H_2O. After 20 minutes at the increased level of PEEP, the following data are obtained:

- Systemic arterial pressure = 110/65 mm Hg
- Pulmonary arterial pressure = 18/8 mm Hg
- Pulmonary artery wedge pressure = 10 mm Hg
- Central venous pressure = 4 mm Hg
- pH_a = 7.39; P_aCO_2 = 42 mm Hg; P_aO_2 = 70 mm Hg; S_aO_2 = 98%
- $pH\bar{v}$ = 7.32; $P\bar{v}CO_2$ = 48 mm Hg; $P\bar{v}O_2$ = 30 mm Hg; $S\bar{v}O_2$ = 65%
- P_ECO_2 = 25 mm Hg; $\dot{V}O_2$ = 230 mL/min; $\dot{V}CO_2$ = 180 mL/min

Interpret these findings.

 Case Study 11-6

Hemodynamic Monitoring: Chest Injury

An 18-year-old man was admitted to the emergency department with a gunshot wound to the chest. He was transferred to the ICU status post left lower lobectomy, splenectomy, and laparoscopy, with bilateral chest tubes. The patient had bullet fragments at T_{12} and at the level of the left hemidiaphragm.

He was placed on jet ventilation with the following settings:

Breathing frequency	150 breaths/min
Pressure	21 cm H_2O
F_IO_2	0.50
T_I	20%
Peak flow	70 L/min
Exhaled V_T	250 mL
pH_a	7.46
P_aCO_2	30.2 Torr
P_aO_2	75.2 Torr
HCO_3^-	21.8 mEq/L
S_aO_2	95%
Hb	9 g%
$S\bar{v}O_2$	81%

The patient was receiving Tracrium (9 µg), dopamine (3 µg/kg/min), Versed (3 µg), dobutamine (6 µg/kg/min), and morphine sulfate (8 µg).

After insertion of a pulmonary artery catheter in the patient, the follow data were obtained:

BSA	1.81 m²
Cardiac output	7.58 L/min
Heart rate	115 beats/min
MAP	107 mm Hg
PAP	35 mm Hg
PAOP	14 mm Hg
CVP	13 mm Hg
Hb	8.2 g%
CI	4.19 L/min/m²
SV	70 mL/beat
SVR	992 dyne × sec × cm⁻⁵
PVR	222 dyne × sec × cm⁻⁵

How would you interpret these data?

Case Study 11-7

ICU and Hemodynamic Assessment

A 72-year-old man is admitted to the intensive care unit, after stabilization in the emergency department, on a nasal cannula at 2 L/min. Arterial blood gases (ABGs) drawn in the emergency department revealed pH = 7.47, P_aCO_2 = 30 mm Hg, and P_aO_2 = 31 mm Hg. The patient was immediately placed on a nonre-breathing mask, and ABGs and vital signs were assessed with the following results:

- pH = 7.48, P_aCO_2 = 32 mm Hg, P_aO_2 = 56 mm Hg
- f = 34 breaths/min, heart rate = 116 beats/min
- Blood pressure = 175/58 mm Hg

The patient was placed on mechanical ventilatory support with the following settings:

- V_T = 850 mL, VC-CMV with rate = 12 breaths/min
- F_IO_2 = 0.5, PEEP = +10 cm H_2O

Hemodynamic monitoring, following successful insertion of a pulmonary artery catheter in the subclavian artery, revealed the following data:

- Cardiac output = 7.98 L/min, CI = 4.41 L/min/m², HR = 81 beats/min
- BP S* = 159 mm Hg, BP D = 64 mm Hg, BP M = 92 mm Hg
- PAP S = 52 mm Hg, PAP D = 18 mm Hg, PAP M = 33 mm Hg
- PAOP = 13 mm Hg, CVP M = 12 mm Hg
- SV = 98.5 mL, SI = 54.4 mL/m², SVR = 802 dynes × cm × s⁻⁵
- PVR = 201 dynes × cm⁻⁵ × s
- Hemoglobin = 14.5 g, Temp = 37° C
- Arterial blood gases (ABGs): pH = 7.362, PO_2 = 80 mm Hg, PCO_2 = 46.2 mm Hg, HCO_3^- = 26.5 mEq/L, S_aO_2 = 95.2%
- Mixed venous blood gases: pH = 7.339, PO_2 = 40 mm Hg, PCO_2 = 50.3 mm Hg, HCO_3^- = 27.4 mEq/L, $S\overline{v}O_2$ = 71.2%
- C_aO_2 = 18.5 vol%, $C\overline{v}O_2$ = 13.8 vol%, $C(a-\overline{v})O_2$ = 4.7 vol%
- O_2 transport = 1476 mL/min, O_2 consumption = 375 mL/min

How would you interpret these findings?

D, Diastolic; *M,* mean; *S,* systolic.
(Modified with permission from Deshpande VM, Pilbeam SP, Dixon RJ: A comprehensive review in respiratory care, Norwalk, Conn., 1988, Appleton & Lange.)

TABLE 11-5	Part I: Hemodynamic Parameters That Can Be Calculated		
Parameter	**Normal Values**	**Formula**	**Use**
Mean arterial blood pressure (MAP)	70-100 mm Hg	(Systolic pressure + diastolic pressure)/3	To calculate systemic vascular resistance; used in hemodynamic monitoring when giving vasoactive drugs
Pulse pressure (systemic)	40 mm Hg	Systolic pressure − diastolic pressure	To estimate the force of the pulse
Stroke volume (SV)	60-100 mL	$\dot{Q}$/HR	Provides information about cardiac performance
Cardiac index (CI)	2.5-4 L/min/m²	$\dot{Q}$/body surface area (BSA)	An important determinant of cardiac performance (removes body size as a variable)
Stroke index (SI)	35-55 mL/beat m²	SV/BSA	An important determinant of cardiac performance (removes body size as a variable)
Systemic vascular resistance (SVR)	900-1500 dyne × sec × cm⁻⁵	([MAP − CVP]/C.O.) × 80	To measure resistance in system circulation; useful in diagnosis of vascular problems
Mean pulmonary artery pressure (MPAP)	10-20 mm Hg	(Pulmonary systolic pressure + pulmonary diastolic pressure)	To calculate pulmonary vascular resistance
Pulmonary vascular resistance (PVR)	100-250 dyne × sec × cm⁻⁵	([MPAP − PAOP]/$\dot{Q}$) × 80	To measure resistance in the pulmonary vascular bed; and useful in the diagnosis of pulmonary vascular problems
Oxygen content of arterial blood (C_aO_2)	20 vol%	([S_aO_2 × Hb] × 1.34)†	To calculate oxygen delivery, cardiac output, and shunt fraction
Oxygen content of mixed venous blood	15 vol%	([$S\overline{v}O_2$ × Hb] × 1.34)†	To calculate cardiac output and shunt fraction
Arterial-to-venous oxygen content difference	3.5-5.0 mL/100 mL or vol%	$C(a-\overline{v})O_2$	Index of tissue oxygenation

Continued

TABLE 11-5	**Part I: Hemodynamic Parameters That Can Be Calculated—cont'd**

Parameter	Normal Values	Formula	Use
Oxygen transport (DO_2)	500-1000 mL/min*	$\dot{Q} \times C_aO_2$	Indicates the amount of oxygen delivered to the tissues
Oxygen consumption ($\dot{V}O_2$)	200-300 mL/min	$\dot{Q} \times (CaO_2 - C\bar{v}O_2)$	Indicates the metabolic rate (i.e., the amount of O_2 used by the body); this can be measured indirectly by noninvasive means but only with great difficulty

Part II: Hemodynamic Parameters That Can Be Measured Directly

Parameter	Normal Values	How Measured	Use
Heart rate (HR)	60-100 beats/min	Pulse rate	Early index of tachycardia and bradycardia
Blood pressure (systemic) (BP)	Systolic: 90-140 mm Hg; diastolic: 60-90 mm Hg	Blood pressure cuff or arterial line	Early index of hypertension or hypotension
Central venous pressure (CVP)	2-6 mm Hg	From CVP catheter or PA three- or four-lumen catheter	To estimate right ventricular preload; also for drug and fluid administration
Pulmonary artery occlusion (PAP)	Systolic: 15-35 mm Hg; Diastolic: 5-15 mm Hg	From PA catheter	To determine PAP and to pressure PVR
Pulmonary artery occlusion pressure (PAOP)	5-12 mm Hg	From PA catheter in the occluded position (balloon inflated)	To estimate left ventricular filling and preload
Cardiac output (C.O.)	4-8 L/min	By thermodilution or dye dilution	An important determinant of hemodynamic function
Partial pressure of oxygen in mixed venous blood ($P\bar{v}O_2$)	40 mm Hg	From blood from the distal port of the PA catheter	Overall parameter for assessment of cardiopulmonary function
Partial pressure of oxygen in arterial blood (P_aO_2)	80-100 mm Hg	From a systemic artery	To assess level of arterial oxygenation

*C.O. $\times$ C_aO_2 = 5000 mL/min $\times$ 20 mL/100 mL = 1000 mL/min.
†Dissolved portion is very small and is not included here (Dissolved O_2 = 0.0031 $\times$ P_aO_2 or $P\bar{v}O_2$).

TABLE 11-6	**Hemodynamic Changes Commonly Seen in Respiratory Diseases**

Disorder	HEMODYNAMIC INDICES											
	CVP	RAP	PAP	PAOP	CO	SV	SVI	CI	RVSWI	LVSWI	PVR	SVR
Chronic bronchitis Emphysema Bronchiectasis Cystic fibrosis	↑	↑	↑↑	—	—	—	—	—	↑	—	↑	—
Pulmonary edema (cardiogenic)	—	↑	↑	↑↑	↓	↓	↓	↓	↑	↓	↑	↓
Pulmonary embolism	↑	↑	↑↑	↓	↓	↓	↓	↓	~↑	↓	~↑	~
Severe adult respiratory distress syndrome (ARDS)	~↑	~↑	~↑	~	~	~	~	~	~↑	~	~↑	~
Lung collapse Flail chest Pneumothorax Pleural disease (e.g., hemothorax)	↑	↑	↑	↓	↓	↓	↓	↓	↑	↓	↑	↓
Kyphoscoliosis	↑	↑	↑	~	~	~	~	~	↑	~	↑	~
Pneumoconiosis	↑	↑	↑↑	~	~	~	~	~	↑	~	↑	~
Chronic interstitial lung diseases	↑	↑	↑↑	~	~	~	~	~	↑	~	↑	~
Lung cancer (tumor mass)	↑	↑	↑	↓	↓	↓	↓	↓	↑	~	↑	~
Hypovolemia	↓↓	↓	↓	↓	↓	↓	↓	↓	↓	↓	↓	↑
Hypervolemia (burns)	↑↑	↑	↑	↑	↑	↑	↑	↑	↑	↑	↑	~
Right-sided heart failure	↑↑	↑↑	↓	↓	~	~	~	~	~	~	~	~

From DesJardins T, Burton GG: Clinical manifestations and assessment of respiratory disease, ed 6, St Louis, 2011, Mosby.
↑, Increase; ↓, decrease; ~, unchanged; *CI*, cardiac index; *CO*, cardiac output; *CVP*, central venous pressure; *LVSWI*, left ventricular stroke work index; *PAOP*, pulmonary artery occlusion pressure; *PAP*, pulmonary artery pressure; *PVR*, pulmonary vascular resistance; *RAP*, right atrial pressure; *RVSWI*, right ventricular stroke work index; *SV*, stroke volume; *SVI*, stroke volume index; *SVR*, systemic vascular resistance.

SUMMARY

- Hemodynamic monitoring can provide a window to observe the effects of various physiological and pharmacologic interventions on cardiovascular function.
- The effective use of hemodynamic monitoring requires knowledge of the basic principles of cardiovascular physiology, as well as an understanding of the physical and technical factors that can influence the measurement conditions.
- Cardiac output is primarily influenced by heart rate and ventricular preload, contractility, and afterload.
- CVP and PAOP can be used to assess right and left ventricular preload, respectively.
- EF is a valuable clinical indicator of ventricular contractility.
- The SVR and PVR are used clinically to describe the afterload to the left and right ventricles, respectively.
- Positioning of a PA catheter can be accomplished by fluoroscopy or by monitoring the pressure tracing generated as the catheter is advanced into the right heart and pulmonary artery.
- Accurate measurements of the PAOP require wedging of the PA catheter in the zone 3 portion of the pulmonary vasculature.

- Pulse pressure is the difference between the systolic and diastolic pressure, and it is influenced by the stroke volume and arterial compliance.
- Cardiac index and stroke index allow the clinician to compare an individual's cardiac output and stroke output with those of healthy individuals of the same weight and height.
- Cardiac index and ejection fraction are important variables used in determining the prognosis of heart failure.
- Cardiac work is primarily influenced by stroke volume and systolic arterial pressure.
- Calculation of oxygen contents requires the measurement of oxygen partial pressures and saturations in arterial and mixed venous blood.
- Oxygen delivery to the tissues is increased in situations where the cardiac output and arterial oxygen content are elevated. It typically is decreased when either of these variables is reduced.
- SVR and PVR represent the impedance or opposition to blood flow offered by the systemic and pulmonary vascular beds, respectively. Vascular resistance influences the force that the ventricular muscle must generate during cardiac contractions.
- Cardiac work provides an estimate of the amount of force that must be generated by the ventricles to achieve a given stroke output.

REVIEW QUESTIONS *(See Appendix A for Answers.)*

1. Tracings from a patient undergoing cardiac catheterization demonstrated a left ventricular systolic pressure of 180 mm Hg and a peak systolic aortic pressure of 110 mm Hg. The patient complained of shortness of breath, fatigue, and syncope (loss of consciousness). Which of the following would you associate with these findings?
   - A. Aortic stenosis
   - B. Mitral regurgitation
   - C. Pulmonary stenosis
   - D. Tricuspid insufficiency

2. Which of the following is **incorrectly** matched for a resting healthy 154-lb (70-kg), 25-year-old sedentary subject?
   - A. Peak systolic left ventricular pressure = 120 mm Hg
   - B. Mean right atrial pressure = 5 mm Hg
   - C. Left ventricular stroke volume = 120 mL
   - D. Left ventricular end-systolic volume = 50 mL

3. The following tracing was obtained during the placement of a pulmonary artery catheter. The contour of the tracing suggests that the catheter is in the
   - A. Right atrium
   - B. Right ventricle
   - C. Pulmonary artery
   - D. Pulmonary wedge position

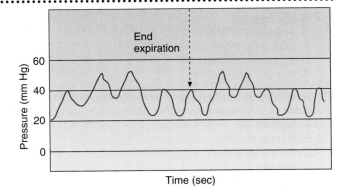

4. For a heart rate of 75 beats/min, the cardiac cycle will last approximately _____ seconds.
   - A. 0.4
   - B. 0.8
   - C. 1.0
   - D. 1.2

5. Which of the following conditions will cause a decrease in cardiac output?
   - A. Exercise
   - B. Hypovolemia
   - C. Increased sympathetic tone
   - D. Fever

6. Which of the following is a characteristic finding in patients with hypovolemia?
   A. Elevated PAOP
   B. Low RAP
   C. Decreased HR
   D. Increased PA pressure

7. Which of the following will cause an elevation in PA pressure?
   A. Hemorrhage
   B. Fluid overload
   C. Administering nitric oxide
   D. Breathing an enriched oxygen mixture

8. Which of the following measurements is a good indicator of left ventricular contractility?
   1. dP/dT
   2. Ejection fraction
   3. Stroke volume
   4. LVEDV
      A. 1 and 2 only
      B. 1 and 3 only
      C. 1, 2, and 3 only
      D. 2, 3, and 4 only

9. Which of the following variables are required to calculate PVR?
   1. Cardiac output
   2. Mean left atrial pressure
   3. Mean pulmonary artery pressure
   4. Mean right atrial pressure
      A. 1 and 2 only
      B. 1 and 3 only
      C. 1, 2, and 3 only
      D. 1, 2, and 4 only

10. Which of the following will typically lead to a **decrease** in cardiac output?
    A. Increase in preload
    B. Increase in afterload
    C. Increase in contractility
    D. Increase in heart rate

11. When properly inserted, the proximal lumen of the pulmonary artery catheter will be positioned in the
    A. Right atrium
    B. Right ventricle
    C. Pulmonary artery
    D. Left atrium

12. The proximal lumen can be used for all of the following **except:**
    A. Monitoring of RA pressure
    B. Fluid administration
    C. Cardiac output injectate insertion
    D. Monitoring of wedge pressures

13. The primary function of the transducer dome in a fluid-filled system is to:
    A. Amplify the weak biological signal
    B. Filter clots from the system
    C. Convert a pressure signal into an electrical signal
    D. Respond to pressure changes in the fluid column

14. If the transducer level is lower than the tip of the catheter during pulmonary artery pressure monitoring,
    A. The readings will be falsely high
    B. An overwedged waveform will appear
    C. The waveform will be dampened
    D. Catheter whip will appear on the waveform

15. The dicrotic notch on the pulmonary artery waveform may disappear in all of the following conditions **except:**
    A. Systemic vasoconstriction
    B. Pulmonary vasodilation
    C. Measurements obtained from a femoral artery
    D. Pulmonary stenosis

16. Left ventricular stroke work is decreased by increases in which of the following?
    A. Mean aortic pressure
    B. Ventricular end-diastolic pressure
    C. Heart rate
    D. Systemic vasodilation

17. Pulmonary hypertension will have which of the following effects?
    A. Increase afterload of the left side of the heart
    B. Increase afterload of the right side of the heart
    C. Decrease preload of the right side of the heart
    D. No effect on myocardial function

18. If a patient has a cardiac output of 5.6 L/min and a BSA of 2.1 m^2, what is the patient's CI?
    A. 2.67 L/min/m^2
    B. 3.50 L/min/m^2
    C. 7.70 L/min/m^2
    D. 11.76 L/min/m^2

19. Which of the following statements is true regarding the effects of mechanical ventilation on hemodynamic measurements?
    A. Lower mean inspiratory pressures present with PSV minimizes the effects of positive intrathoracic pressure
    B. Applied PEEP should be discontinued when making PAOP measurements
    C. PC-IRV is associated with increases in CI and DO_2
    D. PAOP should be measured at the end of a quiet inspiration

20. Which of the following could be used to estimate left ventricular end-diastolic pressure?
    1. PAOP
    2. PA diastolic pressure
    3. PA systolic pressure
    4. RV systolic pressure
       A. 1 and 2 only
       B. 2 and 3 only
       C. 3 and 4 only
       D. 1, 2, 3, and 4

References

1. Bernard GR, Sopko G, Cerra F, et al: Pulmonary artery catheterization and clinical outcomes. *JAMA* 19:2568–2572, 2000.
2. Boron WF, Boulpaep GL: *Medical physiology*, ed 2, Philadelphia, 2008, Saunders-Elsevier.
3. Cairo JM: *Respiratory care equipment*, ed 9, St Louis, 2014, Mosby-Elsevier.

4. Wiedeman HP, Matthay MA, Matthay RA: Cardiovascular-pulmonary monitoring in the intensive care unit. Part 1. *Chest* 85:537–549, 1984.

5. Wiedeman HP, Matthay MA, Matthay RA: Cardiovascular-pulmonary monitoring in the intensive care unit. Part 2. *Chest* 85:656–668, 1984.

6. Agee KR, Balk RA: Central venous catheters in the critically ill patient. *Crit Care Clin* 8:677–686, 1992.

7. Swan HJC, Ganz W, Forrester J, et al: Catheterization of the heart in man with the use of a flow-directed balloon tipped catheter. *N Engl J Med* 75:83–89, 1975.

8. Mathews L, Singh RK: Swan-Ganz catheter in hemodynamic monitoring. *J Anaesth Clin Pharmacol* 22:335–345, 2006.

9. Kacmarek RM, Stoller JK, Heuer AJ: *Egan's fundamentals of respiratory care*, ed 10, St Louis, 2013, Mosby.

10. Brierre SP, Summer W, Happel KI, et al: Interpretation of pulmonary artery catheter tracings. *Clin Pulmon Med* 9:335–341, 2002.

11. Marini J: Hemodynamic monitoring with the pulmonary artery catheter. *Crit Care Clin* 3:551–572, 1986.

12. Pilbeam SP: *Mechanical ventilation, physiological and clinical applications*, ed 3, St Louis, 1998, Mosby.

13. DesJardins T, Burton GG: *Clinical manifestations and assessment of respiratory disease*, ed 6, St Louis, 2006, Mosby-Elsevier.

14. Rubenstein JS, Hageman JR: Monitoring of critically ill infants and children. *Crit Care Clin* 4:621–639, 1988.

15. Morhman DE, Heller LJ: *Cardiovascular physiology*, ed 5, New York, 2002, McGraw-Hill.

16. Rushmer RF: *Cardiovascular dynamics*, ed 4, Philadelphia, 1976, W.B. Saunders.

17. Hoyt JD, Leatherman JW: Interpretation of pulmonary artery occlusion pressure in mechanically ventilated patients with large respiratory excursions in intrathoracic pressure. *Intensive Care Med* 23:1125–1131, 1997.

18. Daily EK: Hemodynamic waveform analysis. *J Cardiovasc Nurs* 15:6–22, 2001.

19. Murphy BA, Durbin CG: Using ventilator and cardiovascular graphics in the patient who is hemodynamically unstable. *Respir Care* 50:262–274, 2005.

20. Sternberg R, Sahebjami H: Hemodynamic and oxygen transport characteristics of common ventilator modes. *Chest* 105:1798–1803, 1994.

21. Chan K, Abraham E: Effects of inverse ratio ventilation on cardiorespiratory parameters in severe respiratory failure. *Chest* 102:1556–1561, 1992.

22. Mercat A, Graïni L, Teboul JL, et al: Cardiorespiratory effects of pressure-controlled ventilation with and without inverse ratio in the adult respiratory distress syndrome. *Chest* 104:871–875, 1993.

23. Pinsky MR: Hemodynamic monitoring in the intensive care unit. *Clin Chest Med* 24:549–560, 2003.

24. Wilkins RL, Dexter JR, Heuer AJ: *Clinical assessment in respiratory care*, ed 6, St Louis, 2009, Mosby-Elsevier.

25. Hardman JG, Limbid LE, Gilman AL: *Goodman and Gilman's the pharmacologic basis of therapeutics*, ed 10, New York, 2001, McGraw-Hill.

26. Libby P, Douglas RO, Mann L, et al: *Braunwald's heart disease: a textbook of cardiovascular medicine*, ed 8, 2010, Saunders.

CHAPTER 2

Methods to Improve Ventilation in Patient-Ventilator Management

KEY TERMS

- Asynchrony
- Hyperosmolar
- Ketoacidosis
- Minute ventilation
- Permissive hypercapnia
- Transpyloric

LEARNING OBJECTIVES   *On completion of this chapter, the reader will be able to do the following:*

1. Recommend ventilator adjustments to reduce work of breathing and improve ventilation based on patient diagnosis, arterial blood gas results, and ventilator parameters.
2. Calculate the appropriate suction catheter size, length, and amount of suction pressure needed for a specific size endotracheal tube and patient.
3. Compare the benefits of closed-suction catheters to the open-suction technique.
4. List the pros and cons of instilling normal saline to loosen secretions before suctioning.
5. List the clinical findings that are used to establish the presence of a respiratory infection.
6. Compare and contrast the protocols for using metered-dose inhalers and small-volume nebulizers during mechanical ventilation.
7. Describe complications associated with using small-volume nebulizers powered by external flowmeters during mechanical ventilation.
8. Discuss the importance of patient-centered mechanical ventilation in the treatment of critically ill patients.
9. Discuss the complications associated with the in-house transport of a mechanically ventilated patient.

Clinicians generally use the first 30 to 60 minutes following initiation of mechanical ventilation to gather information that can be used to evaluate the effectiveness of ventilatory support. As discussed in Chapter 8, these data typically involve vital signs, breath sounds, and assessment of respiratory mechanics (i.e., lung compliance [C_L] and airway resistance [R_{aw}]. Ventilator graphics can also be a valuable resource when evaluating the patient-ventilator interaction (see Chapter 9).

This chapter provides an overview of ventilatory strategies that can be used to manage patients with various acid–base disturbances. It also includes a discussion of airway clearance techniques, aerosol administration, flexible fiberoptic bronchoscopy during ventilation, patient positioning, and techniques used to assess fluid balance. The importance of ensuring patient comfort and safety, as well as in-house transport of the ventilated patient, is also discussed.

Correcting Ventilation Abnormalities

Once an initial physical assessment is performed, an arterial blood gas (ABG) sample should be obtained to evaluate the patient's respiratory and acid–base status. Evaluation of ABG results can be divided into three parts: acid–base status, ventilation, and oxygenation status—pH (alkalinity and acidity), and bicarbonate; P_aCO_2 (partial pressure of carbon dioxide); and oxygenation status— (P_aO_2 [partial pressure of oxygen], S_aO_2 [arterial oxygen saturation], C_aO_2 [arterial content of oxygen], and oxygen delivery [DO_2]). The following discussion focuses on those factors that can alter P_aCO_2 during mechanical ventilation, including **minute ventilation,** physiological dead space, and CO_2 production (Fig. 12-1). Methods to improve oxygenation are reviewed in Chapter 13.

COMMON METHODS OF CHANGING VENTILATION BASED ON P_aCO_2 AND pH

A change in minute ventilation ($\dot{V}_E$) is often required after a patient is placed on mechanical ventilation. It is not uncommon to use full ventilatory support initially and then make adjustments after an initial assessment is performed. The examples provided here represent full support of an apneic patient.

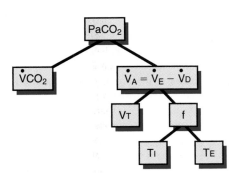

Fig. 12-1 Factors that affect the partial pressure of arterial carbon dioxide (P_aCO_2) during mechanical ventilation. $\dot{V}CO_2$, carbon dioxide production; $\dot{V}_A$, alveolar ventilation; $\dot{V}_E$, minute ventilation; $\dot{V}_D$, dead space ventilation; V_T, tidal volume; T_I, inspiratory time; T_E, expiratory time; f, respiratory rate. (From Hess DR, MacIntyre NR, Mishoe SC, et al: Respiratory care principles and practice, ed 2, Sudbury, Mass., 2012, Jones and Bartlett.)

During mechanical ventilation, adjusting the set tidal volume (V_T) or rate (f) can be used to adjust respiratory alkalosis or acidosis. These changes are based on the following equation*:

$$\text{Known } P_aCO_2 \times \text{Known } \dot{V}_E = \text{Desired } P_aCO_2 \times \text{Desired } \dot{V}_E$$

If we assume that physiological dead space† and CO_2 production (resulting from metabolism) do not change significantly during a short period, then the equation can be modified to read:

Known P_aCO_2 × Known alveolar ventilation per minute ($\dot{V}_A$) = Desired P_aCO_2 × Desired $\dot{V}_A$

If it is appropriate to keep rate (f) constant and change V_T, then the equation becomes:

$$\text{Desired } V_T = \text{Known } P_aCO_2 \times \text{Known } V_T / \text{Desired } P_aCO_2$$

If it is appropriate to keep V_T constant and change f, then the equation is written:

$$\text{Desired } f = \text{Known } P_aCO_2 \times \text{Known } f / \text{Desired } P_aCO_2$$

Respiratory Acidosis: Volume and Pressure Ventilation Changes

When P_aCO_2 is elevated (>45 mm Hg) and pH is decreased (<7.35), respiratory acidosis is present and $\dot{V}_A$ is inadequate. Acute respiratory acidosis is associated with the following:
- Parenchymal lung problems (e.g., pulmonary edema, pneumonia)
- Airway disease (e.g., severe asthma attack)
- Pleural abnormalities (e.g., effusions)
- Chest wall abnormalities
- Neuromuscular disorders (e.g., spinal cord injury, myasthenia gravis)
- Central nervous system (CNS) problems (e.g., drug overdose)[1]

See Chapter 4 for additional information.

In patients receiving mechanical ventilation, respiratory acidosis generally can be corrected by adjusting the set V_T or f to achieve the desired minute ventilation. Regardless of whether the patient is receiving volume-controlled or pressure-controlled ventilation, increasing $\dot{V}_E$ will decrease the P_aCO_2.

Recommended guidelines are to target a V_T of 6 to 8 mL/kg ideal body weight (IBW), while assuring that the plateau pressure ($P_{plateau}$) is maintained less than 30 cm H_2O. As discussed in Chapter 6, tidal volume and breathing frequency adjustments should be based on the patient's pulmonary pathology. It is important to understand that the 6 to 8 mL/kg range is an average. If the V_T is at the upper limit of this range and $P_{plateau}$ is greater than 30 cm H_2O, then V_T may be decreased to achieve a lower $P_{plateau}$.

With PC-CMV, the set pressure is generally adjusted to obtain the targeted V_T. PC-CMV is time cycled. If inspiratory time (T_I) is short, increasing it may also increase volume delivery, without requiring an increase in pressure (P) (Fig. 12-2).

---

*This equation is based on the following: $\dot{V}_A = (0.863 \times \dot{V}CO_2)/P_aCO_2$, where $\dot{V}_A$ is alveolar ventilation, 0.863 is a conversion factor, and $\dot{V}CO_2$ is carbon dioxide production. And, $P_aCO_2 = (\dot{V}CO_2 \times 0.863)/(\dot{V}_E \times [V_D/V_T])$. Assuming dead space and $\dot{V}CO_2$ remain constant, increasing ventilation results in a decreased CO_2.

†Physiological dead space = anatomical dead space + alveolar dead space.

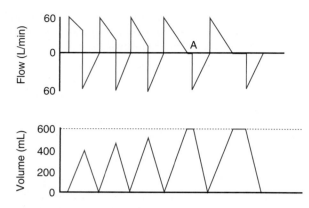

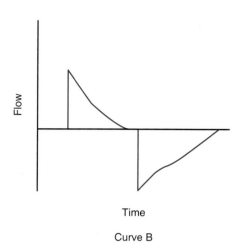

Fig. 12-2 The effect of inspiratory time (T_I) and inspiratory plateau on delivered tidal volume (V_T) in the pressure-controlled ventilation (PCV) mode. Initially, as T_I is increased, V_T increases. Once an inspiratory plateau *(A)* is reached, a further increase in T_I will not increase V_T. (From Wilkins RL, Stoller JK, Kacmarek RM, editors: Egan's fundamentals of respiratory care, ed 9, St Louis, 2009, Mosby.)

Curve B

Clinical Scenario: Adjusting PC-CMV in a Patient with Respiratory Acidosis

A 165-lb (75-kg, IBW) patient is placed on PC-CMV with a rate of 10 breaths/min, a set pressure of 25 cm H_2O, and a measured V_T of 425 mL. The flow–time curve for this patient is shown in *Curve A* below. T_I is 0.7 seconds. The ABGs are as follows: pH = 7.30; P_aCO_2 = 50 mm Hg; HCO_3^- = 23 mEq/L.

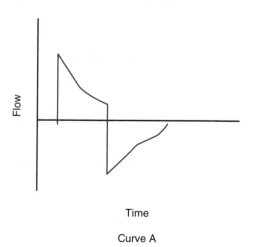

Curve A

To improve ventilation, two things can be adjusted. The T_I can be increased so that the set pressure reaches the alveolar level. This would be apparent when the flow scalar shows a time of zero flow during inspiration *(Curve B)*. This strategy may be tried first. If this does not improve volume delivery sufficiently, the set pressure can be increased.

Clinical Scenario: Respiratory Acidosis: Increasing Tidal Volume

A 50-year-old man with respiratory acidosis is receiving mechanical ventilatory support. He is 6 foot 2 inches tall and weighs 190 lb (81 kg, IBW) (anatomic dead space [$V_{Danat.}$] = 190 mL). Exhaled V_T measured at the endotracheal tube (ET) is 400 mL. His respiratory rate is 16 breaths/min. The patient is receiving VC-CMV. ABGs show a P_aCO_2 of 55 mm Hg and a pH of 7.33. The patient has no pulmonary disease. His desired P_aCO_2 is 40 mm Hg. What ventilator change must be made to decrease the P_aCO_2?

Because the V_T setting is less than 8 mL/kg and the patient has no pulmonary disease, it is appropriate to hold the rate constant and change V_T:

$$\text{Desired } V_T = \text{Known } P_aCO_2 \times \text{Known } V_T / \text{Desired } P_aCO_2$$

$$\text{Desired } V_T = 55 \times 400 / 40 = 550 \text{ mL}$$

The new V_T is set at 550 mL (about 7 mL/kg IBW) to achieve a desired P_aCO_2 of 40 mm Hg. The alveolar ventilation has been increased appropriately to correct the respiratory acidosis.

Clinical Scenario: Respiratory Acidosis: Increasing Rate

A 48-year-old woman who is 5 foot 2 inches tall is receiving VC-CMV and generating no spontaneous breaths. She has a P_aCO_2 of 58 mm Hg; pH is 7.28; V_T at the ET is 425 mL. IBW is 115 lb (52 kg); V_{Danat} is 115 mL. Respiratory rate is 15 breaths/min. How can the ventilator settings be adjusted to achieve a desired P_aCO_2 of 40 mm Hg?

In this case, the patient's V_T is set at about 8 mL/kg, so it is appropriate to change f and not increase V_T.

$$\text{Desired f} = \text{Known f} \times \text{Known } P_aCO_2 / \text{Desired } P_aCO_2$$

Increasing the breathing frequency to 23 breaths/min should decrease the P_aCO_2 to 40 mm Hg. It is important to recognize, however, that setting high respiratory rates may be associated with air trapping because of a reduced expiratory time. (NOTE: It is useful to monitor the flow scalar when setting breathing frequencies greater than 20 breaths/min.)

Clinical Scenario: Changes During Pressure-Targeted Ventilation

During PC-CMV, the same types of adjustments for V_T and rate are made based on ABGs, except that the set pressure is increased or decreased to achieve a desired V_T. Exhaled volume is monitored until the desired V_T is obtained. (Note that it is important to ensure that T_I is long enough to gain the most benefit from the set pressure [see Case Study 12-1].)

A 165-lb (75-kg, IBW) patient with respiratory acidosis is receiving PC-CMV (P_aCO_2 = 59 mm Hg; pH = 7.31; desired P_aCO_2 = 40 mm Hg). At a set pressure of 10 cm H_2O, the exhaled V_T is 400 mL (5.3 mL/kg) and the rate is 16 breaths/min. The patient is not spontaneously breathing. T_I is set so that the flow returns to zero before the end of inspiration and a $P_{plateau}$ period can be measured. What ventilator adjustment must be made to decrease his P_aCO_2? The V_T setting is less than 8 mL/kg, so it is appropriate to hold f constant and change V_T.

$$Desired\ V_T = 59 \times 400/40 = 590\ mL\ or\ about\ 600\ mL$$

A set pressure (P) of 10 cm H_2O results in a V_T of 400 mL (0.4 L); what is an estimated pressure that will achieve a V_T of 600 mL (0.6 L)? Assume that compliance does not change. Remember static compliance (C_S) = $V_T/(P_{plateau} - PEEP)$, C_S = 400/10, and C_S = 40 mL/cm H_2O

$$Desired\ P = Desired\ V_T/C_s$$

$$Desired\ P = 600\ mL/(40\ mL/cm\ H_2O)\ and\ P = 15\ cm\ H_2O$$

$$Desired\ pressure\ is\ 15\ cm\ H_2O.$$

Increasing pressure during PC-CMV will normally increase V_T. Conversely, decreasing pressure decreases V_T for patients with respiratory alkalosis during PC-CMV.

Respiratory Alkalosis: VC-CMV and PC-CMV Changes

When P_aCO_2 is decreased (<35 mm Hg) and pH increases (>7.45), then respiratory alkalosis is present indicating that the alveolar ventilation is excessive. Common causes of respiratory alkalosis include the following[2]:
- Hypoxia with compensatory hyperventilation
- Parenchymal lung disease
- Medications (salicylate, xanthines, analeptics)
- Mechanical ventilation
- Central nervous system disorders (meningitis, encephalitis, head trauma)
- Anxiety
- Metabolic problems (sepsis, hepatic disease)

In mechanically ventilated patients, hyperventilation is often the cause of respiratory alkalosis. To correct respiratory alkalosis in this situation, the clinician should decrease minute ventilation during volume-controlled ventilation by decreasing f, and if necessary, by decreasing V_T. If pressure-controlled ventilation is used, the clinician should decrease f first, and then decrease set pressure, if necessary.

Clinical Scenario: Respiratory Alkalosis: Decreasing the Rate

A 35-year-old man with respiratory alkalosis (P_aCO_2 = 20 mm Hg; pH = 7.60) is on CMV with no spontaneous breaths and a delivered V_T of 550 mL, a rate of 18 breaths/min, and V_{Danat} at 150 mL. His desired P_aCO_2 is 40 mm Hg. IBW is 70 kg. V_T setting is approximately 8 mL/kg. It is appropriate to decrease f and leave V_T constant:

$$Desired\ f = 18 \times 20/40 = 9\ breaths/min$$

A new rate of 9 breaths/min should achieve the desired P_aCO_2 of 40 mm Hg. (NOTE: This case did not state whether this was volume-controlled or pressure-controlled ventilation. It does not matter in this situation, however, because the targeted change was the rate.)

Clinical Scenario: Respiratory Alkalosis: Decreasing the Volume in Pressure-Controlled Ventilation

A 50-year-old woman on PC-CMV originally had a set pressure of 20 cm H_2O, which resulted in a V_T of 450 mL (C_S = 28 mL/cm H_2O). The set rate was 12 breaths/min with no spontaneous efforts. T_I is long enough to provide a slight pause (zero flow) at end inspiration. ABGs on this setting showed a pH = 7.41 and a P_aCO_2 of 44 mm Hg. The patient's IBW is 60 kg.

After 2 days of ventilation on these settings, the pH = 7.51 and the P_aCO_2 = 29 mm Hg. The pressure is still at 20 cm H_2O and V_T is 625 mL (10.4 mL/kg IBW). C_S is now 32 mL/cm H_2O. This is a substantial improvement. The V_T is high, based on IBW. What would be an appropriate target volume for this patient?

$$Desired\ V_T = {\sim}450\ mL$$

How do you set a pressure to get this V_T?

$$Remember\ C_S = V_T/\Delta P,\ so\ P = V_T/C_S$$

and

$$Desired\ P = 450\ mL/(32\ mL/cm\ H_2O) = 14\ cm\ H_2O$$

A decrease in pressure to 14 cm H_2O should achieve the new targeted V_T of 450 mL, which is 7.5 mL/kg IBW for this patient.

Clinical Scenario: Respiratory Alkalosis During Spontaneous Efforts

A 25-year-old man on VC-CMV has a set rate of 14 breaths/min and a V_T of 560 mL. The patient's IBW is 80 kg (176 lb). The patient is triggering the ventilator an additional 4 breaths/min. Total rate is 18 breaths/min; P_aCO_2 is 30 mm Hg; pH is 7.50. What can the respiratory therapist do to improve ventilation? The V_T is 7 mL/kg IBW, which is appropriate for this patient. Suppose the therapist reduces the set f on the ventilator to 10 breaths/min. What impact would this have on ventilation? As long as the patient continues to trigger additional breaths, reducing the set f will have no effect.

Decreasing V_T (or more specifically, pressure during PC-CMV) may be effective in reducing minute ventilation unless the patient increases his spontaneous rate, thus maintaining high alveolar ventilation. In addition, lowering the V_T to less than 7 mL/kg may result in atelectasis from low V_T ventilation.

In this situation, several alternatives are available: (1) reduce the tidal volume but ensure that an adequate level of PEEP is being administered to reduce the potential for atelectasis; (2) institute another mode, such as synchronized intermittent mandatory ventilation (IMV), or pressure-supported ventilation (PSV), to allow the patient to breathe without receiving a mandatory breath with every inspiration; or (3) sedate the patient to control breathing better. Sedation may be needed for patients demonstrating extreme agitation, increased work of breathing (WOB), or patient-ventilator asynchrony. It is important to recognize that sedation may not always be the best choice. Whenever possible, the cause of hyperventilation should be investigated and treated. Common causes of hyperventilation include hypoxemia, pain, anxiety, fever, agitation, and asynchrony.

Head injury that results in a high $\dot{V}_E$ and hyperventilation is sometimes difficult to control, regardless of the mode selected. Some patients with brain injury have a tendency to breathe with a high V_T and f, which is the result of a CNS lesion and cannot be corrected.[3]

METABOLIC ACIDOSIS AND ALKALOSIS

Treatment of metabolic acidosis and alkalosis should focus on identifying those metabolic factors that can cause these acid–base disturbances. Although it may not be apparent, a respiratory component may also be involved, and this possibility should also be addressed.

Metabolic Acidosis

Patients in apparent respiratory distress may present with metabolic acidosis. Blood gases indicate pH = 7.00 to 7.34 and a bicarbonate in the range of about 12 to 22 mEq/L. These patients are often struggling to lower their P_aCO_2 to achieve some degree of hyperventilation to compensate for the metabolic acidosis. As a consequence, these patients are at risk for developing respiratory muscle fatigue. Thus in this situation, mechanical ventilation is indicated to meet the minimum goal of compensated hypocapnia.[4] Whether or not this can be accomplished with noninvasive or invasive ventilation depends on whether the patient meets the criteria for this mode of ventilation (see Chapter 19). If invasive ventilation is required, the risks must be balanced against the temporary benefits.

Causes of metabolic acidosis include the following processes:
- **Ketoacidosis** (alcoholism, starvation, diabetes)
- Uremic acidosis (renal failure to excrete acid)
- Loss of bicarbonate (diarrhea)

- Renal loss of base following administration of carbonic anhydrase inhibitors (e.g., Diamox)
- Lactic acidosis
- Toxins ingested that produce acidosis (salicylate, ethylene glycol [antifreeze], methanol)

Treatment for metabolic acidosis includes initiating effective therapy to address the cause of the acidosis and assessing the need to reverse the acidemia with the administration of an alkalizing agent. Treating the underlying cause of acidemia and making sure vascular volume and cardiac output are normal, in addition to ensuring adequate oxygenation, are essential. These actions allow time for the normal metabolism of organic acids (lactic acid and ketoacids), and allow time for the kidneys to generate bicarbonate to replace losses.[4]

Controversy abounds regarding the benefit of using alkalinizing agents, such as bicarbonate administration in the treatment of metabolic acidosis. Lowering arterial CO_2 is also controversial, but if the patient is losing the struggle to maintain high $\dot{V}_E$ with spontaneous breathing, assisted ventilation may be necessary to avoid respiratory failure. In this situation it is appropriate to keep the pH within normal limits (7.35 to 7.45) (Case Study 12-1).

Case Study 12-1

Hyperventilation

A 190-lb (86-kg), 68-year-old man (IBW = 80 kg) is admitted to the hospital. He is placed on mechanical ventilation for acute respiratory failure compounded by a metabolic acidosis. It is determined that he has a renal disorder. The physician orders peritoneal dialysis. In the interim, the physician asks the respiratory therapist to target a pH of 7.35 with assisted ventilation. Initial assessment of the patient resulted in the following ABG: pH = 7.22; P_aCO_2 = 38 mm Hg; HCO_3^- = 15 mEq/L; P_aO_2 = 98 mm Hg on F_IO_2 = 0.25.

The ventilator settings are: VC-CMV; f = 24 breaths/min; V_T = 600 mL; F_IO_2 = 0.25.

ABG results on this new setting are pH = 7.37; P_aCO_2 mm Hg = 23; HCO_3^- = 13.5 mEq/L; P_aO_2 = 115 mm Hg.

A flow–time graphic shows the following:

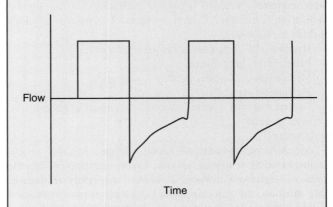

What is the problem, and what would you suggest to correct this problem and still help the patient?

Metabolic Alkalosis

Metabolic alkalosis is present when pH (7.45 to 7.70) and bicarbonate (26 to 48 mEq/L) are elevated above normal. Common causes include the following:

- Loss of gastric fluid and stomach acids (vomiting, nasogastric suctioning)
- Acid loss in the urine (diuretic administration)
- Acid shift into the cells (potassium deficiency)
- Lactate, acetate, or citrate administration
- Excessive bicarbonate loads (bicarbonate administration)

As with metabolic acidosis, treatment involves identifying the underlying cause and reversing those factors leading to the alkalosis. In severe cases carbonic anhydrase inhibitors, acid infusion, and low bicarbonate dialysis may be required.[5]

Uncomplicated metabolic alkalosis is not usually associated with alveolar hypoventilation as a compensatory mechanism, because of the resulting hypoxemia that occurs with severe hypoventilation. For example, P_aCO_2 will usually not rise higher than 55 mm Hg. Remember that the P_aO_2 will fall as the CO_2 rises. Thus hypoventilation is accompanied by hypoxemia in a patient who is breathing room air. The hypoxemia will cause stimulation of the peripheral chemoreceptors, resulting in increased minute ventilation. Only in rare circumstances does full compensation of metabolic alkalosis occur.[5]

MIXED ACID–BASE DISTURBANCES

Some patients with acute respiratory failure have mixed respiratory and metabolic disturbances, such as respiratory acidosis combined with metabolic alkalosis. Notice that the pH may actually be near normal. The following case can be used to illustrate this point. Two additional case studies are also presented to illustrate the management of patients with (1) combined respiratory alkalosis with metabolic acidosis, and (2) combined respiratory acidosis with metabolic alkalosis.

 Clinical Scenario: Mixed Respiratory and Metabolic Disturbances

A 65-year-old patient on mechanical ventilation has a nasogastric tube in place with suction. He is also receiving diuretics for congestive heart failure (CHF). The pH is 7.36, P_aCO_2 is 58 mm Hg, HCO_3^- 31 mEq/L, and P_aO_2 is 111 mm Hg ($F_IO_2 = 0.30$). V_T is 400 mL, and the rate is 12 breaths/min. Is it appropriate to increase $\dot{V}_E$ so that the P_aCO_2 can be returned to 40 mm Hg? In this case it is *not* appropriate to increase $\dot{V}_E$ to decrease the P_aCO_2. This can rapidly result in alkalosis with accompanying cardiac dysrhythmias, seizures, and other neurologic disturbances. The cause of both problems should be determined and corrected.

 Clinical Scenario: Combined Respiratory Alkalosis and Metabolic Acidosis

A 55-year-old man is transported by helicopter to a large metropolitan hospital. His initial diagnosis is acute myocardial infarction. The paramedics intubate the patient, start an intravenous (IV) drip with normal saline, and begin manual ventilation with 100% O_2. After admission to the hospital, the patient has a vascular stent placed in one of the coronary vessels to improve its patency. The patient is stabilized, and mechanical ventilation is initiated with the following settings: IMV 16 breaths/min, V_T = 750 mL (≈10 mL/kg, IBW). No spontaneous breaths are present. No changes are made in the ventilator settings, and the V_T is maintained at ≈10 mL/kg IBW.

Two days later the respiratory therapist obtains a 6:00 AM ABG for this patient. The ventilator settings are still the same. ABG results are as follows:

$$P_aCO_2 = 25 \text{ mm Hg; pH} = 7.42; HCO_3^- = 17 \text{ mEq/L}$$

The patient does not have a history of pulmonary or metabolic disease. His normal P_aCO_2 is about 40 mm Hg. Both the V_T and rate are high for this patient. Because the $P_{plateau}$ is only 20 mm Hg, the therapist decides to reduce the rate initially to begin targeting the patient's normal P_aCO_2.

$$\text{Desired } f = (\text{Actual rate} \times \text{Actual } P_aCO_2)/\text{Desired } P_aCO_2$$

$$\text{Desired } f = (16 \times 25)/40$$

$$\text{Desired } f = 10 \text{ breaths/min}$$

Attempts to reduce ventilator rate to 10 breaths/min result in an increased spontaneous rate of more than 25 breaths/min. The patient is conscious, appears very anxious, and is laboring to breathe. Why is it difficult to reduce the mandatory rate in this situation?

The patient has a compensated respiratory alkalosis. The initial $\dot{V}_E$ was set too high for this patient (set $\dot{V}_E$ = 12 L/min; predicted $\dot{V}_E$ = 10 L/min). After 2 days on these same settings, the kidneys have compensated for an iatrogenic hyperventilation by excreting excess bicarbonate. To allow the reverse process to take place, the mandatory rate will have to be reduced slowly (1 to 2 breaths about every 2 to 4 hours) so the normal ventilation can be restored and the kidneys given time to increase the bicarbonate back to a normal level.

 Clinical Scenario: Combined Respiratory Acidosis and Metabolic Alkalosis

A 35-year-old woman is receiving mechanical ventilation. ABG analysis shows a P_aCO_2 of 60 mm Hg and a pH of 7.41, HCO_3^- = 35 mEq/L. (NOTE: The patient's normal P_aCO_2 is 40 mm Hg.) The fact that the high P_aCO_2 is not reflected in the pH indicates that the patient appears to have a metabolic alkalosis as well as a respiratory acidosis. Before the P_aCO_2 can be corrected with ventilator adjustment, the metabolic alkalosis must be corrected. If the P_aCO_2 were decreased to 40 mm Hg, the pH would increase and the patient would develop a severe alkalosis.

INCREASED PHYSIOLOGICAL DEAD SPACE

If pure respiratory acidosis persists even after alveolar ventilation has been increased, the patient may have a problem that is the result of increased alveolar dead space. Increased alveolar dead space can be caused by a pulmonary embolism or low cardiac output resulting in low pulmonary perfusion.

Increased **alveolar dead space** can also occur when ventilatory support reduces pulmonary blood flow to the lungs by causing high alveolar pressures, such as in the application of high PEEP (Key Point 12-1). Reduced pulmonary perfusion can also be associated with air trapping that results from a high $\dot{V}_E$ or a low inspiratory gas flow (high inspiratory-to-expiratory [I:E] ratio, such as 3:1), or from an uneven distribution of ventilation because of a pathologic lung problem.

In the case of air trapping (auto-PEEP), increasing the flow or decreasing the I:E ratio (to 1:3 or 1:4) may correct the problem (Increasing inspiratory flow can shorten T_I and allow more time for exhalation). Sometimes repositioning the patient so that the disease-compromised lung receives minimal blood flow (nondependent position), while the nondiseased lung receives greater blood flow, can significantly improve gas exchange and help address the problem. (See section on positioning later in this chapter.)

The normal ratio of dead space to tidal volume (V_D/V_T) is 0.2 to 0.4. In critically ill patients, this value can be greater than 0.7. Calculation of V_D/V_T ratio uses the Enghoff modification of the Bohr equation: $V_D/V_T = (P_aCO_2 - P_{\bar{E}}CO_2)/P_aCO_2$, where $P_{\bar{E}}CO_2$ is the partial pressure of CO_2 in the mixed expired gases collected from the patient.* A blood gas sample is collected and the average tidal volume measured while the $P_{\bar{E}}CO_2$ is being measured. Note that although this method of measuring V_D/V_T ratio can provide useful information on mechanically ventilated patients, it typically requires additional equipment and is not routinely performed.

It is more common in ventilated patients to monitor the end-tidal CO_2 (normal $P_{ET}CO_2$ = 35 to 43 mm Hg) and the gradient between arterial and end-tidal CO_2 to determine whether dead space is changing (normal P_aCO_2-to-$P_{ET}CO_2$ gradient = 4 to 6 mm Hg). A decrease in end-tidal CO_2 and an increase in the P_aCO_2-to-$P_{ET}CO_2$ gradient suggest increased dead space. Some clinicians use the mean value of the $P_{ET}CO_2$ instead of measuring mixed expired gas to calculate the V_D/V_T ratio.[6] Advances in capnography using single-breath volumetric CO_2 monitoring offers still another alternative for estimating V_D/V_T. (See Chapter 10 for more details on $P_{ET}CO_2$ and volumetric CO_2 monitoring.)

 Key Point **12-1** Increased alveolar dead space can occur when high levels of PEEP compress pulmonary capillaries and reduce pulmonary blood flow to the lungs.

INCREASED METABOLISM AND INCREASED CARBON DIOXIDE PRODUCTION

Metabolic rate and $\dot{V}CO_2$ are elevated in patients who have fever, burns, multiple trauma, sepsis, **hyperthyroidism,** muscle tremors or seizures, agitation, and in those patients who have undergone multiple surgical procedures. Regardless of the cause, it is clear that $\dot{V}_E$ will be increased and WOB will be elevated. Increasing the

ventilator rate will decrease the patient's WOB, but auto-PEEP may occur. If auto-PEEP is a factor, it may be beneficial to add enough pressure support (PS) for the spontaneous breaths to reduce WOB through the ET and circuit. Other options might include switching to PC-CMV and using sedation to reduce the patient's work.

> ### Clinical Scenario: Increased Metabolism and Increased CO₂ Production
>
> A 25-year-old patient with burns on IMV has a V_T of 0.7 L, rate of 10 breaths/min, P_aCO_2 of 40 mm Hg, and pH of 7.39. The patient has a spontaneous rate of 15 breaths/min and a spontaneous V_T of 600 mL. His P_aO_2 is 88 mm Hg on 0.5 F_IO_2. This patient has a very high total $\dot{V}_E$ (ventilator $\dot{V}_E$ = 7 L/min + patient $\dot{V}_E$ = 9 L/min; total $\dot{V}_E$ = 16 L/min). Given this level of $\dot{V}_E$, one would expect the P_aCO_2 to be lower. The reason that it is not lower may be either an increased $\dot{V}CO_2$ or an increased V_D/V_T.

INTENTIONAL IATROGENIC HYPERVENTILATION

Historically, **iatrogenic** hyperventilation has been used in patients with acute head injury and increased intracranial pressure (ICP). Hyperventilation lowers CO_2 in the blood, which in turn is associated with constriction of cerebral blood vessels, resulting in a reduction in blood flow to the brain. Although this approach was believed by many clinicians to help lower increased ICP, therapeutic guidelines for head injuries with increased ICP do **not** recommend prophylactic hyperventilation (P_aCO_2 <25 mm Hg) during the first 24 hours. Hyperventilation during the first few days following severe traumatic brain injury may actually increase cerebral **ischemia** and cause cerebral hypoxemia (see Chapter 7 section on closed head injury).

Hyperventilation may be required for **brief** periods when acute neurologic deterioration is present and ICP is elevated. Mild hyperventilation (P_aCO_2 30 to 35 mm Hg) may be used for longer periods in situations in which increased ICP is refractory to standard treatment, including sedation and analgesia, neuromuscular blockade, cerebrospinal fluid drainage, and **hyperosmolar** therapy.[7] However, the practice of iatrogenic hyperventilation remains controversial.[8,9] Consider the following example:

> ### Clinical Scenario: Iatrogenic Hyperventilation
>
> A 42-year-old woman who is 5 foot 4 inches tall (IBW = 125 lb, or 57 kg) is on controlled ventilation for 12 hours following a severe cerebral concussion. Her P_aCO_2 is 48 mm Hg, her pH is 7.32, and her V_T is 400 mL. Respiratory rate is 12 breaths/min. What are your recommendations? Current V_T is 7 mL/kg. Is it appropriate to change f? In this case it would be appropriate to increase the f and maintain the P_aCO_2 at normal levels for the first 24 hours.
>
> If we change the rate, the following recommendation would apply:
>
> $$\text{Desired } f = 12 \times 48/40 = 14 \text{ breaths/min}$$

---

*Mixed expired gas includes alveolar gas and gas from the anatomic dead space. Historically, mixed expired analyses were obtained using a large airtight collection bag, such as a Douglas bag. Exhaled gases were collected over a 3-minute period and then a sample of the exhaled gas was analyzed using a standard blood gas analyzer. With most ICU ventilators, mixed expired gas samples can be obtained using rapid responding CO_2 analyzers and computer software incorporated into the ventilator design.

PERMISSIVE HYPERCAPNIA

Occasionally, it becomes impossible to maintain normal P_aCO_2 levels in a patient without risking lung damage from high plateau pressures (>30 cm H_2O) and volumes. Patients with ARDS or status asthmaticus and sometimes patients with chronic obstructive pulmonary disease (COPD) who require ventilatory support are at risk for ventilator-induced injury. Inappropriate ventilator settings can result in severe lung injury, activation of inflammatory mediators, and can even potentially lead to multisystem organ failure.[9] (See Chapter 17 for additional information on ventilator-induced lung injury.)

A technique referred to as *permissive hypercapnia* (PHY) has gained popularity as an alternative form of patient management.[10] PHY is a deliberate limitation of ventilatory support to avoid lung overdistension and injury of the lung. During PHY arterial partial pressures of carbon dioxide (P_aCO_2) values are allowed to rise above normal (e.g., ≥50 and ≤150 mm Hg), and pH values are allowed to fall below normal (e.g., ≥7.10 to 7.30). Patients who do not have renal failure or cardiovascular problems usually tolerate a pH of 7.20 to 7.25. Younger patients may tolerate even lower pH values. Many clinicians who use PHY allow for a gradual rise in P_aCO_2 because an abrupt increase in P_aCO_2 is usually not well tolerated.[11,12]

Alterations in P_aCO_2 and pH can affect multiple organ systems. Researchers often focus on the effects of severe acidosis because of serious consequences associated with it. Although most investigators agree that a pH of 7.25 or greater is acceptable, no one is certain whether a lower pH is acceptable. Survival without complications has been demonstrated in isolated cases in which the pH dropped as low as 6.6 and the P_aCO_2 rose as high as 375 mm Hg when oxygenation was well maintained.[11,13] Similar findings have been shown in studies of patients with ARDS and acute asthma.[14-17]

During hypoventilation increases in P_aCO_2 are accompanied by a decrease in P_aO_2, so O_2 administration must be provided and oxygenation status monitored carefully. Increases in P_aCO_2 and decreases in pH that occur in acute respiratory acidosis also cause a right shift in the oxyhemoglobin dissociation curve. Although this shift in the curve facilitates unloading of O_2 at the tissue level, it also reduces O_2 loading at the lungs and can further compromise gas exchange.

Increases in carbon dioxide have an additional physiological effect. A higher-than-normal P_aCO_2 stimulates the drive to breathe. Therefore it is appropriate to provide sedation to patients with acute lung injury (ALI) in whom permissive hypercapnia is being used. The sedation may improve patient comfort. (It is worth mentioning that extremely high levels of P_aCO_2 can result in an anesthesia effect referred to as *CO₂ narcosis* [Key Point 12-2].)

> **Key Point 12-2** Extremely high levels of P_aCO_2 (>200 mm Hg) can result in an anesthesia effect also known as *CO₂ narcosis*.

Procedures for Managing Permissive Hypercapnia

Efforts to maintain eucapnic breathing (i.e., near a patient's normal level of P_aCO_2) might include removing sources of mechanical dead space and increasing the frequency of mandatory breaths.[18] When the decision is made to allow P_aCO_2 to rise above normal, the following strategy may be used[19]:

| BOX **12-1** | **Protocol for the Implementation of Permissive Hypercapnia** |

When adequate ventilation cannot be maintained within acceptable limits for pressures and volumes, permissive hypercapnia (PHY) can be implemented using the following steps[21]:
1. Hypercapnia should be implemented progressively in increments of 10 mm Hg/h to a maximum of 80 mm Hg/day.
2. If hypercapnia should exceed 80 mm Hg, progress more slowly.
3. F_IO_2 is adjusted to maintain arterial oxygen saturation (S_aO_2) at 85% to 90%. Adequate oxygenation is imperative and can require the intermittent use of 100% O_2.
4. If PHY is used for less than 24 hours, P_aCO_2 can be allowed to decrease by 10 to 20 mm Hg/h, provided that P_aCO_2 is greater than 80 mm Hg. The closer the patient is to normocapnia, the slower the process should be.
5. If PHY is used for more than 24 hours, or if large amounts of buffer agents are used, discontinue PHY even more slowly (in 1 to 3 days).

---

1. Allow P_aCO_2 to rise and pH to fall without changing the mandatory rate or volume. Do nothing other than sedate the patient, avoid high ventilating pressures, and maintain oxygenation.
2. Reduce CO_2 production by using paralytic agents, cooling the patient, and restricting glucose intake.
3. Administer agents such as sodium bicarbonate, *tris*(hydroxymethyl)aminomethane (tromethamine [THAM], an amino buffer), or Carbicarb (a mixture of sodium carbonate and bicarbonate) to keep pH greater than 7.25.

Note that use of these buffering agents remains debatable and not well studied in PHY. A short-term increase in P_aCO_2 might occur when bicarbonate is administered. This is exhaled over time if the level of ventilation is constant. The use of THAM is not associated with an increased P_aCO_2. It produces intracellular as well as extracellular buffering of pH. Whether or not buffers have any effect on the tolerance of permissive hypercapnia is not known.[20] A protocol for the implementation of permissive hypercapnia is provided in Box 12-1.[21]

Contraindications of Permissive Hypercapnia

Carbon dioxide is a powerful vasodilator of cerebral vessels. Thus increasing CO_2 levels can result in cerebral edema and increased ICP, which can aggravate cerebral disorders, such as cerebral trauma or hemorrhage, and cerebral-occupying lesions.[19,21] For this reason the use of PHY is contraindicated in the presence of disorders such as head trauma and intracranial disease. Indeed, it is absolutely contraindicated for those patients who demonstrate intracranial lesions (Key Point 12-3).[22]

> **Key Point 12-3** Permissive hypercapnia is absolutely contraindicated for those patients who demonstrate intracranial lesions.

Permissive hypercapnia is relatively contraindicated in patients with preexisting cardiovascular instability. Circulatory effects of PHY can include decreased myocardial contractility, arrhythmias, vasodilation, and increased sympathetic activity. A common finding in patients receiving PHY is increased cardiac output, a normal systemic blood pressure (BP), and pulmonary hypertension.[20,23] If the patient's sympathetic response is impaired or blocked, or if cardiac function is impaired, then an increase in cardiac output might **not** occur, allowing the vasodilatation to result in hypotension.[19]

The exact response of the cardiovascular system to permissive hypercapnia is difficult to predict; therefore PHY should be used with caution. This is particularly true when working with patients with any of the following cardiovascular conditions: cardiac ischemia, left ventricular compromise, pulmonary hypertension, and right heart failure (Key Point 12-4).[22]

Key Point 12-4 Permissive hypercapnia should be used with caution when treating patients demonstrating cardiac ischemia, left ventricular compromise, pulmonary hypertension, and right heart failure.

Finally it is worth mentioning that elevated CO_2 or decreased pH may affect regional blood flow; skeletal and smooth muscle function; nervous system activity; and endocrine, digestive, hepatic, and renal system functions. Although these effects have not caused significant concern in the clinical setting, further research in these areas is warranted to improve our understanding of this ventilatory strategy.

Clinical Scenario: Permissive Hypercapnia

A 30-year-old man with ARDS has been on ventilatory support for 5 days. Current settings are V_T = 500 mL; f = 12 breaths/min; peak inspiratory pressure (PIP) = 37 cm H_2O; and $P_{plateau}$ = 29 cm H_2O. The patient is 5 foot 8 inches tall and has an IBW of 70 kg. ABGs show pH = 7.24 and P_aCO_2 = 64 mm Hg. What change is appropriate to return his P_aCO_2 to normal? If we tried to increase his V_T, pressures would increase. If we increase f, the desired f would be

$$\text{Desired } f = 12 \times 64/40 = 19 \text{ breaths/min}$$

This equation assumes that we want to maintain a normal P_aCO_2 of 40 mm Hg. One might suspect that the increased rate would also lead to air trapping, an increase in mean airway pressure, and an increased risk of lung injury. However, in patients with ARDS, lung units are more likely to empty quickly (short time constants). We might increase rate slightly and allow P_aCO_2 to remain high (i.e., PHY). To protect the patient from increasing airway pressures, it might be appropriate to use pressure ventilation.

The use of PHY is restricted to situations in which the target airway pressure is at its maximum and the highest possible rates are being used. Although no adverse short-term effects of PHY have been noted for most patients, it is not known whether any long-term effects occur. The risks of hypercapnia are considered by some to be preferable to the high $P_{plateau}$ required to achieve normal CO_2 levels. This represents a significant shift in thinking in regard to ventilator management and ARDS.[24]

Airway Clearance During Mechanical Ventilation

During mechanical ventilation, several techniques can be used to help clear secretions from the airway. These procedures differ somewhat from those used with nonintubated, spontaneously breathing patients. Included in this section are discussions of the following topics: suctioning, aerosol delivery, postural drainage and percussion, and fiberoptic bronchoscopy.* High-frequency percussive ventilation can also assist with secretion clearance.

SECRETION CLEARANCE FROM AN ARTIFICIAL AIRWAY

Clearing secretions from the ET or tracheostomy tube of mechanically ventilated patients is an important component of bronchial hygiene therapy. Although it is not uncommon to see a physician's order read "Suction Q 2 hr," suctioning at fixed intervals is not appropriate and should be performed **only** when necessary (i.e., based on patient assessment findings).

Suctioning a patient's artificial airways involves insertion of a suction catheter into the patient's trachea and the application of negative pressure as the catheter is gradually withdrawn.[25] Suctioning a patient with an artificial airway typically involves **shallow** suctioning, in which the catheter is inserted to a depth that approximates the length of the artificial airways. **Deep** suctioning involves inserting the catheter into the artificial airway until a resistance is met. Once the resistance is encountered, the catheter is withdrawn approximately 1 cm before applying negative pressure.

Two methods of suctioning are typically described based on the type of catheter used: the **open suctioning technique** and the **closed suctioning technique.** The open-circuit technique requires disconnecting the patient from the ventilator; the closed-circuit technique can be performed without removing the patient from the ventilator. With the closed-circuit technique, a sterile, inline suction catheter is incorporated into the ventilator circuit, thus allowing passage of the catheter into the ET and trachea without disconnecting the patient from the ventilator (Key Point 12-5).

Key Point 12-5 Two methods of endotracheal suctioning can be performed based on the type of catheter used: the **open-circuit technique** and the **closed-circuit technique.**

Suction catheters are generally made of transparent flexible plastic that is rigid enough to allow it to be easily inserted into the artificial airway, but flexible enough to negotiate turns and not cause trauma to the airway. Catheters are smooth tipped with two or more side holes near the distal end (Fig. 12-3). (It is thought that these smooth-tipped catheters with side holes may help reduce trauma to the mucosa.)[26]

The proximal end of the catheter connects to a collecting canister via large-bore plastic tube. A thumb port located at the proximal end of the suction catheter allows the operator to control the suction pressure. When it is covered, suction pressure is applied to the catheter and into the airway. The suction pressure applied

---

*Use of kinetic beds is reviewed in Chapter 17.

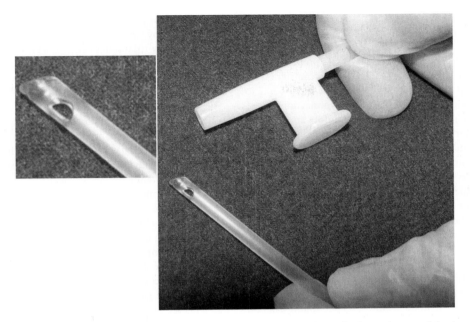

Fig. 12-3 Flexible suction catheter for lower airway suctioning showing rounded tip with side port *(cutaway of photo).*

BOX **12-2**	**Patient Size and Appropriate Suction Levels**

Adults:	−100 to −120 mm Hg	(maximum suction: −150 mm Hg)
Child:	−80 to −100 mm Hg	(maximum suction: −125 mm Hg)
Infant:	−60 to −100 mm Hg	(maximum suction: −100 mm Hg)

BOX **12-3**	**Estimating Correct Suction Catheter Size Based on Endotracheal Tube (ET) Size**

Multiply ET size by 3. This converts the ET size to French units (Fr). Then divide this number by 2 to use half or less of the ET diameter.
  For example: With a size 8 ET, 3 × 8 = 24; 24/2 = 12.
  A size 12 Fr suction catheter would be appropriate.

should be the lowest possible pressure that is required to effectively clear secretions.[25] Box 12-2 provides a list of suggested suction pressure levels. These recommended suction levels are based on current practice, although it is very common to see higher than recommended suction pressures used in many clinical settings. It is important to note that to date no experimental studies are available to support these values.

The catheter length should be long enough to reach a main-stem bronchus. This requires a catheter length of about 22 inches (56 cm).[26] Note that in infants and in patients with recent tracheal reconstructive surgery or pneumonectomy, the suction catheter should not be inserted more than 1 cm below the distal tip of the ET.[27]

Remember that the left main-stem bronchus is narrower and branches at a more acute angle than the right bronchus. Consequently suction catheters often enter the right rather than the left bronchus. A special-tipped suction catheter is available with a bend at the distal end to help facilitate left bronchial suctioning, particularly if the patient is supine or lying on the left side or if the head is turned to the left. Left bronchus suctioning is easier when the patient has a tracheostomy tube in place rather than an ET.[27]

The diameter of the suction catheter selected is governed by the internal diameter of the artificial airway. It is generally accepted that the diameter of the suction catheter should not exceed 50% of the internal diameter of the artificial airway for children and adults and 30% of the internal diameters for infants.[25] Suction catheter sizes are based on French units. French units refer to the circumference of the tube. (NOTE: Circumference equals diameter multiplied by 3.1416 [π].) Because ETs are sized in centimeters and suction catheters are sized in French units, a conversion is required to estimate the correct size (Box 12-3).

Suctioning should be preceded by hyperoxygenation with 100% O_2 for 30 seconds, followed by hyperoxygenation with 100% O_2 for 1 minute after suctioning is complete, especially in patients who are hypoxemic before or during suctioning.[28] This can be done manually with a resuscitation bag, although this approach does not guarantee V_T or pressure, and it has been shown to be ineffective in delivering an F_IO_2 of 1.0.[25] Hyperoxygenation is therefore best accomplished using a temporary oxygen-enrichment program that is available on many microprocessor ventilators.

The duration of suctioning should be brief and must not exceed 15 seconds.[25] Shallow suctioning is recommended over deep suctioning, particularly because deep suctioning has not been shown to be superior and may be associated with significantly greater chance of trauma to the tracheal mucosa. Although there is some debate regarding intermittent versus continuous suctioning, many clinicians choose applied suction intermittently rather than continually as it is withdrawn.[29,30]

Hazards and Complications of Suctioning

Loss of suction pressure may be caused by a leak in the system or because the collection canister is full. All connections should be checked, including ensuring that the suction jar is properly seated and screwed on tightly. In cases where the collection canister is full, a float valve at the top of the canister will close the suction line to prevent the transmission of suction to the wall connection line.

Suctioning can cause a great deal of discomfort and anxiety. Stimulation of the airway with the catheter commonly induces coughing and can result in bronchospasm in patients with reactive airways. Suctioning can also cause hemorrhage, airway edema, and ulceration of the mucosal wall if it is performed improperly.[30]

The severity of the complications associated with suctioning generally is related to the duration of the procedure, the amount of suction applied, the size of the catheter, and whether or not oxygenation and hyperventilation are done appropriately. Reductions in lung volume can occur with suctioning and lead to atelectasis and hypoxemia. Note that to avoid atelectasis, the clinician should limit the duration of suctioning and the amount of negative pressure applied to the patient's airways. Hyperoxygenation and hyperventilation of the patient before and after suctioning can also reduce many of the complications associated with suctioning. It is also important to recognize that there is a temporary loss of applied PEEP when a patient is disconnected from the ventilator, which in turn can increase the severity of hypoxemia.

Cardiac arrhythmias can also occur during aggressive suctioning. Tachycardia is generally attributed to hypoxemia and from the irritation of the procedure; bradycardia can occur if the catheter stimulates vagal receptors in the upper airways.[31] Hypotension may also occur as a result of cardiac arrhythmias or severe coughing episodes. Hypertension may occur because of hypoxemia or increased sympathetic tone resulting from stress, pain, anxiety, or a change in hemodynamics from hyperinflation (see Case Study 12-2).[32,33]

 Case Study 12-2

Assessment During Suctioning

During suctioning of a ventilated patient, the therapist notices a cardiac monitor alarm. The patient's heart rate has increased from 102 to 150 beats/min. What should the therapist do?

See Appendix A for the answer.

Secretion removal is critical in patients with small airways, particularly infants and children, because of the smaller luminal ETs. Suction catheters can even result in pneumothorax in infants if the suction catheter perforates a bronchus.[28] Cross contamination of the airway can occur if suctioning is not performed using sterile conditions.[34]

As previously mentioned patients with closed head injuries usually have increased ICP. The simple process of inserting the suction catheter without suction being applied in patients with severe brain injury can raise the increased mean intracranial pressure (MICP), the mean arterial pressure (MAP), and the cerebral perfusion pressure (CPP).[32,35] This is particularly worrisome in this group of patients. If ICP is being monitored, pressures should be observed before and during suctioning. Oxygenating and

hyperventilating the patient are important in this situation. It may even be appropriate to pretreat the patient with topical anesthetic approximately 15 minutes before the procedure to help reduce the risk of increasing ICP.[36,37]

Closed-Suction Catheters (In-line Suction Catheters)

The closed-suction procedure is considered equally effective as the standard open-suction procedure.[38,39] The closed-suction procedure uses inline catheters that are encased in clear plastic sheaths. The plastic sheaths are attached to special assemblies that connect to a patient's ventilator circuit, near the Y-connector (Fig. 12-4).[40] Notice that inline catheters may add weight and increase the tension on the ET.

The advantage of using the closed-suction technique is that disconnecting the patient from the ventilator can be avoided. This is especially important in patients receiving high F_IO_2 values and PEEP because disconnection increases the likelihood of hypoxia and alveolar collapse. Another advantage of this technique is that it reduces the risk for contaminating the airway and lungs when patients are disconnected from the ventilator. For example, using a manual resuscitation bag may introduce contamination into the patient's lower airways when a single-use disposable suction catheter, which is accidentally contaminated by the handler, is used to suction a patient. Additionally, aerosolized particles from the ventilator circuit can be released into the air during disconnection of the ventilator circuit, thus presenting a potential risk of contamination to the caregiver. Using inline suction avoids these problems and has been shown to reduce the incidence of ventilator-associated pneumonia (VAP).[41] Specific indications for closed-suction catheters are listed in Box 12-4.[42]

Although manufacturers typically recommend that inline catheters be changed daily, studies have shown that there is no increase in mortality, VAP, or length of stay in the hospital when the inline catheters are left in longer.[42-45] Weekly changes do not seem to

---

BOX 12-4 **Indications for Using Closed-Suction Catheter Systems**

Unstable patients who are ventilated (e.g., in acute lung injury or acute respiratory distress syndrome) and have high ventilator requirements:
- High PEEP ≥10 cm H_2O
  - High $\bar{P}_{aw}$ ≥20 cm H_2O
  - Long inspiratory time ≥1.5 sec
  - High F_IO_2 ≥0.6
- Patients who become hemodynamically unstable during suctioning with an open system and ventilator disconnection
- Patients who desaturate significantly (a drop in S_pO_2) during suctioning with an open system and ventilator disconnection
- Patients with contagious infections, such as active tuberculosis, where open suctioning and ventilator disconnect may contaminate health care workers
- Ventilated patients who require frequent suctioning, for example, more than 6 times a day
- Patients receiving inhaled gas mixtures (such as nitric oxide or heliox therapy) that cannot be interrupted by ventilator disconnection

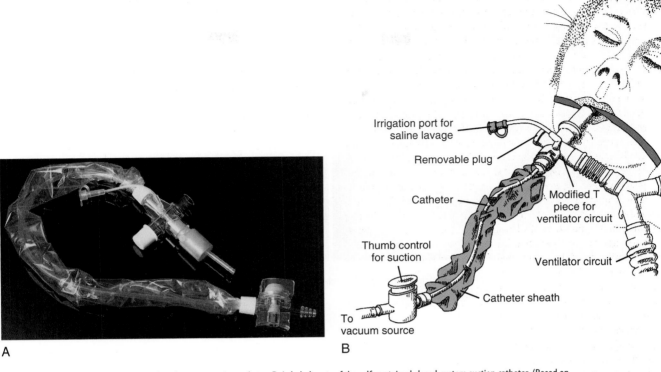

Fig. 12-4 **A,** A closed-system suction catheter. **B,** Labeled parts of the self-contained closed-system suction catheter. (Based on the Kimberly-Clark Ballard Trach Care Closed Suction System.) (**A** from Cairo JM, Pilbeam SP: Mosby's respiratory care equipment, ed 8, St Louis, 2010, Mosby. **B** from Sills JR: The comprehensive respiratory therapist exam review: Entry and advanced levels, ed 5, St Louis, 2010, Mosby.)

increase the incidence of ventilator-associated pneumonia compared with daily changes. In addition, changing less frequently reduces the cost of patient care.[46] (NOTE: Inline suction catheters should be changed more often than weekly if the device mechanically fails or becomes excessively soiled.)

As with regular suctioning, the procedure of hyperoxygenation of the patient is needed when closed-suctioning is performed.[47] Hyperoxygenation is best accomplished using the ventilator as opposed to a manual resuscitation bag. However, different types of problems can occur with inline catheters compared with use of open suctioning methods. Sometimes the catheter remains in the airway following suctioning or migrates into the airway between procedures. The clinician should assure that the suction catheter is withdrawn from the airway following suctioning. During pressure ventilation this increases airway resistance and can affect the patient's V_T delivery. In addition, when the catheter is rinsed with saline following the procedure, there is a risk of accidentally allowing some of the saline to go into the patient's airway.[26] Reduced pressure in the circuit during the suctioning procedure caused by using a very high suction pressure can also cause the ventilator to trigger. Aside from these few problems, the closed-suction catheter is effective and advantageous.

Continuous Aspiration of Subglottic Secretions

Cuffed ETs have been used for years to protect the patient's airway from aspiration. However, even while aspiration of large volumes of material (gastric regurgitation) is generally avoided with a cuff, silent aspiration does occur.

High-volume low-pressure cuffs represent the majority of ETs used in the acute care setting today. These ETs may increase bacterial colonization of the tracheobronchial tree and result in VAP, which is also referred to as *endotracheal tube-associated pneumonia*.[26] (See Chapter 14 for a discussion of VAP.) Silent aspiration and VAP can occur with cuffed ETs for several reasons:

- Injury to the mucosa during insertion and manipulation of the tube following insertion
- Interference with the normal cough reflex
- Aspiration of contaminated secretions that pool above the ET cuff
- Development of a contaminated biofilm around the ET[48]

Silent aspiration occurs in the following manner. Large cuffs can develop longitudinal folds when inflated in the trachea. Liquid pharyngeal secretions leak through these folds (silent aspiration) into the lower airway. Increasing the cuff pressure does not completely eliminate this problem, which in turn can lead to VAP.[26] (It is worth mentioning that the incidence of VAP is between 10% and 60%, and it is associated with increased mortality.)[49]

Specialized ETs have been developed that may reduce the incidence of silent aspiration (e.g., Hi-Lo Evac endotracheal tube, Mallinckrodt, Covidien, Boulder, Colo.; Fig. 12-5, *A*). The Hi-Lo Evac endotracheal tube has a suction port just above the cuff on the dorsal side of the tube (Fig. 12-5, *B*). It was designed to remove secretions above the cuff of the ET and reduce the risk of VAP associated with silent aspiration. The Hi-Lo Evac ET allows for the "continuous aspiration of subglottic secretions" (CASS). The manufacturer currently recommends using 20 mm Hg of continuous

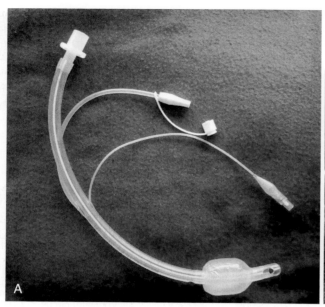
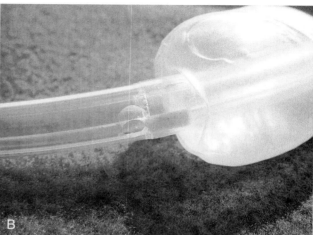

Fig. 12-5 A, Hi-Lo Evac endotracheal tube with endotracheal tube connector *(top),* suction port connector, pilot balloon. **B,** Close-up of the suction lumen above the cuff.

suction. Other advances in ET tube design that have been shown to reduce the incidence of silent aspiration include specially designed ET cuffs made of polyurethane or silicone. These specially designed ET tubes reduce the formation of longitudinal channels in the cuff, which provide openings for secretions to leak around the cuff and enter the lower airways.

Continuous suction tubes are more expensive than standard ETs and as a consequence are not typically inserted in all patients. However, some hospitals have policies to allow insertion of these tubes in emergency departments and during emergency intubations. For patients who may require an extended period on a ventilator with an ET in place, it may be appropriate to change the standard ET tube for the specialized tube.[26] CASS may be most effective in patients requiring intubation for more than 3 days.[50] Although the tube costs more than a standard ET, cost savings can be gained if the patient's length of stay in the intensive care unit (ICU) is reduced. Furthermore, the Centers for Disease Control and Prevention (CDC) has recommended the use of this device because it has been shown to reduce the incidence of nosocomial pneumonias or VAP.[34,50-53] One study showed a fivefold greater likelihood of VAP when CASS was not used.[52]

In general, complications associated with CASS are minimal. Use of CASS can result in severe damage to the airway if the inline catheter is placed in a fixed position. In a case reported in the literature, a fatal tracheal-innominate artery fistula occurred as a result of CASS. In this incident, the inline catheter was fixed to a tooth (the left upper molar), and its position was not changed, resulting in erosion of the tissues.[54]

In addition to silent aspiration, another source of bacterial colonization of the lungs is the presence of a biofilm that forms inside ETs and may serve as a source of bacteria. It is thought that these bacterial colonies can be dislodged from the inner lumen during standard suctioning procedures.[26]

In addition to CASS, another way of avoiding VAP may include decreasing colonization of bacteria in the stomach by maintaining

an acid environment in the stomach and using nonabsorbable antibiotics to reduce the number of growing organisms.[49]

Normal Saline Instillation

An airway clearance technique used by many ICU clinicians involves the instillation 3 to 5 mL of sterile normal saline or half-normal saline into the airway (saline lavage), followed by hyperoxygenation (with 100% O_2) of the patient prior to suctioning. The intent of saline lavage is to loosen secretions and stimulate the patient to cough.[25,55]

Presently there is insufficient evidence to support the practice of instilling normal saline into the ET before suctioning. In fact a number of recent studies indicate that this practice actually may be harmful.[25] Indeed, saline does not thin secretions, and instilling saline may increase the risk of dislodging bacteria-laden biofilm from the ET, which in turn can lead to the development of nosocomial pneumonia.[37,55] Saline instillation may also cause irritation to the airways, resulting in severe coughing episodes and bronchospasm in some patients.

It is also worth noting that less fluid is suctioned compared with the amount instilled into the airway during saline instillation. Additionally, saline instillation can increase the volume of secretions in the airways and potentially add to airway obstruction.[56] It can also reduce oxygenation and increase a patient's sensation of dyspnea, particularly in older patients (i.e., older than 60 years).[57]

Assessment Following Suctioning

The amount, color, odor, and physical characteristics of the sputum should be documented on a ventilator flow sheet along with evaluation of the breath sounds after suctioning. It is also important to check for bilateral breath sounds to assess the effects of suctioning and ensure that the ET has not changed position. It is worth mentioning that right main-stem intubation can occur during these types of procedures and might not always be detected with auscultation.[58] For this reason, some institutions have a standing order for a chest radiograph to be taken every 24 hours to ensure proper tube placement and check for any pathologic changes from the previous film (Box 12-5).[59]

The American Association for Respiratory Care (AARC) has produced an updated Clinical Practice Guideline (CPG) that

outlines the procedure for endotracheal suctioning of mechanically ventilated patients.[25] This CPG provides valuable information regarding patient preparation, the suctioning event and follow-up care, indications, contraindications, hazards and complications, limitations, need and outcome assessments, required resources, types of monitoring that should be used during and after the procedure, and infection-control precautions (Box 12-6).

ADMINISTERING AEROSOLS TO VENTILATED PATIENTS

The delivery of therapeutic aerosols during mechanical ventilation has received considerable attention during the past decade. A number of drugs and agents can be administered to mechanically ventilated patients, including bronchodilators, corticosteroids, antibiotics, mucolytics, and surfactants.[61] Bronchodilators are the most frequently used drug administered by aerosol to mechanically ventilated patients.

| BOX 12-5 | **Routine Chest Radiographs** |

A study conducted by Krivopal and associates found that monitoring daily chest radiographs (CXRs) was not associated with reduced length of stay in the ICU or the hospital, or with a reduction in mortality compared with CXRs taken only when a change in the patient's condition warranted a chest film.[60] New findings on nonroutine CXRs resulted in a significantly greater number of patient interventions. Routine CXRs may not be as important in patient management compared with protocols that recommend the use of a CXR when the patient's condition warrants this evaluation.

| BOX 12-6 | **Excerpts from the American Association for Respiratory Care (AARC) Clinical Practice Guidelines for Endotracheal Suctioning of Mechanically Ventilated Adults and Children with Artificial Airways** |

Indications
The need to remove accumulated pulmonary secretions as evidenced by:
- Patient's inability to generate an effective spontaneous cough
- Changes in monitored flow–volume graphics
- Deterioration of oxygen saturation or arterial blood gas values
- Increased PIP with volume ventilation
- A decrease in V_T with pressure ventilation
- Visible secretions in the airway
- Acute respiratory distress
- Suspected aspiration of gastric or upper-airway secretions

Contraindications
Most contraindications are relative to the patient's risk of developing adverse reactions or worsening clinical condition as a result of the procedure. When suctioning is indicated, there is no absolute contraindication, because abstaining from suctioning to avoid possible adverse reaction may, in fact, be lethal.

Hazards and Complications
- Decrease in dynamic lung compliance and functional residual capacity
- Pulmonary atelectasis: reduction of lung volume
- Hypoxia or hypoxemia
- Hypoxia or hypoxemia: ventilator disconnection and loss of positive end-expiratory pressure (PEEP)
- Tracheal or bronchial mucosal trauma: suction pressures
- Cardiac or respiratory arrest: extreme response to suctioning and ventilator disconnect
- Bronchoconstriction or bronchospasm
- Increased microbial colonization of the patient's lower airways
- Pulmonary hemorrhage or bleeding: trauma to the airways from suctioning
- Elevated intracranial pressure

- Cardiac dysrhythmias
- Hypertension
- Hypotension
- Routine use of normal saline instillation before endotracheal tube (ET) suctioning may be associated with excessive coughing, decreased oxygen saturation, bronchospasm, and dislodgment of bacterial biofilm that colonizes the ET into the lower airways.

Assessment of Need
Qualified personnel should assess the need for endotracheal suctioning as a routine part of a patient-ventilator system assessment.

Assessment of Outcome
- Improvement in the appearance of ventilator graphics and breath sounds
- Decreased PIP with narrowing of PIP-$P_{plateau}$; decreased airway resistance or increased dynamic compliance; increased tidal volume delivery during pressure-limited ventilation
- Improvement in ABG values or saturation as reflected by pulse oximetry (S_pO_2)
- Removal of pulmonary secretions

Monitoring
The following should be monitored before, during, and after the procedure:
- Breath sounds
- Oxygen saturation (S_pO_2)
- F_IO_2
- Respiratory rate and pattern
- Pulse rate, blood pressure, ECG (if indicated and available)
- Sputum (color, volume, consistency, odor)
- Ventilator parameters
- ABGs
- Cough effort
- ICP (if indicated and available)

(From the American Association for Respiratory Care Clinical Practice Guideline: Endotracheal suctioning of mechanically ventilated patients with artificial airways, *Respir Care* 55:758-764, 2010.)

Ventilator related

- Mode of ventilation
- Tidal volume
- Respiratory rate
- Duty cycle
- Inspiratory waveform
- Breath-triggering mechanism

Device related—MDI

- Type of spacer or adapter used
- Position of spacer in circuit
- Timing of MDI actuation

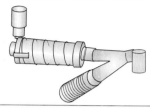

Drug related

- Dose
- Aerosol particle size
- Duration of action

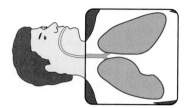

Device related—nebulizer

- Type of nebulizer used
- Continuous/intermittent operation
- Duration of nebulization
- Position in the circuit

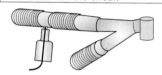

Circuit related

- Endotracheal tube
- Inhaled gas humidity
- Inhaled gas density/viscosity

Patient related

- Severity of airway obstruction
- Mechanism of airway obstruction
- Presence of dynamic hyperinflation
- Patient-ventilator synchrony

Fig. 12-6 Factors that influence aerosol delivery in mechanically ventilated patients: *MDI*, metered-dose inhaler. (Modified from Dhand R, Tobin MJ: Bronchodilator delivery with metered-dose inhalers in mechanically-ventilated patients, Eur Respir J 9:585-595, 1996.)

Figure 12-6 illustrates a variety of factors that must be considered when delivering aerosols to mechanically ventilated patients.[61,62] These factors include the following:

- Type of aerosol-generating device used
- Ventilator mode and settings
- Severity of the patient's condition
- Nature and type of medication and gas used to deliver it

These factors are reviewed in more detail later in this section.

Aerosol administration of bronchodilators to mechanically ventilated patient is indicated for the treatment of bronchoconstriction or increased airway resistance. The decision to administer a bronchodilator should be based on the patient's history and physical assessment findings. Use of ventilator graphics can support these findings (see Fig. 9-6). Box 12-7 summarizes the AARC CPG for the selection of an aerosol device and administration of a bronchodilator to a ventilated patient.[63]

Types of Aerosol-Generating Devices

The most common devices used for administering aerosol are pressurized metered-dose inhalers (pMDIs) and small-volume nebulizers (SVNs). Ultrasonic nebulizers (USNs) and vibrating mesh nebulizers (VMNs) also are available and are becoming more widely used. The primary advantage of using USNs and VMNs is that these devices produce smaller aerosol particles than pMDIs and SVNs without the addition of gas into the ventilator circuit.[64]

Early in vitro and in vivo studies reported that drug deposition rates for aerosolized medications during mechanical ventilation ranged from only 1.5 to 3.0% for SVNs and pMDIs. More recent studies demonstrated that the deposition rates for SVNs can be significantly improved (up to 15%) when optimum conditions are

used.[64] Deposition rates for pMDIs can range from as low as 2.0% to as high as 98%, depending on the delivery technique and whether a spacer is used.

Both pMDIs and SVNs can produce aerosol particles with a mean mass aerodynamic diameter of 1 to 5 μm. Although the physiological response of the patient is similar whether a pMDI or an SVN is used, pMDI doses may need to be adjusted to deliver an adequate amount of medication during mechanical ventilation (i.e., using four or more puffs). This may require doubling the dose that would typically be administered to a spontaneously breathing patient.[62]

Ventilator-Related Factors

As Fig. 12-6 illustrates, various ventilator-related factors can affect aerosol delivery. Table 12-1 lists factors related to the settings on the ventilator.[65-67] Although ventilator settings cannot always be adjusted for aerosol delivery, it can be helpful whenever possible to use low flow rates, higher V_Ts, and lower respiratory rates during the treatment.

The pMDI can be introduced into a ventilator circuit through an elbow adapter or with unidirectional and bidirectional inline chamber and spacer adapters. Elbow adapters are connected directly to the ET. Inline chambers and spacers are placed in the inspiratory limb of the ventilator circuit, as illustrated in Fig. 12-7. Several studies have demonstrated that inline chambers and bidirectional spacers produce considerably greater aerosol delivery than elbow adapters and unidirectional spacers.[65] Elbow adapters, by virtue of their design, create a 90-degree connection with the circuit. Other abrupt angles in the ventilator circuit created by the Y-connector and inline suction catheters can provide points of impact and turbulence that interfere with aerosol delivery

Excerpts from the AARC Clinical Practice Guidelines for Selection of a Device for Administration of a Bronchodilator and Evaluation of the Response to Therapy in Mechanically Ventilated Patients

Indication

Aerosol administration of a bronchodilator and evaluation of response are indicated whenever bronchoconstriction or increased airway resistance is documented or suspected in mechanically ventilated patients.

Contraindications

Some assessment maneuvers may be contraindicated for patients in extremis—for example, a prolonged inspiratory pause for patients with high auto-PEEP. The use of certain medications also may be contraindicated in some patients. The package insert should be consulted for these product-specific contraindications.

Hazards and Complications

- Specific assessment procedures may have inherent hazards or complications, for example, a prolonged inspiratory or expiratory pause.
- Inappropriate selection or use of a device or technique variable may result in underdosing.
- Device malfunction may result in reduced drug delivery and may compromise the integrity of the ventilator circuit.
- Complications may arise from specific pharmacologic agents. Higher doses of β-agonists delivered by pressurized metered-dose inhaler (pMDI) or nebulizer may cause adverse effects secondary to systemic absorption of the drug or propellant. The potential for hypokalemia and atrial and ventricular dysrhythmias may exist with high doses in critically ill patients.
- Aerosol medications, propellants, or cold, dry gases that bypass the natural upper respiratory tract may cause bronchospasm or irritation of the airway.
- The aerosol device or adapter used and the technique of operation may affect ventilator performance characteristics or alter the sensitivity of the alarm systems.
- Addition of gas to the ventilator circuit from a flowmeter or other gas source to power an inline small-volume nebulizer (SVN) may increase volumes, flows, and peak airway pressures, thereby altering the intended pattern of ventilation. The added gas source will also alter oxygen delivery. Ventilator setting adjustments and alarm changes made to accommodate the additional gas flow must be reset at the end of the treatment.
- Addition of gas from a flowmeter to an inline nebulizer in the ventilator circuit may result in the patient becoming unable to trigger the ventilator during nebulization, leading to hypoventilation.

(Modified from American Association for Respiratory Care Clinical Practice Guideline: Selection of a device for administration of a bronchodilator and evaluation of the response to therapy in mechanically ventilated patients, *Respir Care* 44:105-113, 1999.)

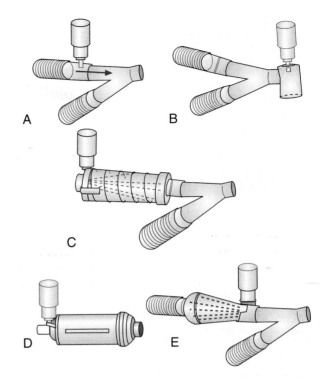

Fig. 12-7 Devices used to adapt a metered-dose inhaler to a ventilator circuit. **A,** Inline device. **B,** Elbow device. **C,** Collapsible chamber device. **D,** Chamber device. **E,** Chamber device in which aerosol is directed retrograde into the ventilator circuit. (Modified from Dhand R, Tobin MJ: Bronchodilator delivery with metered-dose inhalers in mechanically-ventilated patients, Eur Respir J 9:585-595,1996.)

(Key Point 12-6). Recent studies suggest the best position for a pMDI is approximately 7 inches from the Y-connector.[64]

> **Key Point** **12-6** Devices that create abrupt angles between the pMDI and the ET can significantly reduce aerosol delivery to the patient.

Patient-Related Factors

Patients with large amounts of secretions in the ET or who are experiencing severe bronchospasm present a special challenge for aerosol delivery. As airflow obstruction increases, the delivery of aerosol decreases. Thus the patient's condition can affect the aerosol delivery pattern. In patients with COPD and increased airway resistance (R_{aw}), intermittent delivery of nebulized bronchodilators (i.e., during inspiration) may be more effective than continuous delivery.[68] The presence of auto-PEEP (hyperinflation) and patient-ventilator **asynchrony** can also interfere with aerosol delivery.

Circuit-Related Factors

It is generally accepted that larger ETs (≥size 7) permit greater aerosol deposition.[69] This fact is particularly important to remember during pediatric ventilation because the internal diameter of the airway may be between 3 and 6 mm, which can reduce aerosol deposition because of the small size of the ET.[70]

Heated humidifiers can also affect aerosol delivery. Increased humidity increases particle size and is likely to reduce the amount of medication delivered to the patient, regardless of the device.[71,72] However, bypassing the humidifier during a treatment is generally

TABLE 12-1	Ventilator-Related Factors That Influence Aerosol Delivery in Mechanically Ventilated Patients
Ventilator-Related Factor	**Effect on Aerosol Delivery***
Ventilator mode	Spontaneous breaths >500 mL improve aerosol delivery compared with mandatory breaths. VC-CMV is more effective for aerosol delivery compared with PC-CMV.
Tidal volume (V_T)	A set V_T that is large enough to include circuit volume improves aerosol delivery and ensures that dead space is cleared of aerosol.
Respiratory rate	Lower respiratory rates improve aerosol delivery.
Duty cycle or T_I	Longer duty cycle (T_I/TCT) or longer T_I improves delivery.
Inspiratory waveform	SVN medication delivery is lower during PC-CMV (descending flow) than during VC-CMV.

*Metered-dose inhaler medication delivery not influenced by T_I, flow pattern, lung mechanics, or mode (volume-controlled versus pressure-controlled ventilation).

not advisable. In fact, placement of an SVN between the ventilator outlet and the humidifier may improve aerosol delivery from the device.[72,73] Additionally, some nebulizer treatments take up to 30 minutes, and inhalation of dry gases for this amount of time may cause damage to the airway.[61,74]

Delivery of aerosolized bronchodilators is also affected by the delivery gas. Although previous studies stated that helium-oxygen mixtures could not be used to deliver aerosols because helium is a "poor vehicle" for aerosol transport, more recent studies have shown that helium-oxygen mixtures may improve aerosol deposition in patients with asthma by reducing airflow turbulence.[75]

Use of Pressurized Metered-Dose Inhaler (pMDIs) During Mechanical Ventilation

The pMDIs present fewer technical problems than do the SVNs when used during mechanical ventilation. Furthermore, using a pMDI with a spacer has been shown to be more efficient than using a nebulizer in delivering a bronchodilator to the lower respiratory tract[76] (see the section on problems associated with SVNs).

The following procedure is recommended when administering aerosols to mechanically ventilated patients with a pMDI[64]:

1. Review the order, identify the patient, and assess the need for bronchodilator. (Suction airway if needed.)
2. Establish the initial medication dose (e.g., four puffs of albuterol).
3. Shake the pMDI and warm to hand temperature.
4. Place the pMDI in spacer adapter in the inspiratory limb of ventilator circuit.
5. Remove the heat-moisture exchanger (HME). (Do not disconnect humidifier if one is in use.)
6. Minimize the inspiratory flow during VC-CMV; increase T_I (>0.3 seconds) during PC-CMV.
7. Coordinate actuation of pMDI with the precise beginning of inspiration. (Be sure that mandatory breaths are synchronized with a patient's inspiratory effort. V_T must be large enough to compensate for the ventilator circuit, the ET, and the V_{Danat}.)
8. If the patient can take a spontaneous breath (>500 mL), coordinate actuation of the pMDI with a spontaneous breath initiation and encourage a 4- to 10-second breath hold. Otherwise allow passive exhalation.
9. Wait at least 20 to 30 seconds between actuations. Administer total dose.
10. Monitor for any adverse responses to the administration of medication.
11. Assess the patient response to therapy and titrate dose to achieve desired effect.

BOX 12-8	**Factors That Affect Aerosol Deposition with Small-Volume Nebulizers (SVNs) During Mechanical Ventilation**

The performance and rate of aerosol production of SVNs vary by manufacturer and even by production batch.

The volume of liquid (medication + diluent) placed in the SVN before the treatment and the dead volume (amount of medication trapped in the reservoir after the treatment that cannot be nebulized) affect aerosol dose delivery. (Using a 5-mL volume is recommended.)

Position of the SVN in the circuit is important. A better deposition occurs when the SVN is proximal to the humidifier.[72,73] High flows create smaller particles but speed the treatment, resulting in more aerosol being lost during the expiratory phase. Longer delivery time usually increases aerosol delivery. A flow of 6 to 8 L/min is typically recommended.

The duration of nebulization varies from 3 to 5 minutes for continuous nebulization and from 15 to 20 minutes or longer for intermittent nebulization. Continuous nebulization allows the main inspiratory line of the ventilator circuit to fill with aerosol particles during exhalation, although some studies suggest that nebulization only during inspiration may be more efficient because it eliminates aerosol waste during exhalation phase. (NOTE: Nebulization during inspiration can be accomplished only by a nebulizer control that is built into the ventilator.) Continuous nebulization is recommended in patients with status asthmaticus.

12. Reconnect HME.
13. Document clinical outcomes and patient assessment.

Use of Small-Volume Nebulizers (SVNs) During Mechanical Ventilation

Although pMDIs and SVNs are most often used to deliver bronchodilators and corticosteroids, SVNs are commonly used to deliver mucolytics, antibiotics, prostaglandins, and surfactants.[62] Use of an external SVN powered by a separate gas source, such as an O_2 flowmeter, is a common method for delivery of aerosolized medications during mechanical ventilation (Key Point 12-7).[76,77] Figure 12-6 and Box 12-8 illustrate various factors that can affect aerosol deposition with SVNs during mechanical ventilation.[67,78-80]

Key Point 12-7 When a patient requires a larger dose of a beta-agonist, such as a patient with acute severe asthma, a nebulizer (e.g., SVN, USN, and VMN) may deliver more medication into the respiratory tract than a pMDI with spacer.

Technical Problems Associated with Continuous Nebulization Using an External Gas Source

Several problems are associated with adding a nebulizer to a patient circuit. Because the external nebulizer is powered by a continuous external gas source, ventilator function is affected. This is particularly true of the microprocessor ventilators that rely on the monitoring of exhaled gas flows and pressures. For example, expiratory monitors will display higher flows and volumes from previous settings because they will detect the added gas flow from the flowmeter powering the SVN. The high volumes may cause activation of volume alarms that were set when mechanical ventilation was initiated.

When the expiratory valve closes to deliver a positive pressure breath, the added flow increases volume and pressure delivery within the circuit and the patient. This added volume and pressure could be quite significant in infants.[81]

Preset ventilator variables may need to be adjusted during the treatment. In any patient-triggered mode, the patient must inhale (overcome) the flow added to the circuit by the external source to trigger the ventilator. As a result, patients with weak inspiratory efforts may be unable to trigger a machine breath.[82] The apnea alarm will not activate because the expiratory flow monitors detect the flow from the external gas source. Using an external gas source can also alter the F_IO_2 delivery to the patient.

Medications that pass through the expiratory valve and the flow measuring devices may "gum up" these devices, thereby changing their functions. An expiratory gas filter can be used to prevent accumulation of aerosolized medications on the expiratory valves and monitors. However, these filters should be used with caution because as drugs accumulate on the filter, they can increase expiratory resistance and contribute to the generation of auto-PEEP. (NOTE: It is also important to recognize that the increased resistance detected may be the result of a "clogged" expiratory filter rather than from an increase in the patient's R_{aw}.) It may be necessary to change the low V_T, the low $\dot{V}_E$ alarm settings, and the sensitivity setting when adding an external nebulizer so that ventilation is guaranteed during treatment. The clinician must remember to change them back after the treatment is completed.

The use of expiratory filters during mechanical ventilation can also reduce exposure of the staff to the aerosols emanating through the ventilator's expiratory filter and into the environment. (Risk of exposure to second-hand or exhaled aerosol can account for more than 45% of the medication dose administered in addition to droplet nuclei produced by the patient.) Use of ventilators without expiratory filters increases the risk of exposure to aerosol released to the atmosphere from the ventilator, which increases the risk of second-hand exposure for caregivers and families. Without an expiratory filter, aerosol released from the ventilator is more than 160-fold higher than when an expiratory filter is added.[83,84]

Inline SVNs can become contaminated with bacteria and increase the risk of nosocomial infection because these contaminated aerosol particles can be delivered directly into the patient's respiratory tract. The CDC recommends cleaning nebulizers before every treatment. Nebulizers should be removed from the circuit after each use, disassembled, rinsed with sterile water (if rinsing is needed), air-dried, and stored aseptically.[34]

Nebulization Provided by the Ventilator

Several microprocessor-controlled ventilators are equipped with nebulizer-powering systems. It is important to recognize that these ventilators differ in their ability to power nebulizers. Some

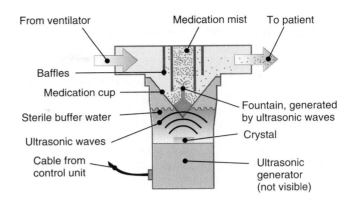

Fig. 12-8 A small-volume ultrasonic nebulizer designed for use with a mechanical ventilator. A vibrating piezoceramic crystal generates ultrasonic waves that pass through the couplant (sterile buffer water) and the medication cup to produce a standing wave of medication, which produces aerosol particles. (Courtesy Aerogen, Inc, Galway, Ireland; http://www.aerogen.com.)

ventilators power the nebulizer only during mandatory breaths on inspiration, whereas other ventilators can power the nebulizer only when inspiratory gas flow is greater than a certain value (e.g., >10 L/min gas flow from the ventilator). In some ventilators the duration of nebulizer flow also changes with the inspiratory flow waveform selected. In still others each breath triggers nebulizer flow, whether mandatory or spontaneous.

Delivery of the aerosol by the ventilator is greater when the pressure powering the nebulizer is ≥3.5 pounds per square inch gauge (psig) to ≤8.5 psig.[67] The clinician must be familiar with the ventilator used to know which ventilator modes can be used with a nebulizer, and the unit's flow requirements and capabilities. Sophisticated algorithms in the software of current ICU ventilators maintain the F_IO_2 and the V_T delivery so that these settings are not altered when the ventilator's nebulizer system is activated.

A growing trend is the use of USNs and VMN devices during mechanical ventilation. These two devices produce particles in the approximate range of 5 to 10 μm. Additionally, they do not require a separate gas source because they are electrically powered. Consequently these devices do not alter volume delivery or oxygen delivery. By comparison, pMDIs, VMNs, and USNs are more efficient than SVNs. For example, mean inhaled percent dose is two to four times greater with a VMN than with a SVN. However, note that when bias flow is present, an SVN or VMN positioned proximal to the ventilator (before the humidifier) delivers more aerosol than when placed at the Y-piece.[85]

The Aeroneb Pro and Aeroneb Solo (Aerogen, Inc, Galway, Ireland) utilize vibrating mesh technology and can be connected to a variety of mechanical ventilators. The aerosol particle characteristics are similar to those of a USN. An example of a ventilator that uses a small-volume ultrasonic nebulizer (USN) is the Servo-i ventilator (Fig. 12-8). Undiluted medication can be injected directly through a membrane at the top of the device so that the nebulizer does not have to be opened to accomplish filling. The mass median diameter of particles produced by the nebulizer is 4.0 μm. The operator sets the amount of time desired for nebulization on the ventilator and nebulization is administered continuously. Other small-volume USNs are also available for mechanical ventilators. See Box 12-9 for protocol for using nebulizers for drug administration.

<table>
<tr><td>

BOX 12-9 | **Protocol for the Administration of Medications with Nebulizers During Mechanical Ventilation**

</td></tr>
</table>

The following procedure is recommended when administering aerosols to mechanically ventilated patients with a small-volume nebulizer (SVN), ultrasonic nebulizer (USN), or vibrating mesh nebulizer (VMN):

1. Review the order, identify the patient, and assess the need for bronchodilator. (Suction airway if needed.)
2. Establish the dose required to compensate for decreased delivery (possibly 2 to 5 times the normal dose for a spontaneous patient when using an SVN).
3. Place the drug in the nebulizer and add diluent to an optimum fill volume (4 to 6 mL).
4. Place the SVN proximal to the humidifier and the USN and VMN in the inspiratory line about 15 cm (7 in.) from the Y-connector.
5. If possible, turn off bias flow or flow trigger that produces a continuous flow through the circuit during exhalation while nebulization is proceeding.
6. Remove the heat and moisture exchange (HME) from the circuit. (Do not disconnect the humidifier.)
7. Turn on the USN or VMN, or set the gas flow to SVN at 6 to 8 L/min. (NOTE: Use the ventilator nebulizer system if it meets the SVN flow needs and cycles on inspiration; otherwise, use continuous flow from an external source.)
8. When possible, adjust the ventilator for optimum medication delivery (high tidal volume [V_T] range, low f range, low flow range, long inspiratory time (T_I >0.3 s), while maintaining appropriate $\dot{V}_E$. (NOTE: Added flow from external source will increase volume and pressure delivery.)
9. In the case of the SVN, adjust the low V_T and low $\dot{V}_E$ alarm, upper pressure limit, and sensitivity to compensate for added flow. With USN and VMN, no changes are required because they do not alter volume, flow, pressure, or oxygen delivery.
10. Check for adequate aerosol generation and manually tap nebulizer periodically during treatment until all medication is nebulized.
11. Monitor for any adverse response to administration of medication.
12. Remove SVN from the circuit, rinse with sterile water, air-dry, and store in safe place. USN and VMN might not require removal or rinsing. The manufacturer's recommendations should be followed with these two devices.
13. Replace HME into circuit.
14. Return ventilator settings to pretreatment values, if changed.
15. Return low V_T, low $\dot{V}_E$, upper pressure limit alarms, and sensitivity setting to original appropriate settings, if changed.
16. Evaluate and assess outcome and document findings.

Use of Nebulizers During Noninvasive Positive Pressure Ventilation

Several points should be mentioned regarding nebulization of medications during noninvasive positive pressure ventilation (NIV). Preliminary studies suggest that both pMDI and SVN can be used to deliver bronchodilators during NIV. For the pMDI and SVN, the greatest aerosol deposition occurs when the nebulizer is placed close to the patient (between the leak port and the face mask), the inspiratory pressure is high (20 cm H_2O), and the expiratory pressure is low (5 cm H_2O).[62] Additional studies will be required to determine the optimum settings to be used with the USN and the VMN during NIV.

Patient Response to Bronchodilator Therapy

Monitoring patient response to bronchodilators can be done by measuring lung mechanics (e.g., compliance, resistance, and ventilating pressures), listening to breath sounds, evaluating vital signs and S_pO_2, and also monitoring pressure–time curves, flow-volume and pressure-volume loops. The following suggest an improvement following therapy:

- Reduced peak inspiratory pressure (PIP)
- Reduced transairway pressure (P_{TA})*
- Increase in peak expiratory flow rate (PEFR)
- Reduction in auto-PEEP levels (if present before the beginning of the treatment)

Figure 12-9 shows before and after flow–volume loops illustrating how both inspiratory and expiratory flow and volume delivery improve following bronchodilator therapy (see also Case Study 12-3).[86,87]

<table>
<tr><td>

 Case Study 12-3

Evaluation of Bronchodilator Therapy
Following the administration of 2.5 mg of albuterol by SVN, the respiratory therapist evaluates pre- and postparameters and notes the following:
Pretreatment: PIP = 28 cm H_2O; $P_{plateau}$ = 13 cm H_2O; P_{TA} = 15 cm H_2O
PEFR = 35 L/min (measured from flow–volume loop)
Posttreatment: PIP = 22 cm H_2O; $P_{plateau}$ = 15 cm H_2O; P_{TA} = 7 cm H_2O
PEFR = 72 L/min
Did the treatment reduce the patient's airway resistance?

</td></tr>
</table>

POSTURAL DRAINAGE AND CHEST PERCUSSION

Although suctioning remains the primary method of secretion clearance for patients with ETs in place, secretions in peripheral bronchi cannot be reached with this procedure. Postural drainage and chest percussions are other techniques that can be used to help clear airway secretions and improve the distribution of ventilation. In ventilated patients, postural drainage involves placing the patient in a number of prescribed positions to drain the affected lung segment. Note that identifying the affected lung segments can be accomplished by analyzing chest radiographs and auscultation of the chest. This procedure is commonly accompanied by percussion of the chest wall using manual techniques or pneumatic percussors.

A study by Takahashi and associates[88] recommended the following positions for ventilated patients based on their findings:
- Supine
- 45-degree rotation prone with left side up

---

*P_{TA} = PIP – $P_{plateau}$.

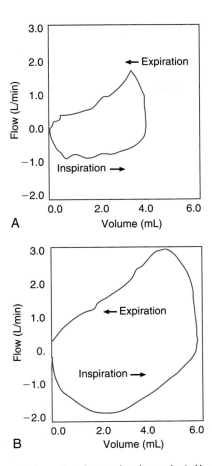

Fig. 12-9 These tidal flow–volume loops are based on mechanical breaths from an infant with a dramatic response to bronchodilator therapy during ventilation. Loop **A**, before bronchodilator. Loop **B**, 20 minutes after bronchodilator. Notice the increase in tidal volume and peak flows after bronchodilator administration. (From Holt WJ, Greenspan JS, Antunes MJ, et al: Pulmonary response to an inhaled bronchodilator in chronically ventilated preterm infants with suspected airway reactivity, Respir Care 40:145-151, 1995.)

- 45-degree rotation prone with right side up
- Return to supine
- Additional patient positions thought to be helpful include 10 degrees right-side-up supine and 45 degrees rotation prone with head raised 45 degrees

Positioning, particularly toward the prone position, is difficult in mechanically ventilated patients and typically requires two or more clinicians to accomplish. Extreme care must be used when moving patients to avoid accidental extubation, or loss, stretching, and kinking of catheters. Patient comfort and safety should always be a primary concern when working with critically ill patients. Because of the potential difficulties that can occur during postural drainage and chest percussions in patients with reduced cardiopulmonary reserve or increased intracranial pressure, other methods, such as use of an oscillating vest (Fig. 12-10), may provide alternative methods for secretion clearance. With the Vest Airway Clearance System (Hill-Rom, St Paul, Minn.), chest wall vibrations are delivered to a vest positioned around the patient's thorax. Vibrations are produced when pressure pulses generated by an air compressor are delivered through tubing to the vest. The pressure settings and frequency of oscillation are adjustable.

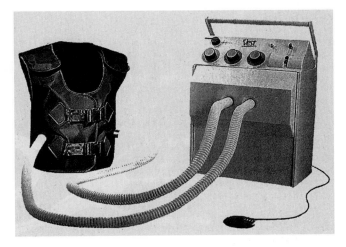

Fig. 12-10 The Vest Airway Clearance System. (Courtesy Hill-Rom, St Paul, Minn.)

Although all the techniques discussed appear to be effective, additional studies are needed to compare the effectiveness of the various airway clearance methods in mechanically ventilated patients, and better define potential complications associated with their use.

FLEXIBLE FIBEROPTIC BRONCHOSCOPY

Bronchoscopy is an invasive procedure used to visualize the upper and lower respiratory tract. It has become an important procedure for the diagnosis and treatment of various types of respiratory disorders, including inflammatory, infectious, and malignant diseases. It can be accomplished using either a flexible fiberoptic or rigid bronchoscope. The flexible fiberoptic bronchoscope consists of a long, flexible tube that contains three separate channels (Fig. 12-11), which are described as follows:

- A light-transmitting channel contains optical fibers that conduct light into the airway.
- A visualizing channel uses optical fibers to conduct an image of the airway to an eyepiece.
- An open multipurpose channel that can be used for aspiration, tissue sampling, or O_2 administration.

Bronchoscopy can be used to inspect the airways, remove objects from the airway, obtain biopsies of tissue and secretion samples, and clear secretions from the airway. Box 12-10 lists the indications and contraindications for fiberoptic bronchoscopy.[89] Newer fiberoptic bronchoscopes like the endobronchial ultrasound (EBUS-TBNA: Olympus, Center Valley, Pa.) allow the use of ultrasound technology to locate specific structures in the lungs and airways, such as lymph nodes, blood vessels, and abnormal structures (e.g., tumors). EBUS-TBNA allows sampling of lymph nodules with real-time view, potentially making lung biopsy less invasive and safer than conventional blind biopsy.

Another fiberoptic bronchoscope, the Electromagnetic Navigation Bronchoscope (superDimension, Inc, i-Logic System, Minneapolis, Minn.) incorporates a computed tomographic image that is reconfigured into a three-dimensional image. The image maps a navigational pathway through the airways to help locate lesions in lung tissue and mediastinal lymph nodes. The scope can navigate to the outer periphery of the lungs to biopsy suspicious findings in the lung fields.

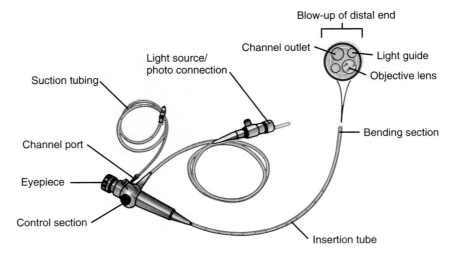

Fig. 12-11 Flexible fiberoptic bronchoscope. (See text for additional information.) (From Wilkins RL, Stoller JK, Kacmarek RM, editors: Egan's fundamentals of respiratory care, ed 9, St Louis, 2009, Mosby-Elsevier.)

Before beginning a bronchoscopy, the respiratory therapist should explain the procedure to the patient, gather the necessary equipment and medications that will be needed, and administer preprocedure medications. An intravenous (IV) line is typically placed for the procedure to administer IV drugs for conscious sedation.

Atropine is sometimes administered 1 to 2 hours before the procedure to reduce secretion production and help dry the patient's airway so that it is easier to visualize. Atropine also blocks the vagal response (e.g., bradycardia and hypotension) that can occur when the bronchoscope enters the upper airway. Conscious sedation typically involves the use of agents such as:

- Opioid analgesics: Sublimaze (fentanyl citrate), Demerol (meperidine hydrochloride), and morphine (hydromorphone hydrochloride)
- Benzodiazepines: Versed (midazolam hydrochloride) or Valium (diazepam)

Narcotics depress the laryngeal cough reflex and alter the respiratory pattern to a slower and deeper pattern. Narcan (naloxone hydrochloride) or Romazicon (flumazenil) should be available if reversal of the sedation is required. In ventilated patients some analgesics and sedatives may already be in use. Therefore obtaining a list of current medications that the patient is receiving is important.

Other useful information to obtain before the procedure includes thoracic imaging reports and laboratory data, particularly clotting factors. A discussion concerning performing the procedure on a spontaneously breathing patient is reviewed elsewhere and is beyond the scope of this text.[90]

Topical anesthesia to the upper airway, which is normally administered to spontaneous nonintubated patients, is usually not required when fiberoptic bronchoscopy is performed on intubated patients. A solution of 2% lidocaine is sometimes instilled into the ET to help reduce coughing when the bronchoscope is introduced.

Performing fiberoptic bronchoscopy generally requires three team members, including a physician, a respiratory therapist or pulmonary function technologist, and an individual trained in conscious sedation (nurse or respiratory therapist). The nurse

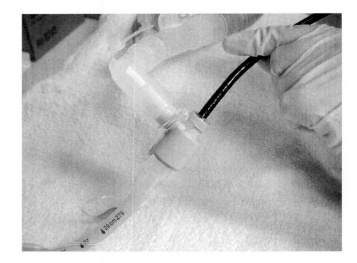

Fig. 12-12 Photograph of an adapter used during fiberoptic bronchoscopy for patients on invasive mechanical ventilation. The adapter is placed between the Y-connector and the endotracheal tube.

typically manages drug administration and keeps records of the drugs used, O_2 saturation, and vital signs. The physician performs the bronchoscopy, and the respiratory therapist or pulmonary function technologist assists the physician by passing different instruments used for biopsy and specimen collection or suctioning the airway. The therapist is also responsible for monitoring the patient and the ventilator.

In patients with artificial airways, choosing the appropriately sized fiberoptic bronchoscope is critical. Once the scope is inserted into the ET, it may occupy 50% or more of the radius of the ET. To help compensate for the tube obstruction, the F_IO_2 is increased to 1.0 during the procedure. To insert the scope, a special adapter like the one shown in Fig. 12-12 is placed between the Y-connector and the patient's ET connector. Once the scope is introduced, the decrease of the ET diameter causes the PIP to increase (during VC-CMV) and the delivered V_T to decrease as some leaking around the scope occurs. Auto-PEEP may occur as well. The respiratory

BOX 12-10   Excerpts from the AARC Clinical Practice Guidelines for: Bronchoscopy Assisting

Indications

The presence of lesions of unknown cause on the chest radiograph or the need to evaluate persistent atelectasis or pulmonary infiltrates

The need to assess upper airway patency or mechanical properties of the upper airways

Suspicious or positive sputum cytology results

The suspicion that secretions or mucous plugs are causing atelectasis

The need to:
- Obtain lower respiratory tract secretions, cell washings, or biopsy samples for evaluation
- Investigate hemoptysis, unexplained cough, wheeze, or stridor
- Evaluate endotracheal or tracheostomy tube problems
- Assist in performing difficult intubations
- Determine the location/extent of inhalation or aspiration injuries
- Remove abnormal tissue or foreign material
- Retrieve a foreign body
- Therapeutically manage ventilator-associated pneumonia
- Achieve selective intubation of a main stem bronchus
- Place and/or assess airway stent function
- Perform airway balloon dilation in the treatment of tracheobronchial stenosis

Contraindications

Absolute Contraindications
- Absence of patient informed consent, unless a medical emergency exists and the patient is not competent
- Absence of an experienced bronchoscopist to perform or supervise the procedure
- Lack of adequate facilities and personnel to care for emergencies, such as cardiopulmonary arrest, pneumothorax, or bleeding
- Inability to adequately oxygenate the patient during the procedure

Perform Only if Benefit Outweighs Risk in Patients with the Following Disorders
- Coagulopathy or bleeding diathesis that cannot be corrected
- Severe obstructive airways disease
- Refractory hypoxemia
- Unstable hemodynamic status including arrhythmias

Relative Contraindications (Recognize Increased Risk)
- Lack of patient cooperation
- Recent myocardial infarction/unstable angina
- Partial tracheal obstruction
- Moderate to severe hypoxemia or any degree of hypercarbia
- Uremia and pulmonary hypertension
- Lung abscess
- Obstruction of the superior vena cava
- Debility, advanced age, and/or malnutrition
- Disorders requiring laser therapy, biopsy of lesions obstructing large airways, or multiple transbronchial lung biopsies
- Known or suspected pregnancy (safety concerns of possible radiation exposure)

Hazards and Complications
- Adverse reaction to medications used before and during the bronchoscopic procedure
- Hypoxemia
- Hypercarbia
- Bronchospasm
- Hypotension
- Laryngospasm, bradycardia, or other vagally mediated phenomena
- Epistaxis, pneumonia, and hemoptysis
- Increased airway resistance
- Infection hazard for health care workers or other patients
- Cross contamination of specimens or bronchoscopes
- Nausea and vomiting
- Fever and chills
- Cardiac dysrhythmias
- Death

Resources
Equipment
- Rigid or flexible fiberoptic bronchoscope
- Bronchoscopic light source and any related video or photographic equipment, if needed
- Specimen collection devices
- Syringes for medication delivery, normal saline lavage, and needle aspiration
- Bite block
- Laryngoscope
- Endotracheal tubes in various sizes
- Thoracotomy tray
- Adaptor with ability to connect mechanical ventilator and bronchoscope simultaneously
- Sterile gauze
- Water-soluble lubricant and lubricating jelly
- Laboratory requisition documentation

Monitoring Devices
- Pulse oximeter
- ECG monitor
- Sphygmomanometer and stethoscope
- Whole-body radiation badge for personnel if fluoroscopy is used
- Capnograph

Procedure Room Equipment
- Oxygen and related delivery devices
- Resuscitation equipment
- Medical vacuum system
- Fluoroscopy equipment including personal protection devices, if warranted
- Adequate ventilation and other measures to prevent transmission of tuberculosis
- Decontamination area equipment
- Medications, including topical anesthetics, anticholinergic agents, sedatives, vasoconstrictor, nasal decongestants, and emergency and resuscitation drugs

Monitoring
Patient monitoring should be performed before, at regular intervals during, and after bronchoscopy until the patient meets appropriate discharge criteria. The level of monitoring required will be influenced by the level of sedation used during the procedure.

Infection Control
- Standard precautions should be used unless disease specific precautions are required
- Centers for Disease Control and Prevention Guideline for Handwashing and Hospital Environmental Control, Section 2: Cleaning, Disinfecting, and Sterilizing Patient Care Equipment
- Hepatitis B vaccination for personnel

(Modified from American Association for Respiratory Care Clinical Practice Guideline: Bronchoscopy assisting, *Respir Care* 52:74-80, 2007.)

therapist will typically have to adjust the ventilator, silence alarms, and monitor S_pO_2 and exhaled V_T during the procedure.[91]

Additional Patient Management Techniques and Therapies in Ventilated Patients

SPUTUM AND UPPER AIRWAY INFECTIONS

Patients on mechanical ventilation with artificial airways in place are at high risk for upper airway infections and VAP. Some of the causative agents for VAP are discussed in Chapter 14.

An elevated patient temperature with an increased white blood cell count (>10,000 per cubic centimeter) may be evidence of an infection. A sputum specimen should be collected and examined for color, quantity, and consistency, and then sent to a laboratory for a culture and sensitivity and wet sputum analyses. Table 12-2 lists sputum color and characteristics that are associated with certain patient problems. Isolating and culturing an organism from the sputum or blood of an infected patient can indicate the causative microbe.

The evaluation of sputum can be correlated with other clinical data such as physical findings and radiographic reports to show a complete picture of a patient's condition in relation to a pulmonary infection. Physical findings might include the presence of crackles, dullness to percussion on physical examination, and purulent sputum. The chest radiograph of an infected patient will typically show evidence of a new or progressive infiltrate, consolidation, cavitation, or pleural effusion, any of which may be consistent with the presence of pneumonia.[92,93]

TABLE 12-2	Sputum Color and Possible Associated Problems
Sputum Color	**Potential Problem**
Yellow	Suggests the presence of pus (white blood cells) and possible infection
Green, thick	Suggests that sputum has been in the airway for a while, because the breakdown of mucopolysaccharides (a component of sputum) results in a green color
Green, foul-smelling	Occurs with *Pseudomonas* infection
Pink-tinged	May indicate fresh blood or can occur after treatment with aerosolized epinephrine, isoproterenol, racemic epinephrine, or isoetharine
Fresh blood present	Suggests airway trauma, pneumonia, pulmonary infarction, or emboli
Brown	Usually indicates old blood
Rust	Might indicate a *Klebsiella* infection
Pink, copious, and frothy	Indicates pulmonary edema

FLUID BALANCE

Positive pressure ventilation can affect fluid balance and urine output, so it is important to monitor fluid input and output. This can be done by comparing daily fluid intake with output (i.e., urine output), and by measuring body weight daily. This information can be used to alert the medical staff of significant changes in a patient's fluid balance.

Normal urine production is about 50 to 60 mL/h (approximately 1 mL/kg/h). Oliguria is a urine output of less than 400 mL/day or less than 20 mL/h. Polyuria is a urine output of more than 2400 mL/day or 100 mL/h.[94]

Decreases in urine output during mechanical ventilation can be due to any of the following:
- Decreased fluid intake and low plasma volume
- Decreased cardiac output resulting from decreased venous return, increased levels of plasma antidiuretic hormone (ADH), heart failure, relative hypovolemia (dehydration, shock, hemorrhage)
- Decreased renal perfusion
- Renal malfunction
- Postrenal problems such as obstruction or extravasation of urinary flow from the urethra, bladder, ureters, or pelvis
- A blocked Foley catheter (one of the most common causes of sudden drops in urine flow, which can be quickly reversed by irrigating the catheter)

Laboratory evaluation of acute renal failure includes tests of blood urea nitrogen (BUN), serum creatinine, BUN-serum creatinine ratio, serum and urine electrolytes, urine creatinine, and glomerular filtration rate. An increase in body weight that is not associated with increased food intake is typically caused by fluid retention. When urine production is reduced and body weight is increased, the cause must be identified and corrected.

Changes in fluid balance may also affect blood cell counts. Fluid retention (overhydration) causes a dilution effect (hemodilution), leading to reduced hemoglobin, hematocrit, and cell counts. Dehydration can cause hemoconcentration and falsely high readings of these same variables.

For a patient receiving positive pressure ventilation, high mean airway pressures ($\bar{P}_{aw}$) can lead to decreased cardiac output and increased plasma ADH. When this occurs, attempts to decrease $\bar{P}_{aw}$ should be made. Pulmonary artery pressure (PAP) monitoring is valuable in this situation. If cardiac output increases when $\bar{P}_{aw}$ is decreased, alterations in fluid balance may be the result of positive pressure ventilation (PPV).

Relative hypovolemia can be caused by dehydration, shock, or hemorrhage. Clinically it causes low vascular pressures (low PAP, low central venous pressure [CVP], and low pulmonary artery occlusion pressure [PAOP]). (See Chapter 11 for additional information on hemodynamic monitoring.) Dehydration commonly results from inadequate fluid intake, vomiting, or diarrhea. It can also be caused by fluid shifting from the plasma to the interstitial space.

Dehydration or relative hypovolemia is evaluated by giving fluid challenges until adequate BP values are restored. Shock is usually treated with fluid administration and appropriate medications such as dopamine, phenylephrine, mephentermine, norepinephrine, or metaraminol, any of which may help to increase BP (Case Study 12-4).

Evaluating Fluid Status

A patient receiving mechanical ventilatory support has elevated red and white blood cell counts. Skin turgor is decreased; urine output has been averaging 40 mL/h; and BP has been lower than the patient's normal value. What is the most likely problem and what would you recommend?

If cardiac output and urine output are decreased, and PAOP is increased, failure of the left side of the heart should be suspected. Chronic failure of the left side of the heart also increases PAP and CVP and is treated with drugs such as digitalis (to increase contractility and cardiac output) and morphine (to decrease venous return to the heart), diuretics (to unload excess fluids through the kidneys), and O_2 (to improve myocardial oxygenation). Sodium nitroprusside can also be used to dilate both arterial and venous vessels, which reduces preload (venous return and end-diastolic volume) and afterload (peripheral vascular resistance). However, the use of this agent must be monitored carefully because of its effects on vascular pressures (i.e., PAOP, PAP, and BP).

Renal failure or malfunction is another common cause of decreased urine production in critically ill patients. Severe hypoxemia, sepsis, and other clinical problems can lead to renal malfunction. The urine is checked for the presence of blood cells and elevated protein or glucose levels, and also for its specific gravity, color, and amount. The presence of abnormal substances in the urine and abnormal BUN levels are indicative of renal malfunction.

Excessive fluid intake can also result from iatrogenic causes. An IV line may malfunction and cause fluids to be administered too rapidly. Another factor that is often overlooked regarding fluid intake and output in mechanically ventilated patients is to account for the water associated with high humidity from heated humidifiers. This additional fluid may represent a considerable portion of a patient's fluid intake, particularly in neonates and infants.

PSYCHOLOGICAL AND SLEEP STATUS

As patients regain consciousness, while on ventilatory support, it is important to show encouragement and explain to the patient why the ventilator and the ET are being used. It is also important to demonstrate to the patient how to communicate his or her needs. Patients should have confidence in the personnel who care for them. Whenever an alarm sounds, the clinician should check the patient first and then check the equipment. It can be very comforting to a patient to have the clinician explain that all is well and that he or she need not be concerned about the alarm.

Critically ill patients typically demonstrate a certain level of sleep disturbance secondary to factors such as pain, medications, staff interruptions, noise, and light. The level of sleep disturbance or sleep fragmentation in mechanically ventilated patients is similar to that seen in patients with obstructive sleep apnea, who have impaired cognitive function and excessive daytime sleepiness.[95]

Relatively little information is available about the relation between patient-ventilator interaction and sleep. In one study, the ventilator mode was noted to alter sleep function in some patients. PSV used during sleep was thought to induce frequent periods of apnea (central apnea) when compared with VC-CMV, which has a set minimum rate. These apneic periods were attributed to longer T_I, deeper V_T, and the subsequent transient lowering of P_aCO_2 values (hypocapnia). In this study, the decreased P_aCO_2 reduced the drive to breathe, and the patient then experienced sleep apnea and sleep disturbance. During the apneic periods, the P_aCO_2 rose to 7 mm Hg above wakeful state P_aCO_2. The apneic periods were also associated with frequent patient arousals from sleep. Repeated arousals can elevate catecholamine levels and blood pressure, and contribute to cardiac arrhythmias and cardiac failure.[95] Practitioners are cautioned against misinterpreting the periods of hypercapnia during sleep in patients being ventilated with PSV.

Patients in the ICU who are deprived of sleep and given a variety of drugs can have many psychological problems. It is not unusual for them to become combative, restless, anxious, depressed, frustrated, angry, and even have hallucinations. Fortunately many patients cannot later recall the time they spent in the ICU. The staff must understand that patients may respond in unusual or atypical ways; it is important to explain this to family members. Whenever possible, allow patients to rest and sleep undisturbed, and give them as much privacy as possible, a concept that is often not practiced in many ICUs.

Members of the health care team should be respectful, kind, reassuring, and keep a positive attitude at all times around the patients for whom they are caring. They should abide by patient confidentiality requirements and protect patients' private information. Being emotionally supportive of patients is vitally important. Addressing patients' psychological needs can be as important as ensuring that their physical needs are met. "Imagine it is your mother you are caring for and your father is paying the bill."[96] This simple sentence reminds the health care team to be loving and compassionate and to give the best possible care with the least amount of pain and discomfort; it is also a reminder not to be wasteful or thoughtless in words and actions.

PATIENT SAFETY AND COMFORT

Practitioners should always keep in mind the primary reasons for initiating ventilatory support. Patients receiving short-term mechanical ventilation include postoperative patients and those with an uncomplicated drug overdose. Patients who may require longer periods of mechanical ventilation (e.g., several days to 1 or 2 weeks) include posttrauma victims and patients with asthma, COPD, pulmonary edema, aspiration, and ARDS. Patients who may require 2 or more weeks of ventilator support typically include those with severe COPD, neuromuscular disorders such as myasthenia gravis, Guillain-Barré, tetanus, botulism, cerebrovascular accidents, cranial tumors, and patients being treated for neurosurgical problems, to name just a few.

Patient Safety

To be ready for emergencies, clinicians should always make sure that several items of equipment are available, including a manual resuscitator with mask, an O_2 source, intubation equipment, an emergency tracheostomy kit, a thoracentesis tray, suction equipment, an emergency cart stocked with the appropriate emergency medication, and ABG kit. Emergency equipment that is readily accessible can provide immediate patient care and protect patient safety.

Staff should rely on keen observation and early detection of problems in both patients and mechanical equipment to assure patient safety and comfort. The patient-ventilator system should be monitored at regular intervals. It is important to try to anticipate problems and trust the assessments made with your senses because the information obtained from monitors may not accurately reflect a patient's true condition or level of comfort.

Patient Comfort

A patient receiving ventilatory support may experience physical discomfort caused by pain from trauma or disease, an awkward body position, distended organs, inadequate ventilation, heavy tubing, restraints, limb boards, the inability to talk or swallow, coughing or yawning, poor oral hygiene, and overcooling or overheating because of environmental conditions. Every effort must be made to keep patients as comfortable as possible.

Feelings of confusion and delirium are commonplace in patients in the ICU.[3] Imagine the sense of vulnerability and isolation that mechanically ventilated patients feel while in the ICU. They cannot talk, they are not surrounded by familiar family faces, and they are not sure when someone will return to their bedside, or what the health care provider will do when they return.

A major problem in many ICUs is the lack of effective methods of communicating with patients. Physicians and other caregivers are often in a hurry to move on to other tasks.[3] If it becomes difficult to communicate with a patient who has a tube in his or her mouth, all too often the caregiver gives up in frustration and leaves the patient no better off emotionally than when the caregiver first walked into the room.

Patients may also suffer from shortness of breath or dyspnea. Restoring ABGs to normal and alleviating patient-ventilator asynchrony may not alleviate dyspnea. Some speculate that using a low V_T for ventilation is associated with discomfort. It may be fair to assume that any volume that is different from what the patient desires produces discomfort and shortness of breath.[3] As an example, patients with muscular diseases seem to desire a large V_T that often results in low P_aCO_2 levels. These volumes can be as high as 1000 mL.

In a study involving reducing sedation in patients on mechanical ventilation in the ICU, researchers found that patients in the group that received continuous infusion of sedation remained awake for 9% of the time, whereas the group that had the sedation discontinued daily spent 85% of their time awake.[97] The decision to use sedatives in mechanically ventilated patients should be based on the patient's psychological and physiological condition. In many cases, the suggestion might be that it is better to be awake most of the time.

Another comment that is often made by clinicians is, "Patients who recover from respiratory failure should be thankful just to be alive. Most have little or no memory of their experience during mechanical ventilation anyway."[3] Several points can be made related to this comment:

- Most of us would not want to experience severe, sustained, and avoidable distress whether we remember it or not.
- Use of sedatives and analgesics needed to produce placidity and amnesia may be excessive and prolong the duration of ventilation and time in the ICU.[96]
- Long-term amnesia may not be as complete or protective as some believe. A high prevalence of anxiety disorders, depression, and posttraumatic stress disorder exist in survivors of ARDS.[97]

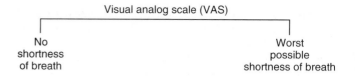

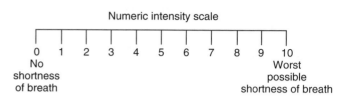

Fig. 12-13 Visual analog and numeric intensity scales. (From Hansen-Flaschen JH: Dyspnea in the ventilated patient: a call for patient-centered mechanical ventilation, Respir Care 45:1460-1464, 2000.)

- Because of a significant lack of research in this area, little is known about the discomfort experienced by ventilated patients.[3] What do patients receiving mechanical ventilation mean when they report shortness of breath?
- How often does dyspnea occur, and how severe is it under different circumstances of mechanical ventilation?
- Can we adjust the ventilator to minimize patient dyspnea and reduce the need for sedation and analgesia?
- Can the incidence or severity of posttraumatic stress disorder be reduced in survivors by minimizing respiratory distress during ventilation?

It has been suggested that a patient's level of dyspnea during mechanical ventilation can be gauged using a visual analog or numeric intensity scale (Fig. 12-13).[98-100] A similar scale, the modified Borg scale, is widely used to measure dyspnea during exercise testing. Dyspnea scores do not correlate with physiological variables.[100] One cannot assume patient comfort just because the numbers look good. Dyspnea must be measured more objectively using tools like those mentioned.

Patient-Centered Mechanical Ventilation

Patient-centered mechanical ventilation should be directed to improving patient safety and survival, while simultaneously reducing patient distress and fear.[3] Patient comfort should be assessed at regularly scheduled intervals, such as when a patient-ventilator system check is performed. Several questions that the clinician can ask patients who are able to respond might include:

1. "Are you short of breath right now?" If the patient indicates that he or she is feeling short of breath then,
2. "Is your shortness of breath mild (#1), moderate (#2), or severe (#3)?" (indicated by holding up fingers)

The clinician may be able to improve patient comfort by adjusting the ventilator flow rate or flow waveform, sensitivity level, pressure target, rise time percentage, and flow cycle criteria (in PSV), or switching modes. As changes are made, the patient can be asked whether one setting is more comfortable than another. When setting changes are completed, the clinician should check S_pO_2, end-tidal CO_2, ABGs, ventilator graphics, and breath sounds to verify that new settings are not resulting in undesirable changes in physiological parameters. If the clinician is unable to improve the patient's comfort level, he or she should communicate with the patient's nurse to determine whether alternative therapies are available. Respiratory therapists are generally successful in complying with this type of dyspnea evaluation protocol.[98] More research is required in the area of assessing dyspnea and comfort levels in mechanically ventilated patients because limited information is currently available.

TRANSPORT OF MECHANICALLY VENTILATED PATIENTS WITHIN AN ACUTE CARE FACILITY

Transporting a seriously ill, mechanically ventilated patient is often required to move the patient from the ICU to a diagnostic or therapeutic area of the hospital. The average duration of patient transport (one way) is between 5 and 40 minutes, and the average time spent at the destination is 35 minutes.[101]

Every effort must be made to ensure that the patient's condition remains stable. This often means continuing the use of medications, which requires transporting vascular lines and pumps. Catheters that may be attached to the patient, including Foley catheters, pleural drainage systems, cardiac and hemodynamic lines, and monitors, will need to be transported. The ventilator, a manual resuscitator and mask, and a reliable O_2 source must also be transported. Box 12-11 lists some of the equipment used during transport of a seriously ill patient.[102] Because of all the equipment and personnel involved, transportation should only be undertaken if the benefits outweigh the risks.[103]

Box 12-12 lists the contraindications, hazards, and complications associated with in-hospital patient transport.[102] Available literature on in-hospital transport of ventilated patients suggests that as many as two thirds of transports performed fail to yield results from diagnostic studies that would have affected patient care.[104]

Three options are available for providing ventilation during transport.
1. The first involves manual ventilation with a self-inflating bag. This option has several risks, including inappropriate ventilation of the patient and contamination of the airway.
2. The second option is to use a transport ventilator that is specifically designed for that purpose. There are very sophisticated microprocessor-controlled transport ventilators that are small, lightweight, and easy to use.
3. Third, most current-generation ICU ventilators can be used for transport. These units are usually large, but most are equipped with backup battery power to maintain function of flow-control valves, displays, alarms, microprocessor systems, and monitors. These ventilators usually require pneumatic power. During transport, these units can operate with cylinder air and O_2.

BOX 12-11 Patient Support Equipment and Monitoring Equipment for Transport of the Ventilated Patient

Equipment
- Emergency airway management supplies
- Stethoscope (for breath sounds and blood pressure)
- Self-inflating manual resuscitator and mask (appropriate size)

Monitors
- Pulse oximeter
- ECG and heart rate monitor and minimum of one channel vascular pressure measurement (a sphygmomanometer should be available if an invasive line and monitor are not present)
- Handheld spirometer for tidal volume monitoring (respiratory rate should be periodically monitored)

Transport Ventilator
If a ventilator capable of transport is used, it should have the following:
- Sufficient portable power (battery and gas) for the duration of transport
- Independent control of tidal volume and rate (tidal volume delivery should be consistent regardless of changing lung compliance or airway resistance)
- CMV or IMV mode capability
- PEEP capabilities
- Disconnect alarm, high-pressure alarm, and low-power (battery) alarm
- Pressure monitoring capabilities
- Provide F_IO_2 (up to 100%)

(From American Association for Respiratory Care Clinical Practice Guideline: In-hospital transport of the mechanically ventilated patient—2002 revision & update, *Respir Care* 47:721-723, 2002.)

BOX 12-12 Excerpts from the AARC Clinical Practice Guidelines for Contraindications, Hazards, and Complications of in-Hospital Transport of the Mechanically Ventilated Patient

Contraindications
Transport should not be undertaken unless all the essential personnel constituting the transport team are present.

Contraindications include the inability to do the following:
- Provide adequate oxygenation and ventilation during transport either by manual resuscitation bag, portable ventilator, or standard ICU ventilator.
- Maintain acceptable hemodynamic stability during transport.
- Monitor the patient's cardiopulmonary status during transport.
- Maintain a patent airway during transport.

Hazards and Complications
- Hyperventilation during manual ventilation, which may result in respiratory alkalosis, cardiac arrhythmias, and hypotension
- Loss of PEEP/CPAP leading to hypoxemia or shock
- Position changes leading to hypotension, hypercarbia, and hypoxemia
- Tachycardia and other arrhythmias
- Equipment failure resulting in inaccurate data, loss of data, and loss of monitoring capabilities
- Accidental disconnection of intravenous access for drug administration resulting in hemodynamic instability
- Disconnection from ventilatory support and respiratory compromise resulting from movement
- Accidental extubation
- Accidental removal of vascular access
- Loss of O_2 supply leading to hypoxemia
- Ventilator-associated pneumonia resulting from transport

(From American Association for Respiratory Care Clinical Practice Guideline: In-hospital transport of the mechanically ventilated patient—2002 Revision & Update, *Respir Care* 47:721-723, 2002.)

Electrically powered transport ventilators rely on battery power during the transport procedure and then plug back into an AC outlet when an outlet is available. The battery power must be checked before beginning the transport process. Battery duration differs considerably between ventilators and may be shorter than that reported in the operator's manual. Clinicians need to be aware that portable ventilator battery life is affected by control settings, lung characteristics, and portable ventilator characteristics.[102] For example, the ventilator settings have an important effect on battery duration. The use of PEEP and pressure-controlled ventilation have the greatest effect on how long the battery will last in electrically powered transport ventilators.[102]

Having the ability to maintain the same V_T delivery during VC-CMV ventilation is another important characteristic of transport ventilators. Of the ventilators tested in one study, most maintained the V_T through the terminal battery testing. At least one reported model did not.[102] Clinicians should evaluate any ventilator by simulating transport conditions before they actually use a machine to transport a patient.

A major disadvantage of pneumatically powered ventilators is that they can consume large volumes of O_2 during operation. It is difficult to determine how long a cylinder of O_2 will last because gas utilization depends on the O_2 setting, $\dot{V}_E$ requirements, lung mechanics, and the operating characteristics of the ventilator. It may be inappropriate to use a ventilator for transporting a patient on noninvasive ventilation because leaks are typically present and ventilator gas consumption will be very high as a result.

Ventilator selection, assembly, preparation of equipment, and personnel training and cooperation are all essential elements in the transport of patients within the acute care facility.

SUMMARY

- Tidal volume and frequency adjustments should be based on the patient's pulmonary condition. Clinicians typically use tidal volumes in a range of 6 to 8 mL/kg while maintaining the $P_{plateau}$ at <30 cm H_2O. Breathing frequencies of 12 to 18 breaths/min are typically acceptable.
- Treatment of metabolic acidosis and alkalosis should focus on identifying those metabolic factors that can cause these acid–base disturbances.

- Permissive hypercapnia is a ventilator technique in which ventilatory support is limited to avoid lung overdistension and injury of the lung. During permissive hypercapnia, arterial partial pressures of carbon dioxide (P_aCO_2) values are allowed to rise above normal (e.g., ≥50 to ≤150 mm Hg), and pH values are allowed to fall below normal (e.g., ≥7.10 ≤ 7.30).
- The use of permissive hypercapnia is restricted to situations in which the target airway pressure is at its maximum and the highest possible rates are being used.
- Clearing secretions from the ET or tracheostomy tube of mechanically ventilated patients is an important component of bronchial hygiene therapy. Suctioning at fixed intervals is not appropriate and should be performed based only on patient assessment findings.
- Two methods of endotracheal suctioning can be performed based on the type of catheter used: the **open-circuit technique** and the **closed-circuit technique.** The duration of suctioning should be brief and must not exceed 15 seconds, and shallow suctioning is recommended over deep suctioning to avoid trauma to the lung.
- There is insufficient evidence to support the practice of instilling normal saline into the ET before suctioning.
- The most common devices used for administering aerosol are pressurized metered-dose inhalers (pMDIs) and small-volume nebulizers (SVNs). Ultrasonic nebulizers (USN) and vibrating mesh nebulizers (VM) also are available but they are used less frequently than pMDIs and SVNs.
- Although pMDIs and SVNs are most often used to deliver bronchodilators and corticosteroids, only SVNs, USNs, and VMNs are used to deliver mucolytics, antibiotics, prostaglandins, and surfactants.
- Numerous ventilator-associated factors can affect the delivery of aerosols, including the mode of ventilation used, the V_T and f, the T_I, and the inspiratory waveform.
- Bronchoscopy has become an important procedure for the diagnosis and treatment of various types of respiratory disorders, including inflammatory, infectious, and malignant diseases.
- A number of routine procedures should be used to ensure that the patient is comfortable and safe during mechanical ventilation.
- Patients on mechanical ventilation with artificial airways in place are at high risk for upper airway infections and VAP.

REVIEW QUESTIONS *(See Appendix A for answers.)*

1. A patient on PC-IMV with no PEEP has the following ventilatory parameters and ABGs: set pressure = 20 cm H_2O; V_T = 400 mL; set rate = 8 breaths/min; spontaneous f = 25 breaths/min; spontaneous V_T = 225 mL; F_IO_2 = 0.4; P_aCO_2 = 58 mm Hg; pH = 7.28; and P_aO_2 = 89 mm Hg. The patient is at IBW of 140 lb (64 kg).
   A. Estimate the patient's total alveolar ventilation (assuming that the dead space changes associated with the ET and V_{Dmech} balance each other).
   B. Calculate the patient's C_S (assuming that flow drops to zero before end inspiration).
   C. Based on ABG results and ventilator data, how do you interpret these data, and what change(s) do you recommend?

2. A 67-year-old man with COPD is being mechanically ventilated with the following settings: V_T = 425 mL (6 mL/kg IBW); f = 6 breaths/min on IMV; F_IO_2 = 0.24. He has a spontaneous f of 25 breaths/min and a spontaneous V_T of 200 mL. PIP = 30 cm H_2O and $P_{plateau}$ = 22 cm H_2O. The following ABGs are obtained: pH = 7.25; P_aCO_2 = 89 mm Hg; P_aO_2 = 55; and HCO_3^- = 38 mEq/L. This patient has a normal P_aCO_2 of 55 mm Hg. What changes would you recommend?

3. A 45-year-old man with Pickwickian syndrome who is 5 foot 4 inches and weighs 280 lb (127 kg) is placed on mechanical ventilatory support following hip replacement surgery. The initial parameters are as follows: $V_T = 1000$ mL; $f = 9$ breaths/min; PIP = 50 cm H_2O; and $P_{plateau} = 35$ cm H_2O. ABGs show pH = 7.41; $P_aCO_2 = 39$ mm Hg; $P_aO_2 = 120$; $HCO_3^- = 24$ mEq/L; and $F_IO_2 = 0.3$. What changes would you recommend?

4. A 22-year-old comatose, apneic man with a closed head injury is being mechanically ventilated. He is also being medically treated for increased ICP. $V_T = 600$ mL (7.5 mL/kg); mode = VC-CMV; $f = 14$ breaths/min; no spontaneous efforts; $P_aCO_2 = 40$ mm Hg; pH = 7.39; $P_aO_2 = 80$ mm Hg on 0.25 F_IO_2. Which of the following changes would be most appropriate?
   A. Make no change at this time.
   B. Increase f to 18 breaths/min.
   C. Increase V_T to 1000 mL (about 12.5 mL/kg).
   D. Switch to the IMV mode of ventilation.

5. A 35-year-old woman with a size 9 ET requires suctioning.
   A. What is an appropriate suction catheter size?
   B. How long should the catheter be?
   C. What is an appropriate suction pressure?

6. Closed-suction catheters may be more appropriate than using open suctioning because of which of the following?
   A. They are less expensive.
   B. They reduce the risk of infections.
   C. There is no risk of the catheter migrating into the ET.
   D. The catheter adds no additional weight to the ventilator circuit.

7. The procedure of instilling normal saline into the ET before suctioning is known to do which of the following?
   A. Effectively thin secretions
   B. Pose no risk to the patient
   C. Increase an elderly patient's sensation of dyspnea
   D. Require a physician's order

8. Silent aspiration and VAP can occur with cuffed ETs as a result of which of the following?
   1. Injury to the mucosa during insertion and manipulation of the tube following insertion
   2. Interference with the normal cough reflex
   3. Aspiration of contaminated secretions that pool above the ET cuff
   4. Rupture of the ET cuff
      A. 1 and 2 only
      B. 1 and 4 only
      C. 1, 2, and 3 only
      D. 1, 2, and 4 only

9. Which of the following is true regarding the special ET that provides continuous aspiration of subglottic secretions?
   A. A pressure of 20 mm Hg is applied continuously to the suction lumen.
   B. The suction port is located just below the cuff on the dorsal side of the tube.
   C. It is most effective in patients requiring intubation for less than 1 to 2 days.
   D. It is no more expensive than a standard ET.

10. A 15-year-old patient with severe acute asthma is being mechanically ventilated. Which of the following methods will deliver the largest quantity of a beta-agonist to the respiratory tract?
    A. pMDI
    B. pMDI with spacer
    C. SVN
    D. Dry powdered capsule

11. When delivering a medication by pMDI to a ventilated patient, the best placement for the device in the ventilator circuit is which of the following?
    A. Between the Y-connector and the ET using elbow connector
    B. On the inspiratory limb attached to the Y-connector using a spacer
    C. On the expiratory limb at the Y-connector
    D. Less than 30 cm from the Y-connector on the inspiratory side of the circuit with spacer

12. Which of the following statements is NOT true when using an externally powered SVN placed in the ventilator circuit?
    A. The added flow will alter monitoring of exhaled V_T and $\dot{V}_E$.
    B. Patient inspiratory efforts may not be sufficient to trigger inspiratory flow from the ventilator.
    C. Use of an expiratory filter may protect the expiratory valve and expiratory monitors from medication deposition.
    D. The HME does not have to be removed from the circuit when using an SVN.

13. The use of atropine in patients who will be having a fiberoptic bronchoscopy is for the purpose of which of the following?
    A. Calming the patient
    B. Reducing respiratory rate and $\dot{V}_E$
    C. Drying the airways
    D. Helping the patient sleep

14. During fiberoptic bronchoscopy of mechanically ventilated patients, the respiratory therapist can anticipate what types of changes in ventilator function?
    A. Increase in volume delivery
    B. Increase in peak pressure
    C. High-rate alarm
    D. High minute volume alarm

15. Postural drainage positions recommended for mechanically ventilated patients include all but which of the following?
    A. Supine
    B. 45-degree rotation prone with left side up
    C. 45-degree rotation prone with right side up
    D. Seated

16. A patient on mechanical ventilation is suctioned for large amounts of foul-smelling green sputum. The patient has a temperature of 39° C and an elevated white blood cell count. The most likely cause of this problem is which of the following?
    A. An overheated cascade humidifier
    B. Cardiogenic pulmonary edema
    C. An allergic reaction to acetylcysteine
    D. A *Pseudomonas* infection

17. Patient-centered mechanical ventilation involves which of the following?
    A. Looking at the patient first and not the machine when a ventilator alarm is activated
    B. Involving the family in making ventilator changes
    C. Asking the patient about his or her level of comfort and dyspnea when making ventilator changes
    D. Involving all members of the health care team in patient management

18. Which of the following must be performed during patient transport to reduce the risk of complications?
    A. Provide adequate oxygenation and ventilation during transport either by manual resuscitation bag, portable ventilator, or standard ICU ventilator
    B. Maintain acceptable hemodynamic stability during transport
    C. Monitor the patient's cardiopulmonary status during transport
    D. All of the above

References

1. Epstein SK, Singh N: Respiratory acidosis. *Respir Care* 46:366–383, 2001.
2. Foster GT, Vaziri ND, Sasson CSH: Respiratory alkalosis. *Respir Care* 46:384–391, 2001.
3. Hansen-Flaschen JH: Dyspnea in the ventilated patient: a call for patient-centered mechanical ventilation, discussion. *Respir Care* 45:1460–1464, 2000.
4. Swenson ER: Metabolic acidosis. *Respir Care* 46:342–353, 2001.
5. Khanna A, Kurtzman NA: Metabolic alkalosis. *Respir Care* 46:354–365, 2001.
6. Cairo JM: *Mosby's respiratory care equipment,* ed 9, St Louis, 2014, Elsevier.
7. Dutton RP, McCunn M: Traumatic brain injury. *Curr Opin Crit Care* 9:503–509, 2003.
8. Go SL, Singh JM: Pro/con debate: Should PaCO₂ be tightly controlled in all patients with acute brain injuries? *Crit Care* 17:202, 2012.
9. Adelson PD, Bratton SL, Carney NA, et al: Guidelines for the acute medical management of severe traumatic brain injury. Chapter 12. Use of hyperventilation in the acute management of severe pediatric traumatic brain injury. *Pediatr Crit Care Med* 4(3 Suppl):S45–S48, 2003.
10. Hess DR: Mechanical ventilation strategies: what's new and what's worth keeping. *Respir Care* 47:1007–1017, 2002.
11. Kollef MH, Schuster DP: Medical progress: the acute respiratory distress syndrome. *N Engl J Med* 332:27–37, 1995.
12. Marini JJ: New options for the ventilatory management of acute lung injury. *New Horiz* 1:489–503, 1993.
13. Potkin RT, Swenson ER: Resuscitation from severe acute hypercapnia: determinants of tolerance and survival. *Chest* 102:1742–1745, 1992.
14. Gillett MA, Hess DR: Ventilator-induced lung injury and the evolution of lung-protective strategies in acute respiratory distress syndrome. *Respir Care* 46:130–148, 2001.
15. Hickling KG, Henderson SJ, Jackson R: Low mortality associated with low volume, pressure limited ventilation with permissive hypercapnia in severe adult respiratory distress syndrome. *Intensive Care Med* 16:372–377, 1990.
16. Darioli A, Perret C: Mechanical controlled hypoventilation in status asthmaticus. *Am Rev Respir Dis* 129:385–387, 1984.
17. Broccard AF, Hotchkiss JR, Vannay C: Protective effects of hypercapnic acidosis on ventilator-induced lung injury. *Am J Respir Crit Care Med* 164:802–806, 2001.
18. Richecoeur J, Lu Q, Vieira SR, et al: Expiratory washout versus optimization of mechanical ventilation during permissive hypercapnia in patients with severe acute respiratory distress syndrome. *Am J Respir Crit Care Med* 160:77–85, 1999.
19. Tuxen DV: Permissive hypercapnic ventilation. *Am J Respir Crit Care Med* 150:870, 1994.
20. Hess DR, Kacmarek RM: *Essentials of mechanical ventilation,* New York, 2002, McGraw-Hill.
21. Feihl F, Perret C: Permissive hypercapnia: how permissive should we be? *Am J Respir Crit Care Med* 150:1722–1737, 1994.
22. Gillette MA, Hess DR: Ventilator-induced lung injury and the evolution of lung-protective strategies in acute respiratory distress syndrome. *Respir Care* 46:130–148, 2001.
23. Feihl F, Eckert P, Brimioulle S, et al: Permissive hypercapnia impairs pulmonary gas exchange in the acute respiratory distress syndrome. *Am J Respir Crit Care Med* 162:209–215, 2000.
24. Tobin MJ: Advances in mechanical ventilation. *N Engl J Med* 344:1986–1996, 2001.
25. American Association for Respiratory Care: Clinical Practice Guideline: Endotracheal suctioning of mechanically ventilated adults and children with artificial airways. *Respir Care* 55:758–764, 2010.
26. Wilson WC, Grande CM, Hoyt DM: *Trauma: critical care,* vol 2, New York, 2007, Informa Healthcare.
27. May RA, Bortner PL, et al: Airway management. In Hess DR, MacIntyre NR, Mishoe SC, editors: *Respiratory care—principles and practices,* Philadelphia, 2003, W.B. Saunders, pp 694–727.
28. Oh H, Seo W: A meta-analysis of the effects of various interventions in preventing endotracheal suction-induced hypoxemia. *J Clin Nurs* 12:912–924, 2003.
29. Spence K, Gillies D, Waterworth L: Deep versus shallow suction of endotracheal tubes in ventilated neonates and young infants. *Cochrane Database Syst Rev* (3):CD003309, 2003.
30. Pedersen C, Rosendahl-Nielsen M, Hjermind J, et al: Endotracheal suctioning of the adult intubated patient—what is the evidence? *Intensive Crit Care Nurs* 25:21–30, 2009.
31. Shim C, Fine N, Fernandez R, et al: Cardiac arrhythmias resulting from tracheal suctioning. *Ann Intern Med* 71:1149–1153, 1969.
32. Brucia J, Rudy E: The effect of suction catheter insertion and tracheal stimulation in adults with severe brain injury. *Heart Lung* 25:295–303, 1996.
33. Stone KS, Bell SP, Preusser BA: The effect of repeated suctioning on arterial blood gases. *Appl Nurs Res* 4:152–158, 1991.
34. Centers for Disease Control (CDC): Guidelines for preventing healthcare-associated pneumonia: Recommendations of the Centers for Disease Control (CDC) and the Healthcare Infection Control Practices Advisory Committee. *MMWR* 53:1–36, 2004. (CDC; U.S. Dept. of Health and Human Services, Atlanta, Ga.) Available at: <www.cdc.gov>.
35. Crosby L, Parsons C: Cerebrovascular response of closed head-injured patients to a standardized endotracheal tube suctioning and manual hyperventilation procedure. *J Neurosci Nurs* 24:40–41, 1992.
36. Brucia J, Rudy E: The effect of suction catheter insertion and tracheal stimulation in adults with severe brain injury. *Heart Lung* 25:295–303, 1996.
37. Branson RD: Secretion management in the mechanically ventilated patient. *Respir Care* 52:1328–1347, 2007.
38. Sills JR: *Respiratory care certification guide,* St Louis, 2000, Mosby.
39. Witmer MT, Hess D, Simmons M: An evaluation of the effectiveness of secretion removal with the Ballard closed-circuit suction catheter. *Respir Care* 36:844–848, 1991.
40. Shilling A, Durbin CG: Airway management. In Cairo JM, editor: *Mosby's respiratory care equipment,* ed 9, St Louis, 2014, Elsevier, pp 113–157.
41. Combes P, Fauvage B, Oleyer C: Nosocomial pneumonia in mechanically ventilated patients, a prospective randomized evaluation of the Stericath closed suctioning system. *Intensive Care Med* 26:878–882, 2000.
42. Branson RD: The patient-ventilator interface: ventilator circuit, airway care, and suctioning. In MacIntyre NR, Branson RD, editors: *Mechanical ventilation,* ed 2, Philadelphia, 2008, Saunders-Elsevier, pp 89–110.
43. Kollef MH, Prentice S, Shapiro SD, et al: Mechanical ventilation with or without daily changes of in-line suction catheters. *Am J Respir Crit Care Med* 156:466–472, 1997.
44. Hess D, Ciano BA, Lemon T, et al: An evaluation of weekly changes of in-line suction catheters (abstract). *Am J Respir Crit Care Med* 82:903, 1998.
45. Ritz R, Scott LR, Coyle MB, et al: Contamination of a multiple-use suction catheter in a closed circuit system compared to contamination of a disposable, single-use suction catheter. *Respir Care* 31:1086–1091, 1986.
46. Stoller JR, Orens DK, Fatica C, et al: Weekly versus daily changes of inline suction catheters: impact on rates of ventilator-associated pneumonia and associated costs. *Respir Care* 49:494–499, 2003.

47. Craig KC, Benson MS, Pierson DJ: Prevention of arterial oxygen desaturation during closed-airway endotracheal suction: effect of ventilator mode. *Respir Care* 29:1013–1018, 1984.

48. Kollet MH, Skubas NJ, Sundt TM: A randomized clinical trial of continuous aspiration of subglottic secretions in cardiac surgery patients. *Chest* 116:1339–1346, 1999.

49. Jaeger J, Durbin CG: Special purpose endotracheal tubes. *Respir Care* 44:661–683, 1999.

50. Collard HR, Saint S, Matthay MA: Prevention of ventilator-associated pneumonia: an evidence-based systematic review. *Ann Intern Med* 138:494–501, 2003.

51. Valles J, Artigas A, Rello J, et al: Continuous aspiration of subglottic secretions in preventing ventilator-associated pneumonia. *Ann Intern Med* 122:179–186, 1995.

52. Rello J, Sonora R, Jubert P, et al: Pneumonia in intubated patients: role of respiratory airway care. *Am J Respir Crit Care Med* 154:111–115, 1996.

53. Mahul P, Auboyer C, Jospe R, et al: Prevention of nosocomial pneumonia in intubated patients: respective role of mechanical ventilation subglottic secretions drainage and stress ulcer prophylaxis. *Intensive Care Med* 18:20–25, 1992.

54. Siobal M, Kallet RH, Draemer R, et al: Tracheal-innominate artery fistula caused by the endotracheal tube tip: case report and investigation of a fatal complication of prolonged intubation. *Respir Care* 46:1012–1018, 2001.

55. Hagler DA, Traver GA: Endotracheal saline and suction catheters: sources of lower airway contamination. *Am J Crit Care* 3:444–447, 1994.

56. Kinloch D: Instillation of normal saline during endotracheal suctioning: effects on mixed venous oxygen saturation. *Am J Crit Care* 8:231–240, 1999.

57. O'Neal PV, Grap MJ, Thompson C, et al: Level of dyspnea experienced in mechanically ventilated adults with and without saline instillation prior to endotracheal suctioning. *Intensive Crit Care Nurs* 17:356–363, 2001.

58. Brunel W, Coleman DL, Schwartz DE, et al: Assessment of routine chest roentgenograms and the physical examination to confirm endotracheal tube position. *Chest* 96:1043–1045, 1989.

59. Conrardy PA, Goodman LR, Lainge F, et al: Alteration of endotracheal tube position: flexion and extension of the neck. *Crit Care Med* 4:7–12, 1976.

60. Krivopal M, Shlobin OA, Schwartzstein RM: Utility of daily routine portable chest radiographs in mechanically ventilated patients in the medical ICU. *Chest* 123:1607–1614, 2003.

61. Duarte AG, Fink JB, Dhand R: Inhalation therapy during mechanical ventilation. *Respir Care Clin N Am* 7:233–260, 2001.

62. Dhand R: Basic techniques for aerosol delivery during mechanical ventilation. *Respir Care* 49:611–622, 2004.

63. American Association for Respiratory Care: Clinical Practice Guideline: Selection of a device for administration of a bronchodilator and evaluation of the response to therapy in mechanically ventilated patients. *Respir Care* 44:105–113, 1999.

64. Fink JB, Ari A: Humidity and aerosol therapy. In Cairo JM, editor: *Mosby's respiratory care equipment*, ed 9, St Louis, 2014, Mosby-Elsevier, pp 158–212.

65. Dhand R, Duarte AG, Jubran A, et al: Dose response to bronchodilator delivered by metered dose inhaler in ventilator supported patients. *Am J Respir Crit Care Med* 154:388–393, 1996.

66. Hess DR, Killman C, Kacmarek RM: In vitro evaluation of aerosol bronchodilator delivery during mechanical ventilation: pressure-control vs volume control ventilation. *Intensive Care Med* 29:1145–1150, 2003.

67. McPeck M, O'Riordan TG, Smaldone GC: Choice of mechanical ventilator influence on nebulizer performance. *Respir Care* 38:887–895, 1993.

68. Yang SC, Yang SP: Nebulized ipratropium bromide in ventilator-assisted patients with chronic bronchitis. *Chest* 105:1511–1515, 1994.

69. Ahrens RC, Ries RA, Popendorf W, et al: The delivery of therapeutic aerosols through endotracheal tubes. *Pediatr Pulmonol* 2:19–26, 1986.

70. Cole CH, Colton T, Shah BI, et al: Early inhaled glucocorticoid therapy to prevent bronchopulmonary dysplasia. *N Engl J Med* 340:1005–1010, 1999.

71. Fink JB, Dhand R, Duarte AG, et al: Deposition of aerosol from a metered dose inhaler during mechanical ventilation: an in vitro model. *Am J Respir Crit Care Med* 154:382–387, 1996.

72. Ari A, Areabi H, Fink JB: Evaluation of aerosol generator devices at 3 locations in humidified and nonhumidified circuits during adult mechanical ventilation. *Respir Care* 55:837–844, 2010.

73. Fink JB, Goody M, Dhand R: Optimizing efficiency of nebulizers during mechanical ventilation: the effect of placement and type in the ventilator circuit. *Chest* 116:312S, 1999.

74. Hess DR: Inhaled bronchodilators during mechanical ventilation: delivery techniques, evaluation of response, and cost-effectiveness. *Respir Care* 39:105–122, 1994.

75. Anderson M, Svartingren M, Bylin G, et al: Deposition in asthmatics of particles inhaled in air or in helium-oxygen. *Am Rev Respir Dis* 147:524–528, 1993.

76. Marik P, Hogan J, Krikorian J: A comparison of bronchodilator therapy delivered by nebulization and metered-dose inhaler in mechanically ventilated patients. *Chest* 115:1653–1657, 1999.

77. Hess DR: Mechanical ventilation strategies: what's new and what's worth keeping? *Respir Care* 47:1007–1017, 2002.

78. Fink JB: Humidity and aerosol therapy. In Cairo JM, Pilbeam SP, editors: *Mosby's respiratory care equipment*, ed 8, St Louis, 2010, Elsevier, pp 88–143.

79. Hughes JM, Saez J: Effects of nebulizer mode and position in a mechanical ventilator circuit on dose efficiency. *Respir Care* 32:1131–1135, 1987.

80. Quinn WW: Effect of a new nebulizer position on aerosol delivery during mechanical ventilation: a bench study. *Respir Care* 37:423–431, 1992.

81. Hanhan U, Kissoon N, Payne M, et al: Effects of in-line nebulization on preset ventilatory variables. *Respir Care* 38:474–478, 1993.

82. Beaty CD, Ritz RH, Benson MS: Continuous in-line nebulizers complicate pressure support ventilation. *Chest* 96:1360–1363, 1989.

83. Ari A, Fink J, Pilbeam SP: Second hand aerosol exposure during mechanical ventilation with and without expiratory filters: an in-vitro study. *Respir Care* 55:1566, 2010.

84. Shults RA, Baron S, Decker J, et al: Health care worker exposure to aerosolized Riboavirin: Biological and air monitoring. *J Occup Environ Med* 38:257–263, 1996.

85. Ari A, Atalay OT, Harwood R, et al: Influence of nebulizer type, position, and bias flow on aerosol delivery in simulated pediatric and adult lung models during mechanical ventilation. *Respir Care* 55:845–851, 2010.

86. Holt WJ, Greenspan JS, Antunes MJ, et al: Pulmonary response to an inhaled bronchodilator in chronically ventilated preterm infants with suspected airway reactivity. *Respir Care* 40:145–151, 1995.

87. Hess DR, Murray R, Rexrod WO: Bronchodilator response during mechanical ventilation. *Chest* 102(Suppl):82, 1992. (abstract).

88. Takahashi N, Murakami G, Ishikawa A, et al: Anatomic evaluation of postural bronchial drainage of the lung with special reference to patients with tracheal intubation: which combination of postures provides the best simplification? *Chest* 125:935–944, 2004.

89. American Association for Respiratory Care: Clinical Practice Guideline: Bronchoscopy assisting. *Respir Care* 52:74–80, 2007.

90. Sachs S: Fiberoptic bronchoscopy. In Hess DR, MacIntyre NR, Mishoe SC, et al, editors: *Respiratory care principles and practice*, Philadelphia, 2002, W.B. Saunders, pp 515–539.

91. Leibler JM, Markin CJ: Fiberoptic bronchoscopy for diagnosis and treatment. *Crit Care Clin* 16:83–100, 2000.

92. Garner JS, Jarvis WR, Emori TG, et al: CDC definitions for nosocomial infections. *Am J Infect Control* 16:128–140, 1988.

93. Rau JL, Pearce DJ: *Understanding chest radiographs*, Denver, 1984, Multi-Media.

94. Balk RA, Bone RC: Patient monitoring in the intensive care unit. In Burton GG, Hodgkin JE, Ward JJ, editors: *Respiratory care: a guide to clinical practice*, ed 3, Philadelphia, 1991, JB Lippincott, pp 705–717.

95. Parthasarathy S, Tobin MJ: Effect of ventilator mode on sleep quality in critically ill patients. *Am J Respir Crit Care Med* 166:1423–1429, 2002.

96. Kress JP, Pohlman AS, O'Connor MF, et al: Daily interruption of sedative infusions in critically ill patients undergoing mechanical ventilation. *N Engl J Med* 342:1471–1477, 2000.

97. Schelling G, Stoll C, Haller M, et al: Health-related quality of life and post-traumatic stress disorder in survivors of the acute respiratory distress syndrome. *Crit Care Med* 26:651–659, 1998.

98. Karampela I, Hansen-Flaschen J, Smith S, et al: A dyspnea evaluation protocol for respiratory therapists: a feasibility study. *Respir Care* 47:1158–1161, 2002.

99. Knebel AR, Janson-Bjerklie SL, Malley JD, et al: Comparison of breathing comfort during weaning with two ventilator modes. *Am J Respir Crit Care Med* 149:14–18, 1994.

100. Powers J, Bennett SJ: Measurement of dyspnea in patients treated with mechanical ventilation. *Am J Crit Care* 8:254–261, 1999.

101. Campbell RS, Johannigman JA, Branson RD, et al: Battery duration of portable ventilators: effects of control variable, positive end-expiratory pressure and inspired oxygen concentration. *Respir Care* 47:1173–1183, 2002.

102. Chang DW, American Association for Respiratory Care: AARC Clinical Practice Guideline: In-hospital transport of the mechanically ventilated patient—2002 Revision & Update. *Respir Care* 47:721–723, 2002.

103. Szem JW, Hydo LJ, Fischer E, et al: High-risk intrahospital transport of critically ill patients: safety and outcome of the necessary "road trip." *Crit Care Med* 23:1660–1666, 1995.

104. AARC Protocol Committee; Subcommittee Adult Critical Care, Version 1.0a (Sept., 2003), Subcommittee Chair, Susan P. Pilbeam, Dallas, Tex. Available at: <www.aarc.org>.

Improving Oxygenation and Management of Acute Respiratory Distress Syndrome

OUTLINE

KEY TERMS

- Absorption atelectasis
- Cytokines
- Deflation point
- Deflection point
- Exudative
- Fibrosing alveolitis
- Independent lung ventilation
- Lower inflection point
- Prone positioning
- Recruitment maneuver
- Thrombotic mediators
- Upper inflection point

LEARNING OBJECTIVES   *On completion of this chapter, the reader will be able to accomplish the following:*

1. Calculate a desired F$_I$O$_2$ required to achieve a desired P$_a$O$_2$, based on current ventilator settings and blood gases.
2. Calculate a patient's pulmonary shunt fraction.
3. Identify indications and contraindications for continuous positive airway pressure (CPAP) and positive end-expiratory pressure (PEEP).
4. List the primary goal of PEEP and the conditions in which high levels of PEEP are most often used.
5. Describe the most appropriate method for establishing an optimum level of PEEP for a patient with acute respiratory distress syndrome (ARDS) using a recruitment–derecruitment maneuver and the deflection point (lower inflection point during deflation or derecruitment).

6. Explain the effects of PEEP/CPAP therapy on a patient with a unilateral lung disease. Describe the problems associated with initiating PEEP in a patient with an untreated pneumothorax.
7. Recommend adjustments in PEEP and ventilator settings based on the physical assessment of the patient, arterial blood gases (ABGs), and ventilator parameters.
8. Compare static compliance, hemodynamic data, and ABGs as indicators of an optimum PEEP.
9. Identify from patient assessment and ABGs when it is appropriate to change from CPAP to mechanical ventilation with PEEP.
10. Identify the severity of ARDS using the P$_a$O$_2$/F$_I$O$_2$ ratio.
11. Recommend an appropriate tidal volume (V$_T$) setting for a patient with ARDS.

12. Identify the maximum $P_{plateau}$ value to use for patients with ARDS.
13. Identify the criteria that should be used to liberate a patient from PEEP or CPAP.
14. Recommend a PEEP setting based on the inflection point on the deflation curve using the pressure–volume loop for a patient with ARDS.
15. Describe the procedure for prone positioning in ventilated patients with adult respiratory distress syndrome.
16. List potential problems associated with placing the patient in a prone position during mechanical ventilation.
17. Discuss several theories that describe how prone positioning improves ventilation-perfusion in adult respiratory distress syndrome.

Improving the ventilatory status of a patient with hypercapnic respiratory failure (i.e., reducing the partial pressure of carbon dioxide [P_aCO_2]) can be accomplished by improving alveolar ventilation, reducing physiological dead space, and reducing carbon dioxide (CO_2) production. Improving oxygenation, on the other hand, involves using various patient management strategies, such as administering supplemental oxygen, applying positive end-expiratory pressure (PEEP) or continuous positive airway pressure (CPAP), and patient positioning.

Although the terms **hypoxia** and **hypoxemia** are often used interchangeably, it is important to recognize that *hypoxia* is defined as a reduction in oxygen in the tissues, whereas *hypoxemia* refers to a reduction in the partial pressure of oxygen in the blood (i.e., P_aO_2 <80 mm Hg and S_aO_2 <95%). Box 13-1 provides a brief description of the four types of hypoxia and Key Point 13-1 provides P_aO_2 and S_aO_2 values typically used to identify mild, moderate, and severe hypoxemia.

inspiratory oxygen [P_IO_2]) can be reversed by having the person breathe an enriched oxygen mixture. When hypoventilation causes hypoxemia, increasing minute ventilation generally improves oxygenation (Case Study 13-1). Serious anemia, on the other hand, is treated with the administration of blood products, which in turn improves the patient's oxygen-carrying capacity (i.e., hemoglobin). Circulatory hypoxia occurs when the patient's cardiac output is reduced. The treatment of this type of hypoxia typically involves fluid resuscitation and pharmacologic interventions, which normalize the patient's cardiac output (e.g., administering drugs that increase ventricular contractility or decrease vascular resistance) and therefore improve oxygen delivery to the tissues. With histotoxic hypoxia, cyanide interferes with a person's ability to utilize oxygen to produce energy (cellular respiration) by uncoupling oxidative phosphorylation (i.e., cytochrome oxidase). Treatment of cyanide poisoning involves administering a cyanide antidote (e.g., hydroxocobalamin) and providing supportive care to maintain oxygenation and acid–base balance.

Key Point 13-1

Levels of Hypoxemia*

Level	P_aO_2 Value	P_aO_2 Range	Saturation (S_aO_2)
Mild hypoxemia	<80 mm Hg	60 to 79 mm Hg	90% to 94%
Moderate hypoxemia	<60 mm Hg	40 to 59 mm Hg	75% to 89%
Severe hypoxemia	<40 mm Hg	<40 mm Hg	<75%

*Values given are for a young adult breathing room air. (NOTE: The levels of hypoxemia defined here may differ depending among clinicians and institutions.)

Case Study 13-1

Myasthenia Gravis

A patient with myasthenia gravis is placed on mechanical ventilation. The chest radiograph is normal. Breath sounds are clear. Initial arterial blood gases (ABGs) on 0.25 F_IO_2 20 minutes after beginning ventilation are as follows: pH = 7.31; P_aCO_2 = 62 mm Hg; bicarbonate = 31 mEq/L; and P_aO_2 = 58 mm Hg. What change in ventilator setting might improve this patient's ABG findings?

The strategy used to treat hypoxia should focus on its cause. For example, hypoxemic hypoxia, which occurs when a person breathes rarefied air at a high altitude (i.e., reduced partial pressure of

Improvement in oxygenation status may require time before the response to treatment is evident. This is particularly evident in cases involving hypoventilation, anemia, and circulatory hypoxia. In these cases, it is appropriate to administer supplemental oxygen until the hypoxemia is relieved.

This chapter begins with a discussion of how to make simple adjustments of F_IO_2 to improve oxygenation. It is followed by a discussion of techniques involving the use of PEEP to improve oxygenation. Achieving optimum PEEP requires close monitoring and the use of either static or dynamic pressure–volume (P-V) loops. Methods used to set optimum PEEP are provided along with a review of P-V loops. Additional uses of PEEP are also discussed in this chapter, along with a description of the effects, complications, and consequences associated with discontinuation of PEEP.

A discussion of the pathophysiology of acute respiratory distress syndrome (ARDS) is included to provide the reader with an understanding of the complexity of this disorder. Patients with

BOX 13-1 Types of Hypoxia

- Hypoxemic hypoxia (lower than normal P_aO_2, ascent to altitude, hypoventilation)
- Anemic hypoxia (lower than normal red blood cell count [anemia], abnormal hemoglobin, carbon monoxide poisoning)
- Circulatory hypoxia (reduced cardiac output, decreased tissue perfusion)
- Histotoxic hypoxia (cyanide poisoning)

ARDS are among the most difficult to oxygenate and manage in the critical care unit. The concept of lung-protective strategies and lung-recruitment maneuvers that are currently being used to improve oxygenation, particularly in patients with ARDS, are included along with three clinical scenarios related to the topics discussed in this chapter.

Basics of Oxygenation Using F_IO_2, PEEP Studies, and Pressure–Volume Curves for Establishing Optimum PEEP

BASICS OF OXYGEN DELIVERY TO THE TISSUES

The most common parameters used to assess the oxygenation status of patients are the F_IO_2, S_pO_2, ABGs, hemoglobin (Hb), the presence of abnormal hemoglobin species, P_aO_2, P_aO_2/P_AO_2, P_aO_2/F_IO_2, shunt, cardiac output, mixed venous oxygen saturation ($S\overline{v}O_2$), and oxygen content of mixed venous blood ($C\overline{v}O_2$). Measuring oxygen delivery (DO_2) to the tissues provides valuable information about oxygen availability to the tissues. Oxygen utilization by the tissues can be determined by measuring arterial-to-mixed venous oxygen content difference ($C[a-\overline{v}]O_2$), oxygen consumption ($\dot{V}O_2$), cardiac output, and $S\overline{v}O_2$. Table 13-1 provides a list of normal values for the parameters used to evaluate a patient's oxygen status. Box 13-2 contains a summary of the equations for calculating parameters that are not directly measured, such as the partial pressure of alveolar oxygen (P_AO_2), C_aO_2, $C\overline{v}O_2$, and DO_2.

Evaluating P_aO_2, S_pO_2, and F_IO_2 in Ventilator Patients

The F_IO_2 should be measured at regular intervals, or continuously if possible, to ensure that the patient is receiving the appropriate concentration of inspired oxygen. When changes in the F_IO_2 are initially made for adults or children, ABGs should be measured

within 15 minutes, although some clinicians choose to obtain a sample after 30 minutes.[1,2]

Every attempt should be made to prevent complications associated with oxygen toxicity by administering an F_IO_2 below 0.6 while maintaining the P_aO_2 between 60 and 90 mm Hg and the C_aO_2 near normal (20 mL/dL). This goal is not always possible, and sometimes a higher F_IO_2 is required. (See section on selection of F_IO_2 or adjusting mean airway pressure.)

The S_pO_2 can be used to titrate F_IO_2 once the relationship between P_aO_2 and S_pO_2 has been established. (After mechanical

---

BOX 13-2 | **Equations Used to Calculate Oxygenation Status: Alveolar Air Equation (Calculation of Alveolar PO_2, P_AO_2)**

$$P_AO_2 = F_IO_2(P_B - P_{H_2O}) - \left[PaCO_2 \times \left\{ F_IO_2 + \left(1 - \frac{F_IO_2}{R} \right) \right\} \right]$$

where P_AO_2 = alveolar partial pressure of oxygen (mm Hg)
F_IO_2 = inspired oxygen fraction
P_B = barometric pressure (mm Hg)
P_{H_2O} = water vapor pressure (at 37° C = 47 mm Hg)
R = respiratory quotient ($\dot{V}CO_2/\dot{V}O_2$; R of 0.8 is commonly used)
With an $F_IO_2 \leq 0.6$ (low value), the effect of R on P_AO_2 is small. To estimate the P_AO_2 for F_IO_2 values <0.6: $P_AO_2 = F_IO_2(P_B - P_{H_2O}) - (1.25 \times P_aCO_2)$
Partial pressure of inspired oxygen: $P_IO_2 = F_IO_2 (P_B - P_{H_2O})$
Arterial oxygen content (C_aO_2): $C_aO_2 = ([Hb \times 1.34] \times S_aO_2) + (0.003 \text{ mL/dL} \times P_aO_2)$
Mixed venous oxygen content ($C\overline{v}O_2$): $C\overline{v}O_2 = ([Hb \times 1.34] \times S\overline{v}O_2) + (0.003 \text{ mL/dL} \times P\overline{v}O_2)$
Oxygen consumption ($\dot{V}O_2$): $\dot{V}O_2$ = Cardiac output (C.O.) $\times (C_aO_2 - C\overline{v}O_2)$
Oxygen delivery (DO_2): $DO_2 = C.O. \times C_aO_2$

TABLE 13-1 | **Measures and Values Used in the Evaluation of Oxygenation Status**

Term	Abbreviation	Normal Value
Partial pressure of arterial oxygen	P_aO_2	80-100 mm Hg
Partial pressure of mixed venous oxygen	$P\overline{v}O_2$	40 mm Hg
Alveolar partial pressure of oxygen	P_AO_2	100-673 mm Hg
		F_IO_2 range: 0.21-1.0
Alveolar-arterial oxygen tension gradient	$P_{(A-a)}O_2$	5-10 mm Hg ($F_IO_2 = 0.21$)
		30-60 mm Hg ($F_IO_2 = 1.0$)
Ratio of P_aO_2 to fractional inspired oxygen (P_aO_2 range = 80-100 mm Hg; $F_IO_2 = 0.21$)	P_aO_2/F_IO_2	380-475
Ratio of P_aO_2 to partial pressure of alveolar oxygen (P_aO_2 range = 80-100 mm Hg; $F_IO_2 = 0.21$)	P_aO_2/P_AO_2	0.8-1.0
Saturation of arterial oxygen	S_aO_2	97%
Saturation of mixed venous oxygen	$S\overline{v}O_2$	75%
Oxygen content of arterial blood	C_aO_2	20 vol%
Oxygen content of mixed venous blood	$C\overline{v}O_2$	15 vol%
Arterial-to-mixed venous oxygen content difference	$C[a-\overline{v}]O_2$	3.5-5 mL/dL
Oxygen delivery	DO_2	1000 mL/min
Oxygen consumption	$\dot{V}O_2$	250 mL/min

ventilation is initiated, an arterial blood gas sample is obtained and the P_aO_2 is compared with the patient's current S_pO_2 to establish this relationship.) A goal for maintaining S_pO_2 at greater than 90% is appropriate. It is important to understand, however, that the S_pO_2 will not always correlate perfectly with P_aO_2. Some patients will have a large discrepancy between S_pO_2 and P_aO_2 and need to be monitored more carefully[3] (see Chapter 10). For example, in patients with chronic obstructive pulmonary disease (COPD), their normal P_aO_2 may be near 55 mm Hg (S_aO_2 ~80%) and the S_pO_2 values may be closer to 88% to 90% on room air.

Although the inspired oxygen percentage can be determined using multiuse oxygen analyzers, most intensive care unit (ICU) ventilators have built-in oxygen analyzers that can provide continuous measurements of F_IO_2. Examples include the Hamilton Galileo (Hamilton Medical, Bonaduz, Switzerland), the Dräger v500 (Dräger Medical, Inc, Telford, Pa.), the Hamilton G5 (Hamilton Medical, Bonaduz, Switzerland), the Puritan Bennett 840 (Covidien-Nellcor Puritan Bennett, Boulder, Colo.), and the Servo-i (Maquet Inc, Wayne, N.J.) to name a few.

Adjusting F_IO_2

The ABGs obtained after mechanical ventilation is initiated are compared with the F_IO_2 being delivered. A linear relationship exists between P_aO_2 and F_IO_2 for any patient as long as the person's cardiopulmonary status remains fairly stable.[4-7] In other words, the minute ventilation, cardiac output, shunt, and V_D/V_T must not change significantly between the time the ABG comparison is made and the F_IO_2 is changed. Most of the time, this is the case because ventilator changes are made quickly after blood gas results are obtained.

Because of this linear correlation, the known P_aO_2 and the known F_IO_2 can be used to select the F_IO_2 necessary to achieve a desired P_aO_2:

$$\frac{P_aO_2(known)}{F_IO_2(known)} = \frac{P_aO_2(desired)}{F_IO_2(desired)}$$

or

$$desired\ F_IO_2 = \frac{P_aO_2(desired) \times F_IO_2(known)}{P_aO_2(known)}$$

This equation provides a reliable method for making appropriate changes in the F_IO_2 to achieve a desired P_aO_2.

Some institutions use the ratio of P_aO_2/P_AO_2 for evaluation of oxygenation and for predicting the inspired oxygen concentration.[7-10] The ratio of P_aO_2 to F_IO_2 (commonly called the *P-to-F ratio* [P_aO_2/F_IO_2]) also has become a very popular way to set F_IO_2 because of its simplicity. To estimate the a change in F_IO_2, for example, if the P_aO_2 is 60 mm Hg with an F_IO_2 of 0.3 and the target P_aO_2 is 80 mm Hg, the calculation of F_IO_2 is as follows:

$$\frac{known\ P_aO_2}{F_IO_2(known)} = \frac{desired\ PaO_2}{F_IO_2(desired)}$$

and $60/0.3 = 80/X$, where X would be the new F_IO_2 setting. In this example, the new setting for F_IO_2 would be 0.4 (Case Study 13-2).[8,9] Making adjustments in F_IO_2 has a greater effect on patients with hypoventilation and reduced $\dot{V}/\dot{Q}$, in which higher alveolar oxygen has better access to pulmonary blood flow than situations of pulmonary shunt. It is worth mentioning that using the **P-to-F ratio** (P_aO_2/F_IO_2) to adjust the F_IO_2 is not as accurate as using the P_aO_2/P_AO_2 because the alveolar PO_2 determination takes P_aCO_2 into account.

Case Study 13-2

Changing F_IO_2

After being supported on a ventilator for 30 minutes, a patient's P_aO_2 is 40 mm Hg on an F_IO_2 of 0.75. Acid–base status is normal and all other ventilator parameters are within the acceptable range. PEEP is 5 cm H_2O. What F_IO_2 is required to achieve a desired P_aO_2 of 60 mm Hg? Is your answer possible? Can you think of another form of therapy to improve oxygenation?

Selection of F_IO_2 or Adjustment of Mean Airway Pressures

Although the exact safe level of F_IO_2 in mechanically ventilated patients is not known at this time, it is generally agreed that maintaining a high F_IO_2 (>0.6) can result in oxygen toxicity.[11] Besides the tissue damage associated with the long-term use of 100% oxygen, it also has an additional complication. Breathing 100% oxygen can lead to **absorption atelectasis** and increase intrapulmonary shunting (i.e., shunt fraction), which further contributes to hypoxemia (Box 13-3).[10,12-14] Thus, F_IO_2 should be kept as low as possible. Although the lower limits of permissive hypoxemia remain controversial, most practitioners agree that a target P_aO_2 of 60 mm Hg and a S_pO_2 of 90% are acceptable lower limits for most adult patients.[12] If the P_aO_2 remains very low while the patient is breathing an enriched oxygen mixture, significant shunting, ventilation-perfusion abnormalities, and/or diffusion defects are present. In these cases, other methods to improve oxygenation, besides increasing F_IO_2, must be considered. One approach that

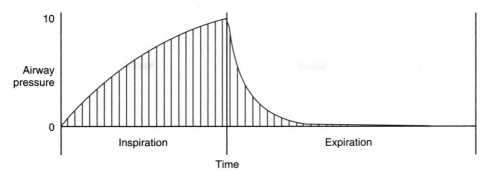

Fig. 13-1 A pressure–time waveform illustrating mean airway pressure ($\overline{P}_{aw}$). Vertical lines under the pressure–time curve represent frequent readings of pressure over the total respiratory cycle. The sum of these pressure readings (i.e., the area under the curve) divided by the cycle time will give the value for mean airway pressure. (See text for additional information.)

BOX **13-4**	Simple Method for Calculating $\overline{P}_{aw}$

$$\overline{P}_{aw} = \frac{1}{2}\left[PIP \times \left(\frac{\text{inspiratory time}}{\text{total respiratory cycle}}\right)\right]$$

When PEEP is used, the equation is as follows:

$$\overline{P}_{aw} = \frac{1}{2}(PIP - PEEP) \times \left(\frac{\text{inspiratory time}}{\text{total cycle time}}\right) + PEEP$$

Fortunately, most ICU ventilators measure pressures and time and perform this calculation automatically.

BOX **13-5**	Inverse Ratio Ventilation (IRV)

IRV is one method for increasing $\overline{P}_{aw}$, in which inspiratory time (T_I) is longer than expiratory time (T_E). IRV can be used either with pressure-controlled or volume-controlled ventilation. The rationale behind increasing T_I is to recruit lung units and avoid overinflating normal units. Keeping alveoli open for extended periods may reduce shunt and $\dot{V}/\dot{Q}$ mismatch.

When an inverse I : E ratio is used with pressure ventilation (PCIRV), a longer T_I increases $\overline{P}_{aw}$. With PCIRV, the PIP and PEEP do not change because these are set values. However, volume delivery varies with changes in compliance and resistance. Exhaled V_T and $\dot{V}_E$ must be closely monitored. (NOTE: Increase in auto-PEEP reduces V_T delivery in PCIRV.) Additionally, using IRV may require sedation and paralysis in a number of patients because an increased I : E breathing pattern is uncomfortable.

Volume control inverse ratio ventilation (VCIRV) is an alternative to PCIRV, but it is seldom used. With VCIRV, V_T is ensured, if this is a desired goal. VCIRV can be accomplished by selecting VC-CMV, using a descending waveform to lengthen T_I or setting a longer T_I if the ventilator is time cycled. T_I can be further lengthened by adding inspiratory pause and by slowing inspiratory flows.

It is important to recognize that IRV can create several risks for patients. Both dynamic hyperinflation (auto-PEEP) and increased $\overline{P}_{aw}$ can increase the risk of lung damage. Furthermore, cardiac output may decrease with increased $\overline{P}_{aw}$. An I : E ratio of 2:1 is therefore rarely exceeded because of adverse hemodynamic consequences.

Manipulating pressures to increase $\overline{P}_{aw}$ may result in injury to the lung from trapped air and overdistention and possibly barotrauma (e.g., pneumothorax). (See Chapter 17 for pulmonary complications of positive pressure ventilation.) High thoracic pressures can reduce venous return and cardiac output.[3] (See Chapter 16 for cardiovascular complications.) Therefore, it is important to monitor the $\overline{P}_{aw}$ and assess the patient's response.

---

can be used to increase the P_aO_2 involves increasing the $\overline{P}_{aw}$. The $\overline{P}_{aw}$ is the average pressure above baseline during a total respiratory cycle (I + E) (Fig. 13-1). Box 13-4 provides an equation to estimate $\overline{P}_{aw}$. As $\overline{P}_{aw}$ increases, the P_aO_2 increases. Factors that affect $\overline{P}_{aw}$ during positive pressure ventilation include peak inspiratory pressure (PIP), total PEEP (i.e., intrinsic PEEP or auto-PEEP plus extrinsic or set PEEP [$PEEP_E$]), inspiratory-to-expiratory (I : E) ratios, respiratory rate (*f*), and inspiratory flow pattern. For example, as the total PEEP increases, the $\overline{P}_{aw}$ increases.

$\overline{P}_{aw}$ is a major determinant of oxygenation in patients with ARDS because it affects mean alveolar pressure ($\overline{P}_{alv}$) and alveolar recruitment and, therefore, oxygenation.[15-19] As such, PEEP is typically used to increase $\overline{P}_{aw}$, although other approaches are also available. For example, high-frequency oscillatory ventilation (HFOV) and airway pressure release ventilation (APRV) can also be used to increase $\overline{P}_{aw}$. (HFOV and APRV are reviewed in Chapter 23.) At one time, inverse ratio ventilation (IRV) was used by many clinicians; however, this strategy is not routinely used today (Box 13-5).[15-24]

INTRODUCTION TO POSITIVE END-EXPIRATORY PRESSURE AND CONTINUOUS POSITIVE AIRWAY PRESSURE

Because PEEP is so frequently used to increase $\overline{P}_{aw}$ and improve and maintain oxygenation, it occupies a key role as a technique for treating acute parenchymal lung injury, such as severe atelectasis associated with various pulmonary pathologic processes. The goal of using PEEP is to recruit collapsed alveoli while avoiding overdistention of already open alveoli.[25] It is important to set an appropriate level of PEEP that avoids overdistention while maintaining alveolar patency and preventing alveoli from collapsing during exhalation of a tidal volume. Both overdistention and repeated collapse and re-expansion of alveoli are associated with ventilator-induced lung injury (VILI) (see Chapter 17 for more details about the effects of PEEP and VILI). The following section reviews the pathophysiology of atelectasis, indications for using PEEP and CPAP, and techniques used to establish an appropriate level of PEEP for a patient.

Pathophysiology of Atelectasis

Atelectasis is the partial or complete collapse of previously expanded areas of the lung producing a shrunken, airless state. It can result from blockage of air passages, shallow breathing (e.g., postoperative atelectasis), or surfactant deficiency. The loss of surfactant can be a result of damage to surfactant-producing cells (type II pneumocytes), leakage of plasma proteins that inhibit surfactant production, or the presence of inflammatory mediators (e.g., **cytokines**). These factors tend to promote atelectasis, particularly in the presence of high O_2 concentrations, pulmonary edema, general anesthesia, mechanical ventilation, chemical toxicity, and ARDS.

The treatment of acute atelectasis involves identifying the cause and then initiating an appropriate corrective action. For mechanical obstruction of the airways, coughing, suctioning, percussion, and therapeutic fiberoptic bronchoscopy may be indicated to clear the obstruction. Therapy with PEEP or CPAP may also be used to help inflate (i.e., recruit) collapsed alveoli.

Goals of PEEP and CPAP

The goals of PEEP/CPAP therapy are:
1. Maintain a $P_aO_2 \geq 60$ mm Hg and S_pO_2 at 90% or greater, at an acceptable pH
2. Recruit alveoli and maintain them in an aerated state
3. Restore functional residual capacity
4. Enhance tissue oxygenation

Achieving these goals may also provide opportunities to reduce the F_IO_2 to safer levels (<0.6). Note that sustaining cardiovascular function and avoiding lung injury are critical requirements for effective PEEP/CPAP therapy.

Terminology

The term *PEEP* as it is commonly used implies that the patient is receiving mechanical ventilatory support and the baseline (i.e., end-expiratory) pressure is above zero cm H_2O. CPAP is pressure above the ambient pressure maintained during spontaneous ventilation. With CPAP, expiratory positive airway pressure (EPAP) and inspiratory positive airway pressure (IPAP) are both positive and equal, albeit the ventilator does **not** provide mandatory breaths.

Technical Aspects of PEEP and CPAP Devices

Generally, PEEP is used when a problem in the lungs results in collapse of alveoli and small airways (atelectasis). If a significant number of alveoli collapse, more areas of the lung are perfused but not ventilated, resulting in a shunt-like situation.

When PEEP is set on a ventilator, the expiratory valve of the ventilator closes when the expiratory pressure drops to the set PEEP level. This traps a certain amount of pressure and volume in the lungs that can prevent or reverse alveolar collapse and reduce the amount of pulmonary shunting.

Although CPAP can also be used to reduce shunting, as mentioned earlier, its application is for patients who are spontaneously breathing. CPAP can be achieved with a mechanical ventilator by setting the mode selection switch to the spontaneous/CPAP mode and then setting the desired level of CPAP (PEEP control). CPAP can also be delivered to spontaneously breathing patients using a freestanding setup (i.e., one without a mechanical ventilator). It is important to recognize that using freestanding CPAP devices carries a potential liability because these devices are usually "homemade" and have not undergone a formal evaluation for approval by an authorized independent agency. (Freestanding CPAP systems are discussed in more detail later in this chapter.)

Application of CPAP and PEEP to the Patient's Airway

The positive pressure employed with CPAP or PEEP is commonly applied to the airway noninvasively with a mask or nasal prongs, or invasively through an endotracheal tube or a tracheostomy tube. Noninvasive CPAP administered with a soft silicon mask eliminates the need for endotracheal intubation in specified groups of patients (see Chapter 5). A variety of tight-fitting masks can be applied to the face or nose, with the pressure adjusted to as high as 15 cm H_2O (see Figs. 19-4, 19-6, and 19-7). Excessive leakage around the mask, however, can create a problem when trying to maintain a desired pressure.

Mask CPAP

Patients receiving mask CPAP are usually alert, awake, and oriented. These patients can protect their lower airways, support work of breathing (WOB), and maintain a normal P_aCO_2 without excessive ventilatory effort. Patients receiving noninvasive mask CPAP should have a P_aO_2/F_IO_2 ratio greater than 200 mm Hg and have a stable cardiovascular status. The hazards and complications of mask CPAP can include vomiting and aspiration, skin necrosis or discomfort from the mask, CO_2 retention, increased WOB, and cerebral hemorrhage at high CPAP levels (infants).

Nasal CPAP

By taking advantage of the fact that neonates are obligate nose breathers, plastic or Silastic nasal prongs can be fitted into an infant's nares. CPAP pressures up to about 15 cm H_2O can be administered with these devices (see Fig. 22-1). Loss of pressure from the system can occur through the mouth at high pressures (>15 cm H_2O) (Case Study 13-3). Problems of nasal CPAP include gastric distention, pressure necrosis, swelling of nasal mucosa, and abrasion of the posterior pharynx. (See Chapter 22 for additional information on nasal CPAP in infants.)

 Case Study 13-3

Problem Solving: Infant CPAP

An infant has been well oxygenated ($S_pO_2 = 97\%$) using nasal CPAP at +6 cm H_2O with an F_IO_2 of 0.4. A nurse readjusts a vascular line and the infant starts crying. Pressures on the manometer drop to 0 to 2 cm H_2O and S_pO_2 drops to 93%. What could cause the drop in S_pO_2?

Endotracheal or Tracheostomy Tubes

Endotracheal intubation or placement of a tracheostomy tube may be necessary to provide an airway for the administration of CPAP for patients who do not meet the criteria for mask or nasal CPAP.

Flow and Threshold Resistors

When PEEP/CPAP is used, the flow or pressure the patient must generate to obtain inspiratory flow for a spontaneous breath or to trigger a mandatory breath depends on the type of system used. High-gas flow systems, pressurized reservoirs, demand valves, and demand flow systems respond to patient flow demand. The more rapidly and easily these devices respond to patient effort, the less WOB is required. Expiratory pressure, on the other hand, is maintained above ambient pressure with PEEP/CPAP and can be accomplished using a variety of devices that are classified as either flow or threshold resistors.

A **flow resistor** achieves expiratory pressure by creating a resistance to gas flow through an orifice. As the diameter of the orifice decreases in size, the pressure level applied increases; conversely as the diameter of the orifice increases, the applied pressure level decreases. Changes in expiratory gas flow also affect the expiratory pressure applied with a flow resistor; that is, the pressure is flow dependent. The higher the expired gas flow, the higher the expiratory pressure generated; the lower the expired gas flow, the lower the pressure. (Positive expiratory pressure [PEP] mask therapy is based on this principle.) An ideal flow resistor is one in which pressure increases linearly with flow.

With **threshold resistors,** a constant pressure is provided throughout expiration regardless of the rate of gas flow (i.e., flow independent). When a threshold resistor is used in the expiratory limb of a ventilator circuit, the exhaled air passes unimpeded until pressure falls to the preset PEEP value. At that time, the expiratory gas flow stops and the system pressure is maintained at the preset PEEP level. The expiratory valves on most ventilators behave as threshold resistors. Note that these threshold resistors are free-floating and provide minimal resistance to exhalation (Key Point 13-2).

Key Point **13-2** Adding any device to the expiratory side of a ventilator circuit that is smaller in diameter than the main expiratory line of the circuit itself will increase expiratory resistance.

Circuitry for Spontaneous CPAP with Freestanding Systems and Mechanical Ventilators

Ventilators can provide CPAP for a spontaneously breathing patient by simply eliminating the mandatory breaths (CPAP/spontaneous mode) and adjusting the PEEP level to the desired pressure. Current ICU ventilators can be used for CPAP because they incorporate inspiratory flow systems that typically respond very quickly to a patient's breathing effort and do not increase WOB.

CPAP can also be provided by a freestanding system without using a ventilator. There are two types of freestanding or stand-alone CPAP or EPAP systems: continuous flow CPAP, which is a closed system, and demand-flow spontaneous CPAP, which is an open system. Both systems can be used only for patients who do not require mechanical ventilation but who might benefit from the effects of CPAP on oxygenation. Patients must be able to comfortably maintain a near-normal P_aCO_2. As mentioned previously, these systems are not used often in the clinical setting. Most institutions simply use a ventilator in the spontaneous/CPAP mode.

PEEP RANGES

Two levels or ranges of PEEP can be employed: minimum or low PEEP, also called *physiological PEEP,* and therapeutic PEEP.

Minimum or Low PEEP

In most situations it is appropriate to use a minimum level of PEEP (3 to 5 cm H_2O) to help preserve a patient's normal functional residual capacity (FRC). FRC usually decreases when a patient is intubated or placed in a supine position.[22-24] The reduction in FRC is due primarily to the abdominal contents moving upward and exerting pressure on the diaphragm. Because only 3 to 5 cm H_2O is applied with minimum PEEP, it is usually not considered a problem in terms of causing complications.

Therapeutic PEEP

Therapeutic PEEP is ≥5 cm H_2O. It is used in the treatment of refractory hypoxemia caused by increased intrapulmonary shunting and ventilation-perfusion mismatching accompanied by a decreased FRC and pulmonary compliance.[25] High levels of therapeutic PEEP (e.g., ≥15 cm H_2O) are beneficial for a small percentage of the patients with ARDS. Because high levels of PEEP are often associated with cardiopulmonary complications, physiological response to therapy must be monitored carefully.

Optimum PEEP

In 1975 Suter[26] and his colleagues coined the term *optimum* (or best) *PEEP.* Since then, other authors have used the terms *therapeutic PEEP* and *preferred PEEP.*[27] Optimum PEEP is the level at which the maximum beneficial effects of PEEP occur (i.e., increased DO_2, FRC, and C_S, and decreased $\dot{Q}_S/\dot{Q}_T$). This level of PEEP is also considered optimal because it is not associated with profound cardiopulmonary side effects, such as decreased venous return, decreased cardiac output, decreased blood pressure (BP), increased shunting, increased V_D/V_T, barotrauma, and volutrauma, and it is accomplished at safe levels of inspired oxygen (F_IO_2 <0.40). It is important to note that optimum PEEP should be correlated with criteria other than arterial PO_2 alone.[27,28] Thus, optimum PEEP has more recently been defined as the PEEP at which static compliance is highest as PEEP is decreased following a **recruitment maneuver** (RM).[29] RMs are discussed later in this chapter.

INDICATIONS FOR PEEP AND CPAP

ARDS remains a prime example of a pathophysiological state in which PEEP is used as an effective means of improving oxygenation. Patients with ARDS do not benefit from mechanical ventilatory support without PEEP. Although collapsed alveoli may open during a positive pressure inspiration, unstable alveoli and airways tend to collapse if the airway pressure returns to ambient pressure during expiration. Because approximately two thirds of the respiratory cycle is spent in expiration, blood passing through these areas of collapsed alveoli during expiration creates a shunt-like state, which perpetuates hypoxemia.

Patients with ARDS benefit from PEEP because it helps to prevent collapse of the small airways and alveoli, and thus it aids

---

BOX 13-6   Indications for Positive End-Expiratory Pressure (PEEP) Therapy

- Bilateral infiltrates on chest radiograph
- Recurrent atelectasis with low functional residual capacity (FRC)
- Reduced lung compliance (C_L)
- P_aO_2 <60 mm Hg on F_IO_2s >0.5
- P_aO_2/F_IO_2 ratio <300 for ARDS*
- Refractory hypoxemia: P_aO_2 increases <10 mm Hg with F_IO_2 increase of 0.2

*The level of applied PEEP will vary depending on the severity of ARDS. See section on Acute Respiratory Distress Syndrome.

---

in recruiting closed lung units. The edema-filled alveoli may also have their volumes partially air-filled with this technique as well, leading to the restoration of FRC. Lung compliance (C_L) and gas distribution are enhanced, thereby reducing the shunt effect of venous admixture and improving oxygenation.[30,31] Box 13-6 lists the indications for PEEP therapy.[32,33]

The indications for initiating CPAP are similar to the criteria used for initiating PEEP; the primary difference between using CPAP versus PEEP is that the patient provides the WOB at all times during CPAP. Thus, if a patient is capable of breathing spontaneously without much difficulty and is able to maintain an acceptable P_aCO_2, then CPAP is appropriate.

Ultimately, PEEP allows for the reduction of F_IO_2 because it improves oxygenation and helps avoid the complications associated with a high F_IO_2 in certain disorders. Examples of disorders that may benefit from the use of PEEP include:

- ARDS
- Cardiogenic pulmonary edema in adults and children
- Bilateral, diffuse pneumonia

INITIATING PEEP THERAPY

Once a patient's clinical condition indicates that PEEP or CPAP therapy is warranted, it is prudent to initiate this form of therapy as soon as possible. High peak pressures (>35 cm H_2O) along with F_IO_2 values of 0.5 or greater may damage alveolar cells (type I and II) in less than 24 hours; therefore, PEEP or CPAP should be initiated early in the course of therapy to avoid lung damage from high pressures, volumes, and F_IO_2 (see Chapter 17 for more information on ventilator-induced lung injury).

SELECTING THE APPROPRIATE PEEP/CPAP LEVEL (OPTIMUM PEEP)

Although some clinicians try to select one specific parameter, such as shunt or C_S, to identify the optimum PEEP for the patient, it is better to analyze several factors simultaneously when deciding if the optimum level of PEEP has been achieved. The medical literature describes several ways of determining when the goals of PEEP have been achieved. The consensus of these different approaches is reviewed here. Additional techniques used in the management of ARDS are discussed later in this chapter.

Application of PEEP Above 5 cm H_2O

For adults, PEEP is usually increased in increments of 3 to 5 cm H_2O. In infants, this range is generally 2 to 3 cm H_2O.[33] Some

clinicians follow specific step increases in F_IO_2 and PEEP when performing a PEEP study using the procedure outlined in the ARDSnet study (Table 13-2).[34] Others follow a more rapidly increasing PEEP-F_IO_2 table from a follow-up study (Table 13-3).[35] Both the low and high PEEP titration techniques for establishing the appropriate PEEP level appear to have similar morbidity and mortality rates.[36]

In addition to using either a moderate (low PEEP increments) or more aggressive (high PEEP incremental changes), other practitioners will use techniques, such as slow or static pressure–volume loops to determine optimum the PEEP level. Still other clinicians use a recruitment maneuver, which may be accompanied by a decremental PEEP study. Pressure–volume loops and recruitment maneuvers will be reviewed later in this chapter.

Regardless of the procedure, an optimal oxygenation point should be targeted that allows adequate tissue oxygenation (optimum oxygen transport) at a safe F_IO_2 and safe ventilating pressures with an acceptable P_aO_2/F_IO_2 ratio[31,32,37,38] (Key Point 13-3). Along with improving oxygenation, cardiovascular status should be monitored to identify adverse side effects of PEEP so they can be managed appropriately by the attending physician. Excessive PEEP must also be avoided because it can result in lung overinflation, stressing pulmonary cells potentially resulting in an inflammatory reaction, and possible barotraumas (see Chapter 17).

Key Point 13-3 Given that a healthy individual's P_aO_2 is approximately 100 mm Hg while breathing room air ($F_IO_2 = 0.21$), then the P_aO_2/F_IO_2 ratio is normally about 500.

Optimum PEEP Study

Performing an optimum PEEP study is a function most often reserved for patients requiring 10 cm H_2O or more of PEEP. For example, in patients with ARDS, PEEP levels greater than 20 cm H_2O of PEEP may be required. Box 13-7 lists the parameters most often monitored during a PEEP or CPAP study. Box 13-3 and Box 13-8 provide information for shunt calculations, which helps monitor PEEP/CPAP when a pulmonary artery catheter is being used (see Chapter 11).

Some common target goals that can be used to assess a patient's response to PEEP include:

- A P_aO_2 of 60 mm Hg to 100 mm Hg on F_IO_2 of 0.4 or less, which represents a S_aO_2 of 90% to 97% at a normal pH. (NOTE: The range of P_aO_2 from the ARDSnet study targeted P_aO_2 from 55 to 80 mm Hg and S_pO_2 from 88% to 95%.[34])
- Optimum oxygen transport is present; normal O_2 transport is about 1000 mL/min of O_2 (5 L/min × 20 vol% × 10). A pulmonary shunt fraction less than 15%, when this parameter is monitored.
- A minimal amount of cardiovascular compromise, which includes adequate systemic BP, a decrease of less than 20% in cardiac output, and stable pulmonary vascular pressures (i.e., PAOP, PVR).
- Improving C_L and improved lung aeration.[31,39]
- A P_aO_2/F_IO_2 ratio >300.
- The point of minimum arterial to end-tidal PCO_2 gradient.[40]
- Optimum mixed venous oxygen values.[40]

In cases of ventilation-to-perfusion ($\dot{V}/\dot{Q}$) mismatch caused by hypoventilation, increasing the F_IO_2 decreases the percentage

TABLE 13-2	Summary of Ventilator Procedures*	
Variable	**Group Receiving Traditional Tidal Volumes**	**Group Receiving Lower Tidal Volumes**
Ventilator mode	*Volume assist/control*	*Volume assist/control*
Initial tidal volume (mL/kg of predicted body weight)[†]	12	6
Plateau pressure (cm of water)	<50	<30
Ventilator rate setting needed to achieve a pH goal of 7.3 to 7.45 (breaths/min)	6-35	6-35
Ratio of the duration of inspiration to the duration of expiration	1:1-1:3	1:1-1:3
Oxygenation goal	P_aO_2, 55-80 mm Hg, or S_pO_2, 88-95%	P_aO_2, 55-80 mm Hg, or S_pO_2, 88-95%
Allowable combinations of F_IO_2 and PEEP (cm of water)[‡]	0.3 and 5	0.3 and 5
	0.4 and 5	0.4 and 5
	0.4 and 8	0.4 and 8
	0.5 and 8	0.5 and 8
	0.5 and 10	0.5 and 10
	0.6 and 10	0.6 and 10
	0.7 and 10	0.7 and 10
	0.7 and 12	0.7 and 12
	0.7 and 14	0.7 and 14
	0.8 and 14	0.8 and 14
	0.9 and 14	0.9 and 14
	0.9 and 16	0.9 and 16
	0.9 and 18	0.9 and 18
	1.0 and 18	1.0 and 18
	1.0 and 20	1.0 and 20
	1.0 and 22	1.0 and 22
	1.0 and 24	1.0 and 24
Weaning	By pressure support; required by protocol when F_IO_2 <0.4	By pressure support; required by protocol when F_IO_2 <0.4

From the Acute Respiratory Distress Syndrome Network: Ventilation with lower tidal volumes as compared with traditional tidal volumes for acute lung injury and the acute respiratory distress syndrome, N Engl J Med 341:1301-1308, 2000 © Massachusetts Medical Society.
*P_aO_2 denotes partial pressure of arterial oxygen, S_pO_2 oxyhemoglobin saturation measured by pulse oximetry, F_IO_2 fraction of inspired oxygen, and PEEP positive end-expiratory pressure.
[†]Subsequent adjustments in tidal volume were made to maintain a plateau pressure of <50 cm of water in the group receiving traditional tidal volumes and <30 cm of water in the group receiving lower tidal volumes.
[‡]Further increases in PEEP, to 34 cm of water, were allowed but were not required.

BOX 13-7	Parameters Measured and Monitored During a PEEP/CPAP Study

Ventilatory Data

V_T, f, $\dot{V}_E$, peak inspiratory pressure (PIP), plateau pressure ($P_{plateau}$), PEEP, C_D, C_S, breath sounds, ABGs (e.g., P_aO_2, C_aO_2, pH, P_aCO_2), $P_{(A-a)}O_2$ or P_aO_2/F_IO_2 ratio, calculated clinical shunt ($\dot{Q}_s/\dot{Q}_t$), arterial minus end-tidal carbon dioxide gradient ($P_{(a-et)}CO_2$).

Hemodynamic Data

Arterial blood pressure (BP), cardiac output (C.O.) (by thermo-dilution or noninvasive techniques), arterial-to-venous oxygen difference $C[a-\overline{v}]O_2$, partial pressure of mixed venous oxygen ($P\overline{v}O_2$, $S\overline{v}O_2$), pulmonary artery pressure (PAP), pulmonary artery occlusion pressure (PAOP), pulmonary vascular resistance (PVR), oxygen transport (C.O. × C_aO_2).

BOX 13-8	Clinical Shunt Calculation

When a patient is breathing 100% O_2, $\dot{Q}_s/\dot{Q}_t$ can be **estimated** with the following equation:

$$\frac{\dot{Q}_s}{\dot{Q}_t} = \frac{(P(A-a)O_2 \times 0.003)}{[(P(A-a)O_2 \times 0.003) + (C_aO_2 - C\overline{V}O_2)]}$$

$\dot{Q}_s/\dot{Q}_t$ is affected by variations in $\dot{V}/\dot{Q}$ mismatching and by fluctuations in mixed venous oxygen saturations ($S\overline{v}O_2$) and F_IO_2.

Using the factor 0.003 in the calculation above converts the reading from mm Hg to vol% (mL/100 mL) so that it becomes $C_{(A-a)}O_2$, or the alveolar-to-arterial content difference.

The $C[a-\overline{v}]O_2$ portion of the equation is the arterial-to-venous content difference. $C[a-\overline{v}]O_2$ is often assigned the value of 3.5 vol%, the approximate arterial-to-venous oxygen content difference in a critically ill patient. Below is an example of a clinical shunt calculation.

TABLE 13-3	Summary of Ventilator Procedures in the Lower- and Higher-PEEP Groups*												
Procedure	**Value**												
Ventilator mode	*Volume assist/control*												
Tidal volume goal	6 mL/kg of predicted body weight												
Plateau-pressure goal	≤30 cm of water												
Ventilator rate and pH goal	6-35, adjusted to achieve arterial pH ≥7.30 if possible												
Inspiration:expiration time	1:1-1:3												
Oxygenation goal													
P_aO_2	55-80 mm Hg												
S_pO_2	88-95%												
Weaning	Weaning attempted by means of pressure support when level of arterial oxygenation acceptable with PEEP ≤8 cm of water and F_IO_2 ≤0.40												
Allowable Combinations of PEEP and F_IO_2†													
Lower-PEEP Group													
F_IO_2	0.3	0.4	0.4	0.5	0.5	0.6	0.7	0.7	0.7	0.8	0.9	0.9	0.9	1.0
PEEP	5	5	8	8	10	10	10	12	14	14	14	16	18	18-24
Higher-PEEP Group (Before Protocol Changed to Use Higher Levels of PEEP)													
F_IO_2	0.3	0.3	0.3	0.3	0.3	0.4	0.4	0.5	0.5	0.5-0.8	0.8	0.9	1.0
PEEP	5	8	10	12	14	14	16	16	18	20	22	22	22-24
Higher-PEEP Group (After Protocol Changed to Use Higher Levels of PEEP)													
F_IO_2	0.3	0.3	0.4	0.4	0.5	0.5	0.5-0.8	0.8	0.9	1.0
PEEP	12	14	14	16	16	18	20	22	22	22-24

From The National Heart, Lung, and Blood Institute ARDS Clinical Trials Network: Higher versus lower positive end-expiratory pressures in patients with the acute respiratory distress syndrome, N Engl J Med 351:4, 2004. ©Massachusetts Medical Society.

*Complete ventilator procedures and eligibility criteria are listed in the Supplementary Appendix (available with the full text of this article at www.nejm.org) and at www.ardsnet.org. P_aO_2 denotes partial pressure of arterial oxygen, S_pO_2 oxyhemoglobin saturation as measured by pulse oximetry, F_IO_2 fraction of inspired oxygen, and PEEP positive end-expiratory pressure.

†In both study groups, additional increases in PEEP to 34 cm of water were allowed but not required after the F_IO_2 had been increased to 1.0 according to the protocol. The combinations of PEEP and F_IO_2 used with PEEP values of less than 12 cm of water were eliminated in the higher-PEEP group after 171 patients had been enrolled in this group.

shunt and increases P_aO_2 because the increased F_IO_2 results in higher P_aO_2. In contrast, for cases where there is an absolute shunt present (i.e., perfusion in the absence of ventilation, for example, atelectasis), the P_aO_2 does not rise with increases in F_IO_2 because there is no improvement in the gas exchange in shunt units, and hypoxemia remains severe. Hypoxemia refractory to increases in F_IO_2 therefore suggests that an absolute shunt exists. The use of PEEP or CPAP may be beneficial in treating hypoxemia associated with atelectasis.

The following is an example of a clinical shunt calculation: barometric pressure (Pb) = 747 mm Hg; hemoglobin (Hb) = 10 g; F_IO_2 = 1.0; P_aO_2 = 85 mm Hg; P_aCO_2 = 40 mm Hg; pH = 7.36; S_aO_2 = 94%; $P\overline{v}O_2$ = 39 mm Hg; $S\overline{v}O_2$ = 70%; respiratory exchange ratio (R) = 0.8.

$$\frac{\dot{Q}_s}{\dot{Q}_t} = \frac{(P(A-a)O_2 \times 0.003)}{[(P(A-a)O_2 \times 0.003) + (CaO_2 - C\overline{V}O_2)]}$$

Step 1: Calculate P_AO_2

$$P_AO_2 = F_IO_2(Pb - 47) - P_aCO_2(F_IO_2 + [1 - F_IO_2/R])$$

$$P_AO_2 = 1.0(747 - 47) - 40(1.0 + [1 - 1.0/0.8])$$

$$P_AO_2 = 700 - 40 = 660 \text{ mm Hg}$$

Step 2: Calculate $P_{(A-a)}O_2 \times 0.003$

$$P_AO_2 = 660$$

$$P_aO_2 = 85$$

$$P_AO_2 - P_aO_2 = 660 - 85 = 575$$

$$P_{(A-a)}O_2 \times 0.003 = 1.73 \text{ vol\%}$$

Step 3: Calculate $C[a - \overline{v}]O_2$

$$C_aO_2 = (P_aO_2 \times 0.003) + (S_aO_2 \times 1.34 \times Hb)$$

$$C_aO_2 = (85 \times 0.003) + (94\% \times 1.34 \times 10)$$

$$C_aO_2 = 0.255 + (0.94 \, [\text{as a fraction}] \times 1.34 \times 10)$$

$$C_aO_2 = 0.26 + 12.6 = 12.86 \text{ vol\%}$$

$$C\overline{v}O_2 = (P\overline{v}O_2 \times 0.003) + (S\overline{v}O_2 \times 1.34 \times Hb)$$

$$C\overline{v}O_2 = (39 \times 0.003) + [0.70 \, (\text{as a fraction}) \times 1.34 \times 10]$$

$$C\overline{v}O_2 = 0.117 + 9.38 = 9.5 \text{ vol\%}$$

$$C[a - \overline{v}]O_2 = 12.86 - 9.5 = 3.36 \text{ vol\%}$$

Step 4: Solve for shunt fraction

$$\frac{\dot{Q}_s}{\dot{Q}_t} = [P(A-a)O_2 \times 0.003]/C(a - \overline{v})O_2 + [P(A-a)O_2 \times 0.003]$$

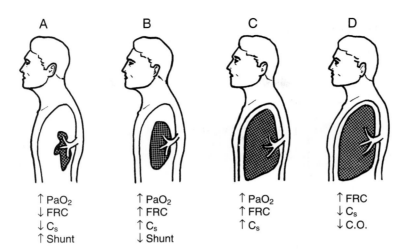

	A	B	C	D
	↑ PaO₂	↑ PaO₂	↑ PaO₂	↑ FRC
	↓ FRC	↑ FRC	↑ FRC	↓ C$_s$
	↓ C$_s$	↑ C$_s$	↑ C$_s$	↓ C.O.
	↑ Shunt	↓ Shunt		

Fig. 13-2 A, The stiff lungs and increased shunt result in a decrease in functional residual capacity (FRC) and arterial oxygen pressure (P$_a$O$_2$). **B** and **C,** As PEEP is increased, C$_s$ and P$_a$O$_2$ improve as the FRC increases, resulting in a lowering of the shunt effect. **D,** Too much PEEP has been added, and C$_s$ and cardiac output decrease as the FRC is increased above the optimum level.

PEEP (cm H₂O)	0	5	10	15	20	25	30
Minutes/time	15	30	45	60	75	90	105
Blood pressure (mm Hg)	117/80	120/85	120/80	110/70	115/75	115/75	90/65
C$_S$ (mL/cm H₂O)	36	36	37	35	40	45	36
PaO₂ (F$_I$O₂ = 1.0)	43	59	65	73	103	152	167
CaO₂ (vol %)	15.3	17.8	18.3	18.9	19.2	19.4	19.6
PaCO₂ (mm Hg)	37	37	38	37	39	37	38
pH	7.41	7.42	7.42	7.42	7.40	7.41	7.41
P(A − a)O₂ (mm Hg)	607	591	585	577	547	498	483
PaCO₂ − P$_{ET}$CO₂ (mm Hg)	16	15	13	10	9	8	15
P$\bar{v}$O₂ (or S$\bar{v}$O₂) mm Hg (or %)	27	37	38	38	39	40	34
C.O. L/min	4.1	4.2	4.0	4.5	4.4	4.4	3.3
C(a − $\bar{v}$)O₂ (vol %)	5.3	5.2	5.4	5.0	4.9	4.9	6.7
PCWP (mm Hg)	3	5	8	11	12	13	18
PAP (mm Hg)	37/21	39/25	41/24	43/25	40/21	38/24	45/30
C.O. × CaO₂ Oxygen transport	627	748	732	851	845	854	647

Fig. 13-3 This figure gives an example of a PEEP study flowsheet including oxygenation and hemodynamic data. Key points to observe when first reviewing a PEEP study are blood pressure (BP), mixed venous oxygen, and O₂ transport. Notice that these three values decline at a PEEP of 30 cm H₂O. BP drops to 90/65, P$\bar{v}$O₂ drops to 34 mm Hg, and oxygen transport drops to 647 mL/min. A more optimum PEEP level is 25 cm H₂O, where these parameters and others indicate that oxygen transport is improving without significant cardiovascular side effects.

$$\frac{\dot{Q}_S}{\dot{Q}_t} = 1.73 \text{ vol\%} / (3.36 \text{ vol\%} + 1.73 \text{ vol\%})$$

$$\frac{\dot{Q}_S}{\dot{Q}_t} = 0.339 \text{ or } 34\% \text{ shunt}$$

Performing an optimum PEEP study. Figure 13-2 illustrates the effects that PEEP might have as it is progressively increases. Figure 13-3 presents a PEEP study check sheet that can be used for monitoring patients receiving PEEP or CPAP therapy. Once the baseline data (0 cm H₂O) is obtained, 5 cm H₂O of PEEP or CPAP is instituted, and PEEP is increased in increments (3 to 5 cm H₂O). (NOTE: Using a baseline of 5 cm H₂O of PEEP as a starting point is also acceptable.) Figure 13-4 shows the effects of PEEP on pressure readings. Approximately 15 minutes after an increase in PEEP, all ventilatory and available hemodynamic parameters are measured and derived variables are calculated.[41]

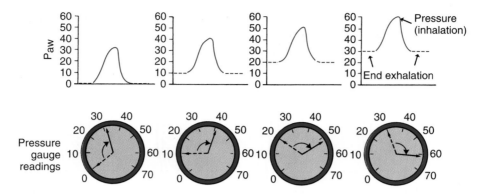

Fig. 13-4 High PEEP levels can be expected to cause PIP and P$_{plateau}$ readings to rise on the ventilator manometer. The baseline reading rises above zero and reflects the increase in FRC.

Patient appearance. A patient's appearance—color (e.g., pale, flushed, cyanotic), level of consciousness, and evidence of anxiety or pain—is checked frequently to ensure that no apparent distress is present. A sudden deterioration in a patient's condition may indicate the onset of cardiovascular collapse or the sudden development of pneumothorax.

Blood pressure. The patient's BP should be checked within the first few minutes after an increment of PEEP is added. A decrease of more than 20 mm Hg systolic is considered significant because a decrease of this magnitude may indicate hypovolemia or obtunded neurologic reflexes that prevent the maintenance of an adequate BP.[42]

Breath sounds. A brief examination of the chest (i.e., auscultation, palpation, and percussion) can indicate barotrauma or any other changes in a patient's lung condition that may have occurred.

Ventilator parameters. Measurement of ventilator parameters, such as $\dot{V}_E$, V_T, f, flow, PIP, and plateau pressure (P$_{plateau}$) can provide valuable information about changes in the patient's C$_L$ and airway resistance (R$_{aw}$).

Measuring $\dot{V}_E$ and V_T are relatively easy. One does not expect $\dot{V}_E$ to change as a direct result of using CPAP or PEEP; P$_a$CO$_2$ is not directly affected. If a patient has been hyperventilating (low P$_a$CO$_2$) because of hypoxemia before the use of CPAP or PEEP, then the relief of the hypoxemia with PEEP/CPAP should be accompanied by a decrease in $\dot{V}_E$ and a rise in P$_a$CO$_2$.[43] P$_a$CO$_2$ may decrease if PEEP improves ventilation to previously perfused alveoli. High levels of PEEP expand the conductive airways, in part because of dilation of terminal and respiratory bronchioles, which increases dead space and leads to an increased P$_a$CO$_2$.

Static compliance. Compliance is considered a good indicator of the effects of PEEP on the lung.[44] As PEEP progressively restores FRC, compliance should increase (Fig. 13-5). Most ICU ventilators allow for the measurement of C$_D$ and calculation of C$_S$. (NOTE: The GE Healthcare Engstrom CareStation [GE Healthcare] has an option that allows for the measurement of FRC [FRC INview—GE Healthcare]). It is important to recognize, however, that when PEEP reaches a point where it overdistends the lung, compliance will decrease. Evidence of this reduction in compliance due to overdistention of the alveoli can be seen in the P-V graphic. A characteristic duck-billed appearance occurs at the top of the P-V

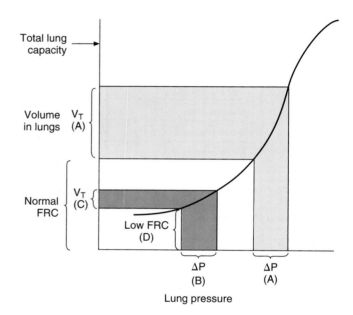

Fig. 13-5 A pressure–volume curve where the x-axis is pressure and the y-axis is volume. Near the section labeled *Volume in lungs* is a corresponding curve that represents normal lung volumes (shaded with *light blue*). A very little change in pressure (ΔP) results in a good tidal volume (V$_T$) *(A)*, at the steepest part of the curve. (Note "Normal FRC.") At the bottom left portion of the curve, the lungs are stiffer (as in ARDS). A change in pressure (ΔP at B) produces a small volume change (V$_T$ at C). FRC is low *(D)*. Theoretically, by placing a patient with stiff lungs on PEEP, the compliance improves (moves upward and to the right—steeper portion) as the FRC increases (shaded with *dark blue*).

loop (Fig. 13-6). (NOTE: When calculating static compliance [C$_S$], calculations of tubing compliance [C$_T$] must be taken into account and include the PEEP value.[45] If auto-PEEP is present, it must be measured and considered part of the end-expiratory pressure when calculating compliance.)

In patients with chest wall injuries or hypovolemia, the use of C$_S$ alone is not a good indicator of optimum PEEP or cardiovascular changes with PEEP, even at low levels of PEEP. More invasive monitoring techniques, such as the placement of a balloon-tipped pulmonary artery catheter, may be needed. For example, if PEEP levels above 15 to 20 cm H$_2$O are used, compliance is not a good indication of cardiovascular function, and monitoring pulmonary

TABLE 13-4	A PEEP Study to Evaluate Use of $P_{(a-et)}CO_2$ not P_aCO_2 for Assessing PEEP in an Experimental Model Involving Oleic Acid Injury					
PEEP	**0**	**5**	**10***	**15**	**20**	**25**
$P_{(a-et)}CO_2$	17	13	8	8	10	14
$\frac{\dot{Q}_s}{\dot{Q}_t}$ (%)	14	3	2	2	2	2
C_S (mL/cm H_2O)	18	20	16	12	7	9
P_aO_2 (on $F_IO_2 = 0.5$)	95	180	>200	>200	>200	>200
O_2 delivery (mL/min)	250	200	300	280	220	180

From Murray JF, Wilkins RL, Jacobsen WK, et al: Chest 85:100, 1984.[26]
*10 cm H_2O represents a PEEP level where all parameters are optimal. With greater increases in PEEP, the $P_{(a-et)}CO_2$ rises and the O_2 delivery and C_S fall. Note that shunt ($\dot{Q}_s/\dot{Q}_t$) remains low and P_aO_2 remains high.

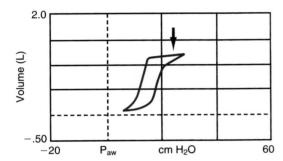

Fig. 13-6 A pressure–volume loop of a patient receiving a volume-targeted breath of 1.2 L with a peak inspiratory pressure of about 30 cm H_2O. The extended upper flat portion of the "beaked" appearance of the curve indicated by the *arrow* suggests overdistention of lung units. (From Wilkins RL, Stoller JK, Scanlan L, editors: Egan's fundamentals of respiratory care, ed 9, St Louis, 2009, Mosby.)

artery pressures may be indicated. Notice that this type of invasive monitoring increases the risk of complications so implementation must be considered very carefully (see Chapter 11).

Arterial PO₂, F₁O₂, and P₂O₂/F₁O₂. The usual approach to the management of F_IO_2 and PEEP is to start with high F_IO_2 and incrementally decrease it as PEEP or CPAP improves oxygenation.[37] A target value for $P_aO_2/F_IO_2 >300$ (e.g., $P_aO_2 = 100$, with $F_IO_2 = 0.33$) is optimum, but not always a realistic goal.

Arterial P₂CO₂ and pH. Adequacy of ventilation is determined by regular evaluation of P_aCO_2 and pH as PEEP is increased. If P_aCO_2 and pH are not being maintained near a patient's normal values, then appropriate adjustments must be made. Depending on the severity of a patient's condition, permissive hypercapnia may be an acceptable alternative. (See Chapter 12 for a discussion of permissive hypercapnia.)

Alveolar-to-arterial oxygen tension (P₍A-a₎O₂). With increases in PEEP, the $P_{(A-a)}O_2$ typically decreases, reflecting improvement in $\dot{V}/\dot{Q}$. This can be further evaluated by calculating P_aO_2/P_AO_2 or P_aO_2/F_IO_2 ratios.

Arterial to end-tidal CO₂ tension gradient (P₍a-et₎CO₂). The arterial to end-tidal CO_2 tension gradient ($P_{(a-et)}CO_2$) is often used as an indirect assessment of the effectiveness of ventilation (i.e.,

dead space to tidal volume [V_D/V_T] ratio). It is lowest when gas exchange units are maximally recruited without being overdistended by PEEP. Normal $P_{(a-et)}CO_2$ gradient is 4.5 ± 2.5 mm Hg. An increase in PEEP that leads to increases in the $P_{(a-et)}CO_2$ gradient above minimum acceptable values signifies that too much PEEP has been added and can be expected to produce a drop in cardiac output and an increase in V_D/V_T.[46] The data shown in Table 13-4 provide an example of changes that might be expected in $P_{(a-et)}CO_2$ with increased PEEP.[46] (See Chapter 10 for a discussion of volumetric CO_2 monitoring.)

Hemodynamic data. In addition to the measurement of arterial BP, hemodynamic monitoring, including the evaluation of $P\overline{v}O_2$ and/or $S\overline{v}O_2$, cardiac output, $C[a-\overline{v}]O_2$, pulmonary artery pressure (PAP), pulmonary artery occlusion pressure (PAOP), pulmonary vascular resistance (PVR), and O_2 delivery (DO₂) may be required. (See Chapter 11 for more details on hemodynamic monitoring.)

Arterial-to-venous oxygen content difference. The arterial-to-mixed venous oxygen content difference ($C[a-\overline{v}]O_2$), which at rest is normally 5 vol%, reflects O_2 utilization by the tissues. An increase in $C[a-\overline{v}]O_2$ with an increase in PEEP may indicate hypovolemia, cardiac malfunction, decreased venous return to the heart, and decreased cardiac output, or increased $\dot{V}O_2$.

A decrease in $C[a-\overline{v}]O_2$ with an increase in PEEP may also be associated with an increase in cardiac output resulting from improved or augmented cardiac function. Reductions in O_2 extraction by the tissues can also result from reduced metabolic rate or histotoxic hypoxia.

Mixed venous oxygen tension or saturation. $P\overline{v}O_2$ is normally about 35 to 40 mm Hg (normal $S\overline{v}O_2 = 75\%$). A $P\overline{v}O_2$ of 28 mm Hg is probably the minimal acceptable level for $P\overline{v}O_2$ and represents an $S\overline{v}O_2$ of about 50%.[45]

As PEEP is increased, it often leads to an improvement in P_aO_2 and $P\overline{v}O_2$ with no net change in $P[a-\overline{v}]O_2$. This indicates that O_2 transport is improving with no apparent change in cardiac output, and the level of shunting is also decreasing.

PEEP may increase P_aO_2 and $P\overline{v}O_2$, decrease net $C[a-\overline{v}]O_2$, and improve O_2 delivery. If $\dot{V}O_2$ is constant, these changes suggest a rise in cardiac output. On the other hand, in patients in whom $P\overline{v}O_2$ decreases with PEEP and $C[a-\overline{v}]O_2$ increases, cardiac output and O_2 delivery may decrease. However, if $P\overline{v}O_2$ was high

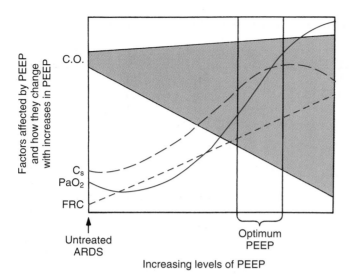

Fig. 13-7 The curves above represent the physiological factors that change during the application of PEEP or CPAP. As the PEEP level is increased, P_aO_2, FRC, and C_S normally increase. Cardiac output (C.O.), represented by the *shaded area*, can increase slightly, stay the same, or decrease. The optimum PEEP level can be expected to occur when P_aO_2, FRC, and C_S are high. C.O. should be maintained near normal so that oxygen transport to the tissues remains high.

TABLE **13-5**	Effects of Increased PEEP on $P\bar{v}O_2$ and Related Parameters				
PEEP (cm H_2O)	0	5	10*	15	20
$P\bar{v}O_2$ (mm Hg)	35	37	39	37	35
$C[a - \bar{v}]O_2$ (mL/100 mL)	3.7	3.7	3.6	3.8	4.1
C.O. (L/min)	7.0	7.0	7.5	6.7	6.5
C.O. $\times$ C_aO_2 (mL/min) (O$_2$ transport)	850	875	950	850	825

*10 cm H_2O of PEEP represents a point where $P\bar{v}O_2$ is nearest normal, and cardiac output (C.O.) and O$_2$ transport are at their highest. Note that as PEEP continues to increase, the $C[a - \bar{v}]O_2$ continues to rise and $P\bar{v}O_2$ falls. The cardiac output falls, reflecting a slower perfusion rate and more time for O$_2$ extraction at the tissues.

to start, and then drops to a normal value, no harmful effects may be present[47] (Case Study 13-4).

Case Study 13-4

Selecting Optimum PEEP

A PEEP study is being performed on a patient. The following data have been specifically selected from all measured parameters to see if you can solve this problem based only on what is provided. What PEEP level appears to be optimum for the patient? Having selected the level, would you make any other changes?

Time	PEEP (cm H_2O)	F_iO_2	P_aO_2 (mm Hg)	BP (mm Hg)	$P\bar{v}O_2$ (mm Hg)
1:00	5	1.0	43	125/90	28
1:30	10	1.0	57	120/85	33
2:00	15	1.0	104	120/85	38
2:30	20	1.0	143	100/70	31

Cardiac output. Cardiac output provides key information about a patient's cardiovascular response to PEEP. Thus, as PEEP improves $\dot{V}/\dot{Q}$ relationships, oxygenation also improves, which may enhance cardiac performance. As intrapleural pressures increase or as the gas exchange units become overdistended, however, venous return decreases and cardiac function is altered; cardiac output then declines and the point of optimum PEEP is no longer present (Fig. 13-7; Table 13-5).[47,48] (NOTE: Cardiac output can be estimated noninvasively using the Respironics NM3 monitor from Respironics, Murrysville, Pa.)

Some clinicians increase vascular volumes with fluid administration (fluid challenge) and give inotropic agents to maintain cardiac function as PEEP is increased. This approach provides a way to ensure that O$_2$ transport and/or delivery are sufficient to meet the O$_2$ demand by the tissues.

USE OF PULMONARY VASCULAR PRESSURE MONITORING WITH PEEP

When PEEP greater than 15 cm H_2O is used, it is important to closely evaluate the patient's hemodynamic status, which may require the placement of a balloon-flotation pulmonary artery catheter. After catheter placement, a chest radiograph is obtained to ensure that the catheter tip is located in a dependent (zone 3) area of the lung. If the catheter is not located in a dependent area of the lung, PAOP may not be a true reflection of pressures on the left side of the heart but rather reflect alveolar or airway pressures (Fig. 13-8). It is important to remember that as PEEP is increased, vascular pressures will also increase. Note that PEEP is not removed to measure vascular pressures because doing so might precipitate severe hypoxemia due to alveolar collapse, which can be difficult to reverse.[49-51] However, there is some controversy about discontinuing ventilation for cardiovascular measurements.[52] If PEEP is removed, the effect of PEEP on the vascular pressures would not be reflected in the measurement. Generally, pulmonary vascular pressures are recorded at end exhalation. (See Chapter 11 for additional information on hemodynamic monitoring.) If the PAOP markedly rises as PEEP is increased, the lungs may be overinflated and PEEP may need to be reduced (Fig. 13-9). Falsely elevated vascular pressures do not give an accurate picture of the true filling of the left side of the heart. On the other hand, when PEEP rises, PAOP may be markedly decreased because pulmonary blood flow is reduced as a result of decreased venous return to the right side of the heart. This situation is often referred to as a *PEEP-induced relative hypovolemia*, and requires either a reduction in the amount of PEEP being used or administration of fluids to increase vascular volume.

Oxygen delivery (cardiac output $\times$ C_aO_2) can be an effective method for evaluating the effect of PEEP and is important because it reflects cardiac and pulmonary functions as well as the carrying capacity of the blood. The normal value for O$_2$ delivery is approximately 1000 mL/min. If cardiac output is low, it may be enhanced by slightly reducing the PEEP level or by using volume loading (administration of fluids) and/or inotropic agents (e.g., dopamine hydrochloride). A low C_aO_2 may be improved by increasing PEEP, F_IO_2, or by normalizing Hb levels (i.e., giving blood, if the patient is anemic).

An example of the effect of PEEP on the cardiovascular responses of a patient with ARDS is shown in Table 13-6. In this example, the P_aO_2 increased substantially with PEEP. Central venous pressure (CVP) increased slightly; cardiac output did not change significantly. The increase in PAOP was matched by an increase in PAP.

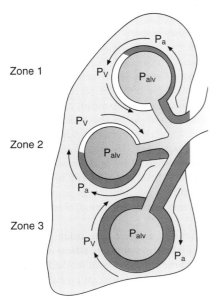

Fig. 13-8 In a normal lung the greatest amount of perfusion and ventilation are to the dependent (lower) lung zones. The zone 3 regions represent lung areas where pulmonary artery pressure (P_a, deoxygenated blood) exceeds pulmonary venous pressure (P_V, oxygenated blood), which exceeds pulmonary alveolar pressure (P_{alv}). In zone 2 lung areas (normally the middle region) pulmonary artery pressure exceeds pulmonary alveolar pressure, which exceeds pulmonary venous pressure ($P_a > P_{alv} > P_v$). In zone 1 lung areas (normally the upper regions), pulmonary alveolar pressure exceeds pulmonary artery pressure, which exceeds pulmonary venous pressure ($P_A > P_a > P_v$). Pulmonary vascular pressure monitoring is most accurate if the catheter is in zone 3.

CONTRAINDICATIONS AND PHYSIOLOGICAL EFFECTS OF PEEP

PEEP, particularly at the levels often needed in patients with ARDS, has contraindications and physiological effects that can impact the patient's safety. Practitioners must monitor the patient for any adverse effects when PEEP is instituted and before instituting lung recruitment maneuvers (described later).

Contraindications for PEEP

PEEP can be detrimental to a patient's cardiovascular status because it can reduce cardiac output and compromise circulation, leading to a reduction in BP. A relative contraindication for PEEP is hypovolemia. A patient who is hypovolemic as a result of hemorrhage or dehydration must be treated and vascular volumes must be replenished before beginning PEEP therapy. Patients can be treated with fluids, volume expanders, or inotropic agents to enhance blood volume and cardiac output.

An absolute contraindication for PEEP is an untreated significant pneumothorax or a tension pneumothorax. Note that this is also true of a lung recruitment maneuver. Increasing positive pressure might further increase the air present in the intrapleural space and cause death. PEEP and recruitment maneuvers must also be used with caution in patients with bronchopleural fistulas or in patients with other types of barotrauma (e.g., pneumopericardium). Additionally, PEEP should be used cautiously in patients

TABLE 13-6	Effects of Increased PEEP on PAOP			
PEEP (cm H_2O)	**0**	**5**	**10**	**15**
P_aO_2 (mm Hg) (F_IO_2 = 1.0)	90	160	280	450
PAP (mm Hg)	39/15	43/18	45/20	47/23
PAOP (mm Hg)	9	13	16	21
CVP (cm H_2O)	9	11	13	14
C.O. (L/min)	4.5	4.8	4.6	4.7

C.O., Cardiac output; *CVP,* central venous pressure; *PAP,* pulmonary artery pressure; *PAOP,* pulmonary artery occlusion pressure; *PEEP,* positive end-expiratory pressure.
P_aO_2 increases substantially. CVP increases slightly. C.O. did not change significantly. The increase in PAOP is matched by an increase in PAP.

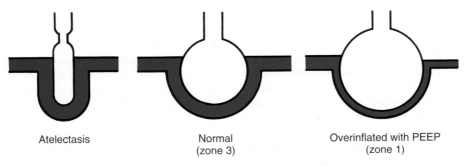

Atelectasis   Normal (zone 3)   Overinflated with PEEP (zone 1)

Fig. 13-9 ARDS creates many lung regions with atelectasis and edema *(left figure).* With PEEP, these affected areas can be re-expanded, creating more zone 3 lung areas *(central figure);* however, overexpansion with PEEP can reduce perfusion to ventilated alveoli and create zone 1 areas of lung *(right figure).*

| BOX **13-9** | **Overdistention or Hyperinflation?** |

There is a difference between overdistention and hyperinflation.[63]

Overdistention, or overstretching lung tissue, increases alveolar wall tension or alveolar distending pressure above normal. Lungs may be overdistended (severe ARDS) and not hyperinflated. Studies have demonstrated that overdistention is associated with the presence of increased levels of inflammatory mediators.

In contrast, **hyperinflation** may be thought of as gas overfilling. As defined by a computed tomography, hyperinflation is a higher-than-normal ratio of gas to tissue. For example, the lungs of an emphysema patient may be hyperinflated but not overdistended.

---

who have recently had lung surgery so that a pneumothorax does not develop. In patients with elevated intracranial pressures (ICP), PEEP may further elevate ICP by increasing CVP. This should not prevent the use of PEEP in these patients, especially if they are severely hypoxemic. The hypoxemia is likely to be fatal if not treated. Thus, if PEEP is used in these patients, ICP should be carefully monitored and treated appropriately.

The beneficial effects of PEEP and lung recruitment occur when they are used to increase FRC by recruiting collapsed alveoli. These effects do not occur, however, in patients with preexisting hyperinflation (e.g., emphysema). Areas of the lung that are already hyperinflated may be further distended, which can lead to compression of adjacent capillaries and the redirecting of blood to areas that are not as well ventilated, resulting in increased shunting, venous admixture, and hypoxemia. The use of low PEEP (3 to 5 cm H_2O) may, however, be beneficial for these patients if it compensates for the reduced FRC resulting from intubation or the supine position or aids in triggering ventilator breaths when auto-PEEP is present (see Chapter 7). Otherwise, use of PEEP in these individuals is not typically beneficial (Key Point 13-4; Box 13-9).

Key Point 13-4 Lungs can be overdistended without being hyperinflated. PEEP can have unexpected and undesirable side effects on blood distribution and lung ventilation if it is used on patients with pathologic conditions that involve only one lung, such as in unilateral pneumonia or lobar pneumonia. For this reason, unilateral lung disorders may represent a relative contraindication to the use of PEEP and may be better managed by using a double-lumen endotracheal tube and unilateral or independent lung ventilation with two ventilators.[53]

Pulmonary Effects of PEEP

The most frequently studied pulmonary disorder in relation to the effects of PEEP is ARDS. ARDS studies provide valuable insight into the behavior of PEEP on various lung units and the advantages of using protective lung strategies. The changes in pulmonary mechanics associated with ARDS cause an uneven distribution of ventilation. In the lungs of a supine patient where the independent zones (ventral areas) receive most of the breath, delivery of a large volume (10 to 15 mL/kg) may cause overexpansion and high ventilating pressures. During patient monitoring, this appears as a decrease in C_L.[15,30,31]

As PEEP is applied in increasing levels, it recruits a certain number of collapsed alveoli. For independent (ventral) portions of the lungs, recruitment is negligible; PEEP simply expands already open lung units. As more PEEP is added, ventral units become overstretched, which decreases their compliance. As a result, the distribution of a V_T breath to this area decreases as PEEP increases. For this reason it has been emphasized that the patient's $P_{plateau}$ should be maintained below 30 cm H_2O.

The same overstretching may occur in the middle portions of the lungs (between the ventral and dorsal regions of supine patients), where it not only stretches alveoli open, but also recruits areas that were previously collapsed. In this situation, two opposing compliance changes are likely to occur. Compliance decreases in some units from overstretching, while the compliance of other units improves as they reopen.[31]

In the dependent (dorsal) areas, fewer lung units are open at FRC (end exhalation; 0 cm H_2O PEEP). But as a sustained high pressure breath is delivered (e.g., recruitment maneuver) or as PEEP is increased, more units are recruited and remain open, increasing compliance in the dependent area and resulting in an enhanced distribution of gas to the dependent units. However, there will be some alveoli that remain collapsed, and these may be scattered throughout the lung. The overall effect is to make the lung more homogeneous when PEEP is increased. An upper limit of PEEP beyond which there is no benefit to lung volume exists for all patients with ARDS. This range usually begins at about 15 cm H_2O and may increase beyond that point.[27,31,54] Results are variable.

Table 13-7 shows one classic case study in which increasing increments of PEEP had no significant effects until 15 cm H_2O was used, at which time the P_aO_2 improved markedly.[55] This represents the point at which alveolar recruitment probably occurred.

Transmission of Airway Pressure to Pleural Space

Transmission of airway pressures to the intrapleural space, the mediastinum, and the thoracic vessels is a concern when positive pressure is applied to the respiratory system. When chest wall compliance is normal and C_L is low, less of the airway pressure ($\overline{P}_{aw}$) is transmitted to the pleural space; however, if C_L is near normal and chest wall compliance is low, then more pressure is transmitted to the pleural space.

Uses of PEEP for Problems Other Than ARDS
PEEP and Congestive Heart Failure

Patients with moderate-to-severe congestive heart failure (CHF) present with reduced cardiac output and impaired cardiac function. They progressively develop pulmonary edema (cardiogenic pulmonary edema) that differs from edema associated with ARDS. The permeability characteristics of the pulmonary vessels and alveoli remain normal, but the pulmonary hydrostatic pressures rise because blood backs up in pulmonary circulation from the left side of the heart. As a result, edema develops in the lungs and the patient becomes hypoxemic. Pulmonary vascular resistance increases and eventually the work of the right side of the heart increases, leading to right heart failure (cor pulmonale) and the presence of peripheral edema.

Patients with untreated CHF admitted to the hospital typically present with pink, frothy secretions and bilateral crackles (rales) indicative of pulmonary edema. These patients usually benefit from positive pressure therapy. Positive pressure reduces the venous return to the heart and the amount of blood that the heart

TABLE 13-7	Data from a Patient with ARDS on Mechanical Ventilation 24 Hours After Admission								
PEEP (cm H_2O)	BP (mm Hg)	HR (beats/min)	PAOP (mm Hg)	C.O. (L/min)	C_s (mL/cm H_2O)	PIP (cm H_2O)	P_aO_2 (mm Hg)	$P\bar{v}O_2$ (mm Hg)
0	130/65	130	16	4.8	28	50	40	27
5	120/55	135	13	4.2	31	58	45	37
10	135/65	125	18	5.8	33	60	50	35
15	130/70	120	19	5.9	36	55	115	37
20	110/50	130	25	4.1	27	63	150	29

Modified from Bone RC: Respir Care 27:402, 1982.
ARDS, Acute respiratory distress syndrome; *BP*, blood pressure; *C.O.*, cardiac output; C_S, static compliance; *HR*, heart rate; *PAOP*, pulmonary artery occlusion pressure; *PIP*, peak inspiratory pressure; $P\bar{v}O_2$, mixed venous oxygen partial pressure; $\dot{V}_E$, minute ventilation.
The following are constant: $V_T = 1100$ mL, f = 6 breaths/min, $\dot{V}_E = 6.6$ L/min, $F_IO_2 = 0.8$. P_aCO_2 and pH do not change significantly.

must pump, which reduces the work of the heart. Increased F_IO_2 values and positive pressure may also help improve myocardial oxygenation and function. It is worth noting that the beneficial effects of PEEP or positive pressure ventilation (PPV) in some patients with CHF is not always predictable. In patients with aortic or mitral valve replacement, PEEP has been associated with changes in V_D/V_T and decreased cardiac index (CI).

Mask CPAP as a Treatment for Postoperative Atelectasis and Hypoxemia

CPAP delivered by mask can be used to help prevent postoperative atelectasis and improve oxygenation. It has been shown to return baseline lung volumes to normal more quickly in patients who had undergone upper abdominal surgery than in patients treated with frequent coughing and deep breathing alone. Levels of CPAP range from about 5 to 15 cm H_2O and are administered for varying intervals (from hourly to every 8 hours) and durations (from 25 to 35 breaths/treatment to continuously for 6 to 10 hours). The exact levels of CPAP required to accomplish the desired results remain undetermined. The effectiveness of CPAP may be similar to the use of a recruitment maneuver in postoperative patients.[56]

Sleep Apnea

Nasal and mask CPAP have been shown to be effective techniques for treating many patients with obstructive sleep apnea. Levels from 5 to 15 cm H_2O can provide a pneumatic splint that helps prevent pharyngeal obstruction. It may also increase FRC in these patients.

Cystic Fibrosis

Application of positive expiratory pressure (PEP) by mask or mouthpiece using a one-way inspiratory valve and a one-way expiratory flow resistor has been shown to be beneficial for the removal of the secretions from patients with cystic fibrosis (positive expiratory pressure [PEP] therapy). PEP devices provide expiratory pressures of 10 to 20 cm H_2O at midexhalation that can be used for 15- to 20-minute periods, three to four times a day to help improve expectoration of secretions, reduce residual volume (less hyperinflation), and improve airway stability.

Airway Suctioning with PEEP

Some patients cannot tolerate the removal of PEEP for the purposes of suctioning. Therefore, it is prudent in these circumstances to use a closed-suction system (see Chapter 12). If this is not

possible, a resuscitation bag equipped with a PEEP valve can be used during the suctioning procedure. The suctioning procedure itself removes air and volume from the lung and can reduce C_S. A recruitment maneuver (RM) following suction may be indicated, but only future studies can determine the role of RM in this circumstance.[57] (Recruitment maneuvers are described later in this chapter.)

WEANING FROM PEEP

The exact length of time that PEEP is needed before the alveoli are stable in patients with ARDS is not known. Premature weaning from PEEP is not without problems. Patients whose P_aO_2 drops to 65 mm Hg or lower with a 5 cm H_2O reduction in PEEP may still need PEEP to maintain lung recruitment (Box 13-10).[58,59]

Several criteria may indicate when a patient is ready for a trial reduction in PEEP. The patient must demonstrate an acceptable P_aO_2 on an F_IO_2 of less than 0.50 and must be hemodynamically stable and non-septic. If ARDS was previously diagnosed, the patient's lung conditions should have improved. For example, if C_L is improved (C_S >25 mL/cm H_2O) and P_aO_2/F_IO_2 ratio is high (>250), then the chances of successfully lowering PEEP are good. A recommended procedure for weaning from PEEP is described in Table 13-8, and Box 13-11 shows some examples of weaning from PEEP.

Acute Respiratory Distress Syndrome

ARDS is one of the most frequently studied pulmonary disorders in terms of how severe hypoxemia is managed. Because of the severity of hypoxemia and shunting encountered in this disorder, selecting the most effective ventilatory strategy remains controversial and a topic of intense discussion. The following discussion addresses some of these pertinent issues related to the pathophysiology and management of ARDS.

ARDS was originally described in a study by Ashbaugh and associates[60] that was published in *The Lancet* in 1967: "The clinical pattern which we will refer to as the respiratory distress syndrome, includes severe dyspnea, tachypnea, hypoxemia that is refractory to oxygen therapy, stiff, low compliance lungs (i.e., reduced C_L) and diffuse alveolar infiltration seen on chest x-ray." Since this initial description of ARDS, several definitions have been proposed and

BOX 13-10 PEEP Withdrawal

It has been known for more than four decades that P_aO_2 drops precipitously when PEEP is withdrawn from patients with acute lung injury. It is now known that this is associated with lung derecruitment. The drop in P_aO_2 and lung volume occurs very quickly.

In a study performed on patients with ARDS in 1970, it was shown that removal of PEEP in patients whose lungs were not stable resulted in an immediate and dramatic drop in P_aO_2 (see figure).

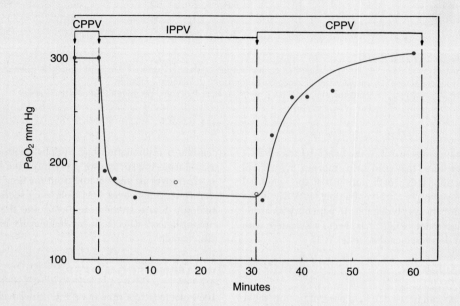

The figure shows the time sequence of P_aO_2 changes with altered ventilation patterns in eight patients. The mean P_aO_2 with CPPV (continuous positive pressure ventilation, now known as CMV + PEEP) at 13 cm H_2O was 304 mm Hg. After changing to IPPV (intermittent positive pressure ventilation, now called CMV without PEEP), it fell 129 mm Hg within 1 minute, and over the next 3 minutes fell 32 mm Hg. Open circles represent mean values of only six patients. (In one patient, a large fall in P_aO_2 required reapplication of CPPV after 6 minutes; a second value was not available because of clotting of the blood sample.) On reapplication of CPPV (i.e., CMV + PEEP), the P_aO_2 gradually rose to its initial value.

(From Kumar A, Konrad JF, Gerrin B, et al: *N Engl J Med* 283:1430, 1970.)

TABLE 13-8 Examples of Weaning Patients from PEEP/CPAP

Example 1

Time (h)	PEEP (cm H₂O)	P_aO₂ (mm Hg)	Blood Pressure (mm Hg)	Static Compliance (mL/cm H₂O)
01:00	12	90	115/65	30
01:03	7	60	120/75	30

Note that P_aO_2 drops significantly. It is better to leave PEEP where it was for several more hours.

Example 2

Time (h)	PEEP (cm H₂O)	P_aO₂ (mm Hg)	Blood Pressure (mm Hg)	Static Compliance (mL/cm H₂O)
02:00	15	98	112/70	32
02:03	10	85	118/70	32

Note that P_aO_2 remains at an acceptable level after the reduction of PEEP. Assuming that the clinical condition of the patient remains stable, PEEP can be reduced to 10 cm H_2O.

used to provide guidance for clinicians treating patients with ARDS, as well as to facilitate clinical trials and resource allocation.[61,62] In 1994, the American-European Consensus Conference (AECC) published a landmark article that provided a list of criteria that could better guide critical care clinicians and researchers caring for individuals afflicted with ARDS.[61] The AECC consensus statement included an overarching definition of acute lung injury (ALI) for patients with a P_aO_2/FiO_2 ratio ≤300 mm Hg with ARDS representing a subset of patients with a P_aO_2/FiO_2 ratio ≤200 mm Hg. The AECC definition also specified that patients demonstrate the presence of bilateral infiltrates on frontal chest radiograph, with no evidence of left atrial hypertension.[61]

BOX 13-11	Procedures for Weaning from PEEP

1. Obtain baseline ABG values and determine that the criteria have been met. Acceptable P_aO_2 (90 mm Hg) on an F_IO_2 of ≤0.40, hemodynamic stability; not septic. Lung compliance is improved (e.g., C_S >25 mL/cm H_2O) and P_aO_2/F_IO_2 ratio >250 to 300.
2. Reduce PEEP by 5 cm H_2O.
3. Monitor S_pO_2 to determine the effect of PEEP reduction. If an ABG is drawn at this time, it is advisable to return the PEEP to the previous level (at step 1) until results from the ABG are obtained. A lung recruitment maneuver may be in order.
4. If S_pO_2 (or P_aO_2) falls by less than 20% of its value at the previous PEEP level, the patient is ready to tolerate the lower PEEP level.
5. If the patient has more than a 20% reduction in S_pO_2 or P_aO_2, the patient is not ready to have the PEEP reduced. PEEP is kept at its previous level.
6. Wait between reductions in PEEP and re-evaluate the initial criteria. If the patient is stable, reduce PEEP by another 5 cm H_2O. This might take only 1 hour or may require as long as 6 hours or more.
7. When a patient is at 5 cm H_2O, then an additional evaluation is necessary. If reducing the PEEP to zero results in a worsening of the patient's condition, then it may be appropriate to leave the patient at 5 cm H_2O until it is time for extubation. The complete removal of PEEP before extubation may not be necessary and may be detrimental to patients with compromised lung-thorax mechanisms, leading to a deterioration of FRC and P_aO_2.

Although the AECC definition provided much needed guidance for clinician and researchers, it became evident that a number of issues required clarification. In 2011, an international consensus group was convened in Berlin, Germany, to update the definition of ARDS to include current epidemiological, physiological, and clinical data.[62] It was proposed that the new definition ("The Berlin Definition") should provide a framework that identifies explicit criteria regarding (1) the time frame of onset of ARDS, (2) criteria for gauging the severity of the syndrome, (3) better clarification of the radiologic and hemodynamic criteria and their role in the diagnosis and treatment of patients, and (4) identification of risk factors for the development of ARDS.[62,63] Table 13-9 provides a comparison of the limitations of the AECC definition and issues addressed in the Berlin definition of ARDS.

The **Berlin Definition** now specifies that the **onset** of ARDS must occur within 1 week of a known clinical insult or the presence of new or worsening respiratory symptoms.[62] A summary of the final draft of the Berlin definition of ARDS is shown in Table 13-10. The definition also provides clarification of radiographic and hemodynamic changes used in the diagnosis of ARDS. Radiographic criteria include bilateral opacities in at least three quadrants for the lung that cannot be fully explained by effusions, lung collapse, or the presence of nodules.[63] Because high pulmonary artery wedge pressure (PAWP) (i.e., pulmonary artery occlusion pressures or PAOP) can coexist with ARDS, the PAWP requirement for identifying the etiology of pulmonary edema has been removed.[61-63] It is noteworthy that the Berlin Definition does not include the term *acute lung injury* (ALI) but relies on a classification of the severity of ARDS based on oxygenation status. The severity of ARDS is determined by using the P_aO_2/FIO_2 ratio value when a defined minimal level of PEEP or CPAP is being administered (e.g., ≥5 cm H_2O of PEEP or CPAP). Lastly, the definition identifies risk factors for the development of ARDS.

TABLE 13-9	The AECC Definition—Limitations and Methods to Address These in the Berlin Definition		
	AECC Definition	**AECC Limitations**	**Addressed in Berlin Definition**
Timing	Acute onset	No definition of acute time frame	Acute time frame specified
ALI category	All patients with P_aO_2/F_IO_2 < 300 mm Hg	Misinterpreted as P_aO_2/F_IO_2 = 201-300, leading to confusing ALI/ARDS term	3 Mutually exclusive subgroups of ARDS by severity
			ALI term removed
Oxygenation	P_aO_2/F_IO_2 ≤300 mm Hg (regardless of PEEP)	Inconsistency of P_aO_2/F_IO_2 ration due to the effect of PEEP and/or F_IO_2	Minimal PEEP level added across subgroups
			F_IO_2 effect less relevant in severe ARDS group
Chest radiograph	Bilateral infiltrates observed on frontal chest radiograph	Poor interobserver reliability of chest radiograph interpretation	Chest radiograph criteria clarified
			Example radiographs created
PAWP	PAWP ≤18 mm Hg when measured or no clinical evidence of left atrial hypertension	High PAWP and ARDS may coexist	PAWP requirement removed
			Hydrostatic edema not the primary cause of respiratory failure
		Poor interobserver reliability of PAWP and clinical assessments of left atrial hypertension	Clinical vignettes created to help exclude hydrostatic edema
Risk factor	None	Not formally included in definition[4]	Included
			When none identified, need to objectively rule out hydrostatic edema

AECC, American-European Consensus Conference; *ALI,* acute lung injury; *ARDS,* acute respiratory distress syndrome; *F$_I$O$_2$,* fraction of inspired oxygen; *P$_a$O$_2$,* arterial partial pressure of oxygen; *PAWP,* pulmonary artery wedge pressure; *PEEP,* positive end-expiratory pressure.
From ARDS Definition Task Force, Ranieri VM, Rubenfeld GD: Acute respiratory distress syndrome: The Berlin definition. *JAMA* 307(3): 2526-2533, 2012.

TABLE 13-10	The Berlin Definition of Acute Respiratory Distress Syndrome
ACUTE RESPIRATORY DISTRESS SYNDROME	
Timing	Within 1 week of a known clinical insult or new or worsening respiratory symptoms
Chest imaging*	Bilateral opacities—not fully explained by effusions lobar/lung collapse or nodules
Origin of edema	Respiratory failure not fully explained by cardiac failure or fluid overload
	Need objective assessment (e.g., echocardiography) to exclude hydrostatic edema if no risk factor present
Oxygenation[†] Mild	200 mm Hg < P_aO_2/F_IO_2 ≤ 300 mm Hg with PEEP or CPAP ≥5 cm H_2O[‡]
Moderate	100 mm Hg < P_aO_2/F_IO_2 ≤ 200 mm Hg with PEEP ≥5 cm H_2O
Severe	P_aO_2/F_IO_2 ≤100 mm Hg with PEEP ≥5 cm H_2O

CPAP, Continuous positive airway pressure; *F$_I$O$_2$,* fraction of inspired oxygen; *P$_a$O$_2$,* arterial partial pressure of oxygen; *PEEP,* positive end-expiratory pressure.

*Chest radiograph or computed tomography scan.

[†]If altitude is higher than 1000 m, the correction factor should be calculated as follows: (P_aO_2/F_IO_2 × [barometric pressure/760]).

[‡]This may be delivered noninvasively in the mild acute respiratory distress syndrome group.

From ARDS Definition Task Force, Ranieri VM, Rubenfeld GD: Acute respiratory distress syndrome: The Berlin definition. *JAMA* 307(3): 2526-2533, 2012.

PATHOPHYSIOLOGY

In ARDS, inflammation of the pulmonary capillary endothelium and alveolar epithelium results in increased permeability of these tissue layers (Fig. 13-10). Injury to the lung parenchyma ultimately leads to leaking of protein-rich plasma out of the capillary, first into the interstitial space (interstitium) and then the alveolar space.

Computed tomography (CT) of the thorax in ARDS shows a gravity-dependent, ground-glass opacification appearance. This is thought to be associated with an active inflammatory process that involves the interstitium and alveoli of both lungs. The inflammation produces abnormal thickening of the alveolar epithelium and incomplete filling of alveolar space with inflammatory cells, cellular debris, and edema.[64,65] Acini are either completely airless or almost airless. Consequently, some alveoli are collapsed (atelectatic) and potentially recruitable.

In general, ARDS produces stiff lungs (reduced lung compliance) and reduced lung volumes (decreased FRC). There appear to be marked regional differences and varying amounts of inflammation present. Parenchymal injury may also affect the airways, particularly the bronchioles and alveolar ducts. As these small airways become narrow and collapse, they may contribute to the reduced ventilation and lead to areas of trapped air.

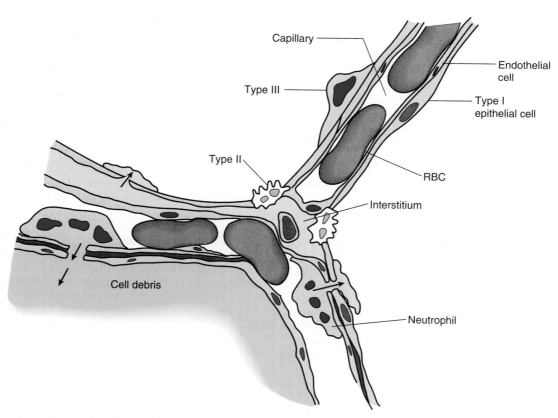

Fig. 13-10 A drawing of the histology of the lung under normal conditions *(top right section)* and during the acute phase of ARDS *(middle and bottom)* showing the following: red blood cell (RBC), white blood cell (WBC), type I pulmonary epithelial cell, pulmonary type II cell (responsible for surfactant production), pulmonary type III cell (macrophage), the capillary, and capillary endothelial cell. During ARDS, leaking occurs into the interstitial space and alveolus. (See text for additional information.)

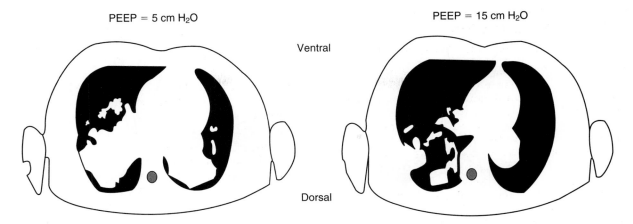

Fig. 13-11 Representative drawings of computed tomographs (CTs) of the thorax of a supine patient. The left CT was taken when the PEEP was set at 5 cm H_2O. The dark areas are aerated lung. These dark areas are in the nondependent portions of the chest near the anterior chest wall (sternum). The greatest densities (white areas) are in the dependent regions of the lung, toward the spine. As PEEP is increased to 15 cm H_2O, the amount of aeration increases. (Redrawn from Gattinoni L, Pesenti A, Bombino M, et al: Anesthesiology 69:824, 1988.)

CHANGES IN COMPUTED TOMOGRAM WITH ARDS

ARDS can be divided into two phases. The first is an acute **exudative** phase characterized by inflammation and alveolar filling. The second is a subacute phase, in which **fibrosing alveolitis** occurs.[65] During the first week, three distinct areas of the lungs can be discerned on chest CT. Initially, normal lung usually appears in nondependent areas (ventral area in the supine patient). Next, a ground-glass appearance is present in the middle area of lung along the vertical axis from sternum to spine. Finally, a consolidated area appears in the dependent region (dorsal in the supine patient). From the ventral to the dorsal area, there is a progressive increase in density (Fig. 13-11).[64]

There is also an increase in density on CT that is seen on a horizontal line in the supine patient from the head area (cephalad) to the base of the spine (caudad). The weight of the heart and the upward push from abdominal pressure may increase the amount of atelectasis in the dorsal area, near the spine, and caudad, near the diaphragm.

Normally, the capillary osmotic pressure tends to pull fluid out of the alveolus and interstitial space and into the microvasculature of the pulmonary circulation. This normal fluid movement is lost in ARDS, resulting in the development of pulmonary edema. The amount of the edema present depends on the pressure gradient between the space inside the pulmonary microvasculature and the space around these vessels (perivascular space). Thus, even when pulmonary blood pressures are normal, edema can still form. This is a result of expanded lung tissue during application of PEEP or high lung volumes pulling on the corner vessels and the adjacent tissue, creating a negative pressure gradient from inside the corner vessel to outside the vessel (Fig. 13-12).

If fluid management is aggressively pursued in patients with ARDS, the pressure in the microvasculature of the lung can increase. The pulmonary capillaries may leak more. This is followed by increased production of biochemical mediators (procollagens and fibronectin).[66] Thus, it is important to use conservative fluid management when possible. The goal of this approach is to reduce extravascular lung water and thus improve oxygenation and reduce morbidity and mortality in ARDS. It is important to mention that the effectiveness of this approach has not been proved.[37] Indeed, some practitioners prefer to use higher volumes of fluid to avoid hypoperfusion of the peripheral tissues and organs.

ARDS AS AN INFLAMMATORY PROCESS

The inflammatory process associated with ARDS involves a complex interaction between platelets, leukocytes, mononuclear cells, macrophages, and epithelial cells.[66] In diffuse lung injury present with ARDS, **cytokines** and other **inflammatory and thrombotic mediators** are released into the bloodstream from the lung. The interaction of these mediators with other body organs can lead to multiple organ failure, also called *multisystem organ failure* and *multiple organ dysfunction syndrome*. ARDS should therefore be viewed as a systemic syndrome and not just a pulmonary problem. Box 13-12 provides a partial list of inflammatory mediators that have been implicated in ARDS.

Two Categories of ARDS

Clinicians sometimes divide ARDS into two categories: *direct* and *indirect*. **Direct** ARDS is also referred to as *primary* or *pulmonary* ARDS and includes disorders of the lung that directly affect lung tissue, such as pneumonia, aspiration, and near-drowning. **Indirect** ARDS is referred to as *secondary* or *nonpulmonary* ARDS because injury to the lung is not the result of a direct lung insult. Nonpulmonary ARDS is associated with an acute systemic inflammatory process, such as acute sepsis and acute pancreatitis.

In primary ARDS (direct), lungs are mostly consolidated. In secondary ARDS (indirect), alveolar collapse is predominant. Note that a lung recruitment maneuver is more likely to improve oxygenation and compliance of the lung in secondary ARDS (see section on Lung Recruitment later in this chapter).[67,68]

CT scans of the lungs of patients with direct ARDS differ considerably from those with indirect ARDS. Primary or direct ARDS tends to be asymmetrical with a mix of parenchymal opacification and ground-glass opacification (Box 13-13).[63,68] Extrapulmonary

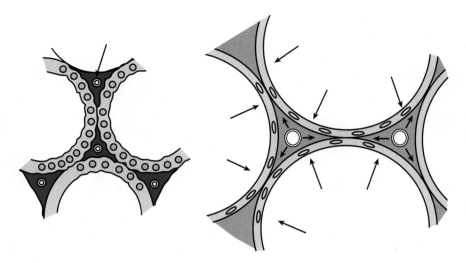

Fig. 13-12 A drawing showing the effect of low lung volume and high lung volume on the pulmonary microvasculature. Note that during low lung volumes *(left)* pulmonary capillaries are most open and corner vessels between the alveoli are most narrow. The reverse is true during high lung volumes. Pulmonary capillaries tend to be compressed and corner vessels increase in diameter. This creates an area of lower pressure around the corner vessel. Edema fluid can build up in this area of the lung. (Courtesy John Marini, MD, Minneapolis, Minn. Redrawn for this text.)

BOX 13-12 **Possible Chemicals That Mediate the Inflammatory Response in ARDS[65]**

- Reactive oxygen species
- Nitric oxide
- Leukotrienes
- Cytokines
- Proteases
- Platelet-activating factor (PAF)
- Cationic proteins
- Interleukins (IL-1, IL-6, IL-8, IL-10)
- Tumor necrosis factor-α (TNF-α)

BOX 13-13 **Terminology of Computed Tomography**

- *Ground glass opacification* is the appearance of a hazy increase in lung density, while the bronchial and vascular margins are preserved.
- *Consolidation* is a homogenous increase in lung density that obscures bronchovascular margins where an air-bronchogram may be present.
- *Reticular pattern* is the presence of many (innumerable) interlacing line shadows that may be fine, intermittent, or coarse.

---

or secondary ARDS CTs have predominantly symmetrical and ground-glass opacification and dorsal consolidation (atelectasis). One problem when trying to be too diligent about classifying ARDS is that the two conditions could coexist. For example, one or more lobes might have had a direct insult, and both lungs may have indirect ARDS at the same time. Thus, a CT cannot reliably be used to distinguish the two.

ARDS: A Heterogeneous Disorder—Normal Lung vs. ARDS

In the late 1980s, Gattinoni and colleagues published a study examining the CT scans of a patient with ARDS.[65] The results of their study showed that the injury in ARDS is scattered (see Fig. 13-11). In fact, the distribution of fluid accumulation and lung collapse appeared to be influenced by gravity (i.e., the involved lung was in the dependent zones).

During the 1980s, it was not uncommon for clinicians to set V_T at 10 to 15 mL/kg for ventilated patients.[69] For patients with ARDS, these large volumes primarily entered the normally aerated tissue in the independent regions. Thus, a relatively small area of the lungs received most of the volume causing overdistention and injury to the alveoli in the independent lung regions. As a result, lung compliance appeared to be low. Gattinoni used the term *baby lung* to describe this phenomenon because it received a large share of the V_T.[64] It is important to note that this is one rationale for using pressure-controlled ventilation in patients with ARDS because it limits the amount of pressure and distention to all lung regions.

Gattinoni and his group also found that PEEP could improve outcomes in ARDS.[68,70] These researchers found that when they increased PEEP from 5 to 15 cm H_2O more of the lung appeared aerated on the CT (see Fig. 13-11).[64,68,70]

Since that time, a number of researchers have compared CTs of patients with normal lungs to patients with ARDS. The findings in normal lungs in supine patients show that there is a normal distribution of densities that occurs throughout the lungs. These densities are related to the thoracic shape, lung weight, and gravitational distribution of blood. The greater densities on CT occur in the dependent areas in supine subjects and are associated with an increase in the pleural pressure from the sternum to the spine. The increase in pleural pressure causes a decrease in the transpulmonary pressure (alveolar pressure minus pleural pressure), which is the distending force of the lungs. Thus, lung units in dependent areas are less open than in nondependent areas (Key Point 13-5).

⊘ *Key Point* **13-5** Transpulmonary pressure is often defined in two ways: (1) alveolar pressure minus pleural pressure and (2) airway pressure minus pleural pressure. In general, when "airway pressure" is used in this situation, it is airway pressure measured during an inspiratory pause. Thus, the airway pressure in this context is an estimate of plateau pressure or alveolar pressure.

The changes noted in ARDS compared with normal lungs are not the thoracic shape or the gravitational distribution of blood, but rather the superimposed weight (pressure) of the lung. In ARDS the weight of the lung is double or triple that of the normal lung. This increased weight is probably caused by inflammation and edema. The increased mass in ARDS leads to "gas squeezing" out of the lung units in the dependent areas.[63] The ventral-dorsal compression can be caused by two factors: interstitial edema can lead to lung collapse and alveoli may be filled with edema. When the superimposed gravitation pressure exceeds the distending pressure, end-expiratory alveolar and small airway collapse increases.[70] Lung collapse can be associated not only with the weight of the lung, but also loss of surfactant and very low $\dot{V}/\dot{Q}$ ratios, which may reach collapse pressures.

In the late stage of ARDS, the CT may show the resolution of the pathologic process. In other patients, when ARDS is present for more than 1 week, the early exudative phase changes to an organized phase. Fluids are reabsorbed from the lung and lung density decreases. As time progresses, pulmonary fibrosis causes an abnormal distortion of the interstitial and bronchovascular markings. Between 1 and 2 weeks, there is an increase in subpleural cysts or bullae. These bullae vary in size. The appearance of these bullae is believed to correlate with the length of mechanical ventilation. These bullae appear in all areas of the lung.[63] Some of these bullae may be caused by cavitation of lung abscesses and some may be caused by ventilator-induced lung injury (VILI) (see Chapter 17 for a discussion of VILI).

In areas of the lung where small airways were narrow early in the disease, this narrowing may contribute to air trapping later in the disease, which may be a factor in later cyst formation that can occur during the healing process.[71,72]

PEEP AND THE VERTICAL GRADIENT IN ARDS

In ARDS, PEEP works by counteracting the superimposed lung pressures caused by the weight of the lung. PEEP must be greater than or equal to the gravitational pressure of the lung weight to keep the dependent regions of the lung open. In contrast, less PEEP is required to keep the lung open in the middle area of the lung because the superimposed pressure is less and no PEEP is required in the nondependent lung region because there is no compression on this lung parenchyma.[63] Overdistention of nondependent areas may be a potential risk of PEEP.

As lungs are maintained in an open position, the dependent lung regions become more compliant. Previously collapsed regions stay open and may increase slightly in volume as they accept more gas. Regional changes in compliance may be one way in which PEEP benefits gas exchange and improves oxygenation.[63] The nondependent regions become less compliant during PPV, probably because of stretching lung units that are already open.

LUNG-PROTECTIVE STRATEGIES: SETTING TIDAL VOLUME AND PRESSURES IN ARDS

To avoid damage from excessive pressures and volumes in patients with ARDS, $P_{plateau}$ must be maintained at less than 30 cm H_2O. The lowest PEEP required to keep the lungs open at end exhalation and provide an acceptable P_aO_2 should be used.[73-76] The PIP (i.e., PEEP plus the inspiratory pressure used to deliver the inspired V_T) should not exceed the **upper inflection point** and total lung capacity.[74]

The ARDS Network trial and other studies provide strong evidence in support of using V_T of 4 to 6 mL/kg and a $P_{plateau}$ less than 30 cm H_2O when ventilating patients with ARDS. Significant differences in survival have been reported when these settings are used compared with using a V_T of 12 mL/kg.[34,62,69,75-82] (NOTE: It is interesting that in spite of the strong support for using low V_T strategies in ARDS, a number of physicians still do not use lung-protective strategies.[82-85]) Adequate levels of PEEP reduce the potential for injury that is associated with repeated reopening and collapsing of lung tissue, keeping the recruited lung open at end expiration.[31] However, many physicians choose not to use levels higher than 10 cm H_2O.[85]

Several basic points should be kept in mind when managing ventilated patients with ARDS using an open-lung or lung-protective strategy:

1. Use of low V_T in ARDS (4 to 6 mL/kg) has been shown to be effective. Clinical studies have confirmed that the use of high V_T can be harmful in ARDS.[69] Use of low V_T should be accompanied by the use of a PEEP level to avoid alveolar collapse.[34,74]
2. PEEP has a protective effect against lung damage, and it helps to keep the lung open.[35,44,86] Maintaining a minimum end-expiratory volume with PEEP helps avoid the widespread alveolar edema, bronchial damage, and shear stress between alveoli that can occur when lung units are repeatedly opened and closed at low lung volumes[34,43,86,87-89] (Box 13-14).
3. As PEEP is increased, P_aO_2 increases. It should be remembered however that using P_aO_2 alone is not always a good indicator of an appropriate PEEP level.[37] P_aO_2 increases because of recruitment of lung tissue in alveoli open in a perfused area (i.e., shunt fraction is reduced). $\dot{V}_A$ increases and P_aCO_2 decreases. When $\overline{P}_{aw}$ increases, cardiac output usually decreases. In addition, blood can be shifted from one area of the lung to another if alveoli become overdistended. Thus, ventilation can be directed to nonperfused areas.
4. PEEP should be applied early (during first 7-10 days after diagnosis of ARDS). The level of applied PEEP should be set 3 to 4 cm H_2O above the upper inflection point of the deflation limb of the P-V curve to help maintain an open lung.[74] This may require a PEEP of 15 cm H_2O or greater.[74,77,90,91] Establishing the **lower inflection point** should be done following lung

| BOX **13-14** | **Measures of Decreased Blood Oxygenation or Lung Injury** |

- Decreased P_aO_2 and S_pO_2
- Decreased P_aO_2/F_iO_2 ratio
- Increased $P_{(A-a)}O_2$
- Increased shunt/venous admixture

recruitment with a slow derecruitment maneuver (Key Point 13-6).[92,93] This may require very small, slow, stepwise decreases in pressure following a deep inflation (recruitment maneuver) (2.5 cm H_2O every 5 to 10 minutes) until the collapse point occurs. Both C_S and P_aO_2 will decrease when significant collapse occurs. During this maneuver, C_S is probably the best single indicator of recruitment and the best indicator of closing point. Note that a rerecruitment maneuver (reinflation of the lung) is required following derecruitment (collapse of the lung).

🌐 Key Point 13-6 "Moreover, because it now seems sensible to titrate PEEP 'from above downward' along the deflation limb of the PV curve to the lowest tolerated level, recruitment maneuvers are an inherent part of this empirical process."[92]

---

5. If it becomes difficult to maintain low pressures during volume-controlled ventilation, switch to pressure-controlled ventilation and monitor V_T delivery.[93,94] If it is necessary to improve P_aO_2, increase the $\overline{P}_{aw}$ by extending inspiratory time (T_I) during pressure ventilation.

6. There is the risk that the areas of the lung that appear normal may become overinflated at end inspiration during tidal breathing as PEEP is increased.[93] Overdistention of alveolar tissues and terminal airways may be avoided by avoiding high transpulmonary pressures; keep $P_{plateau}$ <30 cm H_2O to keep lung volumes lower than TLC.[37,43,63,74,86] When P_aCO_2 increases with increased PEEP (same V_T), lung overdistention is present.

7. When ventilation cannot be maintained at a normal level without risking damage to lung tissue and/or auto-PEEP is present, consider allowing P_aCO_2 to rise (i.e., permissive hypercapnia; see Chapter 12). The need to maintain normal P_aCO_2 has never been demonstrated, especially when pH changes are gradual and oxygenation maintained. Rapid changes in pH, on the other hand, can result in central nervous system dysfunction, increased cerebral perfusion and intracranial hypertension, muscle weakness, cardiovascular dysfunction, and intracellular acidosis.[45,87] When permissive hypercapnia is used, the patient usually requires sedation because it is uncomfortable.

It is unfortunate that many critical care physicians are still reluctant to use PEEP above 10 cm H_2O, despite the fact that low V_T settings without adequate PEEP can result in alveolar derecruitment[69,79] (Key Point 13-7).

🌐 Key Point 13-7 "... the reason to use PEEP in patients with acute lung injury is as part of a lung-protective strategy, rather than simply as a way that we can increase the P_aO_2 and lower the F_IO_2."[36]

Prone positioning is another technique used by some clinicians to improve oxygenation in patients with ARDS. More information about prone positioning can be found in later in this chapter.

LONG-TERM FOLLOW-UP ON ARDS

Some survivors of ARDS show distinct changes in CT of their lungs. These individuals typically demonstrate a reticular pattern in the nondependent areas of the lung. This is the area of the lung that actually possessed normal lung function during the disease process. The appearance of this fibrotic pattern is correlated with the length of mechanical ventilation and whether inverse ratio ventilation was used. Furthermore, this reticular pattern (fibrosis) is generally not seen in the dependent areas, which are probably those areas of the lungs least exposed to high ventilating pressures and high F_IO_2.

Both obstructive and restrictive patterns are seen in long-term follow-up studies of pulmonary function of ARDS patients. Whereas functional exercise is moderately limited in survivors, this limitation was not associated with pulmonary problems and may be a result of muscle weakness and wasting, and abnormal neuromuscular function. The health-related quality of life in ARDS survivors is generally associated with muscle loss and weakness.

Many ARDS survivors have substantial neuropsychological dysfunction. This includes cognitive and affective impairment following hospital discharge that may persist for more than a year. Patients may suffer posttraumatic stress disorder with recollection of traumatic ICU events. Others may experience hallucinations, paranoia, depressed personality, and personality changes.[95] Additional studies are needed to further evaluate ARDS survivors and the best strategies to improve their ICU experience and long-term outcomes.

PRESSURE–VOLUME LOOPS AND RECRUITMENT MANEUVERS IN SETTING PEEP IN ARDS

In addition to protecting the lung in ARDS by restricting tidal volumes and plateau pressures, the clinician also must address the challenge of improving oxygenation. Current strategies for treating hypoxemia in ARDS are directed at recruiting as much lung as possible, which helps restore FRC and improve lung compliance. It also includes setting an appropriate level of PEEP.

In the previous discussion, traditional techniques for managing hypoxemia through increasing PEEP and F_IO_2 were reviewed. This section reviews several other approaches that have received some attention during the past decade. These techniques include recruiting the lung by inflating it to or near TLC and then identifying the optimum level of PEEP, which will maintain the lung as open (recruited) as possible. Methods that will be described include slow or static pressure–volume (SPV) loops and lung recruitment using alternative techniques to the SPV loop.

Patient Evaluation for Lung Recruitment

Before performing a recruitment maneuver (RM), it may be beneficial to obtain a chest CT to rule out the presence of bullae (blebs) or pneumothorax because these conditions are contraindications to recruitment. In addition, an RM is probably not beneficial for unilateral lung conditions, such as unilateral pneumonia. It is also important to perform RMs early in the course of treatment of patients with ARDS. As mentioned earlier, patients with primary ARDS (direct lung injury) are less likely to benefit from an RM than those with secondary or indirect ARDS. Because recruitment procedures require sustained positive pressure, use of sedation is appropriate.

The procedure requires at least two people at the bedside: one to perform the maneuver and monitor the ventilator, the other to monitor the patient and provide sedation. During the procedure,

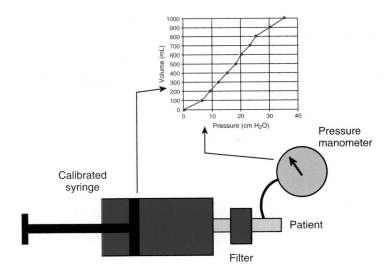

Fig. 13-13 Equipment used to measure a pressure–volume curve using a super syringe. (From Hess DR, Kacmarek RM: Essentials of mechanical ventilation, ed 2, New York, 2002, McGraw-Hill.)

monitoring typically includes evaluation of S_pO_2, C_S, BP, heart rate, ECG, ventilating volumes and pressures, f, and the patient's overall appearance. There is no **gold standard** for evaluating recruitment. In other words, no single parameter provides the best way to monitor the success or failure of the procedure.

Pressure–Volume Loops in Setting PEEP

SPV curves have been used to select an optimum PEEP level and V_T in patients with acute lung injury.[26,96-102] The SPV curve generally has a sigmoid shape. The factors believed to be responsible for the shape include all the individual alveolar P-V curves, plus changes in alveolar duct and airway size, and the elastic forces in the pulmonary parenchyma and chest wall as the lung is inflated.[103] Each of these components has its own time constant that influences curve shape.[66,104]

The purpose of performing a slow or static PV loop is to first recruit the lungs and then to identify the upper inflection point (UIP—also referred to as the *deflection point*) that correlates with the pressure at which major portions of the lung begin to collapse on expiration. Although there are several ways to accomplish an SPV loop measurement, the two most commonly used methods include the super-syringe technique (which is the true "static" PV loop), and the slow-flow technique (also known as the *quasi-static method*).

Super-Syringe Technique

The super-syringe method was originally used in the mid-1990s before ventilators were technically capable of performing an SPV loop. It is performed in the following manner. A calibrated super syringe (3 L) is placed in line with the patient connector[54,77,105] (Fig. 13-13). Notice that a pressure-measuring device (pressure transducer) is also required. The ventilator pressure display can be used for this purpose. The endotracheal tube cuff is completely inflated so no leaks are present.[54,77,106] Note that this procedure cannot be performed accurately in the presence of a bronchopleural fistula. No spontaneous breathing can occur during the testing period. Thus the ventilator rate is set on zero (mode set at CPAP/spontaneous), and the patient is sedated and may require short-term paralysis.

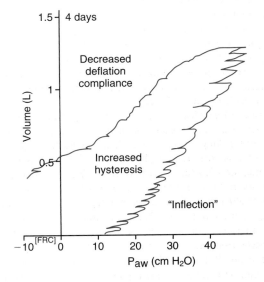

Fig. 13-14 A pressure–volume loop created using the super syringe technique in a patient diagnosed with ARDS (4 days previously). The *scalloped border* of the curve illustrates real-time recording of pressure–volume changes as gas is injected into the patient's lungs. Note the reduced compliance. (From Matamis D, LeMaire F, Harf A, et al: Chest 86:58, 1984.)

Air is injected in volumes of either 50 or 100 mL into the patient's lungs. The resulting $P_{plateau}$ (3- to 10-second pause) is then measured after injection is completed.[107] The resulting P-V values are graphed by hand on paper. Figure 13-14 illustrates a static P-V loop obtained using the super-syringe technique in which the values are continuously monitored. Figure 13-15 shows examples of P-V curves of the respiratory system in a healthy subject and in a patient with ARDS.[74,108-110] The syringe procedure takes about a minute to a minute and a half to perform, excluding set up time and calculations.

Although hypoxemia and hypotension can occur, the procedure is generally considered safe. S_pO_2 values less than 85% and BP less than 90 mm Hg are indications that the procedure is having

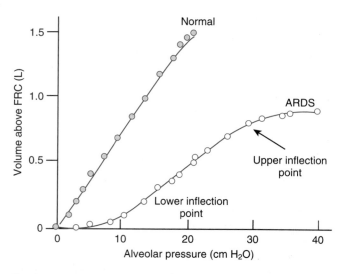

Fig. 13-15 Example of a static, inspiratory pressure–volume curve of the respiratory system in a patient with ARDS compared with a healthy subject. Upper (about 30 cm H_2O) and lower inflection points (about 10 cm H_2O) are present in the patient with ARDS. (From Hess DR, Kacmarek RM: Essentials of mechanical ventilation, ed 2, New York, 2002, McGraw-Hill.)

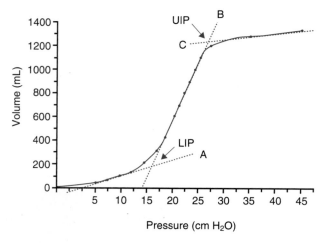

Fig. 13-16 A static pressure–volume curve in a patient with acute respiratory distress syndrome (ARDS). Volume is increased in increments of approximately 100 mL, inspiratory plateau pressure ($P_{plateau}$) is measured, and a pressure–volume curve is plotted. *Straight lines (A, B, and C)* are drawn tangent to the curve, and the lower inflection point (LIP) and upper inflection point (UIP) are identified. The flatter the slope, the less compliant the lung. (From Kacmarek RM, Stoller JK, Heuer AJ (editiors): Egan's fundamentals of respiratory care, ed 10, St Louis, 2013, Mosby.)

adverse effects and should be discontinued.[74,107,109] Notice that the expiratory limb can also be constructed by performing the same procedure to deflate the lung.

The inspiratory portion is intended to recruit the lung and open as many areas of the lung as possible. The deflation curve allows the clinician to determine the point at which the lung begins to collapse. This point would be identified as the point where the curve takes the sharpest downward turn. After the **deflation point** is identified, the lung is reinflated to reopen collapsed areas and the PEEP is set about 2 cm H_2O above the identified deflation pressure point. This marks the optimum level for the patient.

Low-Flow (Quasi-Static) Technique

The low-flow or slow-flow technique (also called the *constant flow technique*) for static P-V measurement uses a single breath delivered at 2 L/min until pressure reaches 45 cm H_2O.[105] It is also referred to as the *quasi-static* PV curve because flow is slow, but not interrupted for measurements, so periods of "no-flow" do not occur. As in the previous techniques, the patient must be sedated and paralyzed. The results of the slow-flow SPV technique are similar to those obtained with the manually performed syringe technique.[111,112] The low-flow inspiratory technique can be used with any ventilator that has a long inspiratory time, a slow constant flow setting, and a screen that will display a P-V loop. Use of slightly higher flows (9 L/min vs. 3 L/min) causes a slight shift to the right of the resulting P-V curve.[113]

Features of the SPV Loop

Several key features of an SPV curve include the following:

- **Lower inflection point on the inspiratory limb (LIPi), some-times called P_{FLEX}.** The LIPi is that point on the curve where the slope of the line changes significantly (Fig. 13-16). It was originally believed that this point represented the opening up of the majority of collapsed alveoli. Clinicians would then set PEEP levels at about 2 cm H_2O above this point. It is now

understood that alveoli open continually along the entire slope of the curve.[98,63]

- **Upper inflection point on the inspiratory limb (UIPi).** The UIPi may not be identified if alveoli are still being recruited in some parts of the lungs.
- The slope of the line between the LIPi and UIPi points represents the respiratory system compliance as alveolar recruitment occurs throughout the inspiratory maneuver.
- **The upper plateau portion of the inspiratory loop representing potential recruitment and possible overdistention of the lungs.** Compliance decreased as areas of the lung are overinflated (overdistended) with pressure. Although pressure can still be increased past the UIP, volume increases very little, if at all. It is advisable not to allow ventilating pressures (pressure from V_T delivery plus PEEP) to exceed the UIP during mechanical ventilation of patients.
- **The upper inflection point on the deflation portion of the curve (UIPd), also called deflection point or deflation point.** The rapid change in slope of the curve during deflation identifies the UIPd during deflation. Current theory suggests that it is more important to set PEEP 2 to 3 cm H_2O above the upper inflection point detected during deflation of the lungs (UIPd).[93,98]

Recently developed software programs, which are now available on ICU ventilators, provide the clinician with an option to perform a slow P-V loop. For example, the Hamilton G5 can perform a slow PV loop. The "PVtool Pro" utilizes a pressure ramping technique to construct a slow P-V loop. The user selects a starting PEEP level, pressurization rise rate, upper pressure limit, and end-expiratory PEEP level. A pause equal to five time constants is automatically applied at the start of the maneuver to allow exhalation to FRC. On completion of the inspiratory and expiratory P-V loop, about 20 seconds, the LIP and UIPd values are automatically displayed with the option to manually identify inflection points. Additionally, the point of the maximal hysteresis is numerically and graphically displayed showing the ability of the lungs to be recruited. If significant inflection points or hystereses are identified, a second maneuver with a pause maneuver can be programmed to perform an automated recruitment maneuver. The user sets the final maneuver PEEP level to that obtained from the inflection points or point of maximal hysteresis to restore and maintain recruitment.

Regardless of the procedure used to establish an appropriate PEEP level, the ventilating pressures should not be allowed to exceed the UIP on the UIPi, because injury to lungs can occur if the lungs become overstretched. The appearance of the UIP on the graphic display may be influenced by the type of recruitment procedure used. For example, in one study when the V_T was set low (5 to 6 mL/kg), the UIP was 26 cm H_2O. However, when the V_T was set at 10 to 12 mL/kg, the UIP was about 22 cm H_2O. These findings suggest that the UIP probably depends on previous tidal alveolar recruitment.

Recruitment Maneuvers

An RM is a sustained increase in pressure in the lungs with the goal of opening as many collapsed lung units as possible.[67] It is performed in the management of patients with ARDS and may also be used in the postoperative treatment of atelectasis in post-anesthesia patients.[114] It is also suggested for use following suctioning maneuvers in some ventilated patients.[57]

Recruitment occurs across the entire range of lung volume from residual volume to TLC. Once the lungs are recruited, they are kept open by maintaining an adequate PEEP above the LIP of an inspiratory maneuver or, preferably, above the UIP of a deflation (expiratory) maneuver (Key Points 13-8 and 13-9).[36,115] Lungs are protected from overdistention by keeping PIP lower than the inspiratory maneuver UIP (Box 13-15).[70,88]

> **Key Point 13-8** Choosing a PEEP level based on the inspiratory portion of the limb is inappropriate. What stays open with PEEP is what has been opened by the preceding inspiratory pressures.[63]

> **Key Point 13-9** "If a collapsed lung is indeed a nidus (center) for further lung injury and inflammation, then a new paradigm in ARDS may be to open the lung with a recruitment maneuver and then keep it open by using PEEP set at a pressure above the level where substantial decruitment begins."[115]

| BOX **13-15** | **PEEP and F_IO_2 Levels with ARDS** |

The ARDSnet study mentioned earlier in this chapter used a table of PEEP-F_IO_2 combinations to guide the setting of PEEP and F_IO_2.[34] In that study, PEEP ranged from 5 to 24 cm H_2O. Some researchers felt that this table progressed too slowly in the application of PEEP. Their opinion was that PEEP should be increased to 15 cm H_2O very early in the management of ARDS.

A subsequent study by the ARDSnet relied on a lung recruitment maneuver and a newer PEEP/F_IO_2 scale that was more aggressive in maintaining PEEP.[35] Either of the tables set by the ARDSnet group may be suitable as clinical guides for setting PEEP.

Illustration of a Recruitment Maneuver

Figure 13-17 illustrates the concept behind a recruitment maneuver. An isolated animal lung is completely collapsed before inflation begins. Corresponding pressure is zero on the P-V loop. Pressure is increased in increments of 4 cm H_2O. The corresponding P-V point is plotted on the graph. It takes 8 to 12 cm H_2O (LIP on the inspiratory limb) before the lung visibly begins to open. The inspiratory LIP is probably at, or slightly above, 8 cm H_2O. At 16 cm H_2O the lung is well inflated. At 20 cm H_2O the lung appears fully inflated. On the P-V loop at 20 cm H_2O the top of the curve begins to flatten out. This portion of the curve has a "beak-like" or "duck-bill" appearance. This decrease in compliance represents overdistention.

During the deflation (expiratory portion) portion of the loop, the pressure is reduced in increments of 4 cm H_2O and the corresponding points are plotted on the P-V loop (see Fig. 13-17, photos below the PV loop). When one compares the photos of the lung during inspiration with those during expiration, it becomes apparent that as more lung tissue is recruited during inspiration, more remains open on exhalation.[116,117] Once the lung units are opened, lung inflation can be maintained with lower pressures.

Lung derecruitment begins at about 8 cm H_2O. Below 4 cm H_2O the lung completely collapses (see Fig. 13-17). Maintaining the PEEP at 11 to 12 cm H_2O (3 to 4 cm H_2O above the deflection point), after the lung is rerecruited, would seem like a reasonable level of PEEP that would maintain the lung in an inflated position. Although this situation represents a lung that is removed from the thorax, it provides a visual image of recruitment and derecruitment as they might occur.

During the deflation stage, at the point during which a significant number of lung units collapses, an accompanying drop occurs in P_aO_2 and in compliance. C_S is probably the best single indicator of the closing point, and it is considerably less expensive to obtain than an ABG at each step in the process.[118]

Following identification of this point, the lung is again reinflated or rerecruited to its maximum capacity (TLC). The pressure is then reduced to a PEEP level 2 to 4 cm H_2O above the deflection point. The lung will remain open only following rerecruitment if an appropriate amount of PEEP is applied to prevent unstable alveoli from collapsing. The superimposed pressure of the lung (and heart) is a key determinant of lung collapse. As long as the applied PEEP is greater than any superimposed gravitational pressures from lung tissue, and PEEP is not interrupted, the alveoli tend to stay open for a longer time.[31,63,119] When gravitational pressure from the lung and heart exceeds PEEP, end-expiratory collapse occurs.[71] Some researchers have suggested that an RM may need to be repeated more than once to gain maximum benefit[63,120] (Key Point 13-10). Others have emphasized the importance of recruiting the lung early to potentially reverse hypoxemia in early ARDS.[121]

> **Key Point 13-10** It is recommended that an RM is performed if PEEP is inadvertently withdrawn because of a circuit disconnect or leak following suctioning, or in cases where significant changes in P_aO_2 occur.

The Function of Lung Recruitment

Figure 13-18 shows a series of CT scans that provide direct evidence that recruitment is "pan-inspiratory"; that is, it occurs throughout inspiration.[63] Note that previously it was thought that recruitment was essentially complete above the LIP.

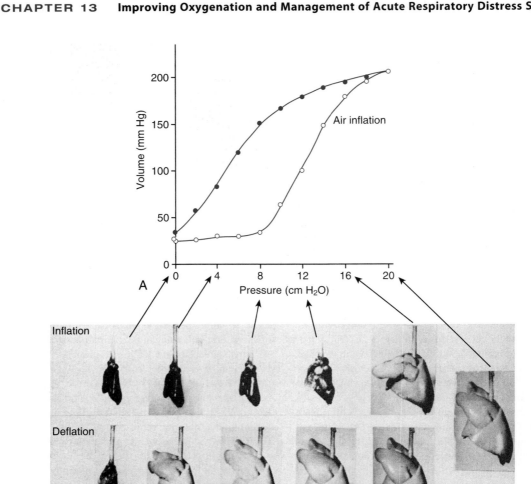

Fig. 13-17 A, Illustration of a pressure–volume loop. **B,** A series of photographs showing a suspended animal lung with progressively increasing pressures during inspiration and progressively different pressures during exhalation. Notice that once the lung is recruited at 20 cm H_2O, when expiration occurs, a high lung volume can be maintained for a similar pressure (expiration versus inspiration). (See text for further explanation.) (**A,** Modified from Radford EP Jr: Recent studies of mechanical properties of mammalian lungs. In Remington JW, editor: Tissue elasticity, Washington, DC, 1957, American Physiological Society. **B,** From Fenn WO, Rahn H, editors: Respiration (vol 1). In Handbook of physiology: a critical, comprehensive presentation of physiological knowledge and concepts, Washington, DC, 1964, American Physiological Society.)

The "sigmoid" shape of the curve suggests that different areas of the lung open at different pressures. Consequently, regional variations exist in opening pressures. The opening pressure for lung units can range from a few cm H_2O to inflation pressures as high as 55 to 60 cm H_2O.[71,115,117] This extreme range of inflation pressures is probably a result of differing types of atelectasis.

The opening pressure required for small airway collapse that is associated with compression atelectasis is in the range of 20 cm H_2O. This type of atelectasis might also be called *loose atelectasis*. One example of compression atelectasis is that which occurs in normal lungs during anesthesia.[63] In contrast, the opening pressure required to recruit alveoli collapsed as a result of "sticky atelectasis," such as might occur with ARDS, is much higher (range, 30 to 40 cm H_2O).[104,122] The true opening pressure for lung units is the transmural pressure; that is, the pressure applied to the airways and alveoli minus pleural pressure.

In addition to selecting an appropriate opening pressure, time is required for recruitment to occur. Indeed, reopening collapsed alveoli takes time, more for some alveoli than for others. In examining the different types of RM used, the reader will see that most RMs are performed with pressure sustained for 40 seconds or more.

Figure 13-19 illustrates how the alveoli might open during an RM. Normal alveoli may become progressively inflated until they are overinflated. Those lung units in the dependent areas of the lung may eventually open and overcome the weight of the overlying lung tissue.

Hazards of Recruitment Maneuvers

Significant increases in thoracic pressure for an extended period (≥40 seconds) can cause a significant decrease in venous return to the thorax, a drop in cardiac output, and a drop in BP. Pressure can

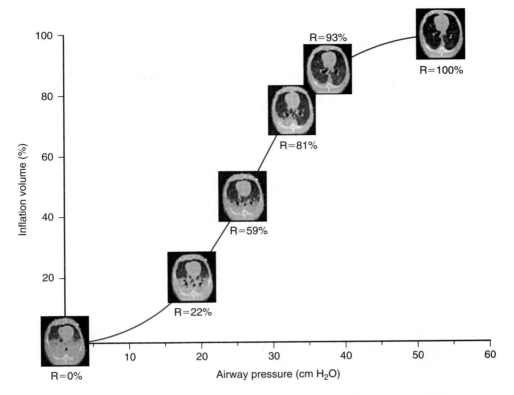

Fig. 13-18 An inspiratory pressure–volume curve in a lung model with acute respiratory distress syndrome (ARDS). Computed tomograms of the lung are shown at varying points along the curve. Note that increased aeration of the lungs occurs along the entire curve. (From Gattinoni L, Pietro C, Pelosi P, et al: Am J Respir Crit Care Med 164:1701, 2001.)

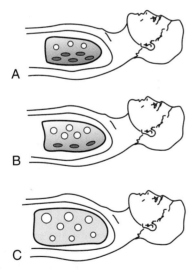

Fig. 13-19 Theoretical model of a recruitment maneuver in a supine patient opening lung units. In **(A)**, only nondependent lung units are open. In **(B)**, as recruitment maneuver (RM) is performed more lung units in the middle area begin to open. In **(C)**, lung units in the dependent zones of the lung open and those in the nondependent zones begin to overexpand from overinflation (overdistention).

also affect the lung unevenly, with some areas receiving more pressure, thus causing a shifting of blood to other areas of the lung.

On the other hand, in patients who respond to an RM, a drop in BP and cardiac output during the maneuver may not occur. In fact, an RM performed with a patient who is hypotensive may

actually improve hemodynamics. One explanation for this phenomenon is that as the alveolar PO_2 improves, pulmonary vessels may open, causing a reduction in pulmonary vascular resistance. This reduces the work of the right side of the heart and may improve cardiac performance.

Variability Among Patients

Recruitment maneuvers can produce varying results among patients. In patients who respond to an RM, P_aO_2 increases, P_aCO_2 decreases, and the change in pressure (ΔP) required to cause an acceptable V_T decreases. In other words, if recruitment improves C_S, a patient can be ventilated with an appropriate V_T at much lower pressures than before recruitment. In contrast, when the RM is not beneficial for the patient, increasing levels of PEEP do not significantly increase lung aeration, and as a result there may be no improvement in P_aO_2, P_aCO_2 or C_S.

Effects of Chest Wall Compliance on Lung Recruitment

Changes in chest wall compliance will affect the pressures needed to open the lungs. Chest wall compliance includes forces from the overlying ribs and muscles, force from the diaphragm, and pressures from abdominal contents that affect the diaphragm. Low chest wall compliance tends to act like a tight vest around the thorax, which increases pleural pressure. Low chest wall compliance (high chest wall elastance) can occur in obese patients, in patients with severe abdominal disease, in patients with abdominal distention (e.g., ascites), and from prone positioning.

In critically ill patients, it is not unusual for abdominal pressures to be higher than normal. Elevated abdominal pressure not only affects the position of the diaphragm but also puts pressure on the vena cava. This augments venous return to the thorax. Thus, with increased abdominal pressure, there is a shift of blood into the thorax. If the lung is injured and leaking, this increases lung fluid.

As chest wall compliance decreases, more lung units collapse and thus affect the recruitment of collapsed alveoli. For example, in an obese patient with peritonitis, an airway pressure of 30 cm H_2O may not be adequate to recruit the lung. As a result, airway pressures might be higher than 40 to 45 cm H_2O to reach a sufficient transpulmonary pressure to open the lung.

To summarize, in ARDS a wide range of airway pressures may be needed to open various alveolar ducts and small airways and overcome the elastic forces in the lung parenchyma and chest wall.[103,115]

Potential Complications During Lung Recruitment

Hypotension has been reported, and brief episodes of hypoxemia can also occur. Most of the time, these changes are not sufficient to discontinue the process. However, if the hemodynamic status becomes significantly unstable with a severe drop in BP, the procedure should be discontinued.[115]

The occurrence of barotrauma, such as pneumothorax, subcutaneous emphysema, and pneumomediastinum, has not been reported as a significant finding compared with patients receiving standard mechanical ventilation.[38] These remain a potential concern, however, when performing an RM. Breath sounds should be evaluated during the procedure if vital signs and ventilatory parameters suggest that a pneumothorax may be present.[115]

Compliance is a good indication of how much of the lung is open in ARDS patients. Monitoring compliance can also help determine the amount of lung that is recruitable. Changes in compliance and P_aO_2 during recruitment and derecruitment are not linear.[29]

If the hemodynamic status of the patient does not change during the procedure, then increases in P_aO_2 and S_pO_2 suggest that there is a decrease in intrapulmonary shunt following recruitment. An improvement in lung compliance is also likely to occur. An effective recruitment maneuver can also be verified with a chest CT, although this is not practical.

Types of Recruitment Maneuvers

In addition to SPV loops, there are several types of RMs that have been used in the clinical setting. These include a sustained high pressure in the CPAP mode, PC-CMV with a single high PEEP level imposed, PC-CMV with progressive increases in PEEP level, and sigh maneuvers.

Sustained inflation. The technique of sustained inflation has received the most attention of the several techniques used. Sustained inflation is accomplished by providing a sustained high pressure. The ventilator is set to CPAP/spontaneous mode (mandatory rate = zero), and CPAP is increased to 30 to 40 cm H_2O for about 40 seconds.[56] PEEP levels as high as 50 cm H_2O have been suggested to recruit the lungs maximally to achieve the lowest possible shunt fraction. However, this approach is not as commonly accepted.[75]

PC-CMV with a high PEEP level. Another technique uses PC-CMV with a set pressure at about 20 cm H_2O above PEEP and a mandatory rate of about 10 to 12 breaths/min. PEEP is then increased so that PIP is at least 40 cm H_2O. The high pressure is

sustained for 40 to 60 seconds and then decreased to a level appropriate to sustain inflation and prevent derecruitment. Ventilation is then continued in the PC-CMV mode.

PC-CMV with increased PEEP. Another RM uses PC-CMV but increases PEEP in increments of about 5 cm H_2O. Each increase is held for several minutes (2 to 5 minutes). For example, the pressure control level might be set to 20 cm H_2O, with the baseline PEEP at 15 cm H_2O; PIP = 35 cm H_2O; mandatory rate of 10 breaths/min; I : E of 1 : 1 or 1 : 2. PEEP is then progressively increased while other parameters are held constant and compliance is monitored. PEEP is then progressively decreased until compliance decreases (derecruitment). The point of decreased compliance represents the UIPd of the lungs. The lung is once again reinflated to allow reopening of lung units. The PEEP once again is decreased until a pressure 2 to 4 cm H_2O above the UIPd is obtained.

Recruitment and decremental PEEP. An alternative technique for recruiting the lung and determining optimum PEEP is called a *decremental PEEP study*.[44] Following a full inflation of the lungs, PEEP is progressively decreased in increments of about 5 cm H_2O (adult) until the compliance of the lungs decreases. This point represents the UIPd for the lungs. Following this maneuver, the lungs are fully reinflated and then the PEEP is set to about 2 to 4 cm H_2O above the UIPd.[44,96]

Sigh techniques. As mentioned in Chapter 12, the use of sigh breaths was originally advocated in the 1960s to prevent atelectasis associated with low-volume, monotonous breathing patterns used during anesthesia. The use of sighs was eventually abandoned, probably because higher V_T settings became popular (V_T 10 to 15 mL/kg) and atelectasis was less likely. Another reason may have been that sigh breaths were set too infrequently and were not of sufficient pressure and length to be effective.[67]

With the use of lower V_T settings (4 to 6 mL/kg) in ARDS, there is a renewed interest in the sigh.[123] A few different sigh techniques have been suggested:

- Three consecutive breaths per min at a $P_{plateau}$ of 45 cm H_2O[121]
- Twice V_T every 25 breaths, with optimum PEEP set[124]
- Holding V_T constant while increasing PEEP from a low level (about 9.5 cm H_2O) to a high level of about 16 cm H_2O for two breaths every 30 seconds.[125] (NOTE: This technique is not as effective in sustaining improvements as continuous application of PEEP at a higher level [16 cm H_2O].)
- Increasing PEEP in a stepwise fashion to 30 cm H_2O while V_T is decreased, resulting in elevated airway pressures over several minutes. (Procedure: each of the following settings is held for a 1-minute interval. The procedure is then repeated a second time.) (NOTE: This sigh technique was shown to modestly sustain improvement in P_aO_2 and respiratory system compliance.)[123]
- Increasing inspiratory pressure to 20 to 30 cm H_2O for 1 to 3 seconds at a rate of 2 to 3 sighs/min. This technique has been used in patients recovering from ARDS who are given pressure support. This type of sigh can be set using such ventilator parameters as the PCV+ mode on the Dräger Evita 4 and Bilevel mode on the Puritan Bennett 840 as examples.[67]
- Use of APRV or HFOV to recruit the lungs. (See Chapter 23 for additional information on APRV and HFOV.)

Derecruitment Maneuver

As mentioned, part of the RM is the deflation or derecruitment to establish the point at which lung collapse is likely to occur. Some clinicians do not perform a derecruitment and simply set PEEP at a high level such as 15 cm H_2O. This is a reasonable target for a minimum PEEP in ARDS.[77]

Derecruitment can be performed in small steps (2.5 to 5 cm H_2O), with each being held for 5 to 10 seconds to evaluate compliance and S_pO_2. P_aO_2 can also be evaluated but obtaining ABGs is more expensive. C_S may be just as effective to determine the point at which significant lung collapse occurs.[126]

The following clinical scenario provides an example of a patient in whom an RM was successful in improving clinical parameters.[115]

Clinical Scenario: Case Report in Lung Recruitment

A 32-year-old woman with ARDS was treated with repeated recruitment maneuvers in an effort to improve oxygenation. The recruitment maneuvers consisted of progressively higher PEEP levels (30, 35, 40 cm H_2O) that were sustained for 2 minutes at each level. At 40 cm H_2O PEEP, the PIP was 60 cm H_2O and $P_{plateau}$ was 55 cm H_2O. The ventilator settings during the maneuvers were PC-CMV at 20 cm H_2O above PEEP, rate of 10 breaths/min and T_I of 3 seconds. The lower inflection point in this patient was in the range of 16 to 18 cm H_2O. Following the maneuvers, PEEP was maintained at 20 cm H_2O.

While oxygenation and V_T delivery improved (increased C_S) after the maneuver, these parameters would progressively decline over the next 2 to 3 hours. Finally, a fourth RM was performed and the PEEP was set at 25 cm H_2O. V_T, oxygenation, and gas exchange remained stable after this maneuver.

Their conclusion was that setting PEEP based on the lower inflection point does not prevent derecruitment of the lung. It may be impossible in some patients to determine an ideal point of recruitment (LIP) or overdistention (UIP). Using the deflation (expiratory) limb of the P-V curve may better identify optimal PEEP to prevent derecruitment of the lung.

- This procedure is generally safe in studies reported to date.[129-132] However, hypotension and hypoxemia can occur during the procedure, and barotrauma is a potential risk.[132]
- Lung recruitment based on CT scan does not produce excessive hyperinflation of the lung.[123,129,131]
- It is important to set the PEEP at a level above UIP on the derecruitment curve to prevent alveolar collapse.[124,133]
- An RM without adequate PEEP can result in unstable alveoli and may ultimately lead to VILI.[119,125]
- RM with PEEP maintained above the deflation point may be even more effective in improving respiratory lung mechanics and oxygenation when combined with prone positioning.[16,130]
- Given the uncertain benefits of improved oxygenation in ARDS and the lack of information about their impact on outcomes, the routine use of RMs cannot be either recommended or discouraged at this time.[134] A number of questions still remain unanswered. Lung units that can be recruited may represent less than 10% of the densities seen on CT. Is it important to recruit this 10%? In addition, some units cannot be kept open at reasonable PEEP levels. For example, at 35 cm H_2O, some lung units are not open. These units probably cannot be recruited. What are the consequences associated with leaving these alveoli collapsed? Must atelectasis be reversed? Is prevention of lung units closing essential? In everyday clinical practice it is common to hear basilar crackles in obese patients. These crackles represent opening and closing of lung units. Is this opening and closing harmful or inconsequential?

While lung recruitment holds promise in the management of ARDS, additional studies are needed to determine whether it really affects outcomes such as morbidity and mortality.[38] To date no significant difference in hospital mortality or barotrauma occurs when compared with an established low V_T ventilator protocol but oxygenation is improved and duration of mechanical ventilation is reduced.[135] Indeed, some clinicians choose not to use RMs as standard practice in the care of patients with ARDS. On the other hand, some find the use of recruitment an important part of patient management (see Key Point 13-11). Figure 13-20 illustrates one protocol that might be used in the management of ARDS.[126]

Key Point 13-11 "Recruitment maneuvers have become an entrenched part of my own practice, as an RM clarifies the extent to which benefit can be expected from higher levels of PEEP and defines the patient's sensitivity to alterations of the heart's loading conditions."[136]

SUMMARY OF RECRUITMENT MANEUVERS IN ARDS

To summarize the current human reports of the use of RMs, the following are noted:

- RMs may improve oxygenation, reduce shunt, and increase lung compliance by opening collapsed lung units.
- Lung recruitment is effective during the early treatment of ARDS and in patients without impaired chest wall mechanics.[127]
- RMs are more effective in patients with secondary (nonpulmonary) ARDS than in primary ARDS.[128]
- RMs may reduce atelectasis in patients following general anesthesia.[56]

THE IMPORTANCE OF BODY POSITION DURING POSITIVE PRESSURE VENTILATION

Hospitalized patients, especially those receiving mechanical ventilatory support, are often immobilized. The rationale for turning these ventilated patients frequently during the day is to help prevent pulmonary complications, such as atelectasis and hypoxemia. Frequent rotation is important because it also reduces the risk of decubitus (skin breakdown).

Kinetic beds automatically turn the patient from side to side on a continuous rotation up to a 45- to 60-degree lateral position. These beds may help reduce the risk of pneumonias and may help mobilize secretions. They are often used in patients who are immobilized because of strokes, spinal injuries, or coma, and in obese

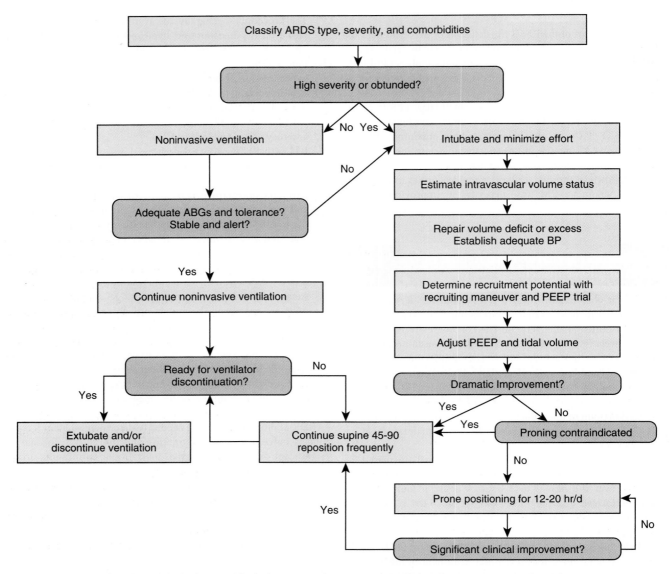

Fig. 13-20 An example of a protocol for the management of a patient with ARDS. (From Marini JJ, Gattinoni L: Crit Care Med 32:250, 2004.)

patients who are otherwise difficult to turn. Precautions are needed with kinetic beds because they can result in stretching and breaking of electrical cords and lines, disconnecting the patient from the ventilator, accidental extubation, and accidental aspiration of condensate from the ventilator circuit.[135]

Other complications associated with kinetic beds include the following:

- Patient agitation and intolerance of the bed
- Worsening of dyspnea and hypoxemia
- Cardiac arrhythmias
- Increased ICP
- Difficulty in examining the patient

Selecting an appropriate body position for a patient may also be beneficial for certain types of pulmonary disorders by ensuring optimum ventilation and perfusion. Positioning is a particularly important issue in two lung pathologies: ARDS and unilateral lung disease.

Positioning in a Patient with ARDS: Prone Positioning

It is well established that body position can affect the distribution of ventilation. Normally during spontaneous breathing, ventilation is higher in the dependent areas of the lungs because the pleural pressure changes during breathing are greater in the dependent areas compared with the independent areas. This may not be true in diseases like ALI and ARDS because edema and injury occur primarily in the dependent (dorsal) lung region of the supine patient.

Placing the patient with ARDS in a prone position may improve oxygenation (increases in P_aO_2 can range from 10 to 50 mm Hg or ≥20%) and decrease the degree of shunt present in the lungs (range in one study from 25% to 12%)[136] (Fig. 13-21). These changes occur in about 75% of patients with ARDS.[136-142] It is important to state that not all patients respond equally well to prone positioning. An improvement of 10 mm Hg in P_aO_2 within 30 minutes of being in

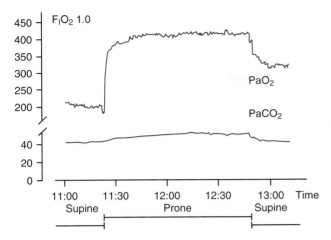

Fig. 13-21 Continuous P_aO_2 and P_aCO_2 values during supine and prone positioning (while on $F_IO_2 = 1.0$) in a patient with ARDS. (From Pappert D, Rossaint R, Slama K, et al: Influence of positioning on ventilation-perfusion relationships in severe adult respiratory distress syndrome, Chest 106:1511, 1994.)

the prone position helps distinguish patients who are responders from nonresponders (i.e., those who do not improve).[143] For some patients, improvement allows the set F_IO_2 and PEEP levels to be reduced. Prone positioning in some patients also results in a decrease in P_aCO_2, suggesting that the V_D/V_T ratio (physiological dead space ratio) is improving.[144]

Potential Mechanisms of Improved Oxygenation in Prone Positioning

The precise mechanisms associated with improvement in $\dot{V}/\dot{Q}$ ratio with prone positioning are not well understood. Within lung tissue, the distribution of the interstitial water and intravascular blood and the anatomical configuration of the lung are all influenced by gravity. As an example, the lungs can be thought of as wet sponges hanging inside the thorax. In a supine patient, hydrostatic pressure is higher in the dependent regions where blood tends to flow. Lung edema formation is more likely in these regions as well. At the same time, the nondependent portions are receiving the greatest amount of ventilation with less perfusion. Note that an important difference between normal subjects and those with ARDS in this aspect is that patients with ARDS have an increased tissue mass compared with what is normal.

When any patient is changed from the supine to prone position, blood redistributes to the gravity-dependent areas, which are now located on the ventral (sternal) side (the "new" dependent region). Blood moves from areas that are not well ventilated in the supine position to areas that are better ventilated in the prone position, resulting in better $\dot{V}/\dot{Q}$ ratios.[139,140] It is believed that partially opened or closed lung units are moved into a position in which they can be distended or recruited (reopened) and better perfused, resulting in improved $\dot{V}/\dot{Q}$.[139] These factors result in an increase in expiratory lung volumes, oxygenation, and pulmonary compliance.[145-149]

Gravity also plays a significant part in gas distribution in supine patients. Areas of lung in nondependent regions overlie lung units in the dorsal (dependent) regions of the chest. In other words, the lung is actually pressing on itself. This pressure is exerted along a vertical gradient from the anterior chest wall to the spine, resulting in lower pulmonary distending pressure in the dorsal alveoli,

which are located in the dependent areas of the supine patient's lungs.[145] This results in collapse of potentially recruitable alveoli in these areas.[146,147] In addition, the heart and great vessels also compress underlying lung tissue and bronchi. Also, abdominal contents press on the lower diaphragm, particularly in paralyzed patients, resulting in abdominal organs encroaching dorsally and into the thorax.[150-152] All these factors contribute to alveolar compression and collapse in the dorsal lung regions of the supine patient.

Prone positioning changes the position of the heart and great vessels so that these structures are no longer pressing on the lungs. Change in the regional movement of the diaphragm also occurs, which may assist in the reopening of collapsed alveoli and areas of atelectasis.

To summarize, the mechanisms believed to improve oxygenation with prone positioning are as follows:

- Blood is redistributed to areas that are better ventilated.
- Blood redistribution may also improve alveolar recruitment in previously closed areas of the lung.
- Redistribution of fluid and gas results in an improved relation between ventilation and perfusion.
- Prone positioning changes the position of the heart so it no longer puts weight on underlying lung tissue.
- Pleural pressure is more uniformly distributed, which could improve alveolar recruitment.
- Prone positioning changes the regional diaphragm motion.

Technical Aspects of Prone Positioning

Before placing a patient in the prone position, potential complications must be weighed against the advantages.[153] Box 13-16 lists some of the contraindications to prone positioning.[154] Moving the patient from the supine to the prone position presents many technical challenges. Adequate sedation is essential. Some patients may even require a brief period of paralysis. The procedure is labor intensive, often requiring the assistance of a team of four individuals, which might include two nurses, a respiratory therapist, and a physician—one team member to turn the head and protect the ET, one to turn the trunk, one to turn the legs, and the fourth to control and move the venous and arterial lines and other catheters.[155]

Care must be taken to avoid accidental extubation, loss of vascular (IV) lines, urinary catheters, and other critical equipment. Box 13-17 outlines a protocol for prone positioning.[156] Once the patient is repositioned, a survey of the ET and all catheters is made to ensure that no displacement has occurred. Special attention should be paid to areas where the skin is in contact with tubes, intravascular lines, and Foley catheters. One of the side effects of prone positioning is facial and eyelid edema, which is resolved once the patient is returned to supine or sitting position.[142] The head requires frequent turning to avoid facial edema. Care must be taken so that the tape securing the ET does not cut into the

BOX **13-16**	**Contraindications to Prone Positioning**

Absolute Contraindication
- Spinal cord instability

Strong Relative Contraindications
- Hemodynamic abnormalities
- Cardiac rhythm disturbances

Relative Contraindications
- Thoracic and abdominal surgeries

BOX 13-17 Protocol for Prone Positioning

Preparation for prone positioning includes the following:
- Adequate sedation of the patient
- Clear assignment of responsibilities between team members
- Moving the patient to one side of the bed
- Checking all lines for length
- Checking the security of the endotracheal tube (ET)
- Endotracheal suctioning prior to turning
- Hyperoxygenation with 100% O_2
- Checking all vital signs

The procedure includes the following:
- Tilting the patient to the side
- Unhooking ECG leads
- Turning the patient prone
- Turning the patient's head toward the ventilator
- Reattaching ECG leads

Care after the prone positioning is accomplished includes the following:
- Checking all lines
- Checking ventilator pressure and volume
- Monitoring vital signs
- Repositioning and recalibrating pressure transducers

Pillow supports should be placed on each side of the patient's chest and forehead so that the ET and head are not compressed.

(From Wilkins RL, Stoller JK, Scanlan CL, editors: Egan's fundamentals of respiratory care, ed 9, St Louis, 2009, Mosby.)

---

corner of the mouth. Most of the body that touches the bed does not have a fat layer to cushion it (e.g., knees, forehead, elbows). Protective cushions are placed under the shoulders, hips, and ankles to help prevent pressure lesions and compression of the abdomen.[109,153-155] Proper arm position is important. The swimmer's position can be used to angle the arm, but a 90-degree angle should be avoided to prevent pressure on the brachial plexus.

Immediately following repositioning, the patient may experience transient hemodynamic instability and oxygen desaturation. This instability can be minimized by preoxygenating the patient with 100% O_2 and using sedatives.[111] Placing the patient in the prone position puts pressure on the chest wall, reducing chest wall compliance.[149] This may actually improve the uniformity of V_T distribution.[138] Moving a patient to the prone position is one procedure in which it is acceptable to ventilate with $P_{plateau}$ higher than 30 cm H_2O because of the reduced anterior chest wall movement. (NOTE: A safe $P_{plateau}$ when ventilating patients in the prone position has not been determined.)

There is no consensus about the length of time a patient can be placed in the prone position. Recommendations range from 2 to 24 hours, although it may require up to 12 hours of positioning daily to improve a patient's oxygenation status.[114] One case study reported a period of 72 hours of prone positioning.[155] It would seem that if prone positioning is to be of benefit, the position needs to be maintained for at least 20 hours/day, allowing return to the supine position for daily nursing care.[154]

The patient must be examined periodically for skin lesions. Patient feeding by the **transpyloric** enteral route may reduce the risk of vomiting and aspiration associated with gastric compression caused by the prone position.[155]

The effect of prone positioning on survival has not been firmly established.[145,158] It continues to be accepted as a safe and effective method to improve oxygenation in ARDS. It may also be indicated for those patients who fail to respond to lung recruitment maneuvers (high levels of PEEP [>12 cm H_2O]) and high inspired O_2 (≥60%).[154]

Patient Position in Unilateral Lung Disease

Two methods are typically used to manage the ventilatory status of patients with unilateral lung disease. The first method involves **independent lung ventilation**, which requires two ventilators and a double-lumen ET. Each lung is ventilated separately. Although it is an effective method to treat unilateral lung disease, not all facilities are able to provide this technique.

Another method that has received a considerable amount of interest is to place the patient in a lateral position so that the "good" lung is in the down, or dependent, position (Fig. 13-22).[159-161] In those cases in which it is difficult or impossible to place the patient in a lateral position, a kinetic bed may be used.

The pathological findings in unilateral lung disease include severe hypoxemia resulting from the persistence of pulmonary blood flow through the consolidated lung. The persistent blood flow through the consolidated lung units occurs because of failure of hypoxic vasoconstriction.

When one lung is affected by a pathologic process (e.g., atelectasis, consolidation, or infiltrates), and the affected lung is in the dependent position (down), the P_aO_2 value is lower than when the normal lung is in the dependent position.[160-162] Normally, the dependent portion of the lung is better perfused. When the affected lung is dependent, the blood flow to it also increases. However, ventilation to this lung does not increase proportionally. The decreased ventilation to the dependent diseased lung could be due to the disease process itself; that is, the alveoli may be filled with exudate. It may also be due to an increased distribution of ventilation to the nondependent areas, particularly if the patient is on positive pressure ventilation (PPV). Lateral positioning dramatically improves gas exchange by improving $\dot{V}/\dot{Q}$ matching without causing any hemodynamic complications, thus potentially allowing a decrease in F_IO_2 (Case Study 13-5).[160]

 Case Study 13-5

Changing Patient Position

A patient with pneumonia involving the right lung is receiving mechanical ventilation. The nurse repositions the patient on the right side for a procedure and the pulse oximetry low-oxygen alarm activates. What is the most likely cause of this problem?

Administration of PEEP in unilateral lung disease can cause an uneven distribution of PEEP to the normal lung when the patient is ventilated with a standard ET. Using PEEP in this case would cause increased shunting of pulmonary blood flow away from the healthy lung as a result of overinflation of the normal lung. If this is coupled with an increased blood flow to the diseased lung, $\dot{V}/\dot{Q}$ and altered gas exchange occur. For this reason, unilateral lung ventilation or proper positioning may be more effective than PEEP to improve oxygenation when compared with standard ventilation in unilateral lung disease.

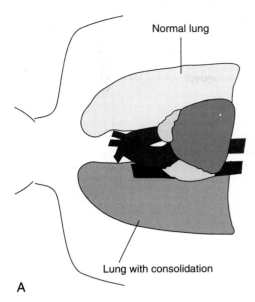

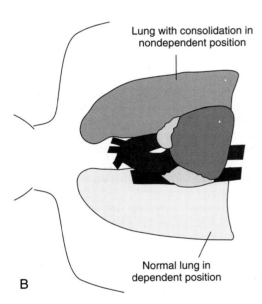

Fig. 13-22 A, Normal lung in the nondependent position and lung with consolidation in the dependent ("down") position. **B,** Normal lung in the dependent ("down") position and consolidated lung in the nondependent position. (See text for additional information.)

Additional Patient Cases

 ### Clinical Scenario: Adult Respiratory Distress Syndrome

In Chapter 7, the case of a 60-year-old trauma victim was presented. He developed severe dyspnea and hypoxemia and required mechanical ventilation. He was later diagnosed with ARDS.

Ventilator settings were VC-IMV + PSV; V_T = 600 mL; f = 16 breaths/min; flow = 100 L/min using a descending ramp waveform; PEEP = +5 cm H_2O; F_IO_2 = 1.0.

The following information relates to the patient after being on ventilatory support with the previous settings for 30 min:

- ABGs: pH = 7.43; P_aCO_2 = 38 mm Hg; P_aO_2 = 189 mm Hg; HCO_3^- = 22 mEq/L on F_IO_2 = 1.0
- Pressures: PIP = 24 cm H_2O; $P_{plateau}$ = 18 cm H_2O; PEEP = +5 cm H_2O; PSV = 10 cm H_2O

A recruitment maneuver is performed. PEEP is set at 2 to 4 cm H_2O above the UIPd measured during derecruitment. The patient is placed on pressure-controlled continuous mandatory ventilation (PC-CMV) with the following settings: F_IO_2 = 0.8; set pressure = 15 cm H_2O; f = 12 breaths/min; PEEP = +15 cm H_2O (PIP = 30 cm H_2O); I:E ratio = 1:2; measured V_T = 525 mL. ABGs on these settings are as follows: pH = 7.36; P_aCO_2 = 48 mm Hg; P_aO_2 = 224 mm Hg; HCO_3^- = 29 mEq/L. At this point the F_IO_2 is decreased to 0.5 to bring it into a safer range. The P_aO_2 will be kept at greater than 60 mm Hg. The acid–base status is acceptable.

The patient is successfully managed over the next 2 weeks, during which ventilator support is progressively reduced. He is eventually discontinued from ventilation and extubated.

Clinical Scenario: Congestive Heart Failure

A patient with CHF has been in the ICU receiving mechanical ventilatory support since admission 2 days ago. Current ventilator parameters and hemodynamic data include volume-control continuous mandatory ventilation (VC-CMV); V_T = 480 mL (7 mL/kg); f = 12 breaths/min; PIP = 23 cm H_2O; $P_{plateau}$ = 16 cm H_2O; PEEP = 0 cm H_2O. ABGs are pH = 7.37; P_aCO_2 = 37 mm Hg; P_aO_2 = 58 mm Hg; HCO_3^- = 23 mEq/L on F_IO_2 = 0.5; PAP = 45/21; PAOP = 26 mm Hg; cardiac index (C.I.) = 2.9 L/min/m². Chest radiographs show increased vascular markings and fluffy infiltrates in a butterfly-like pattern near the hilar region of the lungs. Auscultation reveals bilateral moist crackles. Physical, radiographic, and hemodynamic findings indicate the presence of pulmonary edema. The diagnosis is cardiogenic pulmonary edema.

A PEEP study is performed and the following table shows it in an abbreviated form.

Time	PEEP (cm H_2O)	F_IO_2	P_aO_2 (mm Hg)	CI (L/min/m²)	C_S (mL/cm H_2O)
11:00	5	0.5	65	3.1	24
11:30	10	0.5	78	3.3	31
12:00	15	0.5	123	3.9	35
12:30	20	0.5	153	3.5	30

These findings indicate an improvement in parameters up to a PEEP of +15 cm H_2O. At +20 cm H_2O, PEEP, CI, and compliance became worse, suggesting lung overdistention and decreased cardiac output. The use of PEEP in cardiogenic pulmonary edema can improve O_2 transport not only by increasing P_aO_2 but also by increasing cardiac output in some cases (see Chapter 16).

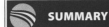
SUMMARY

- The most common parameters used to assess oxygenation status of patients are the F_IO_2, arterial blood gases (ABGs), CO-oximetry, and hemodynamic measurements.

- A linear relationship exists between P_aO_2 and F_IO_2 for any patient as long as the cardiopulmonary status remains fairly constant.

- While the exact level of F_IO_2 that is safe for mechanically ventilated patients is not known at this time, it is generally agreed that maintaining a high F_IO_2 (>0.6) can result in oxygen toxicity.

- Mean airway pressure is a major determinant of oxygenation in patients with ARDS because it affects mean alveolar pressure ($M_{alv}P$) and alveolar recruitment.

- The treatment of acute atelectasis involves identifying the cause and then initiating an appropriate corrective action.

- The goals of PEEP/CPAP therapy are to enhance tissue oxygenation, maintain a P_aO_2 above 60 mm Hg and S_pO_2 ≥90%, at an acceptable pH, recruit alveoli and maintain them in an aerated state, and restore functional residual capacity.

- PEEP as it is commonly used implies that the patient is receiving ventilatory support and the baseline pressure is above zero; CPAP is pressure above the ambient pressure maintained during spontaneous ventilation.

- Two levels or ranges of PEEP can be employed: minimum or low PEEP, also called "physiological PEEP," and therapeutic PEEP.

- Therapeutic PEEP is used in the treatment of refractory hypoxemia caused by increased intrapulmonary shunting and ventilation-perfusion mismatching accompanied by a decreased FRC and pulmonary compliance.

- PEEP is beneficial for the treatment of patients with ARDS because it helps to prevent the collapse of the small airways and alveoli and thus aids in the recruiting closed lung units.

- C_S is considered a good indicator of the effects of PEEP on the lung.

- When PEEP greater than 15 cm H_2O is used, it is important to evaluate the patient's hemodynamic status closely, which may require the placement of a balloon-flotation pulmonary artery catheter.

- Static pressure–volume (SPV) loops have been used to select an optimum PEEP level and V_T in ALI. Current theory suggests that it is more important to set PEEP above the upper inflection point detected during deflation of the lung (UIPd).

- PEEP can be detrimental to a patient's cardiovascular status because it can reduce cardiac output and compromise circulation, leading to a reduction in BP. A relative contraindication for PEEP is hypovolemia.

- Classification of the severity of ARDS is based on the P_aO_2/F_IO_2 ratio. Mild ARDS is defined as a P_aO_2/FiO_2 ratio of between 300 and 200 mm Hg, moderate ARDS is defined as between 200 and 100 mm Hg, and severe ARDS is defined as a ratio of ≤100 mm Hg.

- ARDS can be divided into two phases: an acute exudative phase characterized by inflammation and alveolar filling, and a subacute phase, in which fibrosing alveolitis occurs.

- Clinicians sometimes divide ARDS into two categories: *direct* and *indirect. Direct* ARDS includes disorders of the lung that directly affect lung tissue; *indirect* ARDS is referred to as *secondary* or *nonpulmonary* ARDS because injury to the lung is not the result of a direct lung insult.

- The ARDS Network trial and other studies provide strong evidence in support of using V_Ts of 6 mL/kg or lower and a $P_{plateau}$ less than 30 cm H_2O when ventilating patients with ARDS.

- A recruitment maneuver (RM) is a sustained increase in pressure in the lungs with the goal of opening as many collapsed lung units as possible.

- Recruitment occurs across the entire range of lung volume from residual volume to TLC. Once the lungs are recruited, they are kept open by maintaining an adequate PEEP above the LIP of an inspiratory maneuver or, preferably, above the UIP of a deflation (expiratory) maneuver.

- Lung recruitment maneuvers are more likely to improve oxygenation and lung compliance in patients with secondary ARDS.

- Placing a patient with ARDS in a prone position may improve oxygenation and decrease the degree of shunt in the patient's lungs.

REVIEW QUESTIONS *(See Appendix A for answers)*

1. A 25-year-old woman is recovering from severe pneumonia and has been receiving ventilatory support for 2 days. Current F_IO_2 is 0.6, and the patient's P_aO_2 on this setting is 200 mm Hg. What change in F_IO_2 would achieve a target P_aO_2 of 80 mm Hg?
   A. 0.75
   B. 0.25
   C. 0.50
   D. 0.40

2. CPAP can only be used with patients who have which of the following characteristics?
   A. Have high P_aCO_2 levels
   B. Can breathe spontaneously
   C. Are hypovolemic
   D. Have central sleep apnea

3. A PEEP study is being performed on a patient. When the PEEP is increased from +10 cm H_2O to +15 cm H_2O, cardiac output decreases from 4 L/min to 2 L/min. What would be the next most appropriate step?
   A. Decrease F_IO_2
   B. Administer whole blood
   C. Decrease PEEP to +10 cm H_2O
   D. Make no changes at this time

4. The following table represents a PEEP study for a patient with ARDS. Which PEEP level represents the optimum one for the patient?

	A	B	C	D
PEEP (cm H_2O)	5	8	12	15
$P\bar{v}O_2$ (mm Hg)	35	37	39	34
$C[a-\bar{v}]O_2$ (mL/100 mL)	3.7	3.6	3.8	4.1
C.O.* (L/min)	7.6	7.5	7.6	6.3
C.O. $\times$ C_aO_2 (mL/min) (O_2 transport)	875	865	950	825

*C.O., Cardiac output.

5. During mechanical ventilation with VC-CMV, the PEEP level is set at +10 cm H_2O and PIP is 34 cm H_2O. The PEEP is increased to +15 cm H_2O and PIP rises to 40 cm H_2O. The rise in PIP indicates which of the following?
   A. A normal occurrence when PEEP is increased
   B. A bronchospasm
   C. The presence of a pneumothorax
   D. That compliance had changed

6. A 38-year-old man with ARDS is undergoing mechanical ventilation. The results of an ABG analysis are pH = 7.38; P_aCO_2 = 42 mm Hg; P_aO_2 = 55 mm Hg. The ventilator settings are: F_IO_2 = 0.9; f = 10 breaths/min; V_T = 550 mL; PEEP = +5 cm H_2O. Based on this information, which of the following might be changed to improve the patient's oxygenation status?
   A. V_T
   B. f
   C. Oxygen
   D. PEEP

7. Recent research suggests the way to establish an optimum PEEP level in a patient with ARDS is to do which of the following?
   A. Perform an inspiratory P-V curve maneuver
   B. Progressively increase PEEP until cardiac output decreases
   C. Perform a recruitment–derecruitment maneuver to establish the UIPd during deflation (deflection point)
   D. Monitor $P\bar{v}O_2$

8. Assessment for optimum PEEP is being determined in a mechanically ventilated patient. PEEP is increased progressively from 5 to 10 to 15 cm H_2O. Volume delivery remains constant at 450 mL. P_aO_2 increases progressively from 55 to 63 to 78 mm Hg. BP remains fairly constant. Mixed venous PO_2 goes from 27 to 36 to 30 mm Hg at +15 cm H_2O of PEEP. Based on these findings, the most appropriate action is to do which of the following?
   A. Use a PEEP of 5 cm H_2O
   B. Use a PEEP of 10 cm H_2O
   C. Use a PEEP of 15 cm H_2O
   D. Increase PEEP to 20 cm H_2O and repeat the study

9. A 70-kg man with bilateral viral pneumonia is on VC-IMV. His set V_T is 500 mL; minimum rate is 15 breaths/min with no spontaneous breaths; 40% O_2; +5 cm H_2O of PEEP; and the following ABG values: pH = 7.48; P_aCO_2 = 30 mm Hg; P_aO_2 = 98 mm Hg. Which of the following is appropriate?
   A. Increase PEEP to +10 cm H_2O
   B. Increase F_IO_2 to 0.5
   C. Increase V_T
   D. Decrease f

10. If you could select only one parameter or value that you wanted to evaluate to establish optimum PEEP in a patient, what would you select? Why?

11. The first parameter to measure following the administration of PEEP is which of the following?
    A. HR
    B. BP
    C. PAOP
    D. PAP

12. A patient on CPAP of 10 cm H_2O has f = 36 breaths/min; pH = 7.23; P_aCO_2 = 54 mm Hg; P_aO_2 = 75 mm Hg (F_IO_2 = 0.5). The most appropriate action is to do which of the following?
    A. Increase CPAP to 15 cm H_2O
    B. Increase F_IO_2
    C. Begin mechanical ventilation
    D. Decrease CPAP to +5 cm H_2O

13. A patient has a P_aO_2/F_IO_2 ratio of 150 and severe sepsis. Compliance is reduced and chest radiograph reveals bilateral infiltrates. Which of the following statements are true about this patient?
    1. The patient has moderate ARDS.
    2. This type of patient will probably have an improvement in oxygenation with a recruitment maneuver.
    3. Low V_T and therapeutic PEEP ventilation should be used with this patient.
    4. Protective lung strategies should be started as soon as possible.
       A. 1 only
       B. 2 and 3 only
       C. 1 and 4 only
       D. 1, 2, 3, and 4

14. It is better to use the inspiratory limb of an SPV curve for determining LIP and UIP than to use the deflation limb of the curve.
    A. True
    B. False

15. The purpose of setting an adequate PEEP level in ARDS is to:
    A. Avoid overdistention of the lung
    B. Prevent alveolar collapse at end exhalation
    C. Increase perfusion of the lung
    D. Improve ventilation

16. A patient with ARDS has an ideal (predicted) body weight of 53 kg. An acceptable V_T using a protective lung strategy would be:
    A. 150 mL
    B. 320 mL
    C. 530 mL
    D. 630 mL

17. During mechanical ventilation of patients with ARDS it is strongly recommended that $P_{plateau}$ not exceed 30 cm H_2O.
    A. True
    B. False

18. A 38-year-old woman with ARDS is on +15 cm H₂O of PEEP and an F$_I$O₂ of 0.85. Ventilation is acceptable, but P$_a$O₂ is only 54 mm Hg. What might the respiratory therapist recommend for improving the patient's oxygenation?
    A. Set the F$_I$O₂ at 0.5
    B. Set the PEEP to +10 cm H₂O
    C. Change the patient to the prone position
    D. Recommend an increase in $\dot{V}_E$

19. The improvement in ventilation-perfusion matching and oxygenation seen with prone positioning has been associated with which of the following factors?
    A. Relieving the weight of the heart, great vessels, and part of the abdominal contents from the lungs
    B. Increase in perfusion to the nondependent portion of the lungs when the patient is positioned face down
    C. Clearance of secretion from the airways
    D. Improvement in chest wall compliance in the prone position

20. Which of the following indicates that a patient is ready to be weaned from PEEP/CPAP?
    1. P$_a$O₂ is 80 mm Hg on 30% O₂
    2. The patient is stable and has no active infections
    3. C$_L$ is 37 mL/cm H₂O
    4. P$_a$O₂/F$_I$O₂ ratio is 300
       A. 1 only
       B. 1 and 2 only
       C. 2 and 4 only
       D. 1, 2, 3, and 4

21. The inflection point on the deflation curve (deflection point) using the P-V loop for a patient with ARDS is 8 cm H₂O. At what value would PEEP be set?
    A. 6 cm H₂O
    B. 8 cm H₂O
    C. 10 cm H₂O
    D. Cannot be determined from this information

References

1. American Association for Respiratory Care: Clinical practice guideline: patient-ventilator system check. *Respir Care* 37:882–886, 1992.
2. Sasse SA, Jaffe MB, Chen PA, et al: Arterial oxygenation time after an F$_I$O₂ increase in mechanically ventilated patients. *Am J Respir Crit Care Med* 152:148–152, 1995.
3. Cairo JM: *Mosby's respiratory care equipment*, ed 9, St Louis, 2014, Elsevier.
4. Mithoefer JC, Keighley JF, Karetzkey MS: Response of the arterial PO₂ to oxygen administration in chronic pulmonary disease. *Ann Intern Med* 74:328–335, 1971.
5. Mithoefer JC, Holford FD, Keighley JFH: The effect of oxygen administration on mixed venous oxygenation in chronic obstructive pulmonary disease. *Chest* 66:122–132, 1974.
6. Kacmarek RM: Initiating and adjusting ventilatory support. In Kacmarek RM, Stoller JK, Heuer AJ, editors: *Egan's fundamentals of respiratory care*, ed 10, St Louis, 2013, Elsevier, pp 1088–1130.
7. Maxwell C, Hess D, Shefet D: Use of the arterial/alveolar oxygen tension ratio to predict the inspired oxygen concentration needed for a desired arterial oxygen tension. *Respir Care* 29:1135–1139, 1984.
8. Gilbert R, Keighley JF: The arterial/alveolar oxygen tension ratio: an index of gas exchange applicable to varying inspired oxygen concentrations. *Am Rev Respir Dis* 109:142–145, 1974.
9. Hess D, Maxwell C: Which is the best index of oxygenation—P(A–a)O₂, PaO₂/PAO₂ or PaO₂/FiO₂? *Respir Care* 30:961–963, 1985.
10. Shapiro BA, Cane RD, Harrison RA, et al: Changes in intrapulmonary shunting with administration of 100% oxygen. *Chest* 77:138–141, 1980.
11. Lodata RF: Oxygen toxicity. In Tobin MJ, editor: *Principles and practice of mechanical ventilation*, ed 3, New York, 2013, McGraw-Hill, pp 1065–1090.
12. American Association for Respiratory Care Clinical Practice Guideline: Oxygen therapy for adults in the acute care facility. *Respir Care* 47:717–720, 2002.
13. Rothen HU, Sporre B, Engberg G, et al: Influence of gas composition on recurrent atelectasis after a reexpansion maneuver during general anesthesia. *Anesthesiology* 82:832–842, 1995.
14. Santos C, Ferrer M, Roca J, et al: Pulmonary gas exchange response to oxygen breathing in acute lung injury. *Am J Respir Crit Care Med* 161:26–31, 2000.
15. Marcy TW, Marini JJ: Inverse ratio ventilation in ARDS: rationale and implementation. *Chest* 100:494–504, 1991.
16. Rodriguez-Roisin R, Ferrer A: Effects of mechanical ventilation on gas exchange. In Tobin MJ, editor: *Principles and practice of mechanical ventilation*, ed 3, New York, 2013, McGraw-Hill, pp 851–867.
17. Armstrong BW, MacIntyre NR: Pressure-controlled, inverse ratio ventilation that avoids air trapping in the adult respiratory distress syndrome. *Crit Care Med* 23:279–285, 1995.
18. Neumann P, Berglund JE, Lars G, et al: Effects of inverse ratio ventilation and positive end-expiratory pressure in oleic acid-induced lung injury. *Am J Respir Crit Care Med* 161:1537–1545, 2000.
19. MacIntyre NR, Branson RD: *Mechanical ventilation*, ed 2, Philadelphia, 2007, W.B. Saunders.
20. Mercat A, Graini L, Teboul JL, et al: Cardiorespiratory effects of pressure-controlled ventilation with and without inverse ratio in the adult respiratory distress syndrome. *Chest* 104:871–875, 1993.
21. Sydow M, Burchardi H, Ephraim E, et al: Long-term effects of two different ventilatory modes on oxygenation in acute lung injury: comparison of airway pressure release ventilation and volume-controlled inverse ratio ventilation. *Am J Respir Crit Care Med* 149:1550–1556, 1994.
22. Marini JJ: Weaning techniques and protocols. *Respir Care* 40:233–238, 1995.
23. Hudson LD, Weaver LJ, Haisch CE, et al: Positive end-expiratory pressure: reduction and withdrawal. *Respir Care* 33(7):613–617, 1988.
24. Marini JJ, Tyler ML, Hudson LD, et al: Influence of head-dependent positions on lung volume and oxygen saturation in chronic airflow obstruction. *Am Rev Respir Dis* 128:101–105, 1984.
25. MacIntyre NR: Management of parenchymal lung injury. In MacIntyre NR, Branson RD, editors: *Mechanical ventilation*, ed 2, St Louis, 2009, Saunders-Elsevier, pp 287–296.
26. Suter PM, Fairley HB, Isenberg MD: Optimum end-expiratory airway pressure in patients with acute pulmonary failure. *N Engl J Med* 292:284–289, 1975.
27. Peruzzi WT: The current status of PEEP. *Respir Care* 41:273–279, 1996.
28. Talmor D, Sarge T, Malhotra A, et al: Mechanical ventilation guided by esophageal pressure in acute lung injury. *N Engl J Med* 359:2095–2104, 2008.
29. Maggiore SM, Jonson B, Richard JC, et al: Alveolar derecruitment at decremental positive end-expiratory pressure levels in acute lung injury: comparison with the lower inflection point, oxygenation and compliance. *Am J Respir Crit Care Med* 164:795–801, 2001.
30. Gattinoni L, Pesenti A, Avalli L, et al: Pressure-volume curve of total respiratory system in acute respiratory failure: a computed tomographic scan study. *Am Rev Respir Dis* 136:730–736, 1987.
31. Gattinoni L, Pelosi P, Crotti S, et al: Effects of positive end-expiratory pressure on regional distribution of tidal volume and recruitment in adult respiratory distress syndrome. *Am J Respir Crit Care Med* 151:1807–1814, 1995.
32. Badar T, Bidani A: Mechanical ventilatory support. *Chest Surg Clin N Am* 12:265–299, 2002.
33. Saura P, Blanch L: How to set positive end-expiratory pressures. *Respir Care* 47:279–292, 2002.
34. The Acute Respiratory Distress Syndrome Network (ARDSnet): Ventilation with lower tidal volumes as compared with traditional tidal volumes for acute lung injury and the acute respiratory distress syndrome. *N Engl J Med* 342:1301–1308, 2000.
35. National Heart, Lung, and Blood Institute ARDS Clinical Trials Network: Higher versus lower positive end-expiratory pressures in patients with the acute respiratory distress syndrome. *N Engl J Med* 352:327–336, 2004.

36. Meade MO, Cook DJ, Guyatt GH, et al: Ventilation strategy using low tidal volumes, recruitment maneuvers, and high positive end-expiratory pressure for acute lung injury and acute respiratory distress syndrome. *JAMA* 299:637–645, 2008.

37. Villar J, Pérez-Méndez L, Lopez J, et al: An early PEEP/F$_i$O$_2$ trial identifies different degrees of lung injury inpatients with acute respiratory distress syndrome. *Am J Respir Crit Care Med* 176:795–804, 2007.

38. Hess DR: Mechanical ventilation strategies: what's new and what's worth keeping. *Respir Care* 47:1007–1017, 2002.

39. DesJardin T, Burton GG: *Clinical manifestations and assessment of respiratory disease*, ed 4, St Louis, 2002, Mosby.

40. Nelson RD, Singer M: Supranormal P$\overline{v}$O$_2$ in the presence of tissue hypoxia: a case report. *Respir Care* 28:191–194, 1983.

41. Patel M, Singer M: The optimal time for measuring the cardiorespiratory effects of positive end-expiratory pressure. *Chest* 104:139–142, 1993.

42. Craig KC, Pierson DJ, Carrico JC: The clinical application of PEEP in ARDS. *Respir Care* 30:184–201, 1985.

43. Katz JA: PEEP and CPAP in perioperative respiratory care. *Respir Care* 29:614–629, 1984.

44. Suarez-Sipmann F, Böhm SH, Tusman G, et al: Use of dynamic compliance for open lung positive end-expiratory pressure titration in an experimental study. *Crit Care Med* 35:214–221, 2007.

45. Demers RR, Pratter MR, Irwin RS: Use of the concept of ventilator compliance in the determination of static total compliance. *Respir Care* 26:644–648, 1981.

46. Murray JF, Wilkins RL, Jacobsen WK, et al: Titration of PEEP by the atrial minus end-tidal carbon dioxide gradient. *Chest* 85:100–104, 1984.

47. Nicotra MB, Rogers M, Miller L: Physiologic evaluation of positive and expiratory pressure ventilation. *Chest* 64:10–15, 1973.

48. Sugerman HJ, Rogers RM, Miller LD: Positive end-expiratory pressure (PEEP): indications and physiologic considerations. *Chest* 62(Suppl 2):86S–94S, 1972.

49. Davidson R, Parker M, Harrison RA: The validity of determinations of pulmonary wedge pressure during mechanical ventilation. *Chest* 73:352–355, 1978.

50. Shasby DM, Dauber IM, Pfister S, et al: Swan-Ganz catheter location and left atrial pressure determine the accuracy of the wedge pressure when positive end-expiratory pressure is used. *Chest* 80:666–670, 1981.

51. Weisman IM, Rinaldo JE, Rogers RM: Positive end-expiratory pressure in adult respiratory failure. *N Engl J Med* 307:1381–1384, 1982.

52. Murphy BA, Durbin CG: Using ventilator and cardiovascular graphics in the patient who is hemodynamically unstable. *Respir Care* 50:262–274, 2005.

53. Saura P, Blanch L: How to set positive end-expiratory pressures. *Respir Care* 47:279–292, 2002.

54. Adams AB, Cakar N, Marini JJ: Static and dynamic pressure-volume curves reflect different aspects of respiratory system mechanics in experimental acute respiratory distress syndrome. *Respir Care* 46:686–693, 2001.

55. Bone RC: Complications of mechanical ventilation and positive end-expiratory pressure. *Respir Care* 27:402–407, 1982.

56. Tusman G, Böhm SH, Vazquez de Anda GF, et al: Alveolar recruitment strategy improves arterial oxygenation during general anaesthesia. *Br J Anaesth* 82:8–13, 1999.

57. Almgren B, Wickerts CJ, Hogman M: Post-suction recruitment maneuver restores lung function in healthy, anesthetized pigs. *Anaesth Intensive Care* 32:339–345, 2004.

58. Kumar A, Konrad JF, Gerrin B, et al: Continuous positive pressure ventilation in acute respiratory failure: effects on hemodynamics and lung function. *N Engl J Med* 283:1430–1436, 1970.

59. Amato M: Conventional and pressure limited approaches to ARDS. In *Mechanical ventilation—principles and applications*, St Paul, 1995, University of Minnesota.

60. Ashbaugh DG, Bigelow DB, Petty TL, et al: Acute respiratory distress in adults. *Lancet* 2:319–323, 1967.

61. Bernard GR, Artigas A, Brigham KL, et al: The American-European Consensus Conference on ARDS: definitions, mechanisms, relevant outcomes, and clinical trial coordination. *Am J Respir Crit Care Med* 149:818–824, 1994.

62. ARDS Definition Task Force, Ranieri VM, Rubenfeld GD: Acute respiratory distress syndrome: The Berlin definition. *JAMA* 307:2526–2533, 2012.

63. Fanelli V, Vlachou A, Ghannadian S, et al: Acute respiratory distress syndrome: new definition, current and future therapeutic options. *J Thorac Dis* 5:326–334, 2013.

64. Gattinoni L, Caironi P, Pelosi P, et al: What has computed tomography taught us about the acute respiratory distress syndrome? *Am J Respir Crit Care Med* 164:1701–1711, 2001.

65. Gattinoni L, Pesenti A, Bombino M, et al: Relationships between lung computed tomographic density, gas exchange, and PEEP in acute respiratory failure. *Anesthesiology* 69:824–832, 1988.

66. Piantadosi CA, Schwartz DA: The acute respiratory distress syndrome. *Ann Intern Med* 141:460–470, 2004.

67. Hess DR, Bigatello LM: Lung recruitment: the role of recruitment maneuvers. *Respir Care* 47:308–317, 2002.

68. Gattinoni L, Caironi P, Cressoni M, et al: Lung recruitment in patients with acute respiratory distress syndrome. *N Engl J Med* 354:1775–1786, 2006.

69. Villar J, Kacmarek RM, Hedenstierna G: From ventilator-induced lung injury to physician-induced lung injury: Why the reluctance to use small tidal volumes? *Acta Anaesthesiol Scand* 48:267–271, 2004.

70. Gattinoni L, Mascheroni D, Torresin A, et al: Morphological response to positive end expiratory pressure in acute respiratory failure: computerized tomography study. *Intensive Care Med* 12:137–142, 1986.

71. Crotti S, Mascheroni D, Caironi P, et al: Recruitment and decruitment during acute respiratory failure: a clinical study. *Am J Respir Crit Care Med* 164:131–140, 2001.

72. Kuhlen R, Rossaint R: The role of spontaneous breathing during mechanical ventilation. *Respir Care* 47:296–303, 2002.

73. Girgis K, Hamed H, Khater Y, et al: A decremental PEEP trial identifies the PEEP level that maintains oxygenation after lung recruitment. *Respir Care* 51:1132–1139, 2006.

74. Navalesi P, Maggiore SM: Positive end-expiratory pressure. In Tobin MJ, editor: *Principles and practice of mechanical ventilation*, ed 3, New York, 2013, McGraw-Hill, pp 253–302.

75. Hickling KG: The pressure-volume curve is greatly modified by recruitment: a mathematical model of ARDS lungs. *Am J Respir Crit Care Med* 158:194–202, 1998.

76. Jonson B, Richard JC, Straus C, et al: Pressure-volume curves and compliance in acute lung injury: evidence of recruitment above the lower inflection point. *Am J Respir Crit Care Med* 159:1172–1178, 1999.

77. Amato MBP, Barbas CSV, Medeiros DM, et al: Effect of protective-ventilation strategy on mortality in the acute respiratory distress syndrome. *N Engl J Med* 338:347–354, 1998.

78. Steinberg KP, Kacmarek RM: Should tidal volume be 6 mL/kg predicted body weight in virtually all patients with acute respiratory failure. *Respir Care* 52:556–567, 2007.

79. Stewart TE: Controversies around lung protective mechanical ventilation. *Am J Respir Crit Care Med* 166:1421–1422, 2002.

80. Kallet RH, Katz JA: Respiratory system mechanics in acute respiratory distress syndrome. *Respir Care Clin N Am* 9:297–319, 2003.

81. Haitsma JJ, Lachmann RA, Lachmann B: Lung protective ventilation in ARDS: role of mediators, PEEP and surfactant. *Monaldi Arch Chest Dis* 59:108–118, 2003.

82. Malhotra A: Low tidal-volume ventilation in the acute respiratory distress syndrome. *N Engl J Med* 357:1113–1120, 2007.

83. Young MP, Manning HL, Wilson DL, et al: Ventilation of patients with acute lung injury and acute respiratory distress syndrome: has new evidence changed clinical practice? *Crit Care Med* 32:1260–1265, 2004.

84. Rubenfeld GD, Cooper C, Carter G, et al: Barriers to providing lung-protective ventilation to patients with acute lung injury. *Crit Care Med* 32:1289–1293, 2004.

85. Esteban A, Anzueto A, Alia I, et al: How is mechanical ventilation employed in the intensive care unit? An international utilization review. *Am J Respir Crit Care Med* 161:1450–1458, 2000.

86. MacIntyre NR: Current issues in mechanical ventilation for respiratory failure. *Chest* 128:561S–567S, 2005.

87. Dreyfuss D, Saumon G: Role of tidal volume, FRC, and end-inspiratory volume in the development of pulmonary edema following mechanical ventilation. *Am Rev Respir Dis* 148:1194–1203, 1993.

88. ARDSnet, National Heart, Lung, and Blood Institute, National Institute of Health: Effects of recruitment maneuvers in patients with acute lung injury and acute respiratory distress syndrome ventilated with high positive end-expiratory pressure. *Crit Care Med* 31:2592–2597, 2003.

89. Adams AB: Monitoring and management of the patient in the intensive care unit. In Wilkins RL, Stoller JK, Scanlan L, editors: *Egan's fundamentals of respiratory care*, ed 10, St Louis, 2013, Elsevier, pp 1159–1198.

90. Neumann P, Berglund JE, Mondejar EF, et al: Effect of different pressure levels on the dynamics of lung collapse and recruitment in oleic acid induced lung injury. *Am J Respir Crit Care Med* 158:1636–1643, 1998.

91. Uhlig S: Taking a peep at the upper airways (letter). *Am J Respir Crit Care Med* 168:1026–1027, 2003.

92. Marini JJ: Are recruiting maneuvers needed when ventilating acute respiratory distress syndrome? (letter). *Crit Care Med* 31:2701–2703, 2003.

93. Terragni PP, Rosboch G, Tealdi A, et al: Tidal hyperinflation during low tidal volume ventilation in acute respiratory distress syndrome. *Am J Respir Crit Care Med* 175:160–166, 2007.

94. Papadakos PJ, Lachmann B: The open lung concept of alveolar recruitment can improve outcome in respiratory failure and ARDS. *Mount Sinai J Med* 69:73–77, 2002.

95. Meade MO, Herridge MS: An evidence-based approach to acute respiratory distress syndrome. *Respir Care* 46:1368–1376, 2001.

96. DiRocco JD, Carney DE, Nieman GF: Correlation between alveolar recruitment/derecruitment and inflection points on the pressure-volume curve. *Intensive Care Med* 33:1204–1211, 2007.

97. Marini JJ: Inverse ratio ventilation: simply an alternative or something more? *Crit Care Med* 23:224–228, 1995.

98. Villar J, Kacmarek RM, Pérez-Méndez L, et al: A high positive end-expiratory pressure, low tidal volume ventilatory strategy improves outcome in persistent acute respiratory distress syndrome: a randomized, controlled trial. *Crit Care Med* 34:1311–1318, 2006.

99. Marini JJ: Pressure-targeted mechanical ventilation of acute lung injury. *Semin Respir Med* 14:262–269, 1993.

100. Levy P, Similowski T, Corbeil C, et al: A method for studying the static volume-pressure curves of the respiratory system during mechanical ventilation. *J Crit Care* 4:83–89, 1989.

101. Ranieri VM, Eissa NT, Corbeil C, et al: Effects of positive end-expiratory pressure on alveolar recruitment and gas exchange in patients with adult respiratory distress syndrome. *Am Rev Respir Dis* 144:544–551, 1991.

102. Fernandez R, Blanch L, Artigas A: Inflation static pressure-volume curves of the total respiratory system determined without any instrumentation other than the mechanical ventilator. *Intensive Care Med* 19:33–38, 1993.

103. Schiller HJ, Steinberg J, Halter J, et al: Alveolar inflation during generation of a quasi-static pressure/volume curve in the acutely injured lung. *Crit Care Med* 31:1126–1133, 2003.

104. Vieillard-Baron A, Prin S, Schmitt JM, et al: Pressure-volume curves in acute respiratory distress syndrome. *Am J Respir Crit Care Med* 165:1107–1112, 2002.

105. Branson R: Understanding and implementing advances in ventilator capabilities. *Curr Opin Crit Care* 10:23–32, 2004.

106. Hess DR, Kacmarek RM: *Essentials of mechanical ventilation*, ed 3, New York, 2014, McGraw-Hill.

107. Lee WL, Stewart TE, MacDonald R, et al: Safety of pressure-volume curve measurement in acute lung injury and ARDS using a syringe technique. *Chest* 121:1595–1601, 2002.

108. Harris RS: Pressure-volume curves of the respiratory system. *Respir Care* 50:78–98, 2005.

109. Blanc Q, Sab JM, Philit F, et al: Inspiratory pressure-volume curves obtained using automated low constant flow inflation and automated occlusion methods in ARDS patients with a new device. *Intensive Care Med* 28:990–994, 2002.

110. Maggiore SM, Brochard L: Pressure-volume curve in the critically ill. *Curr Opin Crit Care* 6:1–10, 2000.

111. Albaiceta GM, Piacentini E, Villagra ANA, et al: Application of continuous positive airway pressure to trace static pressure-volume curves of the respiratory system. *Crit Care Med* 31:2514–2519, 2003.

112. Ranieri VM, Giuliani R, Fiore T, et al: Volume-pressure curve of the respiratory system predicts effects of PEEP in ARDS: "Occlusion" versus "constant flow" technique. *Am J Respir Crit Care Med* 149:19–27, 1994.

113. Lu Q, Vieira SR, Richoeur J, et al: A simple automated method for measuring pressure-volume curves during mechanical ventilation. *Am J Respir Crit Care Med* 159:275–282, 1999.

114. Dyhr T, Laursen N, Larsson A: Effects of lung recruitment maneuver and positive end-expiratory pressure on lung volume, respiratory mechanics and alveolar gas mixing in patients ventilated after cardiac surgery. *Acta Anaesthesiol Scand* 46:717–725, 2002.

115. Medoff BD, Harris RS, Kesselman H, et al: Use of recruitment maneuvers and high positive end-expiratory pressure in a patient with acute respiratory distress syndrome. *Crit Care Med* 28:1210–1216, 2000.

116. Fenn WO, Rahn H, editors: Respiration (vol 1). In *Handbook of physiology*, Am Physiol Soc, Baltimore, 1964, Waverly Press.

117. Pelosi P, Goldner M, McKibben A, et al: Recruitment and derecruitment during acute respiratory failure: an experimental study. *Am J Respir Crit Care Med* 164:122–130, 2001.

118. Hickling KG: Best compliance during a decremental, but not incremental, positive end-expiratory pressure trial is related to open-lung positive end-expiratory pressure: a mathematical model of acute respiratory distress syndrome lungs. *Am J Respir Crit Care Med* 163:69–78, 2001.

119. Halter JM, Steinberg JM, Schiller HJ, et al: Positive end-expiratory pressure after a recruitment maneuver prevents both alveolar collapse and recruitment/derecruitment. *Am J Respir Crit Care Med* 167:1620–1626, 2003.

120. Lapinsky SE, Aubin M, Mehta S, et al: Safety and efficacy of a sustained inflation for alveolar recruitment in adults with respiratory failure. *Intensive Care Med* 25:1297–1301, 1999.

121. Borges JB, Okamoto V, Matos GFJ, et al: Reversibility of lung collapse and hypoxemia in early acute respiratory distress syndrome. *Am J Respir Crit Care Med* 174:268–278, 2006.

122. Rothen HU, Spore B, Engberg G, et al: Re-expansion of atelectasis during general anesthesia: a computed tomography study. *Br J Anesth* 71:788–795, 1993.

123. Lim CM, Koh Y, Park W, et al: Mechanistic scheme and effect of "extended sigh" as a recruitment maneuver in patients with acute respiratory distress syndrome: a preliminary study. *Crit Care Med* 29:1255–1260, 2001.

124. Badet M, Bayle F, Richard JC, et al: Comparison of optimal positive end-expiratory pressure and recruitment maneuvers during lung protective mechanical ventilation in patients with acute lung injury/acute respiratory distress syndrome. *Respir Care* 54:847–854, 2009.

125. Foti G, Cereda M, Sparacino ME, et al: Effects of periodic lung recruitment maneuvers on gas exchange and respiratory mechanics in mechanically ventilated acute respiratory distress syndrome (ARDS) patients. *Intensive Care Med* 26:501–507, 2000.

126. Marini JJ, Gattinoni L: Ventilatory management of acute respiratory distress syndrome: A consensus of two. *Crit Care Med* 32:250–255, 2004.

127. Grasso S, Mascia L, Del Turco M: Effects of recruiting maneuvers in patients with acute respiratory distress syndrome ventilated with protective ventilator strategy. *Anesthesiology* 96:795–802, 2002.

128. Tobin MJ, editor: *Principles and practice of mechanical ventilation*, ed 3, New York, 2013, McGraw-Hill.

129. Lim CM, Lee SS, Lee JS, et al: Morphometric effects of the recruitment maneuver on saline-lavage canine lungs: a computed tomographic analysis. *Anesthesiology* 99:71–80, 2003.

130. Kacmarek RM: Strategies to optimize alveolar recruitment. *Curr Opin Crit Care* 7:15–20, 2001.

131. Bugedo G, Gruhn A, Hernandez G, et al: Lung computed tomography during a lung recruitment maneuver in patients with acute lung injury. *Intensive Care Med* 29:218–225, 2003.

132. Suh GY, Yoon JW, Park SJ, et al: A practical protocol for titrating "optimal" PEEP in acute lung injury: recruitment maneuver and PEEP decrement. *J Korean Med Sci* 18:349–354, 2003.

133. Mols G, Hermle G, Fries G, et al: Different strategies to keep the lung open: a study in isolated perfused rabbit lungs. *Crit Care Med* 30:1598–1604, 2002.

134. Fan E, Wilcox ME, Brower RG, et al: Recruitment maneuver for acute lung injury—a systematic review. *Am J Respir Crit Care Med* 178:1156–1163, 2008.

135. Mercat A, Richard JCM, Vielle B, et al: Positive end-expiratory pressure setting in adults with acute lung injury and acute respiratory distress syndrome. *JAMA* 299:646–655, 2008.

136. Voggenreiter G, Neudeck F, Aufmkolk M, et al: Intermittent prone positioning in the treatment of severe post-traumatic lung injury. *Crit Care Med* 27:2375–2382, 1999.

137. Pelosi P, Tubiolo D, Mascheroni D, et al: Effects of the prone position on respiratory mechanics and gas exchange during acute lung injury. *Am J Respir Crit Care Med* 157:387–393, 1998.

138. Pelosi P, Croci M, Calappi E, et al: The prone positioning during general anesthesia minimally affects respiratory mechanics while improving functional residual capacity and increasing oxygen tension. *Anesth Analg* 80:955–960, 1995.

139. Pappert D, Rossaint R, Slama K, et al: Influence of positioning on ventilation-perfusion relationships in severe adult respiratory distress syndrome. *Chest* 106:1511–1516, 1994.

140. Lamm WJ, Graham MM, Albert RK: Mechanism by which the prone position improves oxygenation in acute lung injury. *Am J Respir Crit Care Med* 150:184–193, 1994.

141. Curley MA: Prone positioning in patients with acute respiratory distress syndrome: a systematic review. *Am J Crit Care* 8:397–405, 1999.

142. Hirvela E: Advances in the management of acute respiratory distress syndrome: protective ventilation. *Arch Surg* 135:126–135, 2000.

143. Langer M, Mascheroni D, Marcolin R, et al: The prone position in ARDS patients: a clinical study. *Chest* 94:103–107, 1988.

144. Gattinoni L, Vagginelli F, Carlesso E, et al: Decrease in $PaCO_2$ with prone position is predictive of improved outcome in acute respiratory distress syndrome. *Crit Care Med* 31:2727–2733, 2003.

145. Ward NS: Effects of prone position ventilation in ARDS: an evidence-based review of the literature. *Crit Care Clin* 18:35–44, 2002.

146. Mure M, Domino KB, Lindahl SC, et al: Regional ventilation-perfusion distribution is more uniform in the prone position. *J Appl Physiol* 88:1076–1083, 2000.

147. Tobin MJ: Advances in mechanical ventilation. *N Engl J Med* 344:1986–1996, 2001.

148. Unoki T, Mizutani T, Toyooka H: Effects of expiratory rib cage compression and/or prone position on oxygenation and ventilation in mechanically ventilated rabbits with induced atelectasis. *Respir Care* 48:754–762, 2003.

149. Guerin C, Badet M, Rosselli S, et al: Effects of prone position on alveolar recruitment and oxygenation in acute lung injury. *Intensive Care Med* 25:1222–1230, 1999.

150. Gattinoni L, Pelosi P, Vitale G, et al: Body position changes redistribute lung computed-tomographic density in patients with acute respiratory failure. *Anesthesiology* 74:15–23, 1991.

151. Albert RK, Hubmayr RD: The prone position eliminates compression of the lungs by the heart. *Am J Respir Crit Care Med* 161:1660–1665, 2000.

152. Mutoh T, Guest RJ, Lamm WJ, et al: Prone position alters the effect of volume overload on regional pleural pressures and improves hypoxemia in pigs in vivo. *Am Rev Respir Dis* 146:300–306, 1992.

153. Gaillard GC, Lemasson S, Ayzac L, et al: Effects of systematic prone positioning in hypoxemic acute respiratory failure: a randomized controlled trial. *JAMA* 292:2379–2387, 2004.

154. Kacmarek RM: Ventilatory adjuncts. *Respir Care* 47:319–330, 2002.

155. Flores JC, Imaz A, Lopez-herce J, et al: Severe acute respiratory distress syndrome in a child with malaria: favorable response to prone positioning. *Respir Care* 49:282–285, 2004.

156. Gattinoni L, Taccone P, Mascheroni D, et al: Prone position in acute respiratory failure. In Tobin MJ, editor: *Principles and practice of mechanical ventilation*, ed 3, New York, 2013, McGraw-Hill, pp 1169–1181.

157. Relvas MS, Silver PC, Sagy M: Prone positioning of pediatric patients with ARDS results in improvement in oxygenation if maintained >12 h daily. *Chest* 124:269–274, 2003.

158. Gattinoni L, Tognoni G, Pesenti A, et al: Effect of prone positioning on the survival of patients with acute respiratory failure. *N Engl J Med* 345:568–573, 2001.

159. Froese AB, Bryan AC: Effects of anesthesia and paralysis on diaphragmatic mechanics in man. *Anesthesiology* 41:242–255, 1974.

160. Remolina C, Khan AU, Santiago TV, et al: Positional hypoxemia in unilateral lung disease. *N Engl J Med* 304:523–525, 1981.

161. Zack MB, Pontoppidan H, Kazemi H: The effect of lateral positions on gas exchange in pulmonary disease—a prospective evaluation. *Am Rev Respir Dis* 110:49–55, 1974.

162. Fishman AP: Down with the good lung (editorial). *N Engl J Med* 304:537–538, 1981.

Ventilator-Associated Pneumonia

OUTLINE

KEY TERMS

- Biofilm
- Bronchial alveolar lavage
- Clinical Pulmonary Infection Score
- Deescalation
- Early-onset pneumonia
- Fiberoptic bronchoscopy

- Gastroprotective agents
- Health care–associated pneumonia
- Hospital-acquired pneumonia
- Kinetic therapy
- Late-onset pneumonia
- Multidrug-resistant microorganisms

- Nosocomial infections
- Polymicrobial infection
- Protected specimen brush
- Superinfections

LEARNING OBJECTIVES *On completion of this chapter, the reader will be able to do the following:*

1. Define ventilator-associated pneumonia (VAP) and hospital-acquired pneumonia (HAP).
2. Differentiate between early-onset VAP and late-onset VAP and describe the overall incidence of VAP.
3. Discuss the prognosis, including morbidity and mortality rates, for patients diagnosed with VAP.
4. Identify the most common pathogenic microorganisms associated with VAP.
5. List nonpharmacologic and pharmacologic therapeutic interventions that have been shown to increase the risk of development of VAP.
6. Describe the sequence of events that are typically associated with the pathogenesis of VAP.

7. Discuss the advantages and disadvantages of using clinical findings versus quantitative diagnostic techniques to identify patients with VAP.
8. Briefly describe the criteria for starting empiric antibiotic therapy for patients without evidence of multidrug-resistant (MDR) infections and for those patients with risk of developing MDR infections.
9. Define deescalation of antibiotic therapy and how it can be used to reduce the emergence of MDR pathogens.
10. Discuss how ventilator bundles can be used to prevent VAP and the emergence of MDR pathogens in the clinical setting.

Ventilator-associated pneumonia (VAP) is one of the most frequent hospital-acquired infections encountered in critically ill patients receiving mechanical ventilation. VAP is defined as pneumonia that develops 48 hours after a patient has been placed on mechanical ventilation. It is an important subset of **hospital-acquired pneumonia** (HAP), which is pneumonia that occurs 48 hours or longer after admission to the hospital and results from an infection that was not incubating at the time of admission. HAP is differentiated from **health care–associated pneumonia** (HCAP), which afflicts patients who have resided in a long-term care facility or received acute care in an acute care hospital for a specified time before developing pneumonia (i.e., 2 or more days within 90 days of the infection) (Key Point 14-1).

Key Point 14-1 Ventilator-associated pneumonia (VAP) is one of the most frequent hospital acquired infections in critically ill patients receiving mechanical ventilation.

Most often VAP is caused by bacterial infections, but it can be caused by fungal infections or may be associated with viral epidemics (e.g., SARS [severe acute respiratory syndrome]) (Box 14-1). VAP that develops between 48 and 72 hours following tracheal intubation is usually classified as **early-onset pneumonia,** whereas pneumonia that develops later than 72 hours is considered **late-onset pneumonia.**[1,2]

BOX **14-1**	**Commonly Isolated Pathogenic Organisms from Nosocomial Pneumonias**

Gram-Negative Aerobes
Pseudomonas aeruginosa
Klebsiella pneumoniae
Escherichia coli
Enterobacter spp.
Serratia marcescens
Acinetobacter calcoaceticus
Proteus mirabilis
Haemophilus pneumonia

Gram-Positive Aerobes
Legionella pneumophila
Staphylococcus aureus
Streptococcus pneumoniae

Gram-Negative Anaerobes
Bacteroides fragilis

Fungi
Candida albicans

Others
Severe acute respiratory syndrome (SARS) virus
Influenza A virus

Despite major advances in the management of ventilator-dependent patients, VAP continues to complicate the course of treatment of a significant number of patients receiving invasive mechanical ventilation.[3] Development of VAP is associated with prolonged hospital stays, increased health care cost, and mortality rates that range from 25% to 50%.[3-7]

Guidelines for the management of patients with VAP focus on early diagnosis, appropriate antibiotic treatment, and various strategies to prevent the transmission of pathogenic organisms to patients receiving mechanical ventilation. Although there has been considerable debate among clinicians regarding the most effective means of diagnosing and treating VAP, it is agreed that successful management of VAP requires early diagnosis and appropriate use of antibiotic therapy to avoid the emergence of **multidrug-resistant** (MDR) microorganisms (Key Point 14-2). Effective infection-control procedures and surveillance techniques are also necessary to prevent the transmission of nosocomial infections. Careful handwashing with antimicrobial agents, proper disinfection and sterilization of respiratory therapy equipment along with the adherence to standard and disease-specific precautions, and implementation of clinical protocols, such as "VAP bundles," can significantly reduce the incidence of VAP.[8]

Key Point 14-2 Successful management of VAP requires early diagnosis and appropriate use of antibiotic therapy to avoid the emergence of multidrug-resistant microorganisms.

It is beyond the scope of this text to review every clinical study that has been conducted on VAP. A list of selected articles is provided at the end of the chapter for readers interested in further detail on specific studies about the management of patients with VAP, HAP, and HCAP.

EPIDEMIOLOGY

Ventilator-associated pneumonia is one of the most common **nosocomial infections** encountered in the intensive care unit (ICU).[5] The highest risk for the development of VAP occurs early in the course of the hospital stay. Cook and colleagues estimated that the risk of development of VAP is about 3% per day during the first 5 days of receiving mechanical ventilation, 2% per day for days 5 through 10, and 1% thereafter.[9]

The incidence of VAP ranges from 8% to 28% for all intubated patients.[3,5,10] Clinical studies have consistently demonstrated that critically ill patients with VAP have significantly higher mortality rates than mechanically ventilated patients without pneumonia. The overall attributable mortality rate for VAP ranges from 5% to 48%, depending on the infecting organism(s), underlying disease, comorbidities, and prior antimicrobial therapy.[3,11-15]

The prognosis for patients with early-onset VAP is generally better than those who develop pneumonia later in the course of treatment.[9] The reason for the better prognosis for early-onset VAP is related to the fact that these patients are typically infected with antibiotic-sensitive bacteria, whereas patients with late-onset VAP (i.e., longer than 5 days) are more likely to be infected with MDR pathogens.

Causes and Risk Factors

Ventilator-associated pneumonia has been linked to the aspiration of oropharyngeal secretions and esophageal/gastric contents, direct inoculation of infectious material into the trachea and lungs during endotracheal intubation, inhalation of infected aerosols, embolization of biofilm that can be found in the endotracheal tubes (ETs) of patients receiving prolonged mechanical ventilation, exogenous penetration from the pleural space, and the hematogenous spread of extrapulmonary infections to the lung.[5,16]

Box 14-1 lists the most prevalent aerobic gram-negative and gram-positive bacteria that have been identified as potential pathogens responsible for VAP. Historically, aerobic gram-negative bacilli have accounted for nearly 60% of all VAP infections with *Pseudomonas aeruginosa*, *Klebsiella pneumonia*, *Escherichia coli*, and *Acinetobacter* occurring at the highest frequency (Key Point 14-3).[17] More recent studies have shown that gram-positive bacteria are becoming increasingly more common in VAP, with methicillin-resistant *Staphylococcus aureus* (MRSA) being the predominant gram-positive organism isolated.[3,7,18] **Polymicrobial infections** (i.e., infection by multiple pathogenic microorganisms) constitute nearly 50% of all VAP infections, although pathogenic anaerobic infections are not typically found in these mixed-type infections.[3]

Key Point 14-3 Aerobic gram-negative bacilli have accounted for the majority of all VAP infections.

Various independent factors contribute to the development of VAP or may increase the frequency of complications in these patients. Box 14-2 lists several host-related factors and therapeutic interventions that have been identified as risk factors for VAP. Notice that these factors are generally related to the characteristics of the patient populations affected (e.g., age of the patient, diagnosis at admission, severity of the illness, presence of comorbidities), as well as the impact of using various pharmacologic interventions

BOX 14-2	Conditions and Risk Factors Predisposing to Colonization and Ventilator-Associated Pneumonias[40,45]

Alcoholism	Leukocytosis
Antibiotic therapy	Underlying illness
Diabetes mellitus	Underlying pulmonary
Hypoxemia	disease
Bronchoscopy	Nasal intubation
Intubation	Gastric alkalinization
Tracheostomy	Supine position
Chest tube thoracostomy	Immunosuppression
Hypotension	Radiation/scarring
Nasogastric tubes/enteral	Malignancy
feedings	Coma
Acidosis	Circuit/airway manipulation
Malnutrition	(≤72-hour circuit changes)
Azotemia	Severe illness (Acute
Preceding viral infection	Physiology and Chronic
Leukocytopenia	Health Evaluation
Surgery	[APACHE]) ≥18

BOX 14-3	Common Risk Factors for Multidrug-Resistant Infections[7]

- Antimicrobial therapy in the preceding 90 days
- Current hospitalization for 5 or more days
- High frequency of antibiotic resistance in the community or in the specific hospital unit
- Presence of risk factors for health care–associated pneumonia
- Hospitalization for 2 or more days in the preceding 90 days
- Residence in a nursing home or extended care facility
- Home infusion therapy (including antibiotics)
- Chronic dialysis within 30 days
- Home wound care
- Family member with multidrug-resistant pathogen
- Immunosuppressive disease and/or therapy

and respiratory therapy modalities in the treatment of ventilator-dependent patients.

Older patients are at greater risk for developing VAP than are younger patients. Patients treated for trauma, burns, multiple organ failure, or impaired levels of consciousness typically have the highest risk for development of VAP. The presence of comorbidities may actually predispose patients to infections with specific organisms. For example, patients with chronic obstructive pulmonary disease, or COPD, have an increased risk for *Haemophilus influenza, Streptococcus pneumonia,* and *Moraxella catarrhalis,* whereas cystic fibrosis patients are susceptible to *P. aeruginosa* and *S. aureus* infections.[3] MRSA is particularly prevalent in patients with diabetes, head trauma, and those who have been hospitalized for prolonged periods in the ICU.[7] VAP is also recognized as a major complication of acute respiratory distress syndrome (ARDS). It has been estimated that 35% to 70% of ARDS patients develop pneumonia, which can lead to sepsis and multiple organ failure. The mortality rate for ARDS patients with VAP is significantly higher than patients without VAP.[3,19]

Therapeutic interventions are generally categorized as pharmacologic and nonpharmacologic. Examples of pharmacologic interventions that can lead to the development of VAP or complicate the course of treatment for these patients include concurrent steroid therapy, inappropriate antimicrobial therapy, overuse of sedatives and paralytics for mechanically ventilated patients, and the use of type 2 (H_2) histamine antagonists and **gastroprotective agents,** such as antacids.

Inappropriate use of antibiotics in the hospital setting is particularly troublesome because it has been associated with the selection of MDR pathogens (Key Point 14-4).[3,18,20] It has been suggested that prolonged antibiotic administration to ICU patients for a primary infection may favor selection and subsequent colonization with resistant pathogens responsible for **superinfections.**[3] This is an important issue for patients with late-onset VAP because as mentioned previously, these patients are at a higher risk for being infected with MDR pathogens. Imprudent use of sedatives and paralytics can also increase the incidence of VAP by impairing the patient's level of consciousness, which can ultimately blunt the

patient's cough reflex and increase the chances of aspiration. Box 14-3 lists the most common risk factors for MDR infections.

Key Point 14-4 Inappropriate use of antibiotics in the hospital setting has been associated with an increased emergence of multidrug-resistant pathogens.

Nonpharmacologic interventions that are associated with the increased risk of VAP include the need for an endotracheal ET or tracheostomy tube during ventilation; routine care of ventilator circuits, humidifiers, and nebulizers; and the use of respirometers, reusable electronic ventilator probes and sensors, bronchoscopes, and endoscopes.[5] The most important of these nonpharmacologic factors that has been found to be associated with VAP is the use of an ET or tracheostomy during mechanical ventilation. The incidence of VAP is 6- to 21-fold higher in patients who are intubated receiving mechanical ventilation compared with the incidence in patients receiving noninvasive mechanical ventilation. This has led some clinicians to suggest that "endotracheal intubation-associated pneumonia" might be a more appropriate name for this type of pneumonia.

Respiratory therapy equipment has long been implicated as a source of nosocomial infections. Indeed, epidemics of HAP and VAP are most often associated with contamination of respiratory therapy equipment, bronchoscopes, and endoscopes. Instituting stringent infection-control procedures can reduce the incidence of nosocomial infections in hospitals and other health care facilities; however, ensuring that all of the clinical staff members adhere to the prescribed infection-control policies remains a formidable task. Surveillance of ICU patients at high risk for bacterial pneumonia can also be an important part of determining trends and identifying outbreaks.[21] Additional details on various nonpharmacologic strategies that can be used to reduce the incidence of VAP are presented later in this chapter.

PATHOGENESIS OF VENTILATOR-ASSOCIATED PNEUMONIA

The pathogenesis of VAP most often involves colonization of the aerodigestive tract with pathogenic bacteria, aspiration of contaminated secretions into the lower airways, followed by colonization of the normally sterile lower airways and lung parenchyma with these infectious microrganisms.[15] The upper airways of healthy individuals typically contain nonpathogenic bacteria, such as viridans group of streptococci, *Haemophilus* spp., and anaerobes.[5] Aerobic gram-negative bacilli, most notably virulent forms of *P. aeruginosa* and *Acinetobacter*, are rarely found in the respiratory tract of healthy individuals because of anatomic barriers, the cough reflex, mucociliary clearance mechanisms, and innate cellular and humoral immune factors (e.g., leukocytes, immunoglobulins).

During critical illnesses, particularly in patients with an endotracheal tube and receiving mechanical ventilation, there is a dramatic shift in the flora of the oropharyngeal tract to gram-negative bacilli and *S. aureus*.[5,7] This shift in flora may be attributed to a number of factors that compromise host defense mechanisms, including comorbidities, malnutrition, reduced levels of mucosal immunoglobulin A, increased production of proteases, exposed and denuded mucous membranes, elevated airway pH, and an increased number of airway receptors for bacteria as a result of acute illness and prior antimicrobial use.[5,22-24] Aspiration of the contaminated oropharyngeal secretions and, in some cases, gastroesophageal contents can occur because the patient is unable to protect the lower airways. Impaired level of consciousness, gastroesophageal reflux, a blunted gag reflex, and abnormal swallowing can all contribute to the risk of aspiration.[15] After these offending organisms penetrate and colonize the lower airways, they can overwhelm already compromised pulmonary cellular and humoral immune defense mechanisms and eventually lead to VAP.[15]

DIAGNOSIS OF VENTILATOR-ASSOCIATED PNEUMONIA

The lack of a precise definition for the diagnosis of VAP has caused considerable debate among clinicians.[25-27] It has been suggested that clinical criteria involving patient symptoms and signs, chest radiographs, and baseline hematologic studies can be effective for starting empiric antibiotic therapy; however, simply relying on clinical findings to guide therapeutic interventions can be subjective (i.e., high interobserver variability) resulting in a failure to accurately diagnose VAP and lead to inappropriate antibiotic therapy if the infection is polymicrobial in origin or if a drug-resistant organism is present.

The American Thoracic Society (ATS) and the Infectious Diseases Society of America (IDSA) presented recommendations in 2005 to address these concerns regarding the management of VAP. The ATS/IDSA recommendations provided a list of clinical criteria that could be used in the diagnosis of VAP.[7] The guidelines further advised that invasive microbiologic procedures, such as quantitative cultures of lower respiratory secretions obtained by **bronchial alveolar lavage** (BAL) or **protected specimen brush** (PSB) procedure, are often necessary to ensure effective treatment of patients with VAP.[7]

In 2011, the Centers for Disease Control (CDC) and National Healthcare Safety Network (NHSN) proposed an updated definition that was designed to improve the reporting criteria for VAP used by institutions. Although the CDC surveillance definition incorporates the general features of the ATS/IDSA definition, several points are noteworthy. For example, the CDC surveillance definition uses the term ventilator-associated event (VAE) to describe a range of conditions and complications that occur in mechanically ventilated patients, including VAP.[27] As Table 14-1 shows, a ventilator-associated event can be categorized as a ventilator-associated condition (VAC), an infection-related ventilator-associated complication (IVAC), and possible pneumonia or probable pneumonia. The CDC surveillance definition relies on the use of only objective data, clearly defined time criteria, and the exclusion of

TABLE 14-1	**CDC Surveillance Paradigm for Ventilator-Associated Events**	
Concept	**Name**	**Definition**
New respiratory deterioration	Ventilator-associated condition (VAC)	≥2 Calendar days of stable or decreasing daily minimum positive end-expiratory pressure or daily minimum fraction of inspired oxygen, followed by a rise in daily minimum positive end-expiratory pressure of ≥3 cm of water or a rise in the daily minimum percentage of inspired oxygen by ≥20 points sustained for ≥2 calendar days
New respiratory deterioration with evidence of infection	Infection-related ventilator-associated complication (IVAC)	VAC plus a temperature of <36°C or >38°C or a leukocyte count of ≤4000 or ≥12,000 per cubic millimeter, plus one or more new antibiotics continued for at least 4 days within 2 calendar days before or after onset of a VAC, excluding the first 2 days of mechanical ventilation
New respiratory deterioration with possible evidence of pulmonary infection	Possible pneumonia	IVAC plus Gram's staining of endotracheal aspirate or bronchoalveolar lavage showing ≥25 neutrophils and ≤10 epithelial cells per low-power field, or a positive culture for a potentially pathogenic organism, within 2 calendar days before or after onset of a VAC, excluding the first 2 days of mechanical ventilation
New respiratory deterioration with probable evidence of pulmonary infection	Probable pneumonia	IVAC plus Gram's staining of endotracheal aspirate or bronchoalveolar lavage showing ≥25 neutrophils and ≤10 epithelial cells per low-power field, plus endotracheal aspirate with ≥10⁵ colony-forming units per milliliter or bronchoalveolar-lavage culture with ≥10⁴ colony-forming units per milliliter, or endotracheal-aspirate or bronchoalveolar-lavage semiquantitative equivalent, within 2 calendar days before or after onset of a VAC, excluding the first 2 days of mechanical ventilation

From: Klompas M: Complication of mechanical ventilation—The CDC's new surveillance paradigm, N Engl J Med 368:1472-1475, 2013.

TABLE **14-2**	Clinical Criteria Used in the Diagnosis of Ventilator-Assisted Pneumonia (VAP)[27,29]			
		POINTS		
Variables	*0*	*1*		*2*
Temperature, °C	≥36.1 to ≤38.4	≥38.5 to ≤38.9		≥39 to ≤36
WBC count, µL	≥4000 to ≤11,000	<4000 to >11,000		
Secretions	Absent	Present, nonpurulent		Present, purulent
P_aO_2/F_iO_2	>240 or ARDS	—		≤240 and no ARDS
Chest radiography	No infiltrate	Diffuse or patchy infiltrate		Localized infiltrate
Microbiology	No or light growth	Moderate or heavy growth; add 1 point for same organism on Gram stain		—

From Porzecanski I, Bowton DL: Diagnosis and treatment of ventilator-associated pneumonia, Chest 130:597-604, 2006.
ARDS, Acute respiratory distress syndrome; P_aO_2, arterial oxygen pressure; *WBC,* white blood cell.

radiographic imaging to diagnose the presence of pneumonia in ventilated patients.[26,27]

Clinical Diagnosis

Ventilator-associated pneumonia should be suspected when a mechanically ventilated patient demonstrates radiographic evidence of new or progressive infiltrates and one or more of the following findings: fever, leukocytosis, purulent tracheobronchial secretions, decreased oxygenation, and increased minute ventilation, a decrease in tidal volume, and an increase in respiratory rate.[3] Table 14-2 provides a list of clinical criteria that can be used in the clinical diagnosis of VAP. It is worth mentioning that fever and the presence of pulmonary infiltrates on chest radiographs are nonspecific findings that can be associated with numerous other conditions, including chemical and radiation pneumonitis, atelectasis, pulmonary embolism and infarction, lung contusion, ARDS, and drug or hypersensitivity reactions.[16,25]

Some clinicians emphasize certain findings over others using a "weighted" approach to clinical diagnosis.[25] The **Clinical Pulmonary Infection Score** (CPIS) is an example of this type of approach. The CPIS includes six clinical assessments with each item given a score of 0 to 2 points (see Table 14-1). The assessment criteria include fever, leukocyte count, quantity and purulence of tracheal secretions, oxygenation status, the type of radiographic abnormality, and results of a tracheal aspirate culture and Gram stain. (Note that a modified CPIS in which the endotracheal aspirate culture and Gram stain results are excluded is also available. In this case, the score will range from 0 to 10 instead of 0 to 12).[26-29] When all six criteria are used, a score greater than 6 is considered evidence of the presence of VAP.[27] It is generally accepted that measurements of CPIS should be performed at the beginning of antibiotic therapy and after 2 to 3 days to evaluate the effectiveness of the treatment course. Although some investigators have found considerable inter-observer variability and a lack of specificity to guide antibiotic therapy, a case can be made that measurement of the CPIS may reduce the mortality rate associated with VAP.[28,29] The measurement of CPIS may also provide information that can allow the clinician to aggressively treat patients with VAP while limiting the course of antibiotic therapy and thus controlling for the development of bacterial resistance[25] (Case Study 14-1).

Case Study 14-1

Patient Case—VAP

A 65-year-old man is admitted to the intensive care unit following thoracic surgery. He has an endotracheal tube and has been receiving pressure-controlled mechanical ventilation for 48 hours. The attending physician suspects that the patient may have ventilator-associated pneumonia (VAP). The following clinical data were obtained during an initial assessment. What is his CPIS and does he demonstrate enough evidence of VAP to warrant the initiation of antibiotic therapy?

Temperature = 39.5°C
White blood cell count = 12,000 cells/mm³
Diffuse infiltrates on chest radiograph
Purulent secretions
P_aO_2/F_iO_2 = 300

Bacteriologic (Quantitative) Diagnosis

As mentioned, many clinicians have concerns about simply using clinical findings to guide antibiotic therapy in VAP. They believe this approach can result in the unnecessary use of broad-range antibiotics, which in turn can lead to the emergence of multidrug-resistant strains of microorganisms and higher mortality rates for patients afflicted with VAP. Numerous studies have shown that obtaining quantitative cultures of specimens from the lower respiratory tract by conventional **fiberoptic bronchoscopy** or nonbronchoscopic techniques can significantly improve the diagnosis of VAP and facilitate decision making regarding the management of these patients.[3,30,31]

Fiberoptic bronchoscopy allows the clinician to have direct access to the lower airways. The most common bronchoscopic techniques used to obtain samples from the lower airways and the lung parenchyma involve BAL and PSB sampling. Selection of the sampling site is usually based on the location of the infiltrate on chest radiographs or by direct visualization of inflammation and purulent secretions in the airway.[3,31] Note that relying on chest radiographs when selecting the appropriate sampling area can be challenging if diffuse pulmonary infiltrates are present.

A variety of nonbronchoscopic techniques have been described.[32] The most commonly used nonbronchoscopic techniques include mini BAL, blinded bronchial sampling (BBS), and blinded protected specimen brush (BPSB). The advantages of using these techniques over conventional bronchoscopy are that nonbronchoscopic techniques are noninvasive and less expensive than bronchoscopy, and they can be performed by individuals not qualified to perform fiberoptic bronchoscopy.[3] These techniques also typically do not result in compromised gas exchange, which often occurs during fiberoptic bronchoscopy. The primary disadvantage of using the nonbronchoscopic techniques is that samples are obtained blindly and can therefore increase the chances of a sampling error because of lack of direct visualization of the sampling site.[33]

Once the sample is obtained, it should be processed without delay according to clearly defined procedures for bacteriologic analysis to prevent the loss of viability of the pathogenic organisms or overgrowth by contaminants. Bacteriologic studies include quantitative culture techniques and microscopic analysis of the cultures using an appropriate stain (e.g., Gram stain) to differentiate pathogens from oropharyngeal contaminants.[3] In patients with VAP, pathogens are usually present at concentrations of 10^5 to 10^6 colony-forming units (CFU)/mL, whereas contaminants are generally present in concentrations of less than 10^4 CFU/mL. (Baselski has provided a complete description of the standard laboratory procedures for processing bronchoscopic samples in suspected cases of VAP.)[31] Direct microscopic and histologic examinations of BAL and PBS samples can be used to identify the presence or absence of bacteria in the lower respiratory tract.

TREATMENT OF VENTILATOR-ASSOCIATED PNEUMONIA

The treatment of VAP can be challenging, even under the best of conditions. It should be apparent from the aforementioned issues related to diagnosing VAP that developing an effective strategy for the management of these patients ultimately depends on establishing a reliable diagnosis. Initiating empiric antibiotic therapy should be based on whether the patient has any of the risk factors for the MDR pathogens (Table 14-3). The ATS-IDSA Guidelines for the Management of Adults with HAP, VAP, and HCAP provide a series of pathways to guide clinicians on the initiation of empiric antibiotic therapy, as well as strategies that can be used to reduce the emergence of MDR pathogens. Table 14-3 provides a list of potential pathogens associated with VAP and recommended antibiotics for the management of patients with no known risk factors for MDR, as well as patients with known risk factors for MDR. Table 14-4 contains a list of dosing schedules for several antibiotics that are used in the treatment of nosocomial infections. Information that should also be reviewed when designing an antibiotic regimen includes the predominant pathogens identified for the specific clinical setting and the local patterns of antibiotic susceptibility, the cost and availability of the antibiotics used, and any formulary restrictions.[7]

The algorithm shown in Fig. 14-1 is a summary of the current management strategies that are recommended for patients with suspected VAP. **Deescalation** of antibiotic therapy or, more specifically, focusing the types and duration of antibiotics used (i.e., broad-range antibiotics versus limited-spectrum antibiotics) can be accomplished once quantitative data on lower respiratory tract

and blood cultures are available[7] (Key Point 14-5). It is important to understand that successful treatment of patients with VAP requires serial clinical and microbiologic assessments. More specific information about the use of various antibiotic-dosing schedules, including combination therapy, can be found in the ATS-IDSA Guideline listed in the references at the end of this chapter[7] (Case Study 14-2).

 Key Point 14-5 Deescalating antibiotic therapy can be accomplished once quantitative data on lower respiratory tract and blood cultures are available. Deescalation of antibiotic therapy is an important method that can be used to reduce the incidence of MDR pathogens because it reduces unnecessary use of antibiotics.

Case Study 14-2

Exercise

Patient Case—Methicillin-resistant *S. aureus*

A 55-year-old woman with a 35-pack-year history of smoking cigarettes is admitted into the intensive care unit after a cholecystectomy. She has a history of diabetes mellitus and has been mechanically ventilated via an endotracheal tube for 5 days. Her chest radiograph demonstrates localized infiltrates in the right middle lobe. Her white cell count is 15,000 cells/mm³, and the results of BAL show the presence of methicillin-resistant *Staphylococcus aureus*. Briefly describe the appropriate antibiotic course that should be initiated for this patient.

STRATEGIES TO PREVENT VENTILATOR-ASSOCIATED PNEUMONIA

It is well recognized that establishing well-designed infection-control practices in the ICU can significantly reduce the incidence of VAP. The first step in the development and implementation of an effective program is the recognition that it is a high-priority task. Ensuring that everyone on the clinical staff is familiar with the established infection-control policies and procedures is critical. Staff must consistently follow these procedures for all patients and recognize the consequences of lapses in continuity of care. Adequate physical and human resources must be provided to establish surveillance mechanisms to track the local incidence of VAP and other nosocomial infections. The findings of the surveillance team must be effectively communicated to the clinical staff on a regular basis, and the program must be updated to reflect the most current evidence-based clinical studies, the use of new technology, and changing patterns of disease in the local environment.[2]

Box 14-4 lists a number of strategies can be implemented to prevent VAP. Many of these strategies are incorporated into **ventilator bundles,** which are viewed as evidence-based practices that can significantly reduce the incidence of VAP. As mentioned, these strategies are generally categorized as nonpharmacologic and pharmacologic procedures.[34-37] The following is a brief discussion of each of these strategies that can be used to reduce the incidence of VAP.

TABLE **14-3**	Potential Pathogens Associated with VAP and Recommended Antibiotics for the Management of Patients with Suspected VAP[7]

INITIAL EMPIRIC ANTIBIOTIC THERAPY FOR HOSPITAL-ACQUIRED PNEUMONIA OR VAP IN PATIENTS WITH NO KNOWN RISK FACTORS FOR MULTIDRUG-RESISTANT PATHOGENS, EARLY ONSET, AND ANY DISEASE SEVERITY

Potential Pathogen	Recommended Antibiotic*
Streptococcus pneumoniae[†]	Ceftriaxone
Haemophilus influenzae	or
Methicillin-sensitive *Staphylococcus aureus*	Levofloxacin, monifloxacin, or ciprofloxacin
Antibiotic-sensitive enteric gram-negative bacilli	or
Escherichia coli	Ampicillin/sulbactam or ertapenam
Klebsiella pneumoniae	
Enterobacter spp.	
Proteus spp.	
Serratia marcescens	

*See Table 14-3 for proper initial doses of antibiotics.
[†]The frequency of penicillin-resistant *S. pneumoniae* and multidrug-resistant *S. pneumoniae* is increasing; levofloxacin or moxifloxacin are preferred to ciprofloxacin and the role of other new quinolones, such as gatifloxacin, has not been established.

INITIAL EMPIRIC THERAPY FOR HOSPITAL-ACQUIRED PNEUMONIA, VENTILATOR-ASSOCIATED PNEUMONIA, AND HEALTH CARE–ASSOCIATED PNEUMONIA IN PATIENTS WITH LATE-ONSET DISEASE OR RISK FACTORS FOR MULTIDRUG-RESISTANT PATHOGENS AND ALL DISEASE SEVERITY

Potential Pathogens	Combination Antibiotic Therapy*
Pathogens listed above and MDR pathogens	Antipseudomonal cephalosporin (cefepime, ceftazidime)
Pseudomonas aeruginosa	or
Klebsiella pneumoniae (ESBL[†])	Antipseudomonal carbapenem (imipenem or meropenem)
Acinetobacter spp.[†]	or
	β-Lactam/β-lactamase inhibitor (piperacillin-tazobactam)
	plus
	Antipseudomonal fluoroquinolone[†] (ciprofloxacin or levofloxacin)
	or
	Aminoglycoside (amikacin, gentamicin, or tobramycin)
	plus
Methicillin-resistant *Staphylococcus aureus* (MRSA)	Linezolid or vancomycin[‡]
Legionella pneumophila[†]	

From American Thoracic Society, Infectious Diseases Society of America. Guidelines for the management of adults with hospital-acquired, ventilator-associated, and healthcare-associated pneumonia, Am J Respir Crit Care Med 171:388-416, 2005.
ESBL, Extended-spectrum β-lactamase.
*See Table 14-4 for adequate initial dosing of antibiotics. Initial antibiotic therapy should be adjusted or streamlined on the basis of microbiologic data and clinical response to therapy.
[†]If an ESBL strain, such as *K. pneumoniae,* or an *Acinetobacter* spp. is suspected, a carbapenem is a reliable choice. If *L. pneumophila* is suspected, the combination antibiotic regimen should include a macrolide (e.g., azithromycin), or a fluoroquinolone (e.g., ciprofloxacin or levofloxacin) should be used rather than an aminoglycoside.
[‡]If MRSA risk factors are present or there is a high incidence locally.

Nonpharmacologic Interventions

Handwashing

Routine handwashing with soap and water and alcohol-based hand rubs is the most important prevention strategy to reduce the risk of clinicians transmitting infectious microorganisms from one patient to another or from a contaminated site to a clean site on the same patient[38] (Key Point 14-6). Hand decontamination should be done before and after contact with an intubated patient and before and after performing any procedure where handling contaminated with respiratory secretions can occur.[32] Wearing gloves and gowns reduces the rate of nosocomial infections, but this practice appears to be most effective when used with patients with specific antibiotic-resistant pathogens.[2]

> **Key Point 14-6** Routine handwashing with soap and water and alcohol-based hand rubs is the most important prevention strategy to reduce the risk of nosocomial infections.

TABLE 14-4 Potential Pathogens Associated with VAP and Recommended Antibiotics for the Management of Patients with Risks for Development of Multidrug-Resistant Pathogens[7]

INITIAL INTRAVENOUS, ADULT DOSES OF ANTIBIOTICS FOR EMPIRIC THERAPY OF HOSPITAL-ACQUIRED PNEUMONIA, INCLUDING VAP, AND HEALTH CARE–ASSOCIATED PNEUMONIA IN PATIENTS WITH LATE-ONSET DISEASE OR RISK FACTORS FOR MULTIDRUG-RESISTANT PATHOGENS

Antibiotic	Dosage*
Antipseudomonal cephalosporin	
Cefepime	1-2 g every 8-12 hr
Ceftazidime	2 g every 8 hr
Carbapenems	
Imipenem	500 mg ever 6 hr or 1 g every 8 hr
Meropenem	1 g every 8 hr
β-Lactam/β-lactamase inhibitor	
Piperacillin-tazobactam	4.5 g every 6 hr
Aminoglycosides	
Gentamicin	7 mg/kg per day[†]
Tobramycin	7 mg/kg per day[†]
Amikacin	20 mg/kg per day[†]
Antipseudomonal quinolones	
Levofloxacin	750 mg every day
Ciprofloxacin	400 mg every 8 hr
Vancomycin	15 mg/kg every 12 hr[†]
Linezolid	600 mg every 12 hr

American Thoracic Society, Infectious Diseases Society of America. Guidelines for the management of adults with hospital-acquired, ventilator-associated, and healthcare-associated pneumonia, Am J Respir Crit Care Med 171:388-416, 2005.
*Dosages are based on normal renal and hepatic function.
[†]Trough levels for gentamicin and tobramycin should be less than 1 μg/mL, and for amikacin they should be less than 4-5 μg/mL.
[†]Trough levels for vancomycin should be 15-20 μg/mL.

BOX 14-4 Methods to Reduce the Risk of Nosocomial Pneumonias in Mechanically Ventilated Patients[34-37]

Nonpharmacologic
Noninvasive ventilation
Handwashing and use of accepted infection-control procedures and practices
Semirecumbent positioning of patient
Appropriate circuit changes (when grossly contaminated)
Consider using silver-coated antimicrobial endotracheal tubes
Heat-moisture exchanges when possible
Continuous aspiration of subglottic secretions (CASS)
Appropriate disinfection and sterilization techniques
Kinetic beds
Identifying a dedicated person/group for monitoring nosocomial ventilator-associated pneumonia (VAP) rates
Use of closed-suction catheters and sterile suction technique
Avoiding large gastric volumes
Extubating and removing nasogastric tube as clinically indicated
Avoiding contamination with ventilator circuit condensate
Single patient use of items such as monitors, O_2 analyzers, resuscitation bags
Careful use of in-line small-volume nebulizers
Consider use of expiratory-line gas traps or filters
Oral rather than nasal intubation

Pharmacologic
Stress ulcer prophylaxis with sucralfate instead of histamine type 2 antagonists in high-risk patients for prevention of stress ulcers (still controversial)
Possible prophylactic intestinal decontamination (antimicrobial administration)
Avoid central nervous system depressants

Methods to Improve Host Immunity
Maintain nutritional status
Avoid agents that impair pulmonary defenses (aminophylline, anesthetics, certain antibiotics, corticosteroids, sedative narcotics, and antineoplastic agents)
Minimize use of invasive procedures when possible
Remove or treat disease states that affect host defenses when possible (acidosis, dehydration, hypoxemia, ethanol intoxication, acid aspiration, stress, thermal injury, diabetic ketoacidosis, liver failure, kidney failure, heart failure)

Semirecumbent Patient Positioning and Enteral Feeding

Enteral feeding may predispose a patient to VAP by elevating the gastric pH, which can lead to gastric colonization with pathogenic bacteria and cause gastric distention. This in turn can lead to an increased risk of reflux and aspiration. Following some basic guidelines can reduce aspiration of gastric contents. Routine verification of the proper placement of the enteral feed tube is important.[39,40] Intermittent feedings may also be preferable to continuously feeding because preventing overdistention of the stomach can limit gastropulmonary colonization.[35]

Aspiration occurs more often in patients placed in the supine position than in patients in the semirecumbent position (i.e., 30-45 degrees from the horizontal position).[35,40-42] When it is feasible and the patient can tolerate it, placing a patient in the semirecumbent position is a low-cost, low-risk procedure that is effective in reducing the aspiration of gastric contents when compared with the supine position.

Noninvasive Ventilation

Clinical studies have clearly demonstrated that endotracheal intubation is a modifiable risk factor for the development of VAP. Avoiding ET intubation and use of noninvasive positive pressure ventilation (NIV) has been shown to significantly lower the nosocomial pneumonia rate in select groups of patients (e.g., acute exacerbations of COPD or immunocompromised patients with pulmonary infiltrates and hypoxemic respiratory failure).[7] Using NIV is also associated with a lower rate of other nosocomial infections such as urinary tract infections and catheter-related infections.[43] When it is clinically appropriate, noninvasive ventilation should be preferentially used over invasive ventilation.[36]

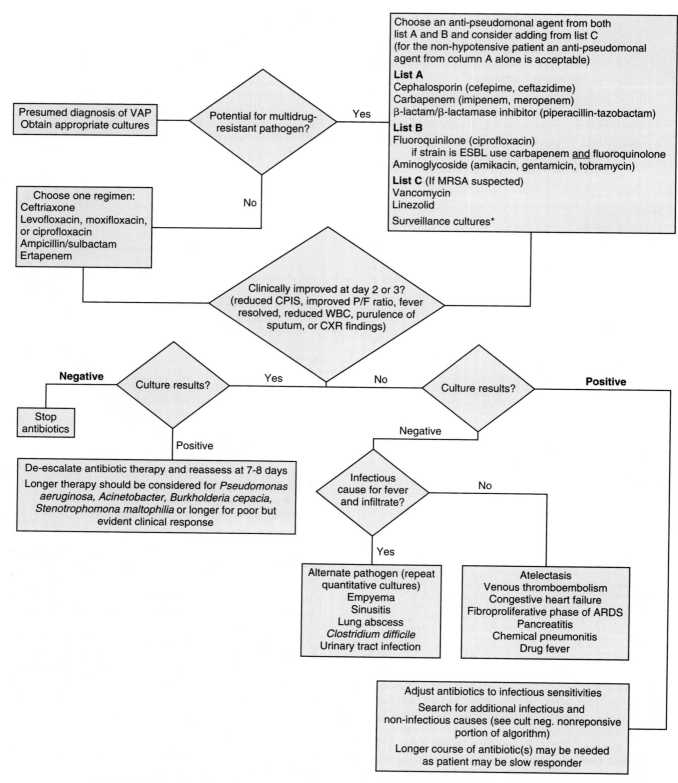

Fig. 14-1 Algorithm illustrating antibiotic regimens used for the management of patients with ventilator-associated pneumonia.[7,52] *Antibiotic choice can be tailored to the pathogens' last sensitivity report if quantitative endotracheal aspirate (QEA) surveillance cultures are obtained twice weekly and if the growth level exceeds 100,000 CFU/mL. Adapted from the *American Journal of Respiratory and Critical Care Medicine*[5] with permission. In Koenig SM, Truwit JD: Ventilator-associated pneumonia: diagnosis, treatment, and prevention, *Clinical Micro Rev* 19(4):637-657, 2006.

Selection, Changing, and Suctioning of the Endotracheal Tube

It is important to recognize that the type of ET selected and the site of insertion are important factors to consider when initiating invasive mechanical ventilation. Advances in endotracheal tube construction have resulted in the development of different cuff materials and shapes that attempt to reduce leakage of secretions around an inflated cuff.[43] Polyurethane and silicon endotracheal tube cuffs decrease the formation of longitudinal channels, which can occur with standard polyvinyl cuffs. Changing the shape of the ET cuff has also been shown to reduce leakage. Tapered or cylindrical designs have been shown to reduce fluid leakage when compared to ET tubes with the standard globular cuff design.[43]

Maintaining adequate ET cuff pressure is also an important factor that must be considered to avoid aspiration of oropharyngeal secretions. There appears to be a higher risk of aspiration pneumonia among patients with persistent intracuff pressures below 20 cm H_2O.[44] Increasing the cuff pressure (e.g., to 20-25 cm H_2O) decreases but does not completely eliminate this aspiration. Furthermore, it is important to recognize that using higher cuff pressure is not without its own problems of potential airway injury (see Chapter 8).

The use of oral rather than nasal intubation is recommended because sinusitis is a particular concern in nasally intubated patients and is associated with VAP.[44] Furthermore, there is an increased risk of VAP when patients are reintubated. The risk and benefits of reintubation should be considered before changing an ET. If the tube is changed, it is important to avoid contamination of the lower airways with oropharyngeal secretions by properly suctioning around the ET cuff before deflating the cuff or replacing the ET. The Centers for Disease Control recommends using a new suction catheter with each open-suction procedure and using sterile water to rinse the catheter when suctioning is performed. The use of sterile gloves is also appropriate for this procedure.[44-47]

Recent studies have demonstrated that antimicrobial-coated ET tubes can reduce the incidence of VAP by delaying bacterial colonization and **biofilm** formation on the tube's inner lining. Laboratory studies have suggested that silver is an ideal coating because it is nontoxic, antimicrobial, and it has antiadhesive properties.[26] It is important to mention, however, that although these devices can delay biofilm formation, the antibacterial efficacy of the coating decreases over time. Additionally, removal of the biofilm can be difficult because routine tracheal suctioning is not effective. Berra and colleagues introduced a novel device called the *Mucus Shaver* to overcome this limitation. The Mucus Shaver consists of an expandable silicon rubber balloon with shaving rings that adhere to the surface of the endotracheal tube. This device has been shown to be effective in the removal of biofilm and thus allows the ET tube to retain its antimicrobial efficacy.[45]

Continuous Aspiration of Subglottic Secretions (CASS)

Secretions that pool around the ET cuff are reservoirs of potentially pathogenic bacteria (Key Point 14-7). Efforts to reduce silent aspiration of secretions above and below the ET cuff have led to the development and use of specialized ETs (see Fig. 14-2). These specialized ETs have a dorsal lumen above the ET cuff that allows for continuous or intermittent suction of tracheal secretions that accumulate above the patient's subglottic area.[49,50] CASS has been shown to reduce the incidence of nosocomial pneumonias.[46] Early studies by Valles and colleagues reported that continuous aspiration of subglottic secretions reduced the incidence of VAP by

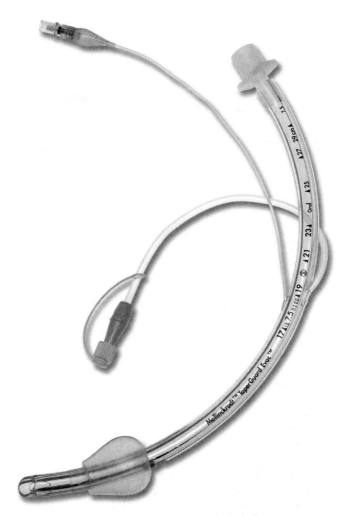

Fig. 14-2 Specialized continuous suction endotracheal tubes.

nearly 50%.[50] Interestingly, these investigators also found that episodes of VAP occurred later in patients receiving continuous aspiration (12.0 ± 7.1 days than in the control patients (5.9 ± 2.1 days).[50] Rello and colleagues also showed a five times greater likelihood of VAP when continuous aspiration of subglottic secretions was not used.[46]

At present, the CDC makes no specific recommendation about how often this system should be changed. Studies have not shown differences in VAP rates between once daily and no routine changes in closed-suction catheters. It may be appropriate to leave the catheter inline until it is visibly contaminated or no longer functional.

🔑 Key Point 14-7 Secretions that pool around the ET cuff are reservoirs of potentially pathogenic bacteria.

Care of the Tracheostomy Tube

Tracheostomy tubes placed by the percutaneous route can predispose the patient to the development of pneumonia, possibly from contamination during the insertion procedure. In cases where the patient has a tracheostomy tube, the caregiver should wear a gown, use aseptic technique, and replace the tube with one that has been sterilized or given high-level disinfection.[44] These types of pneumonia are associated with prolonged ventilation and ICU stay but not with increased mortality. A common pathogen associated with percutaneous tracheotomy is *Pseudomonas* spp.[47]

Ventilator Circuit Management Strategies

Most clinicians agree that reducing ventilator circuits changes is cost-effective and, more important, lessens the risk of VAP.[35,36,48,51] Circuits do not need to be changed unless they are nonfunctional or if they are visibly soiled with secretions or blood.[36,44,51,52]

Using certain types of humidifiers during mechanical ventilation can be another potential source of pathogenic bacteria. Heat and moisture exchangers (HMEs) have the ability to filter bacteria and may be a more effective method of reducing VAP during mechanical ventilation than heated-wire circuits and heated humidifiers.[36,44,47] It is important to recognize that patients with thick, tenacious secretions are not good candidates for using these devices because HMEs might not provide adequate humidification and increase the risk for endotracheal occlusions causing asphyxiation.[36,44,53]

For heated wick or pass-over humidifiers, the CDC recommends the use of sterile water.[47] (NOTE: Although bubble humidifiers are now only rarely used during mechanical ventilation, it is safe to assume that the same advice would be appropriate for these devices too.[53]) Draining of condensate in the ventilator circuits that use heated humidifiers should be performed in a manner that avoids accidentally allowing circuit condensate from spilling into the patient's ET.

Small-volume nebulizers (SVNs) are sometimes used in the ventilator circuit for the administration of medications. Between treatments the CDC recommends that the SVN be disinfected, rinsed with sterile water, and air-dried.[44] Only sterile solutions should be used to fill SVNs and whenever possible unit-dose vials of medication should be used[44] (Key Point 14-8).

 Key Point **14-8** Ventilator circuits do not need to be changed unless they are nonfunctional or if they are visibly soiled with secretions or blood.

Kinetic Therapy

Immobility in critically ill patients can lead to atelectasis and reduced bronchopulmonary secretion clearance. Several investigators have suggested that **kinetic therapy** or the use of automated rotating beds may be effective in reducing the incidence of VAP, particularly in surgical patients or patients with neurologic problems.[39] Whether kinetic beds offer significant advantages over standard ICU patient-turning strategies will require additional studies.[39,44,47] At present, the CDC has no recommendation regarding "kinetic" therapy or continuous lateral rotational therapy.

Pharmacologic Interventions

Oropharyngeal Decontamination

The CDC currently recommends the development and implementation of an oral hygiene program for patients in acute care and long-term care facilities that are at high risk for nosocomial pneumonias. Although there has been a debate regarding the benefits of oral hygiene in preventing VAP, studies have demonstrated that using an oral cleansing agent like chlorhexidine can modulate oropharyngeal colonization and ultimately decrease the incidence of VAP.[54]

Stress Ulcer Prophylaxis

Gastrointestinal bleeding and stress ulcers in critically ill patients are associated with increased morbidity and mortality. Use of prophylactic treatment, such as H$_2$-antagonists and antacids, may reduce the risk of stress ulcers. However, as the acidity of gastric contents decreases, gastric colonization by potentially pathogenic organisms increases (Key Point 14-9). The use of sucralfate may be beneficial in reducing gastric colonization. Sucralfate is a prophylactic agent that does not affect gastric pH.[35,36] Current findings are controversial, and the use of sucralfate is not recommended at this time for patients at high risk for gastrointestinal bleeding.[37] In patients with ARDS, sucralfate was associated with an increased risk of VAP.[37] The CDC currently has no specific recommendations about the use of sucralfate, H$_2$ receptor antagonists, or antacids for stress-bleeding prophylaxis.[47]

Key Point **14-9** Administering type H$_2$ histamine antagonists and antacids may reduce the risk of stress ulcers, but they can also increase the risk of gastric colonization by potentially pathogenic organisms.

Selective Digestive Tract Decontamination

There is substantial interest in topically treating the oropharynx and stomach of patients on mechanical ventilation with antibiotics. The goal is aimed at reducing the number of potentially pathogenic organisms that may colonize the stomach. This, in turn, might reduce the incidence of VAP. Selective digestive tract decontamination may reduce VAP and ICU mortality, when a combination of topical and intravenous prophylactic antibiotics is used. However, this is not without the long-term risk of the development of antibiotic-resistant organisms.[35,36]

Prophylactic Antibiotics

The use of both topical and systemic prophylactic antibiotics may reduce respiratory infections and overall mortality rates in critically ill patients.[36] Inadequate and delayed initial treatment contributes to the risk of VAP and is often associated with a delay in writing the medical order.[55,56]

Antibiotics have a "bimodal" effect in the development of VAP. Within the first days of mechanical ventilation, antibiotics protect against pneumonia development, especially against types caused by endogenous flora. But exposure to antibiotics has a significant risk factor for colonization and infection with nosocomial, MDR pathogens that are associated with significant mortality, such as *P. aeruginosa* and MRSA.[40,55,56]

There are currently no recommendations from the CDC regarding the routine use of systemic antimicrobial agents to prevent VAP or nosocomial pneumonias.[40,47] On the other hand, judicious use of appropriate antibiotics may reduce patient colonization and subsequent infections with multidrug-resistant bacteria.[40]

SUMMARY

- Ventilator-associated pneumonia (VAP) is defined as pneumonia that develops 48 hours after a patient has been placed on mechanical ventilation.
- VAP is the most common nosocomial infection encountered in the ICU.

- Guidelines for the management of VAP focus on early diagnosis, appropriate antibiotic treatment, and various strategies to prevent the transmission of pathogenic organisms to patients receiving mechanical ventilation.
- The prognosis of patients with early-onset VAP is better than those patients with late-onset VAP.
- The most prevalent microorganisms in VAP are gram-negative bacilli. Recent studies have shown an increased incidence of MDR, particularly MRSA.
- Several host-related risk factors can contribute to the development of VAP. These factors are related to the age of the patient, the diagnosis at admission and severity of the illness, and the presence of comorbidities.

- Overuse of sedatives and paralytics, as well as the use of gastroprotective medications for stress ulcers, can increase the risk of VAP.
- Inappropriate use of antibiotics is associated with the emergence of MDR pathogens.
- Nonpharmacologic interventions, such as ETs and routine care of ventilator circuits, are potential sources of infectious material.
- Avoiding ET intubation and using noninvasive mechanical ventilation have been shown to lower the incidence of VAP.
- Ventilator circuits do not need to be changed unless they are nonfunctional or if they are visibly soiled with secretions or blood.

REVIEW QUESTIONS *(See Appendix A for answers.)*

1. What is the incidence of VAP among ICU patients receiving mechanical ventilation?
   - A. 1% to 5%
   - B. 8% to 28%
   - C. 25% to 46%
   - D. 50%

2. Which of the following bacterial infections has been increasingly shown to be associated with VAP?
   - A. *Haemophilus influenzae*
   - B. *Escherichia coli*
   - C. Methicillin-resistant *Staphylococcus aureus*
   - D. *Legionella pneumophila*

3. Which of the following would be considered host-related risk factors for the development of VAP?
   1. Malnutrition
   2. Shift in oropharyngeal flora to gram-negative bacilli
   3. Gastric alkalization
   4. Enhanced gag reflex
      - A. 1 and 2 only
      - B. 2 and 3 only
      - C. 1, 2, and 3 only
      - D. 4 only

4. In patients with VAP, bacterial contaminants are typically less than:
   - A. 10^4 CFU/mL
   - B. 10^6 CFU/mL
   - C. 10^8 CFU/mL
   - D. 10^{12} CFU/mL

5. Which of the following have been implicated in the pathogenesis of VAP?
   1. Colonization of the oropharynx by viridian species of *Streptococcus*
   2. Presence of an endotracheal tube
   3. Impaired level of consciousness
   4. Reduced airway pH
      - A. 1 and 3 only
      - B. 2 and 3 only
      - C. 1, 2, and 3 only
      - D. 1, 2, 3, and 4

6. The CDC definition of probable ventilator-associated pneumonia is based on which of the following criteria?
   1. Oxygenation status
   2. Total leukocyte count
   3. Microbiologic analysis of lower airway secretions
   4. Chest radiographs
      - A. 1 and 2 only
      - B. 2 and 3 only
      - C. 1, 2, and 3 only
      - D. 1, 2, 3, and 4

7. Which of the following would not be considered a risk factor for VAP?
   - A. NIV
   - B. High-frequency use of antibiotic use in the community
   - C. Residence in an extended care facility
   - D. Home wound care

8. Which of the following statement is *false* regarding using sucralfate as a prophylactic agent for the treatment of stress ulcers?
   - A. It does not affect the gastric pH.
   - B. It is the most effective agent to treat stress ulcers in ARDS patients.
   - C. Sucralfate should not be used with patients who are at high risk for gastrointestinal bleeding.
   - D. The CDC does not have specific recommendations for the use of sucralfate in stress-bleeding prophylaxis.

9. Which of these nonpharmacologic strategies has not been shown to reduce the incidence of VAP?
   - A. Semirecumbent positioning of the patient
   - B. Use of closed-suction catheters and sterile suction techniques
   - C. Nasal rather than oral ET intubation
   - D. Maintaining adequate ET cuff pressure

10. Which of the following methods does not improve a patient's immune response to infections?
    - A. Maintain nutritional status
    - B. Relying on the use of invasive procedures when possible
    - C. Avoid agents that impair pulmonary defense (e.g., sedative narcotics, anesthetics, aminophylline)
    - D. Treat disease states that affect host defenses (e.g., acidosis, dehydration, hypoxemia)

References

1. Langer M, Cigada M, Mandelli M, et al: Early onset pneumonia: a multicenter study in intensive care units. *Intensive Care Med* 13:342–346, 1987.
2. Kollef MH: The prevention of ventilator-associated pneumonia. *N Engl J Med* 340:627–634, 1999.
3. Chastre J, Fagon JY: Ventilator-associated pneumonia. *Am J Respir Crit Care Med* 165(7):867–903, 2002.
4. Porzecanski I, Bowton DL: Diagnosis and treatment of ventilator-associated pneumonia. *Chest* 130:597–604, 2006.
5. Safdar N, Dezfulian C, Collard HR, et al: Clinical and economical consequences of ventilator-associated pneumonia: a systematic review. *Crit Care Med* 33:2184–2193, 2005.
6. Safdar N, Crnich CJ, Maki DG: The pathogenesis of ventilator-associated pneumonia: its relevance to developing effective strategies for prevention. *Respir Care* 50(6):725–741, 2005.
7. American Thoracic Society, Infectious Diseases Society of America: Guidelines for the management of adults with hospital-acquired, ventilator-associated, and healthcare-associated pneumonia. *Am J Respir Care Med* 171:388–416, 2005.
8. Kollef MH: Diagnosis of ventilator-associated pneumonia. *N Engl J Med* 355:2691–2693, 2006.
9. Cook DJ, Walter SD, Cook RJ, et al: Incidents of and risk factors for ventilator-associated pneumonia in critically ill patients. *Ann Intern Med* 129:433–440, 1998.
10. Rello J, Ollendorf DA, Oster G, et al: VAP Outcomes Scientific Advisory Group. Epidemiology and outcomes of ventilator-associated pneumonia in large US database. *Chest* 122:2115–2121, 2002.
11. Fagon JY, Chastre J, Hance AJ, et al: Nosocomial pneumonia in ventilated patients: a cohort study evaluating attributable mortality and hospital stay. *Am J Med* 94:281–288, 1993.
12. Stevens RM, Teres F, Skillman JJ, et al: Pneumonia in an intensive care unit: a 30-month experience. *Arch Intern Med* 134:106–111, 1974.
13. Craven DE, Kunches LM, Kilinsky V, et al: Risk factors for pneumonia and fatality in patients receiving continuous mechanical ventilation. *Am Rev Respir Dis* 133:792–796, 1986.
14. Baker AM, Meredith JW, Haponik EF: Pneumonia in intubated trauma patients. Microbiology and outcomes. *Am J Respir Crit Care Med* 153:343–349, 1996.
15. Tejada Artigas A, Bello Dronda S, Chacon Valles E, et al: Risk factors for nosocomial pneumonia in critically ill trauma patients. *Crit Care Med* 29:304–309, 2001.
16. Kollef MH, Micek ST: *Staphylococcus aureus* pneumonia: a superbug infection in community and hospital settings. *Chest* 128:1093–1097, 2005.
17. LaForce FM: Hospital-acquired gram-negative rod pneumonias: an overview. *Am J Med* 70:664–669, 1981.
18. Spencer RC: Predominant pathogens found in European prevalence of infection in intensive care study. *Eur J Clin Microbiol Infect Dis* 15:281–285, 1996.
19. Bell RC, Coalson JJ, Smith JD, et al: Multiple organ system failure and infection in adult respiratory distress syndrome. *Ann Intern Med* 99:293–298, 1983.
20. Kollef MH: Ventilator-associated pneumonia: a multivariate analysis. *JAMA* 270:1965–1970, 1993.
21. National Center for Infectious Diseases, Centers for Disease Control (CDC): Guidelines for preventing health-care-associated pneumonia, 2003 recommendations of the CDC and Healthcare Infection Control Practices Advisory Committee. *Respir Care* 49:926–939, 2004.
22. Salathe M, Wanner A: Nonspecific host defenses: mucociliary clearance and cough. In Niederman M, editor: *Respiratory infections*, Philadelphia, 1994, W.B. Saunders, pp 17–32.
23. Zeiher BG, Hornick DB: Pathogenesis of respiratory infections and host defenses. *Curr Opin Pulm Med* 2:166–173, 1996.
24. Levine SA, Niederman MS: The impact of tracheal intubation on host defenses and risks for nosocomial pneumonia. *Clin Chest Med* 12:523–543, 1991.
25. Porzecanski I, Bowton DL: Diagnosis and treatment of ventilator-associated pneumonia. *Chest* 130:597–604, 2006.
26. Mietto C, Pinciroli R, Patel N, et al: Ventilator associated pneumonia: evolving definitions and preventative strategies. *Respir Care* 58:990–1003, 2013.
27. Klompas M: Complication of mechanical ventilation—The CDC's new surveillance paradigm. *N Engl J Med* 368:1472–1475, 2013.
28. Schurink CAM, Van Nieuwenhoven CA, Jacobs JA, et al: Clinical pulmonary infection score for ventilator-associated pneumonia: accuracy and inter-observer variability. *Intensive Care Med* 30:217–224, 2004.
29. Luyt CE, Chastre J, Fagon JY: Value of the clinical pulmonary infection score for the identification and management of ventilator-associated pneumonia. *Intensive Care Med* 30:844–852, 2004.
30. Singh N, Rogers P, Atwood CW, et al: Short-course empiric antibiotic therapy for patients with pulmonary infiltrates in the intensive care unit: a proposed solution for indiscriminate antibiotic prescription. *Am J Respir Crit Care Med* 162:505–511, 2000.
31. Baselski VS, Wunderink RG: Bronchoscopic diagnosis of pneumonia. *Clin Microbiol Rev* 7:533–558, 1994.
32. Baughman RP: Nonbronchoscopic evaluation of ventilator-associated pneumonia. *Semin Respir Infect* 18:95–102, 2003.
33. Meduri GN, Reddy RC, Stanley T, et al: Pneumonia in acute respiratory distress syndrome. A prospective evaluation of bilateral bronchoscopic sampling. *Am J Respir Crit Care Med* 158:870–875, 1998.
34. Tolentino-DelosReyes AF, Ruppert SD, Shiao SPK: Evidence-based practice: Use of ventilator bundles to prevent ventilator-associated pneumonia. *Am J Crit Care* 16:20–27, 2007.
35. Collard HR, Saint S, Matthay MA: Prevention of ventilator-associated pneumonia: an evidence-based systematic review. *Ann Intern Med* 138:494–501, 2003.
36. Littlewood K, Durbin CG: Evidenced-based airway management. *Respir Care* 46:1392–1405, 2001.
37. Dodek K, Keenan S, Cook D, et al: Evidence-based clinical practice guideline for the prevention of ventilator associated pneumonia. *Ann Intern Med* 141:305–313, 2004.
38. Centers for Disease Control and Prevention: Guideline for hand hygiene in health care settings. *MMWR* 51(RR16):1–45, 2002.
39. MacIntyre NR, Helms M, Wunderink R, et al: Automatic rotational therapy for the prevention of respiratory complications during mechanical ventilation. *Respir Care* 44:1447–1451, 1999.
40. Apostolopoulou E, Bakakos P, Katostaras T, et al: Incidence and risk factors for ventilator-associated pneumonia in 4 multidisciplinary intensive care units in Athens, Greece. *Respir Care* 48:681–688, 2003.
41. Craven DE, Steger KA: Pathogenesis and prevention of nosocomial pneumonia in the mechanically ventilated patient. *Respir Care* 34:85–97, 1989.
42. Hierholzer WJ: Guideline for prevention of nosocomial pneumonia. *Respir Care* 39:1191–1236, 1994.
43. Alcón A, Fabregas N, Torres A: Hospital-acquired pneumonia: etiologic considerations. *Infect Dis Clin North Am* 17:679–695, 2003.
44. Fernandez JF, Levine SM, Restrepo MI: Technologic advances in endotracheal tubes for the prevention of ventilator-associated pneumonia. *Chest* 142:231–238, 2012.
45. Berra L, Curto F, Li Bassi G, et al: Antibacterial-coated tracheal tubes cleaned with the Mucus Shaver: a novel method to retain long-term bactericidal activity of coated tracheal tubes. *Intensive Care Med* 32:888–893, 2006.
46. Rello J, Sonora R, Jubert P, et al: Pneumonia in intubated patients: role of respiratory airway care. *Am J Respir Crit Care Med* 154:111–115, 1996.
47. National Center for Infectious Diseases, Centers for Disease Control and Prevention (CDC): Guidelines for preventing health-care-associated pneumonia, 2003 recommendations of the CDC and the Healthcare Infection Control Practices Advisory Committee. *Respir Care* 49:926–939, 2004.
48. Hess DR: Indications for translaryngeal intubation. *Respir Care* 44:604–609, 1999.
49. Mahul P, Auboyer C, Jospe R, et al: Prevention of nosocomial pneumonia in intubated patients: respective role of mechanical subglottic secretions drainage and stress ulcer prophylaxis. *Intensive Care Med* 18:20–25, 1992.
50. Valles J, Artigas A, Rello J, et al: Continuous aspiration of subglottic secretions in preventing ventilator-associated pneumonia. *Ann Intern Med* 122:179–186, 1995.
51. Han JN, Liu YP, Ma S, et al: Effects of decreasing the frequency of ventilator circuit changes to every 7 days on the rate of ventilator-associated pneumonia in a Beijing hospital. *Respir Care* 46:891–896, 2001.
52. American Association for Respiratory Care: AARC Evidence-Based Clinical Practice Guideline: Care of the ventilator circuit and its relation to ventilator-associated pneumonia. *Respir Care* 48:869–879, 2003.

53. Kelly M, Gillies D, Todd DA, et al: Heated humidification versus heat and moisture exchangers for ventilated adults and children. *Cochrane Database Syst Rev* CD004711, 2010.

54. Panchabhai TM, Dangayach NS, Krishnan A, et al: Oropharyngeal cleansing with 0.2% chlorhexidine for prevention of nosocomial pneumonia in critically ill patients. *Chest* 135:1150–1156, 2009.

55. Markowicz P, Wolff M, Djedaini K, et al: Multicenter prospective study of ventilator-associated pneumonia during acute respiratory distress syndrome. *Am J Respir Crit Care Med* 161:1942–1948, 2000.

56. Koenig SM, Truwit JD: Ventilator-associated pneumonia: diagnosis, treatment, and prevention. *Clin Micro Rev* 19:637–657, 2006.

Sedatives, Analgesics, and Paralytics

OUTLINE

Sedatives and Analgesics
Monitoring the Need for Sedation and Analgesia
Benzodiazepines
Neuroleptics
Anesthetic Agents
Opioids

Paralytics
Monitoring Neuromuscular Blockade
Depolarizing Agents
Nondepolarizing Agents
Summary

KEY TERMS

- Analgesics
- Anesthetic
- Anterograde amnesic
- Depolarizing agents
- Miosis
- Nondepolarizing agents
- Paralytics
- Pruritus
- Ramsay Sedation Scale
- Sedatives
- Train-of-four monitoring

LEARNING OBJECTIVES   *On completion of this chapter, the reader will be able to do the following:*

1. List the most common sedatives and analgesics used in the treatment of critically ill patients.
2. Discuss the indications, contraindications, and potential side effects associated with each of the sedatives and analgesic agents reviewed.
3. Describe the most common method for assessing the need for and level of sedation.
4. Describe the Ramsay scale.
5. Discuss the advantages and disadvantages of using benzodiazepines, neuroleptics, anesthetic agents, and opioids in the management of mechanically ventilated patients.

6. Discuss the mode of action of depolarizing and nondepolarizing paralytics.
7. Explain how the train-of-four method is used to assess the level of paralysis in critically ill patients.
8. Contrast the indications, contraindications, and potential side effects associated with using various types of neuromuscular blocking agents.
9. Recommend a medication for a mechanically ventilated patient with severe anxiety and agitation.

Sedatives, analgesics, and paralytics are often required for the treatment of mechanically ventilated patients in the intensive care unit (ICU). The importance of these drugs in the management of critically ill patients requires critical care therapists to have a working knowledge of the indications and contraindications, mode of action, potential adverse effects, and the most appropriate methods to monitor the effects of these drugs.

Sedatives are used to reduce anxiety and agitation and to promote sleep and anterograde amnesia; **analgesics** are used to lessen pain; **paralytics** are used to facilitate invasive procedures (e.g., surgery, endotracheal intubation), and to prevent movement and ensure the stability of artificial airways. Paralysis may also be used to facilitate less conventional mechanical ventilation strategies.[1-3]

A variety of pharmacologic agents are available for achieving sedation and paralysis of mechanically ventilated patients. The most

common sedative drugs used in the ICU include the following: (1) benzodiazepines (e.g., diazepam, midazolam, and lorazepam), (2) neuroleptics (e.g., haloperidol), (3) anesthetic agents (e.g., propofol), and (4) opioids (e.g., morphine, fentanyl). Paralysis can be achieved with neuromuscular blocking agents (NMBA) that are classified as depolarizing and nondepolarizing, depending on their mode of action. Succinylcholine is the only example of a depolarizing NMBA in widespread use; the most commonly used nondepolarizing NMBAs include pancuronium, vecuronium, and atracurium.

Maintaining an optimal level of comfort and safety for the patient should be a primary goal when administering sedatives, analgesics, and NMBAs. It is important, therefore, to recognize that although these agents can dramatically improve patient outcomes in mechanically ventilated patients, they can also precipitate significant hemodynamic, autonomic, and respiratory consequences in these patients (Key Point 15-1).

> **Key Point** 15-1 Sedatives are used to reduce anxiety and agitation and to promote sleep; analgesics are used to lessen pain.

SEDATIVES AND ANALGESICS

Sedation practices vary considerably because of institutional bias and because the requirements for sedation can vary greatly among patients.[4] As mentioned, sedation is generally prescribed for critically ill patients to treat anxiety and agitation and to prevent or at least minimize sleep deprivation. Agitation and sleep deprivation can result from a variety of factors, including extreme anxiety, delirium, pain, and adverse drug effects. Sedation is also often required for mechanically ventilated patients who are being treated with less conventional modes of ventilation, such as high-frequency ventilation, inverse inspiratory-to-expiratory ratio ventilation, and permissive hypercapnia.[5]

The Joint Commission has defined four levels of sedation: minimal, moderate, deep, and anesthesia (Box 15-1). It is important to recognize that sedation needs may vary considerably during the course of a patient's stay in the ICU. For example, deeper levels of sedation and analgesia may be required during the initial phases of mechanical ventilation, especially in cases in which the patient is asynchronous or "fighting" the mechanical ventilatory mode being used. Conversely, minimal levels of sedation and analgesia are usually required during the recovery phase of an illness. Indeed, weaning a patient from mechanical ventilation can be severely hindered if the patient is oversedated.[6] It should be apparent, therefore, that reliable and accurate methods for assessing the need and level of sedation and analgesia are essential for the successful management of critically ill patients.[7]

BOX 15-1   Levels of Sedation

Minimal Sedation
Patients can respond to verbal commands, although cognitive function may be impaired. Ventilatory and cardiovascular functions are unaffected.

Moderate Sedation (Conscious Sedation)
The patient can perform purposeful response following repeated or painful stimulation. (NOTE: Reflex withdrawal from painful stimulus is not considered a purposeful response.) Spontaneous ventilation is adequate, and cardiovascular function is usually maintained.

Deep Sedation
The patient is not easily aroused but can respond to painful stimulation. Spontaneous ventilation and maintenance of patent airway may be inadequate. Cardiovascular function is usually maintained.

Anesthesia
This level involves general anesthesia, spinal, or major regional anesthesia; local anesthesia is not included. Patient cannot be aroused, even by painful stimulation. Ventilatory assistance is typically required (i.e., artificial airway and positive pressure ventilation). Cardiovascular function may be impaired.

(Modified from the American Society of Anesthesiologists: ASA Standards, Guidelines and Statements, October 2007.)

Monitoring the Need for Sedation and Analgesia

Several techniques have been proposed to assess the level of sedation in adults and children. Examples of scoring systems that have been validated for use in critically ill patients include the **Ramsay Sedation Scale** (RSS), the Motor Activity Assessment Scale (MAAS), the Sedation-Agitation Scale (SAS), and the Comfort Scale. Although considerable debate exists over the best technique, it is generally agreed that patients should be assessed regularly to ensure that they are relaxed and are not complaining of pain (Key Point 15-2).

> **Key Point** 15-2 Pain assessment and response to therapy should be performed regularly and systematically documented.[7]

The RSS is shown in Table 15-1.[8] Notice that it is a graduated single-category scale. The grade assigned by the observer depends on the patient's response to stimuli. The advantages of using this type of single category scale are that it is relatively easy to perform and provides a numerical value that can be used as a target for achieving adequate sedation. For example, a score of 2 to 4 on the RSS indicates adequate sedation. There are several disadvantages associated with using this type of graded scale. Most notably it does not provide any guidance on selection of the most appropriate sedative, and it is a subjective, nonlinear scale that does not allow for consideration of changing physiological and psychological needs of a patient during the course of his or her illness.[1]

Benzodiazepines

Benzodiazepines have been the drugs of choice for the treatment of anxiety in critical care.[1] Preferential use of these drugs by critical care physicians is probably related to their relatively low cost and to the ability of these drugs to produce anxiolytic, hypnotic, muscle relaxation, anticonvulsant, and **anterograde amnesic** effects. Anterograde amnesia relates to preventing the acquisition and encoding of new information that can potentially lead to memories of unpleasant experiences and posttraumatic stress disorder (PTSD).

Benzodiazepines exert their effects through a nonspecific depression of the central nervous system (CNS). This is accomplished when these drugs bind to benzodiazepine sites on the γ-aminobutyric acid (GABA) receptor complex on neurons in the

---

TABLE 15-1   The Ramsay Sedation Scale

Score	Description
1	Patient is awake but anxious, agitated, and restless.
2	Patient is awake, cooperative, oriented, and tranquil.
3	Patient is semi-asleep but responds to verbal commands.
4	Patient is asleep and has a brisk response to a light glabellar tap or loud auditory stimulus.
5	Patient is asleep and has a sluggish response to a light glabellar tap or loud auditory stimulus.
6	Patient is asleep and has no response to a light glabellar tap or loud auditory stimulus.

TABLE 15-2	Selected Sedatives Used for Critically Ill Adult Patients			
Agent	Onset After IV Dose (min)	Half-Life of Parent Compound (hr)	Intermittent IV Dose	Infusion Dose Range (Usual)
Diazepam	2-5	20-120	0.03-0.1 mg/kg q 0.5-6 hr	—
Midazolam	2-5	3-11	0.02-0.08 mg/kg q 0.5-2 hr	0.04-0.2 mg/kg/hr
Lorazepam	5-20	8-15	0.02-0.06 mg/kg q 2-6 hr	0.01-0.1 mg/kg/hr
Propofol	1-2	26-32	—	5-80 µg/kg/min
Haloperidol	3-20	18-54	0.03-0.15 mg/kg q 0.5-6 hr	0.04-0.15 mg/kg/hr

Modified from Jacobi J, Fraser GL, Coursin DB, et al: Clinical practice guidelines for the sustained use of sedatives and analgesics in the critically ill adult, Crit Care Med 30:119-141, 2002.
IV, Intravenous.

brain. Binding of benzodiazepines to the GABA receptor complex increases the chloride permeability of the neuron, which in turn hyperpolarizes the neuron, making depolarization less likely.[9]

Benzodiazepines vary in potency, onset of action, uptake, distribution, and elimination half-life (see Table 15-2 for a comparison of the pharmacologic properties of diazepam, midazolam, and lorazepam). It is worth noting that the intensity and duration of action for the various benzodiazepines can be affected by a number of patient-specific factors, including age, underlying pathology, and concurrent drug therapy. Prolonged recovery from benzodiazepines typically occurs in patients with renal and hepatic insufficiency.[7]

Benzodiazepines generally produce only minimal effects on cardiovascular function; however, they can cause a significant drop in blood pressure when initially administered to hemodynamically unstable patients (e.g., patients with hypovolemic shock). Similarly benzodiazepines normally do not adversely affect the respiratory system; however, they can produce hypoventilation or apnea by causing a reduction in ventilatory drive in patients with chronic obstructive pulmonary disease (COPD) when combined with opioids.

Reversal of the effects of benzodiazepines can be accomplished with flumazenil (Romazicon), which prevents the sedative effects of these drugs by competitively binding to benzodiazepine receptors. It is a short-acting drug that is administered intravenously at doses of 0.2 to 1.0 mg; subsequent doses may be repeated every 20 minutes up to a maximum dose of 3 mg/h. Administration of flumazenil is generally reserved for patients admitted to the emergency department for suspected benzodiazepine overdose. The most common side effects of flumazenil include dizziness, panic attacks, and cardiac ischemia, and it may lead to seizures in patients receiving long-term benzodiazepine or tricyclic antidepressant therapy.

Diazepam

Diazepam (Valium) has a rapid onset of action because of its high lipid solubility and ability to traverse the blood–brain barrier relatively quickly. The average onset of action for diazepam when it is administered intravenously is 3 to 5 minutes.[9] It is metabolized in the liver to active metabolites that have relatively long half-lives (40 to 100 hours). These active metabolites are ultimately eliminated by the kidney. As such, diazepam elimination can be decreased in

older patients, neonates, and patients with compromised hepatic and renal function, resulting in prolonged clinical effects and delayed recovery from sedation.[10]

Intravenous (IV) administration of diazepam is the most reliable method to maintain sedation in critically ill patients because absorption through the oral and intramuscular routes can vary considerably. Continuous infusion of diazepam is not recommended. Instead, a bolus dose of the drug is administered at the start of an infusion, followed by a series of smaller boluses with close titration to produce the desired plasma concentration of the drug.[11]

Midazolam

Midazolam (Versed) has a rapid onset of action and short half-life, making it an ideal sedative for the treatment of acutely agitated patients (Key Point 15-3). Note that although it does have a short half-life, prolonged sedation can occur as a result of the accumulation of the drug and its metabolites in the peripheral tissues when it is administered for longer than 48 hours.[1]

Key Point 15-3 Midazolam and diazepam should be used for rapid sedation of acutely agitated patients.[7]

Midazolam causes a reduction in cerebral perfusion pressure, but it does not protect against increases in intracranial pressure for patients receiving ketamine.[1] Although midazolam does not cause respiratory depression in most patients, it depresses the sensitivity of upper respiratory reflexes, and it can reduce the ventilatory response in patients with COPD and in patients receiving narcotics.[12]

Midazolam typically causes only minimal hemodynamic effects (e.g., lower blood pressure, reduction in heart rate) in euvolemic subjects, and is usually well tolerated in patients with left ventricular dysfunction. It can produce significant reductions in systemic vascular resistance and blood pressure in patients who are dependent on increased sympathetic tone to maintain venous return.[1]

Lorazepam

Lorazepam (Ativan) is the drug of choice for sedating mechanically ventilated patients in the ICU for longer than 24 hours. It has a slower onset of action compared with diazepam and midazolam due to its lower lipid solubility and longer time required to cross the blood–brain barrier. Its lower lipid solubility coupled with decreased distribution in peripheral tissues may account for its longer duration of action in some patients when compared with diazepam and midazolam.[13]

Potential adverse drug interactions are less likely with lorazepam than with other benzodiazepines because it is metabolized in the liver to inactive metabolites. Continual use of lorazepam, however, has been associated with several side effects including lactic acidosis, hyperosmolar coma, and a reversible nephrotoxicity. These latter side effects have been attributed to the use of the solvents propylene glycol and polyethylene glycol in the manufacture of lorazepam.[9] It is also worth noting that lorazepam acts synergistically with other central CNS depressants and should be administered with caution in patients receiving these drugs.[13] Case Study 15-1 provides more information about several potential harmful effects associated with long-term use of lorazepam.

Dexmedetomidine

Dexmedetomidine is an α_2-adrenoreceptor agonist that is used for short-term sedation and analgesia in the ICU. It has been shown to reduce sympathetic tone (i.e., sympatholytic activity), with attenuation of the neuroendocrine and hemodynamic response to anesthesia and surgery.[14,15] It has been shown to reduce the need for anesthetic and opioid requirements.[14] In a randomized controlled study designed to determine the efficacy of dexmedetomidine versus midazolam and propofol in ICU patients, Jakob and colleagues found that dexmedetomidine had similar effects to midazolam and propofol to maintain light to moderate sedation. They also showed that dexmedetomidine appeared to reduce the duration of mechanical ventilation compared to midazolam. When compared to midazolam and propofol, dexmedetomidine reduced the time to extubation. Another interesting finding was that it reduced delirium in patients compared to propofol, and improved patients' ability to communicate pain compared with midazolam and propofol. The study did find, however, that more adverse effects were associated with dexmedetomidine when compared with midazolam and propofol.[15]

Neuroleptics

Neuroleptics are routinely used to treat patients demonstrating evidence of extreme agitation and delirium. Disorganized thinking and unnecessary motor activity characterize delirium; it is often seen in patients who have been treated in the ICU for prolonged periods (i.e., ICU syndrome) (Key Point 15-4).

 Key Point 15-4 The presence of delirium can delay liberation of patients from mechanical ventilation.

Haloperidol is a butyrophenone that causes CNS depression. Although it is the drug of choice for the treatment of delirium in ICU patients, it can cause some potentially serious side effects. It possesses antidopaminergic and anticholinergic effects. It can induce α-blockade, lower the seizure threshold, and evoke Parkinson-like symptoms (i.e., extrapyramidal effects, like muscle rigidity, drowsiness, and lethargy). Dose-dependent cardiac dysrhythmias, including QT prolongation and torsades de pointes,

have also been reported to occur particularly in patients receiving high-dose bolus administration of haloperidol.[16]

Case Study 15-1

Patient Case—Discontinuing Lorazepam

A 50-year-old man with moderately severe pulmonary fibrosis is admitted to the emergency department with an irregular heart rate and signs of agitation. He reports that he is exhausted and unable to get a good night's sleep. He has been treated with lorazepam (Ativan) for anxiety and insomnia for 6 months. He explains to the attending physician that he stopped taking his medication because "it makes me feel too tired to get anything done." What are some common side effects associated with abruptly discontinuing taking the lorazepam?

The onset of action of haloperidol is 3 to 20 minutes after an initial 5-mg dose is administered intravenously. Additional doses of the drug can be administered if the patient continues to be agitated (additional IV doses of 5 mg can usually be administered safely up to a maximum dose of 200 mg). Despite the potential side effects noted above, haloperidol has been demonstrated to be a safe drug for the treatment of delirium in ICU patients.[17]

Anesthetic Agents

Propofol (Diprivan) is an IV, general **anesthetic** agent that possesses sedative, amnesic, and hypnotic properties at low doses, although it has no analgesic properties. It is typically administered as an initial bolus of 1 to 2 mg/kg followed by a continuous infusion at a rate of 3 to 6 mg/kg/hour.

Propofol produces significant hemodynamic effects. Most notably, it causes reductions in systemic vascular resistance with a concomitant fall in blood pressure and bradycardia during the initial induction phase. Propofol reduces cerebral blood flow and intracranial pressure (ICP), making it a useful sedative for neurosurgical patients. In fact, propofol has been shown to be more effective than fentanyl in reducing ICP in patients with traumatic brain injury. Additionally, propofol and morphine administered simultaneously allow greater control of ICP than does morphine alone.[9]

Propofol has a rapid onset and short duration of sedation once it is discontinued. The rapid awakening from propofol allows interruption of the infusion for neurologic assessment. Slightly longer recovery times can occur with prolonged infusion. Clearance appears to be unaffected by renal and hepatic dysfunction (Key Point 15-5).

 Key Point 15-5 Propofol is an ideal sedative when rapid awakening is important, such as when neurologic assessment is required, or for extubation.[7]

Adverse effects associated with propofol administration include hypotension, dysrhythmias, and bradycardia. It has also been shown to cause elevation of pancreatic enzymes. Propofol infusion syndrome in ICU sedation is characterized by severe metabolic acidosis, hyperkalemia, rhabdomyolysis, hepatomegaly, and cardiac and renal failure. Propofol is available as an emulsion in a phospholipid vehicle, which provides 1.1 kcal/mL. This fact is important to keep in mind because propofol is a source of triglycerides and supplemental calories in patients receiving parenteral nutrition.[1] Prolonged use (>48 hours) has also been associated with lactic acidosis and lipidemia in pediatric patients.

Opioids

Opioids (or opiates) are endogenous and exogenous substances that can bind to a group of receptors located in the CNS and peripheral tissues. Opioids are generally classified as naturally occurring, synthetic, and semisynthetic, or as discussed below, may be classified on the basis of their activity at opioid receptors.[1] Morphine sulfate is a naturally occurring opioid agonist; fentanyl citrate is a synthetic analog of morphine.

Although the primary pharmacologic action of opioids is to relieve pain, these drugs can also provide significant secondary sedative and anxiolytic effects, which are mediated through two types of opioid receptors: mu (μ) and kappa (κ) receptors. The μ-receptors are responsible for analgesia, and the κ-receptors mediate the sedative effects of these drugs.

It is well recognized that opioids can cause a number of serious side effects (Box 15-2). The severity of these side effects depends on the dosage administered, as well as the extent of the patient's illness and the integrity of his or her organ function (i.e., renal, hepatic, and hemodynamic function).

Reversal of the aforementioned side effects can be accomplished with the opioid antagonist, naloxone hydrochloride (Narcan). Naloxone has a short onset of action (~30 seconds) and usually lasts about 30 minutes. When used to facilitate opioid withdrawal, a continuous IV infusion is required. It is important to understand that administering smaller doses of naloxone will reverse the respiratory depressant effects of opioids, while not interfering with the analgesic effects of these drugs. Using larger doses will not only reverse respiratory depression, but it will also reduce the analgesic effects.

Morphine

Morphine is a potent opioid analgesic agent that is the preferred agent for intermittent therapy because of its longer duration of action. It can produce significant effects on the CNS and alter the control of breathing even in normal healthy individuals. Some of the potential side effects of morphine include reductions in minute ventilation ($\dot{V}_E$), periodic breathing, and even apnea by altering respiratory activity of the pontine and medullary respiratory centers in the brainstem.[1] Morphine's effects on the CNS also include reductions of cerebral blood flow, ICP, and cerebral metabolic activity, drowsiness and lethargy, **miosis,** and suppression of the cough reflex.[18]

| BOX 15-2 | Side Effects of Opioids |

Nausea, vomiting, constipation
Respiratory depression
Bradycardia and hypotension
Myoclonus (muscle twitching), convulsions
Histamine release, immunosuppression
Physical dependence

The effects of morphine on the gastrointestinal (GI) tract include reduction of lower esophageal sphincter tone and propulsive peristaltic activity of the intestine, which in turn leads to constipation. Morphine can also increase the tone of the pyloric sphincter and ultimately lead to nausea and vomiting by delaying the passage of contents through the GI tract.[1]

Morphine can alter vascular resistance by causing decreases in sympathetic tone and increases in vagal tone. Reduction in vascular tone can lead to significant hypotension in patients who rely on increased sympathetic tone to maintain blood pressure. Increases in serum histamine levels can also occur with the injection of morphine and ultimately add to the peripheral vasodilation and hypotension. Increased serum histamine levels are associated with **pruritus** and bronchospasm in asthmatics and individuals with hypersensitive airways.

In the ICU, the IV route of delivery is the most effective method of administering morphine for sedation. It can be delivered as a bolus or as a continuous infusion when prolonged sedation and analgesia are required. The onset of action of morphine is slower than other opioids because of its lower lipid solubility and slower transit time across the blood–brain barrier. It is metabolized to active metabolites, including morphine-6 glucuronide, which can result in prolonged clinical effects. The presence of renal or hepatic diseases can further impair the clearance of morphine and its metabolites.

Fentanyl

Fentanyl citrate (Sublimaze) is a synthetic opioid that is approximately 100 to 150 times more potent than morphine.[19] Its high lipid solubility and short transit time across the blood–brain barrier produce a rapid onset of action. Fentanyl has a longer half-life than morphine and can accumulate in the peripheral tissues after prolonged infusion. In cases of prolonged infusion, clearance can be delayed, resulting in long-lasting effects (e.g., respiratory depression), particularly in patients with renal failure.

Fentanyl is normally administered as a loading dose followed by a continuous infusion to maintain its analgesic effect because of its short duration of action. Fentanyl transdermal patches are available for patients who require long-term analgesia. Although these patches can provide consistent drug delivery in hemodynamically stable patients, the extent of absorption varies depending on the permeability, temperature, perfusion, and thickness of the patient's skin.[9] Different sites should be used when reapplying patches. It should also be mentioned that fentanyl patches are not indicated for the treatment of acute analgesia because it takes approximately 12 to 24 hours to reach peak effect. Once the patch is removed, a similar lag period occurs before the effects completely disappear.

Fentanyl has minimal effects on the cardiovascular system and does not cause histamine release as does morphine. It also has minimal effects on the renal system compared with other opioids. Therefore fentanyl is the opioid of choice for patients with unstable hemodynamic status and renal insufficiency (Key Point 15-6). It can cause respiratory depression in some patients because of a biphasic elimination response that occurs when the drug is mobilized from peripheral tissues.

Box 15-3 summarizes the agents discussed in this section (Case Study 15-2).

Key Point **15-6** Fentanyl is preferred for patients with hemodynamic instability and renal insufficiency.[7]

BOX 15-3   **Sedatives, Neuroleptics, Anesthetic Agents, and Opioids Used in Mechanically Ventilated Patients**

Sedatives (Benzodiazepines)
Diazepam (Valium)
Rapid onset of action
Relatively low cost
Half-life of 36 hours (or 1 to 3 days); multiple doses result in prolonged effect, especially in older patients and in patients with hepatic dysfunction

Midazolam (Versed)
Onset of action in 2.0 to 2.5 minutes
High cost
Half-life of 1 hour
Prolonged action with impaired hepatic function
Metabolized in the liver

Lorazepam (Ativan)
Onset of action in 5 to 20 minutes
Low cost
Half-life of 6 to 15 hours

Other Sedatives
Chlordiazepoxide (Librium)
Dexmedetomidine (Precedex)
Alprazolam (Xanax)
Triazolam (Halcion)
Flurazepam (Dalmane)

Neuroleptics
Haloperidol (Haldol)
Onset in 3 to 5 minutes
Half-life 18 to 54 hours

Anesthetic
Propofol (Diprivan)
Onset of action in 1 minute
Very high cost
Half-life from <30 minutes to 3 hours

Opioids (Narcotic Analgesics)
Morphine Sulfate
Moderate onset of action
Low cost

Fentanyl Citrate (Sublimaze)
Rapid onset of action
Moderate cost
Short duration of action, but longer half-life than morphine
Less cardiovascular effect than morphine; more potent than morphine; may produce increased muscle tone (e.g., chest and abdominal wall rigidity)

Others
Hydromorphone (Dilaudid)
Rapid onset of action
Moderate cost
Acceptable morphine substitute

 Case Study 15-2

Patient Case—Agitated Patient
A 30-year-old woman admitted to the intensive care unit following a motor vehicle accident is anxious and in obvious pain. She is listed as being in guarded condition because of fluctuation in her arterial blood pressure. She has become increasingly combative to the attending staff, and made several unsuccessful attempts to remove her endotracheal tube. What would be an effective pharmacologic agent to treat this patient's symptoms?

PARALYTICS

The following are the most common reasons for using NMBAs in mechanically ventilated patients:

- Patient-ventilator asynchrony that cannot be corrected by adjusting ventilator settings
- Facilitation of less conventional mechanical ventilation strategies (e.g., inverse I:E ratios, high-frequency ventilation, permissive hypercapnia)
- Facilitation of intubation, ensuring stability of the airway during transport, or repositioning
- Dynamic hyperinflation that cannot be corrected
- Adjunctive therapy for controlling raised ICP
- Reduction of oxygen consumption and carbon dioxide production[1] (Key Point 15-7)

Key Point 15-7 It is important to recognize that ventilator asynchrony may be the result of an inappropriate ventilator setting or the presence of auto-PEEP.

As mentioned earlier, the two classes of NMBAs available for paralyzing mechanically ventilated patients include depolarizing muscle relaxants and nondepolarizing muscle relaxants. **Depolarizing agents** (succinylcholine) resemble acetylcholine in their chemical structure. These drugs induce paralysis by binding to acetylcholine receptors and causing prolonged depolarization of the motor endplate. **Nondepolarizing agents** (pancuronium, vecuronium, atracurium, and cisatracurium) also bind to acetylcholine receptors, but cause paralysis by competitively inhibiting the action of acetylcholine at the neuromuscular junction (Box 15-4 and Case Study 15-3).

Choosing the most appropriate muscle relaxant depends on a number of factors, such as its onset of action and how fast the patient can recover from its effects once it is discontinued, the patient's physical condition and organ function (particularly renal and hepatic function), as well as the pharmacodynamics and cost of the drug.

Regardless of the NMBA used, it is important to understand that these drugs do **not** possess sedative or analgesic properties (i.e., reduce anxiety or provide pain relief), and must therefore be used in conjunction with adequate amounts of sedatives and analgesics to ensure patient comfort. Furthermore, monitoring the effectiveness of neuromuscular blockade is essential to ensure the patient's safety (Key Point 15-8).

 Key Point 15-8 Neuromuscular blocking agents do **not** possess sedative or analgesic properties.

 Case Study 15-3

Patient Case—Asynchrony

A respiratory therapist notes that a patient is using accessory muscle during mechanical ventilation. The ventilator graphics indicate the presence of patient-ventilator asynchrony. The respiratory therapist checks for appropriate settings of flow, sensitivity, and ventilator mode, and rules out the presence of auto-PEEP. After talking with the physician, it is agreed that the patient may require the use of a pharmacologic intervention. What would be appropriate for this patient?

Monitoring Neuromuscular Blockade

Monitoring neuromuscular blockade can be accomplished using visual, tactile, and electronic assessment of the patient's muscle tone. Observing the patient's skeletal muscle movements and respiratory effort can provide an easy method to determine whether the patient is paralyzed; however, more sophisticated electronic monitoring is typically required to determine the depth of paralysis.

A common method used to assess the depth of paralysis is an electronic technique referred to as **train-of-four** (TOF) monitoring.[20,21] With this technique, two electrodes are placed on the skin along a nerve path, often near a hand, foot, or facial nerve. An electrical current consisting of four impulses is applied to the peripheral nerve over 2 seconds, and the muscle contractions (twitches) produced provide information about the level of paralysis (Box 15-5).

Although there has been considerable debate about how to perform the test and interpret the results (i.e., the number of twitches elicited with the TOF stimulation), the Society for Critical Care Medicine (SCCM) recommends that one to two twitches indicate that an adequate amount of NMBA is being administered.[22] It is important to recognize that TOF monitoring can provide valuable information to enable the clinician to maintain the desired depth of paralysis. Variability can occur among individuals performing the test and thus significantly affect the veracity of the

result. When it is performed accurately and in a consistent manner, however, TOF monitoring can reduce the amount of NMBA administered to a patient and thus avoid complications like the development of prolonged paralysis and muscle weakness.[21]

Depolarizing Agents

Succinylcholine

Succinylcholine chloride (Anectine) is the only depolarizing NMBA in widespread use. It is a short-acting (5 to 10 minutes) depolarizing muscle relaxant that has an onset of action of approximately 60 seconds. Succinylcholine (diACh) is most often used to facilitate endotracheal intubation. Its use in the ICU has declined during recent years because of the introduction of newer paralyzing drugs that have minimal cardiovascular side effects. It is important to know, however, that diACh is the recommended drug for inducing paralysis in hemodynamically stable critically ill patients because of its relatively low cost, rapid onset of action, and short duration of action.

Succinylcholine is administered intravenously at a standard dose of 1 to 1.5 mg/kg. Administering large doses (>2 mg/kg) or repeated doses of diACh can produce a desensitization neuromuscular block resulting in a prolonged paralysis.

The most common side effects associated with diACh include transient hyperkalemia; cardiac dysrhythmias; anaphylactic reactions; prolonged apnea; postoperative myalgias; increased intragastric, intracranial, and intraocular pressures; myoglobinuria; and sustained skeletal muscle contraction. (Hyperkalemia induced by the injection of diACh can be particularly problematic in patients with congestive heart failure who are also receiving diuretics and digitalis.) Succinylcholine can also precipitate malignant hyperthermia in susceptible individuals. Malignant hyperthermia is a rare but potentially fatal disorder that that is characterized by sustained skeletal muscle depolarization. It occurs at a rate of 1:50,000 in adults and 1:15,000 in the pediatric population.[20-23]

Succinylcholine is inactivated by the action of pseudocholinesterase. Therefore prolonged action of diACh can occur if the serum pseudocholinesterase concentration is low or inhibited. Low concentrations of the enzyme occur during pregnancy, chronic renal failure, severe liver damage, and following starvation. The enzyme can be inhibited by anticholinesterases, organophosphates, azathioprine, cyclophosphamide, and monoamine oxidase inhibitors.[13]

Nondepolarizing Agents

Pancuronium

Pancuronium (Pavulon) was one of the first nondepolarizing NMBAs used for prolonged paralysis of mechanically ventilated patients in the ICU. Paralysis is achieved by administering a loading dose of 0.08 to 0.1 mg/kg. Sustained muscle paralysis is accomplished by administering a maintenance dose of 0.05 to 0.1 mg/kg/hour.

Pancuronium is a quaternary ammonium compound; more specifically, an aminosteroid muscle relaxant that has a slow onset and prolonged duration of action. It is metabolized by the liver by acetylation and eliminated through the kidney. The most serious side effect attributed to pancuronium includes prolonged paralysis after discontinuation of the drug, particularly in patients with renal and hepatic failure. The prolonged duration of action may be partially explained by the fact that it is metabolized in the liver to an active 3-hydroxy metabolite that retains up to 50% of the activity of the parent compound.[23]

Other significant side effects associated with pancuronium, which result from its vagolytic effect, include tachycardia, increased cardiac output, and elevated mean arterial pressure. Its sympathomimetic activity can also lead to alterations in ventilation-perfusion relationship as a result of pulmonary vasoconstriction.[23]

Vecuronium

Vecuronium bromide (Norcuron) is an intermediate-duration, nondepolarizing aminosteroid NMBA that does not possess the vagolytic properties of pancuronium.[24] The intermediate duration of action for vecuronium may be explained by its metabolism to minimally active metabolites. Sustained paralysis can be achieved following the administration of a loading dose of 0.1 mg/kg by delivering a maintenance dose of 0.05 to 0.1 mg/kg/hour.[19]

Initial data suggested that vecuronium was an effective means of producing prolonged paralysis in patients with renal insufficiency because of its hepatic and biliary elimination. Subsequent reports, however, suggested that prolonged paralysis may occur in patients with renal and hepatic insufficiency due to accumulation of vecuronium and its 3-desacetyl metabolite.[25]

Atracurium/Cisatracurium

Like vecuronium, atracurium besylate (Tracrium) and its stereoisomer cisatracurium besylate (Nimbex) are intermediate-duration, nondepolarizing muscle relaxants that do not have the hemodynamic side effects of pancuronium. Atracurium has been shown to cause mast cell degranulation and histamine release at higher doses, which in turn can lead to peripheral vasodilation and hypotension. Cisatracurium has been shown to cause only minimal mast cell degranulation and subsequent histamine release.[22] The lack of cardiovascular side effects may be explained on the basis that atracurium and cisatracurium are benzylquinolones that are metabolized to hemodynamically inactive metabolites in the plasma by ester hydrolysis and the Hofmann elimination. One of the breakdown products of the Hofmann elimination of atracurium, laudanosine, has been associated with central nervous system stimulation and can precipitate seizures when it accumulates in the plasma.

The pharmacokinetic profiles of atracurium and cisatracurium make these drugs ideal NMBAs for patients with renal and hepatic insufficiency. Recovery from neuromuscular blockade typically occurs in 1 to 2 hours after continuous infusions are stopped. However, long-term use of these drugs can lead to the development of tolerance, which in turn may necessitate significant dosage

increases. Additionally, muscle weakness can occur with prolonged use of these types of agents[13] (Case Study 15-4).

 Case Study 15-4

Patient Case—Neuromuscular Blocking Agent

A 45-year-old man is admitted to the emergency department for injuries sustained from a fall that occurred while he was working to repair the chimney on his house. His admit diagnosis includes a fractured right radius and contusion to his right upper thorax. There is no evidence of head trauma. The patient's respiratory rate is 30 breaths per minute, his blood pressure is 140/85, and his pulse rate is 110 beats per minute. The resident on-call physician requests that a neuromuscular blocking agent (NMBA) is administered to accomplish intubation of this patient. Which NMBA would be appropriate for this patient?

 SUMMARY

- Selection of the most appropriate drug for sedating or paralyzing a patient should be based on several criteria, including the patient's condition, the drug's efficacy and safety profile, as well as the cost of administering the drug over a prolonged period.
- Although historically the selection of sedatives, analgesics, and NMBAs has been based on personal preference, recent clinical practice guidelines have helped to define more clearly the most appropriate drugs and strategies for clinicians treating ICU patients with these drugs.
- Sedation is generally prescribed for the treatment of anxiety and agitation and to prevent or at least minimize sleep deprivation.
- The ideal sedative should have a rapid onset, have a relatively short active effect, and be easily titrated. Its effects should be reversible and have minimal, if any, effects on vital organ function.
- A common reason for using NMBAs is to alleviate patient-ventilator asynchrony that cannot be resolved with ventilator adjustment.
- Two classes of NMBAs are available for paralyzing mechanically ventilated patients: depolarizing muscle relaxants and nondepolarizing muscle relaxants.
- Choosing the most appropriate NMBA depends on the patient's physical condition, as well as the selected drug's onset of action and how fast the patient can recover from its effects once it is discontinued. NMBAs do not possess sedative or analgesic properties and therefore should be used in conjunction with adequate amounts of sedatives and analgesics to ensure patient comfort.
- Maintaining an optimal level of comfort and safety for the patient should be a primary goal when administering sedatives, analgesics, and NMBAs.

REVIEW QESTIONS *(See Appendix A for answers.)*

1. Which of the following is an appropriate short-acting, depolarizing agent to use for intubation of a patient?
   A. Pancuronium
   B. Succinylcholine
   C. Vecuronium
   D. Fentanyl

2. A mechanically ventilated patient exhibits severe anxiety and agitation. Talking with the patient does not successfully relieve his symptoms. The nurse is concerned that the patient is sleep deprived. Which of the following would be an appropriate medication to suggest?
   A. Opioid
   B. Paralyzing agent
   C. Sedative
   D. Neuromuscular blocking agent

3. A patient in the ICU has a Ramsay score of 6. Which of the following is a patient indication resulting from this score?
   A. Patient responds to a painful stimulus.
   B. Patient has irreversible brain injury.
   C. Patient requires an additional dose of paralyzing agent.
   D. Patient is heavily sedated.

4. While performing an assessment of the level of sedation of a patient, the following is observed: Patient is asleep; patient has a brisk response to a light glabellar tap or loud auditory stimulus. These criteria would suggest that the patient would rate a score of _____ on the Ramsay scale.
   A. 1
   B. 2
   C. 4
   D. 6

5. A patient with chronic CO_2 retention and lung cancer is being treated with morphine for pain. She is very anxious and keeps trying to get out of bed, despite the use of restraints. The nurse gives midazolam (Versed) and shortly thereafter notes that the patient's respirations become irregular and periods of apnea occur. Which of the following is the most appropriate treatment for this patient?
   A. Flumazenil (Romazicon)
   B. Caffeine
   C. Noninvasive positive pressure ventilation
   D. Reduction of morphine administration

6. A patient is receiving mechanical ventilation as a result of an apparent tetanus infection. The patient is having tetanic contractions. What medications would be appropriate for this patient?
   1. Paralytic agents
   2. Analgesics
   3. Sedatives
   4. Diuretics
      A. 1 and 2 only
      B. 2 and 3 only
      C. 1, 2, and 3 only
      D. 2, 3, and 4 only

7. A patient receiving morphine postoperatively by a self-actuating morphine pump complains of nausea. Which of the following is the appropriate response?
   A. Nausea is not a common side effect when administering opioids, so you should ignore the patient's complaint.
   B. Notify housekeeping.
   C. The morphine should be stopped.
   D. Contact the nurse and the physician.

8. Which of the following is a nondepolarizing NMBA?
   1. Pancuronium
   2. Vecuronium
   3. Atracurium
   4. Succinylcholine
      A. 1 and 3 only
      B. 2 and 4 only
      C. 1, 2, and 3 only
      D. 1, 2, 3, and 4

9. Which of the following is not correctly matched?
   A. Diazepam, Valium
   B. Propofol, Diprivan
   C. Midazolam, Versed
   D. Fentanyl, Ativan

10. Describe the technique of TOF monitoring.

References

1. Acquilera L, Arizaga A, Stewart TE, et al: Sedation and paralysis during mechanical ventilation. In Marini JJ, Slutsky AS, editors: *Physiological basis of ventilatory support*, New York, 1998, Marcel-Dekker, pp 601–612.
2. Hurford WE: Sedation and paralysis during mechanical ventilation. *Respir Care* 47:334–346, 2002.
3. Frazer GL, Prato S, Berthiaume D, et al: Evaluation of agitation in ICU patients: incidence, severity, and treatment in the young versus the elderly. *Pharmacotherapy* 20:75–82, 2000.
4. Kress JP, Pohlman AS, Hall JB: Sedation and analgesia in the intensive care unit. *Am J Respir Crit Care Med* 166:1024–1028, 2002.
5. Szokol JW, Vender JS: Anxiety, delirium, and pain in the intensive care unit. *Crit Care Clin* 17:821–842, 2001.
6. Blanchard AR: Sedation and analgesia in intensive care. Medications attenuate stress response in critical illness. *Postgrad Med* 111:59–60, 63–64, 67–70, 2002.
7. Jacobi J, Fraser GL, Coursin DV, et al: Clinical practice guidelines for the sustained use of sedative and analgesics in the critically ill adult. *Crit Care Med* 30:119–131, 2002.
8. Ramsay MAE, Savege TM, Simpson BRJ, et al: Controlled sedation with alpaxalone-alphadolone. *Br Med J* 2:656–659, 1974.
9. Gardenshire DS: *Rau's Respiratory pharmacology*, ed 8, St Louis, 2012, Elsevier.
10. Young CC, Prielipp RC: Benzodiazepines in the intensive care unit. In Vender JS, Szokol JW, Murphy GS, editors: *Sedation, analgesia, and neuromuscular blockers in critical care medicine*, 2001, p 843.
11. Arbour R: Sedation and pain management in critically ill adults. *Crit Care Nurse* 20:39–56, 2000.
12. Murphy PJ, Erskine R, Langton JA: The effects of intravenously administered diazepam, midazolam, and flumazenil on the sensitivity of upper airway reflexes. *Anaesthesia* 49:105–110, 1994.
13. Devlin JW, Roberts RJ: Pharmacology of commonly used analgesics and sedatives in the ICU: benzodiazepines, propofol, and opioids. *Crit Care Clin* 25:431–449, 2009.

14. Gertler R, Creighton H, Mitchell DH, et al: Dexmedetomidine: a novel sedative analgesic agent. *Proc (Bayl Univ Med Cent)* 14:13–21, 2001.

15. Jakob SM, Ruokonen E, Grounds RM, et al: Dexmedetomidine vs midazolam or proposal for sedation during prolonged mechanical ventilation. *JAMA* 307:1151–1160, 2012.

16. Metzger E, Friedman R: Prolongation of the corrected QT and torsades de pointes associated with intravenous haloperidol in the medically ill. *J Clin Psychophamacol* 13:128–132, 1993.

17. McNicoll LL, Pisani MA, Zhang Y, et al: Delirium in the intensive care unit: occurrence and clinical course in older patients. *J Am Geriatr Soc* 51:591–598, 2003.

18. Hardman JG, Limbird LE, Gilman AG: *The pharmacologic basis of therapeutics*, New York, 2001, McGraw-Hill.

19. Hill L, Bertaccini E, Barr J, et al: ICU sedation: a review of its pharmacology and assessment. *J Intensive Care Med* 13:174–183, 1998.

20. Stoelting RK: Neuromuscular blocking drugs. In *Pharmacology and physiology of anesthetic practice*, Philadelphia, 1991, Lippincott.

21. Wiklund RA, Rosenbaum SH: Anesthesiology, Part I. *N Engl J Med* 337:1132–1141, 1997.

22. Murray MJ, Cowen J, DeBlock H, et al: Clinical practice guidelines for sustained neuromuscular blockade in the adult critically ill patient. *Crit Care Med* 30:142–156, 2002.

23. Miller RD, Agoston S, Booij LH, et al: Comparative potency and pharmacokinetics of pancuronium and its metabolites in anesthetized man. *J Pharmcol Exp Ther* 207:539–543, 1978.

24. Wierda JM, Maestrone E, Bencini AF, et al: Hemodynamic effects of vecuronium. *Br J Anaesth* 62:194–198, 1989.

25. Smith CL, Hunter JM, Jones JS: Vecuronium infusion in patients with renal failure in an ICU. *Anaesthesia* 42:387–393, 1987.

CHAPTER 16

Extrapulmonary Effects of Mechanical Ventilation

OUTLINE

KEY TERMS

- Cardiac tamponade
- Cardiac transmural pressure
- Oliguria
- Polyneuritis

LEARNING OBJECTIVES *On completion of this chapter, the reader will be able to do the following:*

1. Explain the effects of positive-pressure ventilation on cardiac output and venous return to the heart.
2. Discuss the three factors that can influence cardiac output during positive-pressure ventilation.
3. Explain the effects of positive-pressure ventilation on gas distribution and pulmonary blood flow in the lungs.
4. Describe how positive-pressure ventilation increases intracranial pressure.
5. Summarize the effects of positive-pressure ventilation on renal and endocrine function.
6. Describe the effects of abnormal arterial blood gases on renal function.
7. Name five ways of assessing a patient's nutritional status.
8. Describe techniques that can be used to reduce complications associated with mechanical ventilation.

Effects of Positive-Pressure Ventilation on the Heart and Thoracic Vessels

The physiological effects of mechanical ventilation are well documented. Laboratory and clinical studies have demonstrated that positive-pressure ventilation (PPV) can significantly alter cardiovascular, pulmonary, neurologic, renal, and gastrointestinal function. (See Chapter 17 for information on the pulmonary effects and complications of mechanical ventilation.) As such, every attempt should be made to minimize the adverse effects of PPV. Understanding the physiological effects and potential complications of PPV is therefore essential for clinicians involved with ventilator management.

ADVERSE CARDIOVASCULAR EFFECTS OF POSITIVE-PRESSURE VENTILATION

Positive-pressure ventilation can significantly change physiological pressures in the thorax. The extent of these changes depends on the amount of positive pressure applied to the airways and a patient's cardiopulmonary status (Key Point 16-1).

> **Key Point 16-1** The physiological effects of positive-pressure ventilation depend on the amount of pressure applied to the airways and the patient's cardiopulmonary status.

The Thoracic Pump Mechanism During Normal Spontaneous Breathing and During Positive-Pressure Ventilation

It has been known for several decades that PPV can reduce cardiac output. This phenomenon can be understood in part by comparing intrapleural (i.e., intrathoracic) pressure changes that occur during normal spontaneous or negative pressure breathing with those occurring during PPV.

During spontaneous breathing, the fall in intrapleural pressure that draws air into the lungs during inspiration also draws blood into the major thoracic vessels and heart (Fig. 16-1). With this increased return of blood to the right side of the heart and the stretching and enlargement of the right heart volume, the right ventricular preload increases, resulting in an increased right ventricular stroke volume (i.e., Frank-Starling mechanism). Conversely, during a spontaneous (passive) expiration, intrapleural pressure rises (i.e., becomes less negative), causing a reduction in venous return and right ventricular preload, which in turn leads to a decrease in right ventricular stroke volume. Note that these pressure changes affect left heart volumes in a similar fashion.

The effects on intrathoracic pressures and venous return are quite different when positive pressure is applied to the airway (Fig. 16-2). During inspiration, increases in airway pressure are transmitted to the intrapleural space and to the great vessels and other structures in the thorax. As the airway pressure rises, the intrapleural pressure rises and intrathoracic blood vessels become compressed, causing the central venous pressure (CVP) to increase. This increase in CVP reduces the pressure gradient between systemic veins and the right side of the heart, which reduces venous return to the right side of the heart and thus right ventricular filling (preload). As a result, right ventricular stroke volume decreases.[1,2]

Notice that vascular pressures within the thorax generally increase in proportion to increases in mean airway pressure ($\overline{P}_{aw}$) and intrapleural pressure (i.e., the higher the $\overline{P}_{aw}$, the greater the effects). This phenomenon is particularly evident when one considers the effect of adding positive end-expiratory pressure (PEEP) during PPV. Because PEEP further increases $\overline{P}_{aw}$ during PPV, it is reasonable to assume that reductions in venous return and cardiac output are greater during PPV with PEEP than with PPV alone. Furthermore, the addition of PEEP during an assisted breath decreases cardiac output more than when PEEP is used with intermittent mandatory ventilation (IMV) or continuous positive airway pressure (CPAP) alone.

Increased Pulmonary Vascular Resistance and Altered Right and Left Ventricular Function

During inspiration with high tidal volumes (V_T) or when high levels of PEEP are used, the pulmonary capillaries that interlace the alveoli are stretched and narrowed. As a result, resistance to blood flow through the pulmonary circulation increases (Fig. 16-3). This increases right ventricular (RV) afterload (i.e., pulmonary vascular resistance [PVR] and the resting volume of the RV). In normal healthy individuals, RV stroke volume is maintained in the face of increased PVR because the RV contractile function is not severely impaired. However, in patients with compromised RV function, the RV cannot overcome these increases in PVR, and overdistention of the RV occurs, resulting in a decrease in RV output.

Dilation of the RV can also force the interventricular septum to move to the left. This phenomenon usually occurs when high $\overline{P}_{aw}$ values (>15 cm H_2O) are used and the patient's blood volume is depleted.[3] When this occurs, the left ventricular end-diastolic volume (LVEDV) is encroached upon and left ventricle (LV) stroke volume may decrease because its ability to fill is limited. Septal shifting can significantly decrease cardiac output in patients with compromised LV function or in patients who are volume depleted.[3]

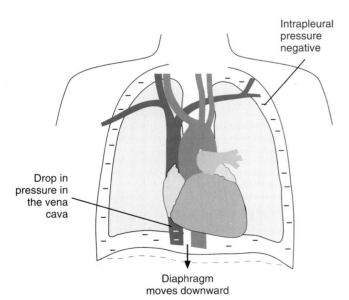

Fig. 16-1 The negative intrapleural pressures that occur during spontaneous inspiration are transmitted to the intrathoracic vessels. A drop in pressure in the vena cava increases the pressure gradient back to the heart and venous return increases.

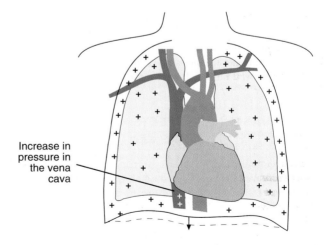

Fig. 16-2 Positive-pressure ventilation increases lung and intrapleural (intrathoracic) pressures. This positive pressure is transmitted to the intrathoracic vessels. A rise in the pressure in the vena cava reduces venous return to the heart.

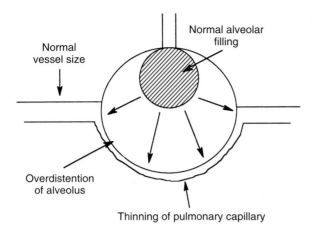

Fig. 16-3 Overfilling of an alveolus. The result is thinning and compression of the pulmonary capillary. Pulmonary vascular resistance is increased.

In this latter group of patients, intravascular volume expansion may help to restore output from the left side of the heart by returning LV preload to normal.

The LV output may also be decreased when high V_Ts are used during PPV because the heart is compressed between the expanding lungs (i.e., **cardiac tamponade** effect). The distensibility of the left side of the heart appears to be directly related to the transmission of positive pressures to the heart from the lung.[2] This effect increases when long inspiratory times and high peak pressures are used.

Coronary Blood Flow with Positive-Pressure Ventilation

In addition to reduced venous return and alteration in ventricular function, lower cardiac output may be caused by myocardial dysfunction associated with reduced perfusion of the myocardium and the resultant myocardial ischemia. The flow of blood into the coronary vessels depends on the coronary perfusion pressure. The coronary artery perfusion pressure gradient for LV is the difference between mean aortic diastolic pressure and left ventricular end-diastolic pressure (LVEDP); the perfusion pressure gradient for the RV is the difference between mean aortic pressure and pulmonary artery systolic pressure.

Reductions in coronary vessel perfusion can result from any factor that decreases this perfusion pressure gradient. Thus, reductions in cardiac output or blood pressure, coronary vasospasms, or direct effect of compression of the coronary vessels caused by increases in intrathoracic pressure during PPV can decrease coronary perfusion and ultimately lead to myocardial ischemia.

FACTORS INFLUENCING CARDIOVASCULAR EFFECTS OF POSITIVE-PRESSURE VENTILATION

The level of reduction in cardiac output that occurs with PPV depends on several factors, including lung and chest wall compliance, airway resistance (R_{aw}), and the duration and magnitude of the positive pressure.

Compensation in Individuals with Normal Cardiovascular Function

Because of compensatory mechanisms, systemic hypotension rarely occurs in individuals with normal cardiovascular function

receiving PPV. Decreases in stroke volume normally result in an increase in sympathetic tone, which leads to tachycardia and an increase in systemic vascular resistance and peripheral venous pressure from arterial and venous constriction, respectively. Additionally, some peripheral shunting of blood away from the kidneys and lower extremities occurs. The net effect is maintenance of blood pressure even with a decrease in cardiac output (Key Point 16-2).[4]

 Key Point **16-2** Systemic hypotension rarely occurs in normal individuals receiving positive-pressure ventilation due to compensatory mechanisms.

It is important to understand that the effectiveness of these compensatory mechanisms in maintaining arterial blood pressure depends on the integrity of the individual's neuroreflexes. Vascular reflexes can be blocked or impaired in the presence of sympathetic blockade, spinal anesthesia, moderate levels of general anesthesia, spinal cord transection, or severe **polyneuritis.** In a patient in whom PPV is being initiated or the ventilatory mode is being changed, it is prudent to measure the blood pressure early to ensure that normal vascular reflexes are intact. The presence of normal vascular reflexes increases the probability that the patient will not experience a significant drop in cardiac output and blood pressure if PPV is initiated. For example, it is unusual to see a reduction in cardiac output in normovolemic patients when low levels of PEEP are used (i.e., 5 to 10 cm H_2O of PEEP). However, decreases in cardiac output can occur in this group of patients if higher levels of PEEP are used (>15 cm H_2O)[4] (Case Study 16-1).

Case Study 16-1

The Effects of Ventilator Changes on Blood Pressure

A patient with chronic obstructive pulmonary disease (COPD) is receiving volume-controlled continuous mandatory ventilation (VC-CMV). The set tidal volume is increased from 700 to 900 mL, and the rate is increased from 10 to 18 breaths/min. The respiratory therapist notices a progressive rise in peak airway pressures. Immediately following the change, the patient's blood pressure drops from 145/83 mm Hg to 102/60 mm Hg. What is the most likely cause of this problem and what should the respiratory therapist recommend?

Effects of Lung and Chest Wall Compliance and Airway Resistance

Patients with very stiff lungs, such as those with acute respiratory distress syndrome (ARDS) or pulmonary fibrosis, are less likely to experience hemodynamic changes with high pressures because less of the alveolar pressure (P_{alv}) is transmitted to the intrapleural space. On the other hand, patients with compliant lungs and stiff (noncompliant) chest walls are more likely to have higher intrapleural pressures with PPV and experience more pronounced cardiovascular effects.

In patients with increased R_{aw}, although peak pressures may be very high, much of the pressure is lost to the poorly conductive airways. As a consequence, high peak airway pressures may not be transmitted to the intrapleural space and the alveoli.

Duration and Magnitude of Positive Pressures

One way to reduce the deleterious effects of PPV is to control the amount of pressure exerted in the thorax. Maintaining the lowest possible $\bar{P}_{aw}$ helps to minimize the reductions in cardiac output that can occur during mechanical ventilation. It is therefore important to understand how peak inspiratory pressure (PIP), inspiratory flow, inspiratory-to-expiratory (I:E) ratios, inflation hold, and PEEP affect $\bar{P}_{aw}$ and, ultimately, cardiac output.

BENEFICIAL EFFECTS OF POSITIVE-PRESSURE VENTILATION ON HEART FUNCTION IN PATIENTS WITH LEFT VENTRICULAR DYSFUNCTION

Although the discussion so far has focused on the adverse effects of PPV, it is important to recognize that positive pressure can also be beneficial for patients with LV dysfunction and elevated filling pressures. For example, PEEP may improve cardiac function by raising the P_aO_2 and improving myocardial oxygenation and performance if the left LV dysfunction is due to hypoxemia. Reductions in venous return decrease the preload to the heart and thus improve length–tension relationships and improve the stroke volume in patients with ventricular overload. Additionally, by raising the intrathoracic pressure, PPV decreases the transmural LV systolic pressure and thus the afterload to the left heart (Critical Care Concept 16-1). Box 16-1 lists some potential effects of PEEP on heart function.[5,6]

 CRITICAL CARE CONCEPT 16-1

Calculating Cardiac Transmural Pressure

The effective filling and emptying of the heart is determined, in part, by the pressure difference between the inside of the heart and the intrathoracic pressure. This is called the **cardiac transmural pressure (P_{TM})**. The more positive the P_{TM} is during diastole, the greater the filling of the heart (preload). The more positive the P_{TM} is during systole, the higher the workload is for the heart (afterload). Keeping this in mind, calculate the P_{TM} during a positive-pressure breath and during a spontaneous breath and compare their values.

Problem 1: Positive-Pressure Breathing

If intrapleural pressure (P_{pl}) is +10 cm H_2O and intraventricular pressure is 150 mm Hg, what is the P_{TM}?

Problem 2: Spontaneous Inspiration

If P_{pl} is −10 cm H_2O and intraventricular pressure is 150 mm Hg, what is the P_{TM}?

MINIMIZING THE PHYSIOLOGICAL EFFECTS AND COMPLICATIONS OF MECHANICAL VENTILATION

As previously stated, the harmful effects of PPV on cardiovascular function occur when high positive pressures are applied to the

---

| **BOX 16-1** | **Potential Effects of PEEP in Left Ventricular Dysfunction** |

- Increased airway pressure ($\bar{P}_{aw}$) and intrathoracic pressure lead to decreased venous return that can reduce preload to a failing heart and improve function.
- Increased functional residual capacity (FRC) that occurs with the application of PEEP leads to increased pulmonary vascular resistance and increased afterload to the right heart, which may shift the intraventricular septum to the left. This does not seem to alter RV contractility until values for PAP are critical.
- Left shift of the intraventricular septum reduces LV volume and decreases the load it must pump. On the other hand, it may also affect LV compliance and either increase or decrease LV function (the response varies).
- The mechanical compression of the heart and aorta by the positive pleural pressure can also alter ventricular function. Vascular pressure in the heart and thoracic aorta are transiently increased relative to the extrathoracic aorta (i.e., LV afterload decreases). This response is not always consistent, and cardiac tamponade from PEEP can negatively alter myocardial compliance as well.
- Improper ventilator settings may lead to increased work of breathing and oxygen demand, which can affect myocardial oxygen supply and result in myocardial ischemia and reduced LV compliance.

---

lungs and transmitted to the intrapleural space. Ventilatory strategies that reduce intrapulmonary pressures during PPV will therefore also reduce the harmful effects on cardiovascular function. Although it may not be obvious, the amount and duration of the pressure applied to the airway, or more specifically the $\bar{P}_{aw}$, ultimately influences the extent of these harmful effects. Thus, the lower the $\bar{P}_{aw}$, the less marked the cardiovascular effects. Figure 16-4 illustrates the airway pressure changes that occur during one respiratory cycle.

Notice in Figure 16-4 that the $\bar{P}_{aw}$ is the area enclosed between the curve and the baseline for one respiratory cycle, divided by the duration of the cycle. Although most of the newer microprocessor ventilators measure, calculate, and display $\bar{P}_{aw}$ with the simple push of a button, it is important to understand how $\bar{P}_{aw}$ is actually calculated. In a constant flow, volume-limited breath, the pressure rise is nearly linear with time and produces essentially a triangular pressure waveform (Fig. 16-5). $\bar{P}_{aw}$ can be estimated by using the following equation: $\bar{P}_{aw} = \frac{1}{2}$ (PIP [inspiratory time/total respiratory cycle]). In this same ventilator mode with PEEP added, the equation is as follows:

$$\bar{P}_{aw} = \frac{1}{2}(PIP - PEEP) \times \left(\frac{Inspiratory\ time}{Total\ cycle\ time}\right) + PEEP$$

The $\bar{P}_{aw}$ generated during PPV varies and may exhibit different waveforms (pressure curves) depending on the ventilator employed, the mode of ventilation used, and the patient's pulmonary characteristics. For example, techniques such as inverse ratio ventilation (IRV) and PEEP produce higher $\bar{P}_{aw}$ compared with conventional PPV.

Mean Airway Pressure and P_aO_2

It should be apparent that $\bar{P}_{aw}$ has clinical importance. For a specific V_T, the P_aO_2 will be predominantly affected by $\bar{P}_{aw}$ and, to a

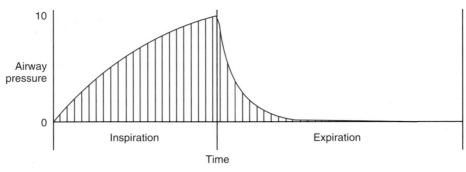

Fig. 16-4 Vertical lines under the pressure curve represent frequent readings of pressure over the total respiratory cycle. The sum of these pressure readings (i.e., the area under the curve) divided by the cycle time will give the $\overline{P}_{aw}$.

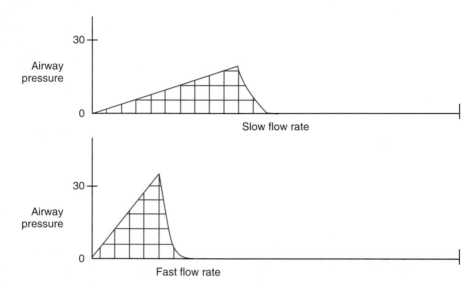

Fig. 16-5 Slower inspiratory flow may reach a lower peak pressure compared with a rapid flow rate, but it may also produce a higher airway pressure ($\overline{P}_{aw}$). Note the number of boxes under each curve.

lesser extent, the ventilator parameters used to achieve the $\overline{P}_{aw}$. This is probably related to an increase in functional residual capacity (FRC) with increased $\overline{P}_{aw}$. Thus, changes in FRC are of importance to increased oxygenation in some pulmonary disorders such as ARDS. (NOTE: The amount of $\overline{P}_{aw}$ required to achieve a certain level of oxygenation may indicate the severity of a patient's lung disease.)

Reduction in Airway Pressure

High $\overline{P}_{aw}$ values suggest the presence of increased intrapleural pressures and the associated problems previously discussed. It cannot be overstated that the level of positive pressure should never be maintained higher or longer than is necessary to achieve adequate ventilation and oxygenation. In the sections that follow, we will discuss how $\overline{P}_{aw}$ can be affected by inspiratory gas flow and pattern, I : E ratio, inflation hold, PEEP, IMV, and the ventilator mode used.

Inspiratory Flow

Although rapid inspiratory flows tend to increase PIP, higher inspiratory flows allow for the delivery of the desired V_T in a shorter time, which in turn produces a lower $\overline{P}_{aw}$ in patients with normal

conducting airways (see Fig. 16-5). Three points must be kept in mind, however, when using high inspiratory flows. First, more pressure will be lost to the patient circuit with higher PIP. Second, more pressure will be required to overcome R_{aw} ($R_{aw} = \Delta P/flow$). And third, uneven ventilation is more likely to occur with high inspiratory flow. If, for example, the right bronchus is partially obstructed, most of the gas flow would go to the left lung because gas flow will follow the path of least resistance. Consequently, a larger volume enters the left lung, creating higher airway pressures in the left lung compared with the right lung. This situation can lead to uneven distribution of gas and contribute to $\dot{V}/\dot{Q}$ mismatching by creating higher intraalveolar pressures in the left lung. These higher intraalveolar pressures may lead to increased dead space ventilation resulting from the high alveolar volume; the elevated alveolar pressures can also reduce capillary blood flow. Additionally, the high volume delivered to the left lung may also increase the risk of alveolar rupture.

The goal should be to use an inspiratory flow that is not too high for the reasons just outlined but also not too low, which may lead to increased work of breathing (WOB) and auto-PEEP. Careful monitoring of the effects of flow changes on volume delivery,

V_D/V_T, $\dot{V}/\dot{Q}$, and transairway pressure (P_{ta}) can help to identify the appropriate inspiratory flow setting. (See Chapter 6 for additional information on setting inspiratory flow.)

Inspiratory: Expiratory Ratio

Another point to consider is the duration of inspiration in relation to expiration. Shorter inspiratory times (T_I) and longer expiratory times (T_E) typically lead to the fewer harmful effects of positive pressure. A range of I:E ratios of 1:2 to 1:4 or smaller in adult patients is considered acceptable. Values of 1:1, 2:1, and higher may result in significant increases in $\overline{P}_{aw}$, air trapping, and significant hemodynamic complications (Key Point 16-3).

Key Point **16-3** Shorter inspiratory times and the longer expiratory times will usually help to minimize the adverse effects of PPV on cardiovascular function.

In patients with poor airway conductance, a longer T_E also allows for better alveolar emptying and less chance of developing auto-PEEP. It is important to mention, however, that using a short I:E of 1:6 or smaller in an apneic patient receiving volume control ventilation may increase physiological dead space due to a T_I that is too short (i.e., T_I <0.5 seconds). It is the responsibility of the clinician to balance the patient's response to variations in I:E ratio and flow rates to achieve the most effective ventilation for that individual.

Inflation Hold

Inflation hold, or **inspiratory pause** was initially proposed as a method to improve oxygenation and distribution of gas in the lungs during volume-targeted ventilation. It was subsequently realized that the inflation hold maneuver could lead to severe consequences if it is used for extended periods of time because it increases T_I and $\overline{P}_{aw}$ (Fig. 16-6). Inflation hold is now used almost exclusively to measure plateau pressure ($P_{plateau}$), which is required to calculate static lung compliance (C_S). It should be kept in mind, however, that because the inflation hold maneuver raises the $\overline{P}_{aw}$ and can potentially cause undesirable hemodynamic side effects, it should be used judiciously.

Positive End-Expiratory Pressure

PEEP increases FRC and improves oxygenation but it also increases $\overline{P}_{aw}$ (Fig. 16-7). As mentioned earlier, inappropriate levels of PEEP that cause overdistention of the lungs can result in a reduction in

cardiac output. It is important to understand, however, that in cases where a patient demonstrates reduced lung compliance (i.e., "stiff" lungs) and a reduced FRC, increased $\overline{P}_{aw}$ with PEEP will not always lead to a decreased cardiac output. In these situations, the application of relatively high levels of PEEP to re-establish a normal FRC does not cause detrimental effects on intrathoracic blood vessels and will therefore have minimal effects on cardiac output.

High Peak Pressures from Increased Airway Resistance

Although high PIP may indicate an increase in $\overline{P}_{aw}$, this increased $\overline{P}_{aw}$ may not always be transmitted to the intrapleural space. For example, increased amounts of pressure are needed to ventilate patients with elevated R_{aw} caused by bronchospasm, mucus plugging, and mucosal edema; but not all of this increased pressure will reach the alveoli because the majority will be transmitted to the conducting airways. Thus, high PIP measured at the upper airway does not always reflect alveolar pressure (P_{alv}). $P_{plateau}$ will be low, and the increase in $\overline{P}_{aw}$ in this case may not result in an improvement in oxygenation. If increased resistance leads to air trapping from inadequate expiratory time or from loss of normal expiratory resistance maneuvers such as pursed-lip breathing, then hazardous cardiovascular side effects are likely to occur (Fig. 16-8). It is worth

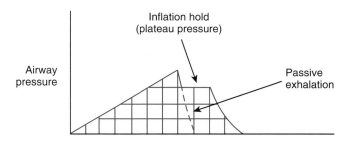

Fig. 16-6 Inflation hold or inspiratory pause may help to improve the distribution of gases in the lungs and increases airway pressure ($\overline{P}_{aw}$). The curve shows an inflation hold compared with a normal passive exhalation.

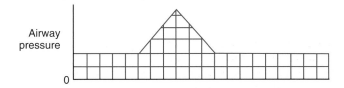

Fig. 16-7 Simplified graphic of PEEP during VC-CMV. PEEP maintains a high baseline pressure and results in an increase of airway pressure ($\overline{P}_{aw}$).

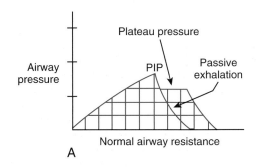

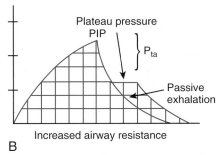

Fig. 16-8 **A,** Normal pressure difference between PIP and $P_{plateau}$, during VC-CMV with a normal R_{aw}. When R_{aw} is increased, the difference between PIP and $P_{plateau}$ is increased (i.e., more pressure goes to the airways [P_{ta}]). **B,** Note that PIP is also increased.

noting that ventilators that calculate $\bar{P}_{aw}$ can show inaccurate $\bar{P}_{aw}$ values in the presence of air trapping (auto-PEEP).

Intermittent Mandatory Ventilation

Another mode of ventilation that can reduce $\bar{P}_{aw}$ in patients requiring PPV is IMV. The cardiovascular complications of high $\bar{P}_{aw}$ can be minimized by reducing the frequency of mandatory breaths and allowing spontaneous breathing to occur at ambient pressure or with PEEP/CPAP between those breaths. It is important to recognize, however, that IMV requires the patient to assume a certain percentage of the WOB. It must be used with caution because IMV can increase the risk of fatigue and add stress to those patients, who may require full ventilatory support.

If the patient's spontaneous respiratory rate between machine breaths is rapid and accompanied by low V_T values, then the patient's WOB is increased and fatigue may result. If the patient's spontaneous respiratory rate is rapid and V_T values are deep in the presence of normal P_aCO_2, then the patient may have some underlying cause for an increased V_D/V_T ratio or increased $\dot{V}CO_2$. It is not uncommon for acutely ill patients, such as those with sepsis, multiple organ failure, severe burns, or trauma, to have higher than normal metabolic rates leading to increased $\dot{V}O_2$ and $\dot{V}CO_2$ and requiring a higher minute ventilation ($\dot{V}_E$). The clinician must decide whether the patient can continue to work this hard or the mandatory rate must be increased. The answer depends on the clinical situation and the ventilatory requirements for each patient. In this situation, pressure-supported ventilation (PSV) at appropriate levels may help solve the problem.

In summary, the most serious complications associated with PPV include alterations in cardiac function, interference with gas exchange, and increased risk of lung injury from overdistention. Procedures that decrease $\bar{P}_{aw}$ may decrease cardiovascular effects, but they may also contribute to uneven ventilation and vice versa (Fig. 16-9). The clinician must evaluate each aspect of the patient's condition and choose the ventilation mode that is most effective.

Effects of Mechanical Ventilation on Intracranial Pressure, Renal Function, Liver Function, and Gastrointestinal Function

EFFECTS OF MECHANICAL VENTILATION ON INTRACRANIAL PRESSURE AND CEREBRAL PERFUSION

The amount of blood flowing to the brain is determined by the cerebral perfusion pressure (CPP), which is calculated by subtracting the intracranial pressure (ICP) from the mean systemic arterial blood pressure (MABP). Because PPV (with or without PEEP) can decrease cardiac output and MABP, it is reasonable to assume that CPP would also decrease during PPV. Consider the following example. If MABP drops from 100 to 70 mm Hg and the ICP is 15 mm Hg, then the CPP would decrease from 85 mm Hg (100 − 15 = 85 mm Hg) to 55 mm Hg (70 − 15 = 55 mm Hg).

Positive-pressure ventilation can also reduce CPP by increasing the CVP. In this situation, CPP is reduced because of a reduction in venous return from the head increases ICP. This can be observed clinically by noting an increase in jugular vein distention. The net result is a potential for cerebral hypoxemia from a reduced perfusion to the brain and an increase in cerebral edema from increased ICP.

With normal intracranial dynamics, patients do not typically develop increased ICP with PPV.[6] The greatest risk of decreased cerebral perfusion occurs in those patients who already have an increased ICP and who may develop cerebral edema, such as patients with closed head injuries, patients with cerebral tumors, or patients who have undergone neurosurgery. Some clinicians advocate using mechanical ventilation to hyperventilate patients with severe, uncontrollable increased ICP. The idea was that the respiratory alkalosis that results from lowering the P_aCO_2 to 32 to 35 mm Hg can constrict cerebral arterial vessels and reduce the ICP, thus increasing the CPP gradient and augmenting cerebral

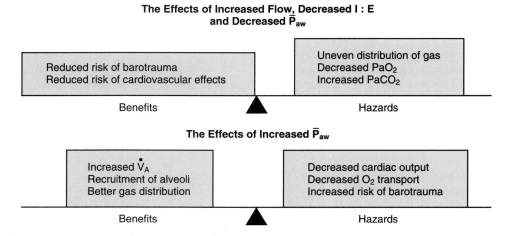

The Effects of Increased Flow, Decreased I : E and Decreased $\bar{P}_{aw}$

| Reduced risk of barotrauma
Reduced risk of cardiovascular effects | Uneven distribution of gas
Decreased PaO2
Increased PaCO2 |

Benefits ▲ Hazards

The Effects of Increased $\bar{P}_{aw}$

| Increased $\dot{V}_A$
Recruitment of alveoli
Better gas distribution | Decreased cardiac output
Decreased O2 transport
Increased risk of barotrauma |

Benefits ▲ Hazards

Fig. 16-9 Balancing the benefits and hazards. The top figure shows the balance between the benefits and hazards of increasing the gas flow rate and decreasing the I : E ratio to reduce the $\bar{P}_{aw}$. The bottom figure shows the balance between the benefits and hazards of increasing the $\bar{P}_{aw}$ to increase alveolar ventilation (by increasing $\dot{V}_A$ and/or respiratory rate) and achieve alveolar recruitment with PEEP and improve gas distribution (by using a slow inspiratory flow rate and a descending waveform). All factors must be considered when treating patients on mechanical ventilatory support.

perfusion. As previously discussed, this effect is temporary and should be used for short periods when ICPs are spiking. Because a considerable amount of controversy exists regarding the actual benefits of this procedure, using hyperventilation as a standard practice in closed head injury is not recommended.[6]

Some patients with traumatic brain injuries require PEEP to treat refractory hypoxemia caused by increased shunting and decreased FRC. When PEEP is used in these patients, it is important to recognize that it can potentially limit CPP by raising ICP. On the other hand, if PEEP is needed to maintain oxygenation, it may be lifesaving and should be used. Regardless of the situation, it is imperative to monitor ICP in this patient group.[4]

RENAL EFFECTS OF MECHANICAL VENTILATION

It has been known for nearly half a century that pressurized breathing can induce changes in renal function.[7-9] These changes can be divided into three areas:

1. Renal responses to hemodynamic changes resulting from high intrathoracic pressures
2. Humoral responses, including antidiuretic hormone (ADH), atrial natriuretic factor (ANF), and renin-angiotensin-aldosterone changes occurring with PPV
3. Abnormal pH, P_aCO_2, and P_aO_2 affecting the kidney

Renal Response to Hemodynamic Changes

Although urinary output remains fairly constant over a wide range of arterial pressures, it becomes severely reduced as the renal arterial pressure decreases below 75 mm Hg. Indeed, urinary output can actually stop in the presence of profound hypotension. Therefore, it would be reasonable to assume that the initiation of PPV would cause a decrease in cardiac output, which in turn would lead to a decrease in renal blood flow and glomerular filtration rates and ultimately a decrease in urine output.[8] However, decreases in urine production seen during PPV may not be caused entirely by a decrease in cardiac output because returning cardiac output to adequate levels is not accompanied by a proportional increase in urinary output. Also, because the arterial blood pressure is usually compensated when PPV is used, decreased blood pressure is probably not a significant factor leading to decreased urinary output during mechanical ventilation.

Redistribution of blood inside the kidney may actually be an important factor that is responsible for changes in kidney function. Flow to the outer cortex decreases, whereas flow to the inner cortex and outer medullary tissue (juxtamedullary nephrons) increases. The net result is that less urine, creatinine, and sodium are excreted. This occurs because the juxtamedullary nephrons near the medulla of the kidney are more efficient at reabsorbing sodium than are those at the outer cortex. As a result of this shift in blood flow, more sodium is reabsorbed, which in turn is accompanied by an increased reabsorption of water.[9] Another possible explanation for this effect may be related to an alteration in renal venous pressure resulting from inferior vena cava (IVC) constriction, changes in IVC blood pressure, or congestive heart failure.

Endocrine Effects of Positive-Pressure Ventilation on Renal Function

Several different types of hormones may also influence urine output during mechanical ventilation. Specifically, these include ADH, ANF, and the renin-angiotensin-aldosterone cascade.

Increases in the release of ADH, also called *arginine vasopressin*, from the posterior pituitary can reduce urine production by inhibiting free water excretion. The major determinant of ADH release is plasma osmolality. Reductions in blood pressure can also cause increased ADH release. Blood pressure changes during PPV may precipitate ADH release through the following mechanism. Within the left atrium are volume receptors that send nerve impulses over a vagal pathway to the hypothalamus, which in turn can stimulate increases or decreases in ADH production and secretion. Baroreceptors in the carotid bodies and along the aortic arch sense changes in pressure and can also raise or lower ADH levels.[10] Because both of these areas are exposed to change in intrathoracic pressures, it follows that PPV can potentially affect ADH secretion. An interesting finding is that negative-pressure ventilation inhibits ADH release and produces a diuretic effect, in contrast to PPV, which enhances ADH release and results in **oliguria.**

Atrial natriuretic factor (also known as atrial natriuretic peptide or ANP) is another hormone that appears to be intimately involved in fluid and electrolyte balance during PPV. ANF is normally released when the atria are distended. When it is released, it causes an increased secretion of sodium (natriuresis) and water (diuresis) in an attempt to reduce the blood volume and stretch on the atria. PPV and PEEP can reduce atrial filling pressure by either causing mechanical compression of the atria or by decreasing right atrial stretch from low venous return. Reducing atrial stretch leads to decreased secretion of ANF. Reduced ANF levels contribute to water and sodium retention during PPV.[5]

Increased sympathetic tone is associated with increases in plasma renin activity (PRA). This appears to be another major factor in sodium and water retention during PPV and PEEP. The increased PRA activates the renin-angiotensin-aldosterone cascade and results in retention of sodium (antinatriuresis) and water (antidiuresis). Renal synthesis of prostaglandin tends to offset these effects but is probably insufficient to completely correct them[8,9] (Key Point 16-4).

Key Point 16-4 Neural and humoral factors play a critical role in fluid and electrolyte balance.

Arterial Blood Gases and Kidney Function

Changes in P_aO_2 and P_aCO_2 changes contribute to the effects of mechanical ventilation on the renal function. Decreasing P_aO_2 values in patients with respiratory failure have been shown to cause a reduction in renal function and a decrease in urine flow. In fact, P_aO_2 levels below 40 mm Hg (severe hypoxemia) can dramatically interfere with normal renal function. Similarly, acute hypercapnia (i.e., P_aCO_2 greater than 65 mm Hg) can also severely impair renal function.

Implications of Impaired Renal Effects

In seriously ill, mechanically ventilated patients, administering positive pressure increases water and sodium retention, resulting in weight gain and in some cases pulmonary edema. To compound this problem, reduced renal function in these patients can complicate fluid and electrolyte management. Additionally, many drugs (e.g., sedatives and neuromuscular blocking agents) and their metabolites are excreted by the kidney. Altered renal function can prolong the effects of these drugs and affect patient care.

EFFECTS OF MECHANICAL VENTILATION ON LIVER AND GASTROINTESTINAL FUNCTION

Some patients on PPV and PEEP show evidence of liver malfunction as reflected by a rise in serum bilirubin (>2.5 mg/100 mL), even when no evidence of preexisting liver disease is present. This may be a result of a drop in cardiac output, an increased diaphragmatic force against the liver, a decrease in portal venous flow, or an increase in splanchnic resistance. Regardless of the mechanism, these changes lead to hepatic ischemia and impaired liver function.[5,11]

Positive-pressure ventilation increases splanchnic resistance, decreases splanchnic venous outflow, and may contribute to gastric mucosal ischemia, which can increase the risk of gastrointestinal bleeding and gastric ulcers. Both of these are complications frequently seen in critically ill patients. These changes are associated with increased permeability of the gastric mucosal barrier. Many patients are treated with antacids or histamine type 2 (H_2)-blocking agents (e.g., cimetidine) to avoid gastrointestinal bleeding from acute stress ulceration. However, as these agents increase gastric pH, they may increase the risk of nosocomial pneumonias. As discussed in Chapter 14, several studies have suggested that oral sucralfate may reduce gastric mucosal bleeding without altering gastric pH, thus reducing the risk of developing nosocomial pneumonias in mechanically ventilated patients. Clinical findings are, however, controversial, and the use of sucralfate is not recommended at this time for patients at risk for gastrointestinal bleeding.[12]

Another problem that is often encountered with patients receiving PPV involves gastric distention. Gastric distention can result from swallowing air that leaks around endotracheal tube cuffs or when PPV is delivered by mask. Use of a gastric tube can remove this air and decompress the stomach.

NUTRITIONAL COMPLICATIONS DURING MECHANICAL VENTILATION

The nutritional status of patients must be carefully monitored and maintained if they are to recover from their illness and be weaned from mechanical ventilation. Both medical and surgical patients are subject to malnutrition during serious illness because of inadequate intake of food and increased metabolic rate associated with fever and wound healing[13] (Key Point 16-5). Many patients who develop respiratory failure already exhibit some form of malnutrition before admission to the hospital, usually caused by a preexisting chronic disease.[14] Furthermore, patients receiving ventilatory support are generally unable to take oral feedings because of the endotracheal tube. Unless special routes for nutritional support are provided, such as nasogastric feedings or intravenous hyperalimentation, these patients will inevitably develop severe malnutrition.

⚡ Key Point **16-5** Critically ill patients are subject to malnutrition because of inadequate intake of food and hypermetabolism associated with fever and wound healing.

Nutritional depletion can cause several deleterious effects on patients (Box 16-2).[14] Malnutrition alters a patient's ability to respond effectively to infection, impairs wound healing, and

---

BOX 16-2	Effects of Malnourishment on Mechanically Ventilated Patients

- Reduced response to hypoxia and hypercapnia
- Muscle atrophy from prolonged bed rest and lack of use; includes respiratory muscles, especially if the patient is apneic and on controlled ventilation
- Muscle wasting, including the respiratory muscles, from lack of nutrition
- Respiratory tract infections from impaired cell immunity and reduced or altered macrophage activity
- Decreased surfactant production and development of atelectasis
- Reduced ability of the pulmonary epithelium to replicate, which slows healing of damaged tissue
- Lower serum albumin levels, which affect colloid oncotic pressures and can contribute to pulmonary edema formation (colloid oncotic pressures <11 mm Hg with normal left atrial pressure)

BOX 16-3	Assessment of Nutritional Status

- Body composition
- Actual versus predicted body weight
- Anthropometric measurements (limb circumference and skin fold measurements)
- Fat versus lean muscle mass
- Protein deficiencies
- Creatinine/height index (24-hour urine creatinine excreted to patient's height in centimeters) <6.0 considered critical protein deficiency
- Visceral protein malnutrition
- Serum albumin <3.5 g/dL
- Transferrin <300 mg
- Immunodeficiency
- Decreased skin test response to known recall antigens

---

severely reduces the ability to maintain spontaneous ventilation from weakened respiratory muscles. It is important to understand that overfeeding can also lead to problems by increasing oxygen consumption, carbon dioxide production, and the need for increased $\dot{V}_E$, resulting in an increase in the WOB. Feedings must be of the appropriate type and in the appropriate amount.[14,15]

Assessment of a patient's resting energy expenditure (REE) provides information about a patient's daily caloric requirements. Box 16-3 lists parameters for assessing nutritional status. Once these have been evaluated, a correct feeding schedule can be instituted.[16] REE can be calculated using standard (i.e., Harris-Benedict) equations that were derived nearly a century ago, or it can measured by indirect calorimetry (see Chapter 10 for a discussion of indirect calorimetry). Indirect calorimetry involves measuring inspired and expired volumes and $\dot{V}O_2$ and $\dot{V}CO_2$.

Nutritional supplements should always be delivered by the most natural route possible. This means oral feedings are the first choice, nasogastric feedings second, and catheters into the gastrointestinal tract third. If enteral (through the gut) feedings are not possible, then parenteral (into a vein) nutrition is provided. Intravenous feedings can be administered via a peripheral vein or a central vein. Feedings should be given in adequate doses to restore the nutritional status of the patient without overfeeding. One final note: intravenous feedings are a potential vehicle for transmitting nosocomial infections and should therefore be carefully handled.

SUMMARY

- Positive-pressure ventilation can significantly alter cardiovascular, pulmonary, neurologic, renal, and gastrointestinal function.
- The degree to which PPV impairs cardiac output depends on the patient's lung and chest wall compliance, airway resistance (R_{aw}), and the $\bar{P}_{aw}$.
- During PPV, the use of high V_T or high levels of PEEP may cause the pulmonary capillaries to be stretched and narrowed resulting in an increased resistance to blood flow through the pulmonary circulation. This in turn leads to an increased right

ventricular afterload and ultimately an increase in the resting volume of the right ventricle.
- Reductions in cardiac output that occur with PPV may be caused by myocardial dysfunction and are associated with reduced perfusion of the myocardium and the resultant myocardial ischemia.
- PPV can alter cerebral perfusion by causing a decrease in cardiac output and mean arterial blood pressure or by causing an increase in CVP, which can cause an increase in intracranial pressure.
- Changes in renal function associated with PPV can be attributed to hemodynamic changes resulting from high intrathoracic pressures, humoral responses, including ADH, ANF, and renin-angiotensin-aldosterone changes occurring with PPV and abnormal pH, P_aCO_2, and P_aO_2.
- Malnutrition alters a patient's ability to effectively respond to infection, impairs wound healing, and severely reduces the ability to maintain spontaneous ventilation from weakened respiratory muscles.

REVIEW QUESTIONS *(See Appendix A for answers.)*

1. Which of the following are potential complications of PPV?
   1. Reduced cardiac output
   2. Reduced urine output
   3. Decreased blood pressure
   4. Increased ICP
      A. 1 only
      B. 1 and 3
      C. 2, 3, and 4
      D. 1, 2, 3, and 4

2. Four days after being placed on ventilatory support, a postoperative abdominal surgery patient has indications of low urine production and a weight gain of 1 kg. Which of the following might have caused these changes?
   1. Kidney failure
   2. PPV
   3. Administration of Lasix (furosemide)
   4. Fluid loading
      A. 1 only
      B. 4 only
      C. 1, 2, and 4
      D. 1, 2, 3, and 4

3. $\bar{P}_{aw}$ can be increased by which of the following?
   1. Adding PEEP
   2. Increasing inspiratory gas flow
   3. Adding an inspiratory pause
   4. Decreasing the I:E ratio
      A. 1 only
      B. 1 and 3 only
      C. 2 and 4 only
      D. 3 and 4 only

4. High V_Ts or high levels of PEEP can result in which of the following?
   A. An increase in resistance to blood flow through the pulmonary circulation
   B. A decrease in right ventricular afterload
   C. A decrease in pulmonary artery pressure
   D. Maintenance of normal RV stroke volume in patients with compromised RV function

5. Reductions in P_aO_2 can decrease renal blood flow and increase sodium and water retention.
   A. True
   B. False

6. To reduce the effects of PPV, the respiratory therapist should evaluate $\bar{P}_{aw}$ and reduce it as much as possible.
   A. True
   B. False

7. Which of the following should be used with caution in a patient with severe hypovolemia?
   1. Administering a plasma volume expander
   2. ≥5 cm H_2O PEEP
   3. Inverse I:E ratio
   4. Short T_I
      A. 2 only
      B. 3 only
      C. 2 and 3 only
      D. 1, 3, and 4 only

8. Briefly explain how PPV can affect cerebral blood flow in patients with closed head injuries.

9. Which of the following should a respiratory therapist measure when assessing the nutritional status of a critically ill patient receiving mechanical ventilation?
   1. Body composition
   2. Actual versus predicted body weight
   3. Arterial PO_2
   4. Urinary nitrogen excretion
      A. 1 and 3 only
      B. 2 and 4 only
      C. 1, 2, and 4 only
      D. 1, 2, 3, and 4

10. Nutritional supplements should always be delivered by the most natural route possible.
    A. True
    B. False

References

1. Tyberg JV, Grant DA, Kingma I, et al: Effects of positive intrathoracic pressure on pulmonary and systemic hemodynamics. *Respir Physiol* 119:171–179, 2000.
2. Steingrub JS, Tidswell M, Higgins TL: Hemodynamic consequences of heart lung interactions. *J Intensive Care Med* 18:92–99, 2003.
3. Pepe PE, Lurie KG, Wigginton JG, et al: Detrimental hemodynamic effects of assisted ventilation in hemorrhagic states. *Crit Care Med* 32:S414–S420, 2004.
4. Griebel JA, Piantadosi CA: Hemodynamic effects and complications of mechanical ventilation. In Fulkerson WJ, MacIntyre NR, editors: *Problems in respiratory care: complications of mechanical ventilation*, Philadelphia, 1991, JB Lippincott, pp 25–33.
5. Stock MC, Perel A: *Handbook of mechanical ventilatory support*, ed 2, Baltimore, 1997, Williams & Wilkins.
6. Hess DR, Kacmarek RM: *Essentials of mechanical ventilation*, ed 2, New York, 2002, McGraw-Hill.
7. Drury DR, Henry JP, Goodman J: The effects of continuous pressure breathing on kidney function. *J Clin Invest* 26:945–951, 1947.
8. Qvist J, Pontoppidan H, Wilson RS, et al: Hemodynamic responses to mechanical ventilation with PEEP. *Anesthesiology* 42:45–55, 1975.
9. Hall SV, Johnson EE, Hedley-Whyte J: Renal hemodynamics and function with continuous positive pressure ventilation in dogs. *Anesthesiology* 41:452–461, 1974.
10. De Backer DD: The effects of positive end-expiratory pressure on the splanchnic circulation. *Intensive Care Med* 26:361–363, 2000.
11. Bonnet F, Richard C, Glaser P, et al: Changes in hepatic flow induced by continuous positive pressure ventilation in critically ill patients. *Crit Care Med* 10:703–705, 1982.
12. Dodek K, Keenan S, Cook D, et al: Evidence-based clinical practice guideline for the prevention of ventilator associated pneumonia. *Ann Intern Med* 141:305–313, 2004.
13. Driver AG, LeBrun M: Iatrogenic malnutrition in patients receiving ventilatory support. *JAMA* 244:2195–2196, 1980.
14. Jenkinson SG: Nutritional problems during mechanical ventilation in acute respiratory failure. *Respir Care* 28:641–644, 1983.
15. Pilbeam SP, Head A, Grossman GD, et al: Undernutrition and the respiratory system. *Respir Ther* 12(Pt I):65–69, 13(Pt II):72–78, 1983.
16. Hodgkin GF, Kwiatkowski CA: Nutritional aspects of health and disease. In Wilkins RL, Stoller JK, Scanlan CL, editors: *Egan's fundamentals of respiratory care*, St Louis, 2003, Mosby, pp 1201–1223.

Effects of Positive-Pressure Ventilation on the Pulmonary System

OUTLINE

KEY TERMS

- Asynchrony
- Barotrauma
- Cardiac tamponade
- Chest-abdominal paradox
- Deep sulcus sign (chest radiograph)
- Hyperinflation
- Hyperventilation
- Hypoventilation
- Multiple organ failure
- Multisystem organ failure (multiple organ dysfunction syndrome)
- Overdistention
- Perivascular
- Volutrauma

LEARNING OBJECTIVES *On completion of this chapter, the reader will be able to do the following:*

1. Recognize the presence of barotrauma or extraalveolar air based on patient assessment.
2. Recommend an appropriate intervention in patients with barotrauma.
3. Evaluate findings from a patient with acute respiratory distress syndrome to establish an optimum positive end-expiratory pressure (PEEP) and ventilation strategy.
4. Identify situations in which chest-wall rigidity can alter transpulmonary pressures and acceptable plateau pressures.
5. Name the types of ventilator-induced lung injury (VILI) caused by opening and closing of alveoli and overdistention of alveoli.
6. Compare the clinical findings associated with hyperventilation and hypoventilation.

7. Recommend ventilator settings for patients demonstrating hyperventilation and hypoventilation.
8. Describe clinical laboratory findings associated with metabolic acid–base disturbances.
9. Identify a patient with air trapping.
10. Provide strategies to reduce auto-PEEP.
11. Suggest methods to reduce the work of breathing (WOB) during mechanical ventilation.
12. List the possible responses to an increase in mean airway pressure in a ventilated patient.
13. Describe the effects of positive-pressure ventilation on pulmonary gas distribution and pulmonary perfusion in relation to normal spontaneous breathing.

There are a number of inherent risks and complications associated with the use of mechanical ventilators. These include ventilator-associated and ventilator-induced lung injury, the effects of positive-pressure ventilation (PPV) on gas distribution and pulmonary blood flow, **hypoventilation** and **hyperventilation**, air trapping, oxygen toxicity, increased WOB, patient-ventilator asynchrony, mechanical problems, and complications of the artificial airway. This chapter reviews the cause and adverse effects of these complications.

LUNG INJURY WITH MECHANICAL VENTILATION

It was not uncommon in the latter part of the 20th century for patients to be ventilated with pressures greater than 45 cm H_2O. Indeed nearly 20% of patients diagnosed with acute respiratory distress syndrome (ARDS) were, at some point in their management, ventilated with pressures of 80 cm H_2O or greater, and volumes in the range of 10 to 12 mL/kg.[1] This is interesting considering that it has been known for more than three decades that using these high levels of pressure and volume can cause lung injury, referred to as *barotrauma* or *volutrauma.*

Barotrauma implies trauma that results from using high pressures. Volutrauma implies damage from high distending volumes rather than high pressures. Evidence suggests that high distending volumes result in **overdistention** and lung injury, whereas high distending pressures alone do not cause lung injury. Overdistention causes the release of inflammatory mediators from the lungs that can lead to multiorgan failure. This latter response has been termed *biotrauma.*

Repeated opening and closing of lung units, also called recruitment/derecruitment, generates shear stress, which results in direct tissue injury at the alveolar and pulmonary capillary level, and the loss of surfactant from these unstable lung units. Shear stress injury and loss of surfactant have been termed *atelectrauma.* The following section provides a summary of these various aspects of lung injury as they relate to mechanical ventilation.

Ventilator-Associated Lung Injury Versus Ventilator-Induced Lung Injury

The terms *ventilator-associated lung injury (VALI)* and *ventilator-induced lung injury (VILI)* have been used frequently in the literature with some inconsistency regarding their meaning. The term *VALI* is generally used when referring to lung injury occurring in humans that has been identified as a consequence of mechanical ventilation.[2] The most common forms of VALI include ventilator-associated pneumonia (VAP), air trapping, patient-ventilator asynchrony, and extraalveolar gas (barotrauma) such as pneumothorax and pneumomediastinum. (See Chapter 14 for a discussion of ventilator-associated pneumonia.)

VILI is lung injury that occurs at the level of the acinus. It is the microscopic level of injury that includes biotrauma, shear stress, and surfactant depletion (atelectrauma). VILI can be specifically studied only in animal models because ventilator strategies that will potentially harm the lung cannot be performed on human subjects during research investigations.

VILI is a form of lung injury that resembles ARDS. It has been studied using animal models and apparently occurs in patients receiving inappropriate mechanical ventilation. VILI is difficult to identify in humans because its appearance is based on radiologic and clinical findings, which overlap with the findings that occur

with the underlying pulmonary pathology such as ARDS. In fact it is reasonable to assume that acute lung injury (ALI) and ARDS may be partially the result of ventilator management rather than the progression of the disease.[3] This supports the idea that mechanical ventilation not only saves lives but also has the potential to worsen preexistent lung injury.[1]

The following section defines and describes the various forms of VALI and VILI (Key Point 17-1).

Key Point **17-1** It is the practitioner's responsibility to do no harm and to use appropriate settings when managing patients on mechanical ventilation.

Barotrauma or Extraalveolar Air

As mentioned, it has been known for some time that PPV increases the risk of *barotrauma*. This type of injury involves the formation of extraalveolar gas, such as subcutaneous emphysema, pneumothorax, pneumomediastinum, pneumoperitoneum, and pneumopericardium.

The risk of rupture to the lung is greater for patients with lung bullae or chest wall injury. A number of conditions can predispose a patient to barotrauma (extraalveolar air). Some of these include the following[4,5]:

- High peak airway pressures with low end-expiratory pressures
- Bullous lung disease such as may occur with emphysema or a history of tuberculosis
- High levels of PEEP with high tidal volumes (V_T)
- Aspiration of gastric acid
- Necrotizing pneumonias
- ARDS

Barotrauma occurs when the delivery of positive-pressure ventilation causes alveolar rupture. Air is forced into the interstitium of an adjacent bronchovascular (**perivascular**) sheath in the area of the distal noncartilaginous airways.[4,6] The "escaped" air moves along the sheath toward the hilum and mediastinum, causing a pneumomediastinum (Fig. 17-1).[4,7] Air can then break through the pleural surface of the mediastinum into the intrapleural space, resulting in a pneumothorax. Pneumothorax may be unilateral or bilateral. Air in the mediastinum also may dissect along tissue planes, producing subcutaneous emphysema. Pneumoperitoneum may follow pneumomediastinum and occurs when air dissects initially into the retroperitoneum. Air that is trapped under the diaphragm in the peritoneum may interfere with effective ventilation.

From its location in the mediastinum, air can also dissect along tissue planes near the heart and form a pneumopericardium.[2] The escaped air can be reabsorbed into adjacent tissues and resolve itself. If it is not reabsorbed by the body, evacuation by a drainage system may be required. Failure to remove this extraalveolar air can lead to life-threatening problems, such as tension pneumothorax or pneumopericardium.

Subcutaneous Emphysema

Subcutaneous emphysema can be easily detected during physical examination. It may be visible as a puffing of the skin in the patient's neck, face, or chest, and may even be present in distal areas such as the feet and abdomen. The skin feels crepitant to the touch. Subcutaneous emphysema typically occurs without complication and tends to clear without treatment as mean airway pressures

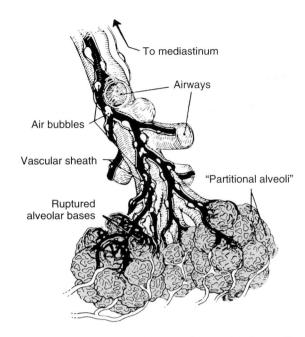

Fig. 17-1 Artist's conception of the development of interstitial emphysema. (From Samuelson WM, Fulkerson WJ: Barotrauma in mechanical ventilation. In Fulkerson WJ, MacIntyre NR, editors: Problems in respiratory care: complications of mechanical ventilation, Philadelphia, 1991, Lippincott Williams & Wilkins.)

are reduced. However, if it is present with dyspnea, cyanosis, and increased peak pressures, it may be accompanied by a pneumothorax.

Pneumomediastinum

Pneumomediastinum can lead to compression of the esophagus, great vessels, and the heart. It usually can be easily identified on chest radiographs. Treatment depends on the severity of the problem and its effect on adjacent structures. In severe cases, pneumomediastinum can cause **cardiac tamponade.** If the air is not removed, cardiac tamponade can ultimately lead to cardiopulmonary arrest.

Pneumothorax

Early clinical studies suggested that the most common clinical manifestation of extraalveolar air was pneumothorax.[8,9] Although studies have shown that the incidence of barotrauma is relatively low (2.9%),[10] results vary from study to study. Interestingly, the reduced incidence of barotrauma may be associated with use of lower V_T and lower airway pressures.

Pneumothorax may lead to lung collapse with mediastinal shifting occurring away from the affected side. Pneumothorax also can be detected by a resonant or hyperresonant percussion note and absence of breath sounds on the affected side, and chest radiographs will indicate lack of vascular markings on the affected side. Treatment usually requires thoracotomy and placement of a chest tube. Because pleural air rises to the highest (nondependent) area of the thorax, the affected area will depend on the patient's position. In the supine patient this is an area over the anterior surface of the lung. When evaluating a chest radiograph taken with the patient supine, detection of a small pneumothorax can be difficult (Case Study 17-1).

Another way of detecting a pneumothorax in patients on mechanical ventilation is to observe progressive changes in peak pressure. Increases in peak pressure occurring within a short period, such as a few minutes to a few hours, may signal the presence of pneumothorax of either rapid onset or one caused by a slow, insidious leak. Physical examination and a chest radiograph should be used to confirm the diagnosis.

⬤ Case Study 17-1

Peak Pressure Alarm Activating

The peak pressure alarm is activated for a mechanically ventilated patient. Assessment of the patient reveals puffing of the skin of the patient's neck and face, which feels crepitant to the touch. The right hemithorax is hyperresonant to percussion and breath sounds are absent. What would be an appropriate action for the respiratory therapist?

Because a simple pneumothorax can develop into a tension pneumothorax, careful monitoring is essential. Administering excessive amounts of positive pressure may aggravate the presence of air in the pleural space, so manual ventilation with a resuscitation bag on 100% oxygen may be advisable until the problem can be treated.[7] However, it is important for the clinician to avoid using excessive pressure with manual compression of a resuscitation bag.[11]

A tension pneumothorax is a life-threatening situation that must be treated immediately. A tension pneumothorax occurs when air enters the pleural space and becomes trapped. Pressure gradually builds, collapsing the affected lung. Mediastinal structures will shift in the thorax, away from the area of tension, and put pressure on the heart and the unaffected lung. Tracheal deviation and neck vein distention are possible signs. Breath sounds will be absent and the percussion note tympanic. A chest radiograph on a patient with a tension pneumothorax is not advisable because it might delay lifesaving treatment. In a chest radiograph of a tension pneumothorax, one diaphragm will be more depressed than the other and may display a **deep sulcus sign,** with air appearing adjacent to the depressed diaphragm.

Treatment for tension pneumothorax involves inserting a 14-gauge needle, or similar device, into the anterior second to third intercostal space on the affected side in the midclavicular line over the top of the rib with the patient in the upright position. This maneuver can be lifesaving. While waiting for trained personnel to be summoned to perform this procedure, the respiratory therapist should decrease mean airway pressures as much as possible while using manual ventilation with a high fraction of inspired oxygen (F_IO_2).

Pneumoperitoneum

Pneumoperitoneum generally follows pneumomediastinum. It occurs when air dissects into the retroperitoneal space. The peritoneum can also rupture, resulting in air moving into the peritoneal cavity. As you might expect, this can be very painful. If a significant amount of air is present, it can interfere with the movement of the diaphragm and reduce effective ventilation.

Barotrauma or Volutrauma

In early studies, researchers tried to determine if the cause of lung injury during mechanical ventilation was the result of the delivery

BOX 17-1	Chest Wall and Transpulmonary Pressures

Transpulmonary pressure (P_L), as defined in Chapter 1, is the difference between the pressure inside the alveolus and the pressure immediately outside, or the intrapleural pressure.[2] It is not uncommon to read scientific journal articles in which transpulmonary pressure is defined as the difference between the static airway pressure measured during a plateau maneuver and the average intrapleural pressure, which is estimated by using an esophageal balloon.[13] Do not be confused by this subtle difference. Both definitions imply alveolar pressure (airway pressure during a plateau) minus intrapleural pressure.

BOX 17-2	Chest Wall Compliance and Protection from Overdistention

The term *chest wall pressure* as used in the clinical setting includes forces or pressures from the overlying ribs and muscles, pressure from the diaphragm, and abdominal pressure. As abdominal pressure increases (>20 cm H_2O is high), an increased amount of pressure is placed on the diaphragm and the vena cava. This added abdominal pressure augments venous return to the thorax as blood shifts into the thorax from the abdominal area. If the lung is injured and leaking, lung fluid is increased. Thus as abdominal pressure increases, more lung collapses. For example, in an obese patient with peritonitis, an airway pressure of 30 cm H_2O may not be adequate to ventilate the patient sufficiently.

of high pressures (barotrauma) or high volumes (volutrauma). Dreyfuss and colleagues coined the term *volutrauma* to describe the injurious effects of mechanical ventilation they observed in laboratory studies using an animal model.[12] They found that it was not high pressure but the relatively large regional volumes that overstretched compliant areas of the lung that resulted in alveolar stretch and edema formation in these areas.[12,13]

It is now generally accepted that using inordinately high tidal volume can lead to lung overdistention and iatrogenic lung injury. Overdistention occurs in those areas of the lungs where high distending pressures—in other words, high transpulmonary pressures (alveolar pressure − pleural pressure [$P_{alv} − P_{pl}$])—are present. Indeed, pressures as low as 30 to 35 cm H_2O have been shown to cause lung injury in animals.[4,12]

Because regional differences in lung compliance and transpulmonary pressures (P_L) occur in most pulmonary disorders, positive pressure applied to the lung tends to produce larger volumes in more compliant lung areas (Box 17-1). The resulting overdistention to these areas causes acute alveolar injury and the formation of pulmonary edema by both increased permeability and filtration mechanisms (e.g., tidal volumes of 10 to 12 mL/kg can cause overdistention of these areas of greater compliance).

Additional animal studies found that when the chest wall movement was restricted by binding the thorax, and pressure was applied to the lungs, less lung injury occurred.[12-14] Thoracic binding prevented severe transpulmonary (alveolar distending) pressure. Furthermore, alveolar stretch and edema formation did not occur under these conditions. In the clinical setting restriction to chest wall movement is present when patients are in the prone position, in severely obese patients, or when heavy dressings are used to manage surgical sites of chest or chest wall injuries (Box 17-2).[15]

To understand the importance of pressure in this setting and its distribution, several circumstances that affect lung pressures must be examined. Pressure at the upper airway is not equal to alveolar pressure (P_{alv}) except when flow is zero and the airway is open. (This is usually termed plateau pressure, or $P_{plateau}$.) To interpret P_{alv}, or $P_{plateau}$, the circumstances in which it is measured should be known. The following are seven of these circumstances:[15]

1. The lungs are normal, but the chest wall is very stiff but relaxed, resulting in high pleural pressures (e.g., 60 cm H_2O).
2. The lungs and chest wall are normal, but the pressure around the chest is high (e.g., pressure on the chest or in the abdomen, such as with obesity).
3. The lungs and chest wall are normal, but the expiratory muscles are actively contracting (e.g., the patient performs a Valsalva maneuver, which causes the pleural pressure to be positive).

4. The lungs are normal, but the abdomen is turgidly overdistended (similar to the first circumstance).
5. The lungs are very stiff, leaving pleural pressure near normal (e.g., 5 cm H_2O).
6. The lungs are normal, but an incorrectly positioned endotracheal tube (ET) expands only one lung to a dangerous degree (e.g., right mainstem intubation with large tidal volumes).
7. Both lungs are dangerously overdistended inside a normal chest wall.

In the first four examples, structures around the lung (e.g., chest wall and abdomen) oppose most of the alveolar pressure; the pleural pressure is high, but the distending pressure is within safe limits. Only the last three examples are situations in which lung distending pressure (i.e., the transpulmonary pressure, or $P_{alv} − P_{pl}$) is abnormally high and thus can cause lung injury. P_{alv} can be high by itself without causing lung damage, but if $P_{alv} − P_{pl}$ is high, lung damage is more likely to occur.

Lung injury from overdistention is much more subtle than air leaks described in the preceding section on barotrauma. Overdistention lung injury causes excessive stretching of alveolar cells, the formation of edema, and the release of inflammatory mediators, also called chemical mediators. As mentioned earlier, the release of these chemical mediators is termed *biotrauma*.

Figure 17-2 shows a pressure–volume curve that indicates the presence of overdistention. The shape of this curve is sometimes said to have a "duck-billed" appearance. Most clinicians now believe that this portion of the curve occurs with overdistention of more compliant areas of the lung, resulting in volutrauma. For the sake of simplicity, the term *barotrauma* will be used in this text to imply the leaking of air into body tissues (extraalveolar air leak) and the term *volutrauma* to describe damage from overdistention that occurs at the alveolar level and involves alveolar and interstitial edema formation, alveolar stretch, and biotrauma.

Atelectrauma

The term *atelectrauma* is used to describe the injuries to the lungs that occur because of repeated opening and closing of lung units at lower lung volumes. Atelectrauma can occur in the management of ARDS when low tidal volumes are used and inadequate levels of PEEP are applied (see Chapter 13). Under these circumstances, alveoli tend to open on inspiration and close on expiration. (This occurs most often in the dependent areas of the lung. In supine patients this would be the dorsal area near the spine.) The repeated opening and closing of lung units in ARDS produces three primary

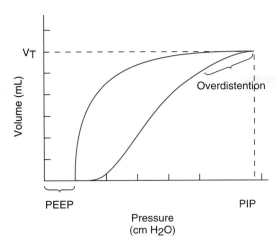

Fig. 17-2 A pressure–volume curve in a patient with acute overdistention of the lung during positive-pressure ventilation. Notice the duck-billed appearance of the top right portion of the curve (overdistention). *PEEP*, Positive end-expiratory pressure; *PIP*, peak inspiratory pressure; V_T, tidal volume.

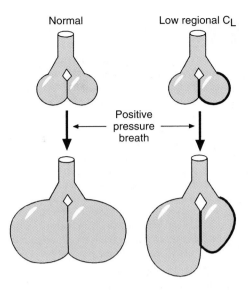

Fig. 17-3 The volume from a positive-pressure breath distributes homogeneously throughout a lung with normal compliance (C_L) *(left)*. In a lung with instability, the volume from a positive-pressure breath distributes preferentially to the regions with more normal C_L *(right)*. Thus a tidal volume (V_T) of normal size in a lung with regions of low C_L can overdistend the healthier regions. This creates shearing between adjacent lung units. (Redrawn from MacIntyre NR: Respir Care 41:318-326, 1996.)

types of lung injury: shear stress, alteration and washout of surfactant, and microvascular injury.[16-18]

Research studies involving animal models showed that ventilating pressures of 30 to 80 cm H_2O produce atelectrauma with resulting reduced compliance and severe hypoxemia. Atelectrauma may be described as alveolar rupture, interstitial emphysema, or perivascular and alveolar hemorrhage, which can eventually lead to death.[12,19-26] Death occurred in experimental animal models in some cases within an hour.

Shear Stress

Shear stress occurs when an alveolus that is normally expanded is adjacent to one that is collapsed (atelectasis) and unstable. As airway pressure increases during inspiration, the normal alveolus inflates, but the collapsed unit does not. In the interstitial space between the two, force is exerted as these two units move or slide against each other. There is a potential zone of risk at the interface of open and closed lung units. This is similar to what occurs when a paper clip is repeatedly twisted; eventually the paper clip breaks. In the lung, the stress pulls normal tissues apart, resulting in physical damage to the alveolar cells, particularly epithelial and endothelial cells (pulmonary microvasculature). The term *shear stress* has been applied to this type of situation. The amount of stress across the entire lung can be estimated by using transpulmonary pressure (Fig. 17-3; Key Point 17-2).[5,27]

Key Point **17-2** Shear stress causes intense strain and rupture of lung tissue, which may lead to an inflammatory response and edema formation.

The importance of shear stress has been known for a number of years. In fact, more than 30 years ago, Mead and colleagues[28] calculated from a model that a transpulmonary pressure of only 30 cm H_2O could result in a stress of 140 cm H_2O being exerted between two adjacent alveoli as one expands and the other unstable unit remains collapsed. Not surprisingly, this force acting on the delicate tissues of the acinus can result in tearing of alveolar epithelium and capillary endothelium along with other structural injury.

Surfactant Alteration

A second consequence of the repeated opening and closing of alveoli involves reorientation of the surfactant molecules lining the alveolar surface. In the alveolus, surfactant forms a molecular layer between the air and the liquid alveolar surface. During alveolar collapse, as the surface area of the alveolus decreases, the surfactant molecules can form together until some actually pop out or get squeezed out at low lung volumes. These "used" lipids do not rapidly spread as the alveolus reopens.[2] Rather it is theorized that newly secreted surfactant replaces surfactant that is lost from the affected area. Reduction in surface area that occurs during exhalation (i.e., lower alveolar volumes) causes a greater number of surfactant molecules to migrate from the affected area. Thus a greater amount of new surfactant is required to stabilize the lung unit.[29] How quickly and for what length of time the alveolar cells can continue to produce an adequate amount of surfactant are uncertain. It is believed that eventually not enough surfactant will be present and the alveolus will become very unstable. Besides the effects of opening and closing of alveoli on surfactant production, it has been suggested that overdistention also reduces surface tension and is believed to alter surfactant function.[5]

Biotrauma

Mechanical stress disrupts normal cell function, strains normal cell configuration, and can also lead to an inflammatory response in the lungs.[13] Current theory suggest that pulmonary cells, particularly epithelial cells, become distorted during mechanical ventilation when they are overstretched (overdistention). This overdistention causes the release of chemical mediators (i.e., cytokines). In addition to epithelial cells, the alveolar macrophages are another important source of inflammatory mediators, which are produced in response to a stretching strain and result in a potential molecular and cellular basis for VILI (Box 17-3).[30-35]

It is important to understand that ARDS does not have to be present for this inflammatory response to occur. However, when

Chemical Mediators, Cytokines, and Chemokines

The production of cytokines and chemokines (i.e., chemotactic cytokines) is increased by harmful ventilator strategies. Pulmonary epithelial and alveolar macrophages are, in part, responsible for the production of these substances, which can occur within 1 to 3 hours of the initiation of an inappropriate ventilatory strategy. Inflammatory mediators, such as platelet activating factor (PAF), thromboxane-B2, tumor necrosis factor-alpha (TNF-α), and interleukin-1B, have also been found isolated from the lungs when low end-expiratory volumes are used. As already discussed, release of these inflammatory mediators is thought to be associated with tidal alveolar reopening and collapse. Neutrophils that migrate into the lung following injury or infection can also release inflammatory mediators.

A number of strategies have been proposed to reduce the adverse effects associated with the production of inflammatory mediators in the lungs. Protective ventilating strategies that were discussed earlier in Chapter 13 can be used to avoid overinflation and the repeated opening and closing of alveoli, and thus reduce the cytokine response. Instilling anti-inflammatory antibodies into the trachea, such as anti-TNF-α, has also been shown to improve oxygenation and lung compliance. Infiltration of leukocytes into the lungs is also reduced. Furthermore the pathologic changes seen in an experimental animal model ventilated with inappropriate settings were reduced when antibodies were administered.

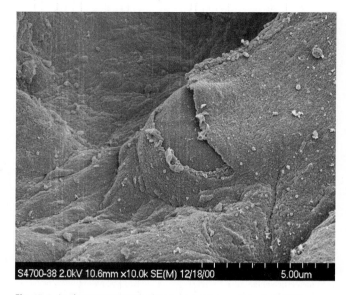

Fig. 17-4 An electron micrograph of the lung showing a red blood cell (RBC) rupturing through the wall of the pulmonary microvasculature. (Courtesy John J. Marini, MD, Minneapolis, Minn.)

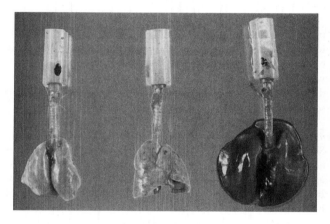

Fig. 17-5 Macroscopic aspect of rat lungs after mechanical ventilation at 45 cm H_2O peak airway pressure. *Left,* Normal lungs; *middle,* after 5 minutes of high airway pressure mechanical ventilation (notice the focal zones of atelectasis, particularly at the left lung apex); *right,* after 20 minutes. (From Dreyfus D, Saumon G: Ventilator-induced lung injury: lessons from experimental studies. Am J Respir Crit Care Med 157:294-323, 1998.)

the inflammatory mediators are released, the lung begins to resemble that of a lung with ARDS. Indeed, the damage that can be caused by ventilator mismanagement may actually be indistinguishable from the underlying disease process of ARDS.[3]

Multiple Organ Dysfunction Syndrome

Chemical mediators produced in the lung can leak into the pulmonary blood vessels. The circulation then carries these substances to other areas of the body and sets up an inflammatory reaction in other organs, such as the kidneys, gut, and liver.[31,36] The release of mediators may therefore lead to **multiple organ failure,** also called **multisystem organ failure** and **multiple organ dysfunction syndrome.**[2,37,38]

Treating patients with ARDS with lung-protective strategies, such as low V_T and therapeutic PEEP, can significantly reduce morbidity and mortality rates in these patients (see Chapter 13).[35,39-41] It also has been suggested that hypercapnia may be beneficial in patients with ARDS (who are difficult to ventilate) because it has an antioxidant effect and may actually reduce inflammation. Therapeutic hypercapnia may actually be a more appropriate name, but additional studies are needed (see Chapter 13).[13,42-44]

Vascular Endothelial Injury

A third problem that can occur with repeated alveolar collapse and reopening involves the pulmonary microvasculature. Recall that during a positive-pressure breath, alveolar capillaries flatten out, but corner micro-alveolar vessels open wider (see Fig. 13-16). The interstitial areas adjacent to the corner vessels develop negative pressure relative to the inside of the vessels. This negative-pressure gradient tends to pull fluid and blood products out of the vessels and into the space. Thus the alveoli and perivascular areas become edematous.

If the vascular pressure of the lung is further increased, at a certain point the vessel can rupture and release red blood cells and other blood components into the alveoli and interstitial space (Fig. 17-4). In Mead's model, a stress of 140 cm H_2O was proposed as occurring between two alveoli as one expanded and the other unit remained collapsed.[28] This pressure could also be transmitted to the pulmonary vessels, which could represent a second cause of vessel rupture. The increased fluid leaking into the lung would create a dramatic increase in lung weight, which may be one of the mechanisms associated with the hemorrhagic appearance of lungs on autopsy in animal models subjected to low V_T ventilation without PEEP (Fig. 17-5).[45] Studies using a canine model have shown that it takes 90 to 100 mm Hg to produce this phenomenon. Perhaps leaving areas of the lung collapsed or at least ventilating them at low pressures might not damage the lung or the vasculature. Whether resting parts of the lung is better than trying to recruit the majority of the lung will require additional studies.

Historic Webb and Tierney Study

Seminal studies conducted by Webb and Tierney[22] in the early 1970s showed that using inspiratory pressures of 45 cm of H_2O without PEEP resulted in the rapid death of normal rats. Their study is frequently cited as evidence of the benefits of using protective ventilatory strategies. Interestingly, their discovery took nearly two decades to be recognized. In a 2003 editorial, Tierney wrote, "… we could hardly believe the results. It was as if we violated a thermodynamic law and got more out of it than we put into it. … Within minutes the rats were cyanotic and appeared moribund. … It took a decade or two for others to conclude that human lungs could be injured by such ventilation. … Our final paragraph 30 years ago suggested management … using protective ventilation and low tidal volumes."[29]

Role of PEEP in Lung Protection

In ALI, PEEP appears to provide some protection from tissue damage when high pressures are used. This is especially true if PEEP levels are greater than the opening pressure for recruitable alveoli. PEEP helps restore functional residual capacity (FRC) by recruiting previously collapsed alveoli. Adequate levels of PEEP prevent repeated collapse and reopening of alveoli and help maintain lung recruitment.[14,27] However, if PEEP overinflates already patent alveoli, then increasing PEEP for a given V_T may maximally stretch alveoli. This situation also may reduce cardiac output. Safely establishing an optimum PEEP level is not an exact science and can be challenging in critically ill patients. (Case Study 17-2; see Chapter 13 for additional information on setting PEEP.)[46]

To summarize, lung injury may occur as a result of either over-distention of the lungs or from repeated opening and closing of lung units throughout the respiratory cycle during mechanical ventilation.[46] These two phenomena can result in shear stress and alveolar injury, edema formation, surfactant washout or alteration, microvascular injury, stretch injury, and biotrauma. Stretch injury and the associated biotrauma produces inflammatory mediators by lung tissue and leaking of these mediators into the circulation, where they have the potential to affect distal organs and ultimately cause multiple organ dysfunction syndrome.[37] Research findings strongly support the concept of maintaining $P_{plateau}$ at less than 30 cm H_2O, setting low V_T, and using enough PEEP to adequately maintain open alveoli in patients with ARDS to avoid lung injury from mechanical ventilation.[47]

Case Study 17-2

Patient Case—Acute Pancreatitis

Two days after admission to the hospital, a 50-year-old man with acute pancreatitis requires mechanical ventilation. Although his minute ventilation is maintained with the ventilator, oxygenation becomes a concern. The P_aO_2 is 70 mm Hg on an F_iO_2 of 0.75. The patient is receiving pressure-controlled continuous mandatory ventilation (PC-CMV) with a set pressure of 20 cm H_2O and a current PEEP setting of 5 cm H_2O. Auscultation reveals bi-basilar crackles and scattered crackles in the posterior basal segments. What is the source of the problem based on auscultation and blood gas findings? What change in therapy might be appropriate?

Ventilator-Induced Respiratory Muscle Weakness

It is clear that delivering high airway pressures and volumes during mechanical ventilation can lead to damage to the lung parenchyma. Recent studies have shown that mechanical ventilation may also cause damage to the respiratory muscles.[45] Specifically, imposing too little stress on the diaphragm during mechanical ventilation by lowering the demands on a patient's respiratory muscles can induce respiratory muscle weakness.[46]

Laboratory studies using animal models have shown that prolonged controlled mechanical ventilation in which complete diaphragmatic inactivity occurs (i.e., no respiratory efforts are made and the mechanical ventilator performs all of the work of breathing [WOB]) can lead to a significant decrease in the cross-sectional area of diaphragmatic fibers.[47] More recent studies by Levine and colleagues involving human subjects support these findings.[48] In their studies, Levine and colleagues obtained diaphragmatic muscle biopsies from mechanically ventilated patients who exhibited complete diaphragmatic inactivity for 18 to 69 hours. Histologic measurements of these muscle samples from the costal diaphragm revealed marked diaphragmatic atrophy. Biochemical analysis of the muscle samples suggested that the atrophy occurred as a result of increased oxidative stress and activation of protein-degradation pathways.[48]

The implications of these findings on clinical management of mechanically ventilated patients are unclear at this time. Additional clinical studies will be required to identify more completely the presence of ventilator-induced respiratory muscle weakness and its effect on weaning and ventilator discontinuation. Although respiratory muscle weakness can result from ventilator injury, it is important for clinicians to recognize that it can be associated with other medical conditions and interventions, such as sepsis and pharmacologic therapy (e.g., antibiotics, corticosteroids, sedatives, and neuromuscular blocking agents.)[46]

EFFECTS OF MECHANICAL VENTILATION ON GAS DISTRIBUTION AND PULMONARY BLOOD FLOW

Ventilation to Nondependent Lung

Early studies of the effects of positive-pressure breathing on the gas distribution in the normal lungs were conducted more than 30 years ago. Froese and Bryan[49] evaluated the movement of the diaphragm in spontaneously breathing, anesthetized adult volunteers. During spontaneous ventilation in the supine position, the greatest displacement of the diaphragm occurs in the dependent region, near the back (Fig. 17-6, A).[49] The dependent lung areas receive a higher portion of ventilation and perfusion (i.e., $\dot{V}/\dot{Q}$ is best matched). When anesthesia is administered but spontaneous ventilation is still present, the diaphragm shifts its movement cephalad (toward the head). The effect of this shift is most pronounced in the dependent (dorsal) regions of the lung, the reverse of normal (Fig. 17-6, B). With anesthesia and the administration of paralytic agents, the contraction of the diaphragm is blocked. When PPV is provided, the diaphragm is most displaced in the nondependent regions of the lung (Fig. 17-6, C). The diaphragm becomes less compliant than the chest wall adjacent to the anterior part of the lungs in the supine patient. This alters the $\dot{V}/\dot{Q}$ ratios by directing the greatest amount of gas flow to the nondependent lung regions, taking the path of least resistance. Unfortunately, this is also the area with the least blood flow.

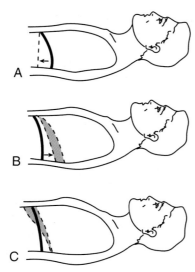

Fig. 17-6 The *solid line* in each figure represents the normal position of the diaphragm. The *dotted lines* represent the position of the diaphragm as it is altered during anesthesia and positive-pressure ventilation. **A,** Normal spontaneous breathing in the supine patient with diaphragm movement primarily in the dependent area of the lungs. **B,** During anesthesia with spontaneous ventilation maintained, the diaphragm shifts cephalad. The shift is most pronounced in the dependent regions. **C,** Anesthesia is sufficient to block spontaneous breaths (paralysis). PPV displaces the diaphragm to the nondependent regions of the lung.

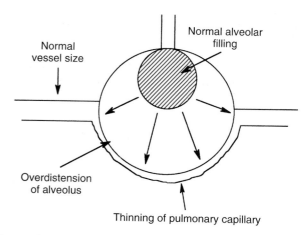

Fig. 17-7 The *shaded area* represents a normal alveolar volume. Overfilling of an alveolus results in thinning and compression of the pulmonary capillary. PVR is increased.

During PPV, alveolar collapse is suspected to most likely occur in the dependent areas with absence of spontaneous diaphragmatic movement. These are also the areas that receive the most blood flow, resulting in increased mismatching of ventilation and perfusion and increased dead space ventilation.[49,50]

Ventilation-to-Lung Periphery

Experimental studies have shown that during spontaneous ventilation, the distribution of gas favors the dependent lung areas and also appears to favor the periphery of the lung closest to the moving pleural surfaces. The peripheral areas receive more ventilation than the central areas.[51,52] However, during a positive-pressure breath with passive inflation of the lung (paralysis), the central, upper airway, or peribronchial portions of the lung are preferentially filled with air.[51] This may be another mechanism by which mismatching occurs during PPV. If spontaneous breathing can be preserved when possible, these changes in $\dot{V}/\dot{Q}$ associated with mechanical ventilation may be reduced. Thus ventilator modes that preserve spontaneous breathing may be beneficial (e.g., pressure support ventilation [PSV]).

Increase in Dead Space

Positive-pressure ventilation (PPV) increases the size of the conductive airways, which in turn increases the amount of dead space ventilation. Additionally, if normal alveoli are overexpanded during PPV and compression of pulmonary vessels results, alveolar dead space will also increase. On the other hand, if an increased V_T is delivered and PPV improves ventilation distribution with respect to perfusion, then PPV will decrease the amount of dead space ventilation.

Redistribution of Pulmonary Blood Flow

Normal pulmonary blood flow favors the gravity-dependent areas and the central, or core, areas of the lungs. However, during PPV, particularly when PEEP is administered, cardiac output may decrease and pulmonary perfusion redistributes to the lung periphery rather than to the center area (i.e., as if the lung had been exposed to a centrifugal force).[53] The clinical significance of this is unknown, but it may influence $\dot{V}/\dot{Q}$ matching.

The increased volume during a positive-pressure breath and PEEP squeezes the blood out of nondependent zones, particularly in areas of normal lung. This further contributes to $\dot{V}/\dot{Q}$ mismatching and physiological dead space by sending more blood into dependent areas, where ventilation is now lower, or into disease-affected areas of the lung, where lung volumes are not substantially increased. This can lead to increased shunting and decreased P_aO_2.[54]

Conversely, improvement in $\dot{V}/\dot{Q}$ matching occurs when PEEP is applied to patients who have refractory hypoxemia resulting from a decreased FRC and increased shunting (i.e., ARDS). PEEP reduces intrapulmonary shunting resulting in an increase in P_aO_2. This increase in P_aO_2 implies improvement in $\dot{V}/\dot{Q}$ matching.[2,6,55,56] A classic and predictable response of gas distribution and pulmonary perfusion during PPV apparently does not exist.

Effects of Positive Pressure on Pulmonary Vascular Resistance

As described previously, pulmonary perfusion may be compromised during PPV, especially when high levels of PEEP are also applied. Increased airway and alveolar pressures can lead to thinning and compression of pulmonary capillaries, decreased perfusion, and increased pulmonary vascular resistance (PVR) (Fig. 17-7). Fortunately, if expiration is prolonged and unimpeded (i.e., PEEP is not applied), the decreased pulmonary perfusion may be offset by normal flow back into the thorax during expiration with no net effect on PVR.

In most patients, severe hypoxia leads to increased PVR. This is caused by constriction of the pulmonary vessels and subsequent pulmonary hypertension. When mechanical ventilation improves oxygenation by opening up these capillary beds, pulmonary perfusion and PVR may actually improve.

At low lung volumes in which FRC is decreased, the addition of PEEP can potentially open collapsed alveoli, recruiting intraparenchymal (e.g., corner) vessels. This improves the $\dot{V}/\dot{Q}$ relations of the lungs. Thus PPV has no clear effect with or without PEEP on PVR. Sometimes positive pressure reduces PVR, whereas at other times, it increases PVR.

RESPIRATORY AND METABOLIC ACID–BASE STATUS IN MECHANICAL VENTILATION

The primary goal of mechanical ventilation is to maintain acceptable arterial blood gas (ABG) values in patients with compromised ventilatory function. Failure to achieve this goal occurs when the ventilator is not optimally adjusted or when adverse effects occur. Ventilatory problems associated with PPV can result in hypoventilation and hyperventilation. Patients may additionally demonstrate metabolic acid–base imbalances that can seriously affect their ventilatory management.

Hypoventilation

Acute **hypoventilation** can occur in patients receiving ventilatory support if adequate alveolar ventilation is not achieved. Hypoventilation will result in an elevated P_aCO_2 (i.e., hypercapnia) and an acidotic pH. Evaluation of clinical signs and symptoms, as well as ABG analysis, will lead to recognition of the problem.

Acidosis causes a right shift in the oxyhemoglobin dissociation curve and reduces the ability of hemoglobin to bind and carry oxygen in the lung. Additionally, in the absence of supplemental oxygen delivery, an increase in P_aCO_2 will lead to proportionate decreases in P_aO_2 and contribute to hypoxemia. If the patient already had hypoxemia, these factors may further reduce oxygenation. On the other hand, a right shift of the curve facilitates unloading of oxygen at the tissue level.

Rapidly rising P_aCO_2 levels and falling pH values can lead to serious problems, including coma. Elevated plasma hydrogen ion levels can contribute to high plasma potassium levels (hyperkalemia), which can affect cardiac function and can lead to cardiac dysrhythmias (Box 17-4). Hypercapnia also increases cerebral perfusion and can lead to increased intracranial pressure, which can be detrimental to patients with cerebral trauma, cerebral hemorrhage, or similar disorders.

On the other hand, in patients with ARDS, ventilation may be difficult to maintain without causing VILI. In these situations, permissive hypercapnia may be appropriate. In addition, hypercapnia may reduce the release of inflammatory mediators (see Chapter 13).[42-44] Ultimately the decision to allow respiratory acidosis to persist must be carefully evaluated on the basis of the patient's condition.

The kidneys normally can compensate for respiratory acidosis within 18 to 36 hours. Obviously it is desirable for the problem to be corrected by increasing alveolar ventilation rather than waiting for renal compensation. Increasing ventilation can be accomplished by increasing the V_T or mandatory rate.

When respiratory acidosis is present, patients receiving controlled mechanical ventilation may try to override the ventilator and take in a breath. They may not be able to trigger the machine or receive adequate flow and will appear to be fighting the ventilator. Increasing the sensitivity or flow will allow the patient to trigger the ventilator and receive an adequate breath. (See the discussion of ventilator asynchrony in this chapter.)

Hyperventilation

Hyperventilation results in a lower than normal P_aCO_2 and a rise in pH. Patient-induced hyperventilation is often associated with hypoxemia, pain and anxiety syndromes, circulatory failure, and airway inflammation. Ventilator-induced hyperventilation is generally caused by inappropriate ventilator settings. Alkalosis causes a left shift in the oxygen dissociation curve, which enhances the ability of hemoglobin to pick up oxygen in the lungs but makes it less available at the tissue level (i.e., the *Haldane* effect). Reduced hydrogen ion concentrations in the blood (i.e., arterial pH) are often accompanied by hypokalemia (low potassium levels), which can lead to cardiac arrhythmias (Box 17-5).

Sustained severe hypocapnia can lead to tetany and also reduces cerebral perfusion, which may contribute to increased cerebral hypoxia. In patients with increased intracranial pressure and cerebral edema, however, this reduced perfusion may be beneficial in reducing acute abnormally high intracranial pressures that cannot be controlled by other methods (see Chapter 7).

Hyperventilation in mechanically ventilated patients reduces the drive to breathe and leads to apnea. This has the advantage of preventing the patient from trying to "fight" the ventilator or

---

BOX **17-4**	Clinical and ECG Changes Associated with Respiratory Acidosis, Hypoxia, and Hyperkalemia

Clinical Signs and Symptoms
- Hypertension (mild to moderate acidosis)
- Hypotension (severe acidosis)
- Anxiety
- Agitation
- "Fighting the ventilator" (ventilator asynchrony)
- Dyspnea
- Attempts to increase minute ventilation
- Headaches
- Hot, moist skin (associated with increased P_aCO_2)

ECG Changes Associated with Hyperkalemia
- Elevated and peaked T waves
- ST-segment depression
- Widened QRS complex
- Long P-R interval

BOX **17-5**	Clinical and ECG Changes Associated with Respiratory Alkalosis and Hypokalemia

Clinical Signs and Symptoms
- Cool skin (decreased P_aCO_2)
- Twitching
- Tetany

ECG Changes Associated with Hypokalemia
- Prolonged Q-T interval
- Low, rounded T waves
- Depressed ST segment
- Inverted T waves
- Inverted P waves
- Atrioventricular block
- Premature ventricular contractions
- Paroxysmal tachycardia
- Atrial flutter

experiencing feelings of dyspnea. The disadvantage is that weaning becomes more difficult if the respiratory alkalosis persists for a prolonged period. With extended periods of hyperventilation, when respiratory muscle activity is absent, respiratory muscle atrophy can occur. In addition, the central chemoreceptors, which respond to changes in PCO_2 and pH, will have an altered function. When respiratory alkalosis occurs, CO_2 diffuses out of the cerebrospinal fluid (CSF) because of the low blood CO_2 level. The hydrogen ion concentration in the CSF decreases and respirations are not stimulated. As long as this condition persists, apnea will remain until the P_aO_2 drops low enough to stimulate the peripheral chemoreceptors.

If chronic hyperventilation and respiratory alkalosis are sustained for an extended period (e.g., typically 18 to 36 hours), renal compensation will occur. The kidneys remove bicarbonate from the plasma and it is excreted in the urine. Simultaneously, bicarbonate is actively transported out of the CSF so that CSF balances with the plasma bicarbonate. The pH is restored to normal in both the plasma and the CSF. The bicarbonate and PCO_2 levels will be lower than normal.

It is important to note that weaning becomes more difficult when a patient has experienced prolonged hyperventilation. As the respiratory rate of the ventilator is reduced, the blood PCO_2 increases and pH falls. The patient tries to maintain a high alveolar ventilation to keep the PCO_2 at the level at which it has been equilibrated. The patient may become fatigued and unable to maintain the high levels of alveolar ventilation. Consequently, the P_aCO_2 continues to rise. The CO_2 diffuses into the CSF, where the pH will fall. This stimulates the central receptors to increase ventilation but the patient may not be able to increase ventilation. Thus weaning is difficult until the patient's normal bicarbonate and P_aCO_2 levels are reestablished and the pH level returns to the patient's normal value (Case Study 17-3).

Case Study 17-3

Appropriate Ventilator Changes

A 60-kg female patient has been maintained on mechanical ventilation for 7 days. The patient's normal baseline ABG values on room air are pH of 7.38, P_aCO_2 of 51 mm Hg, P_aO_2 of 58 mm Hg, and HCO_3^- of 29 mEq/L. Current ABGs on volume-controlled intermittent mandatory ventilation (VC-IMV) at a mandatory rate of 8 breaths/min, V_T of 600 mL, and F_IO_2 of 0.25 at a pH of 7.41, P_aCO_2 of 40 mm Hg, P_aO_2 of 67 mm Hg, and HCO_3^- of 24 mEq/L. The patient is not breathing spontaneously. The VC-IMV mandatory rate is reduced to 4 breaths/min. The patient's spontaneous rate increases to 28 breaths/min, with a spontaneous V_T of 250 mL; S_pO_2 drops from 95% to 91%. The patient appears anxious. What could be the source of this patient's problem?

Metabolic Acid–Base Imbalances and Mechanical Ventilation

When a patient receives adequate alveolar ventilation, P_aCO_2 and pH levels can be expected to be near that patient's normal (i.e., eucapnic breathing). If the P_aCO_2 is near the patient's normal but the pH is not, the cause is probably a metabolic abnormality that should be corrected. Severe metabolic acidosis may require the

TABLE 17-1	Blood Chemistry in Metabolic Acidosis and Alkalosis				
	Serum Sodium	Serum Chloride	Serum Potassium	Arterial Blood pH	P_aCO_2
Alkalosis	→ or ↓	↓	→ or ↓	↑	→ or ↑
Acidosis	→ or ↑	↑	→ or ↑	↓	↓

↑, Increase; ↓, decrease; →, no change.
Normal values: sodium, 135-145 mEq/L; chloride, 98-106 mEq/L; potassium, 3.5-5.0 mEq/L; pH, 7.35-7.45; P_aCO_2, 35-45 mm Hg.

administration of bicarbonate, although its use is controversial. Intravenous administration of bicarbonate is indicated in the presence of life-threatening hyperkalemia either caused by or associated with metabolic acidosis.[56] It is also indicated in cases of salicylate toxicity.[56] When administered, bicarbonate is given slowly and not by bolus. An estimate of the bicarbonate replacement required can be determined by multiplying one third of the patient's body weight in kilograms times the base excess (BE). Generally, only one half of the deficit should be corrected initially (this allows for the patient's compensatory mechanisms to contribute to the correction), so the product is divided by two:

$$HCO_3^- \text{ required} = \frac{(1/3 \text{ kg} \times BE)}{2}$$

If a patient is not being ventilated or cannot increase spontaneous ventilation, the additional bicarbonate will combine with plasma hydrogen ions and increase CO_2 production. If the CO_2 is retained, the acidosis may increase.

Metabolic alkalosis is most often associated with loss of acid from the gastrointestinal tract (e.g., vomiting) or through the kidneys (e.g., diuretic administration). It may also result from excess base that is gained either by oral or parenteral bicarbonate administration, or by administration of lactate, acetate, or citrate. Normally the body will correct a mild to moderate metabolic alkalosis if the cause is removed. On the other hand, if the alkalosis is severe, prompt action is necessary. Administration of carbonic anhydrase inhibitors, acid infusion (ammonium chloride or potassium chloride), or low-sodium dialysis may be necessary.[57] Table 17-1 provides a summary of abnormalities in blood chemistry that are associated with metabolic acidosis and alkalosis.

AIR TRAPPING (AUTO-PEEP)

When airway resistance is increased in spontaneously breathing individuals, both inspiratory and expiratory flows are impeded. Severe airflow obstruction increases the time needed for exhalation. This can occur in patients with severe chronic obstructive pulmonary disease (COPD), status asthmaticus, or similar problems. The loss of structural quality of the conductive airways results in small or medium airways closing off or collapsing during exhalation, increasing FRC. Increased airway resistance reduces the patient's ability to exhale in a normal amount of time (increased time constants).[58]

When air trapping occurs, particularly with PPV, the increased alveolar pressure is transmitted to the intrapleural space creating an undesired PEEP effect. This reduces venous return and cardiac output. Artificially high intravascular pressures result, such as an

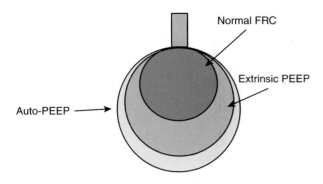

Fig. 17-8 Alveolar filling. The *smallest circle* represents resting FRC under normal conditions. The *second circle* represents the addition of extrinsic PEEP. The *largest circle* shows the resting lung volume with auto-PEEP also present.

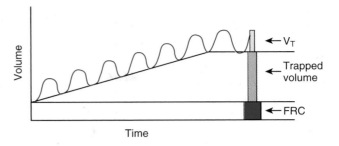

Fig. 17-9 Volume of trapped air above the FRC as a result of auto-PEEP. The gradual rise in volume shows the progressive trapping of air in the lungs. (Redrawn from Tuxen DV: Am Rev Respir Dis 140:5, 1989.)

increase in pulmonary artery occlusion pressure, which normally reflects left heart function.[58] When this occurs during PPV, it is commonly referred to as *auto-PEEP.*

Auto-PEEP is defined as an unintentional PEEP that occurs during mechanical ventilation when a new inspiratory breath begins before expiratory flow has ended. It is an insidious complication that may not be apparent unless the practitioner is looking for it. Auto-PEEP differs from operator-set PEEP (applied or extrinsic PEEP [$PEEP_E$]), which is a selected value at the end of expiration. Total PEEP is the sum of auto-PEEP and $PEEP_E$ and is a measure of the total pressure in the lungs at end exhalation (Fig. 17-8). Auto-PEEP is also referred to as *occult PEEP, inadvertent PEEP, breath stacking,* and *intrinsic PEEP.*

Because air trapping is not typically measured or detectable, its occurrence is an even greater threat. When air trapping occurs in spontaneously breathing, intubated patients, the inspiratory WOB increases, making it more difficult for them to inhale. Auto-PEEP can lead to barotrauma by trapping large volumes of air in the lung at the end of exhalation.[59,60] Alveolar overinflation can be life threatening in patients with acute, severe asthma that are receiving ventilatory support. The risk of tension pneumothorax and circulatory depression is increased in this group of patients.

How Auto-PEEP Occurs

An expiratory time (T_E) of at least three to four time constants is required for the lungs to empty 98% of the inspired volume. When T_E is decreased, complete emptying of the lungs to their normal resting lung volume (FRC) is prevented. For example, suppose T_E is shortened on a ventilated patient so that exhalation is incomplete. For a few breaths, pressure builds and exhaled volume is lower than delivered volume. As a progressively higher FRC is produced, tissue recoil increases so the force (pressure) pushing air out of the lungs increases. This higher pressure helps splint the airways open (diameter increases). The airway resistance to exhaled flow decreases. Within a few breaths the lung volumes stabilize at an elevated FRC. At this point the ventilator V_T delivered can also be exhaled (Fig. 17-9).[58] The result, however, is a higher FRC than normal and higher alveolar pressures at end expiration (auto-PEEP without lung distention).

Physiological Factors That Lead to Auto-PEEP

Auto-PEEP occurs in the following three distinct forms:
1. Auto-PEEP can occur because the expiratory muscles are actively contracting during exhalation. This raises alveolar pressures at end exhalation without increasing the volume at end exhalation (auto-PEEP without lung distention).
2. Auto-PEEP can occur in patients who do **not** have airway obstruction. In patients with normal airway resistance, air trapping can occur with the presence of high minute ventilation, short expiratory times, and mechanical devices that increase expiratory resistance (e.g., small endotracheal tubes [ETs], high-resistance expiratory valves, and certain PEEP devices). Total expiratory resistance across the lungs, ET, and exhalation line and valve is normally less than 4 cm H_2O/L/sec.
3. Auto-PEEP also occurs in patients with airflow obstruction who tend to have airway collapse during exhalation and flow limitation during normal tidal breathing. In these individuals, an increased expiratory effort only increases the alveolar pressure and does not improve expiratory flow.

The last two result in dynamic **hyperinflation,** or the failure of lung volume to return to passive FRC during exhalation by the time inspiration again begins. The level of auto-PEEP cannot be accurately predicted. The following factors increase the risk of auto-PEEP:[58,61-66]

- Chronic obstructive airway disease
- High minute ventilation (more than 10 to 20 L/min) in ventilated patients
- Age greater than 60 years
- Increased airway resistance (e.g., small ET size, bronchospasm, increased secretions, mucosal edema)
- Increased lung compliance (longer time constants)
- High respiratory frequency
- High inspiratory to expiratory ratios, that is short T_E (e.g., 1:1 and 2:1); low inspiratory flow
- Increased V_T, particularly with airflow obstruction

Identifying and Measuring Auto-PEEP

As discussed in Chapter 9, the easiest way to detect air trapping is to evaluate the flow–time curve on the ventilator's graphic display. If the expiratory flow does not return to zero before the next inspiration begins, auto-PEEP is present (Fig. 17-10).[67] Air trapping can also be detected by using flow–volume loops.

Air trapping can be identified during volume ventilation by observing changes in pressure and volume. Peak and plateau pressures will increase, and a transient reduction in exhaled volumes will occur. Physical examination reveals a reduction in breath sounds and an increase in resonance on percussion of the chest wall. Chest radiographs may show increased radiolucency.

The amount of auto-PEEP present in the patient's lungs at end exhalation is normally not registered on the ventilator manometer.

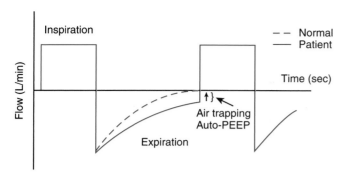

Fig. 17-10 Flow–time waveform showing a normal expiratory flow pattern during exhalation *(dotted line)* compared with a patient with air trapping (auto-PEEP) where flow does not return to zero during exhalation *(solid line)*. *PEEP,* Positive end-expiratory pressure. (From Dhand R: Ventilator graphics and respiratory mechanics in the patient with obstructive lung disease Respir Care [conference proceedings] 50:246-261, 2005.)

During exhalation, the expiratory valve is usually open to atmosphere, assuming no extrinsic PEEP is being used (Fig. 17-11). Pressure in the circuit is zero because the manometer measures atmospheric pressure, but air may still be actively flowing out of the patient's lungs. When inspiration triggers, some of this volume remains in the patient's lungs. This adds to normal FRC. However, this pressure remains undetected.

Many ICU ventilators have end-expiratory pause buttons for measuring auto-PEEP (see Chapter 8). There has been some debate regarding the accuracy of this method of measuring auto-PEEP.[68,69] This technique can provide a reference for the presence of auto-PEEP.

Another method for measuring auto-PEEP uses a Braschi valve (Fig. 17-12). The Braschi valve, which is a T-piece or Briggs adapter, is positioned inline on the inspiratory side of the patient circuit. A manometer is placed near the patient to measure airway pressure. Part of the T-piece has an opening that is normally capped, but is uncapped during auto-PEEP measurement. A one-way valve is another part of the T-piece and allows flow to go from the ventilator to the patient during normal ventilation.

To measure auto-PEEP, the cap is removed during exhalation. When the next breath begins, inspiratory flow from the ventilator is diverted out the uncapped hole and to the room. The expiratory valve is closed during inspiration (normal function of the ventilator during inspiration). The patient continues to exhale, but the expiratory valve is closed. As a result, the pressure equilibrates between the patient's lungs and the ventilator circuit. The pressure can then be read on the manometer. This procedure may be more accurate than occluding the exhalation valve because pressure is measured closer to the patient. One disadvantage is that the measurement is only made during the length of inspiration. If the pressure does not have enough time to equilibrate, the pressure reading may be underestimated.

Detecting auto-PEEP by measuring end-expiratory pressure requires a quiet, relaxed patient on controlled ventilation. The patient cannot be assisting or breathing spontaneously because an actively breathing patient may forcibly inhale or exhale during measurement and alter the results. Whether the patient should be sedated or paralyzed to measure auto-PEEP depends on the patient's pulmonary pathophysiology and the physician's

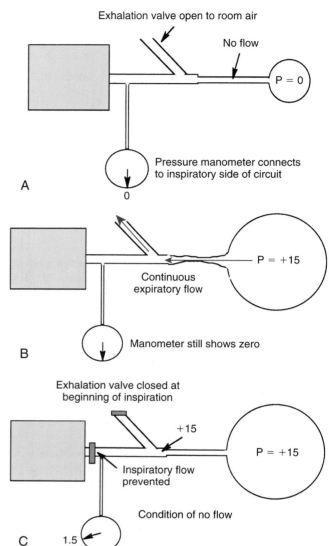

Fig. 17-11 A mechanical ventilator connected to a lung under normal conditions and also when auto-PEEP is present. **A,** Ventilator system during normal exhalation, with no air trapping and no auto-PEEP. The manometer reading is zero. **B,** During exhalation with auto-PEEP present, the manometer still reads zero (ambient) because the exhalation valve is open to room air. **C,** When the exhalation valve is closed and inspiratory flow stopped at end exhalation and before the next breath, a manometer will be able to read the approximate auto-PEEP level in the lungs and circuit. *PEEP,* Positive end-expiratory pressure. (Redrawn from Pepe PE, Marini JJ: Am Rev Respir Dis 126:166, 1982.)

assessment of the patient's condition. In addition, there should be no circuit leaks when making the auto-PEEP measurement.

Effect on Ventilator Function

The presence of auto-PEEP will actually slow the beginning of gas flow during inspiration. If alveolar pressure is higher than ambient at the end of exhalation (auto-PEEP), flow delivery will not start until mouth pressure exceeds this value.[70] The presence of auto-PEEP will also make it more difficult for spontaneously breathing patients to trigger a ventilator breath even when sensitivity settings are appropriate (Case Study 17-4). (See Chapter 7 for a detailed

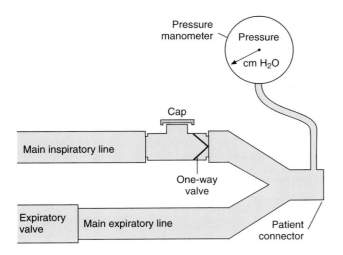

Fig. 17-12 Braschi valve used to measure auto-PEEP. (See text for explanation.)

BOX **17-6**	Pulmonary Changes Associated with Oxygen Toxicity

Decrease in the Following
- Tracheal mucus flow
- Macrophage activity
- Vital capacity
- Surfactant production
- Compliance
- Diffusing capacity
- Pulmonary capillary blood volume

Other Changes
- Capillary injury
- Platelet aggregation in the pulmonary vasculature
- Endothelial cell damage and accompanying increased lung water
- Progressive formation of absorption atelectasis
- Increased $P_{(A-a)}O_2$

discussion of how to adjust ventilator settings to minimize the effects of auto-PEEP).

 Case Study 17-4

Difficulty Triggering in a Patient with COPD

A patient with COPD is receiving volume-controlled continuous mandatory ventilation (VC-CMV) mode. The set tidal volume is increased from 500 to 700 mL, and the rate is increased from 10 to 18 breaths/min. The respiratory therapist notices a progressive rise in peak pressures; tidal volumes transiently are less than 650 mL after the change. Eventually the exhaled tidal volume reads 650 mL. Baseline pressure remains at zero. The patient appears unable to trigger a breath and is using accessory muscles to trigger the breath. What is the most likely cause of this problem?

Measuring Static Compliance with Auto-PEEP

Static compliance values are normally calculated as $V_T/(P_{plateau} - PEEP)$. For this calculation to be accurate, the PEEP value must include the set (applied) PEEP and any auto-PEEP present.[71]

Methods of Reducing Auto-PEEP

To reduce auto-PEEP, higher inspiratory gas flows should be used to shorten inspiratory time and allow a longer time for exhalation (T_E). Longer T_E can also be accomplished by using smaller tidal volumes and decreased respiratory rates. Use of low-resistance exhalation valves, changing partially obstructed expiratory filters, and using large ETs may also reduce air trapping.

Sometimes severe airway obstruction or high minute ventilation demands make reduction of auto-PEEP impossible. Some clinicians recommend hypoventilation (permissive hypercapnia) under these circumstances (see Chapter 12). This may actually be preferable to the complications that occur with auto-PEEP. Another alternative is to use methods of ventilation that allow as much spontaneous ventilation to occur as the patient can tolerate. Synchronized intermittent mandatory ventilation, pressure support, continuous positive airway pressure, and airway pressure release ventilation may be beneficial in these situations.

HAZARDS OF OXYGEN THERAPY WITH MECHANICAL VENTILATION

Oxygen Toxicity and the Lower Limits of Hypoxemia

It is generally agreed that breathing enriched oxygen mixtures for an extended period increases the risk of pulmonary complications. Indeed, adult subjects breathing a gas mixture containing an F_IO_2 of more than 0.6 for prolonged periods (>48 hours), or maintaining a P_aO_2 of more than 80 mm Hg in a newborn or premature infant, can lead to pulmonary oxygen toxicity.[24] Adults can generally breathe an F_IO_2 of up to 0.5 for extended periods without significant lung damage.[72,73]

The use of 100% oxygen can induce pulmonary changes in human beings in as little as 6 hours. Pulmonary changes associated with high oxygen concentrations are listed in Box 17-6.[24,74,75] Exposures for more than 72 hours can result in the development of a pattern that is similar to ARDS.[75] However, resistance to oxygen toxicity varies. In fact, studies suggest normal lung tissues may be more susceptible to oxygen damage than diseased tissue.[74]

The chest radiographs of most patients with acute respiratory failure are abnormal because of their underlying lung pathology. As a result, assessment of the onset of oxygen toxicity is often difficult. If an F_IO_2 of greater than 0.6 is required, then other techniques such as PEEP should be instituted (see Chapter 13). The improvement in oxygenation that occurs when PEEP is initiated often allows the F_IO_2 to be reduced. Prone positioning may also be of value (see Chapter 12).

The lower limits of permissive hypoxemia remain controversial. In general, most clinicians agree that a target P_aO_2 of 60 mm Hg and an S_pO_2 of 90% are acceptable lower limits.[74,76,77]

Absorption Atelectasis

High oxygen concentrations (>70% oxygen) lead to rapid absorption atelectasis, particularly in hypoventilated lung units.[77-80] In one study, 40% oxygen or 100% oxygen was administered after a recruitment maneuver had been performed on patients undergoing general anesthesia. In lungs ventilated with 40% oxygen, lung expansion was sustained. In patients ventilated with 100% oxygen, lung collapse reappeared within minutes.[79] Furthermore, absorption atelectasis has been shown to increase the level of intrapulmonary shunting. In mechanically ventilated patients, this is always a concern when ventilating patients with low tidal volumes.

Depression of Ventilation

In patients with chronic CO_2 retention (e.g., COPD), breathing high oxygen levels can increase P_aCO_2. This is partly caused by the Haldane effect, which increases the unloading of CO_2 from the hemoglobin. It is also caused by an improvement in blood flow to lung units that are not well ventilated. As increased oxygen reduces pulmonary vasoconstriction to these units, CO_2 may increase. Less likely but still possible is a suppression of the hypoxic drive to breathe. However, in mechanically ventilated COPD patients, this should not be a problem if adequate alveolar ventilation is maintained.

INCREASED WORK OF BREATHING

Increased work of breathing (WOB) is another common complication associated with artificial airways and mechanical ventilation systems. Fatigue can result from increased WOB, which can be both intrinsic and extrinsic.[81-86]

System-Imposed Work of Breathing

Until intermittent mandatory ventilation (IMV) became a popular mode of ventilation in the 1970s, WOB was not a major concern for clinicians. Most clinicians assumed that the ventilator performed most, if not all, of the WOB when a patient was receiving continuous mandatory ventilation (CMV). It is now recognized that WOB during VC-IMV can be greater than that required for other modes.[84,87]

During VC-IMV with PSV, when the patient's effort is reduced (e.g., sedation, sleep, high level of assist), the time interval between the onset of the patient's effort and the final ventilator triggering of inspiration increases. In addition, as the mandatory rate is reduced, the patient's inspiratory effort and respiratory rate increase to avoid a decrease in $\dot{V}_E$. The resulting increased drive to breathe during a spontaneous pressure support breath has been found to carry over into the mandatory breath.[86] Thus these patients have patient-ventilator difficulty altering their respiratory effort between breaths that are supported and those that are unsupported.[82,85,88]

Work of Breathing During Weaning

When a patient is being weaned from mechanical ventilation, the amount of work that the patient must perform increases. With a reduction of ventilatory support, the patient's WOB required to move gas through the ventilator circuit and the ET can become too high. A high spontaneous respiratory rate and use of accessory muscles typically indicate increased WOB and may also suggest the presence of auto-PEEP. Patients will also typically report feelings of dyspnea when questioned.[89,90]

When WOB is high (greater than 1.5 J/L or 15 J/L/min), fatigue is more likely to occur (Key Point 17-3). Weaning can be difficult in this circumstance, if not impossible.[89]

> **Key Point 17-3** Normal inspiratory WOB is approximately 0.5 J/L (0.05 kg-m/L).

BOX 17-7	Work of Breathing Performed by the Ventilator

Normal inspiratory WOB is approximately 0.5 J/L (0.05 kg-m/L).

The following equation provides an estimated value for the WOB provided by the ventilator during constant flow, passive inflation of the lungs:

Work = $(PIP - 0.5 \times P_{plateau})/100 \times V_T$ (L)

For example, if PIP is 30 cm H_2O, $P_{plateau}$ is 25 cm H_2O, and V_T is 500 mL (0.5 L),

Work = $[30 - (0.5 \times 25)]/100 \times 0.5 = 0.088$ kg-m

WOB can be reported in either kg-m or J/L.

(From Hess DR, Kacmarek RM: Essentials of mechanical ventilation, New York, 2002, McGraw-Hill.)

Methods to reduce WOB should be pursued in these situations. Imposed WOB can be almost eliminated or even reduced with elimination of auto-PEEP, and the use of low levels of PSV (approximately 10 cm H_2O) or PSV with continuous positive airway pressure.[85] See Chapter 20 for a detailed discussion of ventilator weaning and discontinuation.

Measuring Work of Breathing

Chapter 10 reviewed various methods for evaluating WOB in mechanically ventilated patients. As previously discussed, measurements of WOB can be difficult to obtain. Measuring esophageal pressure, airway pressure, and flow provides a way of estimating the amount of work done by the ventilator and the patient; but esophageal monitoring is rarely performed in a ventilated patient. Most ICU ventilators can calculate and display estimates of WOB. The ability to measure the diaphragm's electrical activity is now available for use in the clinical setting. This tool may provide new insight into the evaluation and measurement of WOB (see Chapter 23). The WOB performed by the ventilator is reviewed in Box 17-7.[89]

Steps to Reduce Work of Breathing During Mechanical Ventilation[86,91]

This section focuses on reducing the WOB by evaluation of the following:

- Reducing work imposed by the artificial airway
- Setting appropriate machine sensitivity, especially in the presence of auto-PEEP
- Ensuring patient-ventilator synchrony and reducing minute ventilation demands

Reducing Work Imposed by the Artificial Airway

One of the simplest approaches to reducing the WOB is to use the largest possible ET that is appropriate for a patient. Long and narrow tubes significantly increase resistance, especially when $\dot{V}_E$ is increased. The ET must be kept free of secretions, kinks, and other types of constrictions. Tracheostomy tubes will have a lower WOB because of their shorter length. The use of PSV and PEEP can also offset the work imposed by the tube. Automatic tube compensation (ATC) has also been shown to reduce the WOB through the ET (see Chapter 20 for a discussion on ATC). In pediatric patients, ETs have a smaller diameter (3 to 5.5 mm), so resistance is a greater concern, even though these tubes are shorter and

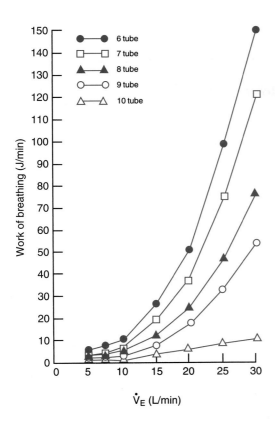

Fig. 17-13 Relations among the size of the endotracheal tube, minute ventilation, and work of breathing. When minute ventilation exceeds 10 L/min, the difference of the WOB through the different-sized tubes is most pronounced. (From Shapiro M, Wilson RK, Casar G, et al: Work of breathing through different sized endotracheal tubes, Crit Care Med 14:1028-1031, 1986.)

the inspired and expired gas flows are lower.[91-94] (The role of ATC may be more important in this population.)

The imposed WOB through an ET in an adult patient is determined by the size of the tube and the minute ventilation of the patient (Fig. 17-13).[92] When large tubes are in place and minute ventilation is low, the imposed work is probably not significant. As shown in Fig. 17-13, unless the minute ventilation is greater than 10 L/min, the work associated with moving gas through the tube is consistent throughout the average range of adult tube sizes. The use of pressure support in ranges of 3 to 20 cm H_2O has been found to reduce the WOB associated with the ventilator and ET.[93,94]

Prolonged spontaneous breathing through an ET is not desired because of the resistance of the tube. However, for short intervals before extubation and to assess extubation readiness (spontaneous breathing trial), the patient can breathe through the ET.[95] In fact, when the WOB was compared during spontaneous breathing before extubation and after the tube was removed, the WOB was similar.[96]

Perhaps more important than a specific value for the work being performed is the effort by the patient. For a similar amount of work, a young, otherwise healthy adult has an easier time maintaining the work than does a chronically ill, older patient. The effort by the older patient will be far greater (higher percent of oxygen cost) than the effort of the young adult, even if the work is the same.

Setting Machine Sensitivity and Inspiratory Flow

Another factor that must be considered when attempting to reduce WOB is to ensure that machine sensitivity is set appropriately. The ventilator must be at its most sensitive level without leading to autotriggering of breaths. It is important to remember that if the ventilator trigger is too sensitive, it will autotrigger. Autotriggering can also be caused by "noise" in the patient circuit, water in the circuit, leaks (e.g., circuit leaks, cuff leaks, chest tube leaks), and cardiac oscillations.[88,97]

Inspiratory gas flow must be adequate to match patient demand. Flows of 60 to 100 L/min are usually adequate. The patient and ventilator should be synchronized. This will depend on flow and sensitivity and possibly the flow pattern and mode. PSV may also be beneficial in reducing WOB if the patient has an intact respiratory center.

Patient-Ventilator Synchrony

Synchronous ventilation occurs when the ventilator responds appropriately to a patient's inspiratory effort and delivers the amount of flow and volume requested by the patient. **Asynchrony** occurs when the patient's inspiratory efforts and flow demands are not accommodated by the ventilator.[88,97] Asynchrony can therefore be very uncomfortable for the patient because WOB increases and the oxygen cost of breathing (effort) is increased. In its most obvious form, the patient appears to be "fighting the ventilator" and displaying noticeable inspiratory efforts and use of accessory muscles. Asynchrony may also be accompanied by tachypnea, chest wall retractions, and sometimes **chest-abdominal paradox.** In some cases, patient-ventilator asynchrony can be subtle and easily overlooked by most clinicians.

Asynchrony is generally identified as follows:

- Trigger asynchrony
- Flow asynchrony
- Cycle asynchrony
- Mode asynchrony
- PEEP asynchrony
- Closed-loop ventilation asynchrony

Trigger asynchrony. Trigger asynchrony occurs when the ventilator sensitivity setting is not appropriate for the patient. With this type of asynchrony, the ventilator does not sense the patient's inspiratory effort and fails to deliver gas flow. A trigger that is too insensitive requires the patient to make a strong, spontaneous effort to achieve gas flow from the ventilator. If pressure triggering is being used, a change to flow triggering may help because flow triggering generally reduces inspiratory WOB. Flow triggering does not require the exhalation valve to close before initiating gas flow, which gives it a faster response time (in general) compared with pressure triggering.[97,98] Recent advances in pressure transducer technology have resulted in ventilators in which either pressure or flow triggering perform comparably.[88]

Another type of pressure triggering, called a "shadow" trigger, is available on Respironic BiPAP ventilators. Shadow triggering may alleviate the problem because it can be quite sensitive to patient efforts. Shadow triggering uses a mathematical model derived from the flow and pressure signals to produce a shadow of the patient's signals (shape signal) (See Fig. 17-14). Although initial studies of shadow triggering were shown to reduce the patient effort required to trigger a breath, its use may also increase the number of autotriggered breaths. Consequently further studies are needed to determine the effectiveness of shadow triggering.[97] (A

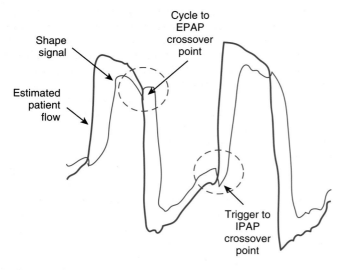

Fig. 17-14 The patient's actual flow waveform *(thick line)* compared with the shadow trigger or shape signal *(thin line)*. A shape signal is produced by offsetting the actual patient's flow signal by 15 L/min and a delay time of 300 msec. This causes the shape signal to be behind the patient's flow. A sudden change in the patient flow (downward movement) crosses the shape signal. Crossover detection begins the inspiratory phase *(right crossover point,* IPAP). The crossover detection also causes the ventilator to end inspiration and cycle to expiration *(left crossover point,* cycle to EPAP). *EPAP,* Expiratory positive airway pressure; *IPAP,* inspiratory positive airway pressure. (Used with permission of Respironics, Inc, Murrysville, Pa.)

more recent form of triggering relies on a neural signal from the diaphragm. It is used with neurally adjusted ventilatory assist [NAVA] mode, described in Chapter 23.)

The presence of auto-PEEP can also make triggering the ventilator more difficult for the patient and result in missed patient triggers. When auto-PEEP is present, the patient's effort may not be transmitted to the sensing mechanism and the ventilator does not provide inspiratory gas flow. Because auto-PEEP is a dynamic condition, it can be present in one breath and absent the next. In fact, in patients normally not suspected of having auto-PEEP, it is probably one of the major contributors to trigger asynchrony, resulting in patient discomfort and increase in the oxygen cost of breathing.[88]

Patients with COPD have a high incidence of auto-PEEP, with trigger asynchrony as a result.[88] Trigger asynchrony in this patient group can be identified by the flow and pressure scalars (Fig. 17-15). In the flow waveform, an ineffective patient effort can be detected during inspiration by an increase in flow on the flow–time curve. During the expiratory phase, ineffective efforts can be detected if an abrupt rise (convex appearance) appears on the flow curve (it appears as a change in expiratory flow).[88] When air trapping is present that cannot be eliminated by normal techniques in patients with COPD, setting low levels of PEEP can make it easier to trigger the ventilator. Applied PEEP set at a level that is less than the auto-PEEP present may therefore reduce the metabolic work of the diaphragm (see Chapter 7).[99,100] However, extrinsic PEEP may not be effective if the minute ventilation is high and not enough time for exhalation is available.

A slight, inherent delay always occurs in the ventilator's response to the patient's effort. Part of this is caused by the delay in the

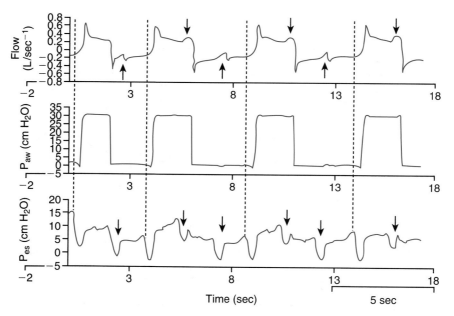

Fig. 17-15 Flow, air pressure (P$_{aw}$) and esophageal pressure (P$_{es}$) in a patient with chronic obstructive pulmonary disease during pressure support ventilation. *Dotted lines* indicate the beginning of an inspiratory effort that triggers ventilator gas flow. *Black arrows* in the P$_{es}$ curve indicate patient efforts that did not trigger ventilatory flow. Note the time delay between the beginning of the effort and ventilator triggering. Ineffective efforts occur during both mechanical inspiration and expiration. During inspiration, the *flow curves* identify ineffective patient efforts and a rise in the inspiratory flow. During expiration, ineffective efforts are identified by *open arrows* showing a small convex shape in the flow curve. Note how no apparent change occurs in P$_{aw}$. (From Kondili E, Prinianakis G, Georgopoulos D: New concepts in respiratory function, Br J Anaesthesiol 91:106-119, 2003.)

patient's spontaneous effort and change in pleural and mouth pressures reaching the ventilator's sensing device. It may also be caused by the time required for the ventilator to respond to the detected signal. Current generation ventilators are much more responsive than older models. Some researchers are exploring the use of monitors that detect contraction of the diaphragm to signal the ventilator. Others are looking at the use of pleural pressure changes to trigger the ventilator. In the future, these may provide quite accurate sensing mechanisms (see Chapter 23).

Flow asynchrony. Flow asynchrony occurs when the patient's flow demand is not met by the ventilator. The type of mode being used often determines how much flow is available. Volume control ventilation with a fixed flow, volume control ventilation with a variable flow, and pressure control ventilation and pressure support ventilation differ from each other.

During volume control ventilation, if flow is constant, the set flow may not match patient demand. This is a fairly common problem.[88] An initial flow of 80 L/min is typically suggested. In this situation the best way to determine if adequate flow is being provided is to evaluate the pressure–time scalar. When the pressure curve appearance changes from breath to breath, the patient is actively breathing. A concave appearance on the inspiratory pressure curve during volume control ventilation indicates active inspiration (Fig. 17-16).[101] (NOTE: Earlier generation ventilators, such as the Puritan Bennett 7200, had fixed flow. In other words, the set flow was the amount the patient received regardless of patient effort. Inadequate flow in this situation could be corrected

by increasing the flow or changing the flow pattern. For example, a descending flow pattern during volume control ventilation may reduce patient WOB as long as the set flow is adequate.)[87]

If the flow varies with patient effort, as occurs with current ICU ventilators (e.g., Servo-i and the CareFusion AVEA), the pressure–time curve will show a slight drop in pressure during inspiration and the flow–time curve will show an increase in flow to accommodate the patient's effort. Thus patient-ventilator synchrony is improved by having the ventilator respond to the patient's demands. This is also true with NAVA, which is available on the Servo-i (see Chapter 23).

During pressure-targeted ventilation, such as PC-CMV and PSV, the ventilator rapidly provides a high flow to achieve and maintain the set pressure. As long as the set pressure is adequate, flow to the patient will be adequate. On the other hand, flow at the beginning of inspiration during pressure-targeted ventilation may be excessive for the patient. A lower rise time or slope may be beneficial in this type of patient (Fig. 17-17).[102]

In general when pressure and rise time are set correctly, pressure-targeted breaths may be more synchronous for patients with high flow demands. If the cause of the high ventilatory demand is a result of anxiety or pain, the patient's condition can be improved by using sedatives such as benzodiazepines or narcotics (see Chapter 14).

Cycle asynchrony. Cycle asynchrony, also called *termination asynchrony,* usually occurs when the patient starts to exhale before the ventilator has completed inspiration. The inspiratory time is

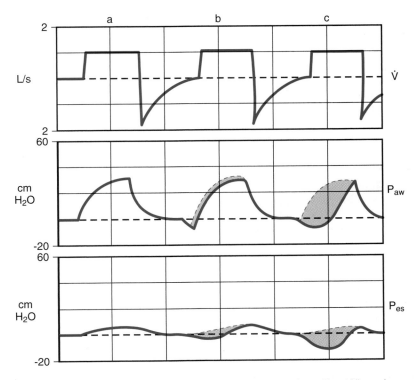

Fig. 17-16 The *upper panel* shows the flow–time curve for constant flow, volume ventilation. The *middle panel* represents the pressure–time curve measured at the upper airway. The *lower panel* is the pressure–time curve for esophageal pressures. Breath **a** is a control breath with no patient effort. Breath **b** is a patient-triggered breath with adequate flow. The *dotted line* mimics a passive breath as in **a**. Breath **c** is a patient-triggered breath with inadequate flow to meet patient demand *(solid line)*. The *shaded area* shows what a curve *(dotted line)* would look like with a control breath. (From MacIntyre NR, Branson RD: Mechanical ventilation, Philadelphia, 2001, W.B. Saunders, 2001.)

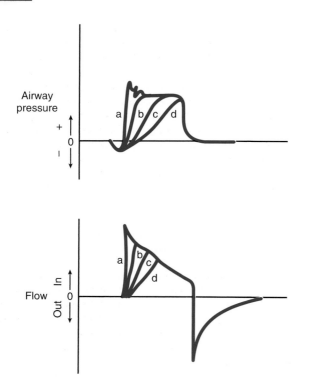

Fig. 17-17 *Upper panel* shows airway pressure over time and the *lower panel* shows flow over time. The *curves* illustrate the changing pressure and flow with different rise time settings. The fastest time *(a)* also has the fastest flow *(a)*. In general, synchrony is optimal when pressure waveform has a smooth square configuration *(curve b)*. Using too much slope may reduce flow and result in asynchrony *(curve d)*. (From MacIntyre NR, Branson RD: Mechanical ventilation, Philadelphia, WB Saunders, 2001.)

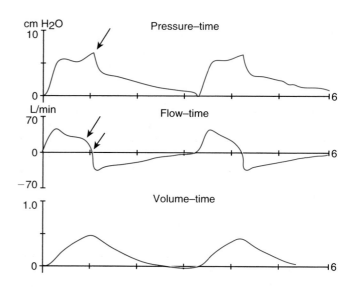

Fig. 17-18 Pressure, flow, and volume scalars illustrating a patient receiving 5 cm H_2O of pressure support. The patient's neural timing precedes the end of the mechanical inflation and results in a pressure spike *(large arrow)* on the pressure waveform. Note the rapid decline in the inspiratory flow waveform at the end of inspiration *(double arrows)* as a result of the patient's active exhalation. (From Nilsestuen JO, Hargett KD: Using ventilator graphics to identify patient-ventilatory asynchrony [conference proceedings], Respir Care 50:202-234, 2005.)

generally set by the practitioner by using an inspiratory time control or basing it on the rate, flow, and volume settings. Cycle asynchrony often occurs when T_I is too long. Increasing the flow in volume control ventilation to shorten T_I, or decreasing the set T_I time in volume control or pressure control may help.

When using older-generation ventilators, as a patient actively exhales during inspiration, such as with a cough, the airway pressure increases. If the pressure exceeds the set maximum, the breath ends and V_T delivery drops. This requires increased work by the patient. One of the strategies now used by ventilator manufacturers to overcome this problem is "floating" or "active" valves. This technology uses closed-loop or servo control of both the inspiratory and expiratory valves. In this system the pressure is maintained at a fairly constant level during inspiration. If the patient were to actively exhale or cough, the expiratory valve would open and keep the pressure at a more consistent level.[98] This improves patient-ventilator synchrony and may decrease the WOB.

Cycle asynchrony can occur with both mechanical (mandatory) and spontaneous breaths. During spontaneous ventilation with PSV, cycle asynchrony commonly occurs when the patient actively tries to exhale before the expiratory flow termination criteria have been met. This is especially common in patients with COPD (Fig. 17-18).[87,103] By changing the flow cycle percentage, this problem can be corrected.[102] However, in patients with COPD, a wide variability in V_T and auto-PEEP can occur.[98] Changes in breath pattern may frequently occur, making cycle asynchrony difficult to manage. Ventilator software programs that evaluate the patient's time constant and the slope at the end of the inspiratory portion of the

pressure–time curve for each breath may provide a way to make automatic adjustments of flow cycle on a breath-by-breath basis.[104]

Mode asynchrony. Mode asynchrony occurs when more than one breath type is delivered by the ventilator. One such mode is VC-IMV. The patient's respiratory center is not able to adjust to the varying breath types and asynchrony results along with increased WOB. When mode asynchrony occurs, the mode must be evaluated and consideration given to changing the mode to PC-CMV or PSV.

PEEP asynchrony. When PEEP levels are too low and atelectasis forms in the lungs, the ventilatory control centers of the brain affect the patient's comfort (dyspnea) and drive to breathe, resulting in PEEP asynchrony. Excessive PEEP may have a similar effect if overdistension of the lungs makes ventilation more difficult and reduces patient comfort.[104] Setting appropriate PEEP levels to avoid overdistension and using pressure support may help decrease the WOB.[105,106] Providing sedation also may be helpful (see Chapter 13 for additional information on setting PEEP).

Closed-loop ventilation asynchrony. Closed-loop ventilation asynchrony can occur in dual control modes of ventilation such as volume support (pressure support with a volume target) and pressure-regulated volume control (PRVC; pressure control with a volume target). Volume support (VS; Servo 300 and Servo-i, Maquet, Wayne, N.J.) and adaptive support ventilation (ASV on the Hamilton G5, Hamilton Medical, Bonaduz, Switzerland) are two examples of pressure support with a volume target. The clinician sets an upper pressure limit not to be exceeded and a target volume. The ventilator delivers pressure to achieve the set V_T (see Chapter 6). Two forms of asynchrony can occur, one that depends on the equipment used and the other that depends on the patient.

For example, with the Servo 300 using VS, if the patient's respiratory rate decreases, or if the ventilator does not detect all the patient's spontaneous efforts (missed triggers), the ventilator detects a decrease in rate and automatically increases the volume delivery up to 150% of the set value to maintain the set minute ventilation. This is a minute ventilation–based unit. However, a larger V_T may not be desirable. This will pose no danger to the patient as long as the high pressure limit has been appropriately set.

The Servo-i also has VS but it is not minute ventilation based. It targets the set V_T and does not make any increase in volume if a slower rate is detected. These two ventilator examples illustrate that ventilator manufacturers can design their device to respond differently to the same circumstance. Clinicians must be aware of the idiosyncrasies of the ventilator they are using.

Another form of asynchrony that can occur with either VS or PRVC has to do with the level of a patient's inspiratory effort. Suppose, for example, in volume support a patient initially receives a V_T of 400 mL with a pressure of 13 cm H_2O. Pulmonary edema then develops from a fluid overload. The patient's inspiratory demand increases to accommodate this decrease in compliance and oxygenation. The ventilator detects the high volume and interprets the high volume as an improvement in compliance or resistance and reduces the pressure. Active inspiration is detected as an improvement in compliance; that is, a large volume is being delivered at the current pressure setting. Consequently the ventilator will decrease the pressure to achieve the target volume. This occurs when the patient requires the most support and the ventilator provides the least.

The dual-control mode that provides pressure control with a target volume is assigned a variety of names. In the Dräger ventilator (Dräger Medical, Telford, Pa.) it is AutoFlow; in the Hamilton G5 it is adaptive pressure ventilation; in the Puritan Bennett 840 it is volume control plus; and in the Servo-i it is PRVC. In this assist/control mode, the practitioner sets a target volume and the ventilator adjusts pressure to achieve the set V_T.

Consider a leak occurring in the patient-ventilator system. If the ventilator compares volume output and volume returned, it may detect the difference, but cannot distinguish a leak from an improvement in lung characteristics (decreased airway resistance or increased compliance) or from an active inspiration. It may increase pressure to try and increase V_T because it detects a drop in V_T.

As described with VS, when PRVC or autoflow is used, active inspiration may be detected as an improvement in compliance. Again the response is a reduction in pressure because the ventilator perceives that the patient is getting a very large V_T for the current pressure. As illustrated with VS, the drop in pressure occurs when the patient may need it the most.

Other types of asynchrony. Other types of asynchrony can occur. The clinician must be alert to changes in the patient's physical characteristics, vital signs, and ventilator graphics to detect and help troubleshoot patient-ventilator asynchrony and avoid increases in the WOB.

Particular attention must be directed at evaluating for and reducing the presence of auto-PEEP. Additional adjustments in ventilator settings that might also improve patient-ventilator synchrony include sensitivity, flow, inspiratory time, mode, and PEEP.

Reducing Minute Ventilation Demands

Perhaps the single most important factor in reducing the WOB is minute ventilation. If $\dot{V}_E$ requirements can be reduced, the overall WOB will decrease. Specifically, this means reducing fever,

agitation, shivering, seizures, pain, and any other factors that can elevate metabolic rate. Careful attention to the patient's WOB and consideration of all possible methods to reduce this work can be beneficial to recovery.

Reducing the patient's airway resistance or improving compliance will also decrease ventilatory demand. Airway resistance can usually be reduced by suctioning the airway or by administering bronchodilators. Lung compliance can be improved using several strategies, including administering diuretics to reduce lung water, pleural drainage to eliminate pleural fluid or air, and placing the patient in a semi-Fowler position, to keep the diaphragm in a downward position, so that visceral organs do not impede diaphragmatic movement.

VENTILATOR MECHANICAL AND OPERATIONAL HAZARDS

Mechanical ventilators are extremely safe to use when monitored and maintained appropriately.[107] As with other types of life-support systems, patient complications can result and sometimes are caused by human error. Equipment malfunction can also occur. Examples of mechanical ventilator failures are listed in Box 17-8. Box 17-9 summarizes the findings from studies done on complications that occurred with mechanical ventilation.[107-110]

In February 2002, the Joint Commission issued a report on deaths or injuries related to long-term ventilation.[111] A total of nineteen injuries resulted in deaths, and four injuries resulted in coma. Sixty percent of these twenty-three reported cases were related to malfunction, misuse of, or inadequate alarm systems. In 52% of cases, the ventilator tubing was disconnected, and in 26% the artificial airway was dislodged. None of the reported injuries was related to ventilator malfunction.

The report cited that the root cause of these mishaps was related to staffing and communication breakdown. It is interesting to note that inadequate orientation and training of staff were found to be important contributing factors in these cases. Indeed, communication breakdown primarily occurred among staff members.[111]

One of the most common problems that occurs during mechanical ventilation involves ventilator disconnection. Box 17-10 summarizes common situations in which ventilator disconnection can occur, and Box 17-11 shows how these disconnections may go

---

BOX 17-8 **Potential Mechanical Failures with Mechanical Ventilation**

- Disconnection from the power source
- Failure of the power source
- Failure of the ventilator to function because of equipment manufacturing problems or improper maintenance
- Failure of alarms due to mechanical failure or failure of personnel to turn them on or use them properly
- Failure of heating or humidifying devices
- Failure of the pressure relief valve to open
- Disconnection of the patient Y-connector
- Leaks in the system, resulting in inadequate pressure or tidal volume delivery
- Failure of the expiratory valve to function, causing a large system leak or causing a closed system with no exit for exhaled air
- Inappropriate assembly of the patient circuit

BOX **17-9** **Complications Associated with Mechanical Ventilation**

Complications Attributed to Intubation, Extubation, or Tube Malfunction
- Prolonged intubation attempts
- Intubation of the right mainstem bronchus
- Premature extubation
- Self-extubation
- Problems associated with tube retaping
- Tube malfunction
- Nasal necrosis
- Sinusitis
- Tube plugging

Complications Attributed to the Operation of the Ventilator
- Mechanical failure
- Inadequate humidification
- Overheating of inspired air

Medical Complications Occurring with Mechanical Ventilation
- Alveolar hypoventilation
- Alveolar hyperventilation
- Massive gastric distention
- Atelectasis
- Pneumonia
- Hypotension
- Pneumothorax, pneumoperitoneum, subcutaneous air

BOX **17-10** **Reasons for Accidental Disconnections in the Patient Circuit**

1. Environmental changes affecting connector performance (e.g., with a heated humidifier, the tubing on the output side can soften and kink from the heat and disconnect/ reconnect use)
2. Weak connection at the endotracheal tube and the Y-connector so it is easy to disconnect for suctioning
3. Inadequate connection force
4. Points of easy disconnection: water traps, temperature probes, oxygen analyzers, humidification systems, capnographs; these act as circuit breakers
5. Incompatible components resulting from nonstandard dimensions, dissimilar materials, inappropriate materials, or reuse
6. High pressure within the circuit
7. Patient movement
8. Deliberate disconnection by patient

BOX **17-11** **Reasons Accidental Disconnections May Elude Detection**

1. Complacency resulting from reliance on alarms
2. Desensitization of the medical staff resulting from frequent false alarms
3. Inappropriate alarm settings
4. Inappropriate sensor location
5. Inadequate understanding of monitor/alarm function
6. Misinterpretation of alarms
7. Incompatible combination of monitors/alarms
8. Disabled alarms
9. Inaudible alarms
10. Malfunctioning alarms

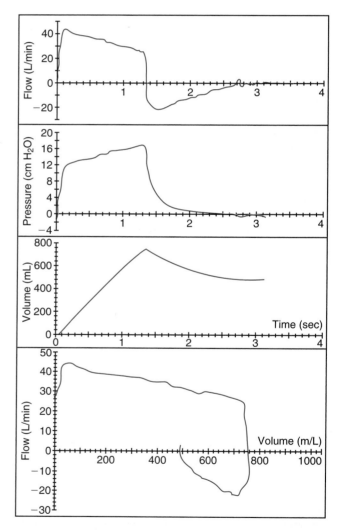

Fig. 17-19 Flow, pressure, and volume curves and a flow/volume loop. An air leak is identified when the expiratory volume waveform does not return to zero volume baseline and the flow–volume loop fails to close (i.e., the expiratory flow does not return to the zero baseline). (From Lucangelo U, Bernabe F, Blanch L: Respiratory mechanics derived from signals in the ventilator circuit [conference proceedings], Respir Care 50:55-65, 2005.)

undetected.[112] Another common problem involves leaks in the ventilator circuit. Figure 17-19 shows waveforms illustrating the presence of a leak.[113] Box 17-12 lists the potential problems associated with humidification systems.[114]

Although dependable equipment, good alarm systems, and sophisticated surveillance systems are beneficial, they cannot replace careful monitoring by trained personnel. By standardizing procedures, keeping records of ventilator maintenance, and familiarizing all essential members of the health care team with equipment function, human error can be kept to a minimum.

BOX 17-12   Hazards and Complications Associated with Use of Humidification Devices

Hazards Associated with Both Heated Humidifiers and Heat-Moisture Exchangers
- Hypothermia
- Hypoventilation and alveolar gas trapping caused by mucus plugging of airways
- Possible increased resistive work of breathing (WOB) caused by mucus plugging of airways
- Possible increased resistive WOB through the humidifier

Hazards Associated with Heated Humidifiers
- Potential for electrical shock
- Thermal injury to the airway from heated humidifiers; burns to the patient and tubing meltdown if heated wire circuits are covered, or circuits and humidifiers are incompatible
- Inadvertent overfilling, resulting in unintentional tracheal lavage
- The fact that when disconnected from the patient, some ventilators generate a high flow through the patient circuit

that may aerosolize contaminated condensate, putting both the patient and the clinician at risk for nosocomial infection
- Potential for burns to caregivers from hot metal
- Inadvertent tracheal lavage from pooled condensate in patient circuit
- Elevated airway pressures resulting from pooled condensation
- Patient-ventilator asynchrony and improper ventilator performance resulting from pooled condensation in the circuit

Hazards Associated with Heat-Moisture Exchangers
- Possible hypoventilation caused by increased dead space
- Underhydration and impaction of mucous secretions
- Ineffective low-pressure alarm during disconnection because of resistance through HME

(From American Association of Respiratory Care, Clinical Practice Guideline: Restrepo RD, Walsh BK: Humidification During Invasive and Noninvasive Mechanical Ventilation: 2012 *Respir Care* 57: 782-288, 2012.)

BOX 17-13   Endotracheal (ET) and Tracheostomy Tube Complications

ET Complications
Damage to the Nasal Passages, Lips, or Eyes
- During insertion: Facial trauma, damage to the nasal structures, lips, or eyes
- While in place: Lip ulceration, pressure necrosis to the soft tissues, erosion of nasal septum, increased airway resistance from a small lumen tube
- During and after extubation: Nasal stricture

Damage to the Oropharynx
- During insertion: Traumatic damage to the oropharyngeal soft tissues, dental accidents, retropharyngeal or hypopharyngeal perforation
- While in place: Grooving of the hard palate from chronic pressure, dental deformities from constant pressure

Damage to the Larynx and Trachea
- During insertion: Soft tissue damage (bleeding and swelling), laryngeal trauma, laryngospasm
- While in place: Laryngeal injury (ulceration, edema, bleeding), laryngeal muscle dysfunction, subglottic edema, necrosis over the arytenoid cartilages and the vocal cords, trauma to mucosa covering the cricoid cartilage in infants, necrosis of tissue leading to the innominate artery and uncontrolled bleeding, tracheal injury (ulceration, edema, bleeding, tracheomalacia, cartilage and mucosal necrosis),

laryngotracheal web formation, laryngotracheal granuloma, tracheal dilation, irritation of the carina, tracheoesophageal fistula, spontaneous dislocation of the tube (into the right mainstem, too high in trachea, extubation), squamous metaplasia of respiratory epithelium
- During and after extubation: Laryngospasm, laryngeal edema, glottic injury, laryngotracheal granuloma, laryngeal stenosis (glottic, subglottic), laryngeal motor dysfunction (vocal cord paralysis), cricoarytenoid ankylosis, tracheomalacia, tracheal dilation, tracheal stenosis, perichondritis, laryngeal chondritis, laryngotracheal web

Complications with Artificial Airways
- During intubation: Intubation of the right mainstem bronchus, bronchospasm, pulmonary aspiration, barotrauma, cardiopulmonary arrest, hypoxemia, cardiac arrhythmias, cervical and spinal cord injuries, patient discomfort
- While in place: Patient discomfort, difficulty in communicating, pain, retching, salivation, malnutrition, sinusitis, otitis media, atelectasis, pneumonia, pulmonary aspiration, decreased mucociliary transport, ineffective cough, contamination of the airway from silent aspiration during suctioning and invasion of the normal lung defenses, bronchial mucosal damage from suctioning

Continued

COMPLICATIONS OF THE ARTIFICIAL AIRWAY

Various problems can arise with the use of artificial airways. These include complications associated with the artificial airway itself, infectious contamination of the patient's airway, excessive heat to the airway from humidification systems, and inadequate or excessive humidification. In addition, an artificial airway alters the geometry

of the upper airway and anatomic dead space, changes resistance to gas flow, increases WOB, and can increase risk of obstruction.[114-116] Box 17-13 summarizes artificial airway complications.

Care must be used during the insertion, maintenance, and removal of artificial airways. High-volume/low-pressure cuffs of good quality used for as short a time as possible will reduce the incidence of complications.

BOX 17-13 **Endotracheal (ET) and Tracheostomy Tube Complications—cont'd**

- During and after extubation: Hoarseness, sore throat, dysphagia, bronchospasm, aspiration, cardiac arrest

Mechanical Problems with Tubes

Disconnection, kinking, obstruction from secretions, patient biting on the tube, displacement of the tube tip into the tracheal endothelial layer or against the side of the trachea or carina

Mechanical Problems Associated with the Cuff

Compression of the tube by the cuff, excessive pressure (>25 mm Hg) from overinflation leading to tracheal necrosis, leaking or rupturing of the cuff causing inadequate ventilation, laceration of the cuff during insertion, leaking around the cuff preventing adequate ventilation, damage to the pilot balloon or connection preventing cuff inflation

Complications Associated with Tracheostomy*

- During the surgical procedure: Bleeding, thyroid injury, inappropriate incision position (too high or too low), injury to the recurrent laryngeal nerve, pneumothorax, tracheoesophageal fistula, subcutaneous emphysema,

mediastinal emphysema, placement of the tube into the pretracheal space, cuff laceration during insertion, cardiac arrest, hypoxia
- While in place: Patient discomfort, infection of the wound or trachea, bleeding (skin vessel, tracheoarterial fistula), tracheal injury (inflammation, bleeding, ulceration, necrosis), tracheal dilation, web formation, perforation of trachea, granuloma formation, pseudomembrane formation, irritation of the carina, tracheoesophageal fistula, sepsis, mediastinitis, atelectasis, pneumonia, aspiration, subcutaneous emphysema, mediastinal emphysema, pneumothorax, decannulation, reduced mucociliary transport, ineffective cough, mechanical problems with the tube or cuff (see ET), squamous metaplasia of respiratory epithelium
- During and after decannulation: Tight stoma making decannulation difficult, patient discomfort, scarring, keloid formation, persistent open stoma, dysphagia, tracheal stenosis, tracheomalacia, tracheal granuloma, tracheal web formation, or tracheal dilation

*(See Chapter 21 for additional information on tracheostomy tubes.)

 SUMMARY

- As with other forms of medical treatment, there are risks and complications associated with mechanical ventilation.
- *Barotrauma* implies trauma that results from using high pressures. *Volutrauma* implies damage from high distending volumes.
- *Ventilator-associated lung injury (VALI)* is the term generally used when referring to lung injury occurring in humans that has been identified as a consequence of mechanical ventilation (e.g., ventilator-associated pneumonia, air trapping, patient-ventilator asynchrony, and extraalveolar gas [barotrauma] such as pneumothorax and pneumomediastinum).
- *Ventilator-induced lung injury (VILI)* is lung injury that occurs at the level of the acinus. It is the microscopic level of injury that includes biotrauma, shear stress, and surfactant depletion.
- Mechanical stress disrupts normal cell function, strains normal cell configuration, and can also lead to an inflammatory response and the release of injurious chemical mediators in the lungs.
- During controlled ventilation in which spontaneous ventilation is absent, alveolar collapse is most likely to occur in the dependent areas of the lung. Because these are the areas that receive the most blood flow, an increased mismatching of ventilation and perfusion and increased dead space ventilation occurs.
- Acute hypoventilation can occur in patients receiving ventilatory assistance if adequate alveolar ventilation is not provided. Hypoventilation will result in an increased P_aCO_2 and an

acidotic pH. Rapidly rising P_aCO_2 levels and falling pH values can lead to serious problems.
- Hyperventilation results in a lower than normal P_aCO_2 and a rise in pH. Patient-induced hyperventilation is often associated with hypoxemia, pain and anxiety syndromes, circulatory failure, and airway inflammation.
- Ventilator-induced hyperventilation is generally caused by inappropriate ventilator settings. Weaning becomes more difficult when a patient has experienced prolonged hyperventilation.
- A number of factors can increase the risk of auto-PEEP, including the presence of COPD, high minute ventilation, increased airway resistance, increased lung compliance, high respiratory frequency, inverse-ratio ventilation, and low inspiratory flow.
- The presence of auto-PEEP will also make it more difficult for spontaneously breathing patients to trigger a ventilator breath even when sensitivity settings are appropriate.
- It is generally agreed that breathing enriched-oxygen mixtures for an extended period can increase the risk of pulmonary complications.
- Patient-ventilator asynchrony occurs when the patient's inspiratory efforts and flow demands are not met by the ventilator. Asynchrony is generally identified as trigger asynchrony, flow asynchrony, cycle asynchrony, mode asynchrony, PEEP asynchrony, and closed-loop ventilation asynchrony.
- Various problems can arise with the use of artificial airways. These include complications associated with the artificial airway itself, infection of the patient's airway, excessive heat to the airway from humidification systems, and inadequate or excessive humidification.

REVIEW QUESTIONS (See Appendix A for answers.)

1. The peak pressure alarm is activated on a patient receiving mechanical ventilatory support. Peak pressures have increased from 25 to 50 cm H_2O in the last 30 minutes. While listening to a patient's breath sounds, the respiratory therapist notices absence of breath sounds over the entire right hemothorax. The patient is unconscious and nonresponsive. Which of the following actions would assist the respiratory therapist in determining the cause of the problem?
   1. Percuss over the right thorax
   2. Increase the pressure limit setting to 60 cm H_2O
   3. Recommend a STAT chest radiograph
   4. Deflate the ET cuff
      A. 1 only
      B. 2 only
      C. 4 only
      D. 1 and 3 only

2. Further evaluation of the patient reveals the following: chest radiograph shows increased radiolucency on the right and absence of vascular markings on the right. The trachea is deviated to the left. Neck veins are distended. The patient is cyanotic. What immediate action(s) should the practitioner take at this time?
   1. Call a physician STAT
   2. Disconnect the patient from the ventilator and manually support ventilations
   3. Increase the pressure limit
   4. Increase the ventilator volume
      A. 1 only
      B. 3 only
      C. 1 and 2 only
      D. 3 and 4 only

3. A patient with ARDS is difficult to oxygenate: F_IO_2 is 0.8, PEEP is 12 cm H_2O, and P_aO_2 is 63 mm Hg. The physician requests that the respiratory therapist perform what maneuver that might help establish an optimum PEEP for the patient?

4. A patient with ARDS requires high PEEP levels. Plateau pressures are approximately 35 cm H_2O and PEEP is 16 cm H_2O. The patient's abdomen is turgidly overdistended. The respiratory therapist is concerned about the high plateau pressure. Should the respiratory therapist reduce the ventilating pressures?

5. VILI is associated with which of the following?
   1. Washout or alteration of surfactant
   2. Shear stress
   3. Damage to pulmonary microvasculature
   4. Possible release of inflammatory mediators from pulmonary cells
      A. 1 only
      B. 4 only
      C. 1 and 3 only
      D. 1, 2, 3, and 4

6. Overdistention injury of the lungs is associated with release of what substances from the lungs into the bloodstream?
   A. Bacterial endotoxins
   B. Surfactant
   C. Cytokines
   D. Mucus

7. During mechanical ventilation, a patient appears to be "fighting the ventilator." He is anxious, agitated, and hypertensive. The patient's skin is hot and moist. The electrocardiogram shows peaked T waves and ST-segment depression. Potassium level is elevated. What further assessment and therapy might be needed for this patient?

8. A patient on PC-CMV has initial ABG findings as follows: P_aO_2 of 101 mm Hg, P_aCO_2 of 60 mm Hg, and pH of 7.30. The respiratory therapist should:
   A. Increase minute ventilation to this patient
   B. Decrease pressure setting
   C. Change the ventilation mode
   D. Very gradually, over several days, increase the minute ventilation to this patient

9. During mechanical ventilation, hyperventilation, particularly in patients with COPD, can cause which of the following?
   1. Muscle twitching and tetany
   2. High pH values
   3. Air trapping
   4. Cardiac arrhythmias
      A. 2 only
      B. 1 and 3 only
      C. 2, 3, and 4 only
      D. 1, 2, 3, and 4

10. During mechanical ventilation with VC-IMV, a respiratory rate of 4 breaths/min and a V_T of 600 mL, a patient has a spontaneous rate of 24 breaths/min between machine breaths. Pressure support is set at 5 cm H_2O. S_pO_2 is 95%. The spontaneous V_T ranges from 175 to 275 mL. The patient is using accessory muscles to breathe. ABG results are within normal range. The patient's ideal body weight is 70 kg. Which of the following might be appropriate?
    A. Increase the V_T setting on the ventilator
    B. Increase the F_IO_2
    C. Decrease the IMV rate
    D. Increase pressure support to 10 cm H_2O

11. Reducing the WOB can be accomplished by using which of the following?
    1. Increased inspiratory flow rates
    2. Increased ventilatory sensitivity
    3. Putting the patient in an upright position
    4. Ensuring the patency of the ET
       A. 1 only
       B. 2 and 3 only
       C. 1, 3, and 4 only
       D. 1, 2, 3, and 4

12. A patient with ARDS is on 15 cm H_2O of PEEP after a recruitment maneuver. F_IO_2 is 0.85. Ventilation is good, but P_aO_2 is only 94 mm Hg. What might the respiratory therapist recommend for improving the patient's oxygenation?
    A. Set the F_IO_2 at 0.5 to avoid oxygen toxicity
    B. Reduce the PEEP to 10 cm H_2O
    C. Change the patient to the prone position
    D. Recommend an increase in minute ventilation

13. Mean airway pressure for a patient is 21 cm H_2O. The respiratory therapist increases mean airway pressure to 25 cm H_2O by increasing PEEP. $P_{plateau}$ is now 35 cm H_2O. This might result in which of the following?
   A. An increase in cardiac output
   B. VILI
   C. A decrease in FRC
   D. An increase in dead space

14. A patient will require 10 to 14 days of mechanical ventilation and is orally intubated with a standard ET. Ventilation and plateau pressures are adequate on VC-CMV with a volume of 450 mL and a rate of 14 breaths/min. ABGs are P_aO_2 of 101 mm Hg, a P_aCO_2 of 41 mm Hg, and a pH of 7.40. What changes might the respiratory therapist recommend at this time?
   A. Make no changes
   B. Increase the V_T
   C. Change the ET to provide CASS
   D. Decrease the F_IO_2

15. What type of problem is indicated in the following figure?

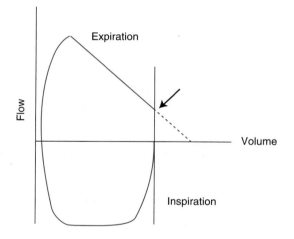

References

1. Branson RD: Enhanced capabilities of current ICU ventilators: do they really benefit patients? *Respir Care* 36:362–376, 1991.
2. Haas CF: Lung protective mechanical ventilation in acute respiratory distress syndrome. *Respir Care Clin North Am* 9:363–396, 2003.
3. Villar J, Kacmarek RM, Hedenstierna G: From ventilator-induced lung injury to physician-induced lung injury: why the reluctance to use small tidal volumes? *Acta Anaesthesiol Scand* 48:267–271, 2004.
4. Samuelson WM, Fulkerson WJ: Barotrauma in mechanical ventilation. In Fulkerson WJ, MacIntyre NR, editors: *Problems in respiratory care: complications of mechanical ventilation*, Philadelphia, 1991, JB Lippincott, pp 52–67.
5. Heulitt MJ, Anders J, Benham D: Acute respiratory distress syndrome in pediatric patients: redirecting therapy to reduce iatrogenic lung injury. *Respir Care* 40:74–85, 1995.
6. Badar T, Bidani A: Mechanical ventilatory support. *Chest Surg Clin N Am* 12:265–299, 2002.
7. Bone RC: Mechanical trauma in acute respiratory failure. *Respir Care* 28:618, 1983.
8. Zwillich CW, Pierson DJ, Creagh CE, et al: Complications of assisted ventilation. A prospective study of 354 consecutive episodes. *Am J Med* 57:161–170, 1974.
9. Fleming W, Bowen J, Hatcher C: Early complications of long-term respiratory support. *J Thorac Cardiovasc Surg* 64:729–738, 1972.
10. Anzueto A, Frutos-Vivar F, Esteban A, et al: Incidence, risk factors and outcome of barotraumas in mechanically ventilated patients. *Intensive Care Med* 30:612–619, 2004.
11. Turki M, Young MP, Wagers SS, et al: Peak pressures during manual ventilation. *Respir Care* 50:340–344, 2005.
12. Dreyfuss D, Soler P, Basset G, et al: High inflation pressure pulmonary edema. Respective effects of high airway pressure, high tidal volume, and positive end-expiratory pressure. *Am Rev Respir Dis* 137:1159–1164, 1988.
13. Marini JJ, Gattinoni L: Ventilatory management of acute respiratory distress syndrome: a consensus of two. *Crit Care Med* 32:250–255, 2004.
14. Caldwell E, Powell R, Mullooly J: Interstitial emphysema: a study of physiologic factors involved in experimental induction of lesion. *Am Rev Respir Dis* 102:516–525, 1970.
15. Pierson DJ, Hildebrandt J: Pierson response to letter from F Piedaliue, (letter). *Respir Care* 39:670, 1994.
16. Gattinoni L, Pietro C, Pelosi P, et al: What has computed tomography taught us about the acute respiratory distress syndrome? *Am J Respir Crit Care Med* 164:1701–1711, 2001.
17. Muscedere JG, Mullen JBM, Gan K, et al: Tidal ventilation at low airway pressures can augment lung injury. *Am J Respir Crit Care Med* 149:1327–1334, 1994.
18. Chiumello D, Prostine G, Slutsky AS: Mechanical ventilation affects local and systemic cytokines in an animal model of acute respiratory distress syndrome. *Am J Respir Crit Care Med* 160:109–116, 1999.
19. Ovensfors CO: Pulmonary interstitial emphysema. An experimental roentgen-diagnostic study. *Acta Radiol Diagn (Stockh)* Suppl 224:1, 1964.
20. Dreyfuss DP, Basset G, Soler P, et al: Intermittent positive-pressure hyperventilation with high inflation pressures produces pulmonary microvascular injury in rats. *Am Rev Respir Dis* 132:880–884, 1985.
21. Kolobow T, Moretti M, Fumagalli R, et al: Lung injury from oxygen in lambs: the role of artificial ventilation. *Am Rev Respir Dis* 135:312–315, 1987.
22. Webb HH, Tierney DF: Experimental pulmonary edema due to intermittent positive-pressure ventilation with high inflation pressures. Protection by positive end-expiratory pressure. *Am Rev Respir Dis* 110:556–565, 1974.
23. Corbridge TC, Wood LDH, Crawford GP, et al: Adverse effects of large tidal volume and low PEEP in canine acid aspiration. *Am Rev Respir Dis* 142:311–315, 1990.
24. Bshouty Z, Ali J, Younes M: Effect of tidal volume and PEEP on rate of edema formation in in situ perfused canine lobes. *J Appl Physiol* 64:1900–1907, 1988.
25. Parker JC, Hernandez LA, Longenecker GL, et al: Lung edema caused by high peak inspiratory pressures in dogs. *Am Rev Respir Dis* 142:321–328, 1990.
26. Dreyfuss D, Soler P, Saumon G: Mechanical ventilation-induced pulmonary edema. Interaction with previous lung alterations. *Am J Respir Crit Care Med* 151:1568–1575, 1995.
27. MacIntyre NR: Minimizing alveolar stretch injury during mechanical ventilation. *Respir Care* 41:318–326, 1996.
28. Mead J, Takishima T, Leith D: Stress distribution in lungs: a model of pulmonary elasticity. *J Appl Physiol* 28:596–608, 1970.
29. Tierney DF: Ventilator-induced lung injury occurs in rats, but does it occur in humans? *Am J Respir Crit Care Med* 168:1414–1415, 2003.
30. Pugin J, Dunn I, Jolliet P, et al: Activation of human macrophages by mechanical ventilation in vitro. *Am J Physiol* 275:L1040–L1050, 1998.
31. Murphy DB, Cregg N, Tremblay L, et al: Adverse ventilatory strategies causes pulmonary-to-systemic translocation of endotoxin. *Am J Respir Crit Care Med* 162:27–33, 2000.
32. Raniere VM, Suter PM, Tortorella C, et al: Effect of mechanical ventilation on inflammatory mediators in patients with acute respiratory distress syndrome: a randomized controlled trial. *JAMA* 282:54–61, 1999.
33. Stüber F, Wrigge H, Schroeder S, et al: Kinetic and reversibility of mechanical ventilation-associated pulmonary and systemic inflammatory response in patients with acute lung injury. *Intensive Care Med* 28:834–841, 2002.
34. Tremblay L, Valenza F, Ribeiro SP, et al: Injurious ventilator strategies increase cytokines and c-fos m-RNA expression in an isolated rat lung model. *J Clin Invest* 99:944–952, 1997.
35. Imai Y, Kawano T, Iwamoto S, et al: Intratracheal anti-tumor necrosis factor-alpha antibody attenuates ventilator-induced lung injury in rabbits. *J Appl Physiol* 87:510–515, 1999.

36. Nahum A, Hoyt J, Schmitz L, et al: Effect of mechanical ventilation strategies on dissemination of intratracheally instilled Escherichia coli in dogs. *Crit Care Med* 25:1733–1743, 1997.

37. Slutsky AS, Tremblay LN: Multiple system organ failure. Is mechanical ventilation a contributing factor? *Am J Respir Crit Care Med* 157(6 Pt 1):1721–1725, 1998.

38. Raniere VM, Giunta F, Suter PM, et al: Mechanical ventilation as a mediator of multisystem organ failure in acute respiratory distress syndrome. *JAMA* 284:43–44, 2000.

39. Imai Y, Parodo J, Kajikawa O, et al: Injurious mechanical ventilation and end-organ epithelial cell apoptosis and organ dysfunction in an experimental model of acute respiratory distress syndrome. *JAMA* 289:2104–2112, 2003.

40. Choi W, Quinn DA, Park KM, et al: Systemic microvascular leak in an in vivo rat model of ventilator-induced lung injury. *Am J Respir Crit Care Med* 167:1627–1632, 2003.

41. Azoulay E, Attalah H, Yang K, et al: Exacerbation by granulocyte colony-stimulating factor of prior acute lung injury: implication of neutrophils. *Crit Care Med* 30:2115–2122, 2002.

42. Broccard AF, Hotchkiss JR, Vannay C, et al: Protective effects of hypercapnic acidosis on ventilator-induced lung injury. *Am J Respir Crit Care Med* 164:802–806, 2001.

43. Shibata K, Cregg N, Engelberts D, et al: Hypercapnic acidosis may attenuate acute lung injury by inhibition of endogenous xanthine oxidase. *Am J Respir Crit Care Med* 158:1578–1584, 1998.

44. Laffey JG, Engelberts D, Kavanagh BP, et al: Buffering hypercapnic acidosis worsens acute lung injury. *Am J Respir Crit Care Med* 161:141–146, 2000.

45. Vassilakopoulos T: Ventilator-induced diaphragm dysfunction. In Tobin MJ, editor: *Principles and practice of mechanical ventilation*, ed 3, New York, 2013, McGraw-Hill, pp 1025–1039.

46. Tobin MJ, Laghi F, Jubran A: Narrative review: ventilator-induced respiratory muscle weakness. *Ann Intern Med* 153:240–245, 2010.

47. Anzueto A, Tobin MJ, Moore G: Effect of prolonged mechanical ventilation on diaphragmatic function: a preliminary study of a baboon model. *Am Rev Respir Dis* 135:A201, 1987.

48. Levine S, Nguyen T, Taylor N, et al: Rapid disuse atrophy of diaphragm fibers in mechanically ventilated humans. *N Engl J Med* 358:1327–1335, 2008.

49. Froese AB, Bryan AC: Effects of anesthesia and paralysis on diaphragmatic mechanics in man. *Anesthesiology* 41:242–255, 1974.

50. Hess DR, Bigatello LM: Lung recruitment: the role of recruitment maneuvers. *Respir Care* 47:308–317, 2002.

51. Watson WE: Observations on the dynamic lung compliance of patients with respiratory muscle weakness receiving intermittent positive pressure respiration. *Br J Anaesth* 34:690–695, 1962.

52. Heironimus TW: *Mechanical artificial ventilation*, ed 2, Springfield, Ill, 1970, Charles C Thomas.

53. Hedenstierna G, White FE, Wagner PD: Spatial distribution of pulmonary blood flow in the dog with PEEP ventilation. *J Appl Physiol Respir Environ Exerc Physiol* 47:938–946, 1979.

54. Tyler DC: Positive end-expiratory pressure: a review. *Crit Care Med* 11:300–308, 1983.

55. Downs JB: Ventilatory patterns and modes of ventilation in acute respiratory failure. *Respir Care* 28:586–591, 1983.

56. Swenson ER: Metabolic acidosis. *Respir Care* 46:342–353, 2001.

57. Khanna A, Kurtzman NA: Metabolic alkalosis. *Respir Care* 46:354–365, 2001.

58. Pepe PE, Marini JJ: Occult positive end-expiratory pressure in mechanically ventilated patients with airflow obstruction. *Am Rev Respir Dis* 126:166–170, 1982.

59. Tuxen DV, Lane S: The effects of ventilatory pattern on hyperinflation, airway pressures, and circulation in mechanical ventilation of patients with severe air-flow obstruction. *Am Rev Respir Dis* 136:872–879, 1987.

60. Tuxen DV: Detrimental effects of positive end-expiratory pressure during controlled mechanical ventilation of patients with severe airflow obstruction. *Am Rev Respir Dis* 140:5–10, 1989.

61. Marini JJ: Should PEEP be used in airflow obstruction? *Am Rev Respir Dis* 140:1–3, 1989.

62. Brown DG, Pierson DJ: Auto-PEEP is common in mechanically ventilated patients: a study of incidence, severity, and detection. *Respir Care* 31:1069–1074, 1986.

63. MacIntyre NR: Respiratory system mechanics. In MacIntyre NR, Branson RD, editors: *Mechanical Ventilation*, ed 2, St. Louis, MO., 2009, Saunders-Elsevier, pp 159–170.

64. Scott LR, Benson MS, Bishop MJ: Relationship of endotracheal tube size and auto-PEEP at high minute ventilations. *Respir Care* 31:1080–1082, 1986.

65. Bergman N: Intrapulmonary gas trapping during mechanical ventilation at rapid frequencies. *Anesthesiology* 37:626–633, 1972.

66. Cartwright DW, Willis MM, Gregory GA: Functional residual capacity and lung mechanics at different levels of mechanical ventilation. *Crit Care Med* 12:422–427, 1984.

67. Dhand R: Ventilator graphics and respiratory mechanics in the patient with obstructive lung disease. *Respir Care* 50:246–261, 2005.

68. Grootendorst AF, Lugtigheid G, Van der Weygert EJ: Error in ventilator measurements of intrinsic PEEP: cause and remedy. *Respir Care* 38:348–350, 1993.

69. Madsen D, Jager K, Fenwick J, et al: Expiratory hold vs clamping/transducing for intrinsic PEEP determination in the Siemens 900C. *Respir Care* 39:623–626, 1994.

70. Rossi A, Gottfried SB, Zocchi L, et al: Measurement of static compliance of the total respiratory system in patients with acute respiratory failure during mechanical ventilation. The effect of intrinsic positive end-expiratory pressure. *Am Rev Respir Dis* 131:672–677, 1985.

71. Cairo JM: *Mosby's respiratory care equipment*, ed 9, St Louis, 2014, Elsevier.

72. Register SC, Downs JB, Stock MC: Is 50% oxygen harmful? *Crit Care Med* 15:598–601, 1987.

73. Pierson DJ: The future of respiratory care. *Respir Care* 46:705–718, 2001.

74. Durbin CG, Wallace KK: Oxygen toxicity in the critically ill patient. *Respir Care* 38:739–750, 1993.

75. Jenkinson SG: Oxygen toxicity in acute respiratory failure. *Respir Care* 28:614, 1983.

76. Lodata RF: Oxygen toxicity. In Tobin MJ, editor: *Principles and practice of mechanical ventilation*, ed 3, New York, 2013, McGraw-Hill, pp 1065–1090.

77. Heuer AJ: Medical gas therapy. In Kacmarek RM, Stoller JK, Heuer AJ, editors: *Egan's fundamentals of respiratory care*, ed 10, St Louis, 2013, Mosby-Elsevier, pp 909–940.

78. Hess DR, Bigatello LM: Lung recruitment: the role of recruitment maneuvers. *Respir Care* 47:308–317, 2002.

79. Rothen HU, Sporre B, Engberg G, et al: Influence of gas composition on recurrent atelectasis after a reexpansion maneuver during general anesthesia. *Anesthesiology* 82:832–842, 1995.

80. McAslan TC, Matjasko-Chiu J, Turney SZ, et al: Influence of inhalation of 100% oxygen on intrapulmonary shunt in severely traumatized patients. *J Trauma* 13:811–821, 1973.

81. Kacmarek RM: The role of pressure support ventilation in reducing the work of breathing. *Respir Care* 33:99–120, 1988.

82. Branson RD, Davis K: Work of breathing by five ventilators used for long-term support: the effects of PEEP and simulated patient demand. *Respir Care* 40:1270–1278, 1995.

83. Marini JJ: The role of the inspiratory circuit in the work of breathing during mechanical ventilation. *Respir Care* 32:419–427, 1987.

84. Marini JJ, Rodriguez RM, Lamb V: The inspiratory workload of patient-initiated mechanical ventilation. *Am Rev Respir Dis* 134:902–909, 1986.

85. Hirsch C, Kacmarek RM, Stanek K: Work of breathing during CPAP and PSV imposed by the new generation mechanical ventilators: a lung model study. *Respir Care* 36:815–828, 1991.

86. Marini JJ: Work of breathing. In Kacmarek RM, Stoller JK, editors: *Current respiratory care*, Philadelphia, 1988, BC Decker, pp 188–194.

87. Leung P, Jubran A, Tobin J: Comparison of assisted ventilatory modes on triggering, patient effort, and dyspnea. *Am J Respir Crit Care Med* 155:1940–1948, 1997.

88. Nilsestuen JO, Hargett KD: Using ventilator graphics to identify patient-ventilator asynchrony. *Respir Care* 50:202–234, 2005.

89. Hess DR, Kacmarek RM: *Essentials of mechanical ventilation*, New York, 2002, McGraw-Hill.

90. Hansen-Flaschen JH: Dyspnea in the ventilated patient: a call for patient-centered mechanical ventilation. *Respir Care* 45:1460–1464, 2000.

91. MacIntyre NR: Weaning from mechanical ventilatory support: volume-assisting intermittent breaths versus pressure-assisting every breath. *Respir Care* 33:121–125, 1988.

92. Shapiro M, Wilson RK, Casar G, et al: Work of breathing through different sized endotracheal tubes. *Crit Care Med* 14:1028–1031, 1986.

93. Brochard L, Rua F, Lorino H, et al: Inspiratory pressure support compensates for the additional work of breathing caused by the endotracheal tube. *Anesthesiology* 75:739–745, 1991.

94. Fiastro JF, Habib MP, Quan SF: Pressure support compensation for inspiratory work due to endotracheal tubes and demand continuous positive airway pressure. *Chest* 93:499–505, 1988.

95. Esteban A, Alia I, Gordo F, et al: Extubation outcome after spontaneous breathing trials with T-tube or pressure support ventilation. The Spanish Lung Failure Collaborative Group. *Am J Respir Crit Care Med* 156:459–465, 1997.

96. Straus C, Louis B, Isabey D, et al: Contribution of the endotracheal tube and the upper airway to breathing workload. *Am J Respir Crit Care Med* 157:23–30, 1998.

97. Hess DR: MacIntyre: Mechanical ventilation. In Hess DR, MacIntyre NR, Mishoe SC, editors: *Respiratory care, principles & practices*, ed 2, Sudbury, MA, 2012, Jones and Bartlett, pp 462–500.

98. Branson R: Understanding and implementing advances in ventilator capabilities. *Curr Opin Crit Care* 10:23–32, 2004.

99. Hess DR: Ventilator waveforms and the physiology of pressure support ventilation. *Respir Care* 50:166–186, 2005.

100. Nava S, Bruschi C, Rubini F, et al: Respiratory response and inspiratory effort during pressure support ventilation in COPD patients. *Intensive Care Med* 21:871–879, 1995.

101. MacIntyre NR: Patient-ventilator interactions. In MacIntyre NR, Branson RD, editors: *Mechanical ventilation*, Philadelphia, 2001, WB Saunders, pp 182–197.

102. MacIntyre NR, McConnell R, Cheng KG, et al: Patient-ventilator flow dyssynchrony: flow-limited versus pressure-limited breaths. *Crit Care Med* 25:1671–1677, 1997.

103. Jubran A, Van de Graaff WB, Tobin MJ: Variability of patient-ventilator interaction with pressure support ventilation in patients with chronic obstructive pulmonary disease. *Am J Respir Crit Care Med* 152:129–136, 1995.

104. Yamada Y, Du HL: Effects of different pressure support termination on patient-ventilator synchrony. *Respir Care* 43:1048–1057, 1998.

105. American Association for Respiratory Care: Positive end expiratory pressure: state of the art after 20 years. *Respir Care* 33:417–500, 1988.

106. Heulitt MJ, Holt SJ, Thurman TL, et al: Effects of continuous positive airway pressure/positive end-expiratory pressure and pressure-support ventilation on work of breathing, using an animal model. *Respir Care* 48:689–696, 2003.

107. Blanch PB: Mechanical ventilator malfunctions: a descriptive and comparative study of 6 common ventilator brands. *Respir Care* 44:1183–1192, 1999.

108. Zwillich CW, Pierson DJ, Creagh CE, et al: Complications of assisted ventilation. A prospective study of 354 consecutive episodes. *Am J Med* 57:161–170, 1974.

109. Benjamin PK, Thompson JE, O'Rourke PP: Complications in mechanical ventilation in a children's hospital multidisciplinary intensive care unit. *Respir Care* 35:873–878, 1990.

110. Abramson RS, Wald RS, Grenvik ANA, et al: Adverse occurrences in intensive care units. *JAMA* 244:1582–1584, 1980.

111. The Joint Commission: Preventing ventilator-related deaths and injuries. *Sentinel Event Alert* 25:2001.

112. United States Department of Health and Human Services: *Accidental breathing circuit disconnections in the critical care setting, Publication No. FDA 90-4233*, Rockville, Md, 1990, HHS, Public Health Service, Food and Drug Administration, Center for Devices and Radiological Health, 1990.

113. Lucangelo U, Bernabe F, Blanch L: Respiratory mechanics derived from signals in the ventilator circuit. *Respir Care* 50:55–65, 2005.

114. Restrepo RD, Walsh BK: Humidification during invasive and noninvasive mechanical ventilation: 2012. *Respir Care* 57:782–788, 2012.

115. Sharar SR: The effects of artificial airways on airflow and ventilatory mechanics: basic concepts and clinical relevance. *Respir Care* 40:257–262, 1995.

116. American Association for Respiratory Care Clinical Practice Guideline. Management of airway emergencies. *Respir Care* 40:749–760, 1995.

Troubleshooting and Problem Solving

OUTLINE

KEY TERMS

- Ascites
- Asynchrony
- Problem
- Pulmonary angiogram
- Thrombolytic therapy

LEARNING OBJECTIVES *On completion of this chapter, the reader will be able to do the following:*

1. Identify various types of technical problems encountered during mechanical ventilation of critically ill patients, and describe the steps that can be used to protect a patient when problems occur.
2. Name at least two possible causes for each of the following alarm situations: low-pressure alarm, high-pressure alarm, low PEEP/CPAP alarms, apnea alarm, low or high tidal volume alarm, low or high minute volume alarm, low or high respiratory rate alarm, low or high F_IO_2 alarm, low-source gas pressure or power input alarm, ventilator inoperative alarm, and technical error message.
3. Determine the cause of a problem using ventilator graphics from a patient-ventilator system.
4. Assess a mechanically ventilated patient experiencing sudden dyspnea and identify the cause of the problem.
5. Describe the signs and symptoms associated with patient-ventilator asynchrony.
6. Explain the correct procedure for determining whether a problem originates with the patient or with the ventilator during patient-ventilator asynchrony.
7. List four ways the addition of a nebulizer powered by an external source gas can affect ventilator function.
8. Recognize abnormalities in ventilator graphics and patient response in the event of inadequate gas flow delivery to a patient.
9. Identify the causes and potential problems related to electrolyte imbalances and their causes.
10. Recognize the signs and symptoms of a respiratory infection.
11. Identify a problem associated with an artificial airway or a mask used for noninvasive positive pressure ventilation.
12. Recognize the presence of auto-PEEP using ventilator graphics.

13. Suggest appropriate interventions for a patient who has experienced a right mainstem intubation and for a patient with a pneumothorax using physical assessment data.
14. Describe the potential problems associated with using a heated humidification system during mechanical ventilation.
15. Use a ventilator flow–volume loop to assess a patient's response to bronchodilator therapy.
16. Make recommendations about ventilator parameters for a patient with acute respiratory distress syndrome (ARDS).
17. Recommend adjustment of flow-cycle criteria during pressure support ventilation based on ventilator graphics.

Troubleshooting, in the context of mechanical ventilation, involves the identification and resolution of technical malfunctions in the patient-ventilator system. Troubleshooting can be thought of as purposeful resolution of inappropriate and potentially dangerous situations.

Previous chapters have reviewed key concepts used in the management of patients receiving mechanical ventilation. This chapter discusses common technical problems encountered during mechanical ventilation and presents basic problem-solving strategies to ensure patient safety.

DEFINITION OF THE TERM *PROBLEM*

A **problem** can be defined as a situation in which a person finds discord or is uncomfortable with a matter that cannot be immediately resolved. Interestingly, a situation that might be uncomfortable for one person may not appear to be a problem for another person. For example, a respiratory therapist in the intensive care unit (ICU) may note that audible and visual alarms have activated for the intravenous pump. Unless it is part of this person's job function, the respiratory therapist might not perceive this as a problem that must be resolved and may simply contact the nurse. In contrast, if a ventilator alarm were activated, the same respiratory therapist would accept the responsibility of going to the patient's bedside to assess the situation and finding a solution to the problem. Individuals therefore must perceive an event as a problem and want to find a meaningful solution; that is, a situation must create discomfort which forces someone perceiving it to take action toward a resolution.

The ability to define a problem is particularly important to clinicians caring for critically ill patients. The lives of patients receiving ventilatory support may ultimately depend on the mechanical ventilator. Indeed, a matter of minutes can mean life or death. Because potential mishaps can occur with the patient-ventilator system, it is essential that clinicians develop the ability to identify and correct associated problems.

Solving Ventilation Problems

The first step in solving any problem is to assess the situation at hand carefully. The next step is to gather and analyze pertinent data, which should point to a number of viable solutions.

When a solution is attempted, the clinician's observations of the patient's response are critical. If the response is positive and leads to the correct remedy, the problem is resolved. If not, the clinician must undo what was attempted and try to determine the reason the particular solution failed before attempting another approach. If the problem cannot be resolved, the clinician should seek help.

Determining the cause of the problem can help prevent its recurrence. Note the steps taken in Box 18-1 to solve the problem shown in Fig. 18-1. Which individual or individuals first perceived it as a problem? What steps were taken to determine the cause? What was the final resolution?

BOX 18-1	Troubleshooting a Problem Using Ventilator Graphics

While doing rounds in the intensive care unit, a pulmonologist notices a ventilator graphic display showing the expiratory portion of the volume curve dropping below baseline (see Fig. 18-1). He contacts the respiratory therapist and inquires about possible causes.

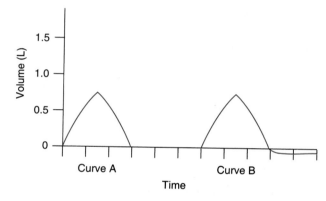

Fig. 18-1 Curve *A* shows a normal volume–time curve. Curve *B* shows the expiratory portion of the volume below the zero baseline.

Notice that the volume delivered by the ventilator (the inspiratory portion of the volume curve) is smaller than the volume exhaled, possibly because the patient is actively exhaling. A patient evaluation reveals that this is not the case.

The respiratory therapist, unable to explain the cause immediately, uses a respirometer to measure the volume coming from the volume delivery port, the patient, and the exhalation valve. The three volumes are equal. Still unable to determine the cause, the respiratory therapist contacts the individual who performs the maintenance checks on the ventilator. The respiratory therapist learns that the expiratory transducer was calibrated for a heated humidifier; however, a heat and moisture exchanger (HME) is being used with this patient. Although recalibrating the transducer would resolve the issue, it is not a life-threatening situation, and therefore no immediate action is required.

PROTECTING THE PATIENT

It is important to understand that ensuring patient safety is the foremost obligation of the clinician. Whenever an alarm activates on a ventilator or monitoring device, the clinician should first make sure that the patient is adequately ventilated and oxygenated. Initially, this can be accomplished by visually assessing the patient's level of consciousness, use of accessory muscles, and chest wall movements. During this initial assessment, the alarm should be checked and silenced. Auscultation of the chest can establish the presence of adequate breath sounds, and checking the S_pO_2 can provide information about the patient's heart rate and oxygen saturation. If the patient is in acute distress, demonstrating labored breathing, pallor, diaphoresis, and apparent anxiety, along with deterioration of breath sounds and a decreasing S_pO_2, immediate action is required. When a serious problem is detected, the patient may need to be disconnected from the ventilator and manually ventilated with a resuscitation bag. (After the patient is stabilized, the clinician can review the cause of the alarm activation and obtain help from other personnel if necessary.)

A self-inflating resuscitation bag can be used temporarily for ventilation of a distressed patient. When it is used properly, the resuscitation bag allows for the assessment of lung characteristics because the clinician can check ("feel") a patient's lung and chest wall compliance and airway resistance manually. Manual ventilation must be performed cautiously to avoid inappropriate patterns of ventilation, excessive pressures (i.e., >40 cm H_2O), and barotrauma.[1,2] Additionally, ventilator disconnection of a patient with ARDS who is ventilated with a high level of PEEP (15 to 25 cm H_2O) can cause derecruitment of the lung, resulting in oxygen desaturation. Manual ventilation must also be used judiciously because disconnecting the patient from the ventilator can also result in contamination of the patient's airway, which in turn can increase the patient's risk of developing ventilator-associated pneumonia (see Chapter 14).

IDENTIFYING THE PATIENT IN SUDDEN DISTRESS

The term *patient-ventilator asynchrony* is typically used to describe the phenomenon that occurs when patients are unable to breathe comfortably with the mechanical ventilator. The phrase "fighting the ventilator" is sometimes used to describe an individual who is apparently doing well while receiving mechanical ventilation but suddenly develops acute respiratory distress.[3,4] This situation is particularly challenging for most clinicians because the patient is unable to verbalize his or her discomfort (Key Point 18-1). (Sometimes clinicians can gain valuable information from patients simply by asking direct ["yes" or "no"] questions.[5])

C **Key Point 18-1** *"The problems we created cannot be solved with the same level of thinking that we had when we created them."—Albert Einstein*

The sudden onset of dyspnea can be identified by observing the physical signs of distress (Fig. 18-2), including tachypnea; nasal flaring; diaphoresis; accessory muscle use; retraction of the suprasternal, supraclavicular, and intercostal spaces; paradoxical or abnormal movement of the thorax and abdomen; abnormal findings on auscultation; tachycardia; arrhythmia; and hypotension.[3,4] Pulse oximetry, capnograph readings, ventilator graphics, peak inspiratory pressure (PIP), plateau pressure ($P_{plateau}$), and exhaled volumes may have changed and may provide information to help identify the cause of the problem.

Patient-ventilator **asynchrony** can be caused by a number of factors. Box 18-2 lists the most common causes of sudden respiratory distress in patients receiving mechanical ventilation. (See the

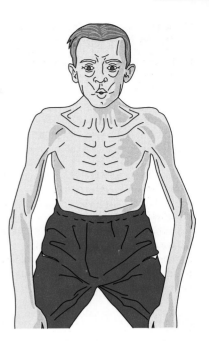

CLINICAL MANIFESTATIONS

- Use of accessory muscles to breathe
- Pursed-lip breathing
- Minimal or absent cough
- Leaning forward to breathe
- Barrel chest
- Digital clubbing
- Dyspnea on exertion (late sign)

Fig. 18-2 Physical signs of severe respiratory distress. (From Copstead LC, Banasik, JL: Pathophysiology, ed 4, Saunders, 2009.)

BOX 18-2	**Causes of Sudden Respiratory Distress in Patients Receiving Mechanical Ventilation**

Patient-Related Causes
- Artificial airway problems
- Bronchospasm
- Secretions
- Pulmonary edema
- Pulmonary embolus
- Dynamic hyperinflation
- Abnormal respiratory drive
- Alteration in body posture
- Drug-induced problems
- Abdominal distention
- Pneumothorax
- Anxiety

Ventilator-Related Causes
- System leak
- Circuit malfunction or disconnection
- Inadequate F_iO_2
- Patient-ventilator asynchrony
  - Inappropriate ventilator support mode
  - Inappropriate trigger sensitivity
  - Inappropriate inspiratory flow setting
  - Inappropriate cycle variable
  - Inappropriate PEEP setting
  - Problems with closed-loop ventilation

(From Tobin MJ: What should a clinician do when a patient "fights the ventilator"? *Respir Care* 36:395-406, 1991.)

BOX 18-3	Management of Sudden Severe Respiratory Distress in a Mechanically Ventilated Patient

1. Disconnect the patient from the ventilator.
2. Begin manual ventilation using a self-inflating resuscitation bag containing 80% to 100% oxygen; maintain normal ventilating pressures, and use a PEEP attachment if the patient has been on high PEEP (≥10 cm H_2O).
3. Manually evaluate compliance and resistance through bag ventilation.
4. Perform a rapid physical examination and assess monitored indexes and alarms.
5. Check the patency of the airway by passing a suction catheter.
6. If death appears imminent, treat the most likely problems: pneumothorax and airway obstruction.
7. Once the patient's condition has stabilized, perform a more detailed assessment and provide any additional treatment required.

(Modified from Tobin MJ: What should a clinician do when a patient "fights the ventilator"? *Respir Care* 36:395-406, 1991.)

BOX 18-4	Causes of Airway Problems That Can Lead to Sudden Respiratory Distress

- Tube migration (flexion and extension of the head and neck can move the endotracheal tube [ET] in the airway an average of 2 cm down and up, respectively)
- Migration of the ET above the vocal cords
- Migration of the ET into the right mainstem bronchus
- Rupture or leakage of the ET cuff
- Kinking of the ET
- Patient biting the ET
- Airway secretions and mucous plugging of airways
- Impingement of the ET on the carina or airway
- Cuff herniation over the end of the ET (less of a problem with the current endotracheal cuffs)
- Development of a tracheoesophageal fistula
- Rupture of the innominate artery

BOX 18-5	Emergency Treatment for Rupture of the Innominate Artery

Rupture of the innominate artery is a potentially serious airway complication and the mortality rate for this condition is high. It usually is seen in the first 3 weeks after a tracheostomy. The immediate indication is blood spurting from the tracheotomy site.

To stop the hemorrhage, the cuff should be overinflated or pressure should be applied internally with a finger inserted through the stoma. The finger is inserted as far as possible toward the carina and then pulled forward in an attempt to compress the artery against the posterior aspect of the sternum.

section in Chapter 17 on steps to reduce the work of breathing [WOB] during mechanical ventilation.)

Evaluation of the ventilator graphics and settings can be used to resolve most of these problems. For example, autotriggering of breaths can occur if the sensitivity setting (inspiratory trigger) is too sensitive, resulting in an excessive number of triggered breaths. Patient-ventilator asynchrony is often associated with a patient's feelings of panic, which can be relieved by encouraging the patient to not "fight the ventilator" and relax while breathing with the ventilator. Selection of the appropriate mode and correct adjustment of the ventilator can eliminate most problems and reduce the need for sedation. (See Chapter 17 for more detailed information on patient-ventilator asynchrony.)

Identifying the cause of patient-ventilator asynchrony can be accomplished using a relatively simple approach (Box 18-3). If the patient is in **severe** distress, the first step is to disconnect the patient from the ventilator and carefully ventilate the patient using a manual resuscitation bag (i.e., avoiding excessive airway pressure). If the patient's distress resolves immediately, the problem is with the ventilator; if the distress does not resolve, the problem is typically due to the patient experiencing anxiety or pain (Key Point 18-2).

> **Key Point 18-2** In cases where patient-ventilator asynchrony is identified, the clinician should disconnect the patient from the ventilator and carefully ventilate the patient using a manual resuscitation bag.

PATIENT-RELATED PROBLEMS

The most common patient-related problems encountered during mechanical ventilation involve the placement and patency of the artificial airway, or the presence of a pneumothorax, bronchospasm, and excessive secretions (see Box 18-2).

Airway Problems

Examples of acute airway problems include kinking of the endotracheal tube (ET), impingement of the tube on the carina, and displacement of the tube upward, above the vocal cords or into the right mainstem bronchus (Box 18-4). Rupture of the innominate artery can also occur (this is usually seen with tracheostomy tubes) (Box 18-5).[4] An unusual case study reported a fatal tracheal-innominate artery fistula caused by fixed positioning of the Hi-lo Evac tube to the left upper molar.[6] (This type of ET is used for continuous aspiration of the subglottic secretions.) Apparently, the continuous suction pressure against the soft tissue of the trachea for an extended period resulted in erosion of the tissue and, eventually, exposure of the innominate artery. This catheter has been redesigned to reduce the risk of this complication.

A quick check of the patient's oral cavity can sometimes reveal whether the ET is kinked or the patient is biting it. The clinician can easily determine whether the tube has been inserted too far or if it is too shallow in the airway by looking at the tube's centimeter markings at the airway opening. A properly positioned oral ET typically shows a centimeter marking at the teeth at approximately 23 cm for men (range, 22 to 24 cm) and 21 cm for women (range, 20 to 22 cm). If the centimeter markings are less than the ranges cited, the tube is too high in the airway. If the marking is greater than the ranges cited, the tube has migrated deeper into the airway.

If a serious airway problem cannot be resolved quickly, the clinician should ventilate the patient manually to assess airway patency. If the patient cannot be ventilated in this manner, an appropriately sized suction catheter should be passed through the artificial airway. If the catheter does not pass freely (and the patient is not biting on the ET), the tube is most likely obstructed. The cuff should then be deflated, which may allow some air to move around the tube in spontaneously breathing patients. If the obstruction cannot be cleared, the tube must be removed immediately and the patient ventilated with a resuscitation bag until reintubation is possible.[7,8]

Pneumothorax

Pneumothorax is another possible problem that must be detected during positive pressure ventilation (PPV) and treated quickly. Pneumothorax can be recognized as increased WOB if a patient is conscious. For example, the patient may demonstrate nasal flaring, use of accessory muscles, uneven chest wall movement, and absence of breath sounds on the affected side. Auscultation and percussion of the chest, cardiovascular assessment, and ventilating pressure evaluations usually can distinguish a pneumothorax from other problems. Table 8-1 provides physical and radiologic findings commonly seen in patients with pulmonary disorders such as pneumothorax, asthma, emphysema, pneumonia, and pleural effusion.

If a tension pneumothorax is strongly suspected and cardiopulmonary arrest is imminent, a 14- or 16-gauge needle is inserted into the second intercostal space at the midclavicular line, over the top of the rib on the affected side. If the patient's condition is stable, a confirming chest radiograph can be obtained with chest tube placement and pleural drainage. The following case study describes the case of a patient with sudden respiratory distress.

◉ Clinical Scenario: A Case of Sudden Respiratory Distress

A 45-year-old woman has been receiving ventilation for 3 weeks for respiratory failure arising from severe asthma. Treatment has included administration of sedatives, antidepressants, and corticosteroids, as well as bronchodilator therapy. Several attempts at weaning her from the ventilator, including a course of noninvasive positive pressure ventilation (NIV), have been unsuccessful. Thirty-six hours after successful placement of a tracheostomy tube, the patient's ventilator high-pressure alarm activates. The respiratory therapist performs an assessment and suctions the patient's airway, which is determined to be patent. Breath sounds are diminished but present bilaterally. Within 10 minutes the high-pressure alarm activates again. The respiratory therapist returns to the room and notes that the patient appears to be coughing forcefully. The patient suddenly develops ventricular tachycardia and loses consciousness. The respiratory therapist finds it extremely difficult to ventilate through the tracheostomy tube. The tube is pulled, and the patient is immediately and successfully reintubated with an oral ET. Unfortunately, the resuscitation effort fails, and a postmortem chest radiograph shows bilateral pneumothoraces.

The clinicians conclude that thickened secretions had blocked the airways, causing air trapping distally, and that increased pressures in the thorax from the patient's forceful coughing caused the bilateral pneumothoraces.

Bronchospasm

Bronchospasm may be manifested as dyspnea, wheezing, evidence of increased WOB (i.e., such as heightened use of accessory muscles), lack of coordination of chest or abdominal wall movement, retraction of the suprasternal, supraclavicular and intercostal spaces, and increased R_{aw} (as evidenced by increased peak inspiratory pressure [PIP] and transairway pressure [PIP − $P_{plateau}$]). Wheezing associated with increased R_{aw} from airway hyperreactivity, such as occurs with asthma, can be treated with bronchodilators and parenteral corticosteroids. Wheezing can also be associated with cardiogenic problems and pulmonary emboli.

Secretions

Evaluation of the patient's secretions can be useful in differentiating a variety of problems. (See Table 12-2 for a list of sputum findings and possible associated problems.) Drying of secretions is most often associated with inadequate humidification (Key Point 18-3). Copious amounts of secretions can occur with pulmonary edema and certain pulmonary disorders (e.g., cystic fibrosis). Depending on their characteristics, secretions may also suggest the presence of a respiratory infection; however, this is not usually a problem with a sudden onset. It is essential that the patient is provided appropriately warmed and humidified air.[8] Suctioning should be performed only when indicated rather than according to a fixed schedule. Bronchial hygiene may include postural drainage and percussion and therapeutic bronchoscopy. (Chapter 12 presents additional information on bronchial hygiene and therapeutic bronchoscopy.)

◑ **Key Point** **18-3** Drying of secretions is most often associated with inadequate humidification.

Pulmonary Edema

Pulmonary edema can be either cardiogenic or noncardiogenic in origin and should be managed accordingly. Cardiogenic pulmonary edema can occur suddenly and often manifests with thin, frothy, white to pink secretions. In cases where cardiogenic pulmonary edema is suspected, the clinician should check for additional evidence of a cardiac problem, such as electrocardiographic findings, elevated blood pressure, evidence of neck vein distention, a history of heart disease, and data from a pulmonary artery catheter, if available (see Chapter 11). Cardiogenic pulmonary edema and heart failure can often be managed successfully with medications that reduce preload, increase contractility, and reduce afterload, such as furosemide (Lasix), digoxin (Lanoxin), enalapril maleate (Vasotec), and morphine.

Noncardiogenic pulmonary edema or pulmonary edema that is caused by an increase in pulmonary capillary permeability (e.g., ARDS) usually develops over a day or two and is not a sudden-onset problem. The management of ARDS is discussed in Chapter 13.

Dynamic Hyperinflation

Auto-PEEP causes dynamic hyperinflation of the lungs and can lead to difficulty with ventilator triggering.[9] Auto-PEEP can also cause cardiovascular problems, such as hypotension and reduced cardiac output. One of the best ways to detect the presence of auto-PEEP is through the evaluation of the ventilator waveforms. Auto-PEEP should be suspected whenever flow does not return to baseline in either a flow–time scalar or a flow–volume loop. Efforts to reduce auto-PEEP can be aided by reducing the inspiratory time (T_I), minute ventilation $(\dot{V}_E)$, and R_{aw}. (Chapter 17 provides additional information on auto-PEEP.) As previously mentioned, auto-PEEP hinders a patient's ability to trigger the ventilator (see Fig. 7-1). (See Chapter 7 for a discussion of how raising the applied PEEP [extrinsic PEEP] can be used to ease breath triggering in patients with chronic obstructive pulmonary disease [COPD] when auto-PEEP cannot be completely eliminated.)

Abnormalities in Respiratory Drive

Inadequate output from the respiratory centers of the brain can occur as a result of heavy sedation, acute neurologic disorders, or neuromuscular blockage.[10] However, these conditions are more likely to reduce respiratory function than to produce sudden respiratory distress. Increased output from the respiratory centers is associated with pain, anxiety, increased peripheral sensory receptor stimulation, medications, increased ventilatory needs, and inappropriate ventilator settings.

Change in Body Position

Changes in the patient's position can be associated with accidental extubation, bending and twisting of the patient circuit, and in some cases alterations in the patient's level of oxygenation. Reductions in oxygenation can occur with repositioning of the patient so that the diseased lung is placed in a dependent position. It can also occur with sudden airway obstruction by a mucous plug, secretions, or clot migration that leads to a pulmonary embolus. (Changing the patient's body position can cause a thrombus to dislodge and migrate, causing a pulmonary embolus.)

Drug-Induced Distress

It is important to recognize that when acute respiratory distress develops in a ventilated patient in the ICU and the cause cannot be readily identified, possible causes may be related to medications the patient takes or possible chemical dependency. For example, intravenous morphine, which is commonly used to relieve pain, can cause nausea, hypotension, disorientation, hallucinations, fever, constipation, and respiratory arrest. This may be especially true in the older patients, whose ability to metabolize and clear medications may be diminished.

Patients with chemical dependency (alcohol, drug, or tobacco) present additional clinical management issues, particularly if the ICU staff is unaware of a patient's chemical dependency. Sudden interruption of use of the chemical by the patient may cause symptoms of withdrawal syndrome, such as anxiety, restlessness, irritability, insomnia, and inability to focus attention.

Abdominal Distention

Abdominal distention can be associated with air being introduced into the stomach (e.g., via a nasogastric tube) and with a number of disorders, including **ascites,** abdominal bleeding or obstruction, and liver or kidney disorders. Some of these conditions have a slower onset than others, but all cause an upward pressure on the diaphragm, restricting its downward movement. This restriction of diaphragm movement can lead to atelectasis in the basilar areas of the lungs, ventilation/perfusion abnormalities, and hypoxemia.

Pulmonary Embolism

Pulmonary embolism (PE) is another acute onset problem that can lead to patient-ventilator asynchrony. The rapid onset of hypoxemia from a large embolus leads to all the signs of distress previously described. The patient typically demonstrates the presence of bilateral breath sounds, indicating that both lungs are being ventilated (i.e., PE interferes with perfusion not ventilation). With PE the heart rate, blood pressure, and respiratory rate are elevated. Even with high ventilator rates and flows, the patient may use accessory muscles to breathe and may become very pale. Checking airway patency and ventilating pressures and increasing the F_IO_2 may not reverse the arterial oxygen desaturation (S_aO_2). Disconnection from the ventilator and manual ventilation will also not help relieve the distress.

Pulmonary embolism is an emergency that often leaves the clinician feeling helpless to determine the cause and treatment (Case Study 18-1). Capnography findings can, however, provide a clue to the presence of a PE. A decrease in the end-tidal carbon dioxide $(P_{ET}CO_2)$ value compared with previous readings and a widening of the arterial-to-end-tidal partial pressure CO_2 gradient $(P_{(a-et)}CO_2)$ may suggest the presence of an embolus. Demonstration of the presence of a PE usually requires a **pulmonary angiogram** and computerized tomography. **Thrombolytic therapy,** such as the use of alteplase (recombinant tissue plasminogen activator [tPA]; Actilyse) or reteplase (Retavase), may be appropriate.

Case Study 18-1

Evaluating Severe Respiratory Distress in a Ventilated Patient

While performing a patient-ventilator check, the respiratory therapist notes that the patient suddenly develops signs of severe respiratory distress. The low-oxygen saturation alarm on the pulse oximeter activates. Breath sounds are equal bilaterally with no change from previous findings. The respiratory therapist disconnects the patient and performs manual ventilation using 100% oxygen. A suction catheter passes through the patient's ET without difficulty; however, the patient's distress continues and oxygen saturation remains low. The therapist notes that the capnometer reading for $P_{ET}CO_2$ has changed from its previous value of 35 mm Hg to 27 mm Hg. Arterial blood gas analysis indicates that the P_aCO_2 has not changed but the P_aO_2 decreased to 20 mm Hg. The $P_{(a-et)}CO_2$ has increased from 6 mm Hg to 14 mm Hg. What is the cause of the patient's respiratory distress?

VENTILATOR-RELATED PROBLEMS

Clinicians typically rely on algorithms to identify problems with the patient-ventilator circuit. A relatively quick way to identify whether the problem is a ventilator-related problem is to determine whether the patient's respiratory distress is relieved by manual ventilation with 100% oxygen via a self-inflating resuscitation bag. If the intervention relieves the respiratory distress, then the problem is probably associated with the ventilator or with the applied ventilator-management strategy.

Leaks

Activation of low-pressure, low-volume, or low $\dot{V}_E$ alarms typically indicates that a leak in the patient-ventilator circuit is present. (As discussed later in this chapter, the presence of a leak can be verified by analyzing the various ventilator graphics that are available on most ICU ventilators.) Leaks are commonly caused by disconnection of the patient from the ventilator; if this is the problem, the ventilator circuit simply needs to be reconnected to the patient's artificial airway.

Leaks can also occur around the cuff of the ET. To determine whether this is the problem, the clinician should auscultate over the tracheal area for abnormal breath sounds during inspiration. To correct a cuff leak, the cuff is reinflated and the cuff pressure is rechecked. If a minimum leak technique is used, the cuff leak and tracheal air sounds should be present at peak inspiration under normal conditions. (See Chapter 4 for more detailed information on checking the circuit and evaluating for leaks.) Small ETs, such as those used with neonates, do not have cuffs and therefore allow for a minimum amount of air to leak around the tube. Migration of the ET into the upper airway, above the vocal cords, is another possible cause of a leak associated with the ET.

Circuit leaks also can occur at junctions in the patient circuit where connections exist. These may include connections at water traps, humidifiers, and HMEs; inline closed-suction catheters; temperature probes; inline metered-dose inhaler chambers; proximal airway pressure lines; capnograph (CO_2) sensors; and unseated or leaking exhalation valves. Another, less common, source of leaks is a pleural drainage system. In this situation, compensation for pleural leaks sometimes can be accomplished by increasing volume delivery to the patient. The amount of air leaking through the pleural drainage system can be determined by comparing the inspiratory and expiratory tidal volume (V_T).

Leak checks are typically performed when equipment is prepared for patient use, but these checks also can be performed while the equipment is in use, for example, if a patient circuit is changed. Newer ICU ventilators can automatically perform the patient-ventilator circuit test. A leak check can also be performed manually if a leak develops during patient ventilation. While the patient is ventilated manually, the clinician changes the ventilator mode to volume-controlled ventilation (VC-CMV) and sets the V_T to 100 mL, the flow to 20 L/minute, the inspiratory pause to 2 seconds, and the pressure limit to maximum. The patient Y-connector is occluded with sterile gauze, and the ventilator is cycled manually. The circuit pressure that develops during inspiration should plateau and hold at that level, falling no more than 10 cm H_2O during a 2-second pause. If the pressure falls more than this, a significant leak is present and must be corrected. If the leak cannot be corrected quickly and easily, a change of equipment may be necessary.

Inadequate Oxygenation

A condition of inadequate oxygenation is usually signaled by activation of a low S_pO_2 alarm. Patients typically demonstrate tachycardia (although bradycardia may also occur) along with other signs of hypoxemia. (See Table 4-1 for the signs and symptoms of hypoxia.) Note that arterial blood gas analysis is required to confirm the presence of hypoxemia. It is important to recognize that worsening hypoxemia can be an ominous sign of deteriorating lung function.

Inadequate Ventilatory Support

Inappropriate $\dot{V}_E$ and ventilator settings can cause an increased WOB, which can ultimately lead to patient-ventilator asynchrony. Respiratory acidosis and hypoxemia may also be seen in cases

where the patient experiences an increased WOB. (Chapter 17 contains more information on the effects of increased WOB.)

Trigger Sensitivity

The ventilator's trigger sensitivity level can be improperly set. Autotriggering is a sign that the trigger sensitivity is set too low. Lack of ventilator response to a patient's inspiratory efforts may be the result of incorrect sensitivity settings, low-flow settings, or a poorly responsive internal demand valve. The trigger sensitivity may also be altered when a nebulizer is being used that is powered by an external gas source, which can blunt the machine's ability to sense a patient breath. Other causes are water in the inspiratory line and the presence of auto-PEEP.

Inappropriate sensitivity can be corrected easily by simply increasing or decreasing the sensitivity setting. If this does not solve the problem, the other causes mentioned must be addressed individually.

Inadequate Flow Setting

A low inspiratory gas flow can be corrected by increasing the flow setting or by changing the flow pattern, such as using a descending ramp rather than a rectangular flow pattern. A concave inspiratory pressure scalar during VC-CMV indicates active inspiration with inadequate flow (Fig. 18-3).[11] Changing the mode of ventilation also may be an effective means of providing adequate flow to the patient. For example, switching from VC-CMV to pressure ventilation with a volume target (e.g., pressure-regulated volume control) can change the flow pattern and sometimes relieve distress.

Other Examples of Patient-Ventilator Asynchrony

In addition to an inappropriate sensitivity setting and inadequate flow, other types of patient-ventilator asynchrony can occur (see Chapter 17). For example, auto-PEEP, an increased ventilatory drive, or the need for sedation may manifest as patient-ventilator asynchrony. In such cases the airway pressure (P_{aw}) usually fluctuates dramatically; the respiratory therapist must determine the cause and correct the problem (Box 18-6).[11,12] For example, with auto-PEEP the patient may have trouble triggering a breath. For patients with COPD with airflow obstruction, setting low levels of PEEP may alleviate the problem (see Box 7-1 and Fig. 7-1, *A* and *B*).[9,13]

Asynchronous breathing may also be seen in patients with COPD when pressure support ventilation (PSV) is used. COPD patients often show active short inspirations and active long expirations.[14] If the patient begins to exhale actively during the inspiratory phase of PSV, the flow may not drop to the necessary cycling value to end inspiration on the pressure-supported breath, resulting in a sudden rise in the scalar at the end of the breath.[15] This problem can be avoided by having these patients use a ventilator with adjustable flow-cycling characteristics.

During PSV another problem may occur in patients with a high-flow demand when pressures are set too low. In markedly distressed patients, the transition to exhalation may be affected by the ventilator's ability to respond quickly and open the exhalation valve.[16]

If all efforts have been made to resolve a patient-ventilator asynchrony problem and a solution cannot be found, medications may be necessary. Sedatives, used either alone or with neuromuscular blocking agents, may be the most effective method to relieve severely distressed patients (see Chapter 15). However, the clinician must make a systematic attempt to find the cause of the

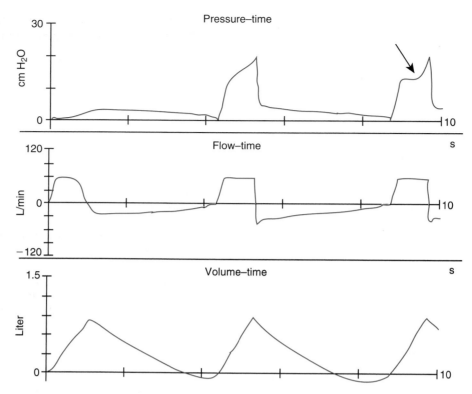

Fig. 18-3 Before the delivery of a mandatory breath (constant flow, volume-controlled continuous mandatory ventilation [VC-CMV]), patient effort reaches the trigger threshold, and a normal breath is delivered (breath on left). The second breath (right) is patient triggered, but the pressure curve *(arrow)* is concave because of the patient's active attempt to inhale. (From Nilsestuen JO, Hargett KD: Using ventilator graphics to identify patient-ventilator asynchrony, Respir Care 50:202-234, 2005.)

| BOX **18-6** | **Resolution of Various Types of Ventilator Asynchrony*** |

- **Trigger asynchrony:** Confirm that the sensitivity level has been set appropriately, that air trapping (auto-PEEP) is not present, and that the patient is not agitated.
- **Flow asynchrony:** Ensure the flow is adequate and the flow delivery curve is appropriate.
- **Cycle asynchrony:** With PSV, ensure that the patient is not exhaling actively; with pressure control ventilation (PC-CMV), make sure the duration set for the T$_I$ is not too long.
- **Mode asynchrony:** Occurs when more than one type of breath is delivered, such as with IMV; another mode may be more appropriate for the patient.
- **PEEP asynchrony:** Causes include overdistention from excess PEEP and atelectasis and atelectrauma from a PEEP setting that is too low; make sure PEEP is set at an appropriate level.
- **Closed-loop ventilation asynchrony:** Closed-loop mode may not be performing as needed for a particular patient. Make sure current settings are appropriate. Consider selecting another mode.

*See Chapter 17 for additional information.

problem and correct it as quickly as possible before recommending medications.

COMMON ALARM SITUATIONS

Ventilators and monitoring equipment have a number of alarms to notify the practitioner of changes in a patient's status. Appropriate use of these alarms is essential for patient safety (see Chapter 7).[17]

Low-Pressure Alarm

As already discussed, low-pressure alarms are most often activated by leaks (Box 18-7).[18,19] When a low-pressure alarm activates, the clinician first should check to ensure the patient is being ventilated. If the alarm occurs because the patient is inadvertently disconnected from the ventilator, then the patient should simply be reconnected. Otherwise, the patient may need to be ventilated with a manual resuscitator until the source of the leak is identified. Once the problem has been identified, the clinician should reset the alarm, making sure that it is set about 5 to 10 cm H_2O below PIP.

High-Pressure Alarm

High-pressure alarms are incorporated into all current ICU ventilators (Box 18-8).[18,19] High-pressure limits usually are set about 10 cm H_2O above PIP. Conditions leading to activation of high-pressure alarms can be categorized as airway problems, changes in the patient's lung characteristics or patient-related conditions, and problems related to the patient-ventilator circuit.

Audible and visible high-pressure alarms are typically activated when a patient coughs or bites on the ET. High-pressure alarms

| BOX 18-7 | Common Causes of Low-Pressure Alarms |

- Patient disconnection
- Circuit leaks
- Disconnection of the inspiratory or expiratory tubing of the ventilator circuit
  - Humidifiers
  - Filters
  - Water traps
  - Inline metered-dose inhalers
  - Inline nebulizers
  - Proximal pressure monitors
  - Flow monitoring lines
  - Exhaled gas monitoring devices
  - Inline closed-suction catheters
- Temperature monitors
- Exhalation valve leaks
  - Cracked or leaking valves
  - Unseated valves
  - Improperly connected valves
- Airway leaks
  - Use of minimum leak technique
  - Inadequate endotracheal tube (ET) cuff inflation
  - Leak in pilot balloon or cut pilot balloon
  - Rupture of ET cuff
  - Migration of ET into upper airway above the vocal cords
- Chest tube leaks

| BOX 18-8 | Common Causes of High-Pressure Alarms |

Conditions Related to the Airway
- Coughing
- Secretions or mucus in the airway
- Patient biting on the ET (oral intubation)
- Kinking of the ET inside the mouth or in the back of the throat
- Impingement of the ET on the trachea or carina
- Changes in the position of the ET (i.e., migration of the tube into the right mainstem bronchus)
- Herniation of the ET cuff over the end of the tube

Conditions Related to the Lungs
- Increased airway resistance (e.g., secretions, mucosal edema, bronchospasm)
- Decreased compliance (e.g., pneumothorax, pleural effusion)
- Patient-ventilator asynchrony

Changes in the Ventilator Circuit
- Accumulation of water condensate in the patient circuit
- Kinking in the inspiratory circuit
- Malfunction in the inspiratory or expiratory valves

also will become activated when secretions build up in the patient's airway. Coughing usually is self-limited and does not require treatment. Use of a bite block or oropharyngeal airway may help prevent unresponsive patients from biting on the ET. Some commercially available ET holders have built-in bite blocks. Conscious and responsive patients can be instructed not to bite on the tube; sometimes they listen. Secretions often can be removed by suctioning.

| TABLE 18-1 | Patterns of Alteration in Thoracic Pressure–Volume Relationships |

PARAMETER	CASE 1* 1 Hour Ago	CASE 1* Now	CASE 2† 1 Hour Ago	CASE 2† Now
Tidal volume (mL)	600	600	600	600
Plateau pressure (cm H$_2$O)	10	10	10	30
Peak pressure (cm H$_2$O)	20	40	20	40
Static compliance (mL/cm H$_2$O)	60	60	60	20
Dynamic characteristic (mL/cm H$_2$O)	30	15	30	15

From Tobin MJ: What should a clinician do when a patient "fights the ventilator"? Respir Care 36:395-406, 1991.
*The plateau pressure has not changed in case 1; therefore an airway problem should be suspected.
†The plateau pressure has increased in case 2, but no increase is seen in the gradient between the peak pressure and the plateau pressure; therefore a pneumothorax, mainstem intubation, or atelectasis should be suspected.

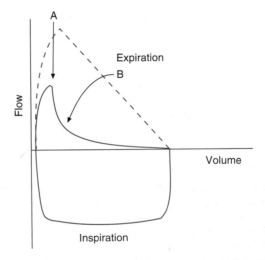

Fig. 18-4 Flow–volume loop. Inspiration occurs below the *x*-axis, and expiration occurs above it. *Arrow A* indicates the peak expiratory flow. *Arrow B* indicates increased expiratory resistance with reduced expiratory flow (*solid line*). The *dashed line* represents the predicted expiratory flow loop for this patient.

Conditions that adversely affect a patient's lung characteristics (e.g., increased airway resistance [R_{aw}] or decreased lung compliance [C_L]) or spontaneous breathing efforts also can trigger high-pressure alarms. Examples of conditions that increase R_{aw} are bronchospasm, secretions, and mucosal edema. Conditions most often seen in the ICU that are associated with decreased C_L include ARDS, pneumonia, pneumothorax, pleural effusions, abdominal distention, and ascites. Identifying R_{aw} and C_L changes can be identified on physical examination by listening to breath sounds and evaluating changes in the PIP and $P_{plateau}$ (Table 18-1) and by interpreting ventilator graphics (Case Studies 18-2 and 18-3; Fig. 18-4).

A high-pressure alarm may also be triggered when a patient actively breathes out of synchrony with the ventilator. PIP rises if the patient actively exhales while the ventilator is in the inspiratory phase, and this can activate the high-pressure alarm. A change in a ventilator setting or in the patient's condition that results in air trapping in the lungs (i.e., auto-PEEP) also causes the PIP to rise and may trigger an alarm.

It is important to recognize that PIP may also be elevated if problems arise in the patient-ventilator circuit. Accumulated water from condensation can lead to oscillations in the gas flow through the circuit and subsequent fluctuations in P_{aw}. Water in the circuit can lead to autotriggering, increased PIP, and sometimes activation of a high-pressure alarm. Kinks in the circuit also can lead to an increased PIP and alarm activation.

Several possible problems should be considered when circuit pressures are rising. For example, nebulized medications can accumulate on the expiratory filter or the exhalation valve, leading to increased resistance to gas flow through the filter or valve. Consequently, the exhalation valve may be unable to open completely. If the valves are malfunctioning, they should be cleaned or replaced, and the sensor should be recalibrated to correct the problem. HMEs also can accumulate excessive secretions, which can lead to increased flow resistance.[20] Notice how slowly the expiratory flow and the expiratory volume return to baseline in Fig. 18-3. This is a graphic example of increased expiratory resistance. (NOTE: A partly obstructed HME can also produce this type of expiratory feature.)

Regardless of the cause of a high-pressure alarm, the patient's safety must always be the clinician's first priority (Key Point 18-4). The clinician must ensure that the patient has a patent airway and is being ventilated and oxygenated.

 Key Point **18-4** Whenever a problem arises, the clinician's first priority must always be the patient's safety.

 Case Study 18-2

Evaluating Peak Inspiratory Pressure (PIP) and Plateau Pressure ($P_{plateau}$) in Volume-Controlled (VC) Ventilation

A 28-year-old man is receiving ventilatory support with VC-CMV. A high-pressure alarm has activated on several occasions over the past 4 hours. The following parameters were noted:

Time	Volume (L)	PIP (cm H$_2$O)	$P_{plateau}$ (cm H$_2$O)
12:00	0.5	25	19
14:00	0.5	34	29
16:00	0.5	39	33

The patient had been admitted 72 hours earlier following a motor vehicle crash in which he sustained chest trauma without pneumothorax. He has been receiving ventilatory support for the past 36 hours because of severe hypoxemia and increased WOB that progressed to acute respiratory failure.

At 16:00 hours the respiratory therapist notes bilateral crackles, particularly in the lung bases, where the percussion note was dull. A chest radiograph shows bilateral infiltrates. What caused the increase in PIP and $P_{plateau}$? Suggest a possible diagnosis for this patient based on the clinical findings.

Low PEEP/CPAP Alarms

Low PEEP/CPAP alarms activate when the airway pressure falls below the desired baseline during PEEP or CPAP. This may occur when the ventilator cannot compensate for a leak in the circuit. Another possible cause of a low-pressure alarm is active inspiration by the patient. Active inspiration can cause the pressure to drop below the alarm setting. The machine sensitivity may not be responsive enough to the patient's effort, or the ventilator demand valve may not open quickly enough in response to flow demand. For example, if inspiratory gas flow is set too low and the demand valve does not respond to the patient's inspiratory effort, the PEEP level drops, which may activate the alarm.

Apnea Alarm

Activation of an apnea alarm may indicate patient apnea or patient disconnection, system leaks, inadequate machine sensitivity, or inappropriately set apnea parameters. An apnea alarm also may be accompanied by a low-pressure or low $\dot{V}_E$ alarm. Some ventilators have a preset apnea period of 20 seconds, whereas others allow the operator to set the apnea period. Ventilators are designed to detect spontaneous and mandatory breaths. Thus, when an apnea alarm sounds, the most obvious cause is patient apnea. After ensuring that the patient is being ventilated, the clinician should check the mandatory breathing rate and the machine's sensitivity. The clinician should also check for possible leaks or patient disconnection. In cases where auto-PEEP is present, patient triggering may be more difficult, resulting in undetected efforts. A ventilator set in a spontaneous mode (e.g., PSV or CPAP) could misinterpret this as apnea.

 Case Study 18-3

Evaluating PIP and Volume in Pressure Control Ventilation

A patient with a history of asthma is receiving mechanical ventilation in the PC-CMV mode following open heart surgery. Occasionally the high-pressure alarm is activated when the patient coughs or appears to try to exhale forcibly. The low V_T alarm is also activated several times. The following values were obtained while monitoring the patient:

Time	Volume (L)	PIP (cm H$_2$O)	f (breaths/min)
09:00	0.75	25	8
10:00	0.68	25	9
11:00	0.6	25	11

Figure 18-4 shows the flow–volume loop measured on the patient at 11:00 hours. Breath sounds reveal bilateral scattered wheezes. What caused the change in volume delivery? What therapy would you recommend?

Some ventilators provide a backup mode of ventilation when the apnea alarm is activated. Backup modes generally provide a minimum safe level of ventilation for the patient until the operator can respond to the alarm and correct the problem. Some ventilators cancel the backup mode once a patient effort is detected (e.g., Puritan Bennett 840, Coviden-Nellcor Puritan Bennett, Boulder, Colo.).

Low-Source Gas Pressure or Power Input Alarm

A low-source gas alarm activates if the gas source fails or the high-pressure line becomes disconnected from the gas source. With ventilators equipped with an air compressor, the operator must ensure that the compressor is operating. (NOTE: Some earlier generation ventilators, such as the Bear 1000 [CareFusion, Viasys Corp, San Diego, Calif.], use an on/off switch that must be turned on; current ICU ventilators, such as the Puritan Bennett 840, automatically turn on the compressor when there is a loss of pressure in the patient-ventilator circuit.) The operator must ensure that the air and oxygen lines are connected to an active gas supply, such as a wall outlet.

Modern microprocessor-controlled ventilators require an electrical power source. If a power-loss alarm activates, the clinician should first confirm that the unit is connected to an active electrical outlet and has not been unplugged. If the electrical outlet is working and the unit fails to start, the line fuse or circuit breaker may need to be replaced or reset. Most ICU ventilators have a reset button near the "power on" switch. In the event of an overall power outage, the ventilator should be plugged into a red electrical outlet (these outlets are connected to emergency generator power supplies). Many ICU ventilators have backup battery power sufficient to operate a unit for 30 minutes to 4 hours, depending on the ventilator and the battery source.

Ventilator Inoperative Alarm and Technical Error Message

With microprocessor-controlled ventilators, an inoperative alarm or a technical error message is displayed if an internal malfunction is detected by the ventilator's self-testing systems. This most often occurs when the ventilator is first turned on. Sometimes simply turning the machine off and then back on corrects the error. If it does not, it may be necessary to replace the ventilator and contact the manufacturer's representative.

Operator Settings Incompatible with Machine Parameters

An error message or alarm (or both) is triggered if the operator tries to select a setting that is outside the range for that parameter or is incompatible with the other selected settings. For example, if the clinician tries to set a V_T of 50 mL and the V_T range for the ventilator is 200 to 2000 mL, the ventilator will indicate that that setting cannot be selected. Another example of an incompatible setting can occur when using volume control ventilation. If the operator sets an inspiratory gas flow that cannot deliver the set V_T within an acceptable time based on the set f, the machine produces an error message asking the operator to correct the flow or reduce the V_T.

Inspiratory-to-Expiratory Ratio Indicator and Alarm

Most current ICU ventilators do not allow the inspiratory-to-expiratory (I:E) ratio to exceed 1:1 unless the operator specifically wants to use an inverse I:E ratio. This generally requires activation of a separate control or touch pad or some similar function that alerts the operator that the ratio is being inverted.

An inverse-ratio alarm may activate if a change occurs in the patient lung's characteristic (i.e., increased R_{aw} or decreased C_L), resulting in a lower inspiratory flow. This does not happen often, however, because most ventilators have enough power to maintain the desired gas flow. Another possibility is a flow setting that is too

low for the desired V_T delivery. The I:E ratio can also change when the selected waveform is changed. For example, changing from a constant flow to a descending ramp waveform may lengthen the T_I in a volume-cycled ventilator. Selection of an inspiratory pause can also lengthen T_I. In pressure-controlled ventilation, a long T_I (depending on the set f) may activate the I:E ratio indicator.

Other Alarms

Additional alarms may be available on many ICU ventilators, including high PEEP/CPAP alarms, low and high V_T alarms, low and high $\dot{V}_E$ alarms, a high f alarm, and low and high F_IO_2 alarms. High PEEP/CPAP alarms often are activated by the same problems that lead to high-pressure alarms. Low V_T and low $\dot{V}_E$ alarms usually activate in situations that cause low-pressure alarms or when the patient's spontaneous ventilation has decreased for some reason. Flow-sensor disconnection, leaks, or malfunction can also cause activation of these alarms.

High V_T, high f, and high $\dot{V}_E$ alarms can activate if the patient's $\dot{V}_E$ has increased, or when the ventilator is too sensitive to patient effort (i.e., autotriggering). High $\dot{V}_E$ alarms also may be activated if a nebulizer powered by a separate external gas source is inline with the main circuit. These problems may be caused by inappropriate calibration, contamination, or malfunction of flow sensors.

Box 18-9 and Fig. 18-5 present several clinical situations that can be associated with alarm activation. It is important that clinicians become familiar with the types of equipment used in their facilities and the various alarm systems available.

USE OF GRAPHICS TO IDENTIFY VENTILATOR PROBLEMS

Ventilator graphic displays can provide valuable information that clinicians can use to evaluate the integrity of the patient-ventilator system (Key Point 18-5). A detailed review of ventilator graphics was presented in Chapter 9, and examples of ventilator-associated problems have been discussed throughout the text. The following discussion provides a summary of how ventilator graphics can be used to identify problems encountered with the patient-ventilator interface.

> **Key Point** 18-5 Ventilator graphic displays can provide valuable information that clinicians can use to evaluate the integrity of the patient-ventilator system.

Leaks

As previously discussed, inadvertent patient disconnection and leaks in the patient-ventilator circuit are common during mechanical ventilation. When these situations arise, low-pressure, low-volume, low $\dot{V}_E$, or apnea alarms usually become activated. Volume–time scalars are one means of identifying leaks, as are pressure–volume and flow–volume loops (see Chapter 9 for more details). In each graphic representation, the most important indicator of a leak can be found using the expiratory volume curve. If the expiratory volume does not return to zero in any of these waveforms, a leak is present in the system (Figs. 18-6 and 18-7; Case Studies 18-4 and 18-5). In some cases the volume tracing may drop below zero; this finding indicates that the equipment needs to be recalibrated (see Fig. 18-1). This also can occur if the patient is actively exhaling.

BOX 18-9   Ventilator Troubleshooting: Response to Alarms and Abnormal Waveforms

If an alarm activates or an abnormal waveform appears:
1. Assess the patient's appearance to evaluate for distress.
2. Ensure that the patient is receiving adequate ventilation and oxygenation.
3. If necessary, and if the patient is suffering severe distress, disconnect the patient from the ventilator and manually ventilate, adding PEEP (if needed, and increase the F_IO_2.)
4. Reassess the patient.
5. Check the activated alarm, and make sure alarm parameters have been set appropriately.
6. Once the cause of problem has been determined, resolve it.
7. If the problem cannot be resolved, change the ventilator or call for help.

Common Alarm Situations
Low-Pressure Alarm
1. Check for patient disconnection.
2. Check for leaks in the patient circuit related to the artificial airway and through chest tubes.
3. Confirm that the proximal pressure line is connected and unobstructed.
4. Low-pressure alarm may be accompanied by a low minute ventilation ($\dot{V}_E$) or low tidal volume (V_T) alarm.

High-Pressure Alarm
1. If the patient is coughing, check to determine whether secretions have built up in the airway or the patient is biting the endotracheal tube (ET).
2. Check for kinking or displacement of the ET; also check the tube's position in the airway (i.e., ensure that the ET is not inserted too far into the trachea).
3. Check whether R_{aw} has increased or C_L has decreased.
4. Ensure that the main inspiratory or expiratory lines are not kinked or obstructed.
5. Check that the patient is breathing synchronously with the ventilator.
6. Determine whether air trapping (auto-PEEP) has developed.
7. Ensure that the expiratory filter and expiratory valve are functioning properly.

Low Positive End-Expiratory or PEEP/CPAP Alarms
1. Check to determine whether the low PEEP alarm is set below the applied PEEP level.
2. Determine whether the patient is actively inspiring below baseline.
3. Determine whether a leak is present.
4. Confirm that the patient has not become disconnected from the ventilator.
5. Ensure that the proximal airway pressure (P_{aw}) line is not occluded.

Apnea Alarm
1. Determine whether the patient is apneic.
2. Check for leaks.
3. Check the sensitivity setting to be sure that the ventilator can detect patient effort.
4. Check the alarm-time interval and the volume setting, when appropriate.

Low-Source Gas Pressure or Power Input Alarm
1. Check the 50 psi gas source (e.g., wall connection, cylinder, or air compressor).
2. Check high-pressure hose connections to the ventilator.
3. Check ventilator's electrical power supply and whether it is plugged into the electrical outlet that is connected to the emergency backup system.
4. Check the line fuse or circuit breaker.
5. Try using the reset button.
6. If alarms continue, replace the ventilator.

Ventilator Inoperative Alarm or Technical Error Message
1. If an internal malfunction message is present and the ventilator is turned on, try turning the ventilator off and restarting it.
2. If alarm continues, follow message instructions or replace the ventilator.

Operator Settings Incompatible with Machine Parameters
1. Error message usually indicates that a parameter must be reset (e.g., flow is not high enough to deliver V_T within an acceptable T_I to keep the I:E ratio below 1:1 [based on f, V_T, and flow]).
2. Adjust the appropriate controls.

Inspiratory-to-Expiratory (I:E) Ratio Indicator and Alarm
1. Usually indicates an I:E ratio greater than 1:1.
2. If inverse I:E ratio is a goal, disable the I:E ratio limit or ignore the audible warning.
3. If normal I:E ratios are a goal, check alarm causes:
   - If increased R_{aw} or decreased C_L has resulted in a lower flow, treat the cause.
   - If the flow setting is too low for the desired V_T delivery, increase flow or change the flow waveform.

Other Possible Alarms
1. High PEEP/CPAP alarms
   - Causes are similar to those for high-pressure alarms.
   - In flow-cycled modes (e.g., PSV), check for system leaks.
2. Low V_T, low $\dot{V}_E$, and/or low f alarms
   - Causes are similar to those for low-pressure alarms.
   - Determine whether spontaneous ventilation has decreased for some reason.
   - Verify that all alarms have been set appropriately.
   - Check flow sensor for disconnection or malfunction.
3. High V_T, high $\dot{V}_E$, or high f alarms
   - Check machine sensitivity level for autotriggering.
   - Check for possible cause of increased patient $\dot{V}_E$.
   - Ensure alarms have been set appropriately.
   - If an external nebulizer is in use, reset the alarm until the treatment is finished, then return the alarm to the appropriate setting.
   - Check the flow sensors for calibration, contamination, or malfunction.
4. Low or high F_IO_2 alarm
   - Check gas source.
   - Make sure built-in oxygen analyzer is functioning properly.

Increased V_T, $\dot{V}_E$, or rate alarm

Low pressure, low PEEP, low V_T, $\dot{V}_E$

(Flowchart A — left side)

Verify patient stability and adequacy of ventilation.

Is patient demand $\dot{V}_E$ increased? — Yes → Check cause of increased $\dot{V}_E$ demand to determine if change is needed.

No ↓

Is the ventilator auto-triggering? — Yes → 1. Check the sensitivity setting. 2. Check the MMV setting.

No ↓

Is an external nebulizer in use? — Yes → Adjust ventilator settings appropriately until treatment is completed.

No ↓

Is the flow sensor malfunctioning? — Yes → 1. Clean and recalibrate the sensor. 2. Clear the sensor line. 3. Check its function and replace as necessary.

No ↓

Is the alarm set too low? — Yes → Adjust the alarm setting.

No ↓

Check the operator's manual and/or contact the manufacturer's technical representative.

A

(Flowchart B — right side)

Verify patient stability and adequacy of ventilation.

Is the patient disconnected? — Yes → Reconnect.

No ↓

Is there a leak in the patient circuit? — Yes → Eliminate the circuit leak.

No ↓

Is there a cuff leak? — Yes → Reinflate the cuff and check its pressure. → Does the leak recur? — Yes → Fix pilot line or reintubate the patient. / No → Resume ventilation.

No ↓

Is there a chest tube leak? — Yes → Contact physician and monitor patient.

No ↓

Is the proximal airway pressure line obstructed? — Yes → Clear the line.

No ↓

Is the flow sensor malfunctioning? — Yes → 1. Clear the sensor and recalibrate it. 2. Clear the sensor line and recheck it. 3. Check sensor function and replace sensor if necessary.

No ↓

Is the alarm set inappropriately? — Yes → Reset the alarm(s).

No ↓

Check the operator's manual and/or contact a trained specialist.

B

Fig. 18-5 Algorithms for troubleshooting activated alarms. **A,** Increased tidal volume (V_T), minute ventilation ($\dot{V}_E$), or rate alarm. *MMV,* Mandatory minute ventilation. **B,** Low-pressure, low positive end-expiratory/continuous positive airway pressure (PEEP/CPAP), low $\dot{V}_E$, low V_T, or low rate alarm.

Continued

Case Study 18-4

Problem Solving Using Ventilator Graphics

The respiratory therapist hears a low-pressure ventilator alarm for a patient receiving VC-CMV. She evaluates the patient and finds that the individual is not in distress and is being ventilated and oxygenated. She checks the activated alarm (i.e., low $\dot{V}_E$), silences it, and saves the graphics display. Figure 18-7 shows the saved graphs. What do these waveforms indicate?

Case Study 18-5

Evaluating a Ventilator Problem

During ventilation of a patient with VC-CMV and 10 cm H_2O of PEEP, the respiratory therapist notices the volume–time graphic shown below. During exhalation the respiratory therapist feels an uninterrupted flow of a small amount of air from the exhalation valve, even though the patient has had no previous evidence of air trapping. What do these findings suggest?

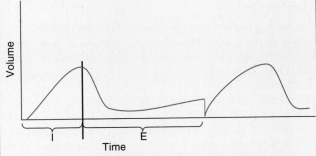

Volume–time curve in which the volume curve descends at the beginning of exhalation and then slowly rises until the start of the next inspiratory phase.

Inadequate Flow

Patient-ventilator asynchrony can occur if a ventilator provides only a fixed flow or an inadequate flow during mechanical ventilation. In such cases the pressure–time graphic is concave and the flow curve is constant (see Fig. 18-3).

Inadequate Sensitivity Setting for Patient Triggering

The ventilator's trigger sensitivity can be set too low for a patient. An inappropriately set sensitivity, like an inadequate flow setting, increases WOB (see Fig. 9-9).

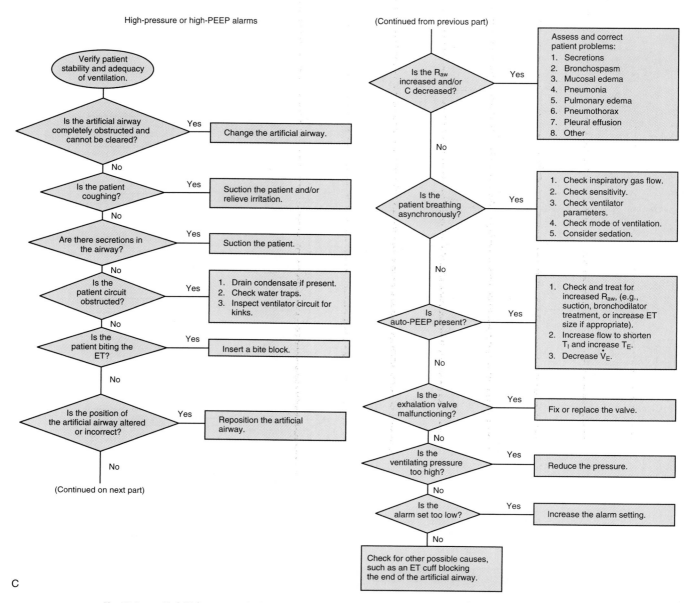

Fig. 18-5, cont'd **C,** High-pressure or high PEEP/CPAP alarm. *ET,* Endotracheal tube; *T_I,* inspiratory time; *T_E,* expiratory time; *C,* Compliance; *R_aw,* airway resistance.

Overinflation

Pressure–volume loops that produce a duck-bill, or "beak," appearance can be used to identify alveolar overinflation (see Fig. 13-6).

Auto-PEEP

Ventilator graphics can be used to detect auto-PEEP. If expiratory flow does not return to zero on a flow–volume loop before the next mandatory breath, auto-PEEP is present (Fig. 18-8).

Inadequate Inspiratory Time During Pressure Ventilation

One goal of pressure-controlled ventilation (PC-CMV) may be to provide a T_I long enough to achieve a slight plateau effect so that the inspiratory flow drops to zero before the end of inspiration (see Fig. 5-2C). Sometimes this plateau is not present because of

changes in the patient's lung characteristics or a short T_I (see Fig. 5-2). The T_I may need to be adjusted, depending on the clinical situation.

Waveform Ringing

When flow and pressure delivery are very high at the beginning of a breath, particularly during a pressure breath, a phenomenon known as *ringing, spiking,* or *overshoot* can result from the oscillation of air in the patient-ventilator circuit and in the upper airway at the beginning of inspiration (Fig. 18-9). This situation, although not life-threatening, does not represent a smooth breath delivery. Current ICU ventilators (e.g., Puritan Bennett 840, Servo-i, Dräger E-4 [Dräger Medical, Inc, Wayne, N.J.] and CareFusion AVEA [CareFusion, Viasys Corp, San Diego, Calif.]) allow adjustment of gas flow and pressure delivery at the beginning of a breath to help taper flow and pressure delivery and reduce overshoot. This feature

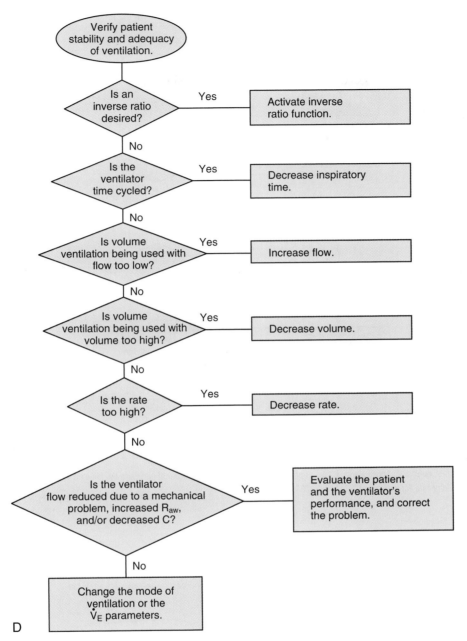

Fig. 18-5, cont'd D, Inverse I : E ratio indicator.   *Continued*

commonly is labeled the *inspiratory rise time*. Oscillation also can occur if condensation is present in the patient circuit. This latter situation can be easily remedied by draining of the circuit.

Expiratory Portion of Volume–Time Curve Below Baseline

In patients with air trapping, active exhalation may cause the expiratory portion of the volume–time curve to drop below baseline. A curve also may descend below baseline if the expiratory flow sensor is out of calibration (see Fig. 18-1).

Patient-Ventilator Asynchrony

Figures 18-3 and 18-10 show graphics for a patient breathing out of synchrony with the ventilator. As mentioned earlier,

patient-ventilator asynchrony can occur when the flow and sensitivity settings are inadequate or when auto-PEEP is present. Adjustment of these parameters or switching to a servo-controlled mode (e.g., pressure-regulated volume control) or to pressure-controlled ventilation may help to alleviate the problem. The patient may also need to be sedated.

UNEXPECTED VENTILATOR RESPONSES

Problems in some microprocessor-controlled ventilators can result from inappropriate use of or idiosyncrasies associated with the machine. The following section discusses a few noteworthy situations; the intent is not to criticize any particular ventilator but rather to make the reader aware of situations that have been

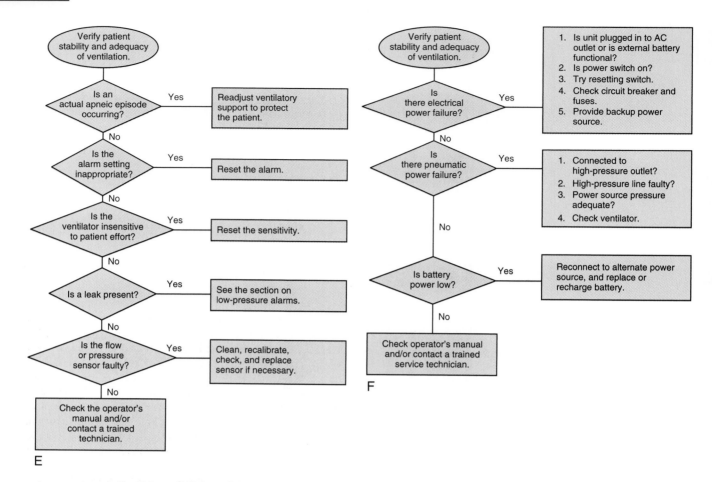

Fig. 18-5, cont'd **E,** Apnea alarm. **F,** Loss of power alarm. *AC,* Alternating current. (From Cairo JM, Pilbeam SP: Mosby's respiratory care equipment, ed 7, St Louis, 2004, Mosby.)

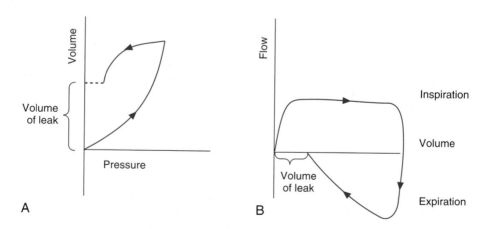

Fig. 18-6 Pressure–volume loop **(A)** and flow–volume loop **(B)** indicating an air leak.

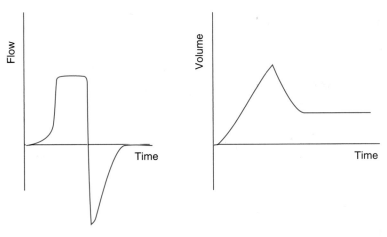

Fig. 18-7 Flow–time curve and volume–time curve demonstrating a problem.

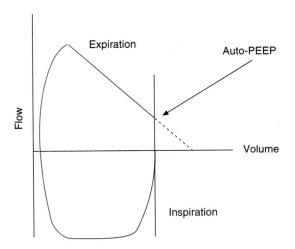

Fig. 18-8 Flow–volume loop reflecting the presence of auto-PEEP. The arrow indicates the amount of flow at the end of exhalation.

reported, including unseating of the exhalation valve, excessive CPAP/PEEP levels, changes in sensitivity, inability to trigger a pressure-supported breath, and altered alarm function.

Unseated or Obstructed Expiratory Valve

The expiratory valve can be unseated if it is blocked to obtain a static compliance (C_S) reading. (This generally is a problem only if the ventilator does not have an inspiratory pause control.) The valve is unseated because a pressure buildup during this procedure causes the exhalation valve to disengage. An unseated expiratory valve may be the cause if the "Venti.In-Op" alarm, a low-pressure alarm, or a low CPAP/PEEP alarm activates and the patient has difficulty breathing. It is important to mention that these same alarms can be activated by other factors, therefore the actual cause must be established.

Expiratory valves may also malfunction if they become obstructed or if their mobility is impaired by an accumulation of residue from medications delivered by small-volume nebulizers. The valves can be protected by placing bacterial filters inline, before the exhalation valve. Expiratory filters must be changed frequently to avoid increased expiratory resistance.

Excessive CPAP/PEEP

Excessive CPAP/PEEP levels (i.e., above those set by the operator) can occur in certain clinical situations. For example, a potential problem that can occur with PSV is a sudden accidental delivery of high flow and pressure because of a leak in the breathing circuit. During PSV on the Bird 8400, increases in PEEP can also occur when a tracheal cuff leak is present. In this latter case, the ventilator attempts to compensate for the leak by increasing flows. Application of high flow to maintain CPAP/PEEP levels can cause the airway pressure to rise, and the patient may develop dyspnea, tachypnea, and tachycardia.[21,22] This problem can typically be solved by eliminating the leak.

Another problem that involves patient-circuit leaks can occur during PSV. This problem was initially reported with the Puritan Bennett 7200 (Covidien-Nellcor Puritan Bennett, Boulder, Colo.).[23] If a leak of more than 5 L/min develops around the cuff of the ET or somewhere in the patient circuit, the set PSV level will be maintained throughout the cycle, causing CPAP to develop in the circuit. A drop in flow to 5 L/min is the normal mechanism that stops the PSV inspiratory phase in this ventilator. All ventilators with PSV now have a safety mechanism. If the T_I exceeds a preset time (approximately 3 to 5 seconds), the ventilator will cycle into expiration.

Nebulizer Impairment of Patient's Ability to Trigger a Pressure-Supported Breath

During PSV the patient must create a slightly negative pressure or drop in flow in the circuit to initiate a breath. When a continuous-flow nebulizer is placed between the patient and the sensing mechanism, the patient often finds it more difficult to generate the effort to trigger the ventilator. Devices that sense ventilator triggering usually are on the inspiratory side of the ventilator. Triggering difficulty is especially apparent in older patients with COPD and weak inspiratory efforts.[24,25] (NOTE: This problem may arise with microprocessor-controlled ventilators whenever a nebulizer powered by an external gas source is used.)

Triggering difficulty may also occur with patients during the VC-CMV when an external nebulizer is added in line. It may not be a significant clinical problem because the set rate and volume ensure the patient will receive an adequate $\dot{V}_E$, even if the patient does not trigger the breath. Unfortunately, there is not a backup rate with PSV and volume support ventilation.[26] Therefore

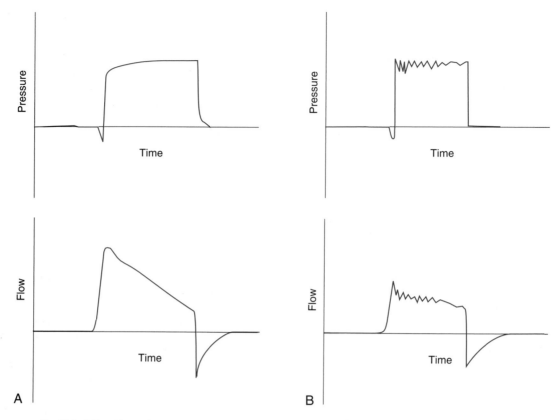

Fig. 18-9 **A,** Flow–time and pressure–time curves demonstrating a normal pressure-supported breath. **B,** Flow–time and pressure–time curves showing ringing (oscillations), a phenomenon that occurs with an overshoot of flow and pressure at the beginning of inspiration.

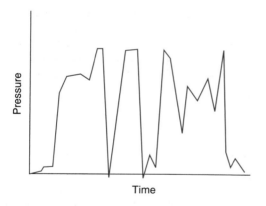

Fig. 18-10 Wide fluctuations can be seen in the pressure–time curve when the patient is actively breathing during mechanical ventilation, but the ventilator is not set up to respond to patient demand; the result is patient-ventilator asynchrony.

clinicians should use only the nebulizer provided by the ventilator's manufacturer. If one is not provided, the practitioner should use an inline metered-dose inhaler (MDI) with a spacer, an ultrasonic nebulizer, or a vibrating mesh nebulizer.

High Tidal Volume Delivery

High V_T delivery can occur when externally powered small-volume nebulizers are used for aerosol delivery. Flowmeters add extra flow to the patient circuit, which can increase the delivered V_T and result in artificially high readings of exhaled $\dot{V}_E$. Although this is not a significant problem in most situations with adults, it can be very significant in neonates, and these devices should not be used for medication delivery during neonatal mechanical ventilation.

High V_T delivery also can occur in a ventilator that allows the patient to receive additional flow during inspiration on demand. For example, current ICU ventilators (e.g., Servo-i) provide additional flow if the airway pressure drops by 2 cm H_2O. This results in a higher V_T delivery than the set value. Set values, therefore, actually represent minimum V_T delivery; patients can receive the volume of air they want.

Altered Alarm Function

Some monitoring devices and ventilator controls operate on optical detectors. When exposed to intense light, such as sunlight through a window, the alarms may sound even though no change has occurred in the patient's status. This may happen with volume monitors, pulse oximeters, and other light-sensitive devices.

Electromagnetic Interference

Electrical devices that emit radio frequencies, such as cell phones, can interfere with the operation of medical equipment. Hospitals generally prohibit the use of cell phones, walkie-talkies, and similar equipment in locations such as the ICU, where problems are likely to occur. These devices have been known to interfere with the function of mechanical ventilators, infusion pumps, smoke detectors, and telemetry equipment. Other medical devices that can be affected include ECG monitors and machines, oxygen and apnea monitors, defibrillators, blood warmers, and dialysis units.[27]

When the purchase of a piece of equipment such as a mechanical ventilator is under consideration, the hospital should determine what built-in safeguards the manufacturer has provided to prevent electromagnetic interference.

Other Ventilator Problems

The operating manuals for microprocessor-controlled ventilators provide information on troubleshooting problems. They also provide information about troubleshooting situations that are unique to their particular ventilator.

SUMMARY

- *Problem solving* can be simply defined as determining a solution to a challenging situation. The first step in solving any problem is to carefully analyze the situation at hand. The next step is to gather and assess pertinent data, which should point to a number of viable solutions.
- The sudden onset of dyspnea can be identified by observing the physical signs of respiratory distress, including tachypnea, nasal flaring, diaphoresis, use of the accessory muscles of breathing, retraction of the suprasternal, supraclavicular, and intercostal spaces, paradoxical or abnormal movement of the thorax and abdomen, and abnormal findings on auscultation.
- Identifying the cause of patient-ventilator asynchrony can be accomplished using a relatively simple approach. If the patient is in **severe** distress, the first step is to disconnect the patient from the ventilator and carefully ventilate the patient using a manual resuscitation bag. When a resuscitation bag is used properly, these devices allow for the assessment of lung characteristics.
- The most common patient-related problems encountered during mechanical ventilation involve the artificial airway or the presence of a pneumothorax, bronchospasm, and excessive secretions.
- Evaluation of the patient's secretions can be useful in differentiating a variety of patient-related problems.
- Changes in the patient's position can be associated with accidental extubation, bending and twisting of the patient circuit, and in some cases alterations in the patient's level of oxygenation.
- Activation of low-pressure, low-volume, and low V_E alarms typically indicates that a leak in the patient-ventilator circuit is present.
- Circuit leaks typically occur at the level of the ET and at junctions in the patient circuit where tube connections exist.
- In addition to an inappropriate sensitivity setting and inadequate flow, other types of patient-ventilator asynchrony can be associated with auto-PEEP, an increased ventilatory drive, or the need for sedation.
- Activation of an apnea alarm may indicate patient apnea or patient disconnection, system leaks, inadequate machine sensitivity, or inappropriately set apnea parameters.
- A low-source gas alarm activates if the gas source fails or the high-pressure line becomes disconnected from the gas source.
- Conditions leading to activation of high-pressure alarms can be categorized as airway problems, changes in lung characteristics or patient-related conditions, and problems related to the patient-ventilator circuit.
- An error message or alarm (or both) is triggered if the operator tries to select a setting that is outside the range for that parameter or is incompatible with the other selected settings.
- Ventilator graphic displays can provide valuable information that clinicians can use to evaluate the integrity of the patient-ventilator system.
- Careful analysis is required to solve patient-ventilator system problems and troubleshoot malfunctions.
- Experience is an important part of the learning process. By using the knowledge gained through experience, practitioners can expand their ability to solve a particular problem.

REVIEW QUESTIONS *(See Appendix A for answers.)*

1. A 25-year-old man receiving mechanical ventilation is rotated from the supine position onto his right side. Immediately after this move, the high-pressure alarm on the ventilator activates. On auscultation, the respiratory therapist hears breath sounds only over the right lung. The centimeter marking of the ET is 25 cm. What should the therapist do to correct this situation?

2. A constant inspiratory flow of 40 L/min is set for a patient receiving VC-CMV. The ventilator I:E ratio indicator shows that I exceeds E. How could this problem be corrected without changing V_E?
   A. Shorten the expiratory time (T_E)
   B. Increase the f
   C. Lengthen the T_I
   D. Increase the inspiratory gas flow setting

3. A patient with COPD is treated with prednisone, theophylline, and furosemide (Lasix). Which of the following is the most important parameter to check regularly?
   A. Clotting times
   B. Calcium levels
   C. Potassium levels
   D. Pupillary response

4. A patient on mechanical ventilatory support is suctioned for large amounts of foul-smelling green sputum. The patient has a temperature of 38° C and a normal white blood cell count. Which of the following is the most likely cause of this problem?
   A. An overheated humidifier
   B. Cardiogenic pulmonary edema
   C. An asthma exacerbation
   D. A respiratory infection

5. Which of the following are potential problems that can result when an externally powered nebulizer is added to a mechanical ventilator circuit?
   1. It increases machine sensitivity.
   2. Expiratory monitor readings increase from previous values.
   3. It may add volume to the delivered V_T.
   4. In a patient-triggered mode, the added flow must be overcome by the patient to trigger the ventilator.
      A. 2
      B. 3
      C. 1 and 4
      D. 2, 3, and 4

6. What is the first step in managing a mechanically ventilated patient in severe distress? How can you tell whether the problem originates with the ventilator or the patient?

7. A 58-year-old man is intubated orally after cardiac arrest. The patient is admitted to the ICU, and ventilatory support is provided using volume control ventilation (VC-CMV) with 100% oxygen. The PIP has been increasing progressively over the past 4 hours. Auscultation of the patient's chest reveals an absence of breath sounds over the left lung and distant breath sounds over the right lung. The left hemithorax is dull to percussion, and the right chest is resonant. The trachea is deviated to the left. No chest radiograph is available. Briefly describe what is causing the problem and how it can be corrected.

8. The low-pressure and low-volume alarms activate on a ventilated patient. Auscultation over the trachea reveals a hiss during the entire mandatory breath cycle. What is the likely problem, and how would you correct it?

9. A patient is undergoing ventilation with bilevel positive airway pressure (bilevel PAP) with a full face mask. Initial pressure readings were an inspiratory positive airway pressure (IPAP) of 12 cm H_2O and an expiratory positive airway pressure (EPAP) of 3 cm H_2O, with a measured V_T of 0.55 to 0.6 L. The measured V_T with the same pressures 3 hours later is 0.3 to 0.45 L. Which of the following could be the cause of the drop in V_T?
   1. Air is leaking around an underinflated ET cuff.
   2. A decrease in the patient's C_L has occurred.
   3. Increase in the patient's R_{aw}.
   4. Ascites is restricting the patient's inspiratory efforts.
      A. 1 and 2 only
      B. 2 and 3 only
      C. 1, 2, and 3 only
      D. 1, 2, 3, and 4

10. While monitoring a patient on mechanical ventilatory support, the respiratory therapist hears the high-pressure alarm and notes that breath sounds are absent over the right lung and diminished over the left lung. The percussion note is tympanic on the right and resonant on the left. The patient's distress is not relieved when the respiratory therapist performs manual ventilation with 100% oxygen. What could cause these findings, and what should be done?

11. A 70-year-old woman with COPD is mechanically ventilated using volume-controlled continuous mandatory ventilation (VC-CMV). Although the sensitivity is at the most sensitive setting, the patient is struggling to breathe (using accessory muscles) and is unable to trigger a machine breath on her own. When breaths are delivered, the ventilator graphics show a concave pressure curve. Expiratory flow does not return to zero before the next mandatory breath is delivered. What is the likely cause of the problem?

12. The low-pressure and low-volume alarms activate on a patient receiving mechanical ventilatory support. The ventilator graphics indicate that the expired volume is lower than the inspired volume. Which of the following could cause this problem? (See Fig. 18-7.)
   1. Pneumothorax
   2. Pulmonary edema
   3. Disconnection from the ventilator
   4. Increased airway resistance
      A. 1 only
      B. 3 only
      C. 1, 2, and 3 only
      D. 1, 3, and 4 only

13. A 26-year-old man who was in a motor vehicle accident is transferred from a rural hospital to the urban trauma center. He is 6 feet 3 inches tall and weighs 200 lb. He suffered trauma to the chest and left leg (fractured left femur). Currently no pneumothorax or hemothorax is present, and he has no head or neck injuries. The artificial airway is a 7-French oral endotracheal tube in the correct position. The patient requires mechanical ventilation. Cuff pressure is 38 cm H_2O to provide the minimum leak technique. Do you think any immediate changes need to be made in the current management of this patient?

14. Difficulty is encountered in the ventilatory management of a patient with acute pancreatitis and ARDS. In PC-CMV, the set pressure is 30 cm H_2O with a T_I of 2 seconds and an I:E ratio of 1:1. The patient is heavily sedated, and the rate is set at 15 breaths/min. P_aO_2 is maintained at 61 mm Hg on an F_IO_2 of 0.5 and 15 cm H_2O of PEEP. However, over the past 4 hours, pH has dropped from 7.31 to 7.22, P_aCO_2 has risen from 45 to 53 mm Hg, and P_aO_2 has dropped to 54 mm Hg as the delivered V_T has steadily decreased. What change in ventilation would you suggest?

15. A respiratory therapist is monitoring a patient receiving CPAP through a freestanding system. The respiratory therapist notes that although a wick-type heated humidifier is in use, no rain-out (condensate) is present in the circuit. Which of the following would be appropriate to do in this situation?
   1. Nothing; this is not unusual
   2. Check that the heater is working
   3. Determine when the system was last changed
   4. Evaluate the system to see if water has been added to the humidifier
      A. 1 only
      B. 2 and 3 only
      C. 1, 2, and 4 only
      D. 1, 2, 3, and 4

16. A patient on VC-CMV receives a bronchodilator by MDI. The flow–volume graphics are shown in the figure below. How would you interpret this ventilator graphic as it relates to the patient's response to therapy?

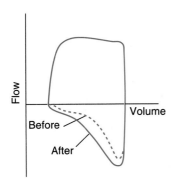

Flow–volume loop for a patient before and after bronchodilator therapy (Question 16).

17. While monitoring a patient on mechanical ventilation following open heart surgery, a respiratory therapist notes that the inspiratory volume is 550 mL and the expiratory volume is 375 mL. The ventilator volume–time and pressure–volume graphics appear in the figure below. Having established that a fairly large leak is present, the therapist checks the cuff and the ventilator circuit and cannot find a leak. What could be another possible source of the leak?

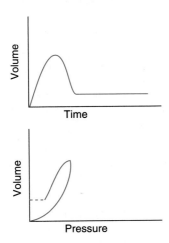

Volume–time curve and pressure–volume loop for a mechanically ventilated patient (Question 17).

18. A patient on PC-CMV has a set pressure of 12 cm H_2O. The pressure–time graphic appears in the figure below. R_{aw} is 12 cm H_2O, and static lung compliance is 30 cm H_2O. The patient is actively inspiring and appears to be "air hungry." What is the likely problem? What is the maximum gas flow available to this patient?

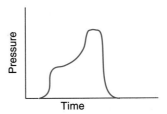

Pressure–time curve (Question 18).

19. A patient on PC-CMV has a set pressure of 30 cm H_2O, a rate of 12 breaths/min, and a T_I of 0.7 sec. Pressure, flow, and volume scalars are shown in the figure below. V_T delivery is 0.5 L, and the patient has respiratory acidosis. The respiratory therapist wants to increase V_T. In this situation, what is the best way to increase the V_T?

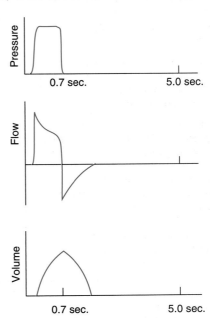

Pressure, flow, and volume scalars (Question 19).

20. During pressure augmentation (P_{Aug}), the clinician notices the pressure–time and flow–time graphics (see the figure below). T_I appears to be longer compared with previous graphic displays for the same patient. How would you interpret these findings?

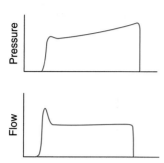

Pressure and flow scalars for a pressure augmentation (P_{Aug}) breath (Question 20).

21. A patient's pressure–volume graphic is shown in the figure below. The patient is using accessory muscles to breathe during inspiration. What could be the source of this problem?

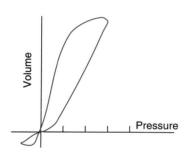

Pressure–volume curve (Question 21).

22. A respiratory therapist increases the mandatory rate to compensate for respiratory acidosis in a patient with COPD on intermittent mandatory ventilation (IMV). After the change, the PIP increases from 38 to 45 cm H_2O and $P_{plateau}$ increases from 27 to 35 cm H_2O. The flow–volume loop also has changed in appearance (see the figure below), and the patient now appears to be in distress. The patient's blood pressure has dropped from 135/95 mm Hg to 125/85 mm Hg. What do you think is the problem, and what is at least one possible solution?

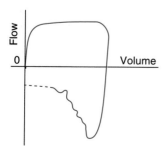

Flow–volume loop (Question 22).

23. PEEP therapy needs to be adjusted for a patient with severe hypoxemia. The pressure–volume loop for this patient appears in the figure below. What would be a reasonable PEEP level to set for this patient, assuming all other parameters are stable?

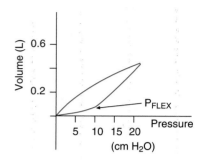

Pressure–volume loop (Question 23).

References

1. Turki M, Young MP, Wagers SS, et al: Peak pressures during manual ventilation. *Respir Care* 50:340–344, 2005.
2. Ricard JD: Manual ventilation and risk of barotraumas: *primum non nocere. Respir Care* 50:338–339, 2005.
3. Tobin MJ: Respiratory parameters for successful weaning. *J Crit Illness* 6:819–837, 1990.
4. Tobin MJ: What should the clinician do when a patient "fights the ventilator"? *Respir Care* 36:395–406, 1991.
5. Hansen-Flaschen JH: Dyspnea in the ventilated patient: a call for patient-centered mechanical ventilation. *Respir Care* 45:1460–1467, 2000.
6. Siobal M, Kallet RH, Draemer R, et al: Tracheal-innominate artery fistula caused by the endotracheal tube tip: case report and investigation of a fatal complication of prolonged intubation. *Respir Care* 46:1012–1018, 2001.
7. American Association for Respiratory Care (AARC) Clinical Practice Guideline: Management of airway emergencies. *Respir Care* 40:749–760, 1995.
8. Hess DR, MacIntyre NR: Mechanical ventilation. In Hess DR, MacIntyre NR, Mishoe SC, et al, editors: *Respiratory care: principles and practices,* ed 2, Sudbury, MA, 2012, Jones and Bartlett, pp 462–500.
9. Tom LR, Sassoon CSH: Patient-ventilator interactions. In MacIntyre NR, Branson RD, editors: *Mechanical ventilation,* ed 2, St Louis, 2009, Saunders-Elsevier, pp 182–197.
10. Khamiees M, Amoateng-Adjepong Y, Manthous CA: Propofol infusion is associated with a higher rapid shallow breathing index in patients preparing to wean from mechanical ventilation. *Respir Care* 47:150–153, 2002.
11. Nilsestuen JO, Hargett KD: Using ventilator graphics to identify patient-ventilator asynchrony. *Respir Care* 50:202–234, 2005.
12. MacIntyre NR: Patient-ventilator interactions: optimizing conventional ventilation modes. *Respir Care* 56:73–84, 2011.
13. Branson RD: Understanding and implementing advances in ventilator capabilities. *Curr Opin Crit Care* 10:23–32, 2004.
14. Parthasarathy S, Jubran A, Tobin MJ: Cycling of inspiratory and expiratory muscle groups with the ventilator in airflow limitation. *Am J Respir Crit Care Med* 158:1471–1478, 1998.
15. Gentile MA: Cycling of the mechanical ventilator breath. *Respir Care* 56:52–60, 2011.
16. Williams P, Muelver M, Kratohvil J, et al: Pressure support and pressure assist/control: are there differences? An evaluation of the newest intensive care unit ventilators. *Respir Care* 45:1169–1181, 2000.
17. The Joint Commission on Accreditation of Healthcare Organizations (JCAHO): Preventing ventilator-related deaths and injuries. *Sentinel Event Alert* 25:2002.
18. Cairo JM, Pilbeam SP: *Mosby's respiratory care equipment,* ed 7, St Louis, 2004, Mosby.

19. MacIntyre N: Ventilator monitors and displays. In MacIntyre NR, Branson RD, editors: *Mechanical ventilation*, St Louis, 2009, Saunders-Elsevier, pp 146–158.

20. Hess D: Prolonged use of heat and moisture exchangers: why do we keep changing things? *Crit Care Med* 28:1667–1668, 2000.

21. Black JW, Grover BS: A hazard of pressure support ventilation. *Chest* 93:333–335, 1988.

22. Monaco F, Goettel J: Increased airway pressures in Bear 2 and 3 circuits. *Respir Care* 36:132, 1991.

23. Fiastro JF, Habib MP, Quan R: Pressure support compensation for inspiratory work due to endotracheal tubes and demand continuous positive airway pressure. *Chest* 93:499–505, 1988.

24. Hess DR, Kacmarek RM: *Essentials of mechanical ventilation*, ed 2, New York, 2002, McGraw Hill.

25. MacIntyre NR, McConnell R, Cheng KG, et al: Patient-ventilator flow dyssynchrony: flow limited versus pressure limited breaths. *Crit Care Med* 25:1671–1677, 1997.

26. Beaty CD, Ritz RH, Benson MS: Continuous in-line nebulizers complicate pressure support ventilation. *Chest* 96:1360–1363, 1989.

27. Marini JJ: Patient-ventilator interaction: rational strategies for acute ventilatory management. *Respir Care* 38:482–493, 1993.

Basic Concepts of Noninvasive Positive-Pressure Ventilation

OUTLINE

KEY TERMS

- Acute cardiogenic pulmonary edema
- Chest cuirass
- Community-acquired pneumonia
- Cor pulmonale
- Delay-time control
- Expiratory positive airway pressure
- Inspiratory positive airway pressure
- Inspissated secretions
- Intermittent positive-pressure breathing
- Intermittent positive-pressure ventilation
- Iron lung
- Nocturnal hypoventilation
- Noninvasive positive-pressure ventilation
- Obstructive sleep apnea
- Pressure-targeted ventilators
- Ramp
- Simethicone agents

LEARNING OBJECTIVES *On completion of this chapter, the reader will be able to do the following:*

1. Define *noninvasive ventilation* and discuss the three basic noninvasive techniques.
2. Discuss the clinical and physiological benefits of noninvasive positive-pressure ventilation (NIV).
3. Identify the selection and exclusion criteria for NIV application in the acute and chronic care settings.
4. Compare the types of ventilators used for noninvasive ventilation.
5. Explain the importance of humidification during NIV application.
6. Describe the factors that will influence the fractional inspired oxygen concentration (F_IO_2) from a portable pressure-targeted ventilator.
7. Identify possible causes of rebreathing CO_2 during NIV administration from a portable pressure-targeted ventilator.
8. Compare the advantages and disadvantages of the various types of interfaces for the application of NIV.
9. List the steps used in the initiation of NIV.
10. Discuss several factors that affect the delivery of aerosols during NIV.
11. Identify several indicators of success for patients on NIV.
12. Make recommendations for ventilator changes based on observation of the patient's respiratory status, acid–base status, or oxygenation status.
13. Recognize potential complications of NIV.
14. Provide optional solutions to complications of NIV.
15. Describe two basic approaches to weaning the patient from NIV.

Noninvasive ventilation (NIV) is defined as the delivery of mechanical ventilation to the lungs using techniques that do not require an endotracheal airway.[1] Until 1960, nearly all mechanical ventilation techniques involved the use of a tank respirator or chest-wrap device that was able to apply subatmospheric (negative) pressure to the body or chest area to ventilate the lungs. Beginning in the early 1960s researchers found that the survival rate for invasive positive-pressure ventilation delivered via an endotracheal or tracheostomy tube was higher than that for negative-pressure ventilation.[1] As a result, invasive positive-pressure ventilation became the standard of practice for the support and management of patients with acute and chronic respiratory failure.

Invasive ventilation is effective and often necessary to support alveolar ventilation; however, it has many associated risks that often result in increased mortality and morbidity and a higher financial cost. NIV is now considered a standard of care for selected patients with acute respiratory failure. Sufficient evidence now proves that application of NIV via a nasal mask, mouthpiece, or full-face mask can reduce the need for intubation and its related complications, reduce mortality rates, and shorten the hospital stay for certain patients requiring mechanical ventilatory assistance.[2-7]

TYPES OF NONINVASIVE VENTILATION TECHNIQUES

The three basic methods of applying noninvasive ventilation are negative-pressure ventilation, abdominal-displacement ventilation (discussed in Chapter 21), and positive-pressure ventilation.

Negative-Pressure Ventilation

Use of negative-pressure ventilators peaked in the 1950s with the polio epidemic. Negative-pressure ventilators, or *body ventilators,* operated on the principle of increasing lung volumes by intermittently applying negative pressure to the entire body below the neck or just to the upper region of the chest. The negative pressure was transmitted across the chest wall, into the pleural space, and into the intraalveolar space. The resulting increase in transpulmonary pressure caused air to enter the lungs. Exhalation was passive and simply depended on the elastic recoil of the lung and chest wall.

The first successful negative-pressure ventilator, known as the ***iron lung***, was designed in 1928 by engineer Phillip Drinker and Dr. Charles McKhann. It consisted of a large metal cylinder that enclosed the patient's entire body below the neck, leaving the head protruding through an airtight rubber neck seal. A simpler and less expensive version of this tank device, which was developed by J.H. Emerson in 1931, became the ventilator that was predominantly used to treat people paralyzed by polio.

The bulk and lack of portability of the iron lung, along with the difficulty in providing routine care for patients, led to the development of smaller, portable negative-pressure devices. The **chest cuirass,** or *shell ventilator,* gained wide popularity during the 1950s. Two versions of this device were primarily used to apply negative pressure to the thorax and upper abdomen. In one version, the patient's chest was covered by a metal shell, which had an air-filled rubber edge that sealed the thorax. Later models used a shell made of plastic, which allowed it to be easier to mold and fit to a patient's chest. Another variation of the chest cuirass used a wraparound piece of plastic over a shell that was powered by a vacuum-cleaner motor (Fig. 19-1).

Positive-Pressure Ventilation

The use of positive-pressure ventilation can be traced as far back as 1780, when the first bag-mask apparatus was designed for resuscitative efforts. Positive-pressure ventilation with a mask was first used clinically in the mid-1940s by Motley et al[8] to treat patients with acute respiratory failure (ARF). **Intermittent positive-pressure ventilation** (IPPV), which used a pressure-targeted ventilator and a mask, later was used primarily to treat ARF complicated by chronic obstructive pulmonary disease (COPD) and asthma. Volume-targeted ventilators and endotracheal tubes were developed in the 1960s and became the standard for providing positive-pressure ventilation in the treatment of respiratory failure. **Intermittent positive-pressure breathing** (IPPB), which used a mask or mouthpiece, became a means of simply delivering aerosolized medication periodically with positive-pressure breaths.

In 1980 clinical studies began to show that the benefits of IPPB were often overstated and could be accomplished using other simpler and more cost-effective therapies.[9] As IPPB lost favor in clinical practice, nasal-mask continuous positive airway pressure (CPAP) began to emerge as a highly effective therapy in the treatment of **obstructive sleep apnea** (OSA).[10-12] Researchers found that

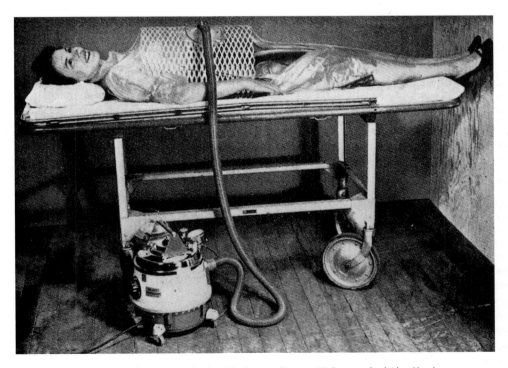

Fig. 19-1 The chest respirator developed by Emerson. (Courtesy J.H. Emerson, Cambridge, Mass.)

application of low levels of continuous airway pressure through a mask interface created a pneumatic splint that prevented airway collapse during sleep.[10]

The use of positive-pressure ventilation via a mask was soon reported to be successful in the treatment of chronic ventilatory insufficiency and muscle weakness in patients with various neuromuscular illnesses.[13-15] In 1989 Meduri et al[16] successfully treated a small sample of patients with ARF using pressure support ventilation through a face mask.

These successes stimulated the production of variable interfaces and small pressure- and volume-targeted ventilators that were lightweight, easy to operate, and ideal for home use. Over the past decade, the use of NIV has increased dramatically, and NIV is now used to treat both acute and chronic respiratory failure in a variety of clinical settings.

GOALS OF AND INDICATIONS FOR NONINVASIVE POSITIVE-PRESSURE VENTILATION

The goals of **noninvasive positive-pressure ventilation** (NIV) and the indications for its use are derived from clinical experiences and systematic research. The following sections review the evidence that supports the use of NIV in various disorders associated with acute and chronic respiratory failure.

Acute Care Setting

NIV is considered by most clinicians to be a lifesaving application for acute respiratory failure. It offers a number of benefits over invasive positive-pressure ventilation (Box 19-1). The most significant benefit is the avoidance of intubation. Endotracheal intubation is associated with complications such as airway trauma, increased risk of aspiration, ventilator-associated pneumonia, and considerable patient discomfort, typically requiring the use of sedatives. Such complications can lead to a longer hospital stay, higher mortality rate, and increased health care costs. Evidence has established that NIV can safely support ventilation, without endotracheal intubation, until the condition leading to the ARF has been reversed. In addition, evidence strongly indicates that NIV reduces the mortality rate, reduces the duration of ventilator use, and shortens the hospital stay in appropriately selected patients. As such, the primary goal of NIV in the acute care setting is to avoid the need for endotracheal intubation and invasive ventilation.

BOX 19-1 **Clinical Benefits of NIV**

Acute Care Setting
- Reduces the need for endotracheal intubation
- Reduces incidence of ventilator-associated pneumonia
- Shortens stay in the intensive care unit
- Shortens hospital stay
- Reduces mortality
- Preserves physiological airway defenses
- Improves patient comfort
- Reduces need for sedation

Chronic Care Setting
- Alleviates symptoms of chronic hypoventilation
- Improves duration and quality of sleep
- Improves functional capacity
- Prolongs survival

The physiological goal of NIV in ARF is to improve gas exchange by resting the respiratory muscles and increasing alveolar ventilation. NIV reduces diaphragmatic pressure swings, which suggests that the respiratory muscles are being rested. In addition, when positive end-expiratory pressure (PEEP) is applied during pressure-supported ventilation (PSV), PEEP helps offset auto-PEEP, thereby reducing the work required to initiate inspiration.[17] Likewise, pressure support (PS) facilitates inspiration, thus increasing the tidal volume (V_T). Resting of the respiratory muscles and improved V_T lead to a lower arterial partial pressure of CO_2 (P_aCO_2), better oxygenation, and decreased respiratory rates.

Acute Exacerbation of Chronic Obstructive Pulmonary Disease

During an acute exacerbation of COPD, increased airway resistance and an increased respiratory rate lead to hyperinflation, development of auto-PEEP (air trapping), and alveolar hypoventilation. As hyperinflation worsens, respiratory muscle activity increases, significantly increasing the oxygen cost of breathing. This becomes a vicious circle of increased demand for ventilation, further air trapping, hypoventilation, and muscle fatigue. Without intervention, ventilatory failure and death may occur. Conventional medical therapy for these patients has included bronchodilators, antiinflammatory agents, judicious use of supplemental oxygen, and antibiotics. If these measures failed, endotracheal intubation and invasive ventilation were the next therapeutic steps. Studies of patients with COPD who have experienced acute exacerbations have shown that NIV reduces inspiratory muscle activity and the respiratory rate and increases V_T and minute volume, allowing for better gas exchange and respiratory muscle rest.[18-21] NIV may help reverse the acute condition when used in conjunction with conventional medical therapy.[18]

The use of NIV in the treatment of ARF caused by COPD exacerbation has been very successful and has been studied more than any other disorder leading to ARF. The strongest evidence from randomized, control trials has confirmed that use of NIV with a face mask significantly reduces the need for intubation, shortens the duration of mechanical ventilation, shortens the patient's stay in the intensive care unit (ICU), and reduces complications and the mortality rate.[2-7]

Compared with patients receiving only conventional medical therapy (e.g., bronchodilators, antiinflammatory agents, supplemental oxygen, and antibiotics), patients receiving NIV have shown significant improvement in vital signs, pH and blood gas values, respiratory rate, and breathlessness within the first hour of application.[3,6,7,19] These results have been compelling enough that NIV is considered a standard of care for the treatment of COPD exacerbation in selected patients[20,21] (Key Point 19-1).

Key Point **19-1** Clinical evidence supports the use of NIV as the standard of care for patients with moderate-to-severe exacerbations of COPD who meet selection criteria.

Asthma

Although the use of NIV in the treatment of severe asthma is controversial, several reports have shown that patients with status asthmaticus complicated by CO_2 retention demonstrate positive outcomes when treated with a trial of NIV. The benefits observed have included improved gas exchange, decreased P_aCO_2 and rapid improvement in vital signs within the first 2 hours of NIV treatment.[22] The benefits of NIV include decreased need for endotracheal intubation and the associated complications, as well as a reduction in mortality rate for these patients.[23] Additionally, NIV decreased the requirement for inhaled bronchodilator when compared with patients receiving conventional medical therapy.[24] Although specific criteria for the selection of asthma patients to receive NIV have not yet been developed, NIV may be appropriate in patients who do not respond to conventional medical treatment, to prevent intubation of patients with mild-to-moderate ARF who do not need immediate invasive mechanical ventilation, or do not have substantial impairment of gas exchange.[25]

Hypoxemic Respiratory Failure and Acute Respiratory Distress Syndrome

Evidence of the efficacy of NIV in the treatment of hypoxemic respiratory failure has been controversial, probably because of the wide variety of non-COPD parenchymal processes that can cause hypoxemic respiratory failure. Several examples include pneumonia, acute respiratory distress syndrome, trauma, and cardiogenic pulmonary edema. These conditions usually result in severe impairment of gas exchange characterized by refractory hypoxemia, an arterial partial pressure of oxygen to fractional inspired oxygen (P_aO_2/F_IO_2) ratio less than 200, and a respiratory rate greater than 35 breaths/min. In several clinical studies, patients who received conventional medical care for hypoxemic acute respiratory failure were compared with patients who received NIV plus the usual medical care.[22,26] In these studies, NIV significantly improved gas exchange, reduced the need for intubation, and reduced the mortality rate in these patients. NIV can be as effective at improving oxygenation within the first hour as invasive ventilation and is associated with fewer complications and a shorter ICU stay.[27] In contrast, other researchers have found no significant improvement in patients' overall condition with NIV unless the patients were also hypercapnic.[28] Although many studies have shown promising results with the use of NIV in hypoxemic respiratory failure, the different causes of hypoxemic respiratory failure make it difficult to apply all of these findings to individual patients.

Community-Acquired Pneumonia

Of the various causes of hypoxemic respiratory failure treated with NIV, pneumonia appears to be one of the most challenging and least consistent for successful outcomes. In a study of patients with COPD and ARF, 38% of the unsuccessful attempts with NIV were associated with the presence of pneumonia.[29] On the other hand, the intubation rate, ICU stay, and mortality rate were reduced when NIV was used to treat patients with severe **community-acquired pneumonia** (CAP).[22,25] In the case of CAP, most of the favorable results were from the subgroup of COPD patients who had pneumonia. In a study by Jolliet et al,[30] 22 of the 24 of non-COPD patients with severe CAP and ARF who received NIV showed initial improvement in oxygenation and a reduced respiratory rate. However, despite the improvement, nearly two thirds of the patients eventually required intubation and mechanical ventilation. Those patients who continued to receive NIV had shorter ICU and hospital stays. Because of the mixed results produced by studies, the current suggestion is that patients with COPD and pneumonia receive an initial trial of NIV. However, caution should be used when non-COPD patients with pneumonia are treated with NIV.

Cardiogenic Pulmonary Edema

Mask CPAP has been shown to be effective in the treatment of **acute cardiogenic pulmonary edema** (ACPE).[16,31] When patients with ACPE do not respond to conventional pharmacologic and oxygen therapy, the use of mask CPAP with oxygen may expand fluid-filled alveoli, resulting in the following:

- Increased oxygenation
- Increased functional residual capacity (FRC)
- Improved lung compliance
- Reduced work of breathing
- Reduced need for invasive ventilation
- Shorter ICU stay
- Improved mortality rate

Several studies have reported similar success in treating ACPE with NIV by mask using PSV plus PEEP.[32-34] In these studies, rapid improvement in gas exchange and pH were noted, along with reduced intubation rates. Patients who were already hypercapnic responded best. A comparison of NIV and CPAP in the treatment of ACPE showed that although patients treated with NIV demonstrated more rapid improvements in P_aCO_2 and pH, the mortality and intubation rates were not significantly different.[35] It is worth mentioning that although NIV and CPAP are equally effective in treating respiratory failure associated with ACPE,[36] CPAP is more cost effective and easier to set up. The current recommendation is to use CPAP (10 to 12 cm H_2O) in the initial treatment of ACPE; NIV should be used in patients who continue to be hypercapnic and dyspneic thereafter[37] (Key Point 19-2).

Key Point **19-2** Patients with ACPE are treated initially with CPAP. If the patient remains hypercapnic and dyspneic with CPAP, a trial of NIV is indicated.

Chronic Care Setting

In chronic respiratory failure, NIV is considered to be a supportive therapy rather than a lifesaving treatment. Most of the clinical disorders that require this level of support are characterized by chronic hypoventilation, nocturnal desaturation, respiratory muscle fatigue, and poor sleep quality. As the disease process progresses, daytime gas exchange worsens and patients often show classic symptoms of chronic hypoventilation (Box 19-2).

Nocturnal use of NIV (4 to 6 hours) can have certain clinical benefits for patients with chronic hypoventilation disorders (see Box 19-1). The most significant of these are improvement of symptoms associated with chronic hypoventilation and an improved quality of life. Although the physiological mechanism underlying these benefits is not well understood, investigators have

BOX **19-2**	Symptoms of Chronic Hypoventilation

- Fatigue
- Morning headache
- Daytime hypersomnolence
- Cognitive dysfunction
- Dyspnea

hypothesized that NIV benefits these patients in one or all of the following ways.[38-41]

- It provides intermittent rest for the respiratory muscles resulting in less muscle fatigue and more efficiency of function.
- It reduces the frequency and severity of sleep-disordered breathing, leading to longer sleep and better sleep quality.
- It eliminates **nocturnal hypoventilation,** making the respiratory centers more responsive to increases in CO_2 and leading to improvement in daytime ventilation.
- It may eliminate auto-PEEP, which would reduce work of breathing required to trigger a breath during NIV.

Restrictive Thoracic Disorders

Restrictive thoracic disorders include chest wall deformities and neuromuscular conditions that result in progressive muscle weakness, hypoventilation, and eventually respiratory failure. Patients with neuromuscular disorders were the first group of patients studied to be successfully converted from invasive ventilation (tracheostomy) to NIV (mouthpiece interface).[38] These patients required continuous support; however, NIV also can benefit patients who only require ventilatory support at night or intermittently during the day. In the short-term use group, daytime gas exchange and respiratory muscle strength improve and symptoms of hypoventilation are alleviated.[39-41] Nocturnal use of NIV also eliminates OSA and oxygen desaturation at night, which are common in patients who use negative-pressure ventilatory support.[41]

Quality of life appears to improve for patients with neuromuscular disorders who use NIV. A high degree of satisfaction, along with improved mental well-being and psychosocial function, have been noted for patients with restrictive thoracic disorders.[42] Long-term follow-up of these patients has shown significantly shortened hospital stays and an overall increased survival time compared with patients who did not receive ventilatory support.[43] For these reasons, the consensus is that NIV is the ventilator mode of choice for chronic respiratory failure caused by restrictive thoracic disorders in patients who can protect their own airway[44,45] (Key Point 19-3).

> **Key Point 19-3** NIV is the ventilator mode of choice for chronic respiratory failure caused by restrictive thoracic disorders in patients who can protect their airways.

Chronic Stable Chronic Obstructive Pulmonary Disease

Evidence of the efficacy of long-term nocturnal NIV is vague and often contradictory in severe stable COPD. Early studies of patients with severe stable COPD focused on the use of intermittent negative-pressure ventilation to rest the muscles of respiration.[46,47] Some investigators reported potential benefits, but most patients could not tolerate the devices used, and the benefits were only temporary. In addition, negative-pressure ventilation actually collapsed upper airway structures during sleep and induced OSA.

A number of studies since have been performed on patients with severe stable COPD who used nocturnal NIV. Results from these studies included reduced daytime P_aCO_2, reduced nocturnal oxygen desaturation and hypoventilation, improved sleep quality, and improved quality of life.[48-50] Other studies have found minimal or no benefit with nocturnal NIV in these patients.[51,52] The discrepancy in these findings could be the result of differing patient selection, methods, or ventilator settings. Closer examination of baseline characteristics of the study participants reveals an important

finding: the greatest benefits from NIV were seen in individuals who had more severe CO_2 retention and more episodes of nocturnal desaturation.

Although the evidence is inconclusive, the current professional consensus and the guidelines from the Centers for Medicare and Medicaid Services (CMS) agree that patients should be considered for NIV if they experience severe daytime CO_2 retention (P_aCO_2 of 52 mm Hg or higher) and nocturnal hypoventilation, despite the administration of nocturnal oxygen therapy.[45]

Cystic Fibrosis

The role of NIV in the treatment of advanced cystic fibrosis has not been precisely defined. In general, NIV increases V_T, reduces diaphragmatic activity, and improves oxygenation in some patients with cystic fibrosis who have acute exacerbations.[53] Intermittent use of NIV could help support these patients for several months while they await lung transplantation.[54-56]

Nocturnal Hypoventilation

Several other disorders associated with nocturnal hypoventilation include central sleep apnea, obesity hypoventilation syndrome, and OSA combined with COPD or congestive heart failure. These disorders also may lead to daytime CO_2 retention. If nocturnal hypoventilation is severe, symptoms will be severe and will manifest during the daytime (see Box 19-2). Without intervention, these symptoms can then progress to overt respiratory failure.

The therapy of choice for OSA is CPAP. However, if these patients continue to hypoventilate despite CPAP therapy, NIV may improve daytime gas exchange and symptoms associated with chronic hypoventilation.[57] Likewise, patients with central hypoventilation or obesity hypoventilation syndrome who do not respond to first-line therapies (e.g., oxygen, respiratory stimulants, weight loss, supplemental oxygen, or CPAP) should be considered for treatment with NIV (Key Point 19-4).

> **Key Point 19-4** Patients with OSA are typically treated initially with CPAP therapy. NIV is indicated if these patients continue to experience hypoventilation and nocturnal desaturation.

OTHER INDICATIONS FOR NONINVASIVE VENTILATION

Facilitation of Weaning from Invasive Ventilation

Reducing the number of days a patient receives invasive mechanical ventilation reduces the risk of infection and other complications, lowers the mortality rate, and reduces health care costs.[58-60] Many respiratory care departments in acute care facilities have devised weaning protocols for discontinuing ventilation and extubating patients as soon as possible. However, many weaning protocols depend on patient tolerance of daily spontaneous breathing trials to determine the likelihood of successful extubation. (See Chapter 20 for information on weaning and spontaneous breathing trials.) After extubation, the excessive work of breathing (WOB) that spontaneous breathing places on the respiratory muscles can lead to fatigue and ultimately reintubation.

NIV provides a viable weaning alternative for patients who demonstrate respiratory muscle fatigue postextubation. It has been suggested that NIV reduces the work of breathing (WOB) and maintains adequate gas exchange as effectively

TABLE 19-1	Indications, Symptoms, and Selection Criteria for NIV in Acute Respiratory Failure in Adults	
Indications	**Symptoms**	**Physiological Criteria**
Acute exacerbation of COPD	Moderate to severe dyspnea	P_aCO_2 >45 mm Hg, pH <7.35
Acute asthma	Respiratory rate >24 breaths/min	**or**
Hypoxemic respiratory failure	Accessory muscle use	P_aO_2/F_IO_2 <200
Community-acquired pneumonia	Paradoxical breathing	
Cardiogenic pulmonary edema		
Immunocompromised patients		
Postoperative patients		
Postextubation (weaning)		
"Do not intubate"		

COPD, Chronic obstructive pulmonary disease; *F_IO_2,* fractional inspired oxygen concentration; *P_aCO_2,* arterial carbon dioxide partial pressure; *P_aO_2,* arterial oxygen partial pressure.

as invasive ventilation.[61] NIV can also shorten the duration of invasive ventilation.[62,63] In one study of a group of patients for whom 3 days of spontaneous breathing trials failed, NIV was shown to reduce the spontaneous WOB, maintain adequate gas exchange, and reduce ICU and hospital stays.[64] NIV has also been shown to reduce the likelihood that patients will need a tracheotomy.[63] Most patients who seem to benefit from NIV during weaning from invasive ventilation suffer from chronic illness (e.g., COPD). Therefore, it is questionable whether the benefits of NIV would apply to patients with other disease processes. Nonetheless, the evidence is strong enough to warrant consideration of NIV in patients for whom spontaneous breathing trials fail and who meet appropriate NIV selection criteria.

"Do Not Intubate" Patients

Patients with terminal or advanced disease who develop ARF are not viewed as good candidates for endotracheal intubation and mechanical ventilation. NIV may be a viable alternative therapy for these patients, although its use with this group of patients remains controversial. Previous studies involving primarily end-stage COPD patients in whom endotracheal intubation was contraindicated found that most of these patients were successfully supported with NIV and eventually weaned from ventilatory support.[65,66] Many of these patients would not have survived the acute process had they not been placed on NIV. Patients with acute pulmonary edema may also benefit from support with NIV. However, survival was not improved in patients with ARF arising from other causes such as pneumonia or cancer.[67]

The argument for using NIV in patients who have "do not intubate" status is that NIV may relieve severe dyspnea and preserve patient comfort. It may also reverse the acute process in disorders such as COPD or pulmonary edema, and allow these patients to live longer.[68] The argument against using NIV in these patients is that it can prolong the dying process, add to patient discomfort, and consume valuable resources.[69] When NIV is used in these cases, the patient and family members should be informed that NIV is a form of life support that can be uncomfortable but that may be removed at any time.[20]

PATIENT SELECTION CRITERIA

The success of NIV and the avoidance of major complications depend on appropriate selection of patients in both the acute and chronic care settings. Evidence gained from the use of NIV in various patient populations and clinical settings has led to the

BOX 19-3	Exclusion Criteria for NIV

1. Respiratory arrest or the need for immediate intubation
2. Hemodynamic instability
3. Inability to protect the airway (impaired cough or swallowing)
4. Excessive secretions
5. Agitated and confused patients
6. Facial deformities or conditions that prevent mask from fitting
7. Uncooperative or unmotivated patients
8. Brain injury with unstable respiratory drive

development of guidelines that promote the highest chance of success (Table 19-1).

Acute Care Setting

In the acute care setting, the selection process must be based on the patient's diagnosis and clinical characteristics, as well as the risk of failure. The assessment process may be viewed as a two-step process. The first step involves establishing the need for ventilatory assistance according to clinical and blood gas criteria. The consensus of studies is that patients who need ventilatory assistance show signs and symptoms of distress, including tachypnea (respiratory rate >24 breaths/min), use of accessory muscles, and paradoxical breathing.[45] Blood gas criteria should reveal a moderate to severe respiratory failure (i.e., a pH <7.35 and P_aCO_2 >45 mm Hg, *or* a P_aO_2/F_IO_2 <200). It is also important to know when NIV is not appropriate. For example, NIV may be unnecessary for patients with mild respiratory distress. NIV may also not be appropriate for a patient who has already deteriorated to severe respiratory failure because it may delay lifesaving intubation and ventilation.

Once the need for ventilatory support is established, the second step is to exclude patients at increased risk of failure and complications (Box 19-3). Such patients include individuals with respiratory arrest, hemodynamic instability, or other major organ involvement; patients with excessive secretions; and patients unable to protect their airway because of impaired cough or swallowing ability. Patients with any of these disorders are at highest risk for aspiration. Finally, agitated and confused patients or those with facial burns or deformities that preclude a good mask fit are excluded.

A final consideration in the selection of patients with ARF is the potential reversibility of the disease process. It has been clearly established that NIV is effective in the treatment of acute exacerbations of COPD. Supportive ventilatory assistance allows time for conventional therapies (e.g., bronchodilators, oxygen, antibiotics) to reverse the acute process so that intubation may be avoided. Other causes of ARF may not be treated as successfully as COPD, but a trial of NIV may be warranted if the patient meets the selection criteria. All patients should be monitored closely so that intubation, if necessary, is not unduly delayed (Key Point 19-5).

> **Key Point** **19-5** The reversibility of the disease process must be considered before NIV is initiated.

Chronic Care Setting

Establishing of the need for intermittent ventilatory assistance in patients with chronic respiratory failure begins with the recognition of typical symptoms of nocturnal hypoventilation and poor sleep quality. These most commonly include the following:

- Excessive fatigue
- Morning headache
- Daytime hypersomnolence
- Cognitive dysfunction
- Dyspnea

Objective criteria, such as blood gases, depend on the rate of progression of the disease process. For patients with restrictive thoracic or central hypoventilation disorders, institution of NIV is recommended when P_aCO_2 is 45 mm Hg or higher or when sustained nocturnal desaturation occurs, as evidenced by an oxygen saturation by pulse oximeter (S_pO_2) under 88% for longer than five consecutive minutes.[44] NIV also may be indicated if a patient with restrictive thoracic disease is symptomatic and has severe pulmonary dysfunction (vital capacity [VC] <50% of the predicted level), even if CO_2 retention is absent.[44] Patients with nocturnal hypoventilation or OSA may require only nocturnal CPAP for splinting the airway open to overcome hypoventilation. However, NIV should be initiated if patients with moderate to severe OSA do not respond to CPAP therapy. Patients who recover from episodes of ARF or who are hospitalized repeatedly for exacerbations of their condition should also be considered for noninvasive ventilatory assistance (Key Point 19-6).

> **Key Point** **19-6** NIV should be considered for patients with severe stable COPD who are symptomatic despite optimal treatment. NIV should also be considered for COPD patients who demonstrate evidence of OSA and are unresponsive to CPAP therapy.

The conflicting findings of studies regarding the use of NIV for severe stable COPD have hampered the development of evidence-based selection guidelines. Studies have demonstrated that COPD patients with severe hypercapnia are likely to benefit from NIV.[50,70] A consensus of medical experts recommended the use of nocturnal NIV in symptomatic yet medically stable patients with COPD whose daytime P_aCO_2 is 55 mm Hg or higher.[44] The term *medically stable* in this instance means that the patient is being optimally

treated, and OSA and CPAP therapy have been considered and ruled out.[44] The consensus statement also recommended a trial of NIV for COPD patients receiving long-term oxygen administration (2 L/min or more) if the P_aCO_2 is 50 to 54 mm Hg and the patient demonstrates evidence of frequent hypopnea episodes and sustained nocturnal desaturation. A history of frequent hospitalizations for acute exacerbations also helps to justify the use of NIV in COPD patients.

As for any patient requiring NIV, the ability to protect the airway is crucial. This is especially important for patients with chronic respiratory failure because most of these individuals live at home or in an extended care setting and may not be monitored closely. Patients with neuromuscular disorders may present an even greater challenge as their disease progresses and they begin to lose oropharyngeal muscle strength and the ability to generate an effective cough. Cough-assisting devices or airway clearance techniques may help these individuals remove secretions and maintain a patent airway.

Patient motivation also must be considered with NIV in the chronic care setting. Very few, if any, therapeutic results are realized if the patient does not comply with the prescribed therapy. Among patients undergoing long-term treatment with NIV, those with COPD and little CO_2 retention were least compliant.[71] This latter point emphasizes the importance of selecting patients who are symptomatic and motivated by the desire for relief of those symptoms. Table 19-2 summarizes the symptoms and selection criteria for chronic respiratory failure disorders.

EQUIPMENT SELECTION FOR NONINVASIVE VENTILATION

The equipment required for NIV generally includes ventilators, humidifiers, and the interfaces or masks.

Types of Ventilators

Successful application of NIV has been achieved using portable homecare ventilators, adult acute care ventilators, and portable pressure support (pressure-targeted) ventilators. The choice of ventilator should be based on the level of support required and the advantages and disadvantages of the appropriate machines.[72]

Pressure-Targeted Ventilators

Portable **pressure-targeted ventilators (PTVs)** are also known as bilevel CPAP ventilators, pressure support ventilators, or bilevel pressure ventilators. These ventilators are microprocessor-controlled, electrically powered units that use a blower to regulate gas flow into the patient circuit to maintain the pre-set pressure levels at the patient connection. Pressure-targeted ventilators have a single-circuit gas delivery system that uses an intentional leak port for patient exhalation instead of a true exhalation valve; this allows the continuous flow of gas through the small leak port to help maintain pressure levels and flush exhaled gases from the circuit.

Pressure-targeted ventilators are pressure-limited, flow- and time-triggered, flow- and time-cycled ventilators. These devices are designed to increase minute ventilation and improve gas-exchange capabilities using the delivery of an **inspiratory positive airway pressure** (IPAP) and an **expiratory positive airway pressure** (EPAP). The calibrated pressure range for IPAP typically is 2 to 30 cm H_2O; the range for EPAP typically is 2 to 20 cm H_2O.[72]

TABLE 19-2	Indications, Symptoms, and Selection Criteria for NIV in Chronic Disorders	
Indication	**Symptoms**	**Physiologic Criteria**
Restrictive thoracic disorders	Fatigue	P_aCO_2 ≥45 mm Hg
Muscular dystrophy	Dyspnea	Nocturnal S_pO_2 ≤88% for 5 consecutive minutes
Multiple sclerosis	Morning headache	MIP <60 cm H_2O
Amyotrophic lateral sclerosis	Hypersomnolence	FVC <50% predicted
Kyphoscoliosis	Cognitive dysfunction	
Postpolio syndrome		
Stable spinal cord injuries		
Severe stable COPD	Following optimal therapy with bronchodilators, O_2, and other therapy, COPD patients must demonstrate:	P_aCO_2 >55 mm Hg
		P_aCO_2 50 to 54 mm Hg + S_pO_2 <88% for 5 consecutive min
	Fatigue	P_aCO_2 50-54 mm Hg + recurrent hospitalizations for hypercapnic respiratory failure (>2 hospitalizations in a 12-mo period)
	Dyspnea	
	Morning headache	
	Hypersomnolence	
Nocturnal hypoventilation	Fatigue	Polysomnographic evidence of OSA not responsive to CPAP
Obstructive sleep apnea	Morning headache	
Obesity hypoventilation	Hypersomnolence	
Idiopathic hypoventilation		

COPD, Chronic obstructive pulmonary disease; *CPAP,* continuous airway pressure; *FVC,* forced vital capacity; *MIP,* maximum inspiratory pressure; *OSA,* obstructive sleep apnea; *P_aCO_2,* partial pressure of arterial carbon dioxide; *S_pO_2,* pulse oximetry saturation.

Manufacturers of pressure-targeted ventilators use variable mode nomenclature, which is often confusing, but most of these units offer the following modes of ventilatory support:

- CPAP (spontaneous)
- PSV (IPAP/EPAP)
- Spontaneous/timed (S/T)

In the CPAP mode the patient breathes spontaneously at a set baseline pressure. The patient controls both the rate and depth of breathing. Flow sensors and pressure transducers respond to the patient's inspiratory and expiratory effort and increase or decrease flow through the circuit to maintain a stable level of pressure.

With the PSV (bilevel) mode, the difference between two pressure levels (IPAP and EPAP) determines the level of pressure support for each assisted breath. A change to the set IPAP occurs only in response to the patient's inspiratory effort. When the patient reaches a predetermined flow threshold, the breath is terminated and the patient exhales to the set EPAP level. There is no set rate; the patient must initiate each breath.

In the S/T mode (older models may use the term *A/C*), the clinician sets the IPAP and EPAP, a respiratory rate, and an inspiratory time (e.g., IPAP%). The patient may initiate breaths that are supported to the IPAP level, as in the PSV mode, but if the patient fails to make an inspiratory effort within a set interval, the machine triggers inspiration to the set IPAP level. IPAP then cycles to EPAP based on the IPAP% period. In all modes, the patient's delivered V_T depends on the gradient between the IPAP level and the EPAP, the inspiratory time, patient inspiratory effort, and the patient's lung characteristics (airway resistance and lung compliance) (Key Point 19-7).

AVAPS (average volume-assured pressure support) is a relatively new technology available on Respironics Philips Healthcare BiPAP devices (e.g., V60 ventilator). AVAPS devices automatically adapt pressure support to match a patient's ventilatory needs by delivering an average tidal volume (V_T range = 200 to 1500 mL) based on the patient's condition. AVAPS may be useful in the treatment of patients with COPD, neuromuscular diseases, obesity hypoventilation, and chronic hypoventilation.

AVAPS devices operate with several modes of ventilation, including CPAP, S/T, spontaneous, timed, and PCV. The Respironics V60 ventilator continually calculates and compensates for the total leak rate (i.e., intentional and unintentional patient leak). The clinician enters the known intentional leak value specific to the mask/patient interface and the circuit's exhalation port so that the ventilator can accurately calculate and display the patient leak using an Auto-Trak sensitivity system.[72] The Auto-Trak+ option allows the clinician to further adjust thresholds that manage trigger and cycling, and the level of Auto-Trak sensitivity. The manufacturer's suggested setting for initiating AVAPS include a target V_T of 8 mL/kg, ideal body weight (IBW), maximum IPAP of 25 cm H_2O (depending on the patient's pathology), minimum EPAP of +4 cm H_2O, respiratory rate 2 to 3 beats/min below resting respiratory rate, and an inspiratory time of 1.5 seconds.[72]

Key Point 19-7 In all modes of bilevel positive-pressure ventilation, the patient's delivered V_T depends on the gradient between the IPAP and EPAP, the inspiratory time, and the patient's inspiratory effort and lung characteristics.

A pressure-targeted ventilator's ability to deliver flow in response to patient demand is equivalent and often superior to that of ICU adult ventilators and portable homecare ventilators. Flow sensors in the pressure-targeted ventilator system continuously monitor and adjust flow (variable up to 180 L/min) based on the set pressure, the patient's inspiratory and expiratory efforts, and the difference between the intentional leak in the leak port and unintentional leaks that might occur around the patient-ventilator interface. The pressure-targeted ventilator's ability to compensate for leaks makes it easier for the patient to flow trigger the unit into inspiration and to reach the inspiratory flow threshold necessary to terminate each pressure-supported breath.

Most units now have adjustable inspiratory and expiratory sensitivity controls that improve synchronization between the patient and the ventilator. Pressure-targeted ventilators also allow adjustment of the amount of time required to reach the IPAP (i.e., rise-time control). Use of the rise-time control may enhance patient comfort, reduce WOB, and improve patient-ventilator synchrony. Two other features of portable PTVs that can enhance patient comfort are the **ramp** and **delay-time controls.** Ramp allows positive pressure to increase gradually over a set interval (delay time). The ramp rate generally can be set in increments of 1, 2, or 3 cm H_2O, and the delay time can be set in 5-minute increments between 5 and 30 minutes. The ramp and delay-time controls are more likely to be used in home or chronic care NIV.

Portable pressure-targeted ventilators have certain limitations that may restrict their use in ARF. For example, oxygen delivery is not standard on most portable pressure-targeted ventilators. When supplemental oxygen is required, it must be bled into the system via the mask or into the circuit near the machine outlet. Therefore, the F_1O_2 can vary and is affected by four factors:

1. Oxygen flow rate
2. Type of leak port in the system
3. Site where oxygen is bled into the circuit
4. IPAP and EPAP

Higher oxygen flow rates result in higher oxygen concentrations. Lower IPAP and EPAP levels also yield higher oxygen concentrations.[73,74] F_1O_2 is also affected by the type of leak port and the site where oxygen is added to the circuit. If the leak port is located in the circuit, higher F_1O_2 values are obtained if the oxygen is bled into the patient's mask. If the leak port is located in the mask, higher F_1O_2 values are obtained if the oxygen is bled into the circuit at the machine outlet.[75] (The lowest levels of oxygen are obtained when the leak port is in the mask and oxygen is bled into the mask.) Because the oxygen concentration delivered is the result of a complex interaction between these variables, a ventilator with an oxygen blender should be used for patients who require a high or precise F_1O_2.

Rebreathing of CO_2 is a concern with any pressure-targeted ventilator that uses a single-circuit gas-delivery system because exhalation occurs through the intentional leak port and depends on the continuous flow of gas in the circuit. If gas flow is inadequate, exhaled gases may not be adequately flushed from the system resulting in the patient rebreathing exhaled CO_2. The flow of gas through the leak port depends on the EPAP setting and the patient's inspiratory-to-expiratory ratio. At low EPAP settings (<4 cm H_2O) and with fast respiratory rates, flow may not be adequate to flush CO_2 from the circuit. Studies have shown that use of an EPAP of 4 cm H_2O or higher improves continuous flow of gas through the system and minimizes CO_2 rebreathing.[76,77] Some have considered adding an isolation-type exhalation valve to the circuit to eliminate CO_2 rebreathing, but these valves tend to increase expiratory airway resistance significantly and increase WOB.

Pressure support ventilators initially were designed for use in the home or in noncritical areas of patient care. Their simple design and ease of operation make them ideal for home or subacute care. However, most of these units have few monitoring capabilities or alarms. With the increased use of NIV to treat ARF and to avoid intubation, pressure-targeted ventilators have been developed with alarms that can detect large leaks, patient disconnection, and mechanical failure. Monitoring capabilities have improved such

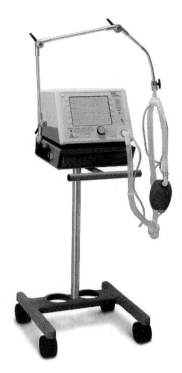

Fig. 19-2 The BiPAP Vision Ventilatory Support System. (Courtesy Philips Respironics, The Netherlands.)

that the respiratory rate and V_T are measured and displayed. Pressure support ventilators, such as the BiPAP Vision (Fig. 19-2) and Hamilton Raphael, provide graphic waveforms, which allow the practitioner to monitor for patient-ventilator asynchrony and make necessary adjustments (Key Point 19-8).

⊃ Key Point 19-8 To prevent CO_2 rebreathing, EPAP level should be set at 4 cm H_2O or higher so that adequate gas flows can flush CO_2 from the breathing circuit.

Portable Homecare Ventilators

Portable homecare ventilators originally were designed for invasive ventilation in the home or extended care facility for patients who required long-term assisted ventilation. These electrically powered, microprocessor-controlled ventilators have the advantages of compact size and the use of three power sources: A/C current, internal D/C battery, and external D/C battery. They are patient- or time-triggered, pressure-limited, and volume- or pressure-cycled.

The first generation of these ventilators had only pressure triggering capabilities, volume cycling, and limited flow delivery during inspiration. This often resulted in increased WOB to initiate breaths and patient discomfort due to unmet flow demands.

Unlike adult critical care ventilators, early portable ventilators have very basic audible and visual alarms, which include low battery, power loss, low pressure, high pressure, power switchover, apnea, and microprocessor malfunction. Older models have no graphic waveforms for monitoring. PEEP can be obtained only by attaching an external threshold resistor to the patient circuit exhalation valve. These units are not equipped with internal blenders, and therefore precise oxygen concentrations are not possible.

As with portable pressure-targeted ventilators, oxygen must be bled into the system through an adaptor from a separate oxygen source. Older portable volume ventilators, if used for noninvasive ventilation, are more likely to be used in patients with chronic respiratory failure resulting from neuromuscular disorders. These patients require higher ventilating pressures that cannot be obtained with portable pressure-targeted ventilators.

With the increased use of NIV, portable homecare ventilators have undergone a revolutionary change. They now include different modes, alarms, and graphic capabilities similar to those of acute care ventilators and portable pressure-targeted ventilators. Previously, these units were strictly volume ventilators, but many (e.g., Pulmonetic LTV 1000 Ventilator [CareFusion, Viasys Corp, San Diego, Calif.] or VerseMed iVent201 [GE Healthcare, Pittsburgh, Pa.] [Fig. 19-3]) now have both volume- and pressure-targeted modes of ventilation, flow triggering, and PEEP capabilities. These ventilators are more responsive to patient flow needs and can be used for either invasive or noninvasive ventilation. Thus, they are ideal for achieving a seamless transition from the extended care facility to the home.

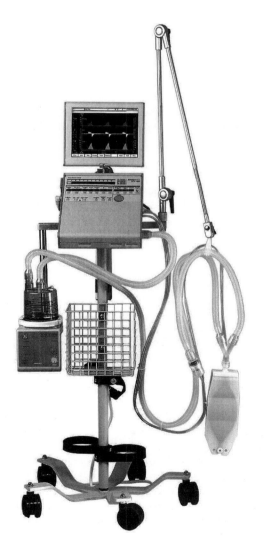

Fig. 19-3 The LTV 1000 ventilator. (Courtesy CareFusion, Viasys, San Diego, Calif.)

Adult Acute Care Ventilators

Ventilators used in adult critical care units offer additional ventilatory support options and alarms, a precise F_IO_2, and more monitoring features than portable pressure-targeted ventilators. These extra features may be advantageous for patients in ARF who require close monitoring and supervision during NIV. Although the pressure support mode is most commonly used to administer NIV, volume- or pressure-controlled modes combined with PEEP can also be administered via mask interface.

The most significant disadvantage of using acute care ventilators is the inability of some machines to compensate for leaks. Leaks at the patient interface interfere with triggering and cycling functions of the ventilator and result in patient-ventilator asynchrony and increased WOB. In the pressure support ventilation mode, air leaks cause gas flow to increase during delivery of the breath, making the cycle threshold difficult to achieve. This may prolong the inspiratory phase or cause the patient to exhale actively against the flow in an effort to terminate the breath. Most ICU ventilators have a flow-cycled mechanism that can be adjusted to terminate the breath sooner if air leaks increase the inspiratory time. The increased flow in the circuit may also cause some ventilators to autotrigger into inspiration or impair the patient's ability to flow trigger the machine into inspiration (trigger asynchrony), resulting in increased muscle activity on inspiration.

When significant leaks are present around the interface, the patient may be more comfortable in a pressure-targeted, time-cycled mode, such as pressure-controlled continuous mandatory ventilation (PC-CMV). In this mode, a rate and inspiratory time can be set according to the patient's rate and inspiratory time during spontaneous breathing. Cycling to exhalation then is a function of time rather than flow, which may improve synchronization with the ventilator and reduce patient respiratory effort.[78]

Although studies have demonstrated no significant differences in gas exchange between volume- and pressure-targeted modes,[78,79] volume control modes are seldom used to deliver NIV in the acute care setting. This is most likely because of the leakage around the interface, which may cause a loss of volume delivery to the patient, resulting in hypoventilation. V_T can be increased to compensate for leaks, but ventilating pressures often increase as well. Volume control modes are more likely to be used in the chronic care setting for patients with neuromuscular disorders who have been taught to "stack" breaths to achieve larger V_T to enhance coughing and secretion clearance.[80]

In response to the growing popularity of NIV, some manufacturers have upgraded acute care ventilators with specific noninvasive modes of ventilation that compensate for leaks in the same manner as portable PTVs. Difficulties with triggering and cycling have improved, but considerable variation in the efficiency of this leak compensation still exists between acute care ventilators.[81,82] As the amount of leakage increases, many of these ventilators still require adjustments of trigger sensitivity and cycling function to maintain patient-ventilator synchrony.

Humidification Issues During Noninvasive Ventilation

Excessive drying of nasal mucosa from the administration of nasal CPAP or NIV has been associated with nasal congestion and increased nasal resistance.[83] This is a leading cause of patient discomfort and noncompliance with the prescribed therapy. Recent studies have shown that using a heated humidifier during administration of nasal CPAP can significantly reduce drying of the nasal mucosa.[84] It is important to recognize that the addition of a humidifier may increase the cost of administering care but humidification leads to improved patient comfort and compliance during NIV.[85] A passover-type heated humidifier should be used because heated bubble humidifiers and heat-moisture exchangers can increase airway resistance in the ventilator circuit and interfere with patient triggering[86] (Key Point 19-9).

Key Point **19-9** Passover heated humidifiers should be used to treat or prevent nasal congestion and improve patient comfort. Bubble humidifiers and heat-moisture exchangers increase airway resistance and will increase inspiratory WOB.

Patient Interfaces

The effectiveness of NIV is greatly influenced by the interface chosen to deliver positive pressure to the airway. A variety of interfaces are available, including nasal masks, oronasal masks, total face masks, helmets, nasal pillows, and mouthpieces with lip seals. All interfaces have advantages and disadvantages (Table 19-3); therefore the clinician must choose one that optimizes patient comfort and compliance with NIV.

Nasal Interfaces

Nasal masks are widely used for both CPAP and NIV (Fig. 19-4). Although nasal masks are available in many sizes and shapes from a number of manufacturers, the basic design is a small translucent, triangular device with a plastic shell and a cushion of soft, supple material that helps provide a seal around the patient's nose. The mask is secured to the patient's head and face by a harness composed of hook-and-loop fastening straps or a soft polyester head cap.

A nasal mask may offer several advantages over a full-face mask. It is much easier to fit and secure to the patient's face, and it may be more tolerable than a face mask to patients who feel claustrophobic. Because the nasal mask covers only the patient's nose, it allows the patient to cough and clear secretions, speak, and possibly eat. Nasal masks have considerably less mechanical dead space than full-face masks; therefore the potential for rebreathing CO_2 is greatly reduced.

The two most common disadvantages of the nasal mask are air leaks and skin irritation. Leaks occur to some degree in all patients receiving NIV with any mask. Nasal masks are more prone to leakage, especially in patients who are primarily mouth-breathers. For these patients, a chin-strap may help hold the mouth closed during administration of NIV. Air leaks around the nasal mask often result in eye irritation. The strap tension required to maintain a snug fit between the nasal mask and the face often creates intolerable skin pressure, especially over the bridge of the nose. If the headgear straps are too tight, leakage may worsen, as does the pressure exerted over the nose. This can lead to redness and irritation of the skin and the potential for ulceration. Clinicians must ensure the tension on the headgear straps is not excessive. The clinician should be able to slip at least one finger between the straps and the patient's face.

Leaks and discomfort commonly occur because the mask is too large for the patient. Most manufacturers now provide mask-specific sizing gauges to aid sizing (Fig. 19-5). For nasal masks, the smallest mask that comes closest to the following contact points should be used:

- The point just above the junction of the nasal bone and cartilage (nasal bridge)
- The skin on the sides of both nares
- The area just below the lowest point of the nose, above the upper lip[87]

TABLE 19-3	Advantages and Disadvantages of the Various Interfaces Used in NIV	
Interface	**Advantages**	**Disadvantages**
Nasal masks	Easy to fit and secure to patient's face	Mouth leaks
	Less feeling of claustrophobia	Eye irritation
	Low risk of aspiration	Facial skin irritation
	Patient can cough and clear secretions	Ulceration over nose bridge
	Maintains ability to speak and eat	Oral dryness
	Less mechanical dead space	Nasal congestion
		Increased resistance through nasal passages
Full-face masks (oronasal masks)	Reduces air leakage through the mouth	Increased risk of aspiration
	Less airway resistance	Increased risk of asphyxia
		Increased dead space
		Claustrophobia
		Difficult to secure and fit
		Facial skin irritation
		Ulceration over nose bridge
		Must remove mask to eat, speak, or expectorate secretions
Nasal pillows or seals Mouthpieces	Same as nasal mask	Pressure sores around nares
	Facilitate communication	Nasal air leaking
	Less feeling of claustrophobia	Hypersalivation
	Low risk of aspiration	Possible orthodontic deformity
	Patient can cough and clear secretions	
	Low risk of CO_2 rebreathing	
	No headgear requirements	

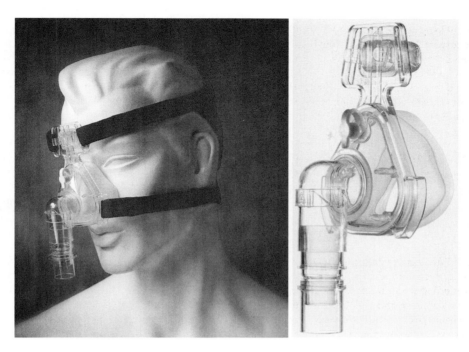

Fig. 19-4 Disposable nasal mask and headgear. (Courtesy Philips Respironics, The Netherlands.)

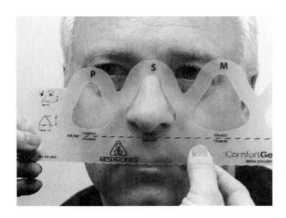

Fig. 19-5 A fitting gauge is used to assure correct fitting of nasal mask. (Courtesy Philips Respironics, The Netherlands.)

Several manufacturers have modified the standard nasal mask to minimize leakage and to enhance patient comfort for chronic use of NIV. One such modification is a mask with gel-filled cushions that seal better and with less pressure exerted over the nose (Fig. 19-6). Other modifications include the use of forehead spacers or an extra-thin plastic flap around the cushion of the mask to permit better sealing of the mask with less pressure and discomfort.

A recently introduced mini-mask incorporates a small lightweight cushion that sits on the tip of the nose, eliminating both the pressure over the bridge of the nose and air leakage into the eyes (Fig. 19-7). For patients who cannot tolerate any of the commercially available masks, a custom-molded mask may be contoured to the patient's face enhancing comfort and reducing air leaks.

Patients who cannot tolerate nasal masks may use nasal pillows or nasal-sealing cushions. These consist of soft rubber or silicone pledgets that fit directly into the patient's nares (or seal the opening) and are held in place by a plastic shell attached to adjustable headgear (Fig. 19-8).

Full (Oronasal) and Total Face Mask and Helmet

The oronasal mask, or full-face mask, covers the nose and the mouth and may be used in NIV for patients who cannot tolerate nasal masks because of large air leaks through the patient's mouth. (Fig. 19-9). This mask has become popular for the treatment of patients with ARF because acutely dyspneic patients tend to breathe more through the mouth as dyspnea increases.

Several concerns arise with the use of the full-face mask. Two important concerns are the potential for aspiration if vomiting occurs and the risk of asphyxia if the ventilator malfunctions. Commercially available masks are now equipped with quick-release mechanisms for simple removal and entrainment valves that open to allow breathing of room air if the ventilator malfunctions. A typical adult full-face mask has an average dead space volume of 250 mL.[88] The presence of dead space raises the concern of possible CO_2 rebreathing. In addition, the full-face mask does not allow the patient to eat or communicate well or to cough and expectorate secretions without removing the mask. Patients may also have a greater tendency to feel claustrophobic with this type of mask. As with the nasal mask, proper size and fit help ensure patient safety, comfort, and compliance with the therapy. Using a sizing gauge for oronasal masks, the clinician should choose the smallest-size mask that comes closest to the following contact points:

• The area just outside the sides of the mouth
• The area just below the lower lip
• The bridge of the nose (Fig. 19-10)

Other alternatives for patients who cannot tolerate nasal or oronasal masks may be the total face mask or helmet. The total face mask consists of a clear, lightweight, plastic faceplate surrounded by a soft inflatable cushion that seals the perimeter of the face and does not obstruct vision (Fig. 19-11). When the mask is connected to a ventilating system, air circulates throughout the entire mask, providing for more comfortable breathing. The incidence of pressure sores is lower because the mask seals the entire face.

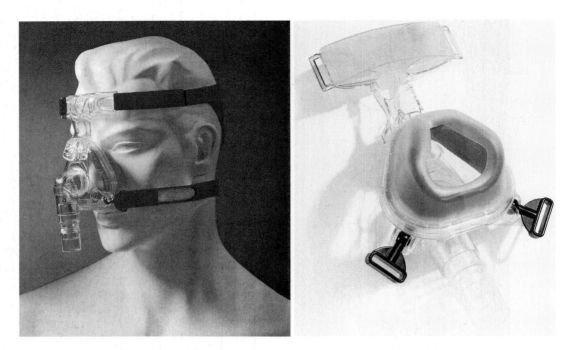

Fig. 19-6 Gel-filled nasal masks. (Courtesy Philips Respironics, The Netherlands.)

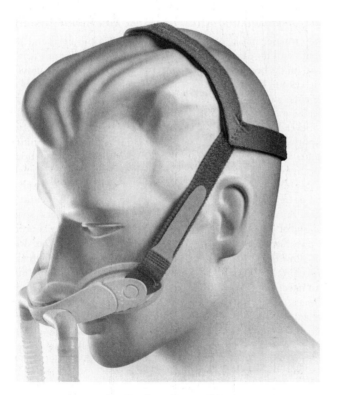

Fig. 19-7 Nasal mini-mask and headgear. (Courtesy Philips Respironics, The Netherlands.)

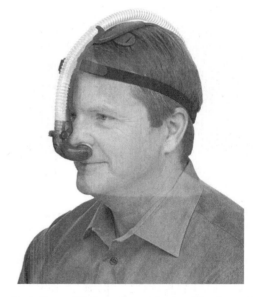

Fig. 19-8 Nasal pillows and headgear. (Courtesy Covidien-Nellcor Puritan-Bennett, Boulder, Colo.)

The concerns discussed for the full-face mask (aspiration, asphyxiation, and rebreathing) also apply to the total face mask. Like the full-face mask, the total face mask is equipped with a quick-release feature and entrainment valve for room air breathing in case of ventilator malfunction.

The helmet is a transparent cylinder of polyvinyl chloride that fits over the patient's entire head. A metallic ring enclosed within a soft silicone collar seats the cylinder at the patient's neck and shoulders and is further secured by straps under each armpit (Fig. 19-12). Two hoses attach to the cylinder to allow for gas entering and leaving the hood. Although this device is not currently approved for use in the United States, it has been used successfully in other countries for the treatment of ARF.[89,90]

The helmet has several advantages compared with the full-face mask: less resistance to gas flow, less need for patient cooperation,

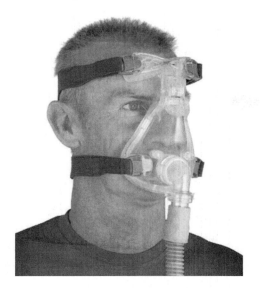

Fig. 19-9 Full-face mask or oronasal mask. (From ResMed, Poway, Calif.)

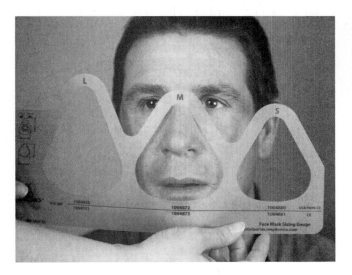

Fig. 19-10 Sizing gauge used to determine proper size of full-face mask. (Courtesy of Philips Respironics, The Netherlands.)

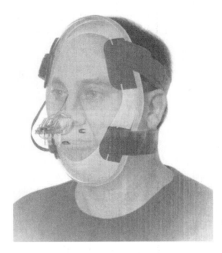

Fig. 19-11 Total face mask. (Courtesy of Philips Respironics, The Netherlands.)

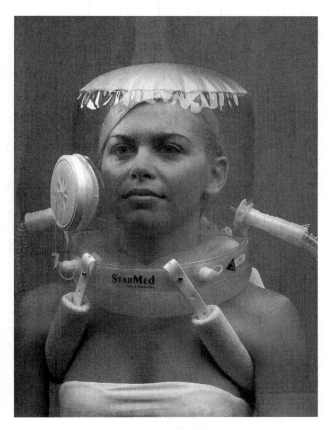

Fig. 19-12 NIV helmet. (Courtesy StarMed Spa, Biomedical CE, Mirondola, Italy.)

less interference with speech or coughing, and less skin breakdown. A primary concern with the use of the helmet is potential for CO_2 rebreathing as a result of the large volume of the cylinder.[91] Studies comparing the use of the helmet to the full-face mask have also shown that the helmet is less efficient in decreasing the inspiratory WOB and increases patient ventilator asynchrony.[91,92]

Oral Interfaces

Mouthpieces and lip seals have been used to provide NIV for many years in patients with chronic respiratory failure (Fig. 19-13). Mouthpieces provide an effective means of ventilation for patients with neuromuscular disorders and may provide an alternative for patients who cannot control mouth leakage during nasal ventilation. Mouthpieces have the advantages of facilitating communication, secretion clearance, and oral intake, and they minimize the problem of CO_2 rebreathing.

Mouthpieces do not usually require the use of headgear or straps. They often can be held in place with the hands or held in the mouth with an orthodontic appliance, especially during daytime hours. Patients with neuromuscular disorders who are confined to a wheelchair often secure their mouthpiece to a gooseneck clamp attached to the chair. It is important to recognize that nasal air leakage is a concern when using mouthpieces and may compromise NIV efficacy. Nose clips may help alleviate this problem. If the mouthpiece is used nocturnally, lip seals can be added over the mouthpiece to prevent leakage during sleep. Also, custom-fitted mouthpieces can prevent leakage and add to the comfort and efficacy of NIV.

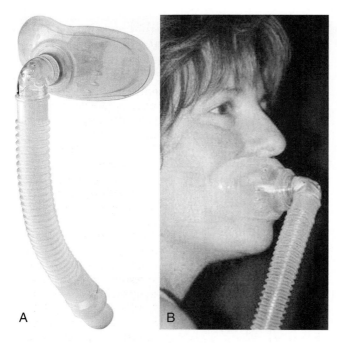

A　　**B**

Fig. 19-13 **A,** Oral mouthseal. **B,** Oral mouthseal position on a patient. (Courtesy Fisher & Paykell Healthcare, Laguna Hills, Calif.)

BOX **19-5**	Predictors of Success with NIV

- Higher level of consciousness
- Younger age
- Less severe illness; no comorbidities
- Less severe gas exchange abnormalities (pH 7.10 to 7.35; arterial partial pressure of carbon dioxide [P_aCO_2] <92 mm Hg)
- Minimal air leakage around the interface
- Intact dentition
- Synchronous breathing efforts with ventilator
- Lower quantity of secretions
- Absence of pneumonia
- Positive initial response to NIV within 1 to 2 hours
  - Correction of pH
  - Decreased respiratory rate
  - Reduced P_aCO_2

BOX **19-4**	Steps for Initiating NIV

1. Place patient in an upright or sitting position. Carefully explain the NIV procedure including goals and possible complications.
2. Using a sizing gauge, make sure a mask is chosen that is the proper size and fit.
3. Attach the interface and circuit to ventilator. Turn on the ventilator and adjust it initially to low-pressure settings.
4. Hold or allow the patient to hold the mask gently to the face until the patient becomes comfortable with it. Encourage the patient in proper breathing technique.
5. Monitor oxygen (O_2) saturation; adjust the fractional inspired oxygen (F_IO_2) to maintain O_2 saturation above 90%.
6. Secure the mask to the patient. Do not make the straps too tight.
7. Titrate the inspiratory positive airway pressure (IPAP) and expiratory positive airway pressure (EPAP) to achieve patient comfort, adequate exhaled tidal volume, and synchrony with the ventilator. Monitor the peak airway pressure delivered.
8. Check for leaks and adjust the straps if necessary.
9. Monitor respiratory rate, heart rate, level of dyspnea, O_2 saturation, minute ventilation, and exhaled tidal volume.
10. Obtain blood gas values within 1 hour.

SETUP AND PREPARATION FOR NONINVASIVE VENTILATION

After selecting the ventilator and interface or interfaces, the respiratory therapist is responsible for initiating NIV (Box 19-4). Effective ventilation absolutely requires patient cooperation and tolerance; therefore the respiratory therapist must gain the

patient's trust and compliance. Carefully explaining the process and repeating the explanations as the process continues can significantly improve patient compliance. The purpose of the interface, goals of the therapy, expected results, and possible complications should be explained clearly using terms that the patient can understand.

The respiratory therapist may want to have several types and sizes of interfaces at the patient's bedside. If a mask is chosen, a fitting gage can aid in ensuring the proper size and fit. After selecting the appropriate interface, the respiratory therapist turns on the ventilator, attaches the interface to the circuit, and sets initial low-pressure settings. Most often, these include an EPAP pressure of 4 to 5 cm H_2O and an IPAP pressure of 8 to 10 cm H_2O.[6] At this point, the alarms are silenced and the patient is allowed to hold the mask to the face before the headgear is secured.

During the setup, the respiratory therapist should reassure the patient and coach the person in the proper breathing pattern. A different interface or mask size may be necessary if excessive leakage or discomfort occurs. Once the patient is comfortable and his or her breathing has become synchronized with the ventilator, the headgear straps are adjusted to ensure a snug, secure fit. The straps should not be too tight because this increases leakage from the mask (as mentioned previously, if the interface has been properly secured, the respiratory therapist should be able to slip at least one finger under the straps). Once ventilation has been established and the patient's comfort is ensured, the respiratory therapist can further assess the patient and the effectiveness of the patient-ventilator system.

MONITORING AND ADJUSTMENT OF NONINVASIVE VENTILATION

Several studies have identified potential indicators of success for patients on NIV in both the acute and chronic care setting (Box 19-5).[93-95] In the acute care setting, NIV is more likely to be successful in patients who are alert and cooperative, can protect the airway, and have not yet developed severe acid–base or gas exchange abnormalities than it is in patients who are limited in any of these. The patient's initial response to NIV may be the most significant indicator of success or failure. For this reason, close bedside monitoring of the patient's vital signs and respiratory status begins as soon as NIV is instituted and continues until the patient's respiratory status has stabilized (Case Study 19-1).

Case Study 19-1

Patient Selection for NIV

A 72-year-old woman with a history of COPD is receiving NIV for ventilatory failure secondary to postoperative pneumonia. The patient is wearing a full-face mask but is having difficulty swallowing and coughing. She appears very weak and has become more agitated and confused in the past hour. The respiratory rate is 24 breaths/min, and the S_pO_2 is 92%. Oxygen is being bled into the patient's mask at the rate of 5 L/min. What action should be taken at this time?

Patient tolerance and comfort with the system are important to ensuring the effectiveness of NIV at alleviating respiratory distress. Clinically, improvement in patient comfort is indicated by a decrease in respiratory rate, reduced inspiratory muscle activity, and synchronization with the ventilator. If these indicators are absent, the respiratory therapist must take steps to ensure patient's comfort, such as refitting or changing the mask to reduce air leakage, encouraging and coaching the patient in the proper breathing pattern, or adjusting ventilator settings (Key Point 19-10).

Key Point 19-10 Improvement in patient comfort is indicated by a decreased respiratory rate, decreased inspiratory muscle activity, and synchronization with the ventilator.

Insufficient IPAP levels often result in sustained or increased respiratory rates caused by inadequate V_T delivery. Slowly increasing the IPAP to maintain the exhaled V_T at 6 to 8 mL/kg may result in a decrease in the respiratory rate.[22] Patient-ventilator synchrony may be improved by adjusting rise time, inspiratory sensitivity, and expiratory flow cycling percentage (if available) and by carefully increasing EPAP to offset possible intrinsic PEEP. If EPAP is increased, IPAP also may need to be increased to maintain the same gradient between IPAP and EPAP and thus ensure adequate V_T delivery. Low doses of sedative may also be necessary to assist patient compliance (Case Study 19-2).

Oxygenation and heart rate are monitored continuously with pulse oximetry. The F_IO_2 is adjusted to maintain S_pO_2 at 90% to 92%. Shortly after initiation of NIV (1 to 2 hours), the adequacy of ventilatory support is determined by arterial blood gas (ABG) measurements. Patients showing an improved pH and P_aCO_2 are more likely to avoid intubation.[94,95] However, the P_aCO_2 may take longer to decrease in some patients, particularly those with chronic hypercapnia. This should not cause alarm as long as the patient is showing clinical improvement in oxygenation and a decrease in respiratory distress.

Case Study 19-2

Monitoring and Adjusting NIV

A 71-year-old, 176-lb (80-kg) man is admitted to the ICU for an acute exacerbation of COPD. On admission he was tachypneic and dyspneic, as evidenced by a respiratory rate of 30 beats/min and the use of accessory muscles of respiration. Arterial blood gas values with nasal oxygen at 2 L/m were as follows: pH = 7.31, P_aCO_2 = 56 mm Hg, P_aO_2 = 49 mm Hg. The attending physician ordered NIV in an attempt to normalize the pH. The respiratory therapist initiates NIV with a full-face mask at the following settings: A/C mode; respiratory rate (f) = 12 breaths/min; IPAP = 10 cm H_2O; EPAP = 4 cm H_2O; and oxygen at 3 L/min bled into the circuit at the machine outlet.

After 1 hour on NIV, the patient complains of some dyspnea and discomfort and has a respiratory rate of 26 breaths/min. The average exhaled tidal volume is approximately 310 mL. The full-face mask appears to fit well, and no significant leaks are detected. Arterial blood gases at this time are as follows: pH = 7.32, P_aCO_2 = 53 mm Hg, P_aO_2 = 59 mm Hg, and S_aO_2 = 90%. What changes, if any, should be made in the current settings to make the patient more comfortable and help to normalize pH?

A patient in ARF is closely observed in an acute care setting (ICU, emergency department) so that if NIV is unsuccessful, other means of support are readily available. Attempts at NIV are terminated in favor of invasive measures if the pH and P_aCO_2 continue to worsen or show no improvement and are accompanied by respiratory distress, worsening level of consciousness, hemodynamic instability, or worsening oxygenation. Other measures of support may be necessary if the patient cannot tolerate any of the types or sizes of interfaces or is unable to clear secretions and protect the airway (Box 19-6).

Some patients require NIV on a long-term, intermittent basis (e.g., as for OSA). The focus of monitoring in these patients is to alleviate the signs and symptoms associated with chronic hypoventilation and impaired sleep, such as fatigue, daytime somnolence, morning headache, and dyspnea. In some cases signs and symptoms of **cor pulmonale** associated with chronic hypoxemia may also be present, such as distended neck veins, enlarged liver, and peripheral edema. Alleviation of these signs and symptoms may take several days or weeks and depend mainly on the patient's comfort, tolerance, and compliance with the NIV system. Efforts

BOX 19-6	Criteria for Terminating NIV and Switching to Invasive Mechanical Ventilation

1. Worsening pH and arterial partial pressure of carbon dioxide (P_aCO_2)
2. Tachypnea (>30 breaths/min)
3. Hemodynamic instability
4. Pulse oximeter oxygen saturation (S_pO_2) less than 90%
5. Decreased level of consciousness
6. Inability to clear secretions
7. Inability to tolerate interface

are made to maximize patient comfort by choosing a well-fitting and comfortable interface and headgear and by initiating short trials of NIV and slowly increasing the patient's time on the system. Once a patient can tolerate the NIV system for 4 to 6 hours per 24 hours, signs and symptoms are likely to improve.

Objective evidence (e.g., continuous nocturnal oximetry, ABGs) may reveal an improvement in gas exchange and a decrease in or complete cessation of the number of sleep-related respiratory events. If no improvement is seen after about 4 to 6 weeks, the clinician should attempt to determine the reasons for failure. These may include lack of motivation and compliance because of discomfort, advanced age, the existence of comorbidities and cognitive defects, or the need for additional therapeutic efforts[72] (Case Study 19-3).

AEROSOL DELIVERY IN NONINVASIVE VENTILATION

The administration of aerosolized bronchodilators is often necessary for patients receiving NIV, especially those with obstructive airway disease. Patients may be removed from the ventilator and given aerosolized medications via nebulizer or metered-dose inhaler (MDI) with a spacer in the traditional manner, but this may cause rapid deterioration of the patient's condition. Bronchodilators given in-line with the NIV single-limb circuit by either a nebulizer or MDI with a spacer are effective, but clinicians should be aware of the factors that affect the efficiency of aerosol delivery (Box 19-7).[96]

Case Study 19-3

Common Complications of NIV

A 68-year-old man with severe stable COPD and OSA has been receiving NIV via nasal mask for approximately 3 months. Follow-up ABG analysis and continuous nocturnal oximetry do not show any significant improvement in gas exchange or the frequency of sleep-related events. When questioned about his use of the NIV system, the patient admits that he uses the system only for about 2 hours because of uncomfortable nasal dryness and sinus pain. The respiratory therapist examines the patient's NIV equipment and notes that it includes an unheated passover humidifier and that the nasal mask appears to fit well without significant leakage. What can be done to increase the patient's comfort and tolerance with the NIV system?

Previous studies have shown that the efficiency of aerosol delivery is similar for either a nebulizer or an MDI when the leak port is located in the circuit and the aerosol device is placed between the

BOX **19-7**	Factors Affecting Aerosol Delivery During NIV

1. Type of aerosol generator (SVN vs. metered-dose inhaler [MDI])
2. Position of the leak port
3. Synchronization of MDI actuation with inspiration
4. IPAP and EPAP levels
5. Presence or absence of a humidifier in the circuit

leak port and the mask[96] (Fig. 19-14). If the leak port is located in the mask, aerosol delivery from an MDI is more efficient than from a nebulizer provided the MDI is actuated at the beginning of inspiration. Regardless of the device used, a greater amount of aerosol is lost through the leak port during the exhalation phase of breathing. Increased aerosol delivery is also more likely when using high inspiratory pressures and low expiratory pressures.[97] This is likely due to a longer inspiratory phase. As expiratory pressures increase, aerosol delivery decreases. Aerosol delivery to the lower airways is less effective when administered through a humidified circuit during invasive ventilation. It is reasonable to suggest that the use of a humidified circuit with NIV would likely give similar results, although this effect has not been studied with NIV.

Nasal masks or full-face masks present additional problems during aerosol delivery. Air leaks in the mask or circuit cause continuous flow in the circuit to increase, which may potentially increase aerosol loss. The volume of the mask itself increases the potential for a larger portion of the aerosol dose to deposit on the face or in the eyes of the patient. For this reason aerosol therapy is not recommended when a total face mask or helmet is being used to administer NIV.[98]

COMPLICATIONS OF NONINVASIVE VENTILATION

NIV is considered much safer than invasive mechanical ventilation. Complications with NIV are usually related to mask discomfort, air pressures, or gas flows. Serious complications can occur, such as aspiration pneumonia, pneumothorax, and hypotension, but they are unlikely if patient-selection guidelines are closely followed. If the NIV is to be successful, the respiratory therapist must be knowledgeable about all potential complications and take the proper course of action to prevent or minimize their occurrence.

Mask discomfort is the most common complication of NIV. Air leaks around the mask often result in eye irritation. In addition, the strap pressure required to maintain an airtight fit often creates excessive pressure over the bridge of the nose and cheek area. Pressure sores may develop, leading to skin breakdown and ulceration of the nasal bridge. To correct this problem, the respiratory therapist first checks the mask for proper size and fit, making sure that the mask is not too large and that headgear tension has been minimized as much as possible. Forehead spacers or wound-care dressing (e.g. Duoderm) or both may alleviate pressure on the nasal bridge and protect the skin. In some cases a change to a different style of mask or headgear system or a complete change of interface may be required. Nasal gel masks, bubble-type masks, and masks with added plastic flaps are designed to facilitate a better seal with lower headgear strap tensions.

Nasal pillows or nasal seals can also be used to relieve pressure on the nasal bridge, but they can become uncomfortable because of pressure on the nares. If this occurs, alternating between interface styles may help, especially when NIV is to be used long term.

Another common complaint from patients who use nasal masks is nasal and oral dryness or nasal congestion from high flows through the mask and air leakage through the mouth. Adding or increasing humidification or irrigating the nasal passages with saline may prove helpful. If congestion persists, topical nasal decongestants or steroids can be used. A chin-strap may help with oral dryness because of air leakage through the mouth for patients who have nasal masks. These straps keep the patient's mouth closed and minimize leakage, thus reducing the airflow to the mask. If

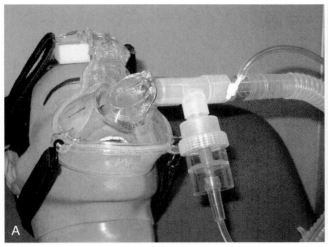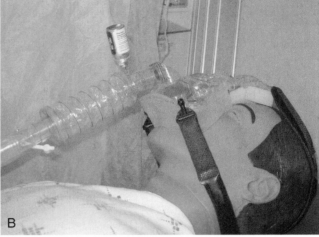

Fig. 19-14 A, Position of small-volume nebulizer between leak port in the circuit and the NIV mask. **B,** Position of MDI spacer between leak port in the circuit and the NIV mask.

chin-straps are not effective at reducing leakage through the mouth, a change to an oronasal mask may be better because it covers both the nose and mouth. However, oronasal masks are subject to the same skin contact problems as nasal masks and may also increase claustrophobic reactions.

Oral interfaces (mouthpieces and lip seals) are associated with minor complications, such as oral discomfort, hypersalivation, and leakage of air from the nose. Most of these problems diminish with fitting adjustments and patient adaptation. If leakage is sufficient to compromise the efficacy of NIV, nose clips may alleviate the problem. Patients who prefer mouthpieces for NIV probably will invest in a custom-made mouthpiece. These may prove to be more tolerable for chronic long-term use of NIV.

Regardless of the interface used, gastric insufflation is a common occurrence in about 50% of all patients using NIV; however, it is rarely intolerable.[86] Gastric insufflation is more likely to occur in patients using volume ventilation.[99] In such cases, gas in the stomach probably is the result of the higher pressure needed for V_T delivery. For the most part, gas insufflation does not cause major problems and usually diminishes in time or with the administration of **simethicone agents.**

A serious potential complication of NIV is aspiration pneumonia, which is most likely to occur if vomitus is retained in the mask when an oronasal mask is used. Some clinicians recommend that a nasogastric tube be used with an oronasal mask, particularly in patients with excessive gastric distention, nausea, and vomiting.[1] As mentioned previously, aspiration is best prevented through careful selection of patients who are able to cough and protect the airway.

Other major complications of NIV include mucus plugging, hypoxemia, hypotension, and respiratory arrest. Mucus plugging is more likely to occur if the patient is dehydrated or has difficulty expectorating secretions or if humidification is inadequate. High oxygen flow rates (up to 40 L/min) have been associated with life-threatening airway obstruction caused by **inspissated secretions.**[100] The risk of mucus plugging can be minimized if patients are kept well hydrated and appropriate adjunct therapies are applied to assist with secretion removal. Patients with neuromuscular disorders who have impaired cough mechanisms may benefit from cough-assistive techniques. Inline aerosolized

bronchodilators and heated humidity may also aid secretion removal in most patients.

Hypoxemia is more likely to occur in patients with hypoxemic respiratory failure who require high oxygen concentrations. Most portable pressure-targeted ventilators cannot achieve consistent F_IO_2 levels above 50% unless oxygen is bled into the system at abnormally high flow rates, which may interfere with patient synchrony and alter the pressure and flow delivery from the ventilator. Mucus plugging, agitation, and failure to keep the mask on the patient's face also have been linked to hypoxemia. The appearance of any of these contributing factors may be an indication to change to invasive mechanical ventilation.

Hemodynamic complications rarely occur during the administration of NIV or CPAP because low inflation pressures are used with these techniques. Hypotension, when it occurs, is usually seen in patients with low intravascular fluid volume or underlying cardiac disease. Hypotension rarely occurs in patients with COPD but may result if high levels of auto-PEEP develop.

Patients with ACPE may benefit from increased intrathoracic pressures, which reduce venous return and subsequently ventricular preload. However, if ventricular preload declines markedly, organ perfusion may be compromised. Careful selection of initial pressures and close monitoring may reduce the risk for cardiac ischemia in these patients. Table 19-4 summarizes the complications associated with CPAP and NIV.

WEANING FROM AND DISCONTINUING NONINVASIVE VENTILATION

The duration of ventilatory assistance with NIV depends on how quickly the cause of respiratory failure can be reversed. In most patients with ARF, successful weaning from NIV may occur within hours or a few days.[22,45] Standard weaning techniques have not been established, but the most common approach involves increasing periods of time off mask ventilation.

Once the patient's condition is stabilized, the mask may be removed for short periods according to the patient tolerance. Supplemental oxygen is administered as necessary during these times off the ventilator. The patient is closely monitored for signs of respiratory distress and fatigue.

TABLE 19-4 Complications Associated with Mask CPAP/NIV Therapy	
Complications	**Corrective Actions**
Mask discomfort	Check mask for correct size and fit
Excessive leaks around mask	Minimize headgear tension
Pressure sores	Use spacers or switch mask style
	Use wound-care dressing over nasal bridge
Nasal/oral dryness or nasal congestion	Add or increase humidification
	Irrigate nasal passages with saline
	Apply topical decongestants
	Use a chin-strap to keep the mouth closed
	Change to full-face mask
Mouthpiece/lip seal leakage	Use nose clips
	Use custom-made oral appliances
Aerophagia, gastric distention	Use lowest effective pressures for adequate V_T delivery
	Use simethicone agents
Aspiration	Adhere to proper selection of patients who can protect their own airway
Mucus plugging	Ensure adequate patient hydration
	Ensure adequate humidification
	Avoid excessive oxygen flow rates (>20 L/min)
	Allow short breaks from NIV to permit directed coughing techniques
Hypotension	Avoid excessively high peak pressures (≤20 cm H_2O)

If signs of respiratory distress occur, the patient is placed back on mask ventilation immediately. Prolonging these periods of ventilator interruption when the patient is experiencing respiratory distress may lead to rapid decompensation and the need for emergency intubation.

In the same manner as spontaneous breathing trials, periods off the ventilator lengthen as the underlying condition improves and the patient shows acceptable vital signs, good gas exchange, and no respiratory distress. (See Chapter 20 for information on spontaneous breathing trials.)

Another approach to NIV weaning is applied in the same manner as weaning from pressure support ventilation during invasive ventilation. IPAP is gradually reduced to a minimum level, allowing the patient to assume more of the WOB. Once the minimum level has been reached, NIV can be discontinued.

Regardless of the weaning method used, the reversibility of the disease process that caused ARF is the most important consideration for successful weaning. Some patients, especially those with chronic hypercapnia and impaired ventilatory function, may continue to use NIV nocturnally after recovering from an acute exacerbation.

PATIENT CARE TEAM CONCERNS

The success of NIV depends on time and commitment from the members of the patient care team. All members of this team must thoroughly understand the indications, benefits, and complications of NIV. As a critical member of this team, the respiratory therapist often must commit considerable time to initiating and monitoring NIV. Studies have shown that more time is required during an initial 8-hour shift to institute NIV than to establish conventional invasive ventilation.[101-103] The extra time is required to fit the patient properly with an interface and to monitor and adjust ventilator settings. Time and patience are also required to remain at the bedside and to instruct patients carefully to obtain

their full cooperation. Once the patient's condition has stabilized, this time requirement usually decreases.

 SUMMARY

- Noninvasive ventilation is an important option for patients requiring mechanical ventilation.
- The three basic methods of applying noninvasive ventilation are negative-pressure ventilation, abdominal-displacement ventilation, and positive-pressure ventilation.
- The physiological goal of NIV in ARF is to improve gas exchange by resting the respiratory muscles and increasing alveolar ventilation.
- The most significant benefit of using NIV in treating ARF caused by COPD is the avoidance of intubation, which in turn can lead to longer hospital stays, higher mortality, and increased health care costs.
- NIV may improve daytime gas exchange and symptoms associated with chronic hypoventilation for patients who continue to hypoventilate despite CPAP therapy.
- NIV can be used to reduce the WOB and maintain adequate gas exchange in patients who show fatigue following extubation.
- Patients with terminal or advanced disease who develop ARF are not good candidates for endotracheal intubation and mechanical ventilation. NIV may relieve severe dyspnea in these patients and help ensure patient comfort.
- In the acute care setting, the selection process for NIV must be based on the patient's diagnosis and clinical characteristics, as well as the risk of failure.
- Establishment of the need for intermittent ventilatory assistance in patients with chronic respiratory failure should begin

with the recognition of the typical symptoms of nocturnal hypoventilation and poor sleep quality.

- NIV should be initiated if patients with moderate to severe OSA do not respond favorably to CPAP.
- Excessive drying of nasal mucosa is a common complaint of patients receiving nasal CPAP or NIV. Proper humidification can prevent or improve mucosal dehydration.
- The type of interface used to deliver positive pressure to the airway can influence the effectiveness of NIV. Nasal masks have considerably less mechanical dead space than full-face masks, thus reducing the potential for rebreathing CO_2.
- NIV is more likely to be successful in the acute care setting for patients who are alert and cooperative, can protect the airway, and have not yet developed severe acid–base or gas-exchange abnormalities.
- Potential complications of NIV include aspiration pneumonia, mucus plugging, hypoxemia, hypotension, and respiratory arrest.

REVIEW QUESTIONS (See Appendix A for answers.)

1. NIV has just been initiated on a patient in respiratory distress with an IPAP pressure of 12 cm H_2O and an EPAP pressure of 5 cm H_2O. Which of the following would indicate clinical improvement of the patient's condition?
   1. Increased respiratory rate
   2. Synchronization with the ventilator
   3. Decreased inspiratory muscle activity
   4. Decreased S_aO_2
      A. 1 and 2 only
      B. 2 and 3 only
      C. 2, 3, and 4
      D. 1, 2, 3, and 4

2. Which of the following patients would **not** be a good candidate for nasal-mask NIV?
   A. A patient with a pH of 7.34
   B. A patient with stable COPD and OSA
   C. A patient with an absent cough reflex
   D. A patient who requires nocturnal NIV only

3. A patient has been on nasal-mask NIV for almost 24 hours. The patient is now complaining of nasal congestion and a dry mouth. Which of the following would you recommend?
   A. Reduce the inspiratory flow
   B. Change to a full-face mask
   C. Begin inline aerosol treatments
   D. Add a heated humidifier

4. A patient may benefit from the nocturnal application of NIV if which of the following symptoms is present?
   1. Morning headache
   2. Daytime hypersomnolence
   3. Aching and stiff joints
   4. Nocturnal desaturation
      A. 1 and 2 only
      B. 1, 2, and 4
      C. 1, 2, 3, and 4
      D. 1 and 4 only

5. A patient has been on NIV with a nasal mask for the past hour. The patient is still experiencing significant leaking around the mask. Which of the following would be the most appropriate action to take at this time?
   A. Change to a full-face mask
   B. Tighten the head straps
   C. Intubate and begin invasive mechanical ventilation
   D. Add a heated humidifier to the circuit

6. The best way to prevent aspiration during NIV is to:
   A. Insert a nasogastric tube before NIV application
   B. Use only a nasal mask for application
   C. Adhere to proper selection guidelines
   D. Use delivery pressures less than 10 cm H_2O

7. Which of the following are reported to be advantages of using a portable pressure-targeted ventilator in the delivery of NIV?
   1. Variable flow delivery capabilities
   2. Leak compensation
   3. Adjustable inspiratory and expiratory sensitivity
   4. Sophisticated alarm systems
      A. 1 and 2 only
      B. 1, 2, and 3
      C. 2, 3, and 4
      D. 1, 2, 3, and 4

8. Which of the following would result in the lowest F_IO_2 during the administration of NIV when oxygen is bled into the circuit of a portable pressure-targeted ventilator?
   A. Bleeding oxygen into the mask when the leak port is located in the mask
   B. Bleeding oxygen into the mask when the leak port is located in the circuit
   C. Bleeding oxygen into the circuit when the leak port is located in the circuit
   D. Bleeding oxygen into the circuit and sealing the leak

9. Which of the following ventilator settings would most likely result in rebreathing of CO_2?
   A. EPAP levels >6 cm H_2O
   B. EPAP levels <4 cm H_2O
   C. IPAP levels >6 cm H_2O
   D. CPAP levels >6 cm H_2O

10. The physiological benefits of NIV include which of the following?
    A. Decrease in P_aCO_2 levels
    B. Decrease in P_aO_2 levels
    C. Decrease in HCO_3^- levels
    D. Increase use of accessory muscles

11. A patient is admitted to the coronary ICU for acute cardiogenic pulmonary edema. The physician wants to use noninvasive ventilatory support in the treatment of this patient's condition. Which mode of ventilatory support would be most appropriate to use at this time?
    A. PSV
    B. IPAP and EPAP
    C. CPAP
    D. PSV and PEEP

12. The highest level of evidence now supports the use of NIV as a standard of care in the treatment of:
    A. Community-acquired pneumonia
    B. Severe but stable COPD
    C. Acute asthma
    D. Acute exacerbations of COPD

13. A patient has been on NIV for 1 hour in the assist mode only. Ventilator settings include IPAP at 8 cm H_2O and EPAP at 4 cm H_2O. Oxygen is being bled into the circuit at 4 L/min. The patient's ABGs after 1 hour reveal pH = 7.34, P_aCO_2 = 62 mm Hg, and P_aO_2 = 62 mm Hg. The patient's respiratory rate is 27 breaths/min and S_pO_2 is 92%. There is minimal leaking around the face mask. What would be the most appropriate ventilator change to make at this time?
    A. Increase EPAP level to 8 cm H_2O
    B. Decrease EPAP level to 2 cm H_2O
    C. Increase IPAP level to 10 cm H_2O
    D. Decrease IPAP level to 6 cm H_2O

14. All of the following may increase CO_2 rebreathing during NIV **except:**
    A. Use of a full-face mask
    B. Low EPAP pressure levels
    C. Patient breathing pattern
    D. High inspiratory flow rates

15. Clinical benefits of NIV in an acute care setting include which of the following?
    1. Lower incidence of ventilator-associated pneumonia
    2. Improved patient comfort
    3. Reducing staff time in the care of patients with COPD
    4. Lower intubation rate
        A. 1 and 2
        B. 2 and 3
        C. 1, 2, and 4
        D. 1, 2, 3, and 4

References

1. Mehta S, Hill NS: Noninvasive ventilation. *Am J Respir Crit Care Med* 163:540–577, 2001.
2. Bott J, Carroll MP, Conway JH, et al: Randomized controlled trial of nasal ventilation in acute ventilatory failure due to chronic obstructive airways disease. *Lancet* 341:1555–1557, 1993.
3. Brochard L, Mancebo J, Wysocki M, et al: Noninvasive ventilation for acute exacerbations of chronic obstructive pulmonary disease. *N Engl J Med* 333:817–822, 1995.
4. Celikel T, Sungur M, Ceyhan B, et al: Comparison of noninvasive positive pressure ventilation with standard medical therapy in hypercapnic acute respiratory failure. *Chest* 114:1636–1642, 1998.
5. Dikensoy O, Ikidag B, Filiiz A, et al: Comparison of non-invasive ventilation and standard medical therapy in acute hypercapnic respiratory failure: a randomised controlled trial at a tertiary health centre in SE Turkey. *Int J Clin Pract* 56:85–88, 2002.
6. Kramer N, Meyer TJ, Meharg J, et al: Randomized, prospective trial of noninvasive positive pressure ventilation in acute respiratory failure. *Am J Respir Crit Care Med* 151:1799–1806, 1995.
7. Plant PK, Owen JL, Elliott MW: Early use of non-invasive ventilation for acute exacerbations of chronic obstructive pulmonary disease on general respiratory wards: a multicenter randomized controlled trial. *Lancet* 355:1931–1935, 2000.
8. Motley HL, Werko L, et al: Observations on the clinical use of intermittent positive pressure. *J Aviat Med* 18:417–435, 1947.
9. The Intermittent Positive Pressure Breathing Trial Group: Intermittent positive pressure breathing therapy of chronic obstructive pulmonary disease. *Ann Intern Med* 99:612–620, 1983.
10. Sullivan CE, Issa FG, Berthon-Jones M, et al: Reversal of obstructive sleep apnoea by continuous positive airway pressure applied through the nares. *Lancet* 1:862–865, 1981.
11. Sullivan CE, Berthon-Jones M, Issa FG: Remission of severe obesity-hypoventilation syndrome after short-term treatment during sleep with nasal continuous positive airway pressure. *Am Rev Respir Dis* 128:177–181, 1983.
12. McEvoy RD, Thornton AT: Treatment of obstructive sleep apnea syndrome with nasal continuous positive airway pressure. *Sleep* 7:313–325, 1984.
13. Ellis ER, Bye PT, Bruderer JW, et al: Treatment of respiratory failure during sleep in patients with neuromuscular disease: positive-pressure ventilation through a nose mask. *Am Rev Respir Dis* 135:148–152, 1987.
14. Bach JR, Alba A, Mosher R, et al: Intermittent positive pressure ventilation via nasal access in the management of respiratory insufficiency. *Chest* 94:168–170, 1987.
15. Kerby GR, Mayer LS, Pingleton SK: Nocturnal positive pressure ventilation via nasal mask. *Am Rev Respir Dis* 136:188–191, 1987.
16. Meduri GU, Conoscenti CC, Menashe P, et al: Noninvasive face mask ventilation in patients with acute respiratory failure. *Chest* 95:865–870, 1989.
17. Carrey Z, Gottfried SB, Levy RD: Ventilatory muscle support in respiratory failure with nasal positive pressure ventilation. *Chest* 97:150–158, 1990.
18. Brochard L, Isabey D, Piquet J, et al: Reversal of acute exacerbations of chronic obstructive lung disease by inspiratory assistance with a face mask. *N Engl J Med* 323:1523–1530, 1990.
19. Lightowler JV, Wedzicha JA, Elliott MW, et al: Non-invasive positive pressure ventilation to treat respiratory failure resulting from exacerbations of chronic obstructive pulmonary disease: Cochrane systematic review and meta-analysis. *BMJ* 326:185, 2003.
20. Hill NS: Noninvasive ventilation for chronic obstructive pulmonary disease. *Respir Care* 49:72–87, 2004.
21. Hess DR: The evidence for noninvasive positive-pressure ventilation in the care of patients in acute respiratory failure: a systematic review of the literature. *Respir Care* 49:810–829, 2004.
22. Meduri GU, Cook TR, Turner RE, et al: Noninvasive positive pressure ventilation in status asthmaticus. *Chest* 110:767–774, 1996.
23. Soroksky A, Stav D, Shpirer IL: A pilot prospective, randomized, placebo-controlled trial of bilevel positive airway pressure in acute asthma attack. *Chest* 123:1018–1025, 2003.
24. Gupta D, Nath A, Agarwall R, et al: A prospective randomized controlled trial on the efficacy of noninvasive ventilation in severe acute asthma. *Respir Care* 55:536–543, 2010.
25. Scala R: Noninvasive ventilation in severe acute asthma? Still far from the truth. *Respir Care* 55:630–637, 2010.
26. Martin TJ, Hovis JD, Costantino JP, et al: A randomized, prospective evaluation of noninvasive ventilation for acute respiratory failure. *Am J Respir Crit Care Med* 161:807–813, 2000.
27. Antonelli M, Conti G, Rocco M, et al: A comparison of noninvasive positive-pressure ventilation and conventional mechanical ventilation in patients with acute respiratory failure. *N Engl J Med* 339:429–435, 1998.
28. Wysocki M, Tric MA, Wolf H, et al: Noninvasive pressure support ventilation in acute respiratory failure. *Chest* 107:761–768, 1995.
29. Ambrosino N, Foglio K, Rubini F, et al: Non-invasive mechanical ventilation in acute respiratory failure due to chronic obstructive pulmonary disease: correlates for success. *Thorax* 50:755–757, 1995.
30. Jolliet P, Abajo B, Pasquina P, et al: Non-invasive pressure support ventilation in severe community-acquired pneumonia. *Intensive Care Med* 27:812–821, 2001.
31. Elliot MW, Steven MH, Phillips GD, et al: Noninvasive mechanical ventilation for acute respiratory failure. *BMJ* 300:358–360, 1990.
32. Hoffman B, Welte T: The use of noninvasive pressure support ventilation for severe respiratory insufficiency due to pulmonary edema. *Intensive Care Med* 25:15–20, 1999.
33. Rusterholtz T, Kempf J, Berton C, et al: Noninvasive pressure support ventilation (NIPSV) with face mask in patients with acute cardiogenic pulmonary edema (ACPE). *Intensive Care Med* 25:21–28, 1999.
34. Nava S, Carbone G, DiBattista N, et al: Noninvasive ventilation in cardiogenic pulmonary edema: a multicenter randomized trial. *Am J Respir Crit Care Med* 168:1432–1437, 2003.
35. Mehta S, Jay GD, Woolard RH, et al: Randomized prospective trial of bilevel versus continuous positive airway pressure in acute pulmonary edema. *Crit Care Med* 25:620–628, 1997.
36. Ferrari G, Olliveri F, De Filippi G, et al: Noninvasive positive airway pressure and risk of myocardial infarction in acute cardiogenic pulmonary edema: continuous positive airway pressure vs noninvasive positive pressure ventilation. *Chest* 132:1804–1809, 2007.
37. Pang D, Keenan SP, Cook DJ, et al: The effect of positive pressure airway support on mortality and the need for intubation in cardiogenic pulmonary edema: a systematic review. *Chest* 114:1185–1192, 1998.

38. Bach JR, Alba AS, Saporito LR: Intermittent positive pressure ventilation via the mouth as an alternative to tracheostomy for 257 ventilator users. *Chest* 103:174–182, 1993.

39. Bach JR, Alba AS: Management of chronic alveolar hypoventilation by nasal ventilation. *Chest* 97:52–57, 1990.

40. Kerby GR, Mayer LS, Pingleton SK: Nocturnal positive pressure ventilation via nasal mask. *Am Rev Respir Dis* 135:738–740, 1987.

41. Ellis ER, Bye PT, Bruderer JW, et al: Treatment of respiratory failure during sleep in patients with neuromuscular disease: positive pressure ventilation through a nose mask. *Am Rev Respir Dis* 135:148–152, 1987.

42. Bach JR: A comparison of long-term ventilatory support alternatives from the perspective of the patient and care giver. *Chest* 104:1702–1706, 1993.

43. Ledger P, Bedicam JM, Cornette A, et al: Nasal intermittent positive pressure: long-term follow-up in patients with severe chronic respiratory insufficiency. *Chest* 105:100–105, 1994.

44. Consensus Conference: Clinical indications for noninvasive positive pressure ventilation in chronic respiratory failure due to restrictive lung disease, COPD, and nocturnal hypoventilation: Consensus Conference Report. *Chest* 116:521–534, 1999.

45. American Respiratory Care Foundation: Consensus Conference: Noninvasive positive pressure ventilation. *Respir Care* 42:364–369, 1997.

46. Braun NM, Marino WD: Effect of daily intermittent rest of respiratory muscles in patients with severe chronic airflow limitation. *Chest* 85:59S–60S, 1984.

47. Cropp A, Dimarco AF: Effects of intermittent negative pressure ventilation on respiratory muscle function in patients with severe chronic obstructive pulmonary disease. *Am Rev Respir Dis* 135:1056–1061, 1987.

48. Elliott MW, Mulvey DA, Moxham J, et al: Domiciliary nocturnal nasal intermittent positive pressure ventilation in COPD: mechanisms underlying changes in arterial blood gas tensions. *Eur Respir J* 4:1044–1052, 1991.

49. Elliott MW, Simonds AK, Carroll MP, et al: Domiciliary nocturnal nasal intermittent positive pressure ventilation in hypercapnic respiratory failure due to chronic obstructive lung disease: effects on sleep and quality of life. *Thorax* 47:342–348, 1992.

50. Meecham-Jones DJ, Paul EA, Carlisle CC, et al: Nasal pressure support ventilation plus oxygen compared with oxygen therapy alone in hypercapnic COPD. *Am J Respir Crit Care Med* 152:538–544, 1995.

51. Meecham-Jones DJ, Paul EA, Jones PW, et al: Nasal pressure support ventilation plus oxygen compared with oxygen therapy alone in hypercapnic COPD. *Am J Respir Crit Care Med* 152:538–544, 1995.

52. Gay PC, Hubmayr RD, Stroetz RW: Efficacy of nocturnal nasal ventilation in stable, severe, chronic obstructive pulmonary disease during a 3-month controlled trial. *Mayo Clin Proc* 71:533–542, 1996.

53. Granton JT, Kesten S: The acute effects of nasal positive pressure ventilation in patients with advanced cystic fibrosis. *Chest* 113:1013–1018, 1998.

54. Hodson ME, Madden BP, Steven M, II, et al: Non-invasive mechanical ventilation for cystic fibrosis patients: a potential bridge to transplantation. *Eur Respir J* 4:524–527, 1991.

55. Hill AT, Edenborough FP, Clayton RM, et al: Long-term nasal intermittent positive pressure ventilation in patients with cystic fibrosis and hypercapnic respiratory failure (1991–1996). *Respir Med* 92:523–526, 1998.

56. Granton JT, Shapiro C, Kesten S: Noninvasive ventilatory support in advanced lung disease from cystic fibrosis. *Respir Care* 47:675–681, 2002.

57. Piper AJ, Sullivan CE: Effects of short-term NIPPV in the treatment of patients with severe obstructive sleep apnea and hypercapnia. *Chest* 105:434–440, 1994.

58. Smyrnios NA, Connolly A, Wilson MM, et al: Effects of a multifaceted, multidisciplinary, hospital-wide quality improvement program on weaning from mechanical ventilation. *Crit Care Med* 30:1224–1230, 2002.

59. Kollef MH, Shapiro SD, Silver P, et al: A randomized, controlled trial of protocol-directed versus physician-directed weaning from mechanical ventilation. *Crit Care Med* 25:567–574, 1997.

60. Chastre J, Fagon JY: Ventilator-associated pneumonia. *Am J Respir Crit Care Med* 165:867–903, 2002.

61. Vitacca M, Ambrosino N, Clini E, et al: Physiological response to pressure support ventilation delivered before and after extubation in patients not capable of totally spontaneous autonomous breathing. *Am J Respir Crit Care Med* 164:638–641, 2001.

62. Nava S, Ambrosino N, Clini E, et al: Noninvasive mechanical ventilation in the weaning of patients with respiration failure due to chronic obstructive pulmonary disease: a randomized controlled trial. *Ann Intern Med* 128:721–728, 1998.

63. Girault C, Daudenthun I, Chevron V, et al: Noninvasive ventilation as a systematic extubation and weaning technique in acute-on-chronic respiratory failure: a prospective, randomized controlled study. *Am J Respir Crit Care Med* 160:86–92, 1999.

64. Ferrer M, Exquinas A, Arancibia F, et al: Noninvasive ventilation during persistent weaning failure: a randomized controlled trial. *Am J Respir Crit Care Med* 168:70–76, 2003.

65. Benhamou D, Girault C, Faure C, et al: Nasal mask ventilation in acute respiratory failure: experience in elderly patients. *Chest* 102:912–917, 1992.

66. Meduri GU, Fox RC, Abou-shala N, et al: Noninvasive mechanical ventilation via face mask in patients with acute respiratory failure who refused endotracheal intubation. *Crit Care Med* 22:1584–1590, 1994.

67. Nelson DL, Short K, Vespia J, et al: A prospective review of the outcomes of patients with "do-not-intubate" orders who receive noninvasive bilevel positive pressure ventilation (abstract). *Crit Care Med* 28(Suppl 12):A34, 2000.

68. Freichels T: Palliative ventilatory support: use of noninvasive positive pressure ventilation in terminal respiratory insufficiency. *Am J Crit Care* 3:6–10, 1994.

69. Clarke DE, Vaughan L, Raffin TA: Noninvasive positive pressure ventilation in terminal respiratory failure: the ethical and economic costs of delaying the inevitable are too great. *Am J Crit Care* 3:4–5, 1994.

70. Benhamou D, Muir JF, Raspaud C, et al: Long term efficiency of home nasal mask ventilation in patients with diffuse bronchiectasis and severe chronic respiratory failure: a case control study. *Chest* 112:1259–1266, 1997.

71. Sittig SE: Transport, home care, and noninvasive ventilatory devices. In Cairo JM, editor: *Mosby's respiratory care equipment*, ed 9, St Louis, 2014, Elsevier, pp 513–597.

72. Lofaso F, Brochard L, Touchard D, et al: Home versus intensive care pressure support devices: experimental and clinical comparison. *Am J Respir Crit Care Med* 153:1591–1599, 1996.

73. Waugh JB, De Kler RM: Inspiratory time, pressure settings, and site of supplemental oxygen insertion affect delivered oxygen fraction with Quantum PSV noninvasive positive pressure ventilator. *Respir Care* 44:520–523, 1999.

74. Thys F, Liistro G, Dozin O, et al: Determinants of F_IO_2 with oxygen supplementation during noninvasive two level positive pressure ventilation. *Eur Respir J* 19:653–657, 2002.

75. Schwartz AR, Kacmarek RM, Hess DR: Factors affecting oxygen delivery with bi-level positive airway pressure. *Respir Care* 49:270–275, 2004.

76. Lofaso F, Brochard L, Touchard D, et al: Evaluation of carbon dioxide rebreathing during pressure support ventilation with airway management system (BiPAP) devices. *Chest* 108:772–778, 1995.

77. Ferguson GT, Gilmartin M: CO_2 rebreathing during BiPAP ventilatory assistance. *Am J Respir Crit Care Med* 151:1126–1135, 1995.

78. Calderini E, Confalonieri M, Puccio PG, et al: Patient-ventilator asynchrony during non-invasive ventilation: the role of expiratory trigger. *Intensive Care Med* 25:662–667, 1999.

79. Restrick LF, Fox NC, Braid G, et al: Comparison of nasal pressure support ventilation with nasal intermittent positive pressure ventilation in patients with nocturnal hypoventilation. *Eur Respir J* 6:364–670, 1993.

80. Bach JR: Mechanical insufflation-exsufflation: comparison of peak expiratory flows and manually assisted and unassisted coughing techniques. *Chest* 104:1553–1562, 1993.

81. Vignaux L, Didier T, Jolliet P: Performance of noninvasive ventilation modes on ICU ventilators during pressure support: a bench model study. *Intensive Care Med* 33:1444–1451, 2007.

82. Ferreira JC, Chipman DW, Hill NS, et al: Bilevel vs ICU ventilators providing noninvasive ventilation: effect of system leaks. *Chest* 136:448–456, 2009.

83. Hayes MJ, McGregor FB, Roberts DN, et al: Continuous nasal airway positive pressure with a mouth leak: effect on nasal mucosal blood flux and nasal geometry. *Thorax* 50:1179–1182, 1995.

84. de Arauja MT, Vieira SB, Vasquez EC, et al: Heated humidification or face mask to prevent upper airway dryness during continuous positive airway pressure. *Chest* 117:142–147, 2000.

85. Massie CA, Hart RW, Peralez K, et al: Effects of humidification on nasal symptoms and compliance in sleep apnea patients using continuous positive airway pressure. *Chest* 116:403–408, 1999.

86. Hill N: Complications of noninvasive positive pressure ventilation. *Respir Care* 42:432–442, 1997.

87. *Mask and accessories: an examination of size, fit and adjustments.* Andover, MA, 1993, Philips Respironics Inc.

88. Turner RE: NIV: Face versus interface. *Respir Care* 42:389–393, 1997.

89. Antonelli M, Conti G, Pelosi P, et al: New treatment of acute hypoxemic respiratory failure: noninvasive pressure support ventilation delivered by helmet—a pilot controlled trial. *Crit Care Med* 30:602–608, 2002.

90. Scandroglio M, Piccolo U, Mazzone E, et al: Use and nursing of the helmet in delivering noninvasive ventilation. *Minerva Anestesiol* 68:475–480, 2002.

91. Fabrizio R, Lorenzo A, Cesare G, et al: Effectiveness of mask and helmet interfaces to deliver noninvasive ventilation in a human model of resistive breathing. *J Appl Physiol* 99:1262–1271, 2005.

92. Navalesi P, Costa R, Ceriana P, et al: Non-invasive ventilation in chronic obstructive pulmonary disease patients: helmet versus facial mask. *Intensive Care Med* 33:74–81, 2007.

93. Lieschring T, Kwok H, Hill NS: Acute applications of noninvasive positive pressure ventilation. *Chest* 124:699–713, 2003.

94. Soo Hoo GW, Santiago S, Williams AJ: Nasal mechanical ventilation for hypercapnic respiratory failure in chronic obstructive pulmonary disease: determinants of success and failure. *Crit Care Med* 22:1253–1261, 1994.

95. Anton A, Guell R, Gomex J, et al: Predicting the result of noninvasive ventilation in severe acute exacerbations of patients with chronic airflow limitation. *Chest* 117:828–833, 2000.

96. Branconnier M, Hess D: Albuterol delivery during noninvasive ventilation. *Respir Care* 50:1649–1653, 2005.

97. Chatmongkolchart M, Guilherme P, Dillman C, et al: In vitro evaluation of aerosol bronchodilator delivery during noninvasive positive pressure ventilation: effect of ventilator settings and nebulizer position. *Crit Care Med* 30:2515–2519, 2002.

98. Hess D: The mask for noninvasive ventilation: principles of design and effects on aerosol delivery. *J Aerosol Med* 20:S85–S98, 2007.

99. Leger P: Noninvasive positive pressure ventilation at home. *Respir Care* 39:501–510, 1994.

100. Wood KE, Flaten AL, Backes WJ: Inspissated secretions: a life-threatening complication of prolonged noninvasive ventilation. *Respir Care* 45:491–493, 2000.

101. Chevrolet JC, Joillet P, Abajo B, et al: Nasal positive pressure ventilation in patients with acute respiratory failure: difficult and time consuming procedure for nurses. *Chest* 100:775–782, 1991.

102. Kramer N, Meyer TJ, Meharg J, et al: Randomized prospective trial of noninvasive positive pressure ventilation in acute respiratory failure. *Am J Respir Crit Care Med* 151:1799–1806, 1995.

103. Nava S, Evangelisti I, Rampulla C, et al: Human and financial costs of noninvasive mechanical ventilation in patients affected by COPD and acute respiratory failure. *Chest* 111:1631–1638, 1997.

Weaning and Discontinuation from Mechanical Ventilation

OUTLINE

KEY TERMS

- Adaptive support ventilation
- Automatic tube compensation
- Mandatory minute ventilation
- Respiratory alternans
- Weaning

LEARNING OBJECTIVES *On completion of this chapter, the reader will be able to do the following:*

1. List the weaning parameters and acceptable values for ventilator discontinuation.
2. Compare the three standard modes of weaning in relation to their success in discontinuing ventilation.
3. Define the closed-loop modes of weaning described in the chapter.
4. Recognize appropriate clinical use of closed-loop modes of weaning from a description of a clinical setting.
5. Identify assessment criteria for discontinuing a spontaneous breathing trial in a clinical situation.
6. Describe criteria used to determine whether a patient is ready for extubation.
7. Recognize postextubation difficulties from a clinical case description.
8. Recommend appropriate treatment for postextubation difficulties.
9. State the first recommendation for weaning a patient from mechanical ventilation established by the task force formed by the American College of Chest Physicians (ACCP), the Society of Critical Care Medicine (SCCM), and the American Association for Respiratory Care (AARC).
10. Describe an appropriate treatment for a patient with an irreversible respiratory disorder that requires long-term ventilation.
11. Name the parameter used as the primary index of drive to breathe.
12. Suggest adjustments to ventilator settings during use of a standard weaning mode based on patient assessment.
13. Explain the appropriate procedure for management of a patient for whom a spontaneous breathing trial has failed.
14. Defend the use of therapist-driven protocols as key components of efficient and effective patient weaning.
15. Explain the function of long-term care facilities in the management of ventilator-dependent patients.
16. Assess data used to establish the probable cause of failure to wean.

Weaning Techniques

Patients require mechanical ventilation when their ability to support ventilatory demands is outweighed by a disease process or when the respiratory drive is inadequate to maintain ventilation because of disease or medications (Fig. 20-1).[1,2] Ventilation can be discontinued after the need for mechanical ventilation has been resolved. This is typically a straightforward maneuver for most patients. The ventilator is simply disconnected from the patient and the endotracheal tube (ET) is removed. About 80% of patients requiring temporary mechanical ventilation do not require a gradual withdrawal process, and can be disconnected within a few hours or days of initial support.[3,4] Examples of this type of temporary ventilation include postoperative ventilatory support for recovery from anesthesia, treatment of uncomplicated drug overdose, and exacerbations of asthma. When the patient has undergone ventilation for less than a week, discontinuation is usually a quick process. However, for a some patients, the process can be lengthy and complex.[5]

The term **weaning** is frequently used to describe the gradual reduction of ventilatory support from a patient whose condition is improving.[1,2,4-7] Some practitioners prefer terms such as discontinuation, gradual withdrawal, or liberation.[1] Regardless of the terminology, the process is the same (Key Point 20-1).

> **Key Point 20-1** Weaning is frequently used to describe the gradual reduction of ventilatory support from a patient whose condition is improving. Other terms that are used describe this process include discontinuation, gradual withdrawal, or liberation.

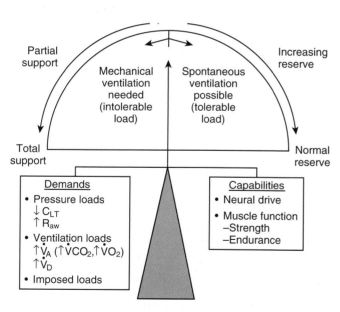

Fig. 20-1 Schematic of the balance between a patient's respiratory capabilities and demands. When demands outweigh capabilities, the balance shifts to the left and a higher level of ventilatory support is needed. As the patient's condition improves, the balance shifts to the right. The clinical challenges are twofold: (1) to recognize when ventilatory assistance is no longer needed and (2) to provide an appropriate level of assistance until that happens. C_{LT}, Compliance of the lungs and thorax; R_{aw}, airway resistance; $\dot{V}_A$, alveolar ventilation; $\dot{V}CO_2$, carbon dioxide production; $\dot{V}O_2$, oxygen consumption; $\dot{V}_D$, dead space ventilation. (Modified from MacIntyre NR: Psychological factors in weaning from mechanical ventilatory support, Respir Care 40:277-281, 1995.)

Several facts must be taken into consideration if ventilation is to be discontinued successfully. First, patients may require ventilatory support during weaning. Second, supplemental oxygen and positive end-expiratory pressure (PEEP) may be required to support oxygenation. Third, some individuals may require maintenance of the artificial airway even after ventilatory support has been discontinued. Fourth, many patients require more than one of these therapeutic interventions. Although each of the first three components mentioned can be treated separately, they are an integral part of the overall process of ventilator discontinuation (Box 20-1).[6,7]

Ventilatory support should be discontinued and the artificial airway removed as soon as possible to avoid the risks associated with mechanical ventilation, such as ventilator-induced lung injury, ventilator-associated pneumonia (VAP), airway trauma from the ET, and unnecessary sedation. However, it is important to recognize that premature withdrawal of ventilatory support or of the airway can result in ventilatory muscle fatigue, compromised gas exchange, and loss of airway protection.[1] Premature discontinuation is also associated with a higher mortality rate.[8-10]

The decision to wean a patient from the ventilator depends on the patient's level of recovery from the medical problems that imposed the need for mechanical ventilation, and the patient's overall clinical condition and psychological state. Therefore the patient's physiological capacity and mental and emotional status must be evaluated before an attempt is made to remove the patient from ventilatory support.

This chapter reviews ventilator techniques used during weaning from ventilatory support, in addition to evidence-based recommendations for determining whether a patient meets the criteria for ventilator discontinuation. A discussion of the process of weaning, clinical conditions that may compromise a patient's ability to be weaned, and the introduction to long-term care when a patient cannot be weaned are also presented.

METHODS OF TITRATING VENTILATOR SUPPORT DURING WEANING

Ventilatory support can be reduced as a patient becomes increasingly able to resume part of the work of breathing (WOB). Three approaches have been commonly used to reduce ventilatory support and gradually place more of the WOB on the respiratory muscles: intermittent mandatory ventilation (IMV), pressure support ventilation (PSV), and T-piece weaning. Until the early 1990s, the three methods were considered equally effective.[11] More recent studies have clearly shown that the weaning process was inordinately prolonged with IMV compared with other weaning techniques.[10,12] Despite these findings, a substantial number of physicians continue to use IMV to wean patients from mechanical ventilatory support.[13]

BOX 20-1	Components of Ventilatory Management and Discontinuation

- Positive pressure ventilation (PPV) to support breathing
- Supplemental oxygen and positive end-expiratory pressure (PEEP) to improve oxygenation
- Artificial airway to protect the airway and to provide invasive ventilation
- Airway management to maintain clear airways (i.e., suctioning; humidification and warming of inspired air; bronchial hygiene; and aerosolized medications)
- Therapy directed at the primary disease process

In addition to these traditional methods, more sophisticated forms of closed-loop ventilation have been introduced for weaning patients. These include volume-targeted PSV (e.g., volume support), automode, **mandatory minute ventilation** (MMV), **automatic tube compensation,** and artificial intelligence systems.

Intermittent Mandatory Ventilation

Intermittent mandatory ventilation (IMV) was first introduced in the 1960s as a method to ventilate infants afflicted with idiopathic respiratory distress syndrome. The first IMV systems used to wean adult patients from mechanical ventilation were introduced in the 1970s. Figure 20-2 shows a diagram of a volume ventilator with an added continuous-flow IMV circuit used for adult patients. A blended gas source is directed into a reservoir bag (3 L anesthetic bag). The IMV circuit connects this reservoir to the ventilator circuit by means of a one-way valve. The one-way valve prevents a positive pressure breath, generated by the machine, from entering the reservoir bag. This system allows a continuous flow of gas from the reservoir bag through the humidifier and the main inspiratory line to the patient. During a positive pressure breath, the high pressure closes the one-way valve, preventing machine air from entering the reservoir bag and allowing the mandatory ventilator breath.

Synchronized intermittent mandatory ventilation (SIMV) was later introduced as a method to synchronize a patient's efforts with the mandatory breaths provided by the ventilator during intermittent mandatory ventilation (IMV). The theory underlying IMV/ SIMV is that the patient's respiratory muscles would work during spontaneous breathing intervals and rest during mandatory breaths.[14] (NOTE: Modern microprocessor ventilators have incorporated this technology into their devices. Consequently the term *IMV* is simply used to describe mechanical ventilators that offer either SIMV or IMV.)

A common weaning practice with IMV is to reduce the mandatory rate progressively, usually in steps of 1 or 2 breaths/min and at a pace that matches the patient's improvement. PSV can be added to unload the spontaneous breaths and reduce the patient's WOB through the ventilator system, circuit, and artificial airway, which in turn can help prevent excessive fatigue (Case Study 20-1). Use of pressure support is especially important when the IMV rate is low (i.e., <4 to 6 breaths/min). The level of PSV used during IMV typically ranges from 5 to 10 cm H_2O; the set pressure usually depends on assessment of the spontaneous tidal volume (V_T) achieved and the apparent work of breathing. Positive end-expiratory pressure (PEEP) of 3 to 5 cm H_2O is also used to help compensate for changes in functional residual capacity (FRC) associated with the use of an ET and the recumbent position.[15,16]

Case Study 20-1

Evaluation of Weaning Attempt

A patient who appears to be ready for discontinuation of ventilatory support is being weaned with IMV. The data below indicate the patient's progress. No pressure support ventilation or continuous positive airway pressure is used to support spontaneous breaths.

Time	Set V_T (mL)	Spontaneous V_T (mL)	IMV Rate (breaths/ min)	Spontaneous Respiratory Rate (breaths/ min)
07:00	800	400-500	6	6
12:00	800	400-500	4	12
16:00	800	350-400	2	18
20:00	800	275-325	1	30

IMV, intermittent mandatory ventilation; V_T, tidal volume.

Do you think the patient is being managed correctly during the weaning process? If not, what would you recommend?

[handwritten note:] add PS ↑ IMV Rate PEEP is acceptable

Continuous Flow Intermittent Mandatory Ventilation

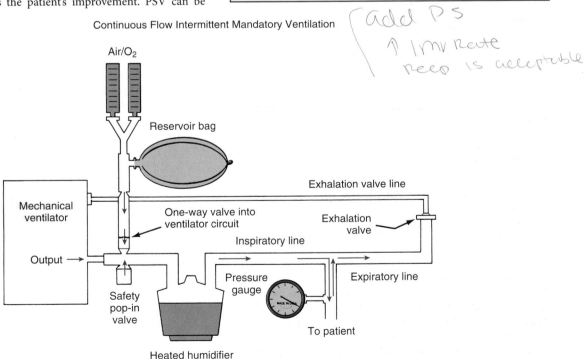

Fig. 20-2 Schematic illustrating the gas flow through a prototype intermittent mandatory ventilation (IMV) circuit. See text for details.

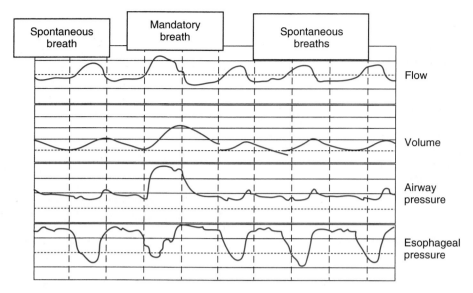

Fig. 20-3 Measurements of flow, volume, airway pressure, and esophageal pressure in a patient ventilated with synchronized intermittent mandatory ventilation (IMV). The esophageal pressure swings reflect the changes in pleural pressure and are the result of respiratory muscle contraction. These pressure swings are nearly as large during a mandatory breath as during spontaneous breaths. (From Hess DR: Mechanical ventilation strategies: what's new and what's worth keeping? Respir Care 47:1007-1017, 2002.)

In reality, the respiratory muscles may perform significant work with both mandatory and spontaneous breaths during IMV (Fig. 20-3). Ventilator asynchrony may occur because the patient's respiratory center does not anticipate whether the next breath from the ventilator will be mandatory or spontaneous.[15] When the mandatory rate is reduced to the point where it provides 50% or less of the required minute ventilation ($\dot{V}_E$), the WOB for the patient actually may be as much as when support is withdrawn completely.[16,17] Consequently the patient's spontaneous respiratory rate may increase significantly.[10,12] (Additional information on IMV can be found in Chapter 5.)

Pressure Support Ventilation

With PSV, the patient controls the rate, timing, and depth of each breath; in other words, PSV is patient triggered, pressure limited, and flow cycled. The sophisticated monitoring and alarm systems available with intensive care unit (ICU) ventilators make this nonvolume-oriented approach a safe and effective mode of weaning. Theoretically PSV allows the clinician to adjust the ventilatory workload for each spontaneous breath to enhance endurance conditioning of the respiratory muscles without causing fatigue.[17,18]

The most practical method of establishing the level of PSV is to base the initial setting on the patient's measured airway resistance. In general, this is a pressure support level of 5 to 15 cm H_2O for patients who meet weaning criteria. Another sound approach involves attempting to reestablish the patient's baseline respiratory rate (15 to 25 breaths/min) and V_T (300 to 600 mL/min). An inappropriate pressure support setting can be identified by the presence of respiratory distress, which manifests as tachycardia, hypertension, tachypnea, diaphoresis, paradoxical breathing, **respiratory alternans** (altering use of the diaphragm to breath and the accessory muscles of respiration), and excessive accessory muscle use.

During weaning with PSV, the clinician gradually reduces the level of support as long as an appropriate spontaneous respiratory rate and V_T are maintained and distress is not evident. When pressure support is reduced to about 5 cm H_2O, the pressure level is not high enough to contribute significantly to ventilatory support. However, this level of support is usually sufficient to overcome the work imposed by the ventilator system (i.e., the resistance of the ET, trigger sensitivity, demand-flow capabilities, and the type of humidifier used).

T-Piece Weaning

T-piece weaning is the oldest of the available techniques. It originally involved removing the ventilator from the patient according to a predetermined schedule. The weaning process started when the patient was able to breathe spontaneously for brief periods without ventilatory support and the criteria for weaning had been met (these criteria are discussed later in the chapter). The original T-piece trial followed a schedule that progressively increased the length of time the patient was removed from ventilatory support. For example, the first period might have been 5 to 10 minutes, after which the patient was returned to the ventilator for the remainder of the hour. This process was repeated once an hour. The time off the ventilator was increased gradually until the patient was off the ventilator for 30 minutes and on for 30 minutes. The off time then was increased to 1 hour and so on.

The setup for a T-piece system includes a heated humidifier with a large reservoir. The humidifier is connected to a blended gas source (air/oxygen) that provides a high flow of gas (at least 10 L/min) at the desired fractional inspired oxygen (F_IO_2). The humidified gas source is connected to a T-piece (Briggs adapter) with large-bore tubing, which is attached to the patient's ET. Another piece of large-bore tubing is attached to the exhalation side of the T-piece (volume of about 120 mL) to provide a reservoir, or as some clinicians refer to it, an afterburner (Fig. 20-4).[19] If the patient

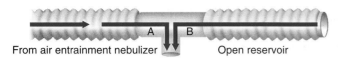

From air entrainment nebulizer   Open reservoir

Fig. 20-4 Use of an open reservoir to enhance oxygen delivery with a T-piece. When the patient inhales, gas at the set fractional inspired oxygen (F_IO_2) is drawn first through the inspiratory side of the circuit from the gas source **(A).** If the patient's flow demand exceeds the output, gas is inhaled from the open reservoir **(B).** Only after the reservoir volume is fully emptied by the patient is room air entrained, compromising F_IO_2 delivery. (From Wilkins RL, Stoller JK, Scanlan CL, editors: Egan's fundamentals of respiratory care, ed 8, St Louis, 2003, Mosby.)

inhales and the gas flow through the tubing from the humidifier is inadequate, some of the patient's inhaled air can be derived from this reservoir and still contain gas at the desired F_IO_2. Patients are seated or semirecumbent for the procedure and should be continuously monitored by a clinician while disconnected from the ventilator. It is important to recognize that this method of weaning requires a high level of staff attention.

When T-piece weaning is accomplished through the ventilator, the ventilatory mode is set to spontaneous/continuous positive airway pressure (CPAP); that is, the mandatory rate is turned off. The advantage of using the ventilator is the availability of alarms; the disadvantage is that the patient's efforts to breathe through the ventilator system may result in an increased workload. However, current ICU ventilators typically provide a bias flow of gas through the system and flow triggering that supports any spontaneous breaths and reduces the patient's WOB. Basically, this is similar to a small amount of pressure support. Thus the T-piece trial using a ventilator provides a means of continuously monitoring the patient. This approach also provides backup apnea alarms or backup ventilator modes to support patients who become apneic.

Patients less likely to tolerate T-piece weaning include those who have severe underlying heart disease, have severe muscle weakness, or who are inclined to panic because of psychological problems or preexisting chronic lung conditions.

Comparison of Traditional Weaning Methods

Studies comparing the IMV, PSV, and T-piece weaning techniques have produced conflicting results.[10,12] Each mode offers particular benefits to certain patients. If one procedure does not work well for a patient, another might work. Ventilator discontinuation is best accomplished when expert, caring staff members work with willing, cooperative patients.

CLOSED-LOOP CONTROL MODES FOR VENTILATOR DISCONTINUATION

In a closed-loop control ventilatory mode, a set variable is compared with a measured control variable.[20] The ventilator uses a feedback signal to adjust the output of the system. Closed-loop modes of ventilation range from simple techniques, such as volume support, to more complex ones, such as **adaptive support ventilation.** Advanced closed-loop control techniques that have been used for weaning include automatic tube compensation (ATC), volume-targeted PSV (e.g., volume support), mandatory minute ventilation (MMV), adaptive support ventilation (ASV), and an artificial intelligence system for weaning.

Automatic Tube Compensation

The WOB may increase when a spontaneously breathing patient breathes unaided through an ET.[20-22] The amount of the increase is directly related to the size of the artificial airway and the $\dot{V}_E$. Reducing the diameter or increasing the length of the tube increases the resistance to flow, as do kinks in the tube. These factors, coupled with high $\dot{V}_E$, increase the spontaneous WOB for the patient (see Chapter 17).

Clinicians often use low levels of pressure support (<10 cm H_2O) to compensate for the increased resistance and WOB associated with breathing through an ET.[21-23] However, the clinician must always keep in mind that a fixed pressure, as with PSV, cannot accurately compensate for the variable flow through the ET because inspiratory flow demand can vary.[24] Therefore a fixed level of pressure support can result in too little support when inspiratory flow is high, or too much support when inspiratory flow is low.[25] In fact, PSV can result in excessive V_T and flow, which is uncomfortable for the patient.[26]

To overcome this problem, some ICU ventilators (e.g., Puritan Bennett 840 [Covidien-Nellcor Puritan-Bennett, Boulder, Colo.], Dräger Evita XL [Dräger Medical, Telford, Pa.]) are equipped with a feature called automatic tube compensation (ATC). ATC was designed specifically to reduce the WOB associated with increased ET resistance.[15] Theoretically ATC delivers exactly the amount of pressure required to overcome the resistive load imposed by the ET for the flow measured at the time. In a sense, this is providing variable PSV with variable inspiratory flow compensation.[24] ATC targets pressure at the tracheal level, adjusting the delivered pressure to try to maintain tracheal pressure at a constant level (Fig. 20-5).[27,28] If the flow-resistive properties of the artificial airway are known, tracheal pressure changes can be determined by measuring inspiratory and expiratory flows.[29]

Automatic tube compensation functions by using a closed-loop control of the ventilator based on calculated tracheal pressures.[27,30] The pressure delivered to the upper airway during ATC increases by an amount equal to the continuously calculated pressure drop across the ET during inspiration.[29] The pressure change required to maintain the flow for a known resistance can be estimated using the following equation:

$$\Delta P = R\dot{V}_E$$

where ΔP is the pressure change, R is resistance, and $\dot{V}_E$ is flow. The equation for calculating tracheal pressure is:

Tracheal pressure = Proximal airway pressure − (Tube coefficient × Flow^2)[31]

In this equation, the tube coefficient relates to the size of the tube and its imposed resistance. (Note: ET resistance is a nonlinear function of flow, especially at higher flows.)[29,32]

To set ATC, the operator selects the ATC function on the ventilator and enters the type of tube (ET or tracheostomy) and the tube size. Some ventilators allow selection of both inspiratory and expiratory ATC.[31,33] Currently it is unclear whether expiratory ATC causes premature closure of unstable airways in patients with chronic obstructive pulmonary disease (COPD)[28] or whether it may, in fact, eliminate dynamic hyperinflation.[34] Further clinical studies are needed to evaluate this issue.

In relation to WOB, ATC may support spontaneous breathing without the overcompensation or undercompensation that occurs with PSV or CPAP.[28,31,35] In addition to the benefit of reduced WOB, patients seem to find ATC more comfortable than PSV.[26,36] (The respiratory discomfort in PSV seems to be related to

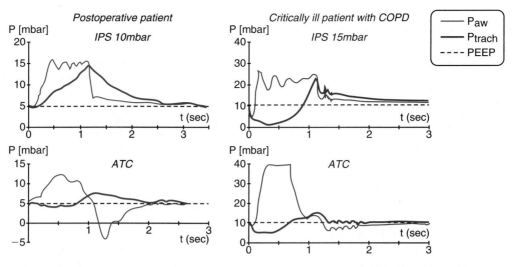

Fig. 20-5 Airway pressure (P_{aw}) and tracheal pressure (P_{trach}) curves using inspiratory pressure support *(upper graphs)* and automatic tube compensation (ATC) *(lower curves)*. Curves on the left are from a patient who had open heart surgery. Curves on the right are from a critically ill patient with chronic obstructive pulmonary disease (COPD). Bottom left, Note that the ventilator lowers P_{aw} during expiration. Control of the expiratory valve keeps P_{trach} above or equal to the positive end-expiratory pressure (PEEP). Bottom right, Note that the patient with acute respiratory insufficiency using ATC generates an inspiratory flow greater than 2 L/sec. This accounts for part of the difference between P_{trach} and PEEP. (From Fabry B, Haberthur C, Zappe D, et al: Breathing pattern and additional work of breathing in spontaneously breathing patients with different ventilatory demands during inspiratory pressure support and automatic tube compensation, Intensive Care Med 23:545-552, 1997.)

| BOX **20-2** | **Potential Advantages of Automatic Tube Compensation** |

Automatic tube compensation may be useful for the following purposes:

- To support or overcome the work of breathing imposed by the artificial airway during spontaneous breathing by a ventilator-supported patient
- To improve patient-ventilator synchrony through variable compensation of inspiratory flow based on patient demand
- To reduce the risk of air trapping caused by expiratory resistance from the endotracheal tube
- To enhance patient comfort
- To preserve the natural, "noisy" breathing pattern
- To facilitate accurate prediction of readiness for extubation
- To unload the inspiratory muscles and increase alveolar ventilation without adverse cardiopulmonary side effects

---

lung overinflation.[26,27,36]) Box 20-2 lists the potential benefits of ATC.[34,37,38]

Arguments against the use of automatic tube compensation. Some clinicians question whether ATC is needed to support a spontaneously breathing, intubated patient. Until a patient's spontaneous $\dot{V}_E$ exceeds 10 L/min, the effect of the ET may not be significant (see Fig. 17-13).[15,20] A high $\dot{V}CO_2$ is seldom required for an intubated patient who is breathing spontaneously; otherwise, the patient would receive ventilatory support.

When an appropriate-size ET is used, the imposed WOB may not be any greater through the tube than it is through the upper airway once the patient has been extubated.[38] In several studies, ATC was found to be the equivalent of pressure support (PS) (5 cm

H_2O) and CPAP (5 cm H_2O) in reducing WOB.[25,39] In some cases, ATC can give the false impression that the patient is ready to be extubated, when in fact the person is dependent on the support supplied by ATC even though it is minimal.[32] In addition, depending on the ventilator model, ATC may not provide sufficient compensation for WOB imposed by the ET.[32,33]

Summary of automatic tube compensation. Automatic tube compensation may reduce resistive WOB and increase patient comfort, depending on the ventilator and the artificial airway used. Additional studies are required, however, to determine whether ATC provides all the benefits for which it was designed. Despite the concerns previously mentioned, ATC may represent another method that can be used successfully to extubate patients who are difficult to wean.[40,41]

Volume-Targeted Pressure Support Ventilation

Volume-targeted PSV was briefly described in Chapter 6. This mode, which is also called volume support (VS) ventilation on the Servo-i ventilator (Maquet Inc., Wayne, N.J.), is basically PSV with a volume target. Volume-targeted PSV provides a set V_T while using PSV criteria (patient triggered, pressure targeted, flow cycled). Although volume-targeted PSV has the advantage of maintaining a target volume, its value in weaning patients from mechanical ventilatory support has not been established.[42] Furthermore, several drawbacks have been noted with using volume-targeted PSV (see Chapter 17 section on closed-loop ventilation asynchrony).

Automode and Variable Pressure Support/Variable Pressure Control

Automode is available on the Servo-i ventilator. A similar mode, called variable pressure support/variable pressure control (VPS/

VPC), is available on the Venturi ventilator (Cardiopulmonary Corp, Milford, Conn.).

When automode (or VPS/VPC) is activated, the ventilator can switch from a time-triggered mandatory breath to a patient-triggered support breath. For example, if a postoperative patient is still recovering from the effects of anesthesia and the ventilator operator has selected volume-controlled continuous mandatory ventilation (VC-CMV) with automode as the operating mode, all breaths are mandatory (time triggered, volume limited, and time cycled). If the patient begins to trigger breaths, the ventilator switches to VS (patient triggered, pressure limited, and flow cycled with a volume target) and remains in this mode as long as the patient is breathing spontaneously. If the patient becomes apneic again or if no patient effort is detected within a certain period, the ventilator switches back to the support mode (VC-CMV). Automode can also be set to switch from pressure-controlled continuous mandatory ventilation (PC-CMV) to PSV, and from pressure-regulated volume control (PRVC) to VS.

Automode has been shown to be an effective weaning technique that typically requires fewer ventilator manipulations than other techniques (e.g., IMV).[43,44] Additional clinical studies are needed to evaluate more completely the performance of automode as a weaning technique.[34]

Mandatory Minute Ventilation

Mandatory minute ventilation (MMV) was first described in 1977 by Hewlett and colleagues.[45] MMV is available on the Dräger Evita XL ventilator. It is a closed-loop system in which the ventilator monitors set parameters and makes adjustments accordingly (i.e., the ventilator adjusts the pressure, frequency, or the V_T to maintain the desired $\dot{V}_E$).

With traditional weaning methods (e.g., IMV and PSV), a constant level of ventilation is not guaranteed. In contrast, MMV automatically increases the level of support if the patient's spontaneous ventilation decreases, thus maintaining a consistent minimum $\dot{V}_E$. Patients who regain the ability to breathe spontaneously can increase their own $\dot{V}_E$, and the machine automatically lowers support without the clinician having to change any specific ventilator settings. Some of the potential benefits of MMV are listed in Box 20-3.[45,46]

Although few clinical studies address the use of MMV as a weaning technique, several guidelines should be kept in mind. The target $\dot{V}_E$ is set slightly below the patient's total $\dot{V}_E$, which includes both mandatory and spontaneous breaths. If a patient is receiving CMV and is neither hypocapnic nor alkalotic, the $\dot{V}_E$ can be appropriately set at 80% of the patient's previous level. A lower $\dot{V}_E$ level (i.e., ≤75%) may be adequate if the patient is slightly alkalotic or

hypocapnic. For patients on IMV, setting the $\dot{V}_E$ at 90% of the mandatory IMV value may be adequate.[45-47]

A potential problem with MMV is that a rapid, shallow respiratory pattern may provide the preset $\dot{V}_E$, but in this situation may result in an increase in dead space ventilation. This type of pattern can result from a decrease in compliance associated with pulmonary congestion, pulmonary edema, pleural effusion, fibrosis, atelectasis, and pneumonia. It can also be associated with abdominal distension or a decrease in ventilatory muscle strength. As a precaution, the high respiratory rate (f) and low V_T alarms must be set appropriately.

Other problems that can occur when using MMV include the development of auto-PEEP, delivery of very high V_T (inappropriately set upper pressure limit), increased dead space ventilation, and inappropriate settings resulting from clinician misunderstanding or misapplication of the mode. Clinicians must be aware of the potential consequences of changing dead space, carbon dioxide (CO_2) production, and patient WOB. The patient's breathing pattern and gas exchange can vary and therefore must be monitored regularly. Although MMV has been available for three decades, research data on the effectiveness of this mode are still lacking.

Adaptive Support Ventilation

Adaptive support ventilation (ASV) is available on the Hamilton G5 ventilator (Hamilton Medical, Bonaduz, Switzerland). Both ASV and its predecessor, adaptive lung ventilation (ALV), were designed to make automatic adjustments from the time ventilation was initiated until ventilation could be discontinued. The technical aspects have been described elsewhere.[48,49] ASV is a patient-centered method of closed-loop mechanical ventilation that increases or decreases ventilatory support based on monitored patient parameters.

Basically ASV provides pressure-limited breaths that target a volume and rate. The rate and V_T are selected by the ventilator's algorithm to provide the minimum WOB for the patient.[50] ASV monitors variables—such as pressure, flow, inspiratory and expiratory time, compliance, resistance, and time constants—to ensure delivery of an acceptable $\dot{V}_E$ based on practitioner settings. These settings include the patient's ideal body weight, the high-pressure limit, PEEP, F_IO_2, rise time, flow cycle, and percentage of predicted $\dot{V}_E$ desired. ASV is designed to minimize WOB and auto-PEEP and is capable of ventilator management in a variety of patient situations, including during thoracic surgery.[51] ASV has also been studied as a strategy for ventilator discontinuation.[52-54] It appears to be as safe and effective as traditional methods of weaning and may find increased use in the future.[34]

Artificial Intelligence Systems

This method of weaning patients from ventilatory support relies on artificial intelligence technology. Presently the only commercial system that is available for clinical use is the SmartCare/PS system, which is offered on the Dräger XL ventilator. The SmartCare/PS system uses predetermined ranges for volume (V), f, and end-tidal CO_2 pressure ($P_{ET}CO_2$) to adjust the inspiratory pressure automatically to maintain the patient in a respiratory "zone of comfort."[23,55] The patient's readiness for extubation is based on achieving the predefined lowest level of inspiratory pressure. Several factors can affect the lowest level of inspiratory pressure, including the type of artificial airway (i.e., ET versus tracheostomy tube), the type of humidifier (i.e., heat-moisture exchange [HME] versus heated humidifier), and the use of automatic tube compensation.

BOX 20-3	**Potential Advantages of Mandatory Minute Ventilation**

- Mandatory minute ventilation may offer greater control of a patient's P_aCO_2 than intermittent mandatory ventilation.
- Acute hypoventilation or apnea does not cause sudden hypercapnia.
- Acute hypoventilation is less likely after administration of sedatives, narcotics, or tranquilizers.
- MMV may provide a smooth transition from mechanical ventilatory support to spontaneous ventilation in patients recovering from a drug overdose or anesthesia.

Once the lowest level of inspiratory pressure is achieved, a period of observation is initiated during which the patient's V_T, f, and $P_{ET}CO_2$ are monitored. If the patient successfully passes this modified spontaneous breathing trial (SBT), the system automatically displays a message suggesting that the clinician should consider separating the patient from the ventilator.[23] It has been suggested that this approach to weaning may be a viable alternative because it reduces the duration of mechanical ventilation and ICU stays.[56,57] Additional clinical trials will be required to better define the use of these systems.

Evidence-Based Weaning

The challenge of successfully liberating a patient from a ventilator has been the subject of considerable debate. Solid evidence on identifying a patient's readiness to wean and ways to accomplish this task remain points of intense discussion among clinicians. In 1999 the federal Agency for Healthcare Policy and Research (AHCPR) asked the McMaster University Outcomes Research Unit to do a comprehensive review of the literature on ventilator withdrawal issues to establish the evidence on which ventilator weaning is based.[58] Using the results of the literature review, a task force of the ACCP, the SCCM, and the AARC created evidence-based guidelines for ventilator weaning for patients requiring more than 24 hours of ventilation.[59] These guidelines (Box 20-4) form the basis for much of the material presented in the remainder of this chapter.[1]

EVALUATION OF CLINICAL CRITERIA FOR WEANING

Three key points have evolved as criteria for weaning:
1. The problem that caused the patient to require ventilation must have been resolved.
2. Certain measurable criteria should be assessed to help establish a patient's readiness for discontinuation of ventilation.
3. A spontaneous breathing trial should be performed to firmly establish readiness for weaning.

RECOMMENDATION 1: PATHOLOGY OF VENTILATOR DEPENDENCE

Although it is often overlooked, the primary pathologic event that led to initiation of ventilatory support must be corrected. The clinician must determine whether this disease process or condition has improved or been reversed. If not, weaning attempts are unlikely to be successful.[59]

The ACCP/SCCM/AARC task force's first recommendation is that a search for all the causes that may be contributing to ventilator dependence should be undertaken for patients who require mechanical ventilation for longer than 24 hours. This recommendation is especially important for patients for whom attempts to be weaned from the ventilator have failed. Reversing all possible ventilator and nonventilator issues is a key part of the ventilator discontinuation process. Box 20-5 provides a summary of factors that must be evaluated to determine a patient's readiness for ventilator disconnection.[6,60,61] Even if the disease process or condition that led to mechanical ventilation has improved or has been reversed, other factors must be considered such as the patient's overall medical condition, a physical assessment of cardiopulmonary reserve and WOB, and the patient's psychological readiness (see Box 20-4).

Box 20-6 lists the clinical factors used to help evaluate a patient's overall condition. Any measured parameter that is outside the normal range may interfere with the patient's ability to breathe spontaneously without ventilatory support. However, occasionally one or more of these criteria may be slightly abnormal and the patient still will be able to support ventilation successfully. This type of situation presents the greatest challenge to clinicians trying to predict whether a patient is ready to be weaned.

Weaning Criteria

When a patient's medical condition is stable and the patient is breathing spontaneously, alert, and cooperative, clinicians typically evaluate certain ventilatory mechanics and gas-exchange values to help assess readiness for weaning (see Box 20-4).[2,59,62,63] These values are often called weaning criteria. About 75% of patients who meet certain weaning criteria tolerate an initial trial of spontaneous breathing in establishing readiness for ventilator discontinuation.[64] It should be mentioned that even among patients who never satisfy weaning criteria, about 30% eventually can be weaned from the ventilator.[65]

Considerable interest has focused on the establishment of specific, measurable criteria for predicting the success of attempts to wean patients from mechanical ventilation. Table 20-1 lists a number of physiological parameters that can be used for weaning and extubation in adults.[2,59,62,63] However, no single measure has yet been established that is uniformly successful in predicting patient ability to be weaned and to have uncomplicated extubation. An ideal weaning index would involve several parameters and might include the requirements listed in Box 20-7.[66]

It is interesting to note that 462 potential weaning predictors have been identified.[11,63] Of those identified, only a few have been found to be reasonably consistent as weaning criteria (see Box 20-4). Although these variables provide information about the patient's potential for liberation from the ventilator, assessments made during a formal, carefully monitored 30- to 120-minute SBT may be the most useful guide for making a decision on discontinuation of the ventilation (Key Point 20-2).[2]

Key Point 20-2 A properly monitored SBT is safe and effective; therefore the other assessments listed under Recommendation 2 (see Box 20-4) and in Table 20-1 may generally be unnecessary.[2]

Patient-Ventilatory Performance and Muscle Strength

For many years several simple measurements have been used to evaluate a patient's ventilatory muscle function before weaning and extubation. These include vital capacity (VC), $\dot{V}_E$, f, spontaneous V_T, and the rapid shallow breathing index (RSBI). VC has not been shown to be a good predictor for ventilator discontinuation, probably because it requires patient cooperation, which is not always consistent. The respiratory rate, V_T, and RSBI can be obtained using a bedside pulmonary function device, a respirometer, or directly through the ventilator. These measurements do not require patient cooperation (see Table 20-1).

The respiratory rate is easy to count and is a fairly reliable guide to a patient's ability to tolerate a ventilatory load.[67] A spontaneous

BOX 20-4 | Selected Recommendations from the American College of Chest Physicians (ACCP)/American Association for Respiratory Care (AARC)/Society of Critical Care Medicine (SCCM) Evidence-Based Weaning Guidelines Task Force

Recommendation 1: Pathology of Ventilator Dependence

All factors that may be contributing to ventilator dependence should be identified for patients requiring mechanical ventilation for longer than 24 hours. This is particularly true if attempts to withdraw the mechanical ventilator have failed. Reversing all possible ventilatory and nonventilatory issues is an important part of the ventilator discontinuation process.

Recommendation 2: Assessment of Readiness Using Evaluation Criteria

A formal patient assessment should be performed to determine whether the criteria have been met for discontinuation of ventilation. The following criteria are recommended:

1. Evidence of some reversal of the underlying cause of respiratory failure.
2. Adequate oxygenation: arterial partial pressure of oxygen (P_aO_2) $\geq$60 mm Hg with fractional inspired oxygen (F_IO_2) $\leq$0.4; ratio of arterial partial pressure of oxygen to fractional inspired oxygen (P_aO_2/F_IO_2) $\geq$150 to 200 mm Hg; required positive end-expiratory pressure (PEEP) $\leq$5 to 8 cm H_2O; F_IO_2 $\leq$0.4 to 0.5; and hydrogen ion concentration (pH) $\geq$7.25.
3. Hemodynamic stability; that is, no clinically important hypotension and no requirement for vasopressors or a requirement only for low-dose vasopressor therapy (e.g., dopamine or dobutamine <5 μg/kg/min).
4. Patient capable of initiating an inspiratory effort.

The decision to use these four criteria must be adapted for each patient. Some patients may not satisfy all the criteria (e.g., patients with chronic hypoxemia below the thresholds cited), but may be ready for attempts at discontinuation of mechanical ventilation.

Recommendation 3: Assessment During Spontaneous Breathing

Formal discontinuation assessments should be done during spontaneous breathing rather than while the patient receives substantial ventilatory support. An initial brief period of spontaneous breathing can be used to assess the patient's ability to perform a formal spontaneous breathing trial (SBT). The criteria used to assess a patient's tolerance of an SBT are (1) respiratory pattern, (2) adequacy of gas exchange, (3) hemodynamic stability, and (3) subjective comfort. Patients who tolerate an SBT of 30 to 120 minutes should promptly be considered for ventilator discontinuation.

Recommendation 4: Removal of the Artificial Airway

For patients whose support from the ventilator has been successfully discontinued, the decision regarding removal of the artificial airway should be based on assessment of airway patency and the patient's ability to protect the airway.

Recommendation 5: SBT Failure

If SBT fails, the causes of the failure and the reasons the patient continues to require ventilatory support should be determined and corrected. Once the reversible causes of failure have been corrected, and if the patient still meets the criteria described in Recommendation 2, an SBT should be performed every 24 hours.

Recommendation 6: Maintaining Ventilation with SBT Failure

Patients receiving mechanical ventilation for respiratory failure who fail an SBT should receive a stable, nonfatiguing, comfortable form of ventilatory support.

Recommendation 7: Anesthesia and Sedation Strategies and Protocols

Anesthesia and sedation strategies and ventilator management should be directed toward early extubation for patients who have had surgery.

Recommendation 8: Weaning Protocols

Protocols for ventilation discontinuation that are designed for clinicians other than physicians should be developed and implemented by intensive care units. These protocols should aim to optimize sedation.

Recommendation 9: Role of Tracheostomy in Weaning

When it becomes apparent that a patient will require prolonged ventilator assistance, tracheotomy should be considered. Tracheotomy should be performed after an initial period of stabilization on the ventilator and when the patient appears likely to benefit from the procedure.

Recommendation 10: Long-Term Care Facilities for Patients Requiring Prolonged Ventilation

Unless evidence of irreversible disease is present (e.g., high spinal cord injury, advanced amyotrophic lateral sclerosis), a patient who requires prolonged ventilatory support should not be considered permanently ventilator dependent until 3 months of weaning attempts have failed.

Recommendation 11: Clinician Familiarity with Long-Term Care Facilities

Critical care practitioners need to be familiar with facilities in their communities or units in their hospital that specialize in managing patients who require prolonged mechanical ventilation. Clinicians need to stay current with peer-reviewed data from long-term ventilation care units.

Patients who fail discontinuation attempts in the intensive care unit (ICU) should be transferred to long-term ventilation care facilities when they are medically stable. These long-term care facilities should have demonstrated competence, safety, and success in accomplishing ventilator discontinuation. These facilities are characterized by less staffing and less costly monitoring equipment; therefore they generate less cost per patient than do ICUs.

Recommendation 12: Weaning in Long-Term Ventilation Units

Weaning of a patient who requires prolonged ventilation should be slow paced and should include gradual lengthening of SBTs.

(Modified from ACCP/AARC/SCCM Task Force: MacIntyre NR: Evidence-based guidelines for weaning and discontinuing mechanical ventilatory support: a collective task force facilitated by the American College of Chest Physicians, the American Association for Respiratory Care, and the American College of Critical Care Medicine, Chest 120(6 Suppl):375S-395S, 2001; Also in: *Respir Care* 47:29-30, 2002; and MacIntyre N: Evidence-based ventilatory weaning and discontinuation, *Respir Care* 49:830-836, 2004.)

| BOX 20-5 | Evaluation of Systems to Determine Etiology of Respiratory Failure |

Neurologic Factors
- The brainstem (controller) should be structurally sound (e.g., absence of a history of cerebrovascular accident (CVA, also known as stroke) or central apnea).
- No electrolyte disturbances should be present, and no sedatives or narcotics should be required that might affect the function of the brain.
- Peripheral nerve failure may be present as a result of structural or metabolic problems or drug use.
- Obstructive sleep apnea may be present and is often overlooked.

Respiratory Factors
- Respiratory muscles weakness (e.g., atrophy from lack of use or injury from overuse).
- Presence of neuropathy and myopathy (neuromuscular blocking agents, aminoglycosides, and corticosteroids can contribute to neuropathy and myopathy).
- Excessive loads may be placed on the ventilatory muscles, possibly as a result of hyperinflation, compliance and resistance changes, and high minute ventilation demands (>10 L/min).
- Increased work of breathing (WOB) increases oxygen consumption and carbon dioxide production. Failure of withdrawal attempts may be related to capacity/load imbalance. These patients tend to have rapid, shallow breathing patterns.
- Wasted ventilation (increased dead space volume [V_D] and arterial partial pressure of carbon dioxide [P_aCO_2]) may be present.

- Impaired gas exchange (e.g., ventilation/perfusion imbalances and shunt) may be a factor.

Metabolic Factors and Ventilatory Muscle Function
- Hypoxic ventilator response and hypercapnic ventilatory response deteriorate under conditions of inadequate nutrition (i.e., semistarvation).
- Overfeeding may lead to increased CO_2 production.
- Electrolyte imbalances, especially phosphate and magnesium deficiencies, are associated with muscle weakness.
- Severe hypothyroidism and myxedema directly impair diaphragmatic function; adequate oxygen delivery also is essential to this process.

Cardiovascular Factors
Patients with susceptible reserves may develop ischemia or heart failure when ventilator support is reduced. Possible causes include the following:
- Increased metabolic demand with increased work of breathing as the patient transitions from mechanical ventilation to spontaneous breathing
- Increased venous return with spontaneous ventilation (negative intrathoracic pressure)
- Increased left ventricular afterload imposed by negative pleural pressure swings

Psychological Factors
- Fear of loss of life support
- Stress
- Poor ambulation
- Loss of sleep

(From Cook DJ, Meade MO, Perry AG: Trials of miscellaneous interventions to wean from mechanical ventilation, *Chest* 120(6 Suppl):438S-444S, 2001.)

| BOX 20-6 | Clinical Factors That Aid Evaluation of a Patient's Overall Condition |

- Acid–base balance
- Anemia or abnormal hemoglobin
- Body temperature
- Cardiac arrhythmias
- Caloric depletion (malnutrition or protein loss)
- Electrolytes
- Exercise tolerance (e.g., up in a chair)
- Fluid balance
- Hemodynamic stability (blood pressure, cardiac output, presence of shock)
- Hyperglycemia or hypoglycemia
- Infection
- Pain (can be minimized without oversedation)
- Psychological condition
- Renal function
- Sleep deprivation (an important and often overlooked problem)
- State of consciousness

| BOX 20-7 | Requirements of an Ideal Weaning Index |

The ideal weaning index should include the following:
- Assessment of the pathophysiological determinants of weaning outcome, including ventilatory muscle function, pulmonary gas exchange (ventilation and oxygenation), and psychological problems
- Accurately evaluate physiological function as it relates to the degree of abnormality present
- Ease of measurement and reproducible measurements
- Minimum patient cooperation
- High positive and negative predictive values

respiratory rate greater than 35 breaths/min in an adult indicates that the patient is not ready to be weaned. Evaluation of the pattern of breathing also is valuable. The clinician should review the patient's sedation history when making these measurements because sedatives can alter breathing patterns.[68]

The RSBI is the most frequently studied and one of the more reliable tests for determining a patient's weaning status. It is calculated by dividing the respiratory frequency (in breaths/min) by the V_T (in liters): f/V_T. This measurement is taken 1 minute after disconnecting the spontaneously breathing patient from the

TABLE 20-1	Physiological Parameters for Weaning and Extubation of Adults

Parameter	Acceptable Value
Ventilatory Performance and Muscle Strength	
VC	>15 mL/kg (IBW)
$\dot{V}_E$	<10-15 L/min
V_T	>4-6 mL/kg (IBW)
f	<35 breaths/min
f/V_T	<60-105 breaths/min/L (spontaneously breathing patient)
Ventilatory pattern	Synchronous and stable
P_{Imax} (up to 20-sec measurement from RV)	< −20 to −30 cm H_2O
Measurement of Drive to Breathe	
$P_{0.1}$	>6 cm H_2O
Measurement and Estimation of WOB	
WOB*	<0.8 J/L
Oxygen cost of breathing*	<15% of total $\dot{V}O_2$
Dynamic compliance	>25 mL/cm H_2O
V_D/V_T	<0.6
CROP index	>13 mL/breaths/min
Measurement of Adequacy of Oxygenation	
P_aO_2	≥60 mm Hg (F_IO_2 <0.4)
PEEP	≤5-8 cm H_2O
P_aO_2/F_IO_2	>250 mm Hg (consider at 150-200 mm Hg)
P_aO_2/P_AO_2	>0.47
$P_{(A-a)}O_2$	<350 mm Hg (F_IO_2 = 1)
% $\dot{Q}_S/\dot{Q}_T$	<20% to 30%

CROP, Compliance, respiratory rate, oxygenation, and inspiratory pressure; *IBW*, ideal body weight; *f*, respiratory rate; *f/V_T*, rapid shallow breathing index; *F_IO_2*, fractional inspired O_2; *P_{0.1}*, pressure on inspiration measured at 100 msec; *P_aO_2*, partial pressure of O_2 in the arteries; *P_aO_2/P_AO_2*, ratio of arterial PO_2 to alveolar PO_2; *P_{(A-a)}O_2*, alveolar-to-arterial partial pressure of O_2; *P_aO_2/F_IO_2*, ratio of partial pressure of O_2 (PO_2) in the arteries to F_IO_2; *PEEP*, positive end-expiratory pressure; *P_{Imax}*, maximum inspiratory pressure; *% $\dot{Q}_S/\dot{Q}_T$*, percent shunt; *RV*, residual volume; *VC*, vital capacity; *V_D/V_T*, ratio of dead space to tidal volume; *$\dot{V}_E$*, minute ventilation; *$\dot{V}O_2$*, oxygen (O_2) consumption per minute; *V_T*, tidal volume; *WOB*, work of breathing.
*Actual measure of WOB.

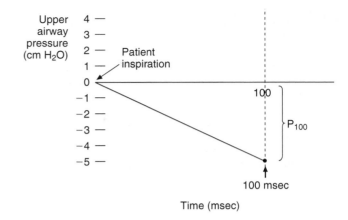

Fig. 20-6 Graphic representation of $P_{0.1}$. The airway is occluded after patient inspiration. Pressure at the mouth is measured at 100 msec, and the airway then is opened. The upper airway pressure at 100 msec is the $P_{0.1}$ value, reported as an absolute number.

Case Study 20-2

Calculation of Rapid Shallow Breathing Index (RSBI)

Which of the following patients has an RSBI that suggests it is time to begin weaning from ventilatory support?
Patient 1: Spontaneous V_T is 0.4 L; f is 10 breaths/min.
Patient 2: Spontaneous V_T is 0.25 L; f is 30 breaths/min.

ventilator and oxygen. Successful weaning is more likely if the RSBI is less than 105 (normal range, 60 to 105). Values above 105 suggest that a patient is not ready for weaning and probably will fail a weaning trial (Case Study 20-2).[63,69,70]

Measurement of the maximum inspiratory pressure (P_{Imax} [or MIP]), also called negative inspiratory force (NIF), was described in Chapter 4 (see Fig. 4-2). For the purpose of weaning, this parameter must be measured with a very specific technique to ensure consistency. P_{Imax} is measured in an occluded airway after 20 seconds.[2] (Note: The procedure should be stopped if oxygen desaturation or arrhythmias occur). A value of P_{Imax} that can be used as a predictor of weaning success or failure has not been firmly established. The ratio of the inspiratory pressure to P_{Imax} and the ratio of the airway occlusion pressure to P_{Imax} may provide other valuable weaning tools, but further study of these parameters is needed.[63,71-73]

Measurement of Drive to Breathe

The inspiratory drive to breathe is established by measurement of the airway occlusion pressure ($P_{0.1}$ [or P_{100}]). The occlusion pressure can be measured by adding special valve systems to a ventilator system; it is available on some ICU ventilators, such as the Dräger Evita Infinity V500 (Dräger Medical, Telford, Pa.).

To obtain the $P_{0.1}$, the airway is occluded during the first 100 milliseconds of inspiration and the pressure at the upper airway is measured (Fig. 20-6). The $P_{0.1}$ is believed to reflect both the drive to breathe and ventilatory muscle strength.[2] The normal range is 0 to −2 cm H_2O.

$P_{0.1}$ is reported as an absolute value even though the pressure generated is below baseline. A value close to normal may indicate that the patient is breathing comfortably. However, a low value may indicate either a weak drive to breathe or muscle weakness, which are not good indicators for readiness to wean.[2] Values below −6 cm H_2O may indicate a high drive to breathe and suggest that weaning is not likely to succeed.[73-76] High occlusion pressures may indicate that the patient is uncomfortable.[2] A high drive to breathe in these situations could lead to fatigue during a ventilator withdrawal challenge. On the other hand, a high $P_{0.1}$ may reflect strong respiratory muscles and a vigorous respiratory drive, which are advantageous if the patient has an intact drive to breathe.[2] Additional studies will be required to evaluate the effectiveness of $P_{0.1}$ as a predictor of weaning success.

Work of Breathing

When a patient has received total ventilatory support for several days or weeks, the respiratory muscles may become weak from lack

BOX 20-8	Physical Signs and Measurements of Increased WOB

- Use of accessory muscles
- Asynchronous breathing (chest wall–diaphragm asynchrony)
- Nasal flaring
- Diaphoresis
- Anxiety
- Tachypnea
- Substernal and intercostal retractions
- Patient asynchronous with ventilator
- Measured WOB >1.8 kg/m/min or >0.8 J/L
- Measured WOB ≥15% of total oxygen consumption

of use. Patients may also be undernourished. As with any other skeletal muscles, lack of nutrition weakens the diaphragm. Therefore, proper nutrition is essential for maintaining respiratory muscle strength and ensuring successful weaning from the ventilator.

The WOB and ventilatory muscle fatigue are both important aspects of ventilator dependency. Unfortunately, a universally accepted normal value for the WOB has not been identified as a predictor of weaning success. In addition, measurement of WOB requires a great deal of expertise and can be both invasive and costly.[2,77,78] Box 20-8 lists signs and measures indicating a high WOB.[78]

Previously mentioned parameters, such as spontaneous f and the f/V_T ratio, allow the clinician to gauge a patient's spontaneous WOB. Less obvious contributors to an increased WOB are a high oxygen cost of breathing, an elevated metabolic rate (high CO_2 production [$\dot{V}CO_2$]), a high ratio of dead space to tidal volume (V_D/V_T) (≥0.6), high airway resistance (R_{aw}), and stiff lungs (low respiratory system compliance).[79] The first three factors require special equipment and are difficult to measure. These parameters are seldom used by clinicians because they require too much respiratory work for a patient to maintain for an extended period (Key Point 20-3).[2,59]

Key Point 20-3 "More complex weaning parameters focused on physiological measurements, such as muscle strength, respiratory system mechanics, metabolic parameters, and work of breathing, add little to the assessment of individual patients for discontinuation potential."[59]

The index that evaluates compliance, respiratory rate, oxygenation, and inspiratory pressure (CROP index) may provide a good assessment of potential respiratory muscle overload and fatigue. The CROP index is calculated as follows:

$$CROP = (CD \times P_{Imax} \times [P_aO_2/P_AO_2])/f$$

where CD is dynamic compliance, P_{Imax} is the maximum inspiratory pressure, P_aO_2 is the arterial partial pressure of oxygen, P_AO_2 is the alveolar partial pressure of oxygen, and f is the respiratory rate. CROP values above 13 indicate the likelihood of successful ventilator withdrawal.[2]

Adequacy of Oxygenation

Mechanical ventilation is rarely used specifically to treat hypoxemia. The notable exception to this is ventilation in patients with acute respiratory distress syndrome (ARDS) (see Chapter 13). If a ventilated patient requires a high F_IO_2, a high level of PEEP, and has low arterial oxygen levels, the underlying pulmonary disease that caused the need for ventilation probably has not resolved sufficiently to allow the patient to breathe without assistance. Several oxygenation parameters can be used to determine whether the underlying disease has resolved; these include the P_aO_2; the ratio of the arterial O_2 partial pressure to the fraction of inspired oxygen (P_aO_2/F_IO_2); the ratio of arterial to alveolar O_2 partial pressure (P_aO_2/P_AO_2); shunt; and the alveolar-to-arterial O_2 partial pressure ($P_{(A-a)}O_2$) (see Table 20-1).[78] Hemoglobin levels must also be sufficient to ensure that oxygen transport is adequate before weaning. Assessment of the patient's hemodynamic status (e.g., blood pressure, heart rate, and cardiac index [CI]) is an important part of the evaluation process.

RECOMMENDATION 2: ASSESSMENT OF READINESS FOR WEANING USING EVALUATION CRITERIA

The ACCP/SCCM/AARC Task Force's Recommendation 2 states that a formal assessment of the patient should be performed to determine whether the criteria have been met for discontinuation of ventilation.[1] Specific criteria for determining weaning readiness are listed in Box 20-4 and Table 20-1.

RECOMMENDATION 3: ASSESSMENT DURING A SPONTANEOUS BREATHING TRIAL

Perhaps the best approach to determining a patient's readiness to wean is a carefully supervised SBT.[1,2] As stated under Recommendation 3 (see Box 20-4), a formal assessment is made during spontaneous breathing rather than while the patient is mechanically ventilated. An SBT typically is conducted when the basic assessment findings suggest that the patient is ready to be weaned, but the clinician nonetheless is uncertain about the patient's ability to sustain breathing without mechanical support. The patient is allowed to breathe spontaneously for a few minutes to determine his or her ability to perform a more extended spontaneous breathing trial. This initial effort is considered a screening phase and usually is conducted before a decision is made to continue an SBT.

During the SBT the patient's ability to tolerate unsupported ventilation is determined by observing his or her respiratory pattern, adequacy of gas exchange, hemodynamic stability, and subjective comfort (see the next section). A patient is considered ready for ventilator discontinuation and assessment for extubation when the person can tolerate an SBT for 30 to 120 minutes (Key Point 20-4). Studies have demonstrated that 77% to 85% of patients who pass an SBT can be successfully weaned and extubated without requiring reintubation.[59,63,80,81]

Key Point 20-4 "The best indicator of ventilator discontinuation potential is the clinical assessment of patients during the 30- to 120-minute spontaneous breathing trial (e.g., respiratory rate, BP, HR, comfort/anxiety, oxygenation, S_pO_2)."[59]

BOX 20-9	Clinical Signs and Symptoms Indicating Problems During a Spontaneous Breathing Trial (SBT)

1. Respiratory rate exceeding 30 to 35 breaths/min (clinicians also should watch for increases of more than 10 breaths/min or decreasing below 8 breaths/min).
2. Tidal volume (V_T) decreasing below 250 to 300 mL.
3. Blood pressure changing significantly, as demonstrated by
   - A drop of 20 mm Hg systolic or
   - A rise of 30 mm Hg systolic or
   - Systolic values >180 mm Hg or
   - A change of 10 mm Hg diastolic (e.g., rise >90 mm Hg)
4. Heart rate increasing more than 20% or exceeds 140 beats/min.
5. Sudden onset of frequent premature ventricular contractions (more than 4 to 6 per minute).
6. Diaphoresis.
7. Clinical signs that indicate deterioration of the patient's condition or that demonstrate the patient is anxious, not ready for weaning, and must be returned to ventilatory support.
8. Deterioration of arterial blood gas values and oxygen saturation measured by pulse oximeter (S_pO_2).[85]

Typically SBTs last at least 30 minutes but not longer than 120 minutes.[1,2,80] The SBT can be accomplished using a low level of CPAP (e.g., 5 cm H_2O), a low level of PSV (e.g., 5 to 8 cm H_2O), ATC, or simply a T-piece.[81,82] Although all these techniques have been shown to be effective for SBTs, it has been suggested that low levels of PSV shorten the length of time on the ventilator and ICU stays compared with a T-tube trial.[83]

The SBT is well established as a key index of a patient's ability to wean from the ventilator and of successful extubation. Studies have shown that successful completion of an SBT reduces ventilatory time, and therefore the cost of patient care, compared with cases in which the 2-hour SBT was not performed.[78,84] Close monitoring of patients undergoing an SBT is critical. Unnecessary prolongation of a failed SBT can result in muscle fatigue, hemodynamic instability, discomfort, or worsening gas exchange. There are no studies suggesting that SBTs contribute to any adverse outcomes if the trial is terminated promptly when signs of failure are recognized. In short, the patient should not be allowed to experience extreme exhaustion during the trial.

A variety of signs, symptoms, and monitored parameters allow clinicians to evaluate patients during the SBT. Patients who are not tolerating the process may show signs of dyspnea, fatigue, pain, anxiety, diaphoresis, pallor or cyanosis, drowsiness, restlessness, or use of accessory muscles. Box 20-9 lists clinical signs and symptoms that should be monitored during an SBT.[81-85] These physical findings provide evidence that some underlying problem is preventing a successful weaning process.

RECOMMENDATION 4: REMOVAL OF THE ARTIFICIAL AIRWAY

When a patient can breathe spontaneously (i.e., has performed an SBT successfully) and ventilator support has been discontinued, a decision must be made about removal of the artificial airway. This decision is based on assessment of airway patency and the patient's ability to protect the airway.[59]

Some practitioners equate ventilator liberation with extubation, which adds to the confusion of defining terms with regard to readiness for discontinuation of ventilation versus readiness for extubation. In most cases, discontinuation of ventilatory support and extubation are a single process. However, in some cases, such as a patient with upper airway burns, or one with copious secretions and a weak cough, the artificial airway may need to be maintained for an extended period after discontinuation of mechanical ventilatory support.

Common risks associated with extubation include potential airway obstruction, aspiration, and inability to clear secretions. Successful extubation is likely if a patient has a strong cough and is able to mobilize secretions, does not have excessive secretions, and has a peritubular leak on cuff deflation (successful cuff leak test).[86]

The cuff leak test is a means of testing for postextubation airway patency. Note that to qualify for this test, the patient must no longer need ventilatory support. To perform this test, the patient is disconnected from the ventilator, the cuff is deflated, and the ET or tracheostomy tube is obstructed. A leak around the cuff (peritubular leak) during spontaneous breathing suggests that the airway caliber is adequate and successful extubation is likely. A leak of less than 110 mL (average of three values on six consecutive breaths) indicates a high risk of postextubation stridor. Treatment with steroids or racemic epinephrine (or both) before extubation may be indicated.[87,88] It is important to recognize that a successful cuff leak test does not guarantee that postextubation difficulties will not arise. Patients without such leaks, however, must be watched more closely.[87,89,90]

Some clinicians are concerned that their extubation attempts might have a high rate of failure and require reintubation. Reported reintubation rates range from as low 4% to as high as 33%. Higher reintubation rates are more common in patients who demonstrate mental status changes and neurologic impairment.[55,91,92] An acceptable reintubation rate has not been determined.[88,93,94] A low reintubation rate (5%) might suggest that clinicians are too conservative in their attempts at extubation and overly exacting in their use of extubation criteria; this gives rise to the risks associated with prolonged intubation (e.g., ventilator-associated pneumonias, ventilator-induced lung injury, and damage to the airway). Conversely, a high percentage of extubation failure (>30%) might indicate that clinicians are too aggressive and too liberal with extubation criteria; this presents the risks associated with reintubation. It has been suggested that an extubation failure rate of 10% to 19% may be clinically acceptable.[62] Box 20-10 lists some of the factors that contribute to extubation failure.[59,91,95]

Reintubation is marked by an eightfold higher risk for the development of nosocomial pneumonia and a sixfold to twelvefold increase in the mortality rate.[55,80,91,92] The risks of continued use of an artificial airway must be weighed against the risks of extubation and its possible failure (Key Point 20-5). Interestingly, up to 80% of patients who intentionally self-extubate do not require reintubation.[62]

> **Key Point** 20-5 Clinicians often are reluctant to remove an ET for fear of having to reintubate the patient.

Box 20-11 briefly outlines the extubation procedure and lists the required equipment. Box 20-12 summarizes some of the key points of the AARC Clinical Practice Guideline for removal of the ET.[96]

Table 20-1 provides a list of physiological parameters that can be used to assess readiness for extubation.

Postextubation Difficulties

Hoarseness, sore throat, and cough are common after extubation. Other postextubation problems include subglottic edema, increased WOB from secretions, airway obstruction, and postextubation laryngospasm.[65]

Postextubation glottal edema can result in partial airway obstruction, causing stridor. This potentially serious condition is commonly treated with a cool aerosol supplemented with oxygen and nebulized racemic epinephrine (0.5 mL, 2.25% epinephrine in 3 mL normal saline). Helium-oxygen mixtures (e.g., 70% He/30% O_2), administered through a nonrebreathing mask, also reduce WOB through the partly obstructed airway. This technique, known as heliox therapy, provides a low-density gas that may aid spontaneous breathing, thus relieving the effects of stridor and temporarily supporting gas exchange. This may allow time for medical treatment (e.g., racemic epinephrine and steroids) to take effect and prevent reintubation.[97] Reintubation may be necessary to prevent the development of respiratory distress if postextubation edema and stridor are severe and refractory to treatment.

Postextubation laryngospasm may occur and usually is transient. Persistent laryngospasm may respond to positive pressure delivered with oxygen (e.g., bag-mask device). If it continues, a neuromuscular blocking agent and reintubation may be necessary.[91]

The risk of aspiration is another potential problem after extubation. Aspiration is associated with a suppressed normal gag or cough reflex, and it is not unusual in patients with central neurologic injury. (Note: In patients who have a neuromuscular or spinal cord injury, a peak cough flow greater than 160 L/min may predict successful extubation or decannulation [removal of the tracheostomy tube].)[1,59] Other factors that may increase the risk of aspiration after extubation include the following:

- Use of muscle relaxants (may also impair the ability to protect the airway)
- Presence of a gastric tube (feedings tubes must be discontinued for 4 to 6 hours before extubation)
- Abnormal paraglottic sensations (usually begin 4 to 8 hours after extubation and can last as long as 8 hours postextubation)
- Inability to close the glottis mechanically (may be impaired postextubation)[7]
- Excessive amounts of secretions (e.g., cystic fibrosis)

BOX 20-10 **Factors That May Contribute to Extubation Failure**

- Type of patient (i.e., medical versus surgical)
- Older age
- Severity of illness at weaning onset
- Repeated or traumatic intubations
- Use of continuous intravenous sedation
- Duration of mechanical ventilation
- Female gender
- Anemia (hemoglobin <10 mg/dL or hematocrit <30%)
- Need for transport out of the intensive care unit
- Initial severity of illness
- Indication for mechanical ventilation (e.g., cause of acute respiratory failure)
- Duration or number of individual spontaneous breathing trials before extubation
- Mode of ventilator support before extubation
- Protocol-directed weaning

BOX 20-11 **Extubation Equipment and Procedure**

Equipment
- Electrocardiogram monitor
- Resuscitation bag, oxygen source, and oxygen mask
- Suctioning equipment, including suction kits and Yankauer suction
- Laryngoscope and additional endotracheal tubes for intubation (if necessary)
- Racemic epinephrine and a small-volume nebulizer (in case postextubation stridor develops)
- A 5-mL unit dose of normal saline or 5-mL syringe for irrigation with normal saline during suctioning (if necessary)
- 10-mL syringe for deflating endotracheal (ET) tube cuff

Procedure
- Position the patient in semi-Fowler or high Fowler position.
- Explain the procedure to the patient.
- Administer 100% oxygen to the patient with a manual resuscitation bag.
- Suction the patient's mouth and pharynx above the cuff. Oxygenate after suctioning.
- Suction the patient to clear the airway as much as possible, and then loosen the tape supporting the tube.
- Squeeze the resuscitation bag while deflating the cuff to force secretions into the mouth from above the cuff for

suctioning (some clinicians cut the pilot balloon). Having the patient cough also helps move the secretions into the mouth.
- Oxygenate and hyperinflate the patient, withdrawing the ET tube when pressure is built up in the lungs at peak inspiration (maximum abduction of vocal cords). An alternate technique is to have the patient breathe in deeply and cough; the tube is removed as the patient coughs (coughing opens the vocal cords). A deep inspiration before cuff deflation, followed by a cough, also helps force secretions into the mouth.
- Have the patient cough after the tube has been removed.
- Administer the same fraction of inspired oxygen (F_IO_2) as before extubation. Some clinicians administer a cool mist after extubation and increase oxygen delivery by 10% if the patient was weaned with positive end-expiratory pressure (PEEP) in use.
- Monitor the patient while encouraging coughing and deep breathing. Listen to the breath sounds, particularly in the neck area. Frequently measure the respiratory rate, heart rate, blood pressure, and oxygen saturation by pulse oximeter (S_pO_2) for 30 minutes.
- Monitor the patient for changes over the next hour. It may be desirable to obtain an arterial blood gas measurement at this time to confirm that the patient's oxygenation and ventilatory status is stable.

| BOX 20-12 | **Summary of the American Association for Respiratory Care Clinical Practice Guideline: Removal of the Endotracheal Tube—2007 Revision and Update** |

Indications

- When airway control provided by the endotracheal (ET) tube is no longer necessary (the patient should be able to maintain a patent airway and generate adequate spontaneous ventilation to maintain normal gas exchange).
- When an acute obstruction of the ET tube cannot be cleared rapidly. Reintubation or other appropriate techniques must be used to maintain effective gas exchange.
- When further medical care of the patient is explicitly declared futile (tube removal is allowed).

Contraindications

- No absolute contraindications to removal of the ET tube have been reported.

Hazards/Complications

- Possible hazards and complications include hypoxemia and hypercapnia from airway obstruction, resulting from edema of the trachea, vocal cords, or larynx, laryngospasm, bronchospasm, aspiration, respiratory muscle weakness, hypoventilation, excessive work of breathing, development of atelectasis, and postextubation pulmonary edema.

Limitations of Methodology

- Predicting an extubation outcome is sometimes very difficult. It is of significant clinical importance because both extubation delay and unsuccessful extubation are associated with poor patient outcomes. The literature on extubation readiness is limited by few validated objective measures to accurately predict the extubation outcome for an individual patient.

Assessment of Extubation Readiness

- Patients should be able to maintain spontaneous ventilation adequately and should not require high levels of positive pressure or oxygenation to maintain adequate arterial blood gas oxygenation (P_aO_2/F_IO_2 >150 to 200 on an F_IO_2 ≤0.4 to 0.5 and low levels of PEEP ≤5 to 8 cm H_2O; pH ≥7.25).

- Successful completion of 30- to 120-minute SBT performed with low level of CPAP (e.g., 5 cm H_2O) or a low level of PS (5 to 7 cm H_2O) demonstrating adequate respiratory pattern and gas exchange.
- Other examples of measurements that can be used to assess extubation readiness include spontaneous respiratory rate, rapid shallow breathing index (RSBI), vital capacity (VC), peak expiratory flow (PEF), transdiaphramatic pressure gradient (Pdi), maximum inspiratory pressure (MIP), work of breathing (WOB), airway occlusion pressure ($P_{0.1}$), maximum voluntary ventilation (MVV), and sustained maximal inspiratory pressures (SMIP).
- Adequate respiratory muscle strength.
- Patients with artificial airways in place to facilitate treatment of respiratory failure should be considered for extubation when they have met weaning criteria.

Assessment of Outcome

- Patient assessment and a physical examination should follow removal of the ET tube to ensure adequate spontaneous ventilation and adequate oxygenation through the natural airway and to ensure that reintubation is not necessary.
- Some patients may require postextubation support or intervention to maintain adequate gas exchange independent of controlled mechanical ventilation. These adjunctive measures may include NIV, CPAP, aerosolized racemic epinephrine, heliox, and possibly diagnostic bronchoscopy.

Monitoring

- Appropriately trained personnel.
- Frequent evaluation of vital signs, assessment of neurologic status, patency of airway, auscultatory findings, WOB, and hemodynamic status.

(Modified from AARC Clinical Practice Guidelines: Removal of the endotracheal tube, 2007 revision and update, *Respir Care* 52: 81-93, 2007.)

- Inability to clear secretions effectively (e.g., inadequate neurologic or muscular function)

Noninvasive Positive Pressure Ventilation After Extubation

Noninvasive positive pressure ventilation (NIV) may be beneficial after extubation for patients who require some degree of ventilatory support to ease the transition from invasive mechanical ventilation to spontaneous breathing. NIV after extubation appears to have the following benefits:[98-103]

- Improves survival
- Lowers the mortality rate
- Reduces the risk of ventilator-associated pneumonia
- Lowers the incidence of septic shock
- Shortens the ICU and hospital stays

Box 20-13 lists potential criteria for the use of NIV after extubation for patients requiring transitional ventilator support.[103] NIV can be administered temporarily for postextubation subglottic edema to give medications that reduce swelling (e.g., corticosteroids) time to take effect. It may also be useful for preventing reintubation when respiratory failure occurs after extubation.[103] However, patient

| BOX 20-13 | **Criteria for Instituting NIV After Failure to Wean from Invasive Mechanical Ventilation in Extubated Patients** |

- Resolution of problems leading to respiratory failure
- Ability to tolerate a spontaneous breathing trial for 10 to 15 minutes
- Strong cough reflex
- Hemodynamic stability
- Minimal airway secretions
- Low F_IO_2 requirements
- Functioning gastrointestinal tract
- Optimum nutritional status

cooperation is essential for successful use of this modality. Unfortunately, NIV tolerance cannot be safely predicted before extubation; therefore deliberate removal of the airway with the intent to switch to NIV carries a high risk of reintubation. (See Chapter 19 for additional information on NIV.)

Factors in Weaning Failure

RECOMMENDATION 5: SPONTANEOUS BREATHING TRIAL FAILURE

As previously mentioned, if a patient fails an SBT, the causes of the failure must be determined and corrected before proceeding with liberation from mechanical ventilation. When the reversible causes of failure have been corrected, and if the patient still meets the criteria for discontinuation of ventilation, an SBT should be performed every 24 hours.[59] It is important to avoid pushing patients to the point of exhaustion during the weaning process because this ultimately can delay liberation from the ventilator. A failed SBT often reflects persistent mechanical abnormalities of the respiratory system, which may not reverse quickly.[77] Other causes or complications may be involved, such as compromised cardiovascular function (e.g., myocardial ischemia), impaired fluid status, acid–base disturbances, inadequate pain control, inappropriate sedation, the need for bronchodilator therapy, nutritional status, and psychological factors.

It is important that clinicians wait 24 hours before attempting another SBT in patients for whom it fails (Key Point 20-6). Frequent SBTs over a single day are not helpful and can lead to serious consequences. Even twice-daily SBTs offer no advantage over testing once a day.[10]

Key Point **20-6** Clinicians should wait 24 hours before attempting subsequent spontaneous breathing trials (SBTs) in patients for whom SBT fails.

NONRESPIRATORY FACTORS THAT MAY COMPLICATE WEANING

The respiratory problems that can lead to unsuccessful weaning attempts are similar to those that often lead to respiratory failure (see Fig. 20-1). Nonrespiratory factors also may contribute to failure of the SBT and are often neglected (Table 20-2).[97] The following sections review the common nonrespiratory factors that can delay or even prevent successful weaning of a patient from mechanical ventilation.

Cardiac Factors

Patients with abnormal cardiac function may develop acute congestive heart failure when abruptly disconnected from mechanical ventilation. The rapid drop in intrathoracic pressures causes two basic problems: (1) sudden increases in negative intrapleural pressure with spontaneous breaths may increase the left ventricular transmural pressure and afterload; and (2) temporary redistribution of blood volume from the systemic venous system to the central veins, which can result in increased right, and subsequently left, ventricular filling. The increased venous return may alter the function and shape of the right and left ventricles, impair left ventricular function, and reduce the stroke volume.[97] With a preexisting heart condition, these acute changes can result in cardiac decompensation, thus contributing to problems in weaning (Case Study 20-3).

 Case Study 20-3

Failed Weaning Attempt

A 76-year-old man with a history of chronic obstructive pulmonary disease has been receiving ventilatory support for 4 days following an acute myocardial infarction. The ventilator settings are V_T: 500 mL; IMV rate: 8 breaths/min; F_IO_2: 0.5; PEEP/CPAP: 5 cm H_2O. ABG results on these settings are: pH = 7.37; P_aCO_2 = 36 mm Hg; P_aO_2 = 78 mm Hg; S_pO_2 = 93%.

The patient currently meets all criteria for weaning and is placed on a T-piece. Within 10 minutes he develops restlessness, tachycardia, rapid, shallow breathing, and diaphoresis. The S_pO_2 drops from 93% to 90%, and the pulmonary artery occlusion pressure rises from 12 to 17 mm Hg. The patient does not complain of chest pain and has no dysrhythmias.

What do you think is responsible for the failed weaning attempt?

Acid–Base Factors

A common reason patients with chronic hypercapnia fail to wean is the presence of relative hyperventilation, respiratory alkalosis, and subsequent renal compensation, leading to a decrease in bicarbonate.[97] Table 20-3 presents an example of this situation. As the table shows, after 3 days of mechanical ventilation, the blood gas values appear normal. However, these results are not normal for this patient. The original state of compensated respiratory acidosis must be restored in 2 to 3 days by gradually reducing ventilatory support before weaning can succeed in this patient.

Even patients without preexisting chronic CO_2 retention can hyperventilate during controlled ventilation. When weaning is attempted, these patients remain apneic until CO_2 levels rise high enough to trigger the respiratory drive. Consequently maintaining a respiratory alkalosis in this type of patient can severely delay the weaning process.

Patients with metabolic acidosis also may not do well during weaning unless the underlying cause of the acidosis is removed. The normal compensatory mechanism for a metabolic acidosis is a respiratory alkalosis (i.e., increased ventilation). Without the ventilator to help support this increased work, the patient is unable to maintain increased $\dot{V}_E$ and may not do well during weaning.

Metabolic Factors

Besides metabolic acidosis, three additional metabolic factors can affect ventilator weaning: hypophosphatemia, hypomagnesemia, and hypothyroidism. Hypophosphatemia, or phosphate deficiency, may contribute to muscle weakness and failure to wean. Values below normal (1.2 mmol/L) may impair respiratory muscle function.

Malnourished patients and those with chronic alcoholism often suffer from hypomagnesemia (low magnesium levels). Magnesium deficiency also has been associated with muscle weakness.

Patients with severe hypothyroidism may have impaired respiratory muscle function. This disorder also blunts the central response to hypercapnia and hypoxemia, which in turn may impair a patient's ability to wean.[97]

TABLE 20-2   **Nonrespiratory Factors in Weaning Patients from Mechanical Ventilation**

Category	Factor	Mechanism	Clinical Presentation
Cardiac status	Acute left ventricular failure	Increased preload because of increased venous return and decreased pulmonary capillary compression as intrathoracic pressure is reduced	Weaning fails, often after patient does well initially for 30-60 min; may develop acute respiratory and/or metabolic acidosis, hypoxemia, hypotension, chest pain, and cardiac dysrhythmias
Acid–base status	Acute alkalosis in patient with underlying CO_2 retention	Loss of preexisting metabolic compensation for hypercapnia; inability to sustain required $\dot{V}_E$ and WOB	Patient with COPD or other cause of chronic respiratory acidosis before acute insult fails weaning after several days of ventilation to a P_aCO_2 lower than the patient's pH-compensated level
	Respiratory alkalosis	Depression of ventilatory drive by hypocapnia and alkalemia	P_aCO_2 rises and pH falls during weaning attempt; patient is said to fail weaning if some arbitrary change in these values (e.g., 10 mm Hg increase in P_aCO_2) is used as a criterion for failure
	Metabolic acidosis	Increase in ventilatory demand to compensate for respiratory alkalosis	Patient may be unable to sustain required increase in $\dot{V}_E$ and WOB to maintain a lower P_aCO_2 to compensate for a lower HCO_3^-
Metabolic status	Hypophosphatemia and hypomagnesemia	Ventilatory muscle weakness	Patient weaning fails because of rapid shallow breathing, respiratory distress, and acute respiratory acidosis; maximal inspiratory pressure is decreased
	Hypothyroidism	Decreased ventilatory drive with possible ventilatory muscle weakness	Rare cause of weaning failure that occurs because of acute respiratory acidosis with or without respiratory distress
Drugs	Narcotics, sedatives, tranquilizers, and hypnotics	Depression of ventilatory drive	Patient fails weaning because of acute respiratory acidosis in the absence of tachypnea and respiratory distress
	Neuromuscular blocking agents	Ventilatory muscle weakness; delayed clearance in patient with renal insufficiency	Patient weaning fails because of rapid shallow breathing, respiratory distress, and acute respiratory acidosis; maximal inspiratory pressure is reduced
		Ventilatory muscle weakness caused by acute myopathy, especially in patients who have received high-dose systemic corticosteroids	Same as above; may have elevated muscle enzymes; can last for weeks or months
	Aminoglycosides	Neuromuscular blockade	Very rare cause of weaning failure that occurs because of rapid shallow breathing, respiratory distress, and acute respiratory acidosis; maximal inspiratory force is reduced
Nutrition	Overfeeding	Increased CO_2 production, especially with excessive carbohydrate calories	Patient fails weaning because of excessive ventilatory demand (high $\dot{V}_E$ requirement to keep P_aCO_2 normal); unusual cause of weaning failure unless very large caloric loads are administered
	Malnutrition	Effects of acute illness; preexisting nutritional deficiencies	May contribute to ventilatory muscle weakness, decreased ventilatory drive, impaired immunologic function, fluid retention, depression; distinguishing this from other factors is difficult
Psychological status	Agitation; "psychological ventilator dependence"	Anxiety, fear, delirium, ICU psychosis, or influence of preexisting personality factors	Patient becomes agitated and panicky during attempt to reduce or discontinue ventilatory support; can be said to cause weaning failure when other factors are absent
	Lack of motivation	Depression, effects of drugs, organic brain dysfunction, or influence of preexisting personality factors	Patient refuses to participate in care (e.g., mobilization, bronchial hygiene, physiological measurements); flat affect and immobility in bed; considered when other factors are absent

From Pierson DJ: Non-respiratory aspects of weaning from mechanical ventilation. Respir Care 40: 263–270, 1995.
COPD, Chronic obstructive pulmonary disease; *HCO$_3^-$,* bicarbonate; *ICU,* intensive care unit; *P$_a$CO$_2$,* partial pressure of carbon dioxide; *pH,* hydrogen ion concentration; *$\dot{V}_E$,* minute ventilation; *WOB,* work of breathing.

TABLE 20-3	Blood Gas and pH Values Reflecting the Effect of Ventilator-Induced Respiratory Alkalosis on Weaning				
Variable	Baseline	Respiratory Failure	On Ventilator	After 3 Days	Weaning
pH_a	7.38	7.24	7.56	7.4	7.24
P_aCO_2 (mm Hg)	58	76	40	40	58
HCO_3^- (mEq/L)	34	36	34	24	26

From Pierson DJ: Respir Care 40:265, 1995.

HCO_3^-, Bicarbonate; P_aCO_2, partial pressure of arterial carbon dioxide; pH_a, hydrogen ion concentration.

Effect of Pharmacologic Agents

As discussed earlier in Chapter 15, the use of sedatives, opioids, tranquilizers, and hypnotic agents can all depress the central ventilatory drive. Use of these agents must be minimized for weaning to be successful. Neuromuscular blocking agents (NMBAs) (e.g., vecuronium bromide and atracurium besylate) cause paralysis and must clear the system before weaning can be initiated. Indeed some patients demonstrate prolonged paralysis even after use of these agents is discontinued. The two primary reasons for prolonged paralysis after withdrawal of NMBAs are: (1) a reduced ability to metabolize and excrete these drugs and (2) the development of an acute myopathy. In the former case, prolonged paralysis occurs as a result of interference with the normal renal or hepatic metabolism and elimination of the NMBAs. Prolonged paralysis occurs in severely ill patients with multiple organ failure secondary to critical illness, especially sepsis.[104] An acute myopathy can develop when high maintenance doses of corticosteroids and continuous nondepolarizing agents (e.g., vecuronium or pancuronium) are used. For example, this is seen in ventilated patients with a history of asthma.[105-107] Muscle biopsies from affected individuals show evidence of muscle destruction.[106] The limbs of affected individuals appear atrophied, and deep tendon reflexes are reduced or absent. Limb paralysis may last from several weeks to months.[107,108]

Nutritional Status and Exercise

Weakening of the respiratory muscles may occur in any patient who does not receive adequate nutrition or who was malnourished before admission. Underfeeding can lead to muscle wasting (including the diaphragm, heart, and other organ tissues), particularly in patients under the stress of an acute, severe illness. Other problems associated with malnutrition include a reduced central response to hypoxemia and hypercapnia and an impaired immune response.

Conversely, overfeeding, particularly with solutions using carbohydrates as the primary calorie source, can cause increases in oxygen consumption, carbon dioxide production, and minute ventilation. The increase in CO_2 production occurs during lipogenesis (i.e., the conversion of carbohydrates to lipids [fats]). Excessive carbohydrate feeding therefore may interfere with weaning from mechanical ventilation because of an increased CO_2 load that the patient must remove during ventilation. Monitoring the patient's metabolic rate and substrate utilization with indirect calorimetry can help minimize this type of problem with parenteral feeding (see Chapter 10).

Feedings must be carefully monitored. Nutritional solutions containing emulsified fats, proteins, carbohydrates, vitamins, and minerals must be provided in appropriate proportions for each patient. Mixed solutions containing emulsified fats do not appear to elevate the metabolic rate and can be used to meet nutritional as well as high-carbohydrate solutions.

Strengthening of respiratory muscles that are weak from lack of use is also important to avoid muscle atrophy and fatigue. Two generally accepted principles apply: First, the clinician must make sure the patient is adequately nourished without being overfed. Second, periods of exercise (spontaneous breathing) are required to strengthen the respiratory muscles, followed by undisturbed rest with sufficient ventilatory support during the night. Even following these principles, it is important to understand that muscle recovery is often unpredictable (see the following Clinical Scenario for an example).[64,109]

⊘ Clinical Scenario: Weaning

A child with C-1 quadriplegia received mechanical ventilation for 1 year. At that time, a phrenic nerve stimulator was inserted into the child's diaphragm. The phrenic nerve stimulator initially produced very low tidal volumes (V_T), which declined dramatically after a short period of diaphragm exertion. The stimulation was stopped, and 1 to 2 days of rest followed. It took at least 48 hours to recover the baseline V_T after the initial exercise of the unconditioned diaphragm. After 2 to 3 weeks, however, the fatigue factor disappeared, and effective V_T could be maintained during several hours of stimulation. This case study illustrates that the response to a well-controlled exercise program for strengthening and reconditioning the diaphragm was unpredictable. It could not be predicted that the initial fatigue problem would be corrected after 3 weeks. In this particular child, recovery was not linear but rather a continually varying process. Although the weaning process often can be unpredictable, respiratory failure that occurs early in weaning probably indicates that the patient needs more rest between spontaneous breathing trials.

Psychological Factors

Although the preceding discussion focused on physiological factors that can affect a patient's ability to be liberated from ventilatory support, it is important to recognize that psychological factors can also influence the success of a weaning trial. Indeed the role of psychological factors on evidence-based weaning protocols remains quite ambiguous. Two intangible psychological factors important must be considered during weaning.[97] Patients that resist being mobilized and are reluctant to assume any responsibility for their recovery can hinder attempts of ventilator liberation. Weaning a patient from mechanical ventilation is typically more successful when the patient is optimistic about his or her illness, motivated to recover, and assists the health care team by being cooperative. Unmotivated patients therefore probably will take longer to wean than those patients who are optimistic about their recovery.

Psychological problems can manifest as fear, anxiety, delirium, ICU psychosis, depression, anger, denial, fear of shortness of breath, and fear of being left alone, among other symptoms. The use of sedatives and many other medications also tends to alter a patient's mental status (see Chapter 15). The attitudes of the nurse, physician, and therapist team and the patient's attitude toward the team can have a huge effect on the outcome of the weaning trial. Patients who are chemically dependent (e.g., tobacco, alcohol, pain medication) may also appear nervous and anxious following withdrawal from these chemical agents.

A number of disease-related issues can also contribute to psychological problems. Two important considerations are the severity and the duration of the illness. For example, older patients with debilitating diseases tend to be more depressed and anxious.[67] Another important issue is sleep deprivation, which commonly is associated with the ICU environment. Patients may report hallucinations and nightmares, express fear of dying or abandonment, and manifest heightened anxiety ascribed to their environment, medical treatment, lack of sleep, and the illness itself.

To allay some of these psychological fears, the clinician must focus on environmental and communication issues. In terms of environment, noise levels should be reduced and an adequate amount of time provided for undisturbed sleep. There are times when it is more important for the patient to receive a good night of sleep rather than obtaining routine vital signs during sleep hours, particularly because continuous monitoring is available. In terms of communication, eye contact, touching, and written or verbal communication efforts can be a valuable means for clinicians to connect with a patient. Health care workers often go into patient areas and perform a clinical procedure or check the equipment and never take the time to communicate with the patient. Establishing effective communication skills is critical for achieving successful clinical outcomes.

A delayed or failed weaning attempt can cause patients and staff to become depressed or anxious. Clinicians must have patience with the process and try to convey a feeling of calm and self-assurance to the patient.

RECOMMENDATION 6: MAINTAINING VENTILATION IN PATIENTS WITH SPONTANEOUS BREATHING TRIAL FAILURE

Patients for whom an SBT fails should receive a stable, nonfatiguing, comfortable form of ventilatory support (see Box 20-4).[59] The clinical focus for the 24 hours after a failed SBT should be on maintaining adequate muscle unloading, optimizing comfort (and thus sedation needs), and preventing complications, rather than on aggressive ventilatory support reduction.[10] The patient may participate in part of the WOB as long as the load is not fatiguing.

As previously mentioned, repeated SBT on the same day is of no benefit. Repetitive and ritualistic attempts at gradual reductions in ventilator settings are not worth the time or effort.[110] To date there is no evidence that a gradual support reduction strategy is

better than providing full, stable support between once daily SBTs.[1] Some factors the respiratory therapist can adjust to improve patient comfort and minimize imposed ventilatory loads include the following:

- Carefully set the sensitivity level (i.e., ventilator triggering system)
- Adjust flow patterns to match patient demand
- Make sure ventilator settings are appropriate to prevent air trapping (auto-PEEP)[1]
- If auto-PEEP is present, use applied PEEP to facilitate breath triggering and counteract the auto-PEEP

An interesting finding of the ACCP/SCCM/AARC task force was how poorly clinicians assess the potential for ventilator discontinuation, especially in patients considered ventilator dependent for longer than several days. This finding emphasizes the need for more focused assessment strategies for these types of patients. The Clinical Scenario below provides an example of a case of weaning failure.[59]

 Clinical Scenario: Weaning Failure

A 47-year-old man is admitted to the ICU with a severe asthma exacerbation. He is intubated and mechanical ventilation is instituted. After 3 weeks of ventilatory support, the medical staff is unable to wean the patient. He has a difficult ventilation history, including the use of sedatives, analgesics, anxiolytics, and multiple bronchodilators. A tracheotomy is performed. About 36 hours later the patient dies, apparently from mucus plugging. A heat and moisture exchanger (HME) had been used with this patient, in whom increased secretions were compounded by a fluid overload. Although no autopsy was performed, excessive, thick secretions may have obstructed the airway and therefore contributed to the potential for the development of mucus plugging.

Final Recommendations

RECOMMENDATION 7: ANESTHESIA AND SEDATION STRATEGIES AND PROTOCOLS

Recommendation 7 states that anesthesia and sedation strategies and ventilator management should be aimed at early extubation in postoperative patients.[59] In these patients a depressed respiratory drive and pain are the main reasons for ventilator dependence. A lower anesthetic/sedation regimen may permit earlier extubation.[59] Ventilator modes that guarantee a certain breathing rate and $\dot{V}_E$ (CMV modes, IMV, and MMV) are important for patients with unreliable respiratory drives. The immediate postoperative patient may be ideally suited for simple automatic feedback modes that provide a backup form of support (e.g., MMV or VS).[47,52]

RECOMMENDATION 8: WEANING PROTOCOLS

Protocols for ventilator discontinuation, which are designed for nonphysician clinicians, should be developed and implemented by ICU staff. They also must be aimed at optimizing sedation.[59] Non-physician protocols often are called therapist-driven protocols (TDPs) or nurse-driven protocols.

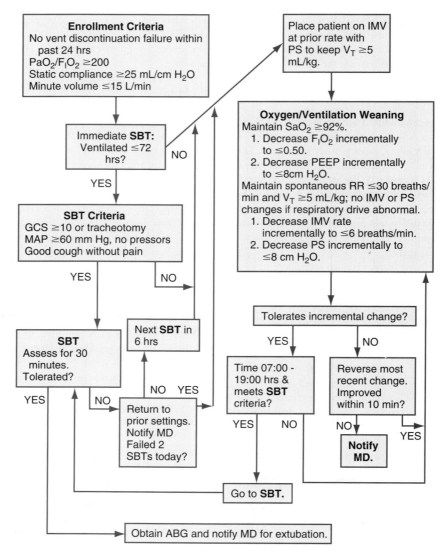

Fig. 20-7 Example of a weaning protocol or ventilator management protocol (VMP). *ABG*, Arterial blood gas; *F$_I$O$_2$*, fractional inspired oxygen; *GCS*, Glasgow Coma Scale; *IMV*, intermittent mandatory ventilation; *MAP*, mean arterial pressure; *P$_a$O$_2$/F$_I$O$_2$*, ratio of partial pressure of oxygen in the arteries to the fractional inspired oxygen; *PEEP*, positive end-expiratory pressure; *PS*, pressure support; *RR*, respiratory rate; *S$_a$O$_2$*, arterial oxygen saturation; *SBT*, spontaneous breathing trial; *V$_T$*, tidal volume. (Redrawn from Marelich GP, Murin S, Battistella F, et al: Protocol weaning of mechanical ventilation in medical and surgical patients by respiratory care practitioners and nurses: effect on weaning time and incidence of ventilator-associated pneumonia, Chest 118:459-467, 2000.)

Therapist-driven protocols for weaning patients from ventilation have been found to be safe and to reduce hospital costs by shortening the time required for ventilatory support.[111,112] A variety of protocols exist; although they can take the form of outlines, tables, and algorithms, their content tends to be similar. Figure 20-7 presents an example of a therapist-driven protocol.[113] It has been suggested that protocols heighten staff awareness of the process and generally promote weaning success.[112]

Protocols implemented by respiratory therapists and associated ICU team members are recognized as efficient, effective approaches to discontinuation of ventilatory support.[54,114-116] Nurses, respiratory therapists, and physicians involved in the patient's care must be informed of the patient's progress so that they can all work toward the goal of successfully weaning the patient from ventilatory support (Key Point 20-7).

Key Point 20-7 Weaning protocols have been shown to be efficient and effective approaches to discontinuation of ventilatory support.

A significant reduction in extubation failures and shorter weaning times are noted when therapist-driven protocols and nurse-driven protocols are used.[11,114] Studies suggest that some physicians may be too conservative when considering whether a patient is ready for SBT or extubation or both.[111,117]

The choice of a specific protocol is best left to the individual institution. Protocols should not replace clinical judgment but complement it. Protocols should be updated regularly to reflect current medical evidence and clinical practice patterns as they evolve. Institutions must commit the resources necessary to develop and implement protocols. Reduced staff levels or inadequate staff training can jeopardize clinical outcomes (Key Point 20-8).

> ⏺ **Key Point** 20-8 *"I believe that a skilled clinician at the bedside does more to facilitate ventilator weaning than any ventilator mode."*[15]

RECOMMENDATION 9: ROLE OF TRACHEOSTOMY IN WEANING

A tracheostomy is considered when it becomes apparent that the patient will require prolonged ventilator assistance.[59] A tracheotomy is performed after the patient is stable on the ventilator and when the person appears likely to benefit from the procedure.[118] The procedure should be performed as soon as possible after the need for extended intubation has been verified, and it should be based on the patient's disease and his or her wishes. The procedure usually is performed within 7 days of the onset of respiratory failure, or sooner in neurologically impaired patients.[118,119] Patients who might benefit from a tracheostomy include the following:

- Those who require high levels of sedation to tolerate ETs
- Those with marginal respiratory mechanics and may have tachypnea as a result
- Those in whom lower resistance (a potential benefit of tracheostomy tubes) may reduce the risk of muscle overload
- Those who may gain psychological benefit from the ability to eat, talk, and have greater mobility
- Those for whom increased mobility may aid physical therapy efforts[120-122]
- Ultimately the most important beneficial outcome of a tracheostomy is the potential to facilitate discontinuation of mechanical ventilatory support.

Despite a lack of data, the general clinical consensus is that patients receiving long-term mechanical ventilation have less facial discomfort when a nasotracheal or orotracheal tube is removed and replaced with a tracheostomy tube. Reduction in WOB and dead space and more effective secretion removal are possible benefits.[122] Interestingly, clinical data do not indicate that the rate of ventilator-associated pneumonia is lower or that the duration of ventilation is shorter for patients with tracheostomies.

A tracheostomy site typically requires 7 to 10 days to mature. If the tracheostomy tube is inadvertently displaced in the first 24 to 72 hours, successful blind tube replacement is highly unlikely.[118]

Removal of a tracheostomy tube is not difficult and can proceed just like extubation. After the tube is removed, the stoma is covered with one or two gauze pads held in place with tape. A stoma is like an open wound, and barring complications, it heals in a few days in most patients. Patients are taught to support the stoma when they cough by applying pressure to the gauze bandage with the flat surface of the hand. The secretions brought to the mouth can be expectorated. A tracheostomy button is recommended if the stoma must remain open because of excessive secretions or for some other reason. This short, hollow tube is inserted into the stoma and is held in place by its inner flanges. It can be capped to occlude the opening if desired.[123]

RECOMMENDATION 10: LONG-TERM CARE FACILITIES FOR PATIENTS REQUIRING PROLONGED VENTILATION

Unless evidence of irreversible disease exists, a patient who requires prolonged ventilatory support should not be considered permanently ventilator dependent until 3 months have passed and all weaning attempts during that time have failed.[59] Those failing to wean may require placement in a long-term care facility.

RECOMMENDATION 11: CLINICIAN FAMILIARITY WITH LONG-TERM CARE FACILITIES

Critical care practitioners must be familiar with facilities in their communities or units in their hospitals that specialize in the management of patients who require prolonged mechanical ventilation.[59] Patients for whom weaning attempts in the ICU fail are transferred to long-term ventilatory care facilities when they are medically stable. These facilities should have demonstrated competence, safety, and success in accomplishing ventilator discontinuation. Often these facilities have fewer staff members and less costly monitoring equipment, which make them less expensive than ICUs.[59]

RECOMMENDATION 12: WEANING IN LONG-TERM VENTILATION UNITS

Patients who are medically stable and able to leave the ICU but who have not been successfully weaned in that environment have several options.[124] Box 20-14 lists alternative sites where these patients can be weaned. The following are the goals for weaning in long-term care facilities[124]:

- To reduce the amount of ventilatory support
- To reduce the invasiveness of support
- To increase independence from mechanical devices
- To preserve and/or improve current function
- To maintain medical stability

Weaning procedures in long-term care units typically are individually designed rather than designed according to a fixed protocol, as in the ICU. In addition, using a variety of techniques may be required because a method that works for one person might not work for another. For example, some patients may not need an artificial airway to maintain airway patency and may only require NIV during the night.[125]

Weaning is slow paced when a patient requires long-term ventilation. Daily SBTs are not performed because patients are unlikely

---

BOX 20-14	**Alternative Sites for Long-Term Ventilatory Support**

- Regional weaning centers
- Noninvasive respiratory care units
- Long-term acute care facilities
- Extended care facilities
- Long-term ventilation units in acute care hospitals
- Home

(From Pierson DJ: Long-term mechanical ventilation and weaning, Respir Care 40:289-295, 1995.)

to be weaned successfully in 24 hours. The medical staff in long-term facilities generally includes registered nurses and registered respiratory therapists who are experienced in the assessment and management of these patients. Staff members understand the need for slow withdrawal of ventilator support and the importance of patience.

Patients with chronic conditions such as amyotrophic lateral sclerosis, muscular dystrophy, severe chronic lung disease, loss of the central drive to breathe, phrenic nerve damage or paralysis, cervical fracture leading to paralysis, and other types of neuromuscular or chronic disorders may require permanent mechanical ventilation. In these cases long-term ventilation refers to a means of support for patients who are not acutely ill but who are presumed to have a permanent need for such support.[124] Ventilator dependence can be challenging but it does not have to be completely confining, and many patients have meaningful lives outside the hospital or medical facility. Chapter 21 discusses long-term ventilation for ventilator-dependent individuals.

ETHICAL DILEMMA: WITHHOLDING AND WITHDRAWING VENTILATORY SUPPORT

The ethical and economic issues related to life support are becoming more important every day as the cost of medical care increases, the availability of payment declines, and the population ages.[126]

Withholding and withdrawal of life support are important ethical issues related to death and dying.

SUMMARY

- Weaning from mechanical ventilator support generally can be easily accomplished for most patients. For those who require more time, several methods are available, including the traditional techniques of IMV, PSV, and T-piece weaning and the more advanced closed-loop modes such as ATC, MMV, and ASV.
- The recommendations established by the ACCP/SCCM/AARC task force have provided a solid foundation upon which clinicians can better approach ventilator discontinuation.
- Verification that the problems leading to mechanical ventilation have been resolved is the first step in successfully liberating a patient from ventilatory support.
- Evaluation of appropriate criteria and the use of therapist-driven protocols or nurse-directed protocols can facilitate the process.
- Long-term care facilities provide a less demanding and less costly approach for patients who require longer ventilatory support and a slower weaning process.

REVIEW QUESTIONS *(See Appendix A for answers.)*

1. Which of the following would suggest that a patient is ready to be weaned from a ventilator?
   A. VC of 8 mL/kg IBW
   B. P_{Imax} of −15 cm H_2O
   C. V_D/V_T of 0.75
   D. f/V_T of 90 breaths/min/L RSBI

2. All of the following are closed-loop weaning modes except:
   A. VS
   B. ASV
   C. MMV
   D. T-piece trials

3. A respiratory therapist would consider ending an SBT under which of the following circumstances?
   A. The respiratory rate increases from 20 to 25 breaths/min
   B. The V_T decreases from 350 mL to 200 mL
   C. The systolic blood pressure decreases from 150 to 135 mm Hg
   D. The heart rate increases from 90 to 100 beats/min

4. You are called to the ICU to extubate a patient who has successfully completed a 120-minute SBT. Which of the following would indicate the potential for airway edema after extubation?
   A. P_{Imax}
   B. VC
   C. Cuff leak test
   D. S_pO_2

5. A patient develops stridor and shortness of breath after extubation. Which of the following is the first appropriate treatment for this problem?
   A. Reintubation
   B. Aerosolized racemic epinephrine
   C. Helium-oxygen by nonrebreathing mask
   D. Noninvasive mask ventilation

6. Which has been shown to be the unquestionably superior weaning technique?
   A. IMV
   B. PSV
   C. T-piece trials
   D. None of the above

7. State the ACCP/SCCM/AARC Task Force's first recommendation in weaning a patient from mechanical ventilation.

8. A patient with amyotrophic lateral sclerosis has a tracheostomy tube in place. He has been unable to perform an SBT successfully and has been on mechanical ventilation for 4 months. An appropriate recommendation for this patient might be which of the following?
   1. Transfer to a long-term care facility
   2. Evaluation for use of NIV
   3. Termination of ventilation
   4. Waiting until the primary cause of respiratory failure has been resolved
      A. 1 and 2 only
      B. 2 and 3 only
      C. 1, 2, and 3 only
      D. 1, 2, and 4

9. Once a patient has been successfully weaned from ventilatory support, assessment of the airway for extubation would include all of the following except:
   A. Ability to mobilize secretions
   B. Presence of a strong cough
   C. Presence of a peritubular leak on cuff deflation (successful cuff leak test)
   D. Normal breath sounds

10. MMV is appropriate for which of the following situations?
    1. During weaning from mechanical ventilation
    2. For patients who can partly assume WOB
    3. During cardiopulmonary resuscitation
    4. When a patient's ventilation is variable
       A. 1 and 2 only
       B. 2 and 3 only
       C. 3 and 4
       D. 1, 2, and 4

11. A physician wants to evaluate a male patient for discontinuation of ventilatory support. The patient is 70 kg and is receiving VC-IMV. He has no spontaneous respiratory efforts. Important parameters are: $V_T = 500$ mL; $f = 6$ breaths/min; $F_IO_2 = 0.4$; pH $= 7.3$; $P_aCO_2 = 58$ mm Hg; $P_aO_2 = 75$ mm Hg. The most appropriate ventilator change at this time is
    A. Implement PEEP
    B. Increase V_T
    C. Increase f
    D. Begin an SBT

12. Which of the following are reported advantages of MMV?
    1. The machine responds automatically to changes in V_E.
    2. Abrupt changes in CO_2 from a drop in spontaneous ventilation can be avoided.
    3. Alveolar ventilation is monitored.
    4. A much lower F_IO_2 can be used.
       A. 1 and 2
       B. 2 and 3
       C. 1, 2, and 3
       D. 2, 3, and 4

13. If the patient fails an SBT, the clinician should
    A. Determine the causes of the failure and correct them when possible
    B. Place the patient on full support and repeat the SBT in 8 hours
    C. Obtain an arterial blood gas analysis
    D. Switch to an artificial intelligence system for weaning

14. Assessment of WOB is not commonly performed before weaning because:
    A. It is not a reliable indicator of weaning success.
    B. It can be difficult to perform and requires expensive equipment.
    C. It can be easily determined by monitoring the respiratory rate.
    D. It is more appropriately viewed as an indication for ventilation than as a criterion for weaning.

15. When weaning is unsuccessful for a patient who successfully performs an SBT, which of the following factors should be assessed?
    1. Cardiac factors
    2. Nutritional status and respiratory muscle strength
    3. Acid–base status
    4. Psychological factors

A. 1 and 3
B. 2 and 4
C. 2, 3, and 4
D. 1, 2, 3, and 4

16. Sedatives can alter a patient's respiratory rate and V_T, thus affecting the assessment for ventilator discontinuation.
    A. True
    B. False

17. All of the following are true for nonphysician protocols except:
    A. They are more efficient than physician-directed weaning.
    B. They are more costly than conventional weaning techniques.
    C. They shorten weaning time.
    D. They significantly reduce extubation failures.

18. A tracheotomy is indicated for which of the following types of patients receiving mechanical ventilation?
    A. Those requiring low levels of sedation to tolerate ETs
    B. Those with strong respiratory mechanics who rarely exhibit tachypnea
    C. Those who may gain psychological benefit from the ability to eat, talk, and have greater mobility
    D. Those with good mobility and easy tolerance of physical therapy efforts

19. Patients who fail weaning attempts in the ICU for 3 months are:
    A. Transferred to long-term ventilatory care facilities when they are medically stable
    B. Given a tracheostomy
    C. Transferred to an ICU stepdown unit for physical therapy
    D. Recommended for termination of ventilatory support

20. Automatic tube compensation can best be described as
    A. Variable PS with variable inspiratory flow compensation
    B. Low-level PS with fixed flow-cycling criteria
    C. MMV
    D. Adaptive support using PS

References

1. MacIntyre NR: Evidence-based ventilatory weaning and discontinuation. *Respir Care* 49:830–836, 2004.
2. MacIntyre NR: Respiratory mechanics in the patient who is weaning from the ventilator. *Respir Care* 50:275–286, 2005.
3. Slutsky AS: Mechanical ventilation. American College of Chest Physicians' Consensus Conference. *Chest* 104:1833–1859, 1993.
4. MacIntyre NR, Leatherman NE: Ventilatory muscle loads and the frequency–tidal volume pattern during inspiratory pressure–assisted (pressure-supported) ventilation. *Am Rev Respir Dis* 141:327–331, 1990.
5. Esteban A, Alia I, Ibanez J, et al: Modes of mechanical ventilation and weaning. A national survey of Spanish hospitals. The Spanish Lung Failure Collaborative Group. *Chest* 106:1188–1193, 1994.
6. Pierson DJ: Weaning from mechanical ventilation: why all the confusion? *Respir Care* 40:228–232, 1995.
7. Sharar SR: Weaning and extubation are not the same thing. *Respir Care* 40:239–243, 1995.
8. Epstein SK: Etiology of extubation failure and the predictive value of the rapid shallow breathing index. *Am J Respir Crit Care Med* 152:545–549, 1995.
9. Esteban A, Alia I, Gordo F, et al: Extubation outcome after spontaneous breathing trials with T-tube or pressure support ventilation. The Spanish Lung Failure Collaborative Group. *Am J Respir Crit Care Med* 156:459–465, 1997.
10. Esteban A, Frutos F, Tobin MJ, et al: A comparison of four methods of weaning patients from mechanical ventilation. Spanish Lung Failure Collaborative Group. *N Engl J Med* 332:345–350, 1995.

11. Meade MO, Guyatt GH, Cook DJ: Weaning from mechanical ventilation: the evidence from clinical research. *Respir Care* 46:1408–1415, 2001.

12. Brochard L, Kauss A, Benito S, et al: Comparison of three methods of gradual withdrawing from ventilatory support during weaning from mechanical ventilation. *Am J Respir Crit Care Med* 150:896–903, 1994.

13. Esteban A, Anzueto A, Alia I, et al: How is mechanical ventilation employed in the intensive care unit? An international utilization review. *Am J Respir Crit Care Med* 161:1450–1458, 2000.

14. Kirby R, Robinson E, Shultz J, et al: Continuous-flow ventilation as an alternative to assisted or controlled ventilation in infants. *Anesth Analg* 51:871–875, 1972.

15. Hess DR: Mechanical ventilation strategies: what's new and what's worth keeping? *Respir Care* 47:1007–1017, 2002.

16. Marini JJ: Weaning techniques and protocols. *Respir Care* 40:233–238, 1995.

17. MacIntyre NR: Respiratory function during pressure support ventilation. *Chest* 89:677–683, 1986.

18. Leith DE, Bradley M: Ventilatory muscle strength and endurance training. *J Appl Physiol* 41:508–518, 1976.

19. Heuer AJ: Medical gas therapy. In Kacmarek RM, Stoller JK, Heuer AJ, editors: *Egan's fundamentals of respiratory care*, ed 10, St Louis, 2013, Elsevier, pp 887–944.

20. Chatburn RL, Mireles-Cabodevila E: Closed-loop control of mechanical ventilation: description and classification of targeting schemes. *Respir Care* 56:85–102, 2011.

21. Shapiro M, Wilson RK, Casar G, et al: Work of breathing through different sized endotracheal tubes. *Crit Care Med* 14:1028–1031, 1986.

22. Wright PE, Marini JJ, Bernard GR: In vitro versus in vivo comparison of endotracheal tube airflow resistance. *Am Rev Respir Dis* 140:10–16, 1989.

23. Brochard L, Rua F, Lorino H, et al: Inspiratory pressure support compensates for the additional work of breathing caused by the endotracheal tube. *Anesthesiology* 75:739–745, 1991.

24. Kuhlen R, Rossaint R: The role of spontaneous breathing during mechanical ventilation. *Respir Care* 47:296–303, 2002.

25. Oczenski W, Kepka A, Krenn H, et al: Automatic tube compensation in patients after cardiac surgery: effects on oxygen consumption and breathing pattern. *Crit Care Med* 30:1467–1471, 2002.

26. Mols G, Rohr E, Benzing A, et al: Breathing pattern associated with respiratory comfort during automatic tube compensation and pressure support ventilation in normal subjects. *Acta Anaesthesiol Scand* 44:223–230, 2000.

27. Fabry B, Haberthur C, Zappe D, et al: Breathing pattern and additional work of breathing in spontaneously breathing patients with different ventilatory demands during inspiratory pressure support and automatic tube compensation. *Intensive Care Med* 23:545–552, 1997.

28. Kacmarek RM: Ventilatory adjuncts. *Respir Care* 47:319–330, 2002.

29. Guttman J, Eberhert L, Fabry B, et al: Continuous calculation of intratracheal pressure in tracheally intubated patients. *Anesthesiology* 79:503–513, 1993.

30. Fabry B, Guttman J, Eberhard L, et al: Automatic compensation of endotracheal tube resistance in spontaneously breathing patients. *Technol Health Care* 1:281–291, 1994.

31. Branson R: Understanding and implementing advances in ventilator capabilities. *Curr Opin Crit Care* 10:23–32, 2004.

32. Elsasser S, Guttmann J, Stocker R, et al: Accuracy of automatic tube compensation in new-generation mechanical ventilators. *Crit Care Med* 31:2619–2626, 2003.

33. Fujino Y, Uchiyama A, Mashimo T, et al: Spontaneously breathing lung model comparison of work of breathing between automatic tube compensation and pressure support. *Respir Care* 48:38–45, 2003.

34. Branson RD, Johannigman JA: What is the evidence base for the newer ventilation modes? *Respir Care* 49:742–760, 2004.

35. Haberthur C, Elsasser S, Eberhard L, et al: Total versus tube-related additional work of breathing in ventilator-dependent patients. *Acta Anaesthesiol Scand* 44:749–757, 2000.

36. Guttmann J, Bernhard H, Mols G, et al: Respiratory comfort of automatic tube compensation and inspiratory pressure support in conscious humans. *Intensive Care Med* 23:1119–1124, 1997.

37. Guttmann J, Haberthur C, Mols G, et al: Automatic tube compensation (ATC). *Minerva Anestesiol* 68:369–377, 2002.

38. Straus C, Louis B, Isabey D, et al: Contribution of the endotracheal tube and the upper airway to breathing workload. *Am J Respir Crit Care Med* 157:23–30, 1998.

39. Haberthur C, Mols G, Elsasser S, et al: Extubation after breathing trials with automatic tube compensation, T-tube, or pressure support ventilation. *Acta Anaesthesiol Scand* 46:973–979, 2002.

40. Guttman J, Haberthur C, Mols G: Automatic tube compensation. *Respir Care Clin N Am* 7:475–501, 2001.

41. Hess DR, Branson RD: Ventilators and weaning modes. Part II. *Respir Care Clin N Am* 6:407–435, 2000.

42. Branson RD, Johannigman JA, Campbell RS, et al: Closed-loop mechanical ventilation. *Respir Care* 47:427–451, 2002.

43. Roth H, Luecke T, Lansche G, et al: Effects of patient-triggered automatic switching between mandatory and supported ventilation in postoperative weaning period. *Intensive Care Med* 27:47–51, 2001.

44. Holt SJ, Sanders RC, Thurman TL, et al: An evaluation of automode, a computer-controller ventilator mode, with the Siemens Servo 300A ventilator using a porcine model. *Respir Care* 46:26–36, 2001.

45. Hewlett AM, Platt AS, Terry VG: Mandatory minute volume. A new concept in weaning from mechanical ventilation. *Anaesthesia* 32:163–169, 1977.

46. Quan SF, Parides GC, Knoper SR: Mandatory minute ventilation (MMV): an overview. *Respir Care* 35:898–905, 1990.

47. Davis S, Potgieter PD, Linton DM: Mandatory minute volume weaning in patients with pulmonary pathology. *Anaesth Intensive Care* 17:170–174, 1989.

48. Cairo JM: *Mosby's respiratory care equipment*, ed 9, St Louis, 2014, Elsevier.

49. Campbell RS, Branson RD, Johannigman JA: Adaptive support ventilation. *Respir Care Clin N Am* 7:425–440, 2001.

50. Otis AB, Fenn WO, Rahn H: Mechanics of breathing in man. *J Appl Physiol* 2:592–607, 1950.

51. Weiler N, Eberle B, Heinrichs W: Adaptive lung ventilation (ALV) during anesthesia for pulmonary surgery: automatic response to transitions to and from one-lung ventilation. *J Clin Monit Comput* 14:245–252, 1998.

52. Linton DM, Potgieter PD, Davis S, et al: Automatic weaning from mechanical ventilation using an adaptive lung ventilation controller. *Chest* 106:1843–1850, 1994.

53. Petter AH, Chiolero RL, Cassina T, et al: Automatic "respiratory/weaning" with adaptive support ventilation: the effect on duration of endotracheal intubation and patient management. *Anesth Analg* 97:1743–1750, 2003.

54. Strickland JH, Hasson JH: A computer-controlled ventilator weaning system. A clinical trial. *Chest* 103:1220–1226, 1993.

55. Rose L, Presneill JL, Cade JF: Update in computer-driven weaning from mechanical ventilation. *Anaesth Intensive Care* 35:213–221, 2007.

56. Lellouche F, Mancebo J, Jolliet P, et al: A multicenter randomized trial of computer-driven protocolized weaning from mechanical ventilation. *Am J Respir Crit Care Med* 174(8):894–900, 2006.

57. Rose L, Presneill JL, Johnston L, et al: A randomized, controlled trial of conventional versus automated weaning from mechanical ventilation using SmartCare/PS. *Intensive Care Med* 34:1788–1795, 2008.

58. Cook DJ, Meade MO, Guyatt GH, et al: *Weaning from mechanical ventilation. For the McMaster Evidence Based Practice Center*, Rockville, Md, 2000, Agency for Healthcare Research and Quality. Contract No. 290-97-0017, Task order no. 2.

59. MacIntyre NR, Cook DJ, Ely EW, Jr, et al: ACCP/AARC/SCCM Task Force: evidence-based guidelines for weaning and discontinuing mechanical ventilatory support: a collective task force facilitated by the American College of Chest Physicians; the American Association for Respiratory Care; and the American College of Critical Care Medicine. *Chest* 120(6 Suppl):375S–395S, 2001; Also in: *Respir Care* 47:29–30, 2002.

60. Cook DJ, Meade MO, Guyatt G, et al: Trials of miscellaneous interventions to wean from mechanical ventilation. *Chest* 120(6 Suppl):438S–444S, 2001.

61. Cook D, Meade M, Perry AG: Qualitative studies on the patient's experience of weaning from mechanical ventilation. *Chest* 120(6 Suppl):469S–473S, 2001.

62. Campbell RS: Extubation and the consequences of reintubation. *Respir Care* 44:799–806, 1999.

63. Meade M, Guyatt G, Cook D, et al: Predicting success in weaning from mechanical ventilation. *Chest* 120(6 Suppl):400S–424S, 2001.

64. Epstein SK: Weaning from mechanical ventilation. *Respir Care* 47:454–466, 2002.

65. Ely EW, Baker AM, Dunagan DP, et al: Effect on the duration of mechanical ventilation of identifying patients capable of breathing spontaneously. *N Engl J Med* 335:1864–1869, 1996.

66. Tobin MJ: Predicting ventilator independence. *Semin Respir Med* 14:275–280, 1993.

67. MacIntyre NR: Psychological factors in weaning from mechanical ventilatory support. *Respir Care* 40:277–281, 1995.

68. Khamiees M, Amoateng-Adjepong Y, Manthous CA: Propofol infusion is associated with a higher rapid shallow breathing index in patients preparing to wean from mechanical ventilation. *Respir Care* 47:150–153, 2002.

69. Yang KL, Tobin MJ: A prospective study of indexes predicting the outcome of trials of weaning from mechanical ventilation. *N Engl J Med* 324:1445–1450, 1991.

70. Lee KH, Hui KP, Chan TB, et al: Rapid shallow breathing (frequency-tidal volume ratio) did not predict extubation outcome. *Chest* 105:540–543, 1994.

71. Yang KL: Inspiratory pressure/maximal inspiratory pressure ratio: a predictive index of weaning outcome. *Intensive Care Med* 19:204–208, 1993.

72. El-Khatib MF, Baumeister B, Smith PG, et al: Inspiratory pressure/maximal inspiratory pressure: does it predict successful extubation in critically ill infants and children? *Intensive Care Med* 22:264–268, 1996.

73. Capdevila XJ, Perrigault PF, Perey PJ, et al: Occlusion pressure and its ratio to maximum inspiratory pressure are useful predictors for successful extubation following T-piece weaning trial. *Chest* 108:482–489, 1995.

74. Sassoon CSH, Te TT, Mahutte CK, et al: Airway occlusion pressure. An important indicator for successful weaning in patients with chronic obstructive pulmonary disease. *Am Rev Respir Dis* 135:107–113, 1987.

75. Scott GC, Burki NK: The relationship of resting ventilation to mouth occlusion pressure. An index of resting respiratory function. *Chest* 98:900–906, 1990.

76. Sasson CSH, Mahutte CK: Airway occlusion pressure and breathing pattern as predictors of weaning outcome. *Am Rev Respir Dis* 148:860–866, 1993.

77. Jubran A, Tobin MJ: Pathophysiologic basis of acute respiratory distress in patients who fail a trial of weaning from mechanical ventilation. *Am J Respir Crit Care Med* 155:906–915, 1997.

78. Stoller JK: Establishing clinical unweanability. *Respir Care* 36:186–198, 1991.

79. Mitsuoka M, Kinninger KH, Johnson FW, et al: Utility of measurements of oxygen cost of breathing in predicting success or failure in trials of reduced mechanical ventilatory support. *Respir Care* 46:902–910, 2001.

80. Esteban A, Alia I, Tobin MJ, et al: Effect of spontaneous breathing trial duration on outcome of attempts to discontinue mechanical ventilation. Spanish Lung Failure Collaborative Group. *Am J Respir Crit Care Med* 159:512–518, 1999.

81. Esteban A, Alia I, Gordo F, et al: Extubation outcome after spontaneous breathing trials with T-tube or pressure support ventilation. Spanish Lung Failure Collaborative Group. *Am J Respir Crit Care Med* 156:459–465, 1997. (erratum in *Am J Respir Crit Care Med* 156:2028, 1997).

82. Cohen JD, Shapiro M, Grozovski E, et al: Automatic tube compensation-assisted respiratory rate to tidal volume ratio improves the prediction of weaning outcome. *Chest* 122:980–984, 2002.

83. Matic I, Majeric-Kogler V: Comparison of pressure support and T-tube weaning from mechanical ventilation: randomized prospective study. *Croat Med J* 45:162–166, 2004.

84. Vallverdu I, Calaf N, Subirana M, et al: Clinical characteristics, respiratory functional parameters, and outcome of two-hour T-piece trial in patients weaning from mechanical ventilation. *Am J Respir Crit Care Med* 158:1855–1862, 1998.

85. Salam A, Smina M, Gada P, et al: The effect of arterial blood gas values on extubation decisions. *Respir Care* 48:1033–1037, 2003.

86. Coplin WM, Pierson DJ, Cooley KD, et al: Implications of extubation delay in brain-injured patients meeting standard weaning criteria. *Am J Respir Crit Care Med* 161:1530–1536, 2000.

87. Marik PE: The cuff-leak test as a predictor of postextubation stridor: a prospective study. *Respir Care* 41:509511, 1996.

88. Meade MO, Guyatt GH, Cook DJ, et al: Trials of corticosteroids to prevent postextubation airway complications. *Chest* 120(6 Suppl):464S–468S, 2001.

89. Fisher MM, Raper RF: The "cuff-leak" test for extubation. *Anaesthesia* 47:10–12, 1992.

90. Engoren M: Evaluation of the cuff-leak test in a cardiac surgery population. *Chest* 116:1029–1031, 1999.

91. Epstein SK: Extubation. *Respir Care* 47:483–492, 2002.

92. Epstein SK, Ciubotaru RL, Wong JB: Effect of failed extubation on the outcome of mechanical ventilation. *Chest* 112:186–192, 1997.

93. Meade MO, Guyatt G, Butler R, et al: Trials comparing early versus late extubation following cardiovascular surgery. *Chest* 120(6 Suppl):445S–453S, 2001.

94. Rady MY, Ryan T: Perioperative predictors of extubation failure and the effect on clinical outcome after cardiac surgery. *Crit Care Med* 27:340–347, 1999.

95. Solh E, Bhat A, Gunen H, et al: Extubation failure in the elderly. *Respir Med* 98:661–668, 2004.

96. AARC Clinical Practice Guideline: Removal of the endotracheal tube. *Respir Care* 52:81–93, 2007.

97. ACCP, AARC, ACCCM: Taskforce: Evidence-based guidelines for weaning and discontinuing ventilatory support. *Respir Care* 47:69–90, 2002.

98. Girault C, Daudenthun I, Chevron V, et al: Noninvasive ventilation as a systematic extubation and weaning technique in acute-on-chronic respiratory failure: a prospective, randomized controlled study. *Am J Respir Crit Care Med* 160:86–92, 1999.

99. Nava L, Ambrosino N, Rubini F, et al: Survival and prediction of successful ventilator weaning in COPD patients requiring mechanical ventilation for more than 21 days. *Eur Respir J* 7:1645–1652, 1994.

100. Hill NS, Lin D, Levy M, et al: Noninvasive positive pressure ventilation (NPPV) to facilitate extubation after acute respiratory failure: a feasibility study (abstract). *Am J Respir Crit Care Med* 161:A263, 2000.

101. Ferrer M, Esquinas A, Arancibia F, et al: Noninvasive ventilation during persistent weaning failure: a randomized controlled trial. *Am J Respir Crit Care Med* 168:70–76, 2003.

102. Navalesi P: Weaning and noninvasive ventilation: the odd couple (editorial). *Am J Respir Crit Care Med* 168:5–6, 2003.

103. Sassoon CSH: Noninvasive positive-pressure ventilation in acute respiratory failure: review of reported experience with special attention to use during weaning. *Respir Care* 40:282–288, 1995.

104. Mathewson HS: Prolonged neuromuscular blockade (editorial). *Respir Care* 38:522–523, 1993.

105. Douglass JA, Tuxen DV, Horne M, et al: Myopathy in severe asthma. *Am Rev Respir Dis* 146:517–519, 1992.

106. Griffin D, Fairman N, Coursin D, et al: Acute myopathy during treatment of status asthmaticus with corticosteroids and steroidal muscle relaxants. *Chest* 102:510–514, 1992.

107. Segredo V, Caldwell JE, Matthay MA, et al: Persistent paralysis in critically ill patients after long-term administration of vecuronium. *N Engl J Med* 327:524–528, 1992.

108. Hansen-Glaschen J, Cowen J, Raps EC: Neuromuscular blockade in the intensive care unit. More than we bargained for (editorial). *Am Rev Respir Dis* 147:234–236, 1993.

109. Stoller JK: Physiologic rationale for resting the ventilatory muscles. *Respir Care* 36:290–296, 1991.

110. MacIntyre NR: Bringing scientific evidence to the ventilator weaning and discontinuation process: evidence-based practice guidelines (editorial). *Respir Care* 47:29–30, 2002.

111. Wood G, MacLeod B, Moffatt S: Weaning from mechanical ventilation: physician-directed vs a respiratory therapist-directed protocol. *Respir Care* 40:219–224, 1995.

112. Domini L, Wallace P, Pilbeam SP: Weaning protocol in ICU can save money. *AARC Adult Acute Care Section Bulletin* 1996. Winter.

113. Marelich GP, Murin S, Battistella F, et al: Protocol weaning of mechanical ventilation in medical and surgical patients by respiratory care practitioners and nurses: effect on weaning time and incidence of ventilator-associated pneumonia. *Chest* 118:459–467, 2000.

114. Ely EW, Meade MO, Haponik EF, et al: Mechanical ventilator weaning protocols driven by nonphysician health-care professionals: evidence-based clinical practice guidelines. *Chest* 120(6 Suppl):454S–463S, 2001.

115. Ely EW, Bennett PA, Bowton DL, et al: Large scale implementation of respiratory therapist-driven protocol for ventilator weaning. *Am J Respir Crit Care Med* 159:439–446, 1999.

116. Kollef MH, Shapiro SD, Silver P, et al: A randomized, controlled trial of protocol-directed versus physician-directed weaning from mechanical ventilation. *Crit Care Med* 25:567–574, 1997.

117. Stoller JK, Mascha EJ, Kester L, et al: Randomized controlled trial of physician-directed versus respiratory therapy consult service–directed respiratory care to adult non-ICU inpatients. *Am J Respir Crit Care Med* 158:1068–1075, 1998.

118. Littlewood K, Durbin CG: Evidenced-based airway management. *Respir Care* 46:1392–1405, 2001.

119. Harrop JS, Sharan AD, Scheid EH, et al: Tracheostomy placement in patients with complete cervical spinal cord injuries: American Spinal Injury Association Grade A. *J Neurosurg* 100:20–23, 2004.

120. Heffner JE: The role of tracheotomy in weaning. *Chest* 120(6 Suppl):477S–481S, 2001.

121. Maziak DE, Meade MO, Todd TR: The timing of tracheotomy: a systematic review. *Chest* 114:605–609, 1998.

122. Jaeger JM, Littlewood KA, Durbin CG: The role of tracheostomy in weaning from mechanical ventilation. *Respir Care* 47:469–480, 2002.

123. Bortner PL, May RA: Artificial airways and tubes. In Eubanks DH, Bone RC, editors: *Principles and applications of cardiorespiratory care equipment*, St Louis, 1994, Mosby, pp 117–145.

124. Pierson DJ: Long-term mechanical ventilation and weaning. *Respir Care* 40:289–295, 1995.

125. Curtis JR: The long-term outcomes of mechanical ventilation: what are they and should they be used? *Respir Care* 47:496–505, 2002.

126. Wilson ME, Azoulay E: The ethics of withholding and withdrawing ventilatory support. In Tobin JJ, editor: *Principles and practice of mechanical ventilation*, ed 3, New York, 2013, McGraw-Hill.

Long-Term Ventilation

OUTLINE

KEY TERMS

- Chest cuirass
- Decannulation
- Erosive esophagitis
- Gastrostomy or jejunostomy tubes
- Ileus
- Pneumobelt
- Respite care
- Rocking bed

LEARNING OBJECTIVES *On completion of this chapter, the reader will be able to do the following:*

1. State the goals of mechanical ventilation in a home environment.
2. List the criteria for selection of patients suitable for successful homecare ventilation.
3. Name the factors used to estimate the cost of home mechanical ventilation.
4. Describe facilities used for the care of patients requiring extended ventilator management in terms of type of care provided and cost.
5. Identify the factors used when considering selection of a ventilator for home use.
6. Compare the criteria for discharging a child versus discharging an adult who is ventilator dependent.
7. Explain the use of the following noninvasive ventilation techniques: pneumobelt, chest cuirass, full-body chamber (tank ventilator), and body suit (jacket ventilator).
8. List follow-up assessment techniques used with home-ventilated patients.
9. Describe some of the difficulties families experience when caring for a patient in the home.
10. Identify pieces of equipment that are essential to accomplishing intermittent positive pressure ventilation in the home.
11. Name the specific equipment needed for patients in the home who cannot be without ventilator support.
12. Name the appropriate modes used with first-generation portable/homecare ventilators.
13. On the basis of a patient's assessment and ventilator parameters, name the operational features required for that patient's home ventilator and any additional equipment that will be needed.
14. Discuss the instructions given to the patient and caregivers when preparing a patient for discharge home.
15. List the items that should appear in a monthly report of patients on home mechanical ventilation.
16. Describe patients who would benefit from continuous positive airway pressure by nasal mask or pillows.
17. Recommend solutions to potential complications and side effects of nasal mask continuous positive airway pressure.
18. Recognize from a clinical example a potential complication of negative pressure ventilation.

19. Name three methods of improving secretion clearance besides suctioning.
20. List the advantages of using mechanical insufflation-exsufflation in conjunction with positive pressure ventilation.
21. List five psychological problems that can occur in ventilator-assisted individuals.
22. Explain the procedure for accomplishing speech in ventilator-assisted individuals.
23. Compare the functions of the Portex and the Pittsburg speaking tracheostomy tubes.
24. Name one essential step required by the respiratory therapist when setting up a speaking valve for a ventilator-assisted individual.
25. List six circumstances in which speaking devices may be contraindicated.

Most patients receiving mechanical ventilation require ventilatory support for less than 7 days. Approximately 5% of those patients requiring more than 7 days cannot be successfully weaned from ventilatory support and require long-term mechanical ventilation (LTMV). For these patients, weaning is slow paced and may not always result in ventilator discontinuation.[1]

Patients requiring LTMV can be divided into two groups: those recovering from an acute illness and unable to maintain adequate ventilation for prolonged periods, and those with chronic progressive cardiopulmonary disorders. Patients who have an acute, severe illness may not recover sufficiently to be weaned from ventilation while in an acute care facility and are generally transferred to special units on mechanical ventilation within the hospital, long-term care facilities, or their homes. Chronic progressive disorders that require LTMV include ventilatory muscle disorders, alveolar hypoventilation, obstructive lung diseases, restrictive lung diseases, and cardiac diseases (e.g., congenital cardiac diseases).[2]

Mortality rates for patients receiving LTMV are high (2-year mortality rate of 57%; 5-year mortality rate range of 66% to 97%).[3-5] Patients who are successfully liberated from the ventilator and decannulated have the best chance of survival.[4]

The number of ventilator-assisted individuals (VAIs) being discharged to homes or alternative care sites has increased during the past three decades[6] (Key Point 21-1). Approximately 11,419 VAIs were in the United States in 2002, with care requiring an annual cost of almost $3.2 billion. Most of the cost for VAIs is absorbed by acute care hospitals, where reimbursement is often inadequate. As a consequence of rising costs and falling reimbursements, specialized respiratory care units in acute, intermediate, and chronic care facilities were developed. However, recent growth of these specialty units has slowed, again because of limited funding and reimbursement.[4,7]

Key Point 21-1 Long-term ventilator-assisted patients are defined by the American College of Chest Physicians (ACCP) as individuals requiring mechanical ventilation for at least 6 hours per day for 21 days or more.[6]

Five major factors have added to this upsurge in numbers of VAIs:
1. First, continued advances in pulmonary medicine and technology have contributed to increased survival rates of critically ill adults and children. Many of these patients can be saved, stabilized, and sent home or to alternative sites for continued ventilator support.[8]
2. Second, an increased emphasis has been placed on reducing the cost of medical care through earlier discharge of patients from acute care hospitals. These patients can be transferred to less costly facilities for continued care.
3. Third, noninvasive positive pressure ventilation (NIV) such as bilevel mask ventilation is an effective alternative to invasive ventilation, both as an initial mode of treatment and as a long-term alternative to managing ventilator-dependent patients.
4. Fourth, simpler and more versatile equipment is available for home use.
5. Fifth, an increase in medical equipment agencies and the availability of homecare services that provide ventilator care outside the hospital. These latter services allow the patient to benefit from the psychological advantages of being in the family setting or in a nonacute care environment.

An excellent example of a VAI who not only survived but lived a quality life is Christopher Reeve, an actor and active sportsman who sustained a high cervical fracture as a result of a horseback riding accident that left him a quadriplegic. With his determination and the support of his wife, family, and caregivers, he was able to have a productive life while being maintained on LTMV for 10 years. During this time, he directed films, became a public speaker, raised awareness of spinal cord injury, and became a strong advocate for stem cell research.[9]

The number of elder Americans is increasing, along with an increase in the number of people with chronic illnesses. Given these trends and the demand for more stringent methods of controlling healthcare costs, the number of VAIs discharged to home or alternative care sites will continue to increase. LTMV has been shown to be a safe and effective alternative to acute care institutionalization. The home is generally the least expensive environment and the one that provides the greatest level of patient independence and family support. A large part of this chapter is devoted to a discussion of home mechanical ventilation.

GOALS OF LONG-TERM MECHANICAL VENTILATION

The overall goal of LTMV at home or other alternative care sites is to improve the patient's quality of life by providing the following environmental attributes[2,10]:
- Enhancing the individual's living potential
- Improving physical and physiological level of function
- Reducing morbidity
- Reducing hospitalizations
- Extending life
- Providing cost-effective care

Because patients require different levels of care, it is desirable for every patient to progress to his or her point of maximum activity and take an active role in his or her own care. If this is accomplished, then his or her psychosocial well-being will also improve.

SITES FOR VENTILATOR-DEPENDENT PATIENTS

The terminology used to describe facilities for VAIs is not standardized. Sites can be grouped in three general categories: acute care, intermediate care, and long-term care.[1]

Acute Care Sites

Acute care sites include the following:

- Intensive care units (ICU) or critical care units (CCU), which provide invasive monitoring, extensive care, and a higher ratio of practitioners to patients. These units are more expensive and provide the least amount of patient independence and quality of life.
- Specialized respiratory care units, which have fewer resources and are generally designed for more stable VAIs. These are often designated units within a hospital and may be called *pulmonary specialty wards,*[11] *respiratory special care units,* and *chronic assisted ventilator care units.*[12]
- General medical-surgical care units, which typically are located on general patient floors of the hospital. Nursing and allied health staff working on these general medical-surgical units often require additional preparation and training to manage these VAIs.
- Long-term acute care hospitals, which are specifically designed to care for patients who require extensive monitoring and care, such as daily physician visits, continuous monitoring, intravenous therapy, wound care, and isolation. These patients may still be acutely ill but no longer require the intensive care provided in a critical care unit in the hospital.[12] Long-term ventilator hospitals fall in this category.

VAIs in specialized units located within a hospital typically have the following characteristics:

- A longer hospital stay
- Lower hospital mortality rates
- Higher weaning rates
- Higher likelihood of being discharged to their homes
- Longer life expectancy after discharge
- Greater independence in daily activities

Success revolved around the strong leaderships of pulmonologists, who were dedicated to the care of these individuals.[13]

Intermediate Care Sites

Intermediate care sites usually include subacute care units, long-term care hospitals, and rehabilitation hospitals. Intermediate care sites are not as expensive as acute care sites and provide somewhat more patient independence and quality of life.

Subacute care units may be located in acute care hospitals. They often admit patients who require physiological monitoring, intravenous therapy, or postoperative care.

Long-term care hospitals are designed to provide care for long-term invasive ventilator-dependent patients (i.e., length of stay usually exceeds 25 days). These patients may still require high levels of positive end-expiratory pressure (PEEP) or fraction of inspired oxygen (F_IO_2). Once they are liberated from the ventilator or switched to a noninvasive method of support, these patients can then be transferred to a congregate living center or home.

Admission to a rehabilitation hospital is based on the patient's specific rehabilitation goals. Current standards include the requirement for nursing rehabilitation care and at least two additional rehabilitation needs, such as physical therapy, occupational therapy, or speech therapy. After a 10-day trial period, patients must be able to participate for 3 hours of therapy per day.

Long-Term Care Sites

Long-term care sites include skilled nursing facilities, congregate living centers, and single-family homes. These sites do not have the resources to treat acutely ill patients. They are **not** the ideal site for weaning a patient from ventilation. However, they are the least expensive and provide a better quality of life and more independence for the patient.

Skilled nursing facilities include nursing homes, extended care facilities, and convalescent centers. A greater number of VAIs are being admitted in these locations.

Congregate living centers are commonly large private residences, apartments, foster homes, or homes with as many as six to 10 patients. These sites are more common in Europe than in the United States.[10]

Homes are the preferred environment for caring for ventilator-dependent patients. The quality of life for patients living at home is enhanced, and they are less costly than most other sites, perhaps with the exception of skilled nursing facilities. The family usually provides most of the support, both financial and medical.

Increasing pressure from managed care and utilization review is resulting in more rapid discharge from ICUs and acute care facilities. Intermediate- and long-term care sites provide newer and less costly approaches to patient care.[14-21] Treatment objectives are generally met at specific facilities. For example, weaning may occur in acute or intermediate care facilities, but it is usually inappropriate in the home.[10]

PATIENT SELECTION

Patient selection is the key to success for any long care ventilation program. Although many factors must be considered in this selection, they can be broadly grouped into three areas:

1. Disease process and clinical stability
2. Psychological evaluation of patient and family
3. Financial considerations

Disease Process and Clinical Stability

Previous studies have shown that some patients with disorders requiring LTMV may be more successfully managed than others.[22-25] The following three categories can be used to describe ventilator-dependent patients.[1,10]

1. Patients recovering from acute illnesses and acute respiratory failure that do not respond to repeated attempts at liberation from the ventilator. These patients may need mechanical ventilation for an extended period and will require several weeks to months for recovery but are likely to recover. Some of these patients may sustain several hours of unsupported spontaneous breathing but generally will fatigue when challenged with longer periods of ventilator disconnection.
2. Patients with chronic disorders who only require mechanical ventilation for a part of the day, such as at night, but can support spontaneous ventilation on their own for several hours each day.
3. Patients requiring continuous ventilatory support to survive, that is, patients diagnosed as having complete loss of ventilatory function with absent or severely impaired spontaneous breathing efforts. These patients are unable to sustain spontaneous ventilation and depend on life support from the ventilator.

BOX 21-1	Patient Groups Requiring Long-Term Mechanical Ventilation

1. Patients recovering from acute illnesses and acute respiratory failure who do not respond to repeated attempts at liberation from the ventilator. This group might include patients who have had a major insult to the respiratory system caused by a severe medical illness, such as acute respiratory distress syndrome or severe pneumonia; patients who had a catastrophic postoperative event; and patients in whom an acute illness develops superimposed on a chronic disorder (e.g., malnutrition, advanced age, heart disease, systemic infection, COPD).

2. Patients with chronic disorders who only require mechanical ventilation for a portion of the day, such as at night, but can support spontaneous ventilation on their own for several hours each day, such as severe COPD, kyphoscoliosis, and severe or progressing neuromuscular disorders, such as amyotrophic lateral sclerosis.

3. Patients requiring continuous ventilatory support to survive, that is, those patients diagnosed as having complete loss of ventilatory function with absent or severely impaired spontaneous breathing efforts. Examples include intracranial hemorrhage, cerebrovascular accidents, central alveolar hypoventilation syndrome, and diaphragmatic paralysis. This group also includes patients with severe respiratory muscle failure such as those with a high spinal cord injury, end-stage pulmonary interstitial fibrosis, and end-stage neuromuscular disorders.

BOX 21-2	Medical Conditions Appropriate for Long-Term Mechanical Ventilation

Central Nervous System Disorders
- Arnold-Chiari malformation
- Central nervous system trauma
- Cerebrovascular disorders
- Congenital and acquired central control of breathing disorders
- Myelomeningocele
- Spinal cord traumatic injuries

Neuromuscular Disorders
- Amyotrophic lateral sclerosis
- Congenital childhood hypotonia
- Guillain-Barré syndrome
- Infant botulism
- Muscular dystrophy
- Myasthenia gravis
- Phrenic nerve paralysis
- Polio and postpolio sequelae
- Spinal muscular atrophy
- Myotonic dystrophy

Skeletal Disorders
- Kyphoscoliosis
- Thoracic wall deformities
- Thoracoplasty

Cardiovascular Disorders
- Acquired heart diseases
- Congenital heart diseases

Respiratory Disorders
Upper Airway
- Pierre Robin syndrome
- Tracheomalacia
- Vocal cord paralysis

Lower Respiratory Tract
- Bronchopulmonary dysplasia
- COPD
- Complications of acute lung injury
- Cystic fibrosis
- Complications of infectious pneumonias
- Pulmonary fibrotic diseases

(From Make BJ, Hill NS, Goldberg AI: Mechanical ventilation beyond the intensive care unit: report of a consensus conference of the American College of Chest Physicians, *Chest* 113:289S-344S, 1998.)

Their disorder is inexorably progressive. (Box 21-1 lists the disorders grouped in each category.)

Patients with neuromuscular conditions, skeletal disorders, central hypoventilation syndromes, and stable chronic lung diseases are more likely to have long-term success than patients with disorders causing failure of gas exchange. Disease processes affecting other organ systems besides the pulmonary system are associated with a higher risk of complications. Patients affected with these types of conditions are not suitable for long-term ventilation in most extended care facilities and require a long-term acute care facility. Box 21-2 lists medical conditions appropriate for long-term ventilation.[10,6,25]

Individuals who are considered candidates for LTMV in the home or in extended care facilities must be clinically and physiologically stable to the degree that they are free from any medical complications for at least 2 weeks before discharge. Proof of medical stability must include stable cardiovascular and renal function; no evidence of uncontrolled hemorrhage or coma or, if comatose, prognosis for improvement; acceptable arterial blood gas (ABG) values; freedom from acute respiratory infections and fever; stabile F_IO_2 requirements; and ventilator settings which do **not** result in high inspiratory pressures or high levels of PEEP (Case Study 21-1).

Other considerations include the ability to clear secretions (either spontaneously or by suctioning), the ability to tolerate and meet criteria for a face mask or nasal mask for NIV, or the presence of a tracheostomy tube (TT) for invasive positive pressure ventilation (IPPV). Additionally, major diagnostic tests or therapeutic interventions should not be anticipated for at least 1 month after discharge. Box 21-3 lists selection criteria for children.[26]

Psychosocial Factors

The psychological stability and coping skills of the patient and family are critical to the success of long-term ventilation. The family must be made aware of the patient's prognosis and the advantages and disadvantages of LTMV.

In cases where the patient will be going home, a detailed psychological evaluation may be necessary to determine the ability of the patient and family to cope with stress.[10,22] If the requirements for patient care exceed the family's capabilities, professional assistance is essential. The availability of other support systems such as home health agencies, **respite care,** and psychological consultants are often critical to the success or failure of homecare candidates. The need for support and counseling is assessed before discharge and reassessed periodically while the patient remains on mechanical ventilatory support.[27,28]

Selection Criteria for Children to Be Ventilated at Home

Infants and children being considered for home mechanical ventilation may have additional criteria besides clinical stability and financial resources that must be fulfilled. These criteria include the following:

- Positive trends in weight gain and growth curve
- Stamina for periods of play while ventilated
- Family determined to be suitable candidates, as shown by their awareness of potential stresses of long-term home care and commitment to implementing the program
- Adequate family support from home nurses, homemaker aids, and family and friends

(From American Thoracic Society Board of Directors Official Statement, *Am Rev Respir Dis* 141:258-259, 1990.)

 Case Study 21-1

Patient Case—Difficulty Weaning

A 48-year-old male patient with stable amyotrophic lateral sclerosis (requiring nocturnal ventilation only) develops chest pain and is taken to the emergency department by his family. An electrocardiogram reveals an anterior myocardial infarction. The patient is intubated with a 7.5-Fr endotracheal tube and placed on appropriate ventilatory support.

The patient is stabilized and after 2 days on ventilation, a spontaneous breathing trial (SBT) is attempted. The patient fails the SBT. He also fails SBTs evaluated over the next week. A tracheostomy is placed.

After 4 weeks in an acute care setting, the patient is medically stable but requires continuous ventilation. Why has it become so difficult to wean this patient? Would you recommend transferring this patient to another facility?

Financial Considerations

Regardless of the location in which it is provided, mechanical ventilation is an expensive treatment modality. Note that mechanical ventilation in an ICU and acute care unit is the most expensive option of the facilities previously mentioned, whereas homecare ventilation is the least expensive.[14-17] It is important to recognize that despite the significant savings accrued when a patient receives ventilatory care in the home, the overall cost can strain family budgets, even for those who are insured.

A variety of factors can also influence the total cost associated with delivering LTMV. These factors include the following patient characteristics[11,20]:

- Diagnosis
- Age
- Level of acuity
- Need for rehabilitation services (e.g., occupational therapy, physical therapy)
- Type of ventilator selected
- Need for monitoring
- Supplemental oxygen
- Medications

For example, patients with chronic obstructive pulmonary disease (COPD) may require a higher level of care than patients with neuromuscular disorders because of the need for additional care such as suctioning, bronchopulmonary drainage, bronchodilator therapy, and anxiolytic and antibiotic administration. Children younger than 10 years may also require higher costs because of special needs compared with adults.

For homecare patients, ventilator equipment can be bought at a reasonable price; however, in many cases, families may choose to rent the ventilator because regular service, maintenance, and 24-hour emergency services are available as part of the rental contract. Unfortunately, the costs of accessory medical supplies, including items such as suction catheters, skin lotions, and absorbent underpads, may be difficult to estimate and can significantly increase the total cost of care.

The major factor affecting the cost of home care is the need for professional or skilled caregivers. This cost depends on the availability of family members and how much they are willing and able to do. Cost also depends on patient independence and self-care abilities and the number of hours and level of care required from others.[21]

It is important to recognize that inadequate third-party coverage for supplies and equipment, which is almost always passed on to the patient and family, must be factored into the costs of providing LTMV in the home. An estimate of the actual cost to the patient must be determined as accurately as possible and presented to the patient and family before discharging the patient from the care facility to the home.

PREPARATION FOR DISCHARGE TO THE HOME

Respiratory therapists who are assigned to prepare a ventilator-assisted patient for transfer to another facility or home must ensure that the receiving site can accommodate the patient's and family's needs. Although similarities in discharge planning exist between an acute care and an intermediate care facility, the transfer from either of these facilities to the patient's home requires particular attention.[28,29]

When the VAI is being transferred home, preparation is extremely important. Preparation of the home begins almost simultaneously with home and patient assessment and includes the process of equipment selection. The coordinated efforts of the multidisciplinary health care team, a comprehensive discharge prescription, and an educational program for the patient and caregivers are developed to ensure a safe transition from hospital to home or alternate care site (Key Point 21-2).

Key Point 21-2 A discharge plan should contain the basic components of assessment, education, training, and a plan of care.[10]

The discharge process may be complex and time-consuming depending on the patient's medical condition, needs, and goals. Consequently, it is initiated as early as possible before transfer to make it as smooth as possible. This often requires a minimum of a 7- to 14-day period before the patient is discharged because this much time may be needed to obtain insurance verification and authorization and equipment procurement. In other words, the plan may begin almost as soon as the patient is admitted to the acute care facility or as soon as he or she is identified as a VAI.

The discharge planning process ensures patient safety and optimal outcome in the new environment.

The goal of the discharge planning team is to identify all patient care issues that need to be addressed before discharge and develop a plan of care to facilitate transfer.[10,29,30] The health care team generally consists of the patient and family, the patient's primary physician, a pulmonary physician, a nurse, a respiratory therapist, and a social worker/hospital discharge planner. Depending on the patient's level of care, other specialists, such as a physical therapist, a psychologist, an occupational therapist, a speech pathologist, and a clinical dietitian, may also be included. The durable medical equipment (DME) supplier will also be a crucial member of this team, and equipment should be selected as soon as possible. A coordinator should be designated if a hospital-based discharge planner is not available.[31]

Team members must communicate regularly to discuss the patient's progress and address any issues that may hinder the discharge process. A thorough review of the patient's hospital record is also important to determine the patient's history and established medical condition. Ventilator settings are discussed to ensure that the DME supplier can provide a ventilator that can accommodate the desired settings. An assessment of the financial status of the patient is imperative to ensure that additional assistance can be pursued for gaps that exist between third-party reimbursement and actual cost.

Geographic and Home Assessment

The geographic area where the patient will reside should also be considered. This is done to ensure that a home health agency or DME provider is near the patient's home and is available to provide assistance. A hospital emergency department should also be within a reasonable driving distance.

As part of the discharge plan, the medical supplier or practitioner assesses the patient's home environment to see whether any modifications must be made before the patient goes home. In general, this assessment includes a home visit to view the size of the patient care area and determine whether it is adequate for the prescribed equipment. Areas should be available for storage as well as for cleaning and disposal of supplies. Judging the accessibility into and out of the home and between rooms is important and should not be overlooked. The home should also be assessed for safety (e.g., fire extinguishers and smoke detectors and alarms). The family needs to have telephone service. The number of people in the home may be a factor in the size of the space, and, of course, the primary caregivers must be identified.

The electrical system must provide adequate amperage for the ventilation, suction equipment, oxygen concentrator if needed, and other necessary electrical devices. An important step is counting the number and type of electrical outlets and determining the amperage requirements of the equipment (Box 21-4). This may be accomplished by the family, or it may require an electrician.[32]

When modifications in the home are recommended, they will not be covered by health insurance, which means that they will be out-of-pocket costs for the family. Therefore only absolutely necessary modifications should be made.[33]

Family Education

A written educational program is provided to caregivers and includes measurable performance objectives. At least three caregivers should be selected, with one being trained at a high enough level to be able to train and instruct other caregivers. Each

---

BOX 21-4	**Mapping Electrical Circuits in the Home**

1. Place a number by each of the circuit breakers or fuses in the main electrical panel.
2. On a piece of paper for each room in the home, draw a square representing the room and mark each receptacle or light in the room.
3. Make sure each receptacle has a small appliance or light plugged into it. Turn on all the lights and small appliances plugged into an electrical outlet.
4. Turn off the first circuit and note the appliances affected (they will be off). Mark the circuit number by the receptacles and lights in that room on the drawing for that room.
5. Turn that circuit back on and turn off the next circuit in the numbering sequence.
6. Continue until all appliances or lights in all rooms have been assigned to a circuit.

(From May D: Rehabilitation and continuity of care in pulmonary disease, St Louis, 1990, Mosby.)

---

discharge team member is responsible for educating the caregivers in specific areas of the management of the ventilator-dependent patient. The education component includes providing detailed instructions on the operation of the ventilator, cardiopulmonary resuscitation, the use of manual resuscitators, aseptic suctioning techniques, tracheostomy care, tracheostomy collars and humidification systems, methods of disinfecting equipment, bronchial hygiene therapies such as chest physiotherapy, aerosolized medication administration, bowel and bladder care, and bathing. The family is also taught to recognize the early signs and symptoms of a respiratory infection (assessment) and what action must be taken if such a situation arises. Part of this process requires that the caregivers stay in the acute care facility for 24 to 48 hours before discharge, providing total care to the patient under the supervision of the medical staff. Additionally, a written protocol with directions for respiratory treatments and other aspects of care is included.

Not all caregivers will be able to tolerate performing some procedures, such as suctioning, bladder and bowel management, or bathing. Not surprisingly, working with a ventilator-dependent patient can be intimidating. Patience is essential in family training. In some cases, additional family members or outside caregivers are needed. An adequate number of caregivers should be identified and trained to allow the family time for sleep, work, and relaxation. Outside caregivers may include the immediate family as well as extended family, friends, nonprofessional paid caregivers, volunteers, and paid licensed health professionals.

The respiratory therapist is charged with the responsibility to teach caregivers the skills necessary for airway maintenance (suctioning and tracheostomy care), ventilator settings, circuit maintenance, infection control, troubleshooting the equipment, and emergency measures. A basic checklist of these skills is given to the patient and family and used to guide the educational process. All family members involved in the patient's care need to demonstrate adequate hands-on performance of all aspects of patient care before the patient is discharged. Figure 21-1 is an example of a caregiver assessment sheet. Once these tasks are learned and competencies are demonstrated, the patient is placed on the home

**QUALITY CARE HEALTH AGENCY
CAREGIVER CHECK-OFF SHEET**

I, (caregiver name) _____ , have received adequate instruction and demonstration from a homecare instructor, and have successfully returned the demonstration of the following procedures:

RESPIRATORY CARE SKILL	Inst Date	Demo. (initial)	Return Demo.	Not Applic.
Airway Suctioning Procedure				
- Manually hyperinflate/hyperoxygenate with resuscitation bag prior to suctioning.				
- Airway suctioning (ET or TT), selecting suction pressure, duration, etc.				
- Aseptic technique and assessment of patient during procedure.				
- Post-suctioning manual hyperinflation/hyperoxygenation				
- Follow-up assessment of patient				
- Equipment cleaning and maintenance				
Ventilator Management				
- Prescribed settings and confirmation of settings				
- Alarm settings, conditions, and responses				
- Circuit changes and equipment cleaning				
- Safety precautions				
- Emergency response (e.g. electrical power loss, emergency weather conditions [hurricane evacuation, etc.])				
- Troubleshooting situations (e.g. frequent high pressure alarms, ventilator failure [manual ventilation], airway occluded, etc.)				
- Patient assessment: for respiratory infections, for pneumothorax, for early signs of respiratory distress, etc.				
Additional Management Procedures				
- Aerosolized medication administration				
- Chest physiotherapy				
- Patient ambulation				
- Others				

Caregiver signature: _____

I feel comfortable that the above named caregiver can provide the skills listed for (patient name _____).

Homecare Instructor: (name/signature) _____

Date: _____

Fig. 21-1 An assessment sheet used for evaluating caregiver skill performance.

ventilator several days before discharge, allowing family members to become comfortable with the process.

Additional Preparation

The primary physician usually makes arrangements with a local physician and nursing service if the patient lives far away. The local hospital emergency department should be designated for emergency care, with an emergency plan clearly outlined. The local power company must be notified in writing of the patient's condition. The patient's home will need a priority status for electrical power service in case of a power failure.

The family and patient must also be prepared for emergency situations such as fires, hurricanes, tornados, flooding, and so forth. A contingency plan must be in place if power loss occurs from any of these disasters. A disaster may require evacuating the patient from the home to a special-needs shelter. Because of these possibilities, local fire departments, emergency medical teams, utility companies, police departments, and the local hospital emergency department should all be aware of the patient's urgent medical needs.

FOLLOW-UP AND EVALUATION

Before the patient is discharged, equipment and supplies are set up in the patient's home or another care site and checked for proper placement and function. Members of the discharge planning team assist with the transfer from the acute care facility to the intermediate care facility or from the intermediate care facility to home or another alternative long-term care facility.

When a transfer to home is being coordinated, practitioners from the homecare company must be present. They can assist with the transfer to the ambulance and from the ambulance to the home. Homecare practitioners must be present when the patient arrives home to reassure the patient and family and alleviate any apprehensions.

Part of the assessment of the patient involves how the patient feels about his or her interaction with the ventilator once he or she arrives home. Simple but key questions to ask include the following[34]:

- Are you feeling anxious?
- Are you getting a deep enough breath?
- Does the breath last long enough?
- Is it too deep?
- Do you have enough time to get all your air out?
- Do you need more breaths? Do you need fewer breaths?

Initially patients may require frequent home visits or daily calls until they are stable and adjusted to a routine of care. Once this routine is established, only formal monthly visits are necessary to evaluate the patient and report on progress. Box 21-5 reviews follow-up and evaluation of infants and children. Evaluations during home visits may include patient assessment parameters such as bedside pulmonary function studies, vital signs, and pulse oximetry. Assessment in the home does not generally include ABG studies.

Assessment may also include observation of the home environment and assessment of the equipment and any other problems the patient or family members may have. In some cases other health care providers may need retraining. For example, a homecare nurse may be disposing of the TT after each weekly visit not realizing this was not appropriate. Another example involves a family member calling the homecare respiratory therapist because of a

BOX 21-5	**Follow-up and Evaluation for Infants and Children Ventilated in the Home**

Ventilator requirements of infants and children change because of their growth and development. Periodic (once every 2 to 3 months) in-hospital evaluations may be necessary for the first 2 years of life and twice yearly thereafter until age 4 or 5 years.

frequent high-pressure alarm. In this latter example, the family needs retraining about how to identify when suctioning is needed.

A written report is completed after the monthly visit, and copies are sent to the patient's physician, homecare agency, and other members of the health care team. This report might include the following:

- Identification of company, servicing location, date, and time
- Patient name, address, phone, e-mail
- Patient diagnosis
- Physician and phone number
- Prescribed equipment and procedures
- Assessment (vital signs, breath sounds, sputum evaluation, oxygen saturation (S_pO_2), ventilator parameter and alarm settings, functioning of ancillary equipment)
- Caregiver and patient (if possible) comprehension of equipment and procedures
- Compliance with plan of care
- Recommendations of DME company representative

The task of caring for ventilator-dependent patients often creates frustration and anxiety for family members who are the primary caregivers. If problems are identified during home visits, the patient's physician should be notified. It may be necessary to provide psychological counseling to family members or suggest an alternative means of care (e.g., respite care) to allow family members time to rest.

Adequate Nutrition

Another aspect that must not be ignored is the nutritional status of the patient. Food intake is critical in avoiding problems associated with poor nutrition, such as increased risk of infection (e.g., pneumonia) and weakened muscles, including the diaphragm.[35] Caregivers should have a general idea of the patient's food and fluid intake as well as output. Constipation and bowel impaction need to be avoided. Some patients are at risk for aspiration when taking food by mouth, in which case a preferred feeding route might be through a **gastrostomy tube** or a **jejunostomy tube.**

Family Issues

Despite all efforts to discharge patients successfully to home, some factors may be difficult to manage. Significant delays in discharge from the hospital may occur if organizing the discharge plan or providing adequate funding is not possible.[4,33] Often one or more family members will lose employment time when a patient is discharged to home. This can worsen the family's financial position. Planned funding may have been based on the family's budget before discharge.

In addition, the respite for family caregivers may not be adequate. Getting extended family members and friends to help will not be successful unless these individuals are adequately trained in the care of the VAI. When caregivers from outside the family are in the home 24 hours a day, this erodes family privacy and can also be stressful.[36] When external caregivers take vacation or sick days,

| BOX 21-6 | Primary Components of a Discharge Plan for Sending the Patient Home on Long-Term Ventilation |

Preparation of the Patient for Discharge
- Stabilization of the patient's medical condition
- Evaluation and development of realistic goals
- Rehabilitation planning to set the stage for training
- Physical rehabilitation training plan to increase the patient's strength and endurance

Discharge Plan Implementation
- Appointment of a discharge planning team and a team leader
- Assignment of team member responsibilities
- Communication among team members
- Education of the caregivers and the patient
- Review of the patient's chart and ventilator orders
- Geographic survey of patient's home location
- Assessment of the home environment
- Review of the electrical system in the home
- Provision of a written education program and instructions
- Demonstration by caregiver(s)
- Primary physician and nursing service arrangements
- Planning for emergencies

the family caregivers often have to step in to provide additional coverage.

Careful, well-planned, timely preparation is absolutely essential to success in discharging a VAI from an acute care facility to home or a skilled nursing facility. Patient and home assessment, caregiver education and training, and demonstration of care by caregivers are all important elements. Box 21-6 lists the primary components of a discharge plan for sending the patient home on long-term ventilation.[33]

EQUIPMENT SELECTION FOR HOME VENTILATION

When patients are transferred to their home, equipment setup, instructions, and planning are especially important. Families must have immediate access to all required equipment and supplies. Box 21-7 provides a preliminary checklist of equipment for care of the mechanically ventilated patient in the home.[10,21]

It should be apparent that the most important equipment to be selected is the ventilator. Selection depends on the goals for the particular patient. Ventilation can be provided by invasive positive-pressure ventilation to patients with a tracheostomy tube. Invasive positive pressure ventilation is indicated for patients who have persistent symptomatic hypoventilation. It is also indicated for patients who do not meet selection criteria for NIV or who are unable to tolerate NIV or negative pressure ventilation (NPV).

This section reviews ventilator selection for IPPV and NPV and the use of noninvasive devices, such as the rocking bed and the pneumobelt, continuous positive airway pressure (CPAP) devices, and noninvasive devices for secretion clearance. The use of NIV is discussed in Chapter 19.

Tracheostomy Tubes

The use of TTs is essential for invasive LTMV. Generally a tracheotomy is performed as soon as possible after the need for extended

intubation is verified and it appears the patient is likely to benefit from the procedure. This usually occurs when a patient is stabilized on the ventilator in an acute care hospital within about 7 days of the onset of respiratory failure or sooner in patients who are neurologically impaired.[37-39] Chapter 20 reviews the role of tracheostomy in ventilator discontinuation. The use of speaking tubes and devices for patients with long-term tracheostomies is explained later in this chapter.

Ventilator Selection

Many types and models of ventilators are available for home use. Some of these are quite sophisticated, offering an array of modes, alarm systems, and other complex ventilatory characteristics. Although these machines may occasionally be necessary for medical stability outside the hospital, simple technology should be the goal of ventilator selection when it is possible.[34,40]

The most important factors in choosing a ventilator are the following:
- **Reliability.** The ventilator must be mechanically dependable and trouble free for extended periods without breaking down or requiring costly maintenance.
- **Safety.** The ventilator must be safe to operate in oxygen-enriched environments and have an adequate alarm system to warn of low ventilating pressure, high ventilating pressure, patient disconnection, and mechanical failure.
- **Versatility.** The ventilator should be portable or able to be adjusted for travel outside the home, necessitating the use of reliable internal and external battery sources and alarms.
- **User-friendly.** Ventilator controls should be easy to understand and manipulate. The circuit should be simple and easy to change.
- **Easy patient cycling.** The ventilator should be easy to cycle in the volume-controlled continuous mandatory ventilation (VC-CMV) mode for patients able to make spontaneous efforts.

For all home ventilator patients, backup ventilatory support must be available in case of electrical failure or malfunction. A self-inflating manual resuscitator should be readily available and caregivers should be instructed on proper use of these devices. If a patient can maintain spontaneous ventilation for four or more consecutive hours, a manual resuscitator may be all that is necessary as a backup.[32,41] For patients who are totally dependent on ventilatory support or those who live far from medical support, a second mechanical ventilator is necessary as a backup. Those patients who require supplemental oxygen also should have a concentrator and an E-cylinder as a backup.

Examples of Homecare and Transport Ventilators

A positive pressure ventilator is the most commonly used device for providing ventilatory support for the homecare patients. Unlike the large and sophisticated positive pressure ventilators used in the ICU, homecare ventilators have an array of advantages; notably they are compact, lightweight, and portable. Most of these homecare units are designed to use three different power sources: normal AC current, internal DC battery, and external DC battery. Ventilators that use an external DC battery can be mounted relatively easily on a wheelchair or placed in a motor vehicle, enhancing a patient's capability of mobility and participation in other activities.

Many homecare positive pressure ventilators have been developed in the past three decades. This text cannot completely describe all of the available features of each ventilator, but a brief review is provided. Most of these units are described elsewhere.[41,42]

BOX 21-7   **Respiratory Care Plan Equipment Checklist for Ventilator-Dependent Patients at the Home Site**

Mechanical Ventilator and Related Equipment
- Primary ventilator with operating instructions
- Prescription for ventilator parameter and alarm settings, specific time on and off ventilator, critical values
- Circuits (disposable or nondisposable with instructions for cleaning and assembly)
- Connectors, PEEP valves (as needed with instructions)
- Humidifier, heater, bracket, and heat-moisture exchanger (and instructions for use and cleaning)
- Temperature probes (if heater is used)
- Power supply, including external 12-volt battery and connecting cable
- Backup ventilator (for patients who cannot be without ventilator support)
- Manual resuscitation bag
- Tracheostomy attachments
- Replacement ventilator circuit filters
- Patient monitor and alarms (if not incorporated in ventilator), including instructions
- Communication aids (e.g., call button, bell, intercom, infant audio-visual monitor)
- Test lung for ventilator
- Noninvasive patient interfaces with head gear and chin-strap (as indicated)

Airway Management Equipment
- Suction machine (portable, with instructions)
- Suction container
- Appropriately sized catheters
- Connecting tube(s)

- Latex gloves
- Instructions for tracheostomy tubes (TT), including name, type, and size of artificial airway with instructions for care
- Replacement TTs (appropriately sized with one size smaller and instructions)
- Disposable inner TT cannulas (as indicated)
- Tracheostomy care kits (with instructions)
- Speaking valve for tracheostomy (as indicated with instructions)
- Appropriate cleaning solution, sterile saline, or water solution
- Water-soluble lubricant
- Syringes
- Antibiotic ointment

Oxygen Administration Equipment
- Oxygen concentrator
- E-cylinder backup
- Oxygen tubing
- Tracheostomy collar or T-tube adaptor
- Large-bore tubing
- Nasal cannula

Disinfectant Solution
- Vinegar/water 1:3
- Quaternary ammonium compound

Miscellaneous
- Compressor for aerosolized medications
- Spacers for metered-dose inhaler medications
- Wheelchair
- Hospital bed
- Bedside commode

First-generation portable volume ventilators. Most of the first-generation portable ventilators are no longer manufactured; however, many are still used in this country and around the world. This is due to their simplicity and reliability. First-generation ventilators are lightweight (average, 30 lb) and can serve as both transport ventilators and ventilators for long-term care sites. In general, they are easy-to-operate, piston-driven ventilators that can provide VC-CMV mode and volume-controlled intermittent mandatory ventilation (VC-IMV). They also have high- and low-pressure alarms, ventilator malfunction, and power-loss alarms. Some offer additional alarms such as "setting error" (e.g., Aequitron LP6 Plus and LP10 (Covidien-Nellcor Puritan Bennett, Boulder, Colo.) and Lifecare PLV-100 and PLV-102 (Philips Respironics, The Netherlands)).

These units generally operate from a standard 115- to 120-volt AC electrical outlet. Although they possess an internal battery, these batteries have limited capabilities (15 to 60 minutes). The battery capacity varies depending on the ventilator settings and by the type of ventilator being used.[43] Most portable ventilators can be connected to a 12-volt DC, deep-cycle marine-type battery as an external power source. These batteries are heavy (30 to 40 lb) but can provide extended power for several hours depending on the workload (respiratory rate [f] and tidal volume [V_T]) set on the ventilator.

To provide an intermittent mandatory ventilation (IMV) system for home use, practitioners used to add an external H-valve

assembly to home ventilators. However, the additional equipment increased the cost and complexity of home ventilatory support. Consequently, manufacturers designed subsequent models to provide the IMV/synchronized IMV (SIMV) mode without the need for added circuitry. Example ventilators include the LP10 and LP20 ventilators (Fig. 21-2 includes a functional diagram of the LP10 ventilator). Although these ventilators simplify the IMV circuitry, demand or continuous-gas flow systems are not incorporated into their design. During spontaneous breathing, the patient must draw gas from an air-intake valve in the piston chamber or through the exhalation valve of the ventilator circuit. As a result, the inspiratory work of breathing can be significant.[10,44] Therefore, IMV/SIMV is not recommended for long-term ventilation with these ventilators (Key Point 21-3).[10,43-45]

Key Point **21-3** "The SIMV mode found on *(older generation)* home-care ventilators is not recommended without modification of the gas delivery system with a one-way valve in the inspiratory limb to allow inspiration from the atmosphere. A continuous high gas flow system may also be used, but is not preferred in the long-term home setting."[10]

When the patient requires an F_IO_2 greater than 0.21, oxygen must be bled into the system. This can be done after the outflow valve from the ventilator by using a separate oxygen source

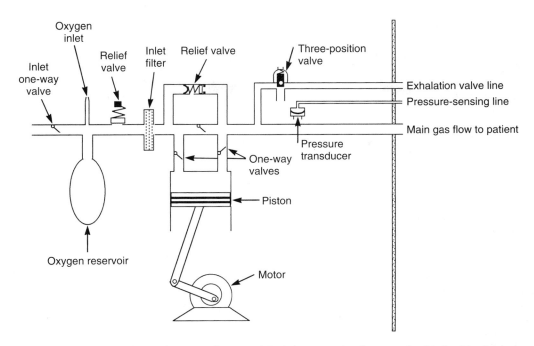

Fig. 21-2 A functional diagram of the LP10 ventilator internal circuit. A one-way valve allows gas to flow into the piston during the backstroke that occurs during exhalation. This valve closes during inspiration and flow is directed to the patient. Note the oxygen reservoir before the piston chamber, which allows for an increased F_IO_2. F_IO_2, Fraction of inspired oxygen. (Courtesy Covidien-Nellcor Puritan Bennett, Boulder, Colo.)

(concentrator or cylinder oxygen). It is important to recognize that adding additional flow to the inspiratory limb of the ventilator may make it more difficult for the ventilator to sense a patient's inspiratory effort. Ventilators with a sensitivity setting (patient triggering) may need the sensitivity reset. Another option is to use a reservoir bag or mixing chamber primed with oxygen that can be added to the ventilator's air intake. Sometimes this procedure can increase the F_IO_2 to more than 0.4, depending on the ventilator in use.

Some units have a system to provide up to 100% oxygen-enriched gas to the patient. A reservoir or optional elbow attachment is connected to the machine's patient outlet to allow a flow of oxygen to be introduced into the patient circuit. These systems deliver up to 100% oxygen-enriched gas, depending on the flow of the gas and changes in a patient's minute ventilation ($\dot{V}_E$). In general, a patient's F_IO_2 requirements should be less than 0.40. The need for an F_IO_2 greater than 0.40 indicates clinical instability that requires more respiratory care than is available at home.

On most portable ventilators, PEEP can be obtained by attaching an external threshold resistor to the patient circuit exhalation valve. These PEEP valves add to circuit complexity and may become dislodged from the exhalation valve or cause V_T loss.[33,46] They may also increase a patient's work of breathing, especially if the machine sensitivity is not properly adjusted.[33] PEEP should not be used for patients ventilated at home unless absolutely necessary. Its use also often indicates clinical instability, especially when adequate oxygenation must be maintained.[33]

First-generation ventilators have provided dependable service in a variety of environments for many years. Although these devices are considered reliable devices by some patients, a second generation of ventilators with a variety of improvements in SIMV delivery, patient triggering, PEEP, and F_IO_2 administration is now available.

BOX 21-8   Transport and Homecare Ventilators

First-Generation Portable Volume Ventilators
- LP-6 Plus, LP-10, LP-20 (Puritan Bennett Covidien Ltd) Lifecare PLV 100, and PLV 102 (Phillips Respironics)
- TBird Legacy (CareFusion Corp.)

Second-Generation Portable Ventilators
- Achieva, Achieva PS, and PSO$_2$ (Covidien-Nellcor Puritan Bennett, Boulder, Colo.)
- iVent (VersaMed/GE Healthcare) Newport HT-50 (Newport Medical, Newport, Calif.)
- Pulmonetics LTV series (CareFusion Corp.)

Current generation portable ventilators. Current portable positive pressure ventilators are primarily microprocessor-controlled and piston-driven machines. Note that some manufacturers offer units that are turbine driven or use a rotary compressor. These second-generation portable ventilators may be patient or time triggered; pressure or volume targeted; and pressure, volume, flow, or time cycled. Examples of second-generation units are listed in Box 21-8.

Current generation homecare ventilators are much more advanced in their design and provide a greater number of advanced features (e.g., CareFusion LTV 1000, 1200 ventilators (CareFusion, Viasys Corp. San Diego, Calif.)). The LTV series ventilators are electrically-powered units that use an internal rotary compressor to generate gas flow. The LTV 1000 model ventilator is small enough to be portable (Fig. 21-3). The LTV 1000 model offers enough features and alarms to allow it to be used in the acute care setting (Fig. 21-4). LTV ventilators provide ventilation in the following modes: CMV, IMV, CPAP, apnea backup ventilation, and NIV. The IMV provided is more advanced than SIMV used in first-generation ventilators and the work of breathing associated with it is not as high.

Other second-generation ventilators, like the Achieva PSO_2 (Covidien-Nellcor Puritan Bennett, Boulder, Colo.) can provide a

variety of features (Fig. 21-5). Some features include volume- or pressure-targeted mandatory breaths, continuous gas flow for IMV, F_IO_2 control, and internal PEEP control. These are lightweight and small, with built-in batteries that can last up to 4 hours. Additional features may include flow triggering, backup ventilation, leak compensation, pressure support ventilation (PSV), rise time, and flow termination criteria for PSV.

Standard audible and visual alarm controls incorporated into newer homecare ventilators include alarms for low battery power, power loss, low pressure, high pressure, power switchover, apnea, oxygen fail, and microprocessor malfunction. The power switchover alarm is activated whenever the ventilator switches from a higher to a lower power source (e.g., from an AC power source to a DC power source). A secondary alarm, such as a remote alarm, may be necessary if patient disconnection is likely to produce serious adverse effects.[45]

Second-generation ventilators have introduced a greater flexibility of ventilator settings for portable and home use. Respiratory

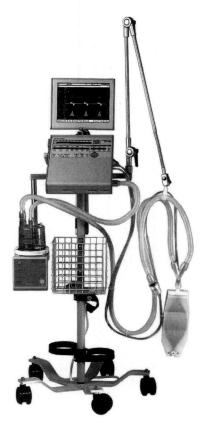

Fig. 21-3 The CareFusion LTV 1000 ventilator with patient circuit, humidifier, and monitoring screen. The screen would not be required for home ventilation. (Courtesy CareFusion, Viasys, San Diego, Calif.)

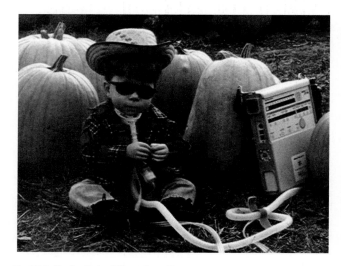

Fig. 21-4 The CareFusion LTV ventilator. (Courtesy CareFusion, Viasys, San Diego, Calif.)

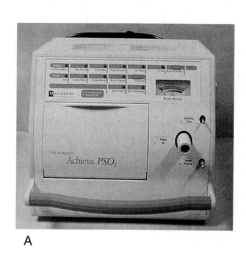

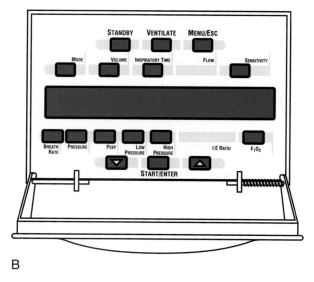

A   B

Fig. 21-5 **A,** The Achieva PSO_2 ventilator with front panel closed. **B,** A drawing of the front panel controls of the Achieva. (Courtesy Covidien-Nellcor Puritan Bennett, Boulder, Colo.)

therapists must familiarize themselves with all units used by their organization because functions and features can vary considerably from one unit to another. Even different models of the same ventilator and upgraded versions of the same model can have different features.

It is important to recognize that versatility is important when selecting a long-term ventilator. However, quality, reliability, and safety are the most important factors that must be considered when selecting an appropriate homecare and transport ventilator.

COMPLICATIONS OF LONG-TERM POSITIVE PRESSURE VENTILATION

In addition to the potential failure or malfunction of the ventilator or artificial airway, complications of long-term positive pressure ventilation (PPV) may also include the following:

- Pulmonary complications
- Complications to the cardiovascular system, the airway, the gastrointestinal (GI) tract, and neurologic complications
- Problems associated with immobility
- Psychological dysfunction

The pulmonary, cardiovascular, and GI problems in long-term VAIs are similar, in many respects, to those seen in critically ill ventilated patients. (see Chapters 16 and 17 for additional information on complications of mechanical ventilation.) Figure 21-6 compares airway problems in the acute care setting (acute complications) with the long-term care facility (chronic complications). Complications to the airway in VAIs are listed in Box 21-9.[3] Unlike nosocomial infections in the ICU setting, ventilator-associated pneumonia in VAIs is often caused by enteric gram-negative bacteria such as *Enterobacter* spp., *Escherichia coli, Klebsiella* spp., and *Pseudomonas aeruginosa*.[3] These organisms are often resistant to a variety of antibiotics. In patients receiving home mechanical ventilation by NIV, *Staphylococcus aureus* has been cited as a common contaminant of the ventilator circuit and the nasal mask. Colonization of this organism has also been found in patients' nostrils.[47]

GI disorders may occur in VAI from chronic illness, resulting in system breakdown. GI problems in VAIs may include the following:

- Damage to the GI mucosa from stress
- Swallowing dysfunction and aspiration

BOX 21-9   Complications to the Airway in Long-Term Ventilation

Nasopharyngeal Injury
- Sinusitis
- Otitis
- Injury to the nasal septum
- Ulceration to the nose, mouth, lips, and pharynx

Laryngeal Injury
- Damage to the laryngeal cartilages (e.g., arytenoid cartilage, cricoid cartilage)
- Glottic and subglottic stenosis
- Vocal cord injury or paralysis

Tracheal Injury
- Infection or bleeding of the stoma
- Granuloma formation
- Tracheal stenosis, malacia, or dilation
- Tracheoinnominate or tracheoesophageal fistula formation

(From Chatila WM, Criner GJ: Complications of long-term mechanical ventilation, *Respir Care Clin N Am* 8:631, 2002.)

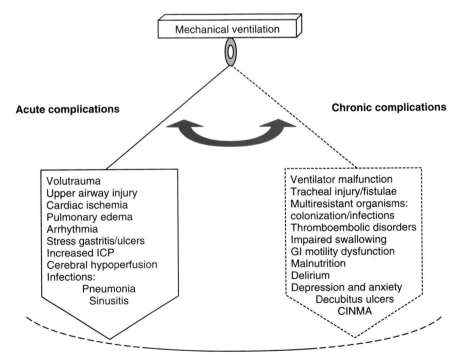

Fig. 21-6 Acute and chronic complications of mechanical ventilation. *CINMA,* Critical illness neuromuscular abnormality; *GI,* gastrointestinal; *ICP,* intracranial pressure. (From Chatila WM, Criner GJ: Complications of long-term mechanical ventilation, *Respir Care Clin N Am* 8:631, 2002.)

- Hypomotility of the GI tract causing constipation and **ileus**
- In addition, placement of nasogastric tubes or the occurrence of reflux can cause **erosive esophagitis,** which may occur in as many as 50% of VAIs.[48]

Approximately 45% of patients who transfer to long-term care facilities on mechanical ventilation have some type of neurologic disorder, which is generally the primary cause of their ventilator dependence.[48] Neurologic or neuromuscular dysfunctions can also be caused by patients' chronic morbidities or follow an acute severe illness. Determining the major contributing neuropsychological problem is not always possible.[48]

To avoid some of the complications of long-term ventilation, early mobilization, as part of the rehabilitation process, can help reduce muscle and skeletal wasting and reduce the risk of decubitus ulcers.

Psychological problems in VAIs can be attributed to a host of causes, including the following[48]:

- Severity of illness
- Longevity of illness
- Multiple medications (sedatives, analgesics, psychotropics, steroids [see Chapter 15])
- Sleep disruption
- Delirium
- Anxiety
- Depression

Critically ill patients who cannot be easily weaned from ventilatory support after recovery of the acute illness are more susceptible to complications of mechanical ventilation.[48] Consequently, the patients' well-being and survival are adversely affected. Efforts must be aimed at preventing these complications to have a better chance of discontinuing ventilation and improving the patient's quality of life.

ALTERNATIVES TO INVASIVE MECHANICAL VENTILATION AT HOME

In addition to NIV by nasal mask and IPPV through a TT, alternative methods of ventilation for VAIs include NPV, noninvasive breathing support devices, nasal CPAP for treating obstructive sleep apnea (OSA), and glossopharyngeal breathing.

Noninvasive Positive Pressure Ventilation

For years NPV and IPPV were the only mechanical ventilation systems available for people with moderate to severe chronic respiratory failure. Since the early 1980s, a number of alternative methods to conventional methods of mechanical ventilation for use in the home and acute care facility have been introduced. The effectiveness of NIV through a nasal mask, nasal pillows, a mouthpiece or mouth seal, or CPAP through a nasal mask have been examined in several studies of patients with neuromuscular disorders, chest wall defects, obstructive and restrictive intrinsic lung diseases, and OSA.[49-58] These studies found that NIV or CPAP can prevent episodes of severe hypoxemia and hypercapnia in selected groups of patients. In addition, daytime P_aO_2 and P_aCO_2 improved in the studies' subjects. Improvement in respiratory muscle strength and stabilization of lung volumes were also reported.[59] Patients also reported subjective improvement in symptoms such as headaches and daytime somnolence and an increase in their ability to perform activities of daily living. Abundant evidence now supports the effectiveness of NIV and CPAP assistance in the homecare setting.

Chapter 19 provides an extensive discussion of NIV as an alternative method for support of ventilation in both the acute care and long-term care of patients.

Negative Pressure Ventilation

Negative pressure ventilation is durable, easy to use, and dependable. It is used less often than IPPV or NIV but is occasionally used for long-term ventilation. NPV can provide support to a patient without requiring an artificial airway; thus, patients can speak, eat, and drink while avoiding the complications associated with artificial airways.

Use of NPV is preferable for patients with disorders such as neuromuscular disease, spinal cord injuries, chest wall disorders, or central hypoventilation syndromes.[60-64] Nighttime use in patients with COPD is another example of their application, although some of these patients find NPV difficult to tolerate.[60,61] However, for the treatment of **acute** respiratory failure in patients with COPD, NIV is the mode of choice.[65]

If excessive airway secretions, decreased pulmonary compliance, or increased airway resistance are present, or if the patient is at risk for aspiration, NPV is not recommended (see Chapter 2 for additional details about the physiology of NPV). NPV is available in three basic designs: the iron lung (tank ventilator), the cuirass, and the body suit or jacket ventilator.[66,67]

Tank Ventilators/Iron Lungs

Iron lung ventilators enclose the patient's whole body (except for the head) and seal around the neck. They are sometimes referred to as *body tanks*. The Emerson iron lung and the NEV-100 (Philips Respironics, The Netherlands) are two examples.

Tank ventilators work by transmitting negative pressure across the chest wall, into the pleural space, and finally to the alveolar level. The resulting increase in transpulmonary pressure causes air to enter the lungs. Exhalation is passive and depends on the elastic recoil of the lung and chest wall.[66,67]

Tank ventilators have several disadvantages: they are large (3 m long and 136 kg) and cumbersome and make bronchial drainage, intravenous therapy, and physical contact with the patient difficult. In some patients, negative pressure applied to the abdominal area as well as the thorax results in a pooling of blood in the abdominal vasculature, which leads to a decrease in venous return to the heart and, subsequently, a reduction in cardiac output. If a patient is hypovolemic, this results in hypotension. Some patients, on the other hand, have augmented venous return to the thorax and an improvement in cardiac output.[1] If the patient has excessive secretions or a depressed (obtunded) epiglottic reflex response, airway management becomes a problem and requires an artificial airway.

Because older tank ventilators are controllers, they allow little, if any, adjustments if the patient makes spontaneous efforts. V_T is determined by the amount of negative pressure applied and the characteristics of the lung. V_T must be measured during setup and throughout use of the tank ventilator. Newer models allow for patient-triggered ventilation.[61]

The Porta-lung (Philips Respironics, The Netherlands) is a portable version of the iron lung that is smaller (2 m) and lighter weight (50 kg).[42] Current models allow for a ventilator rate (f) range of 12 to 24 breaths/min and a pressure range of −15 to −45 cm H_2O.

Starting NPV in the treatment of chronic respiratory failure is carried out in a manner similar to IPPV. For example, typically pressures of −12 to −25 cm H_2O are sufficient to generate an

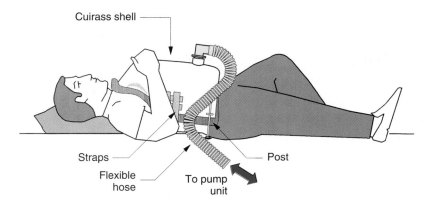

Cuirass shell

Straps
Flexible
hose
To pump
unit
Post

Fig. 21-7 Cuirass shell used for negative pressure ventilation. Patient is placed in supine position, and cuirass is stabilized with the use of straps and posts. (From Dupuis Y: Ventilators: theory and clinical application, ed 2, St Louis, 1992, Mosby, 1992.)

adequate V_T. Adjustments are based on the achieved V_T, blood gases, and pulse oximetry evaluation during use. It is important to understand that NPV may induce or exacerbate OSA.[67,68] If a patient has or develops OSA, the use of NPV, regardless of how it is applied, is contraindicated because it may aggravate the associated airway closure.[69]

The Chest Cuirass

The **chest cuirass,** or chest shell, partially compensates for some of the problems that occur with tank ventilators. The cuirass is a rigid shell that is placed over the patient's chest, touching the upper abdomen (Fig. 21-7). A space exists between the shell and the chest wall. This design restricts most of the negative pressure to the thoracic area, thus relieving most of the abdominal area from exposure to negative pressure. Some models have a trigger device that detects changes in flow or pressure at the nostrils. When a patient's inspiratory effort is detected, an assist breath is delivered. These sensing devices are not as efficient as those used with positive pressure ventilators; therefore the patient's inspiratory work to achieve a ventilator response is greater.

The chest cuirass and the body suit or body wrap (see section on The Body Suit below) are attached by hoses to an external pump that generates the alternating negative pressure. The chest cuirass is the least efficient NPV device and may not be adequate for severely compromised patients. Pressures of −35 to −60 cm H_2O may be necessary to achieve sufficient V_T with the chest cuirass.[10] Sometimes sufficient negative pressure cannot be achieved. This may be attributable to leaks in the system, particularly with older sealing materials. Plastic wrapping that is placed around the shell and newer custom-made shells can help eliminate the leakage problem. Other problems with the cuirass include patient discomfort and skin abrasions at points of contact. In patients with severe chest wall deformities, a custom-made cuirass may be required. Despite some difficulties, the chest cuirass is still being successfully used in the treatment of patients.[70,71]

The Body Suit

A third type of NPV is the body suit, which is a rigid chest grid that, in some models, attaches to a flat back plate. The rigid portion is fitted with a rain jacket or poncho wrap with fittings at the neck, wrists, waist, and ankles, depending on the style (Fig. 21-8). Two of the currently available models are the Pulmo-Wrap (Lifecare International Inc., Lafayette, Colo.) and the Poncho-Wrap (Emerson JH, Cambridge, Mass.).[61]

The body wrap is more portable than the tank ventilator. It also allows the patient to sleep in his or her own bed. However, it is less efficient and hard to completely seal. Negative pressure is also applied to a smaller surface area than with the tank ventilator. Because it restricts movement and patient positioning, it can cause muscular and joint pain, particularly back pain.[61]

NPV is not used nearly as much as portable PPV for long-term ventilation. However, it still has an occasional place in patient support. For example, a patient may be able to be in a wheelchair during the day and use a portable volume ventilator with a mouthpiece as an interface.[71] At night, the patient could use NPV. Both techniques allow noninvasive ventilation and avoid the necessity of a tracheostomy.

Additional Noninvasive Devices

Two additional noninvasive techniques for assisting ventilation are the rocking bed and the pneumobelt.[67,71-73] Both devices operate by the principle of moving the abdominal contents and diaphragm to aid in breathing. They both rely on the compliance of the abdomen and chest wall and are not appropriate for obese patients, those with severe chest wall deformities, or patients with intrinsic lung disease.[1]

The **rocking bed** (Fig. 21-9) is all but obsolete but continues to be used as an alternative form of noninvasive ventilatory support.[1,74] For example, in one reported case, a 40-year-old woman with muscular dystrophy required nocturnal ventilatory support. Eventually, as her muscle weakness progressed, she had difficulty setting up her NIV circuit. The rocking bed turned out to be a successful alternative form of support.[75]

Another situation in which the rocking bed has been shown to be effective is in patients with bilateral diaphragmatic paralysis.[76] This condition can occur as a potential postoperative complication of cardiac surgery.

The rocking bed is a motorized bed that continuously moves in a longitudinal plane. The patient is placed in a supine position in the bed. As Fig. 21-9 shows, the patient's head and knees can be elevated, which may improve patient comfort and help prevent sliding. The bed supports ventilation by rhythmically moving through an arch of 40 to 60 degrees (Trendelenburg to the reverse Trendelenburg position). The rate of rocking is 12 to 22 times/min. The optimal range is approximately 12 to 16 times/min.[1] Expiration is assisted when the head is in the down position and the abdominal contents and diaphragm are moved by gravity toward the thorax (cephalad). When the feet are in the down position (reverse

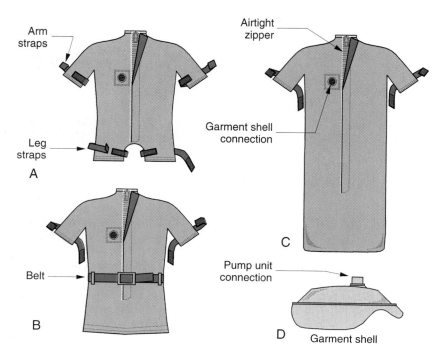

Arm straps

Leg straps

A

Airtight zipper

Garment shell connection

C

Belt

B

Pump unit connection

D Garment shell

Fig. 21-8 Airtight garments used for negative pressure ventilation. **A,** Garment is sealed at neck, arms, and legs. **B,** Garment is sealed at neck, arms, and waist. **C,** Patient is placed in bag sealed at neck and arms. **D,** Shell fitted with pump connection extending through garment opening is used to keep garment off patient's chest and enhance ventilation. (From Dupuis Y: Ventilators: theory and clinical application, ed 2, St Louis, 1992, Mosby Year-Book.)

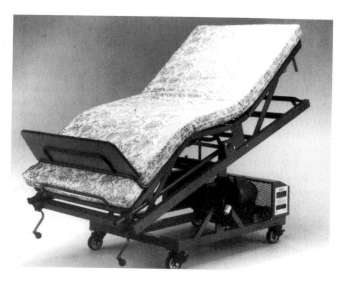

Fig. 21-9 The rocking bed. (Courtesy Emerson Company, Boston, Mass.)

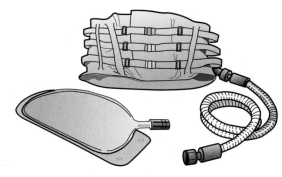

Fig. 21-10 The pneumobelt with positive pressure generator. (From Cairo JM, Pilbeam SP: Mosby's respiratory care equipment, ed 8, St Louis, 2010, Mosby.)

BOX **21-10**	**Conditions in Which the Rocking Bed Is Not Effective or Should Be Used with Caution**

- Obesity
- Excessively thin patients
- Severe chest wall abnormalities
- Infants
- Intrinsic lung disease

Trendelenburg position), the diaphragm and abdominal contents move toward the feet (caudad) and inspiration is assisted. The rocking bed generally does not cause motion sickness, probably because it rotates only in one plane.[1] Box 21-10 lists conditions in which the rocking bed should be avoided.

The **pneumobelt** (Fig. 21-10), also referred to as an *intermittent abdominal pressure ventilator,* contains an inflatable bladder that fits between the umbilicus (below the xiphoid process) and the pubic arch (over the abdomen) and is held in place by a nylon corset. The upper edge of the belt just overlaps the lower end of the rib cage. The patient must be in a seated position (45 degrees or

more) to use this device. It is ineffective if the head is lower than 30 degrees from horizontal.[73] The pneumobelt should fit snugly in place but must not impede spontaneous ventilation. A motor inflates the bladder, which pushes the abdominal content up, moving the diaphragm upward (cephalad) to assist exhalation. Deflating the bladder allows the diaphragm to return to the resting position, allowing inhalation. The device is not very powerful. A positive pressure ventilator able to generate pressure of approximately 50 cm H_2O and an inspiration-expiration ratio of 1:2 can be used to power the device.[10] The inflation rate is set to approximate the patient's spontaneous rate (12 to 22 breaths/min). Pressure is increased from approximately 30 cm H_2O upward until a satisfactory V_T is achieved or until the patient reports discomfort.

The pneumobelt is best used for daytime use and, like the rocking bed, may be effective for patients with bilateral diaphragmatic paralysis as well as patients with high spinal cord lesions. The pneumobelt can be used as adjuncts with other forms of assisting ventilation. Some patients can sleep in the upright position. In these cases, it also can be used during the night.

Diaphragm Pacing

Some patients with respiratory failure caused by high spinal cord lesions or central hypoventilation can benefit from diaphragmatic pacing. With this therapeutic intervention, the phrenic nerve is electrically stimulated through surgically implanted phrenic electrodes connected to an implanted receiver. The receiver obtains signal transmissions from an extracorporeal radiofrequency transmitter and antenna.

This technology has limited application. Not all patients will respond to this type of intervention because of inadequate phrenic nerve and diaphragm function. In addition, some patients experience obstructive apnea and a drop in S_pO_2 during sleep when using this technology. Diaphragmatic pacing systems do not have alarms, although failure can occur. This technology is also expensive, with initial costs in excess of $300,000.[10]

Although diaphragmatic pacing equipment is much smaller than a portable ventilator, it does not provide many additional advantages. Patients can learn to talk and eat with a TT in place by using a portable ventilator. The use of phrenic pacing is probably best reserved for children with high spinal cord injuries or central hypoventilation who cannot use other noninvasive methods to assist ventilation.[10]

Continuous Positive Airway Pressure for Obstructive Sleep Apnea

Clinicians should be aware of the fact that some patients who require some form of noninvasive support may also have OSA and need additional assistance to treat this disorder. An accepted method of treating patients is the application of CPAP via a face mask or nasal mask.

The decision to use CPAP depends on the degree of upper airway obstruction that the patient demonstrates and his or her respiratory muscle strength. For those patients who have adequate respiratory muscle strength and do not require mechanical ventilation but become hypercapnic and hypoxemic during sleep, nasal CPAP may be all that is necessary to alleviate hypoxemia and alveolar collapse. This is especially true for patients with OSA. CPAP levels can be titrated to increase expired lung volumes during sleep and reduce inspiratory and expiratory resistance, resulting in improvement of P_aO_2, decreased respiratory rate, and prevention of air trapping. The diagnosis of OSA and the procedure for establishing the appropriate level of CPAP for the patient are typically performed in a sleep study laboratory.[41]

CPAP systems. A nasal CPAP system for home care consists of two main elements: an air blower unit and a nasal mask system.[75]

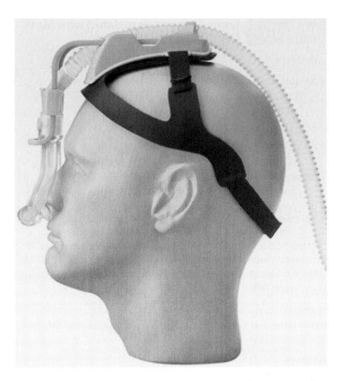

Fig. 21-11 The Aura nasal interface for the Aura CPAP system, fitted with specially designed nasal pillows. (Courtesy AEIOMed, Inc., Minneapolis, Minn.)

The blower incorporates an electrically powered motor, fan assembly or turbine, and a mechanism for setting and controlling the pressure delivered to the circuit. Air from the blower is delivered to the nasal mask through a lightweight 21-mm-diameter corrugated plastic hose that is attached to a one-way valve or a whisper swivel valve. These specialized valves prevent expired gas from flowing into the inspiratory limb and typically include a fixed leak.

The nasal mask system usually includes a soft, translucent mask. The mask is available in a variety of sizes designed to custom fit faces (see Figs. 19-4 through 19-7).[77] Other alternatives to the nasal mask include the nasal pillow (Fig. 21-11; see also Fig. 19-8) and the oral mask. Nasal pillows are short silicone tubes that fit the patient's nares to eliminate excessive leaks. A small opening in the nasal interface allows for exhalation of gases. The oral mask is a soft silicone mouthpiece with an inner flap that fits inside the mouth and in front of the teeth. An outer silicone flap is positioned on the outside of the mouth, sealing the lips. Nasal masks, nasal pillows, and oral masks are secured to the face by lightweight, adjustable headgear.

Levels of CPAP ranging from 2.5 to 20 cm H_2O are available on most homecare units. Home CPAP units incorporate electronic pressure transducers that sense pressure changes in the circuit and regulate the amount of flow into the circuit. As the patient inhales and the circuit pressure decreases, the pressure transducers increase the blower speed, allowing more air to move into the circuit. As the patient begins to exhale and circuit pressure increases, the amount of air flowing into the circuit decreases. The increase and decrease of airflow in response to circuit pressure changes allow the patient to inhale and exhale against the same pressure.

Operation of these CPAP units by patients and their family simply involves turning the "on/off" switch to the "on" position. The level of prescribed CPAP is set by the respiratory therapist or

TABLE 21-1	Complications Associated with Mask CPAP or NIV Therapy
Problem	**Possible Solution**
Aerophagia—gastric distention	Lower peak inspiratory pressure (<20-25 cm H_2O)
	Use PSV
	Alter sleeping position
	Use abdominal strap
Hypoxemia/desaturation	Correct mouth leaks
	Increase CPAP levels
Nasal dryness or congestion	Increase humidification
	Spray nasal passages with saline
Eye irritation	Correct mask leaks
	Use other interfaces
Patient discomfort from head straps	Alternate other interfaces
Nasal or dental pain, dental deformities	Alternate other interfaces

Compiled from Bach JR, Saporito BA: Indications and criteria for decannulation and transition from invasive to noninvasive long-term ventilatory support, Respir Care 39:515-528, 1994.
CPAP, Continuous positive airway pressure; *PSV,* pressure support ventilation.

by the medical supplier during installation of the unit in the home. Most current devices have "hidden" menus and controls that prevent access by the user. Once the prescribed levels are set, a panel conceals the controls.

Potential complications of CPAP. All forms of positive pressure ventilation have associated risks and complications. However, the risk of such problems occurring is greatly reduced by using CPAP compared with conventional mechanical ventilation. Complications associated with CPAP by nasal mask are reviewed in Chapter 19 and are summarized in Table 21-1.[56,77-80]

Glossopharyngeal Breathing

Glossopharyngeal breathing, or "frog" breathing, is a technique for assisting alveolar ventilation in patients with poor respiratory muscle strength. Patients who may benefit from learning this technique include those with spinal cord injury or **postpolio syndrome.** The technique requires good tongue strength, an intact gag reflex, absence of tracheostomy, and the ability to close the nasal passages and larynx and to swallow.[81]

Glossopharyngeal breathing is performed as follows. Approximately 50 to 100 mL of air is trapped in the oropharynx when the mouth and nasopharynx are closed. Then the jaw and larynx are raised while the continued forward motion of the tongue forces air from the larynx into the trachea. Then the glottis is closed and the technique is repeated. Approximately 10 to 15 rapid swallows are repeated in approximately 10 seconds, during which time the volume of air going into the lungs increases. The larynx is then opened and the patient exhales passively. A well-trained patient can perform 10 to 12 such breaths per minute, accomplishing adequate minute ventilation.[10]

The technique is difficult to learn but once it is mastered it can significantly increase inspiratory capacity and expiratory flow sufficient to generate effective coughs. It also may allow VAIs increased time off the ventilator and security in the event of ventilator failure during sleep.[81]

EXPIRATORY MUSCLE AIDS AND SECRETION CLEARANCE

Patients with neuromuscular disorders, restrictive intrinsic lung disease, and COPD may use NIV techniques for as long as 24 hours a day, thus avoiding tracheostomy (see Chapter 19). However, one of the major difficulties with this type of support is the management of airway secretions, especially when respiratory infections are present. Adequate respiratory muscle function is critical for clearing airway secretions. Most VAIs do not have sufficient strength to produce an effective cough. That is, they cannot generate a vital capacity (VC) of more than 1.5 L or a peak cough expiratory flow (PCEF) of more than 3 L/s.[82] Some form of cough assistance is necessary if pulmonary complications are to be avoided. The following techniques have successfully improved lung volumes and reversed arterial desaturation from secretions and mucus plugging: assisted coughing, chest wall oscillation, and mechanical insufflation-exsufflation.

Assisted Coughing

Assisted coughing is a technique of applying abdominal thrusts or compression to a patient's anterior chest wall during the expiratory phase of breathing. The purpose is to increase expiratory gas flow. This maneuver requires a well-coordinated effort between the patient and caregiver. Before applying the thrusts, the patient is instructed to take a deep breath to maximum inspiratory capacity. If the patient's VC is less than 1.5 L, a positive pressure deep insufflation is administered before expiratory thrusts. A manual resuscitator can be used for this purpose. The expiratory thrusts can increase patient's expiratory flow to approximately 5 L/s provided that the patient is cooperative and the caregiver has adequate physical effort and coordination.[82] Manually assisted coughing is usually not effective for severe scoliosis or obesity and is contraindicated for those patients with osteoporosis. It should not be performed on patients after they have consumed a meal.

Mechanical Oscillation

High-frequency mechanical oscillation is a technique in which rapid pressure pulses are applied to the chest wall or upper airway. The purpose is to assist in the mobilization of secretions. The Vest (Advanced Respiratory, Hill-Rom, Corp, St Paul, Minn.) and the Hayek Oscillator (Breasy Medical Equipment Ltd, London, UK) are devices used to deliver high-frequency external chest wall oscillation.[41] With these devices, chest wall vibrations are delivered to a vest placed around the patient's thorax. Vibrations are produced through a series of air pressure pulses delivered to plastic bladders located on the inner walls of the vest. The air pressure pulses are produced by an air compressor connected to the vest by large-bore, corrugated tubing. For some VAIs, airway clearance with chest wall oscillation may be more effective than chest physical therapy or oscillating valve devices (e.g., Flutter device or Acapella). Additional studies are needed to support these findings.[83]

Mechanical Insufflation-Exsufflation

The theory of operation of mechanical insufflation-exsufflation (MI-E) involves inflating the patient's lungs via a mouthpiece, mask, or tracheostomy, and then providing forced exsufflation as the positive pressure rapidly decreases to subatmospheric pressure.

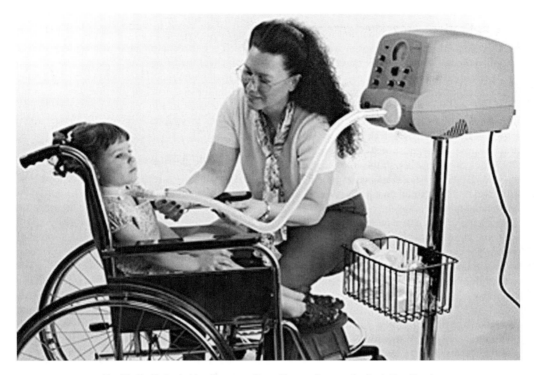

Fig. 21-12 Mechanical insufflator-exsufflator. (Courtesy Emerson Co., Cambridge, Mass.)

The insufflator-exsufflator (JH Emerson Co., Cambridge, Mass.) shown in Fig. 21-12 allows manual cycling between positive and negative pressure so that caregiver-patient coordination is optimized. Its use is typically reserved for patients in whom manually assisted coughing is inadequate.

Pressures can be adjusted from +65 to −65 cm H_2O, but pressures of ±30 to ±40 cm H_2O are the most commonly effective and best tolerated pressure ranges.[10,82] These ranges represent a 60 to 90 cm H_2O change in pressure over a 0.2-second period. One treatment consists of approximately five cycles of positive to negative pressure swings followed by short periods of normal breathing or positive pressure ventilation to allow the patient to rest. The cycles can be repeated every 10 to 15 minutes as needed.

The MI-E may be the most effective alternative for generating optimal PCEF and clearing airway secretions. PCEF has increased to as much as 6 to 10 L/sec during therapy and can be increased more if a manual abdominal thrust can be synchronized with exsufflation.[82] MI-E does not cause the airway irritation and discomfort associated with tracheal suctioning and may actually decrease the production of airway secretions. Abnormal VC values, flows, and arterial oxygen saturation (S_aO_2) values can also significantly improve with clearing of mucus plugs by MI-E.[82] No significant complications have been reported with the use of this device. However, it is contraindicated in patients with bullous emphysema or pulmonary disorders that predispose a patient to barotrauma.[1]

TRACHEOSTOMY TUBES, SPEAKING VALVES, AND TRACHEAL BUTTONS

As mentioned, the use of TTs is an important part of long-term ventilation. When a TT is used, methods for allowing the patient to talk should also be pursued if possible. When it is time for **decannulation** (removal of the TT), the option of using a tracheal button can be evaluated.

BOX **21-11**	**Advantages of Early Tracheostomy Tube Placement in Ventilator-Dependent Patients**

- Improved patient comfort
- Increased potential for speech
- Ability to eat by mouth
- More effective airway suctioning
- Decreased airway resistance
- Enhanced patient mobility
- A more secure airway
- Improved ventilator weaning times
- Reduced risk of ventilator-associated pneumonia
- Improved likelihood of transfer of ventilator-dependent patients from the ICU

Tracheostomy Tube Selection and Benefits

As discussed in Chapter 20, placement of a TT is essential when long-term ventilation is required. Early placement of a TT in VAIs has several advantages (Box 21-11).[84,85] The type of TT used depends on the needs of patient. In patients at risk for aspiration and who are unable to speak, a cuffed tube is appropriate. For those who might aspirate but are able to speak, a specialized TT that allows for speech may be considered (see below). Using a cuffless tube or deflating the cuff may also promote speech for patients who have no trouble swallowing and who have the ability to speak.[1,86] Cuffless tubes are also recommended for children younger than 8 years. Fenestrated TTs can be used for transitioning from a cuffed tube to decannulation. However, they are not recommended for long-term use because granulomatous tissue can grow into the fenestrations. When discontinuing a TT after long-term use, a general practice is to insert progressively smaller TTs. In this way, greater expiratory flow can be directed through the vocal cords, allowing for speech.[84,85]

Loss of Speech

The use of an artificial airway for patients requiring mechanical ventilation produces the sudden loss of the spoken word, which makes communication difficult. The ability to speak also has a profound effect on the quality of life for VAIs.

Patients in the ICU usually attempt to communicate by mouthing words, using gestures, and nodding the head,[87] but for VAIs, loss of speech can make emotional adjustments to a difficult life even more challenging, leading to anxiety, fear, and depression.[12] The ability to communicate through speech can dramatically improve a patient's outlook on life. Although the emotional aspect of providing speech to VAIs has not been extensively studied, those who work with VAIs notice a substantial change in patients' attitudes when they are able to talk.[88]

For an infant requiring a TT, its use may have to be extended into the period when the child learns the skill of speaking a language. For this reason, professional evaluation of the child's language and vocal skills is important.[89] Children are at risk for delays in their communication skills development if therapeutic intervention does not occur.[89]

Various techniques and devices have been investigated that allow speech in patients with tracheostomies. This includes techniques of cuff deflation during ventilation with VC-CMV, bilevel PPV, and CPAP and the use of different devices that allow speech in patients who have normal-functioning oral and laryngeal structures. These devices include allowing for speech with a TT in place, electronically activated devices, self-activated pneumatic systems, speaking TTs, and one-way valves for speaking (e.g., Passy-Muir valve, Irvine, Calif.).

Speaking with Tracheostomy Tubes During Ventilation

In patients who can tolerate deflation of the TT cuff during ventilation or CPAP, speech can be accomplished. For speech to occur, tracheal pressures of approximately 2 cm H_2O are required to vibrate the vocal cords and produce a quality voice.[90] (Normal speaking pressure is 5 to 10 cm H_2O.)

With cuff deflation during PPV, air is allowed to flow around the cuff and through the vocal cords during the inspiratory cycle of the ventilator. During exhalation, with the cuff deflated, most of the exhaled air will exit the ventilator's expiratory valve and speech is interrupted.[91] If PEEP is applied, it impedes expiratory flow through the ventilator's expiratory valve so that air flows through the larynx. This occurs because most ventilators will increase flow during exhalation to maintain the set PEEP level when a leak (deflated cuff) is present. In this way, flow may pass through the larynx during exhalation as well. In addition, by using both a longer T_I and PEEP, an additive effect is produced that increases speaking time and speech quality.[91,92]

For patients receiving CPAP, the cuff can be deflated without substantial loss of pressure (median, 1 cm H_2O at CPAP of 7.5 or 10 cm H_2O). This allows patients to speak without clinically significant changes in heart rate, respiratory rate, or S_pO_2 levels.[86]

Cuff deflation of VAIs is not without potential problems. The size of the TT and its position in the airway may increase resistance of air movement and increase the patient's WOB (work of breathing). Additionally, if the upper airway becomes occluded, the result will be hyperinflation of the lungs, a drop in cardiac output, and possible barotrauma. During PSV, where the breath is flow cycled, the cycling of the ventilator may be affected by cuff deflation and the leak that results. The CareFusion LTV series ventilator has an option of time cycling a pressure support breath, which would assist with cycling in the presence of a leak. Cuff deflation for speech is not recommended with critical care ventilators because it can affect their function.

Patients who require the use of a TT for prolonged periods may have multiple defects in the swallowing mechanism. Before a cuff is deflated to allow speech, patients need to be evaluated for the ability to swallow, protect the airway, and avoid the risk of aspiration.[91,93]

Electrically Activated Speaking Devices

The handheld electronic larynx allows speech when the device is held against the outside of the neck and is frequently used by patients with laryngectomies to facilitate speech. The electronic larynx produces an unnatural vocal quality, which some patients find frustrating. It also requires hand coordination, which may be difficult for some physically impaired individuals.

Electronic resonators are also available. With this device, a small tube is placed in the mouth, which activates a resonator as the patient attempts to speak. Notice that because the tube is inside the mouth, the patient may not be able to speak clearly.[94]

Speaking Tracheostomy Tubes

Three specialized TTs that allow for speech are the Portex Speaking TT (Smiths Medical, St Paul, Minn.), the Pitt speaking TT (National Catheter Corp, division of Mallinckrodt, St. Louis, MO), and the voice tracheostomy tube (VTT). The Portex Speaking TT has an opening in the posterior portion above the cuff (Fig. 21-13). Through this opening an external flow of air is directed through the vocal cords and allows speech. The patient controls flow by covering the port on the air connecting line (Fig. 21-14).[95,96]

The Pitt speaking TT (Fig. 21-15) uses an extra lumen through which gas can be directed either continuously or intermittently.[97]

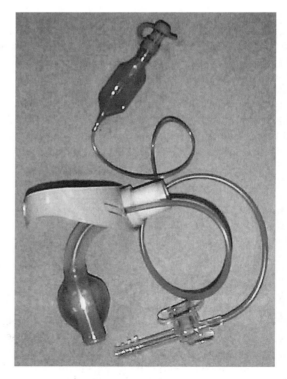

Fig. 21-13 The Portex speaking tracheostomy tube. (From Hess DR, MacIntyre NR, Mishoe SC, et al: Respiratory care principles and practice, Philadelphia, 2002, WB Saunders.)

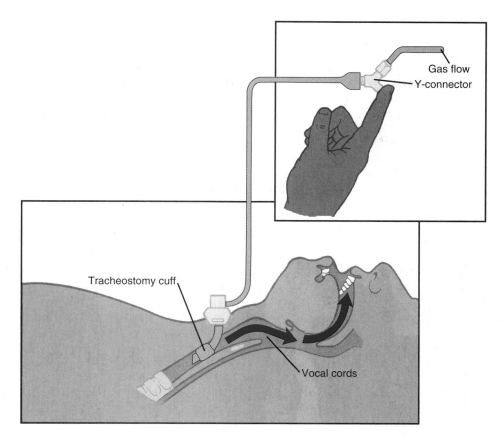

Fig. 21-14 A "talking" tracheostomy tube, in which gas flow to the airway is directed from an opening in the tracheostomy tube above the cuff and through the larynx when the patient obstructs the open port with the finger. (From Wilkins RL, Stoller JK, Scanlan CL: Egan's fundamentals of respiratory care, ed 9, St Louis, 2009, Mosby.)

The gas flows upward through the larynx and allows speech.[98] These specialized tubes may require flows of 6 to 8 L/min to be effective and voice quality can still be poor. In addition, the port above the cuff can also become occluded during use. The added flow for talking TTs may also result in throat dryness.[89]

The VTT cuff, which was reported in the medical literature in 2004, inflates during the inspiratory phase of positive pressure and deflates during exhalation.[99] The VTT apparently allows patients to speak during ventilation while maintaining adequate alveolar ventilation, without aspiration and without damage to the tracheal mucosa. Additional studies may demonstrate the effectiveness of the VTT (Case Study 21-2).[88]

 Case Study 21-2

Patient Case—Communication Difficulty
A 74-year-old male patient is being support by IPPV through a tracheostomy tube. The patient has a history of progressive muscular dystrophy and COPD. He is in a long-term ventilator care hospital. The patient is on SIMV with a rate of 6 breaths/min, V_T of 750 mL, and PEEP of 5 cm H_2O. His F_IO_2 is 0.3. He is alert and cooperative. The patient expresses frustration with his inability to communicate with his wife. What might the respiratory therapist suggest to help reduce the patient's frustration and allow him to speak?

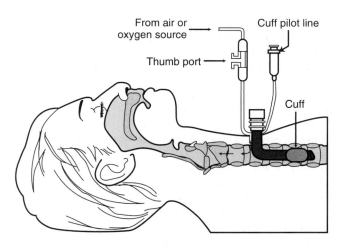

Fig. 21-15 A Pitt speaking tracheostomy tube. (From Cairo JM, Pilbeam SP: Mosby's respiratory care equipment, ed 8, St Louis, 2010, Mosby.)

Tracheostomy Speaking Valves

Speaking valves are used to allow speech in patients with a TT in place. Examples of speaking tracheostomy valves include the Passy-Muir, the Shiley (Mallinckrodt, Pleasanton, Calif.), the Shikani (The Airway Company, Forrest Hill, Md.), and the Montgomery (Stuart K. Montgomery, Westborough, Mass). Note that the Passy-Muir is currently the only valve that has approval

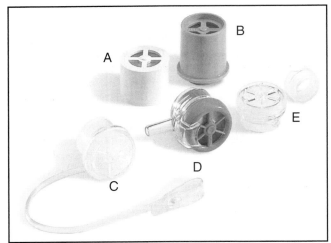

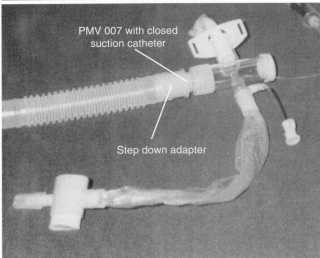

PMV 007 with closed suction catheter

Step down adapter

Fig. 21-16 *Top,* Examples of Passy-Muir speaking valves (PMVs). **A,** PMV 005 (white); **B,** PMV 007 (aqua); **C,** PMV 2000 (clear) with the PMV Secure-It; **D,** PMV 2001 (purple) with the PMA 2000 oxygen adapter; **E,** PMV 2020 (clear) with the PMA 2020-S adapter. *Bottom,* The valve in-line during mechanical ventilation. (Courtesy Passy-Muir, Inc., Irvine, Calif.)

from the Food and Drug Administration for use inline with a ventilator.

Speaking valves do not require a separate air source; therefore the patient does not have to occlude a valve with the finger to speak. This could be an obvious advantage for some patients.[100] Speaking valves have a 15-mm inner-diameter connector that fits over the proximal end of any standard tracheostomy tube. These valves are generally connected between the TT connector and the Y-connector.[100] A piece of 22-mm-diameter flexible, corrugated tubing can be placed between the speaking valve (attached to the tracheostomy connector) and the ventilator's Y-connector.[101] This may add a small amount of mechanical dead space to the circuit but can also add flexibility to the circuit attachment (Fig. 21-16).

For the valve to work, the cuff of the TT must be deflated. With the Passy-Muir valve the one-way valve opens on inspiration, allowing gas to flow to the lungs. During exhalation the valve closes and air is directed to the larynx and upper airway (Key Point 21-4). The Passy-Muir valve has been shown to improve speech flow, reduce speech hesitancy, and increase speech time.[102] The

Passy-Muir valve has also been shown to reduce aspiration during swallowing.[103-106]

Key Point **21-4** A heat-moisture exchanger (HME) should not be used when a Passy-Muir or similar device is used. Expired gas must pass through the heat-moisture exchanger for it to function properly.

Speaking valves can be used on ventilator-dependent patients or spontaneously breathing patients with TTs. They can also be used to help wean patients from TTs by allowing them to adjust to air moving through the upper airway again (Key Point 21-5). When using a speaking valve for the first time, the patient should be evaluated to be sure no untoward side effects occur. For example, if the space between the TT and the tracheal wall does not allow adequate exhalation, or if the tracheostomy is in place because of tracheal stenosis, the patient may be unable to exhale effectively. This can lead to air trapping and hyperinflation of the lungs with the potential complications of pneumothorax and subcutaneous emphysema.[89] One method to test for air trapping is to remove the speaking valve and listen for a "puff" of air. The "puff" may occur as air that could not be exhaled through the mouth passes through the TT.[89] On the other hand, airway pressures may increase because of exhalation through the oropharynx, which causes a low level of PEEP. This may allow the readjustment of the set PEEP. If peak pressures rise above allowable limits, however, the valve needs to be immediately removed.[107] Initial evaluation of valve placement includes checking respiratory rate, heart rate, S_pO_2, changes in respiratory pattern or effort, increased coughing, increased peak pressures, and expressions of patient discomfort.

Key Point **21-5** A child with a TT in place should never be left unattended when a speaking valve is in place.[89]

Before a speaking valve is attached to a ventilated patient, the following steps are performed:
1. The upper airway and the pharyngeal area above the cuff and the trachea are suctioned.
2. Peak inspiratory pressure and V_T are checked.
3. The TT cuff is deflated.
4. The V_T setting may need to be increased to maintain adequate ventilation.
5. The peak pressure alarm and disconnect alarms are adjusted.
6. The patient's heart rate, respiratory rate, S_pO_2, effectiveness of cough, passage of air into the oral cavity, and subjective expression of comfort are monitored.[101]

If the cuff is deflated during mechanical ventilation, some air will leak. For patients who are dependent on a set volume delivery, the V_T setting can be increased. Activation of the peak pressure alarm may indicate poor exhalation (through the mouth) and buildup of pressure. Water condensate from the ventilator circuit can obstruct the valve. The volume must be readjusted and the cuff reinflated when a speaking valve is removed to avoid overinflation or hyperventilation. After use, ventilator parameters should be rechecked and the patient assessed. Currently the Puritan Bennett 760 ventilator has a speaking valve setup to accommodate the use of a speaking valve.[108]

Patients have reported feeling better and more motivated about their own care when a speaking valve is used. This is illustrated in the Clinical Scenario below.[100,109]

Clinical Scenario: A Patient's Experience with the Passy-Muir Valve

Brooke Ellison is a young woman who is quadriplegic and ventilator dependent. She presented an inspiring lecture during the American Association for Respiratory Care's 50th Anniversary International Congress in New Orleans, La. In part of her presentation she mentioned her first opportunity to speak, although she has a TT. Her mother, Jean Ellison, describes in their book, *The Brooke Ellison Story*. This is an excerpt from that book:

"When can we start weaning Brooke off the ventilator?" I asked the RT when he arrived to change Brooke's ventilator tubing.

"We'll be working on that," he said, but in a way that seemed to indicate that it was not on his list of priorities as it was on mine.

"What do you think about trying to speak, Brooke?" He asked, in a way that I couldn't tell whether he was just making conversation or whether he knew something that I didn't know.

"What?" Ed (Brooke's father) said, not really sure of what he had just heard.

"Would you like to speak, Brooke?" he asked again, pulling a small circular piece of blue plastic out of his pocket and holding it up for us all to see.

"What's that?" I asked.

"It's a Passy-Muir valve," he said.

"A what?" Ed asked again, not really understanding what he was saying.

"It's a Passy-Muir valve. We can put it in Brooke's ventilator tube to redirect her exhaled air over her vocal cords, and as a result, allow her to speak. Would you like to try it, Brooke?" he said.

Brooke, in excited disbelief, moved her lips and said, "Yes."

"How does it feel?" I said, after the RT fit it in her tube.

Brooke stared back and didn't say anything. She looked scared and confused as if she had forgotten how to speak.

"Brooke, Love, can you say something?" Ed said anxiously.

After a long pause, Brooke said: "This … feels … weird," in a raspy, breathy voice.

She wasn't used to how it worked, so each word she spoke came out slowly, separated by a breath or two from her ventilator. Ed and I looked at each other and started to cry.

"I … sound … that … bad?" she said in the same raspy, staccato voice when she saw us crying.

"Oh, my God, no," I said. "It's the most beautiful sound I've ever heard."

(From Ellison B, Ellison J: The Brooke Ellison Story, New York, 2001, Hyperion.)

Concerns with Speaking Tubes and Valves

Some precautions are needed with speaking valves. The cuff must be deflated when it is attached. Whenever a cuff is deflated, regardless of the reason, an increased risk of aspiration may exist. Increased resistance to breathing through the valve, the TT, or between the tube and the wall of the trachea may occur during spontaneous breathing and speech. If more than 10 cm H_2O of pressure is required for the patient to generate a breath through the tube, WOB may dramatically increase.

Supplemental oxygen may be required when using speaking tubes if a significant amount of room air is entrained and the S_pO_2 of the patient decreases. Speaking devices may be contraindicated in the following circumstances[89]:

- Comatose or unconscious patient
- Foam cuff in place or cuff that must remain inflated
- Increased or thick secretions
- Severe upper airway obstruction
- Increased airway resistance and increased compliance that may cause air trapping (e.g., COPD)
- Endotracheal tube in place (not TT)
- Reduced lung compliance
- Laryngeal and pharyngeal dysfunction

Tracheal Buttons and Decannulation

The need to constantly keep a TT in place may eventually end. When concerns exist about a patient's ability to tolerate decannulation, the procedure is best observed on an inpatient basis. This can be done in a non-acute care setting. However, a nurse, respiratory therapist, and physician should be immediately available during the procedure.[110] The airway is inspected to ensure that the airway lumen is of an appropriate size and is not affected by scarring, narrowing, or obstruction. This can be accomplished with a flexible fiberoptic endoscope.

A protocol can be used that progressively downsizes the TT. The patient is observed during the size reduction process to be sure it is tolerated. Eventually the tube is capped. Once capping of the tube is well tolerated, the tube can be removed and the tracheotomy wound covered with an occlusive dressing. Most of the time the tracheotomy wound will heal without further intervention.

Occasionally a stoma must be maintained because the patient will require additional surgical procedures, such as head, neck, or maxillofacial surgery. The stoma can be kept patent by using a tracheal button. Tracheal buttons may also be used to preserve the site for patients with OSA treated by tracheotomy.[78,110] The button consists of two pieces, a hollow inner cannula and an external cap (Fig. 21-17). The inner cannula fits between the outside of the patient's neck and the inside of the trachea. To determine the appropriate depth before insertion, a toothpick-sized measuring device, which resembles a small golf club, is used to determine the depth of insertion of the cannula. The short L-shaped end is inserted in the stoma and hooked on the edge of the trachea. The clinician then places a gloved fingertip at the outside edge of the measuring device to mark the external point at the neck and then unhooks the distal end from the edge of the tracheal wall and removes the device. The distance from the fingertip to the end of the instrument is the cannula depth needed. To adjust cannula size, various rings can be added to the outer (proximal) part of the cannula. The cannula is then inserted. This is followed by placement of the cap. When the cap is inserted all the way, the flanges at the distal end of the cannula flare outward, locking the button in place inside the trachea. It is recommended that the button be

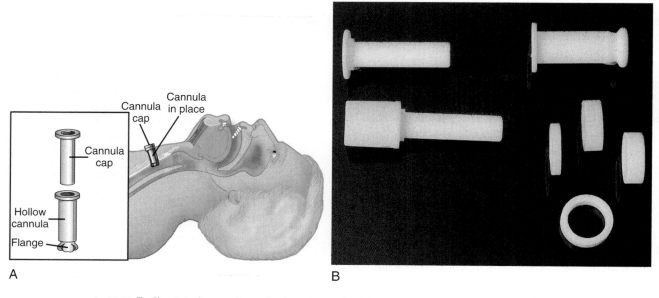

Fig. 21-17 The Olympic tracheostomy button showing various sized rings for adjusting the depth of the button in the tracheal wall. (**A,** From Cairo JM: Mosby's respiratory care equipment, ed 9, St Louis, 2014, Elsevier. **B,** From Kacmarek RM, Stoller JK, Heuer AJ: Egan's fundamentals of respiratory care, ed 10, St Louis, Mosby, 2013.)

rotated approximately one-quarter turn daily to prevent tissue growth into the flange. A 15-mm adaptor is available to allow manual bag ventilation if needed.

Most patients will be anxious about removal of the TT. They are usually concerned about their ability to breathe, clear secretions, and protect their airway when the TT is no longer in place.[110] These concerns need to be addressed and the procedure performed in a safe and comfortable environment.

ANCILLARY EQUIPMENT AND EQUIPMENT CLEANING FOR HOME MECHANICAL VENTILATION

In addition to the mechanical ventilator, a patient ventilated at home requires various supplies for general daily care, including supplies for airway care, humidification, supplemental oxygen, disposable circuits, and an emergency backup ventilator. The type and quantity of medical equipment necessary in the home depend on the patient's clinical status, age, and mode of mechanical ventilation. Patients receiving mechanical ventilation through noninvasive methods obviously require less equipment than patients with tracheostomies requiring continuous invasive mechanical ventilation. Box 21-7 lists the potential equipment and supplies that may be necessary for patients requiring continuous ventilatory support.

Disinfection Procedures

The presence of an artificial airway in a compromised ventilator-assisted patient makes the potential for infection from contaminated equipment a risk in the home setting, so infection control and decontamination procedures are taught to all persons involved in caring for the patient at home. Infection control measures emphasize avoiding person-to-person and object-to-person contamination. Family members and other caregivers are instructed to wash their hands thoroughly before and after touching the patient or equipment. The use of gloves (nonsterile) is encouraged when performing tasks such as suctioning or tracheostomy care.[111]

Ventilator Circuit Disinfection

As previously discussed, when circuits are changed less frequently, the risk of ventilator-associated pneumonia decreases.[112-115] The National Center for Infectious Diseases suggests that circuits need not be changed unless they are nonfunctional or if they are visibly soiled with secretions or blood.[116] Changing the circuit less frequently is also less costly. The rates of ventilator-associated pneumonia in long-term ventilated patients in long-term acute care hospitals and the home environment have been reported to be much lower when compared with ventilator-associated pneumonia rates in acute care facilities when national Centers for Disease Control and Prevention (CDC) guidelines are followed.[117-119]

When equipment is to be cleaned, it is first disassembled and rinsed with tap water. Then it is washed in a mixture of lukewarm water and mild detergent to remove all foreign matter. It is then rinsed thoroughly with tap water. The parts are then soaked in an effective disinfectant solution for approximately 10 minutes.[1] Finally, it is rinsed thoroughly, air-dried, and placed in a plastic bag. Ideally a patient should have at least three circuits so that one can be in use while the other is being disinfected and the third drying.

Because Medicare does not reimburse for most disposable supplies or will reimburse for only a limited number of disposable supplies, many homecare patients are taught to clean and reuse supplies when possible. Suction catheters, for instance, are often cleaned and reused in the home. This is safe as long as the procedure for cleaning is followed carefully (Box 21-12). The American Association for Respiratory Care (AARC) provides a clinical practice guideline for suctioning of the patient in the home.[111]

White vinegar mixed with distilled water (acetic acid content of 1.25%) is an adequate disinfectant solution but should be discarded after use and not reused.[120,121] Activated glutaraldehydes and quaternary ammonium compounds can also be used at home

| BOX **21-12** | **Procedure for Reusing Suction Catheters** |

1. Wash two plastic containers in warm water and detergent solution. Rinse them under running water and soak in disinfectant solution for 10 minutes. Allow to air-dry. Store one container for later use and use the second container to store suction catheters between uses.
2. After a suction procedure is completed, tap water should be aspirated through the catheter to clear the inside. The outside of the catheter is wiped with a clean gauze or sponge.
3. The catheter is disconnected from the connecting tubing and placed inside the plastic container. The lid is then closed.
4. Catheters are removed from the container, to be reused as needed.
5. The catheter and plastic container are changed after 8 hours of use.
6. The dirty catheter is rinsed with cold tap water to remove all mucus.
7. The catheter is washed with a solution of warm water and detergent, rinsed under running water, and the excess water shaken off.
8. The catheter is then soaked in disinfectant solution for a minimum of 10 minutes.
9. Afterwards the catheter is removed, rinsed, and air-dried on a clean paper towel.
10. After drying the catheter completely, it is placed in a plastic bag and closed until ready for use.
11. The procedure in step 1 is followed to clean and disinfect the plastic container.

| BOX **21-13** | **Guidelines for Disinfecting Home Ventilator Equipment** |

Preparation
1. Choose a clean, dry area.
2. Have all supplies ready for use.
3. Wash hands (gloves may be worn).

Procedure
1. Disassemble circuit completely. Wipe small tubes with clean, damp cloth.
2. Rinse large-bore tubing, connectors, humidifiers, and exhalation valve with cold tap water.
3. Soak equipment in warm, soapy water for several minutes.
4. Scrub equipment with a small brush to remove dirt and organic material.
5. Rinse thoroughly to remove any soap residue and drain off excess water.
6. Place equipment parts in disinfectant solution. Be sure that all parts are submerged.
7. After 15 minutes, rinse equipment thoroughly.
8. Drain off excess water, hang tubes to dry, and place small parts on a clean surface to dry.
9. When equipment parts are dry, reassemble circuit and store it in a clean plastic bag.

following manufacturer's recommendations.[111] Although these may be the disinfectant solutions of choice, their cost and availability are limiting factors. Whatever method is used, equipment must be processed in a clean, dry space separate from food preparation areas.

Water to be used as a diluent or in humidifiers needs to be boiled for 30 minutes and stored in a sterile container in a refrigerator. After 24 hours, the water should be discarded. Box 21-13 reviews a procedure for cleaning ventilator-related equipment in the home.[122,123]

Humidifiers

The CDC recommends the use of sterile water in the humidifier used for long-term ventilation. Because heated humidifiers are often used, condensate will normally build in the circuit. The condensate can pool in the dependent limbs of the circuit and make it difficult both to trigger the ventilator into inspiration and to exhale. For this reason, the condensate should be removed from the circuit regularly. When handling the circuit, efforts must be made to avoid accidentally allowing circuit condensate to spill into the patient's airway.[11,116]

 SUMMARY

- LTMV is required by two categories of patients: those recovering from an acute illness and those with chronic progressive disorders.

- The overall goal of LTMV at home or other alternative care sites is to improve the patient's quality of life.
- LTMV can be administered in acute care units, intermediate care facilities, and long-term care sites, including the home environment.
- Discharging VAIs to the home or an alternate care site is a complex process that involves careful patient selection, adequate financial resources, a knowledgeable and dedicated health care team, and a patient and family willing and able to take the responsibility for self-care management at home.
- The respiratory therapist assumes a large responsibility for selecting and placing primary and ancillary equipment, evaluating the home or alternative care site, coordinating in-hospital training of patients and caregivers, assisting in patient discharge and transfer, and following up with continuing care.
- Many types and models of ventilators are available for home use. Some of these are quite sophisticated, offering an array of modes, alarm systems, and other complex ventilatory characteristics.
- The most important factors in choosing a ventilator are its reliability, safety, versatility, whether its controls are easy to understand and manipulate, and whether it can be easy to cycle in the VC-CMV mode for patients with some spontaneous effort.
- The pulmonary, cardiovascular, and GI problems in VAIs are similar, in many respects, to those seen in critically ill ventilated patients.
- In addition to the mechanical ventilator, a patient undergoing ventilation at home requires various supplies for general daily care, including supplies for airway care, humidification, supplemental oxygen, disposable circuits, and an emergency backup ventilator.
- Perhaps one of the more important roles that the respiratory therapist must fill when caring for patients receiving long-term

mechanical ventilation is that of an educator. The ability to teach the patient and caregivers how to use the equipment properly and safely and alleviate the patient's fears and apprehension of ongoing care and emergency management is essential to the success of any home mechanical ventilation program.

- LTMV in the home environment is more likely to be successful when the patient and family are highly motivated, maintain hope, and communicate effectively.
- This increased awareness of the effectiveness of LTMV suggests that it is a desirable method of managing patients requiring long-term ventilatory support.[124]

REVIEW QUESTIONS *(See Appendix A for answers.)*

1. All the following are realistic goals of home mechanical ventilation **except**
   A. To extend life
   B. To improve the physical, psychological, and social functions of the individual
   C. To reverse the disease process
   D. To reduce the amount of hospitalizations

2. According to the criteria for patient selection, which of the following conditions would be most suitable for successful homecare ventilation?
   A. A patient with fibrotic lung disease on continuous ventilatory support with high F_IO_2 values and PEEP
   B. A patient with progressive muscular dystrophy
   C. A patient with severe COPD, cor pulmonale, and recurrent respiratory tract infections
   D. A patient with terminal lung cancer who is postpneumonectomy

3. Which of the following factors must be considered when estimating a patient's cost of home mechanical ventilation?
   1. Type of ventilator selected
   2. Accessory medical supplies
   3. Need for professional caregivers
   4. Adequacy of third-party coverage
   A. 1 and 2
   B. 1 and 3
   C. 2, 3, and 4
   D. 1, 2, 3, and 4

4. In terms of cost and patient independence, the facility that is generally the least expensive and provides the most patient independence is
   A. A long-term acute care facility
   B. An extended care facility
   C. The patient's home
   D. An in-hospital pulmonary step-down unit

5. Which of the following factors must be considered when selecting a ventilator for homecare ventilation?
   1. Electrical adequacy of the patient's home
   2. Ventilator versatility to accommodate the patient in all areas of the home
   3. Sophisticated and elaborate alarm system
   4. Ease of ventilator operation for caregivers
   A. 1 and 2
   B. 1, 2, and 3
   C. 2, 3 and 4
   D. 1, 2, and 4

6. Additional considerations for discharging a child to home mechanical ventilation include which of the following?
   A. Re-evaluation because of growth
   B. Stamina for periods of play while ventilated
   C. Well-educated family with good financial outlook
   D. A large number of siblings to assist as caregivers

7. Which of the following NPVs is most efficient for providing ventilatory assistance but is cumbersome?
   A. Pneumobelt (intermittent abdominal pressure ventilator)
   B. Chest cuirass
   C. Full-body chamber
   D. Body suit (jacket ventilator)

8. Follow-up assessment of a home-ventilated patient on a regular service schedule generally includes which of the following?
   1. Vital signs
   2. ABG evaluation
   3. S_pO_2
   4. Portable chest radiograph
   A. 1 only
   B. 2 only
   C. 1 and 3
   D. 1, 2, 3, and 4

9. Which of the following are experienced by family members caring for VAIs in the home?
   1. Loss of work time
   2. Loss of privacy when outside caregivers are in the home 24 hours a day
   3. Financial stress
   4. Transmission of nosocomial infections from patient to family
   A. 1 and 3
   B. 2 and 4
   C. 1, 2, and 3
   D. 1, 2, 3, and 4

10. Which of the following pieces of equipment, besides the ventilator, is essential to accomplish IPPV in the home?
    A. TT
    B. Good-fitting nasal mask
    C. Capnograph
    D. Tracheal button

11. Which of the following should be available for patients who require continuous ventilatory support?
    A. A 12-volt DC battery for backup power
    B. A backup ventilator
    C. A manual resuscitation bag
    D. All the above

12. Which of the following ventilator modes is **not** recommended for VAIs when using a first-generation portable/homecare ventilator?
    A. VC-CMV
    B. SIMV (volume targeted)
    C. Pressure support
    D. Volume-targeted control (apneic patient)

13. A patient with stable COPD has been selected for homecare ventilation. His ABG values are stable while on a volume ventilator with VC-CMV with the following settings: VT of 500 mL, f of 10 breaths/min, and F_IO_2 of 0.3. What operational features need to be considered when selecting his home mechanical ventilator?
    A. Optional modes of operation
    B. Capabilities for the addition of oxygen
    C. Low and high minute ventilation alarm
    D. High and low F_IO_2 alarm

14. A patient with high spinal cord injury has been selected for home mechanical ventilation. The patient has a tracheostomy and is on VC-CMV with room air. In addition to this patient's ventilator, what other equipment will be needed?
    1. Backup ventilator
    2. Tracheostomy care kits
    3. Concentrator
    4. Portable suction unit
    5. Manual resuscitator
       A. 1, 2, and 4
       B. 1, 2, 3, and 5
       C. 1, 2, 4, and 5
       D. 1, 2, 3, 4, and 5

15. While preparing a patient for discharge home, the respiratory therapist should instruct the patient and family to do what?
    A. Wash and dry the ventilator equipment as necessary
    B. Soak the equipment in warm soapy water, rinse, and towel dry twice daily
    C. Soak the equipment in warm soapy water, scrub to remove organic material, rinse, and place in disinfectant solution and rinse again
    D. Boil the equipment in water for 10 minutes then allow it to air-dry before packaging

16. A patient with a progressive neuromuscular disorder has been selected for home mechanical ventilation. What should the health care team include in the discharge plan?
    1. Instruct family and caregivers on aseptic suction procedures
    2. Give detailed instructions on cardiopulmonary resuscitation
    3. Provide a written protocol with directions for respiratory treatments and other aspects of care
    4. Assess the caregivers as they demonstrate techniques they have learned
       A. 1 only
       B. 3 only
       C. 2 and 4
       D. 1, 2, 3, and 4

17. All the following should be considered when preparing a patient for home mechanical ventilation **except**
    A. The family's critical care experience
    B. The family's ability to operate the ventilator adequately
    C. The availability of financial resources
    D. The electrical safety and available space in the patient's home

18. A written report should be completed monthly during the follow-up and evaluation of patients on home mechanical ventilation. Which of the following conditions should this monthly report include?
    1. ABG analysis
    2. Patient and family apprehensions
    3. Proper functioning of the equipment
    4. Compliance with the therapeutic plan
       A. 3 and 4
       B. 1, 2, and 3
       C. 1, 2, and 4
       D. 1, 2, 3, and 4

19. Which of the following patients would benefit from CPAP by nasal mask or nasal pillows?
    A. A patient with progressive neuromuscular disease requiring a chest cuirass at night only
    B. A patient diagnosed with congestive heart failure who has good respiratory muscle strength
    C. A patient with stable COPD requiring nocturnal ventilation
    D. A patient with kyphoscoliosis who has episodes of hypercapnia and hypoxemia at night

20. A potential complication of providing NPV with a chest cuirass to a patient with COPD is
    A. Increased cardiac output
    B. OSA
    C. Hyperventilation
    D. Barotrauma from excessive pressures

21. Alternative methods of assisting ventilation noninvasively include which of the following?
    1. NIV
    2. Pneumobelt
    3. Rocking bed
    4. NPV
       A. 1 and 4
       B. 2 and 3
       C. 2, 3, an 4
       D. 1, 2, 3, and 4

22. A patient is receiving ventilatory support at night by NPV with a body suit. The suit is unable to achieve the normal target pressure of -30 cm H_2O. The most likely cause of the problem is
    A. The shell is not attached correctly to the back plate.
    B. There is a leak in the system.
    C. This device cannot achieve a pressure of -30 cm H_2O.
    D. The patient is too small for the device.

23. A patient on nasal mask CPAP reports dried, irritated nasal passages. All the following will be beneficial in remedying this problem **except**
    A. Readjusting the nasal mask for better fit
    B. Periodically irrigating the nasal passages with normal saline
    C. Using a chin-strap
    D. Adding a humidifier to the circuit

24. The advantages of using MI-E in conjunction with PPV include
    1. It generates optimal PCEF for clearing airway secretions.
    2. It does not cause airway irritation or discomfort.
    3. It may decrease the production of airway secretions.
    4. It may improve VC and S_aO_2 associated with mucus plugging.
       A. 1 and 2
       B. 2, 3, and 4
       C. 2 and 4
       D. 1, 2, 3, and 4

25. Methods for improving secretion clearance, besides suctioning, might include
    A. Assisted coughing
    B. Mechanical oscillation
    C. MI-E
    D. All the above

26. List five factors that can contribute to psychological problems that can occur in VAIs.

27. Speaking can be accomplished in VAIs who are on non–critical care ventilators by deflating the cuff and making what ventilator adjustments?

28. The Portex and the Pittsburg speaking tracheostomy tubes require the patient to perform what function?

29. What step is absolutely essential when using a speaking valve?

30. List six circumstances in which speaking devices may be contraindicated.

References

1. MacIntyre NR: Evidence-based ventilatory weaning and discontinuation. *Respir Care* 49:830–836, 2004.
2. Kohorst J, Blakely P, Dockter C, et al: AARC Clinical Practice Guideline: Long-term invasive mechanical ventilation—2007 revision and update. *Respir Care* 52:1056–1062, 2007.
3. Lone NI, Walsh TS: Prolonged mechanical ventilation in critically ill patients: epidemiology, outcomes, and modelling the potential cost consequences of establishing a regional weaning unit. *Crit Care* 15:R102, 2011.
4. Engoren M, Arslanian-Engoren C, Fenn-Buderer N: Hospital and long-term outcomes after tracheostomy for respiratory failure. *Chest* 125:220–227, 2004.
5. Stoller JK, Xu M, Mascha E, et al: Long-term outcomes for patients discharged from a long-term hospital-based weaning unit. *Chest* 124:1892–1899, 2003.
6. MacIntyre NR, Epstein SK, Carson S, et al: National Association for Medical Direction of Respiratory Care: Management of patients requiring prolonged mechanical ventilation: report of a NAMDRC consensus conference. *Chest* 128(6):3937–3954, 2005.
7. Gracey DR: Cost and reimbursement of long-term ventilation. *Respir Care Clin N Am* 8:491–497, 2002.
8. Amin RS, Fitton CM: Tracheostomy and home ventilation in children. *Semin Neonatol* 8:127–135, 2003.
9. Massachusetts RTs remember Christopher Reeves. *AARC Times* 28:52, 2004.
10. Make BJ, Hill NS, Goldberg AI, et al: Mechanical ventilation beyond the intensive care unit: report of a consensus conference of the American College of Chest Physicians. *Chest* 113:289S–344S, 1998.
11. Aloe K, Faffaniello L, Williams L: Creation of an intermediate respiratory care unit to decrease intensive care utilization. *J Nurs Adm* 39:494–498, 2009.
12. Wijkstra PJ, Avendano MA, Goldstein RS: Inpatient chronic assisted ventilatory care: a 15-year experience. *Chest* 124:850–856, 2003.
13. Criner GJ: Long-term ventilation: introduction and perspectives. *Respir Care Clin N Am* 8:345–353, 2002.
14. Grenard S: *Essentials of respiratory home care*, Springfield, Ill., 1986, Glenn Educational Medical Services.
15. Feldman J, Tuteur PG: Mechanical ventilation: from hospital intensive care to home. *Heart Lung* 11:162–165, 1990.
16. American Association for Respiratory Care: Clinical practice guideline: Long-term invasive mechanical ventilation in the home—2007 revision and update. *Respir Care* 52:1056–1062, 2007.
17. Bach JR, Intintola BA, Augusta S, et al: The ventilator-assisted individual: cost analysis of institutionalization vs. rehabilitation and in-home management. *Chest* 101:26–30, 1992.
18. Downes JJ, Sharon PL: Chronic respiratory failure—controversies in management. *Crit Care Med* 21:S363–S364, 1993.
19. American Association for Respiratory Care: *Home respiratory care services. An official position statement by the AARC*, Irving, TX, 2010, American Association for Respiratory Care.
20. Goldberg A, Leger P, Hill N, et al: Clinical indications for noninvasive positive pressure ventilation in chronic respiratory failure due to restrictive lung disease, COPD, and nocturnal hypoventilation—a consensus conference report. *Chest* 116:521–534, 1999.
21. O'Donohue WJ, Giovannoni RM, Keens TG, et al: Long-term mechanical ventilation: guidelines for management in the home and at alternate community sites. *Chest* 90(1 Suppl):1S–37S, 1986.
22. Sivak ED, Crodasco EM, Gipson WT, et al: Home care ventilation: the Cleveland experience from 1977 to 1985. *Respir Care* 33:294–302, 1986.
23. Splaingard ML, Frates RC, Harrison GM, et al: Home positive pressure ventilation: twenty years experience. *Chest* 84:376–382, 1983.
24. Gilmartin ME: Long-term mechanical ventilation: patient selection and discharge planning. *Respir Care* 36:205–216, 1991.
25. Gonzalez C, Ferris G, Diaz J, et al: Kyphoscoliotic ventilatory insufficiency: effects of long-term intermittent positive-pressure ventilation. *Chest* 124:857–862, 2003.
26. American Thoracic Society Board of Directors Official Statement: Home mechanical ventilation of pediatric patients. *Am Rev Respir Dis* 141:258–259, 1990.
27. Smith CE, Mayer LS, Parkhust MN, et al: Adaptation in families with a member requiring mechanical ventilation at home. *Heart Lung* 20:349–356, 1991.
28. Beach SR, Schulz R, Williamson GM, et al: Risk factors for potentially harmful caregiver behaviour. *J Am Geriatr Soc* 53:255–261, 2005.
29. Warren ML, Jarrett C, Senegal R, et al: An interdisciplinary approach to transitioning ventilator-dependent patients to home. *J Nurs Care Qual* 19:67–73, 2004.
30. AARC Clinical Practice Guidelines: Discharge planning for the respiratory care patient. *Respir Care* 40:1308–1312, 1995.
31. Plummer AL, O'Donohue WJ, Petty TL: Consensus conference on problems in home mechanical ventilation. *Am Rev Respir Dis* 140:555–560, 1989.
32. May D: *Rehabilitation and continuity of care in pulmonary disease*, St Louis, 1990, Mosby–Year Book.
33. Gilmartin ME: Transition from the intensive care unit to home: patient selection and discharge planning. *Respir Care* 39:456–477, 1994.
34. Schonhofer B: Choice of ventilator types, modes, and settings for long-term ventilation. *Respir Care Clin N Am* 8:419–445, 2002.
35. Ambrosino N: Long-term mechanical ventilation and nutrition. *Respir Med* 98:413–420, 2004.
36. Margolan H, Fraser J, Lenton S: Parental experience of services when their child requires long-term ventilation. Implications for commissioning and providing services. *Child Care Health Dev* 30:257–264, 2004.
37. Cox CE, Carson SS: Prolonged mechanical ventilation. In MacIntyre NR, Branson RD, editors: *Mechanical ventilation*, ed 2, Philadelphia, 2009, Saunders-Elsevier, pp 324–338.
38. Littlewood K, Durbin CG: Evidenced-based airway management. *Respir Care* 46:1392–1405, 2001.
39. Harrop JS, Sharan AD, Scheid EH, et al: Tracheostomy placement in patients with complete cervical spinal cord injuries: American Spinal Injury Association Grade A. *J Neurosurg* 100(1 Suppl):20–23, 2004.
40. Goldberg AI: Home mechanical ventilation. *Am J Nurs* 110:13–14, 2010.
41. Cairo JM: *Mosby's respiratory care equipment*, ed 9, St Louis, 2014, Elsevier.

42. King A, McCoy R: Home respiratory care. In Hess DR, MacIntyre NR, Mishoe SC, et al, editors: *Respiratory care, principles and practices*, Philadelphia, 2012, Jones & Bartlett Learning, pp 559–588.

43. Campbell RS, Johannigman JA, Branson RD, et al: Battery duration of portable ventilators: effects of control variable, positive end-expiratory pressure, and inspired oxygen concentration. *Respir Care* 47:1173–1183, 2002.

44. Kacmarek R, Stanek KS, McMahon K, et al: Imposed work of breathing during synchronized intermittent mandatory ventilation provided by five home care ventilators. *Respir Care* 35:405–414, 1990.

45. Make B: AACP guidelines for mechanical ventilation in the home setting. *AARC Times* 11:56, 1987.

46. Gietzen JW, Lund JA, Swegarden JL: Effect of PEEP-valve placement on function of home-care ventilator. *Respir Care* 36:1093–1098, 1991.

47. Gonzalez-Moro R, Vivero A, de Miguel Diez J, et al: Bacterial colonization and home mechanical ventilation: prevalence and risk factors (in Spanish). *Arch Bronconeumol* 40:392–396, 2004.

48. Chatila WM, Criner GJ: Complications of long-term mechanical ventilation. *Respir Care Clin N Am* 8:631–647, 2002.

49. Hill NS: Noninvasive ventilation for chronic obstructive pulmonary disease. *Respir Care* 49:72–87, 2004.

50. Bach JR, Augusta SA: Management of chronic alveolar hypoventilation by nasal ventilation. *Chest* 97:52–57, 1990.

51. Leger P, Bedicam JM, Cornette A, et al: Nasal intermittent positive pressure ventilation: long-term follow-up in patients with severe chronic respiratory insufficiency. *Chest* 105:100–105, 1994.

52. Ellis ER, Grunstein RR, Chan S, et al: Noninvasive ventilatory support during sleep improves respiratory failure in kyphoscoliosis. *Chest* 94:811–815, 1988.

53. Ellis ER, Bye P, Bruderer JW, et al: Treatment of respiratory failure during sleep in patients with neuromuscular disease. *Am Rev Respir Dis* 35:148–152, 1987.

54. Kerby G, Mayer L, Pingleton S: Nocturnal positive pressure ventilation via nasal mask. *Am Rev Respir Dis* 135:738–740, 1987.

55. Leger P, Jennequin J, Gerard M, et al: Home positive pressure ventilation via nasal mask for patients with neuromuscular weakness or restrictive lung or chest-wall disease. *Respir Care* 34:73–77, 1989.

56. Leger P: Noninvasive positive pressure ventilation at home. *Respir Care* 39:501–510, 1994.

57. Simonds AK, Elliot MW: Outcome of domiciliary nasal intermittent positive pressure ventilation in restrictive and obstructive disorders. *Thorax* 50:604–609, 1995.

58. Mohr CH, Hill NS: Long-term follow-up of nocturnal ventilatory assistance in patients with respiratory failure due to Duchenne-type muscular dystrophy. *Chest* 97:91–96, 1990.

59. Linder K, Lotz P, Ahnefeld F: CPAP effect on FRC, VC and its subdivisions. *Chest* 92:66–70, 1987.

60. Cordova FC, Criner GJ: Negative-pressure ventilation: who, when, how? *Clin Pulm Med* 8:33–41, 2001.

61. Corrado A, Gorini M: Long-term negative pressure ventilation. *Respir Care Clin N Am* 8:545–557, 2002.

62. Splaingard ML, Frates RC, Jefferson LS, et al: Home negative pressure ventilation: report of 20 years of experience in patients with neuromuscular disease. *Arch Phys Med Rehabil* 66:239–242, 1985.

63. Holtakers TR, Loosborck LM, Gracey DR: The use of the chest cuirass in respiratory failure of neurologic origin. *Respir Care* 27:271, 1982.

64. Corrado A, Gorini M: Negative pressure ventilation. In Tobin MJ, editor: *Principles and practice of mechanical ventilation*, New York, 2013, McGraw-Hill, pp 417–433.

65. Sauret JM, Guitart AC, Rodriguez-Frojan G, et al: Intermittent short-term negative pressure ventilation and increased oxygenation in COPD patients with severe hypercapnic respiratory failure. *Chest* 100:455–459, 1991.

66. Hill NS: Clinical applications of body ventilators. *Chest* 90:897–905, 1986.

67. Back J: Respiratory assistance: why, what, when, and how to begin. In Robert D, Make BJ, Leger P, et al, editors: *Home mechanical ventilation*, Paris, 1995, Arnette Blackwell.

68. Bach JR, Penek J: Obstructive sleep apnea complicating negative pressure ventilatory support in patients with chronic paralytic/restrictive ventilatory dysfunction. *Chest* 99:1386–1393, 1991.

69. Cropp A, DiMarco AF: Effects of intermittent negative pressure ventilation on respiratory muscle function in patients with severe chronic obstructive pulmonary disease. *Am Rev Respir Dis* 135:1056–1061, 1987.

70. Klonin H, Bowman B, Peters M, et al: Negative pressure ventilation via chest cuirass to decrease ventilator-associated complications in infants with acute respiratory failure: a case series. *Respir Care* 45:486–490, 2000.

71. Bach JR: *Management of patients with neuromuscular disease*, Philadelphia, 2003, Hanley and Belfus-Elsevier.

72. Plum F, Whedon GD: The rapid-rocking bed: its effect on ventilation of poliomyelitis patients with respiratory paralysis. *N Engl J Med* 245:235–241, 1951.

73. Adamson JP, Stein JD: Application of abdominal pressure for artificial respiration. *JAMA* 169:1613–1617, 1959.

74. Gilmartin ME: Body ventilators: equipment and techniques. *Respir Care Clin N Am* 2:195–222, 1996.

75. Corican LJ, Higgins S, Davidson AC, et al: Rocking bed and prolonged independence from nocturnal non-invasive ventilation in neurogenic respiratory failure associated with limb weakness. *Postgrad Med J* 80:360–362, 2004.

76. Abd AG, Braun NM, Baskin MI, et al: Diaphragmatic dysfunction after open heart surgery: treatment with a rocking bed. *Ann Intern Med* 111:881–886, 1989.

77. Jones DJ, Braid GM, Wedzicha JA: Nasal masks for domiciliary positive pressure ventilation: patient usage and complications. *Thorax* 49:811–812, 1994.

78. Bach JR: Adding muscle to non-invasive ventilation. *Progress notes: a publication for Puritan Bennett customers* 6:27, 1994.

79. Bach JR, Saporito BA: Indications and criteria for decannulation and transition from invasive to noninvasive long-term ventilatory support. *Respir Care* 39:515–528, 1994.

80. Bergofsky EH, Gregg J, Galchus R: Management of respiratory failure in neuromuscular diseases. *Cur Rev Respir Ther* 21:163, 1981.

81. Bach JR, Alba AS, Bodofsky E, et al: Glossopharyngeal breathing and non-invasive aids in the management of post-polio respiratory insufficiency. *Birth Defects* 23:99–113, 1987.

82. Bach JR: Mechanical insufflation-exsufflation: comparison of peak expiratory flows with manually assisted and unassisted coughing techniques. *Chest* 104:1553–1562, 1993.

83. Scherer TA, Barandun J, Martinez E, et al: Effect of high-frequency oral airway and chest wall oscillations and conventional chest physical therapy on expectoration in patients with stable cystic fibrosis. *Chest* 113:1019–1027, 1998.

84. Heffner JE: The role of tracheotomy in weaning. *Chest* 120(6 Suppl):477S–481S, 2001.

85. MacIntyre NR, Cook DJ, Ely EW, Jr, et al: ACCP/AARC/SCCM Task Force. Evidence based guidelines for weaning and discontinuing mechanical ventilatory support: a collective task force facilitated by the American College of Chest Physicians; the American Association for Respiratory Care; and the American College of Critical Care Medicine, 2001. *Chest* 120(Suppl 6):375S–395S, 2001; *Respir Care* 47:69–90, 2001.

86. Conway DH, Mackie C: The effects of tracheostomy cuff deflation during continuous positive airway pressure. *Anesthesia* 59:652–657, 2004.

87. Happ MB, Tuite P, Dobbin K, et al: Communication ability, method, and content among nonspeaking, nonsurviving patients treated with mechanical ventilation in the intensive care unit. *Am J Crit Care* 13:210–218, 2004.

88. Gudsteinsdottir E, Powell C: Passy-Muir valve helps ventilator patients speak. *Adv Respir Care Pract* 17:31, 2004.

89. Orringer MK: The effects of tracheostomy tube placement on communication and swallowing. *Respir Care* 44:845–853, 1999.

90. Draper MH, Ladefoged P, Whitteridge D: Expiratory pressures and air flow during speech. *Br Med J* 1:1837–1843, 1960.

91. Hoit JD, Banzett RB, Lohmeier HL, et al: Clinical ventilator adjustments that improve speech. *Chest* 124:1512–1521, 2003.

92. Prigent H, Samuel C, Louis B, et al: Comparative effects of two ventilatory modes on speech in tracheostomized patients with neuromuscular disease. *Am J Respir Crit Care Med* 167:114–119, 2003.

93. Peruzzi WT, Logemann JA, Currie D, et al: Assessment of aspiration in patients with tracheostomies: comparison of the bedside colored dye assessment with video fluoroscopic examination. *Respir Care* 46:243–247, 2001.

94. Sparker AW, Robin KT, Newland GN, et al: A prospective evaluation of speaking tracheostomy tubes for ventilator-dependent patients. *Laryngoscope* 97:89–92, 1987.

95. Altobelli N: Airway management. In Kacmarek RM, Stoller JK, Heuer AL, editors: *Egan's fundamentals of respiratory care*, ed 10, St Louis, 2013, Elsevier, pp 732–786.

96. May RA, Bortner PL: Airway management. In Hess DR, MacIntyre NR, Mishoe SC, et al, editors: *Respiratory care—principles and practices*, Philadelphia, 2003, WB Saunders.

97. Shilling AM, Durbin C: Airway management devices and advanced cardiac life support. In Cairo JM, editor: *Mosby's respiratory care equipment*, ed 9, St Louis, 2014, Elsevier, pp 113–157.

98. Jaeger JM, Durbin CG: Special purpose endotracheal tubes. *Respir Care* 44:661–683, 1999.

99. Nomori H: Tracheostomy tube enabling speech during mechanical ventilation. *Chest* 125:1046–1051, 2004.

100. Manzano JL, Lubillo S, Henrizuez D, et al: Verbal communication of ventilator-dependent patients. *Crit Care Med* 21:512–517, 1993.

101. Jackson D, Albamonte S: Enhancing communication with the Passy-Muir valve. *Pediatr Nurs* 20:149–153, 1994.

102. Passy V, Baydur A, Prentice W, et al: Passy-Muir tracheostomy speaking valve on ventilator-dependent patients. *Laryngoscope* 103:653–658, 1993.

103. Gross RD, Mahlmann J, Grayhack JP: Physiologic effects of open and closed tracheostomy tubes on the pharyngeal swallow. *Ann Otol Rhinol Laryngol* 112:143–152, 2003.

104. Elpern EH, Okonek MB, Bacon M, et al: Effect of the Passy-Muir tracheostomy speaking valve on pulmonary aspiration in adults. *Heart Lung* 29:287–293, 2000.

105. Stachler RJ, Hamlet SL, Choi J, et al: Scintigraphic quantification of aspiration reduction with the Passy-Muir valve. *Laryngoscope* 106:231–234, 1996.

106. Dettelbach MA, Gross RD, Mahimann J, et al: Effect of the Passy-Muir valve on aspiration in patients with tracheostomy. *Head Neck* 17:297–302, 1995.

107. *Passy-Muir tracheostomy and ventilator speaking valves instruction booklet*. Irvine, Calif., 1989, Passy-Muir.

108. Pilbeam SP: Mechanical ventilators: general use devices. In Cairo JM, Pilbeam SP, editors: *Mosby's respiratory care equipment*, St Louis, 2004, Elsevier, pp 409–642.

109. Ellison B, Ellison J: *The Brooke Ellison story*, New York, 2001, Hyperiod.

110. Reibel JF: Decannulation: how and where. *Respir Care* 44:856–859, 1999.

111. AARC Clinical Practice Guideline: Suctioning of the patient in the home. *Respir Care* 44:99–104, 1999.

112. Hess DR: Guidelines for preventing health-care-associated pneumonia, 2003: buyer beware! (editorial). *Respir Care* 49:891–896, 2004.

113. Littlewood K, Durbin CG: Evidenced-based airway management. *Respir Care* 46:1392–1405, 2001.

114. Han JN, Liu YP, Ma S, et al: Effects of decreasing the frequency of ventilator circuit changes to every 7 days on the rate of ventilator-associated pneumonia in a Beijing hospital. *Respir Care* 46:891–896, 2001.

115. American Association for Respiratory Care: AARC Evidence-Based Clinical Practice Guideline: care of the ventilator circuit and its relation to ventilator-associated pneumonia. *Respir Care* 48:869–879, 2003.

116. National Center for Infectious Diseases, Centers for Disease Control and Prevention (CDC): Guidelines for preventing health-care-associated pneumonia, 2003 recommendations of the CDC and the Healthcare Infection Control Practices Advisory Committee. *Respir Care* 49:926–939, 2004.

117. Walkey AJ, Reardon CC, et al: The epidemiology of ventilator-associated pneumonia in long-term acute care hospital setting. *Am J Respir Crit Care Med* 179:A1742, 2009.

118. Chenoweth CE, Washer LL, et al: Ventilator-associated pneumonia in the home care setting. *Infect Control Hosp Epidemiol* 28:910–915, 2007.

119. Baram D, Hulse G, Palmer LB: Stable patients receiving prolonged mechanical ventilation have a high alveolar burden of bacteria. *Chest* 127:1353–1357, 2005.

120. Chatburn RL: Decontamination of respiratory care equipment: what can be done, what should be done. *Respir Care* 34:98–109, 1989.

121. Chatburn RL, Kallstrom TJ, Bajaksouzian S: A comparison of acetic acid with quaternary ammonium compound for disinfection of hand-held nebulizers. *Respir Care* 33:801–808, 1988.

122. AARC Home Care Consensus Report, Part 2: product standards and infection control. *AARC Times* 14:57, 1990.

123. American Respiratory Care Foundation: Guidelines for disinfection of respiratory care equipment used in the home. *Respir Care* 33:801–808, 1988.

124. Ceriana P, Delmastro M, Rampulla C, et al: Demographics and clinical outcomes of patients admitted to a respiratory intensive care unit located in a rehabilitation center. *Respir Care* 48:670–676, 2003.

125. Chao DC, Scheinhorn DJ: The challenge of prolonged mechanical ventilation: a shared global experience (editorial). *Respir Care* 48:668–669, 2003.

Neonatal and Pediatric Mechanical Ventilation

ROBERT M. DiBLASI, CHRISTINE KEARNEY

OUTLINE

KEY TERMS

- Bronchomalacia
- Bronchopulmonary dysplasia
- Choanal atresia
- Cleft palate
- Extracorporeal membrane oxygenation
- Meconium aspiration syndrome
- Neonate
- Patent ductus arteriosus
- Pediatric
- Prophylactic therapy
- Rescue therapy
- Tracheoesophageal fistula
- Tracheomalacia

LEARNING OBJECTIVES *On completion of this chapter, the reader will be able to do the following:*

1. Discuss the clinical manifestations of respiratory distress in neonatal and pediatric patients.
2. Identify differences in the level of noninvasive ventilatory support.
3. Describe device function and settings for different mechanical respiratory support strategies.
4. Identify the primary and secondary goals of ventilatory support of newborn and pediatric patients.
5. Explain some key areas of assessment that influence the decision on whether to initiate ventilatory support.
6. Recognize the indications, goals, limitations, and potentially harmful effects of continuous positive airway pressure (CPAP) in a clinical case.
7. Describe the basic design of nasal devices used to deliver CPAP to an infant.
8. Compare and contrast a mechanical ventilator equipped with a CPAP delivery system to a freestanding CPAP system.
9. From patient data, recognize the need for mechanical ventilatory support in newborn and pediatric patients.
10. Identify the essential features of a neonatal and pediatric mechanical ventilator.
11. Explain how the advanced features of a ventilator enhance its usefulness over a wide range of clinical settings.
12. Relate the major differences between older-generation neonatal ventilators and modern microprocessor controlled mechanical ventilators.
13. Distinguish demand flow from continuous flow, and discuss other modifications that have been made to the basic infant ventilator.
14. Select appropriate ventilator settings based on the patient's weight, diagnosis, and clinical history; also discuss strategies and rationale for ventilator settings.
15. Discuss newborn and pediatric applications, technical aspects, patient management, and cautions for the following ventilatory modes: pressure-controlled ventilation, volume-controlled ventilation, dual-controlled ventilation, pressure support ventilation, airway pressure release ventilation, and neurally adjusted ventilatory assist.
16. Discuss the rationale and indications for high-frequency ventilation in newborn and pediatric patients.
17. Compare the characteristics and basic delivery systems of the following high-frequency ventilation techniques: high-frequency positive pressure ventilation, high-frequency jet ventilation,

high-frequency flow interruption, high-frequency percussive ventilation, and high-frequency oscillatory ventilation.
18. Explain the physiological and theoretic mechanisms of gas exchange that govern high-frequency ventilation, and defend the mechanism believed to be most correct.

19. Explain how settings of a given high-frequency technique are initially adjusted, the effect of individual controls on gas exchange, and strategies of patient management.
20. Discuss the physiological benefits of inhaled nitric oxide therapy, and suggest recommended treatment strategies.

RECOGNIZING THE NEED FOR MECHANICAL VENTILATORY SUPPORT

Mechanical ventilation of newborn and pediatric patients involves the use of devices that recruit and maintain lung volumes, improve gas exchange and lung mechanics, assist in overcoming the resistive properties of an artificial airway, and reduce the work of breathing. These devices may provide continuous positive airway pressure (CPAP), assist spontaneous ventilation (e.g., noninvasive positive pressure ventilation [NIV], bilevel positive airway pressure [BiPAP] units), or support part or all of the patient's ventilatory requirements (e.g., invasive mechanical ventilation).

Currently there are no well-defined, disease-specific criteria available to guide the decision on when to initiate mechanical ventilatory support in newborns and pediatric patients in respiratory distress. In fact, many institutions with desirable outcomes prefer to implement ventilatory support before the onset of severe respiratory illness, making the process of initiating support even more complicated. The ongoing clinical management of patients requiring ventilatory support also remains an elusive practice that is based more on experience and clinician preference, and less on experimental data obtained from large randomized controlled trials.

This chapter focuses on the best available clinical and experimental evidence for initiating and managing neonatal and pediatric respiratory support. For the purpose of this discussion, a **neonate** will be defined as any infant less than 44 weeks of age and **pediatric** will include any patient beyond the neonatal period and up to adolescence.

Clinicians caring for neonatal and pediatric patients must understand the causes and pathophysiology of the various diseases and conditions that affect the airways and lung parenchyma of these patients.

They must also be knowledgeable about the theory of operation and limitations of the different ventilatory support devices used. Additionally, clinicians must be able to interpret physiological data derived from the history and physical assessment, laboratory studies, and radiographic findings to evaluate properly the effectiveness of the ventilatory support provided. Keep in mind that although these data are a critical part of the decision-making process, other factors must be considered when initiating mechanical ventilation in these patients. In many cases, the approach to initiating ventilatory support may have to be individualized for neonates and pediatric patients, because anatomical structure, size, and disease severity can vary widely from one patient to the next.

Clinical Indications for Respiratory Failure

Respiratory failure is defined as the inability to establish or maintain adequate gas exchange. Respiratory failure can present at birth and persist throughout the neonatal period or following a catastrophic event. Many pediatric patients encounter respiratory failure as a chronic condition (e.g., bronchopulmonary dysplasia). Although lung disease is the most common cause of respiratory failure, there are many extrinsic factors that can predispose patients

to this life-threatening event. For example, hemodynamic conditions and congenital cardiac anomalies can also contribute to respiratory failure. Neonatal and pediatric patients have smaller lungs, greater airway resistance, lower lung compliance, less surface area for gas exchange, and lower cardiovascular reserve than do adults, making them more vulnerable to rapid deterioration. In fact, respiratory failure is a major cause of cardiac arrest in neonatal and pediatric patients. As such, clinicians must act quickly to limit the potential adverse outcomes associated with respiratory failure by observing clinical signs and symptoms. These factors can guide timely intervention well before respiratory failure develops into cardiopulmonary arrest.

Neonate

Neonates experiencing respiratory distress typically present with tachypnea, nasal flaring, and intercostal, substernal, and retrosternal retractions. The chest wall during infancy is composed primarily of cartilage, making the chest wall compliance much greater than that of the lungs. As the resistance and compliance worsen, neonates have to generate higher pleural pressures during inhalation, causing the "floppy" chest wall to collapse inward creating retractions. On exhalation, the neonatal chest wall lacks the necessary recoil to counteract the inward forces of the lungs, and thus the lungs are prone to premature collapse. Infants will attempt to maintain a back pressure in the lungs, to preserve the functional residual capacity, by narrowing the glottis and maintaining respiratory muscle activity (active exhalation). This results in vocalization during exhalation or "grunting," which is often mistaken for infants' crying. Grunting can usually be heard without auscultation and is a useful clinical sign of impending respiratory failure. The Silverman-Anderson respiratory scoring system is a useful clinical tool to assess the degree of respiratory distress in neonates (Fig. 22-1).

Although this tool has been available in the clinical setting for nearly three decades, it has recently been reintroduced in a number of institutions to better evaluate patient response to settings changes during CPAP and mechanical ventilation.

Premature neonates can become apneic due to underdeveloped neural respiratory centers, and may or may not be stimulated to reestablish spontaneous breathing. Infants that do not respond to gentle stimulation and caffeine therapy often require immediate respiratory assistance using a manual resuscitator and, when necessary, invasive mechanical ventilation.

Pediatric

Pediatric patients experiencing respiratory distress can present with some of the same clinical manifestations as neonates. However, larger pediatric patients have ossified or "stiffer" chest walls and are able to sustain longer periods of higher work of breathing (WOB) than neonates. Nonetheless, clinicians should be well versed in recognizing age-specific normal and abnormal respiratory and hemodynamic parameters prior to implementing mechanical respiratory support.

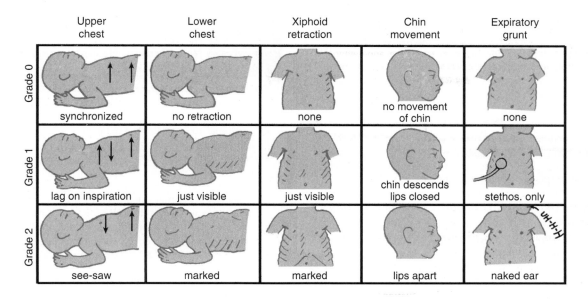

	Upper chest	Lower chest	Xiphoid retraction	Chin movement	Expiratory grunt
Grade 0	synchronized	no retraction	none	no movement of chin	none
Grade 1	lag on inspiration	just visible	just visible	chin descends lips closed	stethos. only
Grade 2	see-saw	marked	marked	lips apart	naked ear

Fig. 22-1 The Silverman-Anderson score for assessing the magnitude of respiratory distress. (Modified from Silverman WA, Anderson DH: Pediatrics 17:1-10, 1956; Wilkins RL, Stoller JK, Kacmarek RM: Egan's fundamentals of respiratory care, ed 10, St Louis, 2013, Elsevier.)

Determining Effective Oxygenation and Ventilation

Arterial blood gas (ABG) analysis is considered the gold standard for determining oxygenation, ventilation, and acid–base balance in neonates and pediatric patients with respiratory failure. It is important to recognize that frequent ABGs can deplete the circulating blood volume of small patients. Noninvasive techniques (i.e., pulse oximetry [S_pO_2] and transcutaneous CO_2 measurements) are alternative methods for trending gas exchange in most patients. Interpretation of ABG or noninvasive gas exchange values must also be coupled with data obtained from physical assessment and other clinical and laboratory data. For example, observing the color of the skin and mucous membranes can be used to assess tissue oxygenation; oxygen delivery and tissue perfusion can be evaluated clinically by noting capillary refill. Indeed, close attention to vital signs and physical assessment findings can help prevent deterioration of ABG/acid–base status.

Patients with certain congenital heart defects often require a high pulmonary vascular resistance to prevent excessive pulmonary blood flow and maintain adequate systemic circulation and cardiac output; thus abnormal values are acceptable in this patient population before surgical correction. Additionally, allowing carbon dioxide levels to rise and pH levels to fall to abnormal levels has become a common standard for lung protection during mechanical ventilation. If necessary, an individualized or standardized approach for managing gas exchange during ventilatory support should be identified early in management.

Chest radiographic evaluation is another important tool that can add to the overall clinical assessment of patients with respiratory failure or those receiving respiratory support. Because lung volumes are difficult to measure in neonatal and pediatric patients, chest radiographs can provide valuable insight into the approximate level of lung expansion in patients susceptible to developing atelectasis or hyperinflation. Many clinicians use the chest radiograph to guide the setting of ventilator parameters. It is important to realize the limitations of chest radiographs and understand that frequent radiography may expose patients to unnecessary high levels of radiation. The following sections provide more in-depth information about clinical and laboratory indications for mechanical ventilatory support.

GOALS OF NEWBORN AND PEDIATRIC VENTILATORY SUPPORT

The goals of mechanical ventilatory support in newborn and pediatric patients are:
- To provide adequate ventilation and oxygenation
- To achieve adequate lung volume
- To improve lung compliance
- To reduce WOB
- To limit lung injury

One may argue that avoiding mechanical ventilatory support altogether or minimizing the duration of support should be the first goal because even short-term ventilation can result in ventilator-induced lung injury (VILI).

Maintenance of an appropriate functional residual capacity (FRC) ensures optimum lung mechanics, which leads to reduced WOB and reduced lung injury. To move gas into and out of the lungs, the patient must generate relatively high intrathoracic pressures to balance the resistive and elastic components that resist lung inflation. Positive pressure ventilation can significantly reduce this burden and improve recovery in patients with lung disease. In fact, some patients receive chronic mechanical ventilatory support as a means of reducing caloric utilization by the respiratory muscles. These patients are often able to breathe spontaneously, but at a significant caloric cost. Mechanical ventilatory support can help promote normal function and development of the respiratory system, especially in neonatal patients with lung disease.

NONINVASIVE RESPIRATORY SUPPORT

Continuous positive airway pressure (CPAP) is used in spontaneously breathing patients and may be applied **with** or **without** an artificial airway. CPAP provides a **continuous distending pressure** to the lungs, which increases FRC and thus helps improve lung compliance (C_L). Often airway resistance (R_{aw}) is also reduced and the patient's WOB dramatically decreases with the use of CPAP.[1] CPAP is most commonly applied noninvasively to the nasal airway opening and has become very popular over the last decade in the neonatal population as a strategy to avoid intubation and invasive mechanical ventilation. In this discussion, the term *CPAP* refers to *nasal CPAP* in neonates. CPAP often is recommended for patients who have adequate alveolar ventilation, and yet are hypoxemic despite receiving an FIO_2 greater than 0.5. CPAP may be used to prevent atelectasis and to reduce WOB in patients who have been weaned and extubated from the ventilator.

Noninvasive Nasal Continuous Positive Airway Pressure in Neonates

Indications and Contraindications

When introduced in 1971, CPAP was touted as the "missing link" because it could provide oxygen treatment while avoiding mechanical ventilation in the neonate.[2] Used appropriately, CPAP is a less invasive and less aggressive form of therapy than other forms of ventilatory support. Newborns with retained lung fluid, atelectasis, insufficient surfactant production, or respiratory distress syndrome (RDS) are good candidates for CPAP. Such patients include very low birth weight (VLBW) and premature infants.[3] CPAP also can be used successfully in infants with respiratory distress arising from other causes, including transient tachypnea of the newborn, **meconium aspiration syndrome,** primary pulmonary hypertension, pulmonary hemorrhage, and paralysis of a hemidiaphragm. CPAP is also used following surgical repair of diaphragmatic hernias, congenital cardiac anomalies, congenital pneumonias, respiratory syncytial virus (RSV), bronchiolitis, apnea of prematurity, and congenital and acquired airway lesions.[4]

Box 22-1 lists the indications for CPAP in neonates originally established by the American Association for Respiratory Care (AARC).[5]

Compared with standard oxygen therapy, CPAP reduces grunting and tachypnea, increases FRC and arterial oxygen partial pressure (P_aO_2), decreases intrapulmonary shunting, improves lung compliance, aids in the stabilization of the floppy infant chest wall, improves distribution of ventilation, and reduces inspiratory WOB.[4] CPAP is believed to reduce the severity and duration of central and obstructive apneas by mechanically splinting the upper airway, promoting better alveolar recruitment, oxygenation, and stimulation of the infant to breathe.[6]

Although there is no consensus on how best to manage neonates on CPAP, two general approaches are currently being used to minimize the use of invasive mechanical ventilation and better protect the fragile neonatal respiratory system. Early CPAP involves implementing therapy in the delivery room or neonatal intensive care unit (NICU) only after the infant is stabilized and is effectively breathing on his or her own. This is performed prophylactically even if the neonate is not exhibiting respiratory distress or apnea. The goal is to recruit air spaces and maintain lung volumes early to promote gas exchange and reduce the likelihood that respiratory failure and apnea will occur. This approach is beneficial for premature infants that lack lung surfactant and are at risk for developing atelectasis. Breathing at low lung volumes can result in unnecessary lung injury (atelectotrauma), which can hinder surfactant production. Many premature neonates can be managed successfully using CPAP without ever requiring endotracheal intubation and mechanical ventilation. If the patient does develop respiratory failure, then

BOX 22-1 Indications for Continuous Positive Airway Pressure (CPAP) in Newborns Via Nasal Prongs, Nasopharyngeal Tube, or Nasal Mask

Abnormalities on Physical Examination
- Increased work of breathing (WOB), as indicated by a 30% to 40% increase above the normal respiratory rate (f)
- Substernal and suprasternal retractions
- Grunting and nasal flaring
- Pale or cyanotic skin color
- Agitation
- Inadequate arterial blood gas (ABG) values:
  - Inability to maintain a partial pressure of arterial oxygen (P_aO_2) above 50 mm Hg with a fraction of inspired oxygen (F_IO_2) of 0.6, provided minute ventilation $\dot{V}_E$ is adequate, as indicated by a partial pressure of arterial carbon dioxide (P_aCO_2) of 50 mm Hg and a pH of 7.25 or higher
- Poorly expanded and/or infiltrated lung fields on a chest radiograph
- Presence of a condition thought to be responsive to CPAP and associated with one or more of these:
  - Respiratory distress syndrome (RDS)
  - Pulmonary edema
  - Atelectasis
- Apnea of prematurity
- Recent extubation
- Tracheal malacia or other abnormality of the lower airways
- Transient tachypnea of the newborn
- Very low birth weight infants at risk for the development of RDS as an early intervention along with surfactant administration
- Administration of controlled concentrations of nitric oxide in spontaneously breathing infants

(Modified from AARC Clinical Practice Guidelines: Application of continuous positive airway pressure to neonates via nasal prongs or nasopharyngeal tube or nasal mask, *Respir Care* 49:1100-1108, 2004.)

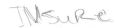

he or she is intubated, given lung surfactant, and then promptly weaned from the ventilator and extubated. This approach is a drastic departure from the previous approach that has been used over the last 20 years, in which neonates would be intubated and placed on a ventilator for weeks or even months until they were a certain size or weight. Centers that implement early CPAP report a very low incidence of infants developing chronic lung disease or bronchopulmonary dysplasia (BPD) because the lungs are not being subjected to the relatively large inflation pressures that are observed during mechanical ventilation.[7,8] A recent clinical trial in premature neonates demonstrated that this early CPAP approach resulted in less need for intubation and fewer days of mechanical ventilation, and infants were more likely to be alive and free from the need for mechanical ventilation after a week than were neonates intubated for surfactant and supported with mechanical ventilation for at least 24 hours.[9]

Another clinical approach implements elective intubation, prophylactic surfactant administration, short-term lung-protective ventilation, and rapid extubation to CPAP within hours of birth. (NOTE: This approach is also known as InSURE [Intubate, SURfactant, Extubation], and is implemented shortly following birth.[10])

The InSURE approach assures that all premature infants will receive at least one dose of surfactant, but it does not eliminate the potential that even short-term ventilation can result in some degree of lung injury. The InSURE approach has been associated with lower incidences of mechanical ventilation, air-leak syndromes, and BPD than an approach that administers surfactant and embraces prolonged mechanical ventilation support.[11]

The major question that remains is whether these two disparate approaches impact long-term survival and the development of chronic complications (e.g., BPD). Another important outcome related to these different approaches is the incidence of CPAP failure and subsequent ventilation requirements among neonates. Approximately 25% to 40% of infants with birth weights between 1000 and 1500 g may fail early CPAP and require intubation and mechanical ventilation, whereas 25% to 38% of infants with similar birth weights may fail CPAP using the InSURE approach.[4] Some institutions use a combination of these approaches wherein smaller premature neonates (<28 weeks' gestational age), with lower surfactant production, will be supported initially using InSURE and larger neonates are supported using the early CPAP strategy. Both these strategies strive to minimize invasive mechanical ventilation and have redefined the approach to supporting premature infants at risk for developing respiratory failure. Minimally invasive ventilation strategies, such as CPAP, have likely been a major reason why premature neonates are able to survive at a lower gestational age and with fewer complications than ever before.

Any neonate that has recently been extubated from mechanical ventilation is at risk for developing hypoxemia, respiratory acidosis, and apnea. Extubation to CPAP, regardless of whether surfactant was administered, has been associated with a reduction in the incidence of respiratory failure and the need for additional ventilatory support in neonates.[12]

Infants with certain congenital heart diseases reportedly benefit from CPAP. Cardiac anomalies that increase pulmonary blood flow can reduce C_L and FRC, thus increasing WOB and worsening hypoxia. The most common defects associated with increased pulmonary blood flow are ventricular septal defects, atrial septal defects, atrioventricular (AV) canal, and patent ductus arteriosus. Positive intrathoracic pressure produced by a CPAP system can mechanically reduce pulmonary blood flow while restoring FRC.[13,14]

Use of CPAP is not appropriate and is potentially dangerous in infants who show signs of nasal obstruction or severe upper airway malformation, such as choanal atresia, cleft palate, or tracheoesophageal fistula.[13] CPAP has been used in patients with bronchiolitis, but its use in these patients has been controversial and may be contraindicated in some cases.[5,15,16] More recent evidence suggests, however, that CPAP can result in favorable outcomes in infants affected with bronchiolitis by reducing carbon dioxide levels and eliminating the need for mechanical ventilation.[17]

Patients who have severe cardiovascular instability, severe ventilatory impairment (pH <7.25, P_aCO_2 >60), refractory hypoxemia (P_aO_2 <50 Torr on >0.6 F_IO_2), frequent apnea that does not respond to stimulation or intravenous caffeine therapy, or patients who are receiving high levels of sedation may require intubation and mechanical ventilation rather than CPAP.[13] CPAP or any form of noninvasive positive pressure to the airway should not be used in infants with untreated congenital diaphragmatic hernia; these infants should be intubated to prevent gastric insufflations and distention, and further compromise of the heart and lungs.[15] Some surgeons discourage the use of CPAP in infants after any surgical procedure involving the gastrointestinal tract.

Most commonly, CPAP is applied via nasal prongs; however, some clinicians prefer to use CPAP in intubated neonates while weaning from mechanical ventilation to observe whether the infant is experiencing apnea. Prolonged support using this approach should be discouraged whenever possible because it is has been associated with an increased need for reintubation after the breathing tube has been removed.[12]

Application of Nasal CPAP

Because newborns are obligate nose breathers, nasal CPAP can be applied in several ways. Previously a short endotracheal tube (ET) was placed into one of the nares and taped to the face to provide nasopharyngeal tube CPAP. A snug-fitting set of short binasal prongs is the most commonly used interface. Neonatal nasal masks are also available and are gaining popularity among some clinicians. It is common practice to alternate between these two nasal airway interfaces. Both devices are effective, but the distending pressure they provide can be lost when the infant cries or breathes through the mouth. Binasal prongs and masks may be more beneficial than a nasopharyngeal tube because they are less invasive and provide the least amount of resistance to gas flow, and hence lower imposed (or resistive) WOB, and facilitate mobilization and oral feeding.[14,18] Additionally, short binasal prongs were found to be more effective than using a single nasopharyngeal tube in reducing the rate of reintubation in premature neonates supported with CPAP.[19]

Nasal prongs and masks must be fitted correctly so that they do not leak or cause trauma to the patient. Nasal prongs and masks usually are made of a latex-free material, such as silicone. Molded into a manifold or attached to one, the prongs are placed just inside the infant's nares (Fig. 22-2). Prongs are available in a variety of sizes. The fit of the prongs is critical; they must fit snugly into the nares, but must not be so tight as to cause skin blanching. If a nasal mask is used instead of prongs, it too must be carefully selected for proper size and fit. Masks can cause pressure injury to the skin if improperly fitted, and they may not seal if they are too large or small.

The entire CPAP apparatus is stabilized on the patient's head with headgear or a fixation system consisting of a bonnet, cap, or straps (Fig. 22-3). Many commercial system configurations are available. The correct size of straps and head coverings must be carefully chosen and adjusted so that no part of the infant's head is subjected to squeezing or occlusive pressure points. After the CPAP delivery device has been attached to the CPAP manifold, the CPAP level and F_IO_2 are set. The CPAP system is assessed frequently to ensure effective delivery. The patient's nose is checked regularly for signs of pressure necrosis, and the prongs must be checked routinely for patency.

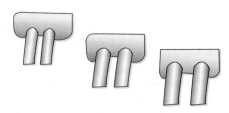

Fig. 22-2 Infant prongs for continuous positive airway pressure (CPAP) (see text for additional information). (Redrawn from Fisher & Paykel Healthcare, Inc., Laguna Hills, Calif.)

If you have a diaphragmatic hernia it should be intubated

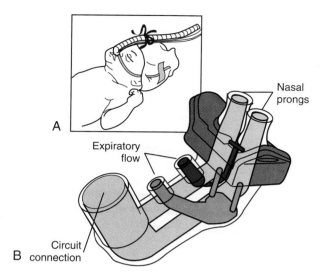

Fig. 22-3 A, Infant flow generator used with the Hamilton Arabella continuous positive airway pressure (CPAP) system. **B,** Infant flow generator mounting system. (From Cairo JM, Pilbeam SP: Mosby's respiratory care equipment, ed 8, St Louis, 2010, Mosby.)

The CPAP system functions primarily to regulate gas flow during inhalation and exhalation, and to maintain a consistent pressure at the nasal airway opening. The CPAP system consists of five essential components:

1. A heated/humidified blended gas source
2. A nasal interface
3. A patient circuit
4. The pressure regulation mechanism
5. A means for monitoring and limiting the airway pressures[4]

Numerous studies have compared differences in gas exchange, WOB, and requirement for (re)intubation with the available CPAP devices; however, it is important to note that no single device has been shown to be superior to another when major outcomes (i.e., mortality and morbidity) in neonates are considered (Key Point 22-1).[4]

> **Key Point 22-1** The success by which CPAP is applied to neonates is probably based more on the clinicians' abilities to understand the system and identify pathophysiological changes in response to settings changes than is the type of CPAP device or nasal interface being used.

Over the last three decades, the most common CPAP system that has been applied noninvasively has been accomplished using a mechanical ventilator. Ventilator CPAP has also been referred to as *conventional CPAP* in the clinical setting. Ventilator CPAP is convenient because it has traditionally been used following extubation from mechanical ventilation and does not rely on having to use a separate device to apply therapy. Many ventilator manufacturers have designed specific noninvasive CPAP modes into the ventilator platform exclusively for neonates. The clinician can set the CPAP level, and the exhalation valve regulates the pressures accordingly. Another advantage of these modes is that the ventilator may be able to deliver noninvasive "backup breaths," based on a preset apnea interval, when the neonate has stopped breathing. One potential limitation of ventilator CPAP is that the demand

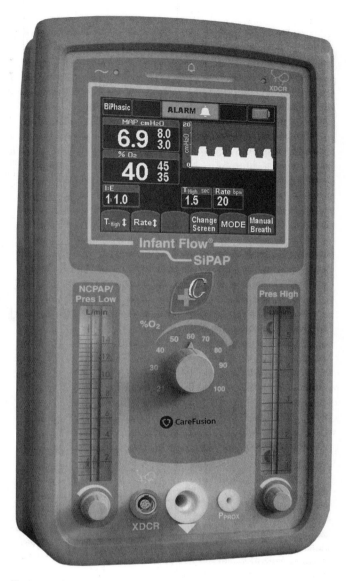

Fig. 22-4 Infant flow "sigh" positive airway system (SiPAP) System. (Courtesy CareFusion, San Diego, Calif.)

flow system may not be able to respond adequately to changes in patient respiratory efforts because pressure is being measured at the ventilator and not at the patient's airway. Additionally, new evidence suggests that the expiratory resistance of newer neonatal ventilator's exhalation valves may impose additional resistance and hence increase the WOB during spontaneous breathing.[20]

Two commercially available, freestanding CPAP devices that use fluidic gas principles are widely used to provide CPAP to infants. The Hamilton Arabella (Fig. 22-3, *A* and *B*) and the CareFusion Infant Flow SiPAP System (Fig. 22-4) are favored by some clinicians. The overall function of these fluidic devices to generate CPAP at the airway is similar. Both devices have a fully integrated flow controller, a delivery circuit, different-sized nasal prongs that attach to a gas delivery manifold, and a bonnet with Velcro straps to secure the manifold and prongs. The manifold incorporates a fluidic flip-flop mechanism at the infant's nasal airway opening to regulate flow to match the infant's inspiratory demand and provide a consistent pressure level (see Fig. 22-3, *B*). The controller provides gas flow with an adjustable F_IO_2 and also

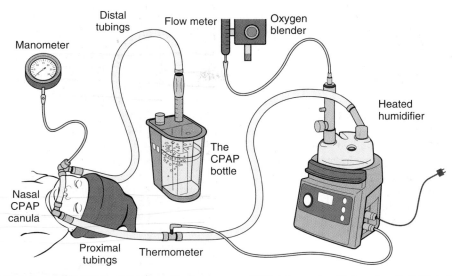

Fig. 22-5 Diagram of the bubble continuous positive airway pressure (CPAP) delivery system. (Redrawn from Aly H, Milner JD, Patel K, El-Mohandes AA: Does the experience with the use of nasal continuous positive airway pressure improve over time in extremely low birth weight infants? Pediatrics 114:697-702, 2004.)

monitors CPAP pressure. Turbulence caused by continuous flow has been eliminated in these systems to make exhalation easier and reduce the WOB. The manufacturers have attempted to provide better-fitting, easier-to-secure nasal prongs to make CPAP more effective and patient care easier. These devices are particularly effective at reducing WOB in VLBW infants. CPAP is better tolerated in these patients, which helps to avert the need for positive pressure ventilation.[21]

Bubble CPAP (B-CPAP) is a technique for delivering CPAP via a simple freestanding system (Fig. 22-5). It has been used in certain forms for more than 30 years and is again gaining favor over other CPAP techniques. In the United States, two B-CPAP devices are now available (B&B Medical, Fischer Paykel), but most centers that implement B-CPAP have done so using homemade systems consisting of a blended and humidified gas source, ventilator circuits, nasal prongs, pressure manometer, and a water column. The blended gas flow is adjusted at 5 L/min, and the CPAP level is regulated by varying the depth of the distal ventilator circuit below the water surface (i.e., 5 cm = 5 cm H_2O CPAP). Higher pressures than those anticipated by the submersion depth of the distal tubing have been observed when using higher flows,[22,23] thus clinicians will use the lowest flow possible to maintain constant bubbling throughout the respiratory cycle. An additional safeguard involves measuring the pressure at the nasal airway interface using a pressure manometer and limiting excessive pressures with a safety pop-off valve during B-CPAP.

Tiny vibrations or oscillations in the airway pressure created by gas bubbling through the water column may assist in enhancing gas exchange and lung recruitment. Anecdotal reports made by clinicians have observed the chest walls of intubated premature neonates supported by B-CPAP oscillating at frequencies similar to those provided by high-frequency ventilation, but these ventilation effects have never been quantified in neonates using leaky nasal prongs.[24]

Initial pressures for CPAP are commonly set at about 4 to 6 cm H_2O.[25] The CPAP level requirements are likely to fluctuate throughout the course of treatment, and the optimal level is one that results in adequate lung inflation without overdistending the lung

parenchyma.[4] If little clinical improvement is seen, the level is gradually increased to 10 cm H_2O in increments of 1 to 2 cm H_2O.[10] The response is considered adequate when the required F_IO_2 is 0.6 or less and the P_aO_2 is at least 50 mm Hg.[26] Adequate oxygenation usually is accompanied by reduced WOB, as manifested by a 30% reduction in the respiratory rate and a decrease in retractions, grunting, and nasal flaring. In some cases the chest radiograph indicates improvement by showing better aeration and increased lung volumes (Key Point 22-2).[27] Continuous noninvasive monitoring of transcutaneous CO_2, pulse oximetry, and Silverman-Anderson respiratory scores can provide reliable trending of physiological response in patients when adjustments are made to the CPAP level.

Key Point 22-2 Regardless of the type of nasal prongs or nasopharyngeal (NP) tube used for CPAP, the clinician must always verify the patency of the device and strive to reduce injury by frequently assessing the proper fit.

Complications of CPAP

CPAP can cause pulmonary overdistention and can lead to ventilation/perfusion mismatching, decreased pulmonary blood flow, increased pulmonary vascular resistance, and decreased cardiac output.[28] Marked overdistention can increase WOB and cause CO_2 retention.[29] Air-leak syndromes have also been reported.[30] The clinician must be aware that the CPAP system can cause abdominal distention and gastric insufflation, which can lead to aspiration if not detected and corrected early.[31] Perforations of the gastrointestinal tract, although rare, are possible.[14] Excessive pressure from the application devices can injure the nose and nasal mucosa, and inadequate humidification can contribute to injury.

Noninvasive Positive Pressure Ventilation in Neonates

As noted in the previous discussion, a large percentage of neonates supported by CPAP still develop severe respiratory failure requiring endotracheal intubation and mechanical ventilation. Recent evidence suggests that invasive mechanical ventilation contributes to the development of BPD and other complications in neonates.[32]

It is unclear whether this is related exclusively to the VILI or whether the presence of the ET in the airway is also a contributing factor. The neonate can experience endotracheal intubation as a traumatic and painful procedure, especially if proper sedation levels are not achieved. Intubation is accompanied by significant hemodynamic instabilities, airway injury, colonization of the trachea, reduced ciliary movement, secretions, high resistance to air flow, and increased WOB.[33]

Also known as "CPAP with a rate," noninvasive positive pressure ventilation (NIV) is an established form of ventilatory support in adults and pediatric patients. It is accomplished by using superimposed positive pressure inflations with CPAP. NIV is becoming a new intermediary approach between CPAP and invasive mechanical ventilation to re-expand atelectatic areas, improve gas exchange, reduce respiratory distress, prevent apnea, and potentially avoid the need for invasive mechanical ventilation. NIV is used as an initial form of respiratory support and following extubation from invasive mechanical ventilation.[34] Like CPAP, NIV assists spontaneous breathing patients only, and thus neonates with persistent apnea cannot be supported by this method of mechanical ventilator support. Furthermore, not all neonates can be supported by NIV alone, and intubation is indicated for severe ventilatory impairment (pH <7.25, P_aCO_2 >60), refractory hypoxemia (P_aO_2 <5 0 Torr on >0.6 F_1O_2), and frequent apnea that does not respond to stimulation or intravenous caffeine therapy.[35] The same complications that arise during CPAP and mechanical ventilation can be observed during noninvasive positive pressure ventilation (NPPV).

Most commonly NIV is applied using short binasal prongs or a nasal mask and a fixation technique similar to that of CPAP. As improvements in nasal airway interfaces and ventilator devices have evolved, clinicians have begun implementing different forms of NIV in neonates with little experimental evidence to support their use. The following section discusses the most common methods and approaches for applying NIV in neonates.

Nasal Intermittent Mandatory Ventilation in Neonates

Nasal synchronized and intermittent mandatory ventilation, or *nasal IMV* (IMV or N-IMV), is the most commonly used form of NIV in neonates, and pressure control is the most common mode for providing NIV in neonates. Like nasal CPAP, it requires placement of a nasopharyngeal tube or snugly fitting nasal prongs or mask. In addition to the CPAP effect of the ventilator, the patient's spontaneous breaths are assisted by patient-triggered or machine-triggered, time-cycled, positive pressure inflations. Although ventilators, equipped with proximal flow sensors, have been used for patient-triggered nasal IMV, appropriate triggering is difficult to obtain because of the large leaks that can occur between the patient airway and nasal interface.

Traditionally the most commonly used device for patient-triggered nasal IMV in neonates has been the Stars Synch abdominal capsule used with the Infrasonics Infant Star ventilator (Infrasonics Mallinckrodt, Inc., St Louis). The Infant Star ventilator is no longer being supported by the manufacturer; thus machine-triggered, N-IMV breath types are being used with apparent success. In two recent publications there were no clinically relevant differences in WOB and gas exchange or rate of patent ductus arteriosus, intraventricular hemorrhage, periventricular leukomalacia, retinopathy of prematurity, necrotizing enterocolitis, or death/BPD in neonates, comparing patient-triggered with machine-triggered breath types during N-IMV.[36,37] Suggested initial N-IMV settings in

neonates are inspiratory pressure of 16 to 20 cm H_2O, positive end-expiratory pressure (PEEP) of 4 to 6 cm H_2O, inspiratory time of 0.35 to 0.45 seconds, rate 40 to 60 breaths/min, and F_1O_2 adjusted to keep saturations 90% to 96%.[38] Subsequent adjustments in peak inspiratory pressure (PIP) are made to improve chest rise, and ventilator rate is adjusted to maintain CO_2 levels. Pressure support ventilation is typically not provided to assist spontaneous breaths because of large airway leaks and ineffective triggering.

Compared with standard CPAP approaches, N-IMV has been shown to improve chest wall stabilization and synchrony, reduce WOB and apnea, and promote better gas exchange. These physiological differences are likely related to the use of higher mean airway pressures and the ability to provide active stimulation and sighs to recruit airspaces and prevent apneic episodes during N-IMV.[39] In two separate clinical trials, premature neonates supported with patient-triggered N-IMV had fewer requirements for endotracheal intubation and less BPD than those supported by CPAP.[38,40] However, this form of support remains controversial. In a recent study, comparing N-CPAP to N-IMV in extremely low birth weight infants, the rate of survival to 36 weeks of age without bronchopulmonary dysplasia did not differ between the two forms of noninvasive support.[41] Additionally, there have been no reported risks of gastrointestinal insufflation or perforation related to the use of N-IMV in neonates. It has been suggested that the reduction in BPD from previous trials may be related to the absence of an ET and the natural pressure release created at the neonate's mouth and nasal airway, which may limit excessive pressure transmission to the distal airways during N-IMV.

Nasal "Sigh" Positive Airway Pressure in Neonates

Nasal "sigh" positive airway pressure (SiPAP, CareFusion, Viasys, San Diego, Calif.) (nasal SiPAP) (see Fig. 22-4) is a relatively new form of N-IPPV that is being used more frequently to assist spontaneously breathing infants in the NICU. Nasal SiPAP is different from other forms of NIV because it allows the neonate to breathe continuously at CPAP and during a sustained sigh breath to recruit lung units at two different lung volumes. Simply put, the neonate is able to breathe at a high and a low CPAP setting. The sum of alveolar ventilation depends on both the neonate's spontaneous minute ventilation and the minute ventilation created by nasal SiPAP when transitioning between the two preset CPAP levels. The higher CPAP level is generally set at 2 to 4 cm H_2O higher than the baseline CPAP pressure (4 to 6 cm H_2O), the breath hold at the higher CPAP level is set at 0.5 to 1 second, and the respiratory rate controls the frequency of the machine-triggered sigh breaths. The same nasal prongs, masks, and fluid-flip mechanism as the infant flow nasal CPAP is used during SiPAP. Several small preliminary clinical studies in neonates following extubation have demonstrated that SiPAP provides better gas exchange and results in less need for invasive mechanical ventilatory support than conventional CPAP without causing additional lung injury.[42,43] Compared with similar mean airway pressures as nasal continuous positive airway pressure (N-CPAP), SiPAP does not improve CO_2 removal or oxygenation. Thus it may be important to set the mean airway pressure higher than CPAP when using this form of support, especially if a patient is failing conventional CPAP.[44]

Noninvasive Nasal High-Frequency Ventilation in Neonates

Nasal high-frequency ventilation (N-HFV) has been used more commonly as a form of NIV in clinical practice over the last 5 years.

Unlike N-IMV and nasal SiPAP, N-HFV uses smaller pressures, higher frequencies, and may be more lung protective than other NIV devices that apply higher pressure to the lungs. The most common ventilator that has been used to apply N-HFV is the Infrasonics Infant Star ventilator. The N-HFV is applied using either a nasopharyngeal tube or binasal prongs with fixation. Unfortunately N-HFV is such a new form of NIV that there are very few published papers to suggest a strategy for long-term management of neonatal patients. Initial mean airway pressure is usually set to equal the previous level of CPAP, frequency is set at 10 HZ, and amplitude is adjusted to obtain visible chest wall vibration and increased every 30 minutes by 4 to 6 units, if necessary, to maintain clinically appropriate chest wall vibration or blood gases.[45] In one study, researchers demonstrated a significant reduction in P_aCO_2 in neonates that were transitioned from CPAP to short-term nasal HFV.[45] There is also potential that nasal HFV could provide better carbon dioxide elimination than N-IMV.[46] Another short-term study showed that nasal HFV promotes better alveolar growth and development in preterm lungs than invasive mechanical ventilation.[47,48] This research has stimulated a tremendous amount of interest in using nasal HFV as an initial form of ventilatory support for neonates failing CPAP and following extubation from mechanical ventilation. Although the widespread use of nasal HFV is not common, much-needed research will be required to evaluate whether nasal HFV reduces the need for intubation and the incidence of BPD in neonates with respiratory distress.

Continuous Positive Airway Pressure and Bilevel Positive Airway Pressure in Pediatric Patients

Although CPAP is used less often for pediatric patients than for adults, it is useful in children to restore FRC and reduce WOB with acute hypoxemia, neuromuscular disorders, and conditions that cause abdominal distention. It also is used to relieve the airway obstruction associated with obstructive sleep apnea or airway lesions like laryngotracheal malacia. The use of CPAP for many of these purposes follows the guidelines established for adults (see Chapters 13 and 19).

Some clinicians recommend the use of ventilator CPAP trials to help evaluate an intubated patient's readiness for extubation after a weaning period during mechanical ventilation. The intent of the CPAP trial is to evaluate spontaneous breathing. However, WOB can increase markedly when CPAP is provided through a small ET. When spontaneous breathing evaluations are performed, enough pressure support to overcome ET resistance should be provided, or ET resistance compensation, a feature found on some ventilators, should be used. This approach is explored in more detail in the chapter on weaning and discontinuation of mechanical ventilation (Chapter 20).

In addition, CPAP may be provided effectively through a tracheostomy tube. Patients who fatigue easily because of neuromuscular weakness, or who are susceptible to lung collapse seem to tolerate CPAP by tracheostomy tube, especially if continuous or nearly continuous support is needed.

In nonintubated patients, nasal prongs, a nasal mask, or a full face mask can be used in children through the toddler years. Nasal prongs that are designed for neonates are unable to be used in larger infants and toddlers. Furthermore, these patients may not be able to trigger the demand flow systems effectively in these devices. These factors pose a unique challenge for clinicians and manufacturers considering CPAP in this patient population. Children who

are 3 years old or older, who require CPAP, generally are encouraged to use a nasal mask. Some of these patients are better managed with a full face mask, especially if they require CPAP only intermittently. Pediatric patients with airway obstructions often benefit from CPAP. Certain obstructions, such as **tracheomalacia or bronchomalacia**, can make weaning from ventilation and extubation difficult. A decision may be made early in a patient's course to perform a tracheotomy and to apply CPAP on a 24-hour basis. Other patients with less severe obstructions may have difficulty breathing only when they are sleeping. These patients can avoid a tracheotomy and continue to rely on CPAP provided by nasal prongs. Many patients with obstructive lesions require surgery, and CPAP often is necessary until correction is complete.

Some patients have mechanical obstruction of the upper airway caused by soft tissue or excessive loss of muscle tone during sleep (i.e., obstructive sleep apnea [OSA]). OSA involves obstruction by either the tongue or the soft palate. Often CPAP can stent open these obstructions and dilate the oropharynx during sleep and reduce apnea.

The BiPAP system (Philips, Respironics, The Netherlands) delivers CPAP by nasal or full face mask to children and adolescents. This device is useful for patients with higher inspiratory flow rates and can overcome leaks at the mask by increasing flow. It also can monitor the tidal volume (V_T) and minute ventilation, and it provides high and low alarms, and high F_iO_2 levels.

Also CPAP systems are available for home use in patients who require chronic support. These units are recommended for nasal CPAP using nasal prongs, or a mask in older children and adults. Bilevel positive airway pressure units (e.g., Respironics BiPAP ST and S/T-D and Vision) also can be set to deliver CPAP. These units are recommended for adults and children older than 1 year who require little or no supplemental oxygen. Like home CPAP systems, these units are intended to be used with nasal prongs (pillows) or masks held in place by adjustable headgear.[47] The BiPAP unit can easily be switched from CPAP to BiPAP without modifications for patients who need additional support (Case Studies 22-1 and 22-2).[47]

The use of BiPAP systems and NIV, using critical care ventilators, has gained considerable popularity in the pediatric intensive care unit (PICU) settings as an alternative to invasive mechanical ventilation to support spontaneously breathing patients with acute respiratory failure and acute exacerbations of chronic lung disease. It is also being used to support patients, following extubation, who are difficult to wean from the ventilator, or are thought to have difficulties following extubation. Patients with acute exacerbation of asthma, acute respiratory distress syndrome (ARDS), cystic fibrosis, neuromuscular disorders, and respiratory infections (e.g., pneumonia) have been supported successfully using this approach.

Case Study 22-1

Assessment and Treatment of a Newborn

About 30 minutes ago, a 3.5-kg male infant was born prematurely. The footling breech presentation was delivered at term by cesarean section following 24 hours of labor. He currently is in the neonatal intensive care unit receiving blow-by oxygen. His respiratory rate ranges from about 67 to 83 breaths/min, he has a Silverman-Anderson score of 7, and his fingers and toes have a blue tinge. He periodically shows mild retractions. What steps would you take in the respiratory care of this infant?

Case Study 22-2

Adjustments to Home Therapy

A 2-year-old girl with spinal muscular atrophy (SMA) is on BiPAP at home. She has a gastrostomy tube, and her parents are the primary caregivers. She is taken to the emergency department for moderate respiratory distress. Breath sounds reveal coarse crackles throughout both lung fields. The S_pO_2 is 87% to 91% on room air; the respiratory rate is in the low 50s (breaths/min) and shallow, and the heart rate is 130 beats/min. The patient is afebrile.

The parents state that the patient was not tolerating the BiPAP because of a weak, persistent cough. They say she occasionally coughs up small amounts of thick white secretions. The father says that every time he applied the BiPAP mask, she began to cough and fight the BiPAP machine.

The respiratory therapist (RT) is asked to evaluate the patient and make recommendations. How should the RT proceed?

Suction, CPT - coughassist

Both BiPAP and NIV have been shown to improve gas exchange and reduce the need for invasive ventilation by 40% in pediatric patients with acute respiratory failure.[49] Inspiratory positive airway pressure (IPAP) settings are initially set very low and increased slowly to provide time for the patient to become comfortable and allow the clinician to assess accurately the reduction in WOB. The PEEP or EPAP settings are usually set between 4 and 10 cm H_2O. The maximum inspiratory pressure or IPAP level is dependent on patient size and lung pathology. Older pediatric patients may tolerate inspiratory pressure as high as 20 cm H_2O, but in all cases, a nasogastric or orogastric tube should be placed and small amounts of sedation should be considered to improve comfort. Gastric insufflation has been observed in pediatric patients (>1 year old) using inspiratory pressure greater than 15 cm H_2O with a full face mask.[50] However, larger patients may tolerate higher inspiratory pressure, but the patient should have a gastric tube and be monitored frequently for abdominal distention. In patients who do not tolerate this strategy, or continue to develop severe respiratory failure and poor gas exchange, invasive mechanical ventilation is indicated.

CONVENTIONAL MECHANICAL VENTILATION

Conventional mechanical ventilation or *invasive* mechanical ventilation involves the use of positive pressure inflations in intubated patients who are breathing spontaneously or who are heavily sedated or paralyzed. Many of the techniques for managing neonatal and pediatric patients during conventional mechanical ventilation have been based on adult strategies. Neonatal and pediatric patients present with a multitude of respiratory diseases that warrant fundamentally different ventilator approaches. There have been no large randomized clinical trials in this patient population to suggest that a particular ventilator mode or ventilator brand is preferable over another in managing different lung diseases. However, there is overwhelming agreement among clinicians that the management of such patients should be to avoid invasive ventilation whenever possible to minimize VILI. This section discusses the techniques most widely practiced in neonatal and pediatric

ventilator management. Clinicians working with children should always keep guidelines in mind, but they should also be able to "think outside the box" when faced with the unique challenges these patients sometimes present.

Indications for Ventilatory Support of Neonates

New advances in noninvasive ventilatory support have resulted in less frequent use of invasive ventilation; however, mechanical ventilation is a lifesaving intervention that remains an essential tool for managing neonates with respiratory failure. Infant mortality caused by respiratory distress syndrome in the United States decreased from ≈268 in 100,000 live births in 1971 to 98 in 100,000 live births in 1985[51] and 17 in 100,000 live births in 2007.[52] The decrease in mortality from 1971 to 1985 was in large part a result of the development and widespread availability of mechanical ventilators designed to work well in neonates. Approximately 2% of neonates born in the United States require mechanical ventilatory support at or shortly after birth.[52] About 75% of these patients are either VLBW neonates (i.e., weighing <1500 g), or are low birth weight (LBW) neonates (weighing 1500 to 2500 g).[53] As a result, ventilator care of the newborn is often an integral part of the broader management of premature infants.

Most newborns who require full ventilatory support are placed on infant ventilators or infant-through-adult ventilators specifically designed to respond to even the smallest patients. The indications for ventilation of neonates are listed in Box 22-2.[54]

Infants with very low Apgar scores who do not respond to initial resuscitation efforts may require early intubation and ventilatory support. Intubation and mechanical ventilatory support are usually necessary when an infant has been diagnosed with congenital anomalies that are likely to interfere with normal ventilatory function (e.g., diaphragmatic hernia, cardiac structural defects). The decision to provide mechanical ventilation for infants who do not have any of the previously described conditions is more subjective. The degree of respiratory distress is a valuable indicator even when ABG values are within acceptable ranges. Intercostal and substernal retractions, grunting, and nasal flaring are classic warning signs of impending ventilatory failure. Increasing supplemental oxygen requirements may be a sign that gas exchange is worsening. These indicators, along with the patient and maternal histories, often are more persuasive for initiation of ventilatory support than are laboratory data. Infants who are intubated for reasons other than respiratory failure often are sedated and mechanically ventilated for at least a short period. In many such cases, airway protection is the only indication for intubation. In other situations, sedation is required to alleviate discomfort during certain procedures. Whenever ETs are placed, the WOB from airway resistance can increase markedly. Even when these patients have sufficient drive to breathe spontaneously, minimum positive pressure or pressure support can help overcome ET resistance and help prevent lung collapse.

Indications for Ventilatory Support of Pediatric Patients

In contrast to premature infants, term infants and older pediatric patients have a wider variety of conditions requiring mechanical ventilatory support. One of every six term infants and children who are admitted to an intensive care unit (ICU) requires some form of mechanical ventilation. Airway obstruction is a common cause of intubation and ventilation. A study by the Pediatric Lung Injury and Sepsis Network found that 13.5% of children requiring

BOX 22-2	Clinical Indications for Invasive Mechanical Ventilation in Neonates[54]

The presence of one or more of the following conditions constitutes an indication for mechanical ventilation:

- Respiratory failure despite the use of continuous positive airway pressure (CPAP), noninvasive positive pressure ventilation (NPPV), and supplemental oxygen (i.e., fractional inspired oxygen [F_IO_2] of 0.6 or higher)
- Respiratory acidosis with a pH <7.25
- Partial pressure of arterial oxygen (P_aO_2) <50 mm Hg
- Abnormalities on physical examination:
  - Increased work of breathing, demonstrated by grunting, nasal flaring, tachypnea, and sternal and intercostal retractions
  - Pale or cyanotic skin and agitation
- Neurologic alterations that compromise the central drive to breathe
  - Apnea of prematurity
  - Intracranial hemorrhage
  - Congenital neuromuscular disorders
- Impaired respiratory function that compromises the functional residual capacity (FRC) as a result of decreased lung compliance and/or increased airway resistance, including but not limited to:
  - Respiratory distress syndrome
  - Meconium aspiration syndrome
  - Congenital pneumonia
  - Bronchopulmonary dysplasia
  - Bronchiolitis
  - Congenital diaphragmatic hernia
  - Sepsis
- Impaired cardiovascular function
  - Persistent pulmonary hypertension of the newborn
  - Postresuscitation state
  - Congenital heart disease
  - Shock
- Postoperative state characterized by impaired ventilatory function

BOX 22-3	Indications for Use of Mechanical Ventilation in Pediatric Patients[57]

Respiratory Failure
- Partial pressure of arterial carbon dioxide (P_aCO_2) over 50 to 60 mm Hg
- Partial pressure of arterial oxygen (P_aO_2) under 70 mm Hg

Neuromuscular or Hypotonic Disorder
- Muscular dystrophies
- Spinal muscular atrophy
- Guillain-Barré syndrome
- Myasthenia gravis

Intrinsic Pulmonary Disease
- Viral/bacterial pneumonia
- Aspiration pneumonia
- Asthma

Increased Intracranial Pressure
- Direct trauma
- Diabetic ketoacidosis

Near-drowning
Infection
Neurologic Disorders
- Seizure disorders

Postoperative Management
- Surgical procedures involving the head, neck, chest, or abdomen

mechanical ventilation for longer than 24 hours were intubated as a result of airway obstruction.[19] The most frequently diagnosed cause of respiratory failure in children under 1 year old was bronchiolitis; in children older than 1 year, pneumonia was most often the cause.[55,56]

Recognizing the need for ventilatory support in older pediatric patients involves many of the same criteria used to assess adult patients. Compared with adults, children have a limited capacity for compensation of acute illness and are more likely to develop respiratory distress with apnea and hypoxemia early. In pediatric patients, ventilation that is insufficient to provide adequate gas exchange is determined primarily by ABG results and additional clinical assessments. This clinical condition has many possible causes (Box 22-3).[57]

The Pediatric Ventilator

Ventilators designed for infants and small children have been available since the late 1960s. Even with the availability of neonatal care units, many clinicians used adult models for neonates and small pediatric patients through the 1970s and early 1980s. They were more familiar with adult units and often found it difficult to justify

financially the purchase of a ventilator that could be used only for a limited number of patients. Most current-generation, microprocessor-controlled ventilator platforms can provide seamless ventilation for any size of patient, from premature newborns to adults. A single ventilator for all patient sizes and age ranges may provide several advantages related to institutional cost, training, and patient safety. Commercially available neonatal and pediatric ventilators should incorporate the essential features described in Box 22-4.

Current-generation ventilators also provide several choices of modes, including volume-controlled continuous mandatory ventilation (VC-CMV), pressure-controlled continuous mandatory ventilation (PC-CMV), volume-controlled intermittent mandatory ventilation (VC-IMV), pressure-controlled intermittent mandatory ventilation (PC-IMV), CPAP, and pressure support ventilation (PSV). In the last decade other forms of volume-targeted or hybrid modes of ventilation, known as dual-controlled CMV (DC-CMV), dual-controlled IMV (DC-IMV), and dual-controlled PSV (DC-PSV), have been used successfully.

For nearly 30 years, infants were ventilated with infant-specific, time-cycled, pressure-limited, intermittent mandatory ventilation (TCPL/IMV) breaths. Unlike current microprocessor-controlled ventilators, these TCPL/IMV ventilators used a preset continuous flow of an oxygen–air mixture. The patient could breathe from the flow during spontaneous breaths but was unable to trigger mandatory breaths from the ventilator (Fig. 22-6, *A*). In this design, a machine-triggered positive pressure breath resulted when the machine's exhalation valve closed, permitting the gas mixture to flow to the patient (Fig. 22-6, *B*). When a preset inspiratory pressure was reached, the pressure was maintained until the ventilator time cycled into expiration (Fig. 22-6, *C*). When the exhalation valve opened, the expiratory phase began. As long as the exhalation

Essential Features for Commercially Available Neonatal/Pediatric Ventilators[47]

- Pressure-controlled ventilation (PC), volume-controlled ventilation (VC), pressure support ventilation (PSV), and dual-controlled ventilation (DC) modes
- Continuous mandatory ventilation (CMV), intermittent mandatory ventilation (IMV), and continuous spontaneous ventilation (CSV)
- Flow or pressure triggering
- Visible and audible alarms for high and low pressures and volumes
- High-pressure release to ambient capability
- Visible and audible alarms for low and high oxygen concentrations
- Visible and audible alarms for loss of power and gas source
- Servo-regulated humidifier with low-compressible-volume water chamber and continuous-feed water supply system
- Low compliance ventilator circuit and/or capability for ventilator to measure and subtract compressible volume from delivered and monitored volume displays
- Proximal flow sensor (essential for neonatal patients) or compliance factor (sufficient for larger patients)
- Mechanism to drain water condensate from circuit or heated inspiratory/expiratory circuit limbs

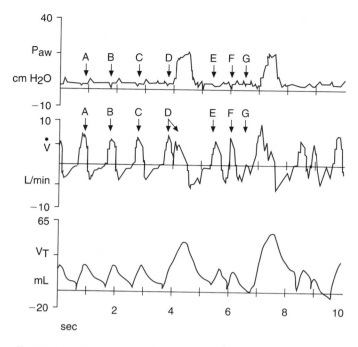

Fig. 22-7 Time-triggered, pressure-limited, time-cycled ventilation (TPTV) with inadequate patient triggering of mechanical breaths (see text for explanation). (From Wilson BG, Cheifetz IM, Meliones JN: Optimizing mechanical ventilation in infants and children, Palm Springs, Calif., 1995, Bird Products.)

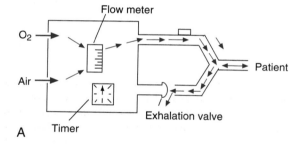

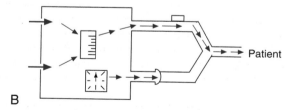

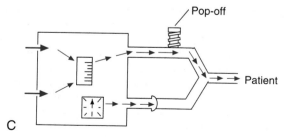

Fig. 22-6 Schematic for a continuous flow neonatal ventilator circuit. **A,** Spontaneous phase. **B,** Inspiratory phase. **C,** Pressure-limiting phase. (From Koff PA, Gitzman D, Neu J, editors: Neonatal and pediatric respiratory care, ed 2, St Louis, 1993, Mosby.)

valve remained open, a constant flow of the gas mixture passed by the patient's airway and was available for spontaneous breathing.[57] The ventilator's inability to permit patient triggering of mandatory breaths during spontaneous respiratory efforts led to asynchrony in spontaneously breathing patients. Nonetheless, the operation of previous TCPL/IMV ventilators still serves as a simple conceptual model for explaining the fundamental operation of neonatal mechanical ventilators and the major advances in pediatric mechanical ventilation.

Neonates that exhibit asynchrony during TCPL/IMV are at an increased risk for developing intraventricular hemorrhage and possibly pneumothorax. Heavy sedation and paralytic drugs (e.g., pancuronium) may reduce these risks, but these drugs also pose potential complications that may prolong ventilator support.[58] In Fig. 22-7, initial patient efforts (breaths *A, B,* and *C*) appear to be synchronous; however, when a mandatory breath (breath *D*) is delivered on top of a spontaneous breath, the ensuing spontaneous breaths (breaths *E, F,* and *G*) are asynchronous. A mandatory breath delivered in the middle of a spontaneous breath can result in breath stacking. When flow triggering is used, mandatory breaths can be delivered between spontaneous breaths, resulting in better patient-machine synchrony with a reduction in WOB and caloric and sedation requirements (Fig. 22-8).[59] Although some current pediatric ventilators still allow the option to use a preset continuous flow during PC-CMV and VC-CMV, machine-triggered TCPL/IMV has been replaced with patient-triggered PC-IMV.

Major improvements in ventilator technology now provide the ability for even the smallest patients to be able to control sophisticated demand flow systems to improve triggering and synchrony with mandatory ventilator breaths. Patients can trigger breaths based on a pressure or flow change that is sensed by the ventilator.

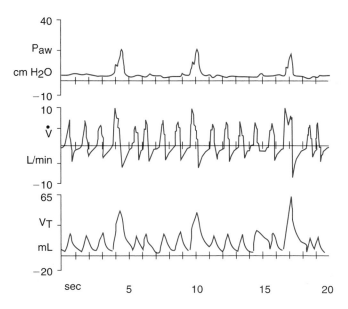

Fig. 22-8 Same patient as in Figure 22-6; flow triggering has improved patient-ventilator synchrony. (From Wilson BG, Cheifetz IM, Meliones JN: Optimizing mechanical ventilation in infants and children, Palm Springs, Calif., 1995, Bird Products.)

Flow sensing is more sensitive and allows better synchronization than pressure triggering in neonates.[60,61] Additionally, patient triggering may reduce the need for heavy sedation and paralytics during mechanical ventilation. Compared with earlier forms of nontriggered ventilation, patient-triggered ventilation is associated with a shorter duration of ventilation.

Because all ventilators now provide patient-triggered ventilation, the term *PC-IMV* has replaced the previously used TCPL/IMV constant-flow mode. As such, synchronized intermittent mandatory ventilation, or SIMV, and assist/controlled, or A/C, have been replaced with IMV and CMV, respectively.[62] Additionally, mandatory breaths denote fully supported ventilator breaths (i.e., PC-CMV, VC-CMV), and can be initiated by the patient or by the ventilator and terminated based on time, whereas spontaneous breaths are always initiated and terminated by the spontaneously breathing patient (i.e., CPAP, PSV). During CMV every breath from the ventilator is mandatory, or fully supported, whereas during IMV the patient can breathe using both mandatory and spontaneous breath types. Each manufacturer may use completely different names to differentiate modes and breath types, and as a result, there is great confusion among clinicians, educators, researchers, and manufacturers about mode classification. Efforts are being made to standardize ventilator mode classification based on the approach used in this discussion.[62]

Another important advancement in neonatal and pediatric ventilators has been the development of the accurate measurement of airflow and tidal volumes in very small patients. This allows possible improved methods for measuring dynamic compliance, static compliance, airway resistance, and airway waveform graphics on mechanical ventilators. A complete understanding of lung mechanics and airway graphics may eliminate a lot of conjecture in managing patients on a mechanical ventilator. Tidal volume and airway graphics are usually obtained by using proximal airway sensors that measure airflow at the connection of the ventilator's circuit and the patient's artificial airway. It has been shown that ventilators

that do not measure tidal volume with a sensor at the proximal airway produce measurements that are not sufficiently accurate to use for managing the ventilator in neonates.[63] Thus the most useful neonatal-capable ventilators are those that have proximal airway flow sensors for accurate determination of tidal volume, lung mechanics, and airway graphics. The use of a proximal flow sensor also allows more precise flow triggering and graphics monitoring than those provided at the ventilator valve. It is important to mention that a major limitation of proximal flow sensors is that condensation and secretions can form on the flow-sensing elements. Clinicians must remain wary of this limitation and replace or clean flow sensors when changes in the airway graphics are observed.

Additional features or enhancements can make ventilators more useful in a wide range of clinical situations (Box 22-5). Many ventilators have advanced features that allow clinicians to modify the gas flow within the breath to fine-tune or improve patient-ventilator synchrony and gas delivery. The slope, or *rise-time*, setting is an advanced feature that can be used during pressure control, dual-control, and pressure support ventilation to adjust the aggressiveness of initial gas delivery at the start of the breath. A fast rise time and rapid pressurization may reduce asynchrony in patients with high flow requirements, and a slow rise provides slower and hence more laminar gas delivery during inhalation (Fig. 22-9).

Flow cycling is another feature that allows patients to terminate the breath based on flow rather than on time. Flow cycling is described in greater detail later in this chapter. Sophisticated leak-compensation algorithms are available for invasive and

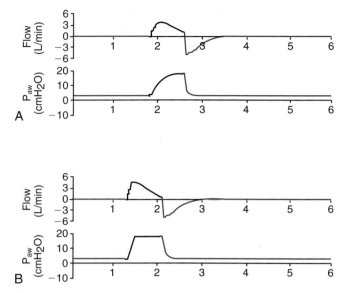

Fig. 22-9 A, Shows a child receiving pressure-controlled continuous mandatory ventilation (PC-CMV) with a slow rise to peak inspiratory pressure because the slope setting on the CareFusion AVEA is set to 9. **B,** In the same child, there is a rapid rise to peak inspiratory pressure because the slope setting is set on 1. The set inspiratory pressure is the same for both breaths.

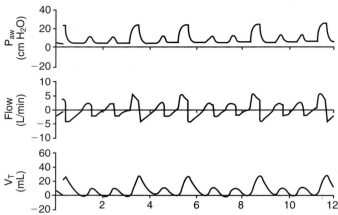

Fig. 22-10 This graphical waveform shows pressure, flow, and tidal volume in a neonate receiving patient-triggered pressure-controlled intermittent mandatory ventilation (PC-IMV) (larger inspiratory pressure breaths) with the addition of PS breaths (smaller inspiratory pressure breaths).

noninvasive ventilation. When this option is activated, loss of end-expiratory pressure caused by an ET leak triggers the addition of flow to the ventilator circuit to maintain constant PEEP. Some ventilators have also incorporated leak compensation during inhalation to provide stable volume delivery in the presence of large ET leaks. The potential advantages of this feature are discussed in a later section.

As respiratory monitoring has grown more comprehensive and sophisticated, sensing adapters at the proximal airway have become necessary. With some ventilator models, monitoring of end-tidal CO_2 and flow–volume loops require two airway sensors. These sensors add extra weight to the ET, which can lead to excessive tube movement and possibly accidental extubation. These devices can also add dead space to the system, resulting in excessive accumulation in carbon dioxide at the airway and consequent increases in ventilation requirement. Ventilator and monitor manufacturers have addressed this clinical problem and are including integrated end-tidal CO_2/volume monitoring sensors in the mechanical ventilator.

Pressure Control Mode

This section discusses PC-CMV and other applications of ventilator modes commonly used in pediatric settings (see Chapter 5 for a detailed description of ventilator modes.) Disease-specific management strategies, using these modes, will be described in a later section.

The most widely used mode of ventilation in neonates and pediatric patients is PC-CMV. The PC-CMV breath can be triggered by pressure or flow and is terminated based on time. Because pressure is constant, the tidal volume delivery can vary widely as a result of changes in lung mechanics and respiratory effort. PC-IMV is very similar to TCPL/IMV with some subtle but clinically important differences. It usually is not incorporated into a continuous-flow generator, although a small bias flow might be

present to allow flow-triggered (or patient-triggered) breaths. The major difference is that inspiratory flow is variable and can be much greater in this mode, resulting in an almost immediate rise to peak pressure. Furthermore, if a patient generates spontaneous inspiratory efforts within the breath, the demand valve opens to provide additional flow to maintain constant inspiratory pressure for the duration of the inspiratory time. Additionally, the demand valve will also provide additional flow in the presence of leaky ETs to maintain airway pressure constant. This mode has long been preferred for pediatric and adult patients in clinical situations in which ventilation or oxygenation (or both) is particularly difficult. Because there is a rapid rise to inspiratory pressure, the mean airway pressure tends to be higher than volume control where peak pressure varies and reaches a maximum in the last part of the breath. The theoretical advantage of PC-CMV lies in the characteristics of its inspiratory phase. Lungs with varying time constants may benefit from an early rise to peak pressure by rapid inspiratory flow and a subsequent period of decreased flow, which allows gas to be distributed more evenly to areas of the lung with both long and short time constants. In this way, improved gas distribution to underventilated areas can be achieved with limited distention of well-ventilated areas.

Most ventilators that provide PC-IMV also provide pressure-supported breaths for spontaneously breathing patients. This combination, sometimes called *mixed-mode ventilation,* allows patients to assume the breathing load better when lowering the frequency of mandatory breaths during the weaning phase (Fig. 22-10). The results of one study suggest that the addition of pressure support as a supplement to PC-IMV may play a role in reducing the duration of mechanical ventilation and oxygen dependency in VLBW neonates.[64]

In PC-CMV, minimizing $\overline{P}_{aw}$ is essential in patients with exceptional oxygenation. The ventilator frequency should only be high enough to reach the desired P_aCO_2, and inspiratory pressure is adjusted in increments of 1 to 2 cm H_2O to keep the monitored exhaled tidal volume values within an acceptable range. The I:E ratio initially should be 1:3 to 1:2. Changes in blood gas values often take time with PC-CMV; only a few setting changes are made at one time, and sufficient time is allowed before the patient's response is evaluated.

Inspiratory Pressure

This section discusses the controls, monitoring systems, and alarms used in pressure control mode. Some of these principles can also be applied to other modes of ventilation.

While ventilating a child with a manual resuscitator or T-piece device with an airway pressure manometer inline, it is good practice for the clinician to evaluate bilateral lung aeration and chest movement and to note the average inspiratory pressure required. This average is the starting point for placing the child on the ventilator, especially if manual ventilation at this inspiratory pressure has optimized the child's skin color and oxygen saturation. Traditionally, the inspiratory pressure has been adjusted based on adequate chest rise and blood gas values. Today, the patient is connected to the ventilator circuit and exhaled tidal volume is evaluated as a guide for further inspiratory pressure adjustments. This practice has resulted in less need for blood gases because the rate is the primary adjustment for CO_2 elimination. Once the inspiratory pressure is set to deliver a preferred tidal volume, the rate is the primary adjustment for CO_2 elimination. Pressure–volume loops are helpful in setting the optimum inspiratory pressure. The rising inspiratory pressure produces an almost linear increase in volume; therefore a peak appears in the loop's configuration at the point where inspiration ends and expiration begins. However, if the volume rise of the loop begins to flatten with a continued increase in the inspiratory pressure, overdistention is likely (Fig. 22-11). If this occurs, the inspiratory pressure should be reduced until little or no flattening of the loop occurs. Because lung mechanics can change rapidly, this graphic display should be rechecked routinely and the inspiratory pressure adjusted as necessary.[65] When the set inspiratory pressure is lowered, PEEP may need to be increased to maintain acceptable oxygenation. However, when PEEP is increased, it is important to observe the effect of this action on the exhaled tidal volume and the pressure–volume loop relationship. (See Chapter 9 for more information on pressure–volume loops.)

Positive End-Expiratory Pressure

Positive end-expiratory pressure, or PEEP, is used to establish the FRC and prevent alveolar collapse. In some conditions, such as asthma, increasing PEEP may reduce airway resistance and provide better patient triggering. The appropriate level of PEEP can greatly improve oxygenation, reduce ventilation/perfusion ($\dot{V}/\dot{Q}$), mismatching, and transpulmonary shunting, and increase compliance. Because of the transmission of pressure to the intrapleural space, excessive PEEP can increase pulmonary vascular resistance, which

can lead to reduced venous return to the heart, reduced cardiac output, and an increase in dead space (see Chapter 13). The increase in dead space alerts the clinician that the PEEP level might be excessive. The patient's P_aCO_2 may increase even though the minute ventilation ($\dot{V}_E$) remains unchanged. High PEEP levels and consequent hyperinflation may contribute to traumatic lung injury, such as pulmonary interstitial emphysema (PIE) and other air-leak syndromes (see Chapter 17). The effects of PEEP should be closely monitored, especially when lung mechanics improve. PEEP usually is set initially at 4 to 7 cm H_2O. PEEP levels above 7 cm H_2O occasionally are necessary, but they should be used with caution in infants who have diseases with obstructive components, such as bronchiolitis or meconium aspiration syndrome (MAS). Careful inspection of chest radiographs for adequate lung inflation and signs of hyperinflation are vital to monitoring the effects of PEEP.

The clinician should consider increasing the PEEP level when the oxygen requirement exceeds an F_IO_2 of 0.6 to maintain a P_aO_2 greater than 50 mm Hg. Long before this point, however, the chest radiograph may show decreasing lung volumes. Therefore the need for higher PEEP levels may be recognized before worsening ABG values are seen. Patients who undergo surgical procedures that result in high abdominal girths often require higher than usual levels of PEEP to restore baseline lung volumes.

In patients with surfactant deficiency syndromes (e.g., IRDS; ARDS), the pressure–volume loop of a positive pressure breath may show a rapid rise in pressure with a delayed rise in volume (Fig. 22-12, A). Increasing the PEEP may result in a more immediate rise in volume for the pressure delivered (Fig. 22-12, B).[65] This improvement in volume delivery is associated with the critical opening pressure of various lung units. As more PEEP is applied, progressively more lung units may be opened and recruited.

Ventilator graphics, particularly the pressure–volume loop (Fig. 22-13), show how appropriately applied levels of PEEP can improve compliance. Favorable responses to increasing PEEP levels include a shift of the loop to the left, an increase in V_T at the same inspiratory pressure, and an increase in P_aO_2.[59]

Inspiratory Time, Expiratory Time, and Inspiratory-to-Expiratory Ratio

Lung mechanics must be considered when the inspiratory time (T_I), expiratory time (T_E), and I:E ratio are set, especially for patients with surfactant deficiency. These patients are likely to have a low C_L with normal R_{aw}; therefore the T_I must be short. Because R_{aw} usually is normal in this scenario, allowing extra time for

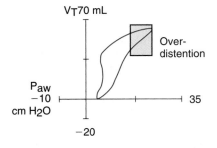
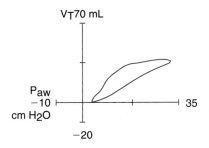

Fig. 22-11 Pressure–volume loop showing overdistention. In the pressure–volume loop on the left, the increase in volume begins to lose its linearity as the inspiratory pressure approaches its set limit. The shaded area indicates a small increase in volume even though pressure continues to increase. In the example on the right, a more linear waveform exists without evidence of overdistention. (From Nicks JJ: Graphics monitoring in the neonatal intensive care unit, Palm Springs, Calif., 1995, Bird Products.)

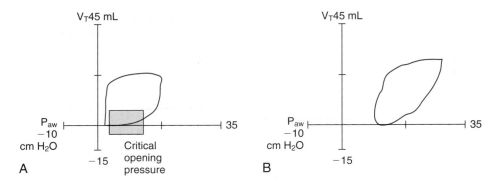

Fig. 22-12 Effects of an increase in positive end-expiratory pressure (PEEP) on critical opening pressure. **A,** Volume delivery is delayed until the pressure has increased significantly, indicating a high critical opening pressure. **B,** When PEEP is increased, volume delivery begins earlier in the inspiratory phase. P_{aw}, Airway pressure; V_T, Tidal volume. (From Nicks JJ: Graphics monitoring in the neonatal intensive care unit, Palm Springs, Calif., 1995, Bird Products.)

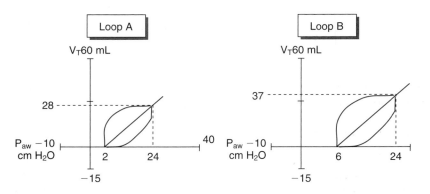

Fig. 22-13 Effect of increasing positive end-expiratory pressure (PEEP) on pressure–volume loop slope and tidal volume (V_T) (see text for more information). P_{aw}, Airway pressure. (From Wilson BG, Cheifetz IM, Meliones JN: Optimizing mechanical ventilation in infants and children, Palm Springs, Calif., 1995, Bird Products.)

inspiratory gas to traverse the airways is not necessary. However, because compliance is low, small volumes must be used to inflate the lungs quickly. Because elastic forces are high, expiration is also relatively fast. Lungs with these mechanical characteristics are said to have short time constants (see Chapter 1). One time constant is calculated by multiplying the R_{aw} by the C_L (Box 22-6). Historically, neonates and pediatric patients with short time constants (e.g., in RDS, ARDS) have been ventilated using long T_I, and hence, higher mean airway pressure, to promote better oxygenation. Although this approach may work well in chemically paralyzed and sedated patients, long T_I may cause an inspiratory breath hold to occur when the patient is breathing spontaneously. In a summary of studies conducted in neonates with restrictive lung disease, long T_I was associated with a significant increase in air leak and mortality.[66]

A prolonged T_I can be identified, using airway graphics, as a period where inspiratory flow decays to zero and pressure is held in the lung during a PC-CMV breath (Fig. 22-14). This subtle phenomenon is often overlooked and is a major cause of asynchrony during PC-CMV. A breath hold can be avoided by reducing the inspiratory time so that the breath is terminated just before zero inspiratory flow. Newer ventilators allow the clinician to set an adjustable flow cycle parameter during PC-CMV (Fig. 22-15). Flow cycling essentially allows an otherwise time-cycled, PC-CMV breath to cycle to flow, much like a PSV breath, and T_I can be

---

BOX 22-6 Calculation of a Time Constant

If airway resistance (R_{aw}) is 30 cm H_2O/L/sec and lung compliance (C_L) is 0.004 L/cm H_2O, the time constant (TC) is calculated as follows:

$$TC = R_{aw} \times C_L$$
$$TC = 30 \text{ cm } H_2O/L/sec \times 0.004 \text{ L/cm } H_2O$$
$$TC = 0.12 \text{ sec}$$

---

monitored during spontaneous breathing. At times a patient-triggered exhalation or flow cycling can result in a dramatic reduction in WOB and P_aCO_2. Some clinicians will leave the flow cycle parameter on, whereas others will disable it and use the previously measure T_I as the new T_I setting during PC-CMV. It is important to realize that time constants in the lungs can change rapidly; thus flow cycling during PC-CMV may change the inspiratory time dramatically as compliance is reduced, resulting in lower mean airway pressure and lower tidal volume delivery.

Conditions that result in airflow limitation generally have longer inspiratory and expiratory time constants, which can be a factor in the inability to deliver the desired V_T and $\dot{V}_E$ (see Fig. 22-15) during PC-CMV. In severe asthma, for example, gas-flow limitation can affect inspiratory and expiratory flow as well as V_T

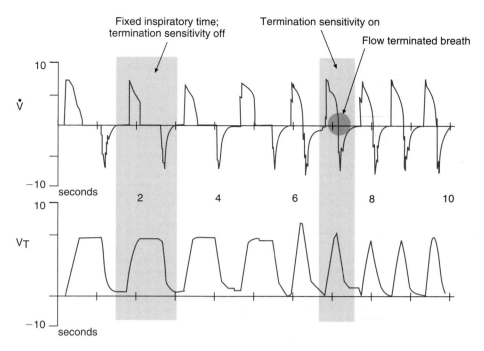

Fig. 22-14 Assist/control (A/C) pressure-controlled ventilation using the flow cycle feature. The flow cycle is off for the first four breaths, and each breath is time cycled. When flow cycle is activated, the breath terminates when a predetermined decrease in flow is sensed at the airway. V_T, Tidal volume. (Modified from Nicks JJ: Graphics monitoring in the neonatal intensive care unit, Palm Springs, Calif., 1995, Bird Products.)

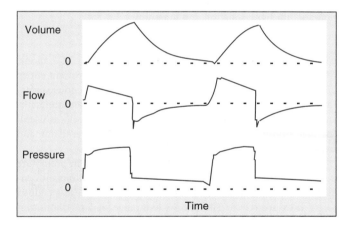

Fig. 22-15 Pressure-controlled ventilation with severe inspiratory airflow limitation. Note that with each breath, the peak pressure is reached and the inspiratory phase time cycles before flow can decelerate to zero.

volume delivery. Because as much time as possible must be allowed for the expiratory phase in such clinical situations, the clinician often must keep T_I at 25% to 33% of the total cycle time (TCT). In doing so the limitation of inspiratory flow may be so great that the flow does not decelerate to zero as it normally does, which means that the inspiratory phase would time limit, delivering a smaller V_T than if the flow had been permitted to taper to zero. Such a phenomenon, called *flow chop* by some clinicians, is unavoidable in some situations, especially if a longer TCT (and thus a lower $\dot{V}_E$) cannot be tolerated. Many clinicians advocate a permissive hypercapnia ventilation strategy in severe reactive airway disease (discussed later). To accomplish this, a small V_T is selected, in addition to a low $\dot{V}_E$, a low rate, an inspiratory time sufficient to

eliminate flow chop, and an expiratory time sufficient to achieve zero or near-zero expiratory flow. However, this strategy and the recommended settings are controversial and may not be suitable for some patients, leaving no alternative but to accept the presence of some flow chop. Because airway dynamics can change quickly and dramatically and changes in V_T and $\dot{V}_E$ are directly affected, flow chop must be monitored carefully (Case Study 22-3).

Case Study 22-3

Patient Case—Acute Status Asthmaticus

A 7-year-old boy in acute status asthmaticus has not responded to treatment consisting of continuous albuterol aerosol therapy, intravenous (IV) Solu-Medrol, IV terbutaline, and two injections of magnesium sulfate. He has just been intubated with a 5-mm internal diameter (ID) endotracheal tube and placed on a CareFusion AVEA ventilator. He has been paralyzed and sedated and is being ventilated in the pressure control mode with a 60/40 helium-oxygen mixture. Ventilator settings are: PIP/PEEP = 24/5 cm H_2O, respiratory rate = 16 breaths/min, inspiratory time = 0.9 seconds.

The patient's expired V_T is 3 mL/kg. The end-tidal partial pressure of carbon dioxide ($P_{ET}CO_2$) is 92 mm Hg, and the S_pO_2 is 88%. The RT has increased inspiratory pressure in increments of 2 cm H_2O to 32 cm H_2O, but the V_T has not changed. An ABG sample has been sent to the laboratory.

What additional monitoring should the RT consider with this patient? What other setting changes should the RT recommend?

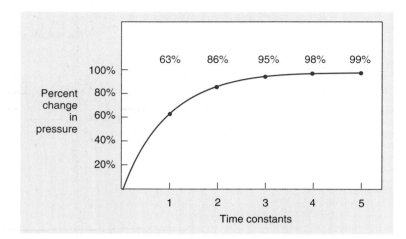

Fig. 22-16 Percentage change in pressure in relation to time (in time constants) allowed for equilibration. As the time allowed for equilibration increases, so does the percentage change in pressure. The same applies to the equilibration for changes in volume.

Nearly complete equilibration of alveolar pressures (P_{alv}) occurs in 3 to 5 time constants (Fig. 22-16). In infant lungs with normal mechanics, equilibration occurs in at least 0.6 seconds (time constant $\times$ 5 = ($R_{aw} \times C_L$) $\times$ 5 = (30 cm H_2O/L/sec $\times$ 0.004 L/cm H_2O) $\times$ 5 = 0.6 sec). Less time is needed for lung inflation in surfactant-deficient lungs, in which the time constant is shorter. Therefore the T_I can be set for a short interval and the respiratory frequency can be set high with less concern for breath stacking and hyperinflation.[67]

The concept of time constants can easily be related to the clinical situation by evaluating the spontaneous ventilatory pattern of a premature infant with RDS. The patient's spontaneous WOB is high because of low C_L and high alveolar surface tension. The spontaneous rate may be high and V_T low. T_I and T_E are very short, and inspiratory flow is high. Short time constants are responsible for this familiar ventilatory pattern and are considered when the ventilator's T_I and T_E are set. However, ventilator settings should not simulate a patient's spontaneous breathing pattern, particularly when the TCPL mode is used. It is estimated that infants with RDS can have time constants as short as 0.05 second, which means that the ideal T_I is 0.25 second.[67] On the other hand, when acute lung disease makes adequate oxygenation difficult, lengthening the T_I and increasing the $\overline{P}_{aw}$ can increase the P_aO_2.[68] **Bronchopulmonary dysplasia** (BPD) is an example of a pulmonary disease of infants in which high R_{aw} is a major component. Time constants for BPD are estimated to be as high as 0.5 seconds.[67] The longer time constants associated with this disorder require careful manipulation of ventilator controls to provide for long inflation and even longer deflation times. Although a patient's compliance and R_{aw} cannot be measured precisely, characteristics of the disease are used to guide the clinician in matching ventilator settings with a patient's inherent ventilatory pattern and in promoting better patient-ventilator synchrony.

With time constants in mind, the I : E ratio usually is set between 1 : 2 and 1 : 3 in surfactant deficiency syndromes. If an infant's gas exchange does not improve with these ratios, other techniques may be considered, such as high-frequency ventilation. Inverse ratios are rarely used in PC-CMV because of the risk of hyperinflation and lung trauma. Waveform monitoring is useful for determining the most appropriate T_I and T_E ventilator settings. The expiratory flow waveform does not return to baseline before the next positive pressure breath is delivered in patients with increased expiratory resistance (Fig. 22-17). Although treatment (e.g., bronchodilator therapy) may improve the patient's expiratory flow, manipulation of the I : E ratio to extend the T_E may also permit lung emptying before the next breath. Recognizing this problem and taking the appropriate steps to correct it are important for reducing the potential for hyperinflation and lung injury.[69]

Tidal Volume

Tidal volume is not a set parameter in the PC-CMV mode. Mechanical V_T depends on T_I, lung mechanics, and patient effort. Changes in compliance after administration of exogenous surfactant are almost immediately reflected in direct V_T measurements. In addition, noting trends in an infant's spontaneous V_T is useful for determining readiness for weaning from the ventilator and extubation.

Cuffless ETs are still used in neonates, especially in premature patients. Leaks around the tube are common. Most clinicians consider small leaks (<20%) acceptable and even desirable as an added safety pressure release site and as assurance that no significant inflammation is present around the tube. When leaks are present, the V_T monitor can be used to assess the difference between delivered and expired V_T (V_{Texh}). This loss of volume often is expressed as the *percent leak,* which can be calculated with the following formula:

$$\text{Percent leak} = [(V_{Tinsp} - V_{Texh})/V_{Tinsp}] \times 100$$

where V_{Tinsp} is the inspired V_T and V_{Texh} is the expired (exhaled) V_T.

Some ventilators calculate and display the percent leak. Other monitors display V_{Tinsp} and V_{Texh}. Volume monitoring also provides an important safety measure by alerting clinicians to sudden drops in expired $\dot{V}_E$. A small leak or an obstructed ET is more easily detected when these monitors are used. Low-pressure alarms, although important, are not as sensitive to all alarm conditions involving a reduction of effective ventilation. High pressure and respiratory rate in addition to low tidal volume, and low exhaled $\dot{V}_E$, may also alert clinicians to serious conditions that arise during ventilation.

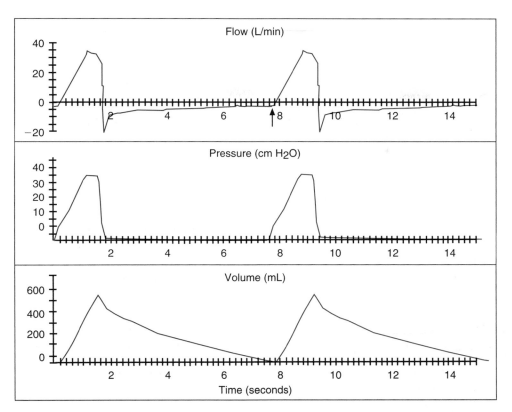

Fig. 22-17 Prolonged expiratory flow pattern in a patient with auto-positive end-expiratory pressure (auto-PEEP). Prolonged expiratory flow can lead to breath stacking and hyperinflation. Expiratory gas flow shows an initial spike downward and then changes to a low level of flow, which continues throughout the expiratory phase. Expiratory flow does not return to baseline before the next breath. (From Wilkins RL, Stoller JK, Kacmarek RM: Egan's fundamentals of respiratory care, ed 9, St Louis, 2009, Mosby.)

Frequency

The initial frequency setting can be gauged, while the infant is manually ventilated before being connected to the ventilator, just as an initial inspiratory pressure can be determined by clinical assessment. Trying out different frequencies can help determine the initial setting to achieve the best S_pO_2 and vital signs. Airway graphics are a very helpful resource in determining the proper frequency setting. Higher rates can result in gas trapping, thus complete exhalation should be noted on flow scalars when setting the initial frequency and with subsequent adjustments. However, a blood gas or a transcutaneous CO_2 monitor that correlates well with P_aCO_2 is the standard method used to adjust frequency. Noting the patient's $\dot{V}_E$ and relating it to the P_aCO_2 is important. Once the initial P_aCO_2 is known, it, along with the desired P_aCO_2, can be used to calculate an appropriate change in V_T or frequency. These calculations may not work well for all clinical purposes, but they serve well in larger pediatric patients. (These calculations are discussed in Chapter 12.)

Although pulse oximeters have replaced transcutaneous monitors as noninvasive means of monitoring oxygenation in infants, transcutaneous CO_2 monitors can provide trending information about alveolar ventilation. Even though transcutaneous CO_2 may not correlate all of the time, a rapid change in transcutaneous CO_2 could warn clinicians to a serious condition, whereas a blood gas may take time to get results. For instance, a gradual reduction in transcutaneous CO_2 following surfactant administration may alert the clinician to observe exhaled tidal volumes and compliance, and possibly wean inspiratory pressures during PC-CMV. Monitoring of the transcutaneous partial pressure of carbon dioxide ($P_{tc}CO_2$) gives the clinician valuable baseline and trending information before a switch is made from a conventional ventilator to a high-frequency ventilator. This information, which is particularly valuable in patients with severe lung disease, can be used to stabilize the patient on high-frequency ventilation (see the section on high-frequency ventilation later in the chapter).

Mean Airway Pressure

Conventional ventilators do not have a $\overline{P}_{aw}$ setting; rather this is a monitored parameter that must be closely watched. Increases in $\overline{P}_{aw}$ can greatly improve oxygenation, but can also reduce venous return and cardiac output. $\overline{P}_{aw}$ levels greater than 12 cm H_2O have been associated with lung injury. The $\overline{P}_{aw}$ is directly affected by PIP and PEEP, inspiratory hold, frequency, T_I, and flow.

Inspired Oxygen Concentration

An F_IO_2 higher than 0.6 is avoided as much as possible in pediatric patients to prevent oxygen toxicity. This concern is even greater for premature infants because of the role of oxygen in developing retinopathy of prematurity. Tissue oxygen delivery is as important as

F_1O_2 in ventilator management. Maintaining a hematocrit of more than 40%, even in premature infants, maximizes the blood's oxygen-carrying capacity and augments the oxygenating effects of PEEP, $\bar{P}_{aw}$, and F_1O_2.

P_aO_2 should be maintained above 50 mm Hg in infants and above 70 mm Hg in pediatric patients, but clinicians often accept lower limits, especially when a patient's oxygenation fails to improve despite high $\bar{P}_{aw}$ values and an F_1O_2 of 0.6.

One ventilator (AVEA, CareFusion, Viasys Corp, San Diego, Calif.) has implemented a closed-loop F_1O_2 algorithm wherein the ventilator automatically titrates the F_1O_2 based on a measured oxygen saturation and preset oxygen range (i.e., 88% to 92%). This may be a useful system for managing oxygenation in patients, but few trials have evaluated the effectiveness of closed-loop F_1O_2 in reducing adverse outcomes in patients during mechanical ventilation. At the time of writing, closed-loop F_1O_2 was not FDA approved.

Volume Control Mode

Older children and adults have been ventilated with VC-CMV mode over the past several decades. Although this mode was not commonly used for neonates in the recent past, with improvements in ventilator performance and V_T monitoring, clinicians are now using it in the smallest of patients. In the late 1960s and early 1970s, the Bourns LS-104-150 infant ventilator, a linear-driven piston volume ventilator with an IMV option, was commonly used for infants. However, this practice was hampered by technological limitations, which resulted in air leaks and BPD in neonates. Today most ventilators can target a preset tidal volume as low as 2 mL and measure small volumes with great accuracy. These improvements in technology and the improved understanding of the effects of volume overdistention of the lung as a primary cause of VILI has led clinicians to favor VC-IMV/CMV in pediatric patients with ARDS and premature neonates with RDS. A discussion of preferred settings and management is reviewed in greater detail in the section on Lung-Protective Strategies in Conventional Ventilation.

Volume-targeted ventilation permits V_T, rather than inspiratory pressure, to be set. As such, the measured inspiratory pressure will vary based on lung mechanics and patient effort. T_I is a function of the set V_T and inspiratory flow. During VC-CMV, some ventilators require the clinician to set the inspiratory time, and the calculated flow will be delivered to obtain the preset V_T, whereas other ventilators require the clinician to set the flow and the T_I is dependent on the preset flow and volume. The constant flow profile provided during VC-CMV is a square waveform. It has been speculated that a square flow profile may not be as effective as a decelerating flow profile when considering gas distribution in the lungs. Based on this, manufacturers have incorporated the option to change from a traditional square flow waveform to 50% decelerating flow waveform. Because the flow is calculated or preset, constant flow is frequently associated with asynchrony, especially when the flow is insufficient to meet the patient's inspiratory flow requirements. Increasing the flow or reducing the T_I setting can alleviate asynchrony. Some ventilator systems incorporate an advanced setting that allows patients to transition to a variable flow pattern during VC to meet higher flow requirements by the patient. The volume-targeted mode can be used with CMV and IMV, or VC-CMV and VC-IMV, respectively.

Breaths can be patient triggered by flow or pressure, or machine triggered if the patient is not assisting the ventilator. Every volume-targeted breath is a positive pressure breath of the same V_T, flow, and T_I. During VC-IMV, PSV breaths can be added to support spontaneous breaths, but during VC-CMV all the breaths are supported with the preset V_T. Patients receiving VC-CMV should be monitored closely for clinical signs of hypocapnia and hyperinflation, especially when the patient is agitated or autotriggering the ventilator as a result of a large ET tube leak. In theory V_T does not vary with changing lung compliance or airway resistance during VC-CMV; however, V_T may decrease if the ventilator cannot correct for volume losses resulting from gas compression in the patient circuit. Delivered V_T volume may also be affected by leaks from cuffless ETs. When ventilating a larger patient, the volume loss may be negligible; however, in a small child or infant it may be a significant portion of the delivered V_T. Failure to consider this volume loss may result in hypoventilation and hypercapnia of the patient.[63]

Infants who undergo cardiothoracic or abdominal surgery are often placed on VC-IMV because changes in C_L and abdominal distention do not affect V_T delivery. Unlike pressure-controlled ventilation, there is a slower rise to the peak inspiratory pressure during volume-controlled ventilation, and hence lower mean airway is obtained for the same tidal volume. Transitioning from pressure-controlled ventilation to volume-controlled ventilation may be preferable in patients that have hemodynamic compromise or do not tolerate higher mean airway pressure.

Pressure Support Ventilation

PSV is strictly a spontaneous mode or form of continuous spontaneous ventilation (CSV) that is used to augment a patient's V_T by means of a clinician-set inspiratory pressure. As mentioned, PSV can also be used during IMV to assist with weaning. During PSV the patient controls frequency and T_I, and patient triggering is based on either pressure or flow. Cycling occurs when flow from the ventilator decays to a preset point. If the cycling flow is not reached because of a leak around the ET, a backup time-cycling mechanism activates. Furthermore, if a patient becomes apneic, based on a preset apnea interval, the ventilator will provide backup ventilation.

PSV is very useful in pediatric patients who have stable ventilatory drives and acceptable ventilatory mechanics but who must remain intubated for other reasons. These patients may show asynchrony with mandatory breaths and appear more comfortable with PSV. The small diameter of pediatric ETs can significantly contribute to a patient's WOB. The goal of PSV in this situation is not only to provide inspiratory pressure sufficient to overcome tube resistance, but also to allow the patient's lung and chest wall mechanics to determine V_T. Analysis of a patient's pressure–volume and flow–volume loops while on PSV provides some indication of the effort required to overcome artificial R_{aw} (Fig. 22-18). Although some patient effort may be desirable to condition ventilatory muscles, other considerations may require minimization of ET resistance by increasing the level of pressure support (Fig. 22-19).[59]

Initially a higher level of pressure often is needed to enable these patients to achieve V_T in the range of 4 to 7 mL/kg. Over time the PSV level can be reduced if the patient maintains a satisfactory V_T, respiratory rate, and S_pO_2. Some clinicians periodically reduce the pressure below the minimum level as a means of reconditioning ventilatory muscles. Once pressure support can be reduced

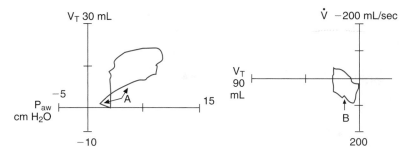

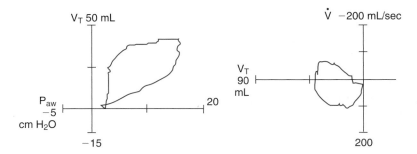

Fig. 22-18 Flow asynchrony arising from inadequate pressure support. Note the "figure 8" pattern *(double arrow)* in the pressure–volume loop **(A)** and the notching on the inspiratory limb *(arrowhead)* in the flow–volume loop **(B)**. These signs indicate that gas flow is inadequate to overcome artificial airway pressure (R$_{aw}$). The pressure support level is 6 cm H$_2$O. P_{aw}, Airway pressure; $\dot{V}$, flow; V_T, tidal volume. (From Wilson BG, Cheifetz IM, Meliones JN: Optimizing mechanical ventilation in infants and children, Palm Springs, Calif., 1995, Bird Products.)

Fig. 22-19 Same patient as in Figure 22-18; flow synchrony has improved with the appropriate level of pressure support. Pressure support has been increased to 13 cm H$_2$O. The figure 8 pattern in the pressure–volume loop *(left)* and the notching on the inspiratory limb in the flow–volume loop *(right)* have been eliminated. P_{aw}, Airway pressure; $\dot{V}$, flow; V_T, tidal volume. (From Wilson BG, Cheifetz IM, Meliones JN: Optimizing mechanical ventilation in infants and children, Palm Springs, Calif., 1995, Bird Products.)

to a minimum level appropriate for the ET's internal diameter, most patients can breathe spontaneously through the tube until extubation.

Small-diameter ETs, particularly those less than 4.5 mm, may provide excessive resistance during pressure support, and pressurization of the ventilator circuit may occur before sufficient flow enters the patient's airway (see Fig. 18-9). When that happens, rapid deceleration of flow may prematurely end the inspiratory phase; this is sometimes called *premature pressure support termination (PPST)*. With PPST, the desired augmentation of V_T does not occur, and patient-ventilator asynchrony may result. When PPST is suspected, a slower rise time can be adjusted, and this may reduce or eliminate it. This problem was frequently seen in the past when adult ventilators were used in pediatric patients, but is less of a problem when using ventilators that are designed for infants through adults.

Another common problem with PSV in pediatric patients is failure to flow cycle because of ET or tracheostomy tube leaks. The clinician has some control over the length of backup time cycling on most ventilators providing PSV. Establishing and relying on time cycling rather than on flow cycling is sometimes desirable if the tube leak is so excessive that the patient cannot trigger the next breath. If both triggering and cycling are problems, the artificial airway may need to be changed to a larger size so that the leak is reduced. Cycling issues are rarely sufficient reason to change to a cuffed airway (Case Study 22-4).

Case Study 22-4

Recommending Changes in Ventilator Settings

A 1-month-old prematurely born baby boy with a diagnosis of respiratory syncytial virus (RSV) pneumonia is being ventilated with the PC-CMV. The patient's initial measured V_T was about 5 mL/kg with a respiratory rate of 40 to 60 breaths/min, the S$_p$O$_2$ was 95% on an F$_I$O$_2$ of 0.3, and $\dot{V}_E$ was 0.28 L. Over several hours V_T diminishes to about 2 to 3 mL/kg, and the respiratory rate increases to over 100 breaths/min. The S$_p$O$_2$ decreases to about 92%, but the $\dot{V}_E$ remains unchanged. What change in ventilator settings is necessary for this patient?

Dual-Control Mode

The dual-control mode is an adaptive form of pressure-controlled ventilation that can also be used with CMV, IMV, and PSV breaths. It combines the best features of pressure and volume modes to provide a minimum V_T during ventilation. Dual-control breaths can be patient triggered based on flow or pressure, or machine triggered if the patient does not have a spontaneous respiratory effort. The dual-control breath can be cycled to exhalation based on time or once the peak flow has decelerated to a preset value. The

V_T is preset, and the inspiratory pressure level will vary based on changes in patient effort, respiratory system mechanics, and measured V_T. Dual-control modes provide variable, decelerating inspiratory flow waveforms. The ongoing inspiratory pressure adjustments are servo-controlled based on volume and compliance measurements made at the proximal flow sensor or back at the ventilator. Adaptive algorithms vary based on the different modes provided by manufacturers. Depending on the mode, the inspiratory pressure level will readjust on a breath-to-breath, or within-the-breath basis to target a minimum V_T. The ventilator may take time to incrementally adjust the inspiratory pressure level to target the tidal volume, especially when the patient is breathing erratically.

This can result in disparities between the set and delivered V_T. Many manufacturers have incorporated a preset volume limit, which limits excessive V_T delivery during dual-control ventilation. An important concept that some clinicians fail to recognize during dual control is that V_T may decrease if the ventilator cannot correct for volume losses resulting from gas compression in the patient circuit. Delivered V_T may also be affected by leaks from cuffless ETs. It may be very difficult for dual-control modes to provide a precise V_T with ET leaks of more than 30%. In these cases, clinicians may change the mode or reintubate with a larger ET tube. The latest ventilator manufacturers have incorporated new algorithms to target a theoretic delivered V_T after the leak has been calculated, and adjust inspiratory pressure based on this value, rather than the measured inspiratory or expiratory V_T.

The following sections provide only a brief explanation of commercially available dual-control modes. Further descriptions of these modes can be found in Chapters 5 and 23.

Pressure-regulated volume control. A widely used form of dual-control ventilation in neonates and pediatric patients is pressure-regulated volume control (PRVC). PRVC is commonly used in patients with CMV or IMV breath types. V_T, frequency, PEEP, and T_I are preset by the operator. The ventilator initially performs a test breath sequence, which measures dynamic or static system compliance. Subsequent adjustments in pressure or V_T are made on the basis of the previous breath or a historical average of breaths. Some ventilators initiate a test breath sequence during PRVC by implementing a brief inspiratory pause during a volume-controlled breath. The static pressure measured during the pause will be the pressure control level for the next breath. The following breaths will increase or decrease the pressure control level by a maximal value of 3 cm H_2O to try to achieve the set V_T with the lowest possible inspiratory pressure (Fig. 22-20). Within a few sequential breaths, the V_T goal may be reached. Certain conditions can restart the test breath sequence for optimal accuracy, including high-pressure limitation, V_T in excess of 150% of the set V_T, and after-settings changes.[63] It should be noted that during PRVC, the inspiratory pressure is usually adjusted based on the monitored inspiratory V_T. In the presence of substantial ET leaks and patient effort, PRVC may reduce the level of support provided, which may result in underinflation and consequent hypercapnia (Fig. 22-21).[70]

Alarms should be adjusted properly, and patients should be monitored frequently for signs of respiratory distress. Additionally, in some ventilators, inspiratory tidal volumes are measured at the airway using a proximal flow sensor, but inspiratory pressure is being regulated based on a volume measurement at the ventilator.

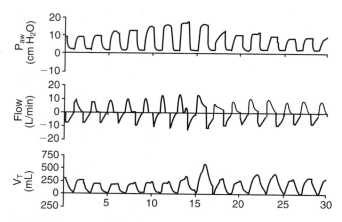

Fig. 22-20 Pressure-regulated volume control (PRVC) mode being used in a pediatric patient with acute respiratory distress syndrome (ARDS). The flow and pressure vary from breath to breath, with changes in respiratory system compliance as the ventilator attempts to maintain a minimum tidal volume.

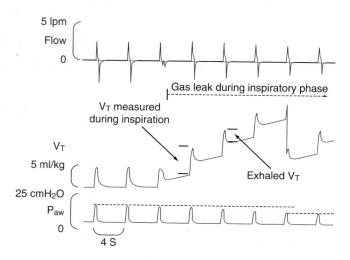

Fig. 22-21 Effects of leaks during the inspiratory phase of pressure-regulated volume-controlled (PRVC) ventilation. (From Claure N, Bancalari E: Methods and evidence on volume-targeted ventilation in preterm infants, Curr Opin Pediatr 20:125-131, 2008.)

In this case, the V_T may need to be readjusted in neonates with reduced compliance to eliminate underventilation from compressible volume loss in the circuit. Generally speaking, ventilator-displayed V_T, without circuit compensation, generally overestimates true-delivered V_T, and with circuit compensation, generally underestimates true-delivered V_T.[71] If a proximal flow sensor is not available in neonates, then a tubing compliance factor should be used to improve V_T delivery.

Volume guarantee. Volume guarantee is yet another variation of PRVC that is used primarily in neonates. Available on the Dräger Babylog models 8000plus and VN500 (Dräger Medical, Inc. Luebeck, Germany), the volume guarantee setting allows a set V_T target while maintaining either the pressure control mode or PSV mode and its characteristic waveforms. Volume guarantee with the Dräger Babylog models 8000plus adjusts inspiratory pressure on a

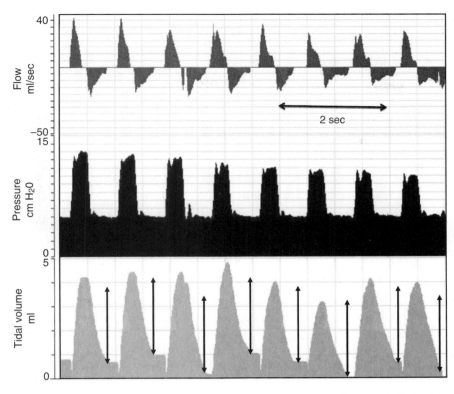

Fig. 22-22 Volume guarantee breaths illustrating flow, pressure, and tidal volume waveforms for triggered inflations during volume-controlled continuous mandatory ventilation (VC-CMV). The vertical arrows show the set tidal volume (V_T). Notice that the expired V_T is larger than the set V_T for all breaths and the peak inspiratory pressure (PIP) is reduced for each subsequent breath. (From Klingenberg C, Wheeler KI, Davis PG, Morley CJ: A practical guide to neonatal volume guarantee ventilation, J Perinatol 31:575-585, 2011.)

breath by breath average based on an expiratory V_T measurement obtained from a hot-wire flow sensor at the patient. Similar to time cycle, pressure-limited/IMV ventilators, the operator must set a continuous flow to maintain pressure and V_T delivery. This setting may need to be readjusted throughout the ventilator course with changes in lung mechanics and ET leaks.

The microprocessor assesses an eight-breath historical average of expired V_T and will increase pressure on the basis of these measurements up to the pressure limit to deliver the target volume (Fig. 22-22).[72]

If lung mechanics improve dramatically, then the ventilator will terminate breath delivery if the delivered V_T exceeds 130% of the set V_T. Pressure will also wean as the result of improving compliance-based V_T on the breath average. Because the ventilator makes manipulations on the basis of expiratory V_T, this mode can correct for compressible volume loss of inspired gases and small ET leaks, and is useful in the neonatal population. The practitioner should exercise some caution when using this mode with excessive ET leaks because there are concerns that this system will falsely underestimate the actual V_T delivered to the lung and overcompensate the subsequent breaths with excessive V_T.

When volume guarantee is used according to accepted guidelines, the inspiratory pressures required to provide effective ventilation have been statistically lower than those used without volume guarantee[73] (Case Study 22-5).

A new form of volume guarantee provided by the Dräger Babylog VN500 (Dräger Medical, Inc. Luebeck, Germany) uses an algorithm that adjusts inspiratory pressure based on a calculated leak during inhalation. As such, infants with ET tube leaks >50% could be supported by volume guarantee on the VN500 more effectively than a ventilator that uses inspiratory or expiratory tidal volumes to guide pressure adjustments. Also when an infant contributes to volume delivery during a triggered inflation, the inspiratory pressure is lower than the untriggered breaths. This may prevent overdistension of the lungs (Fig. 22-23).[74]

This mode requires the clinician to set a maximum inflation pressure limit (P_{max}) that alarms once a pressure of 25 to 30 is being met. If the patient volume exceeds the inspiratory preset V_T (due to agitation or improvement in the lung condition), inspiratory pressures will wean (Fig. 22-24).[75] In some cases, the inspiratory pressure could be equal to the PEEP level. If the pressure is consistently low and the patient appears stable, then clinicians may assess for weaning; otherwise, if the patient has high WOB with low inspiratory pressures and is not ready for extubation, increasing the V_T gradually in small increments may reduce the WOB and stabilize the patient. This phenomenon is prevalent when the V_T has not been adjusted as the patient grows, or when the patient develops chronic lung disease. It is important to update the patient weight at least on a weekly basis so that measured tidal volumes reflect the appropriate tidal volumes in mL/kg. If the WOB still continues to be high, placing the patient onto PC mode may be a better option. However, some ventilators allow a minimum pressure setting during DC-CMV or DC-PSV.

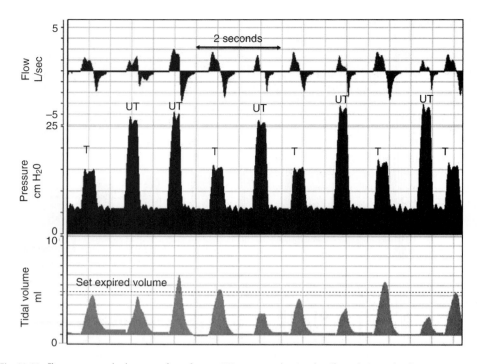

Fig. 22-23 Flow pressure and volume waveforms from an 850-g neonate showing the effects of triggered and spontaneous inflations. Notice that the breaths occur close to each other because the ventilator backup rate is set too close to the neonate's spontaneous rate. The untriggered breaths are indicated as UT. The inflating pressure for each breath depends on the expired tidal volume of the preceding inflation. Notice that a large difference exists between inflation pressures although there is a relatively small difference in tidal volume delivery. (From Klingenberg C, Wheeler KI, Davis PG, Morley CJ: A practical guide to neonatal volume guarantee ventilation, J Perinatol 31:575-585, 2011.)

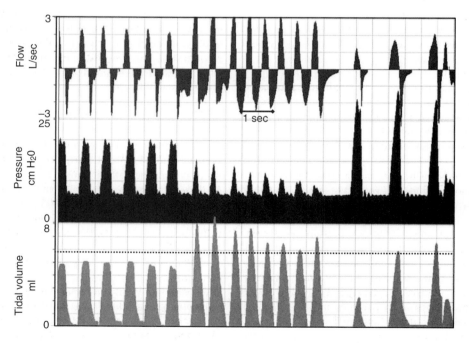

Fig. 22-24 Pressure-controlled continuous mandatory ventilation (PC-CMV) with volume guarantee of a 1000-g neonate illustrating the effect of the large spontaneous breaths. During the first six breaths, the baby is breathing quietly and triggering each breath. During the next eight breaths, the baby demonstrates increased inspiratory efforts and the inspired tidal volume (V_T) exceeds the set V_T shown by the horizontal dotted line. During the remaining three breaths, the baby stops making inspiratory efforts and three backup ventilator (timed) breaths are delivered. (From Klingenberg C, Wheeler KI, Davis PG, Morley CJ: A practical guide to neonatal volume guarantee ventilation, J Perinatol 31:575-585, 2011.)

Case Study 22-5

Evaluation of PRVC Dual-Control Mode

A respiratory therapist is setting PRVC on a premature neonate patient who is recovering from RDS breathing spontaneously. The neonate is stable while receiving PC-CMV on the Servo-i ventilator. The peak inspiratory pressure is 20 cm H$_2$O. The patient has a large ET leak (60%). The ventilator is switched to PRVC with a V$_T$ of 5 mL/kg. Within 2 hours, the patient's respiratory rate increases to 80 beats/min and the F$_I$O$_2$ is increased by 40% to maintain adequate oxygen saturations. What are some reasons why the patient is doing poorly on PRVC mode?

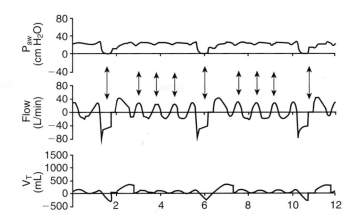

Fig. 22-25 A 50-kg patient with severe acute respiratory distress syndrome (ARDS) breathing spontaneously during airway pressure release ventilation (APRV). The *large arrows* indicate pressure releases and the *small arrows* indicate spontaneous breathing at P$_{high}$.

Volume Support Ventilation

Volume support ventilation (VSV) is well suited for infants and pediatric patients. Its use in infants is similar to PSV in that both ventilator triggering and cycling are patient controlled. However, VSV has additional features that may make it preferable to PSV. In most ventilator models, VSV targets a preset V$_T$ or $\dot{V}_E$ or both, whereas PSV does not. If apnea occurs, many ventilators switch automatically to a mode with a mandatory rate (e.g., PRVC, PC-CMV, or VC-CMV). The ventilator measures changes in compliance, such as might occur after administration of surfactant, and automatically adjusts the required PIP. This is essentially a self-weaning mode. However, as with other spontaneous modes, sizeable ET and tracheostomy tube leaks make VSV difficult to use.

In pediatric patients, VSV can be used instead of PSV. The advantages are essentially the same as for infants: the target V$_T$ is maintained, and self-weaning is possible. Muscle reconditioning can be promoted by reducing the target volume; this allows pressures to decrease and requires the patient to participate actively if a higher V$_T$ is to be achieved by patient effort. Some practitioners prefer switching to CPAP or PS modes for reconditioning periods.

Airway Pressure Release Ventilation

Improvements in exhalation valve performance have made possible new forms of ventilation. Airway pressure release ventilation (APRV) mode is similar to inverse I:E ratio ventilation, a mode previously used in patients to promote higher mean airway pressures and improve oxygenation. APRV differs from this approach by allowing spontaneous breathing throughout the entire respiratory cycle; hence, less sedation or paralytics are required. The mode has been referred to as *CPAP with releases* (Fig. 22-25). The clinician sets a high pressure (P$_{high}$) slightly greater than the measured mean airway pressure, inspiratory pressure, or plateau pressure during conventional ventilation, and the low pressure (P$_{low}$) is set between 0 and 5 cm H$_2$O. The frequency controls the rate of rapid pressure releases from the P$_{high}$ and P$_{low}$, which in combination with spontaneous ventilation, aids in alveolar ventilation and breathing at P$_{high}$ and allows recruitment of air spaces. The P$_{high}$ is held in the lung for up to 2 seconds for neonates and 4 seconds for pediatric patients.[75] Spontaneous breathing at a higher pressure not only aids in alveolar recruitment, but also through the application of pleural pressure change makes improvements in the distribution of lung volume to diseased lung units that improve FRC and pulmonary compliance.[63,76] APRV has been used in neonatal, pediatric, and adult forms of respiratory failure, but few studies have been performed in neonates and pediatric patients to ascertain specific management protocols.

Neurally Adjusted Ventilatory Assist

Neurally adjusted ventilator assist (NAVA) allows the patient full neurologic control of the triggering, magnitude, and timing of the mechanical support provided, regardless of changes in respiratory drive, mechanics, and muscle function.[77] NAVA uses a nasogastric tube with specialized sensors that obtain signals from the electrical activity of the diaphragm to control the timing and pressure of the ventilation delivered.[78] In theory, this form of triggering and support is particularly useful in patients with severe gas trapping and auto-PEEP because it bypasses the effort required in these patients to trigger a ventilator breath. This form of triggering is not affected by leaks and secretions; therefore auto-cycling and hypocapnia in newborns can be potentially avoided. In neonates this mode has been shown to provide better comfort and less need for sedation than PRVC.[79] However, this modality is invasive and placement of the nasogastric tube must be evaluated to ensure proper function of this modality. More information about NAVA can be found in Chapter 23.

Lung-Protective Strategies in Conventional Ventilation

As mentioned in previous sections, avoiding or limiting the amount of time a patient is exposed to invasive mechanical ventilation is the primary means of avoiding VILI. Premature neonates are particularly susceptible to developing VILI because the lungs are fluid-filled, critically underdeveloped, and lack mature surfactant. Additionally, the pliable chest wall of neonates is less able than ossified chest walls in larger pediatric patients to limit lung overinflation. Thus the goal of any lung-protective strategy is to:

1. Avoid repetitive opening and closing of small airways (atelectrauma)
2. Limit overinflation during inhalation (volutrauma)
3. Reduce gas trapping during exhalation (auto-PEEP)
4. Alleviate pulmonary inflammation (biotrauma)

The standard approach to providing the best lung-protective strategy in neonates embraces low V$_T$ or pressures and higher PEEP settings, or an open lung approach. However, it is also important to realize that different neonatal lung diseases warrant different approaches. Table 22-1 provides some evidence-based lung-protective strategies for initiating and managing infants with different lung disorders during neonatal mechanical ventilation.

TABLE 22-1	Lung-Protective Ventilation Strategies for Neonatal Lung Disorders	
Lung Disease	**Ventilator Settings**	**Blood Gas or S$_p$O$_2$ Targets**
Respiratory distress syndrome (RDS)	1. PC, VC, or DC ventilation to target tidal volume 4-6 mL/kg 2. Rapid rates ≥60 breaths/min 3. Moderate PEEP (4-5 cm H$_2$O) 4. Short inspiratory time 0.25-0.4 sec	1. pH 7.25-7.35 2. P$_a$CO$_2$ 45-55 mm Hg 3. P$_a$O$_2$ 50-70 mm Hg 4. S$_p$O$_2$ 88%-94%
Meconium aspiration syndrome (MAS)	1. PC, VC, or DC ventilation with lowest PIP to maintain adequate chest excursion 2. Relatively rapid rates (40-60 breaths/min) 3. Moderate PEEP (4-6 cm H$_2$O) 4. Short inspiratory time to allow exhalation time (0.5-1 sec) 5. Sedation, neuromuscular paralysis, and inhaled NO (20 ppm)	Without PPHN 1. pH 7.3-7.4 2. P$_a$CO$_2$ 40-50 mm Hg 3. P$_a$O$_2$ 70-80 mm Hg 4. S$_p$O$_2$ >90% With PPHN 1. pH 7.30-7.4 2. P$_a$CO$_2$ 35-45 mm Hg 3. P$_a$O$_2$ 80-100 mm Hg 4. S$_p$O$_2$ >95%
Congenital diaphragmatic hernia (CDH)	1. PC, VC, or DC ventilation with lowest PIP to maintain adequate chest excursion 2. Rapid rates (40-80 breaths/min) 3. Moderate PEEP (4-5 cm H$_2$O) 4. Short inspiratory time (0.3-0.5 sec)	1. pH >7.25 2. P$_a$CO$_2$ 45-55 mm Hg 3. P$_a$O$_2$ 50-70 mm Hg 4. S$_p$O$_2$ >95%
Persistent pulmonary hypertension of the newborn (PPHN)	1. PC, VC, or DC ventilation with lowest PIP to maintain adequate chest excursion 2. Higher rates (50-70 breaths/min) 3. Low PEEP (3-4 cm H$_2$O) 4. Inspiratory time (0.3-0.5 sec) 5. Inhaled NO (20 ppm)	1. pH 7.35-7.45 2. P$_a$CO$_2$ 30-40 mm Hg 3. P$_a$O$_2$ 70-100 mm Hg 4. S$_p$O$_2$ >95%
Bronchopulmonary dysplasia	1. PC, VC, or DC ventilation to maintain tidal volume (5-8 mL/kg) 2. Slow rates (20-40 breaths/min) 3. Moderate PEEP (4-6 cm H$_2$O) 4. Inspiratory time (0.4-0.7 sec)	1. pH 7.25-7.35 2. P$_a$CO$_2$ 45-55 mm Hg 3. P$_a$O$_2$ 50-70 mm Hg 4. S$_p$O$_2$ range

Sources: Logan JW, Cotten CM, Goldberg RN, Clark RH: Mechanical ventilation strategies in the management of congenital diaphragmatic hernia, Semin Pediatr Surg 16:115-125, 2007; Goldsmith JP: Continuous positive airway pressure and conventional mechanical ventilation in the treatment of meconium aspiration syndrome, J Perinatol 28 Suppl 3:S49-55, 2008. Review; Vitali SH, Arnold JH: Bench-to-bedside review: Ventilator strategies to reduce lung injury lessons from pediatric and neonatal intensive care, Crit Care 9:177-83, 2005; Ambalavanan N, Schelonka RL, Carlo W: Ventilatory Strategies. In Goldsmith JP, Karotkin EH, editors: Assisted ventilation of the neonate, ed 4, pp 249-259 Philadelphia, 2004, WB Saunders, pp 249-259.
DC, Dual-controlled ventilation; *PC,* pressure-controlled ventilation; *PEEP,* positive end-expiratory pressure; *PIP,* peak inspiratory pressure; *VC,* volume-controlled ventilation.

As previously discussed, compelling evidence now suggests that volutrauma created by excessive volumes, and not necessarily barotrauma, is chiefly responsible for instigating VILI.[80,81] Even short-term exposure to volutrauma during mechanical ventilation initiates lung inflammation in premature infants, which can occur after only a few minutes of manual resuscitation.[82] Ventilation for 15 minutes with a V$_T$ of 15 mL/kg has been shown to cause an injurious process in the preterm lung.[83] As few as three overdistending breaths at birth have been shown to compromise the therapeutic effect of subsequent surfactant replacement in an animal model of prematurity.[84] Critical underinflation, using small V$_T$ (atelectrauma) can also contribute to VILI.[85] Furthermore, VILI can put premature neonates with RDS at a greater risk for arrested lung growth and development.[86]

Over the last decade, volume-targeted strategies have been at the forefront of clinical investigation. Volume-targeted ventilation strategies, using a preset V$_T$, are usually implemented using dual-control or volume control modes, whereas some clinicians still prefer to use pressure control and guide the inspiratory pressure based on measured V$_T$.

In a recent review of all clinical trials comparing pressure-targeted to volume-targeted modes, neonates supported with volume-targeted modes had significantly lower duration of ventilation, pneumothorax, hypocarbia, severe intraventricular hemorrhage, periventricular leukomalacia, and the combined outcome of death or BPD than infants supported with pressure control modes.[87,88]

In the acute phase of lung disease, it has been suggested that the initial strategy should use CMV mode rather than IMV mode to deliver volume-targeted breath types so that every breath that the infant receives is volume-targeted and without PSV. With use of IMV, infants were shown to be more tachypneic and to have faster heart rates and consistently lower oxygen saturations, suggesting substantially higher WOB compared with VC-CMV.[89] During weaning and when applicable, it has been suggested that volume-targeted strategies be implemented using PS so that infants can determine their own inspiratory time.[6]

At present, it is unclear what the absolute target V$_T$ or target range should be used in infants and whether this V$_T$ needs to be adjusted according to varying levels of disease severity. Generally the consensus among clinicians is to use V$_T$ target around 4 to

6 mL/kg in LBW neonates.[90] One study evaluated lung injury response in 30 preterm infants with RDS using V_T of 3 mL/kg or 5 mL/kg. The 3 mL/kg group showed significantly higher levels of lung inflammation and longer duration of ventilation than the 5 mL/kg.[91] A V_T target of 3 mL/kg has also been associated with increased alveolar dead space, tachypnea, and higher transcutaneous carbon dioxide in preterm infants compared to higher V_T targets (5 mL/kg).[92]

Larger infants and pediatric patients with acute lung injury and ARDS are susceptible to lung injury and hyperinflation when placed on mechanical ventilatory support. The most common causes for respiratory distress in these patients are pneumonia, bronchiolitis, trauma, seizures, sepsis, and pulmonary edema.[57] Studies have reported reduced mortality in adults when lung-protective strategies are used.[93,94] Reduction of barotrauma, volutrauma, and atelectrauma are thought to be the reasons (see Chapter 17).[95] Repeated collapse and inflation result in stress injury to alveolar and pulmonary vascular tissue, and loss or alteration of surfactant.[95]

Adult studies have had a dramatic impact on the management of pediatric patients with ARDS. Central to these strategies is the use of a V_T less than 6 mL/kg, plateau pressures ($P_{plateau}$) less than 30 cm H_2O, and appropriate levels of PEEP in patients with ARDS. PEEP itself has been shown to have lung-protective effects during mechanical ventilation (Case Study 22-6).[80]

Mechanical ventilation has the potential to create dynamic hyperinflation (auto-PEEP) in patients affected by diseases of airflow limitation (e.g., asthma, bronchiolitis, or ARDS). These patients often have a prolonged expiratory time because of early collapse or obstruction of smaller airways. As auto-PEEP dynamic hyperinflation occurs, trapped air increases in the lung and peak pressures gradually increase during VC-CMV in a spontaneously breathing patient. In assisted ventilation, WOB usually increases. The lung-protective strategy for minimizing the effects of both VILI and dynamic hyperinflation is to use a lower V_T, appropriate PEEP levels, and low $P_{plateau}$, and to allow permissive hypercapnia (i.e., an increased P_aCO_2). Maintaining adequate PEEP, low inspiratory pressures ($P_{plateau}$ <30 cm H_2O), and low volumes also reduces alveolar shear injury and overdistention. Additionally, using a short T_I and prolonging the expiratory phase of each mechanical breath allows more time for exhalation but results in a low respiratory rate. Incorporation of all these strategies usually makes an increase in P_aCO_2 unavoidable.

Case Study 22-6

Interpretation and Response to Monitored Data

A 7-month-old girl with a diagnosis of bronchiolitis is being ventilated. The machine's pressure control settings are PIP = 26 cm H_2O, PEEP = 6 cm H_2O, inspiratory time = 0.8 second, and respiratory rate = 16 breaths/min. The F_IO_2 is 1.0. ABG values are: P_aO_2 = 55 mm Hg, P_aCO_2 = 73 mm Hg, and pH = 7.19. An inline Cosmo Plus monitor shows a $\dot{V}CO_2$ of 83 mL/min. (See Chapter 11 to review volumetric CO_2 monitoring.)

Guided by chest radiographic findings, the attending physician and the respiratory therapist decide to increase the PEEP to 8 cm H_2O. Soon after making the change, they note that the $\dot{V}CO_2$ has risen and is now at 85 mL/min. What action should the physician and respiratory therapist take?

Extensive experience has shown that ventilated patients usually tolerate moderate hypercapnia and often some degree of hypoxemia if the patient does not experience shock, hemodynamic complications, or anemia during the clinical course. Patients with severe cardiac disease or elevated intracranial pressure are not good candidates for permissive hypercapnia. Experience has shown that permitting the P_aCO_2 to rise has little deleterious effect as long as the pH is maintained above 7.2. As mentioned earlier, maintaining a higher than normal CO_2 may actually have an anti-inflammatory effect. (NOTE: Inflammation is the biochemical complication associated with overstretching of the lung [see Chapter 17].)[96-100]

HIGH-FREQUENCY VENTILATION

Emerson introduced the first high-frequency ventilator in 1959, and many attempts have been made since to apply various forms of this type of ventilation to a wide range of patients.[101] With technological advances, sophisticated devices have been introduced and continue to improve. Interest in high-frequency techniques for neonates was sparked primarily by two complications of conventional mechanical ventilation: pulmonary air leaks and the development of BPD. Before high-frequency ventilators became widely accepted, about 24% of infants with RDS who required ventilatory support developed air leaks.[102] Among LBW infants who survived RDS, 25% to 33% eventually developed BPD.[61]

Minton, et al used the term *pulmonary injury sequence (PIS)* to describe the issue of prematurity and pulmonary disease, or the "continuum of disease."[103] The continuum of PIS includes RDS, PIE, pulmonary air-leak syndrome, oxygen toxicity, and BPD. The extent to which high-frequency ventilation can reduce the incidence of PIS remains unclear. However, the consensus is that the high pressures sometimes used with conventional ventilation are contributory factors. With high-frequency techniques, lung-volume recruitment can be accomplished with a higher $\overline{P}_{aw}$ than with conventional ventilation. Even at a higher $\overline{P}_{aw}$, lung injury is less likely because high peak pressures can be avoided.

High-frequency ventilation can be used in conjunction with surfactant therapy. Studies have demonstrated that lung injury can be reduced with high-frequency ventilation if early recruitment of optimal lung volumes is achieved and maintained after surfactant administration.[104] This has prompted some clinicians to apply an early intervention strategy to the management of premature infants: high-frequency ventilation is initiated and the first dose of exogenous surfactant is given within the first few hours of life.

Another problem with conventional ventilation, not only in LBW infants but also in older pediatric patients, is ineffective gas exchange despite extremely high settings. This most often occurs in acute lung injury (ALI) and is clearly attributable to the limitations of conventional devices. Experience with high-frequency techniques has shown that improved gas exchange is possible without excessive $\overline{P}_{aw}$ not only in newborns, but also in older children and adults (Box 22-7; also see Chapter 23).

Indications for High-Frequency Ventilation

High-frequency ventilation (HFV) should be considered for patients with heterogeneous lung disease (e.g., ALI/ARDS) if the $\overline{P}_{aw}$ on conventional ventilation exceeds 15 cm H_2O. A change from conventional ventilation to HFV may be seriously considered at a lower $\overline{P}_{aw}$ if the patient's clinical picture is worsening and the settings on the conventional ventilator are rising. HFV also should be

---

BOX 22-7 **Conditions for Which High-Frequency Ventilation Is Used in Infants and Children**

- Homogenous lung disease requiring conventional $\overline{P}_{aw}$ over 15 cm H_2O
- Respiratory distress syndrome (RDS)
- Pneumonia
- Aspiration syndromes
- Pulmonary hemorrhage
- Acute respiratory distress syndrome (ARDS)
- Persistent pulmonary hypertension of the newborn (PPHN)
- Air-leak syndromes
- Pulmonary interstitial emphysema
- Pneumothorax/bronchopleural fistula
- Pneumomediastinum
- Pneumoperitoneum
- Pulmonary hypoplasia
- Impaired cardiac function
- Bronchoscopy and airway-thoracic surgery

---

used as an early intervention (i.e., before high conventional settings are used) for premature infants or patients who have air-leak syndromes. Patients with an oxygen index of 40 (which in some centers meets the criterion for extracorporeal life support) should have a trial of HFV if possible. A trial of HFV also may be considered for patients with sepsis, persistent pulmonary hypertension of the newborn, or congenital diaphragmatic hernia when a high $\overline{P}_{aw}$ is required for effective alveolar ventilation on a conventional ventilator.

Contraindications and Complications of High-Frequency Ventilation

No absolute contraindications to HFV have been reported, but patients with obstructive airway disease (e.g., asthma) have historically been considered poor candidates for HFV because of the risk of overinflation. However, some recent data suggest that high-frequency oscillatory ventilation (HFOV), a form of HFV, may be safe and effective in patients with small airways disease (e.g., bronchiolitis), hyperinflation, and hypercapnia. Overinflation of one or both lungs is a possible complication with any patient receiving HFV. Overinflation can occur as a consequence of inadequate lung unit emptying or remarkably fast reductions in alveolar surface tension that dramatically reduce compliance.

A chest radiograph should be taken within 2 hours of initiation of HFV and at least daily thereafter to check for lung hyperinflation. Frequent radiographs may be necessary for patients at greater risk for overinflation. Placement of the ET tip is checked on every chest radiograph because the position of the tube can affect lung volumes when high-frequency techniques are used.

Focal obstruction of the lungs caused by mucus plugging is a potential complication of HFV. Plugging is not necessarily caused by the high-frequency technique; rather the small V_T cannot traverse plugging obstructions in addition to the higher V_T delivered in conventional ventilation. Loss of chest movement sometimes is seen when an obstruction develops. Infants with meconium aspiration and other aspiration syndromes may require frequent and aggressive suctioning with ET lavage and chest vibration. However, mucus plugging rarely responds to suctioning, and a brief period on conventional ventilation may be necessary. Increased mucus

production in the airways is associated with overdistention and volutrauma, and could be problematic if conventional ventilation was used before HFV. Mucus plugging can be caused by inadequate humidification, especially if prolonged manual ventilation took place with a heat and moisture exchanger humidifier.

Impaired cardiac output has been observed as a complication of HFV, particularly in HFOV and with techniques that require high lung volumes and $\overline{P}_{aw}$. In addition, crystalloids and colloids are more often necessary over the first 24 hours in these situations than they are with conventional ventilation. Infants in particular depend on sufficient intravascular volume for adequate pulmonary perfusion and left atrial filling. Monitoring of the blood pressure (BP), heart rate (HR), and central venous pressure for adverse hemodynamic effects is very important. Echocardiograms are useful for evaluating and maximizing myocardial function and blood volume status.

Intraventricular hemorrhage (IVH) has been reported to be higher in premature infants receiving HFOV than in those receiving conventional ventilation.[64] Presumably this is caused by elevated intrapleural pressure and fluctuations in cerebral vascular pressures. Fewer cases of IVH are seen with the combination of HFOV and surfactant therapy than with conventional treatment.[61] Recent data have indicated that when HFOV is used as an initial ventilation strategy, neurodevelopmental outcomes were actually improved.[105] Some have suggested that a low P_aCO_2 is a primary cause of IVH in premature infants.[62] A possible explanation is that HFV can dramatically reduce the P_aCO_2 before the clinician is aware of this development.[106] This is why trending P_aCO_2 levels, as will be discussed later in this section, are essential during HFV.

High-Frequency Ventilation Techniques

As its name implies, HFV is a form of mechanical ventilation that uses high respiratory rates, or *frequencies*. Frequencies usually are specified in hertz (Hz) or cycles per second; 1 hertz equals 60 cycles/min or 60 breaths/min. Under guidelines established by the U.S. FDA, HFV is any form of mechanical ventilation in which the breath frequency exceeds 150 breaths/min. HFV has evolved into five basic types: high-frequency positive pressure ventilation, high-frequency flow interruption, high-frequency percussive ventilation, high-frequency oscillatory ventilation, and high-frequency jet ventilation. Each type has been somewhat successful in improving outcomes in the management of severe lung disease.

High-Frequency Positive Pressure Ventilation

High-frequency positive pressure ventilation (HFPPV) is a modified form of conventional ventilation that uses high frequencies and low V_T values. HFPPV usually is delivered by conventional ventilators with low-compliance circuits. Until jet ventilators and oscillating devices became readily available, HFPPV was a reasonable alternative for LBW infants with RDS when the combined problems of severe hypoxemia and respiratory acidosis did not respond to more conventional methods. HFPPV also was effective for pediatric patients with surfactant deficiency syndromes. This type of ventilation, which was developed by Sjöstrand and colleagues in the late 1970s, originally was intended to minimize the cardiovascular effects of PPV.[106] It was discovered that HFPPV sometimes could also improve gas exchange while keeping airway pressures ($\overline{P}_{aw}$) lower than they would be with the low frequency/high V_T technique. HFPPV does not technically fit the FDA definition of HFV because it uses frequencies up to 150 breaths/min.

Rates up to this limit are attainable on most of the conventional ventilators currently in use.

Two potential problems are associated with HFPPV: (1) the high rate and short T_I may prevent adequate V_T delivery; and (2) because expiration is entirely passive, breath stacking can occur, causing pulmonary hyperinflation as a consequence of insufficient time for emptying of all lung units.[107] Both problems can be managed by careful application of HFPPV and close monitoring of ventilatory waveforms and chest radiographs. The use of HFPPV has diminished with the availability of other types of high-frequency devices and with clinicians' tentative acceptance of permissive hypercapnia in pediatric patients.

High-Frequency Flow Interruption

Flow interruption is similar to jet ventilation (discussed later in the chapter) in that the V_T is created by a device that interrupts a gas flow or a high-pressure source at frequencies as high as 15 Hz. High-frequency flow interruption (HFFI) can be used either with a jet catheter in the airway or as a bulk flow device connected directly to the artificial airway. The most often discussed flow interrupter device is the one invented by Emerson, which consists of a conduit through which gas flow is directed. The conduit contains a ball that has a flow port in its center. An electric motor moves the ball back and forth in the conduit at a frequency of up to 200 cycles/min, interrupting the outflow of gas. As with a high-frequency jet ventilation system, the high-pressure streams of gas can entrain more static gas supplied by an added bias flow to augment the delivered V_T. This type of HFV was among the early models developed, and it currently is used mostly for investigational purposes.

High-Frequency Percussive Ventilation

Forrest M. Bird, a pioneer in mechanical ventilation technology, developed high-frequency percussive ventilation (HFPV). Bird's intent was to incorporate the most effective characteristics of jet and conventional ventilation into one device. HFPV can be used with a mask or mouthpiece as a therapeutic device to percuss the chest internally to remove secretions, or it can be used intermittently or before extubation of intubated patients to help mobilize secretions. It also can be used as a continuous mode of ventilation. HFPV has been used successfully as a continuous mode in children and has served as a prophylactic measure to prevent pneumonia and atelectasis in patients with thermal injury.[108]

The VDR-4 (Bird Space Technology, Sandpoint, Idaho) is a high-frequency percussive generator that is used to superimpose high-frequency breaths onto conventional breaths. The device can be compared with time-cycled, pressure-limited ventilation, except that high-frequency pulsations (as high as 600 cycles/min [10 Hz]) are injected throughout the inspiratory phase. At the heart of the device is a sliding Venturi (Fig. 22-26) with a jet orifice at its mouth. The jet is surrounded by a continuous bias flow of warmed, humidified gas. On inspiration, a diaphragm connected to the Venturi fills with gas and slides it forward toward the patient's airway, blocking the expiration ports. At the same time, the jet begins delivering short, percussive pulsations. A large amount of air is entrained so that flow to the patient is very high; this is the result of the large pressure gradient between the patient connection and the jet. When the gradient begins to decrease during inspiration, air entrainment and total flow also begin to slow, but the jet pulsations continue. When the time limit for inspiration is reached, the jet cycles off. The diaphragm, no longer pressurized, collapses, and

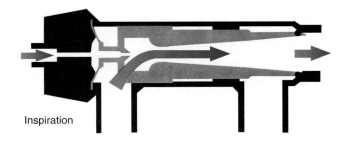

Inspiration

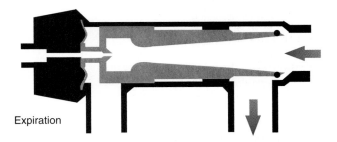

Expiration

Fig. 22-26 Design of the sliding Venturi for the high-frequency percussive generator. (See text for additional information.)

the Venturi slides back, opening the expiratory ports. A counter flow of gas sufficient to maintain a set PEEP is directed toward the airway during the expiratory phase. A schematic of the HFPV system is shown in Fig. 22-27.

High-Frequency Oscillatory Ventilation

High-frequency oscillatory ventilation (HFOV) has become the most widely used high-frequency technique for infants and pediatric patients. It differs from other high-frequency techniques in several important ways:

- Both inspiration and expiration are active.
- Gas flow is sinusoidal rather than triangular.
- Bulk flow, rather than jet pulsations, is delivered.
- V_T is less than dead space.

An HFOV device can be powered by a reciprocating pump, diaphragm, or piston. Although they are not true oscillators, flow interrupters can be assimilated into ventilators called *pseudo-oscillators* that provide the effect of an oscillator.[109] Another type of HFOV device has been implemented by Dräger (Babylog VN500, Luebeck, Germany) and combines HFOV with volume guarantee. This device shows promise in its ability to measure V_T. However, it is currently unavailable in the United States.

Oscillators and at least one pseudo-oscillator have been in use since the late 1980s. An example of a commonly used oscillator is the Sensor Medics 3100A (SensorMedics, a division of Viasys, San Diego, Calif.). This oscillator uses a diaphragm-shaped piston that is driven magnetically, similar to the action of a stereo speaker (Fig. 22-28). The 3100A has a rigid plastic circuit into which a warmed, humidified bias flow of gas is introduced just in front of the piston (Fig. 22-29). The bias gas flows through the circuit and exits from a restricted orifice and mushroom valve assembly that maintain the set $\overline{P}_{aw}$. The $\overline{P}_{aw}$ control is used to set the tension on the diaphragm, which oscillates the flow. The V_T, or amplitude, is set by the power control and is determined by the forward and backward excursion

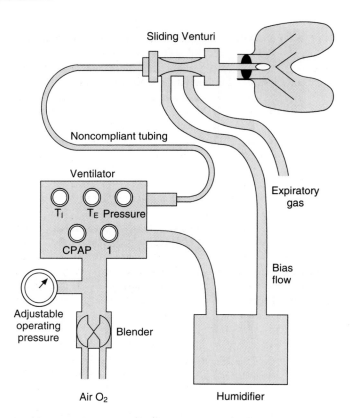

Fig. 22-27 Schematic of a high-frequency percussive ventilation (HFPV) system. (Modified from Branson RD, Hess DR, Chatburn RI: Respiratory care equipment, Philadelphia, 1995, JB Lippincott.)

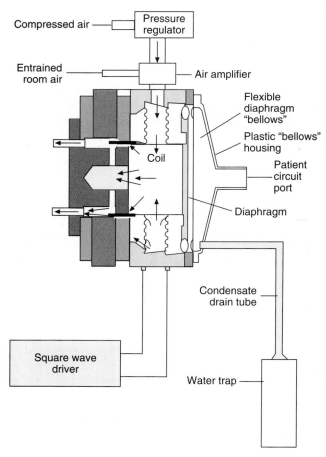

Fig. 22-28 Drive mechanism for the SensorMedics 3100A oscillator. A timer *(square wave driver)* signals the motor to drive the piston toward and away from the patient circuit port, making both inspiration and expiration active. Because the movement of the piston generates extreme heat, compressed air and entrained room air are introduced around the motor's coil to provide cooling. (Courtesy SensorMedics, Corp., Yorba Linda, Calif.)

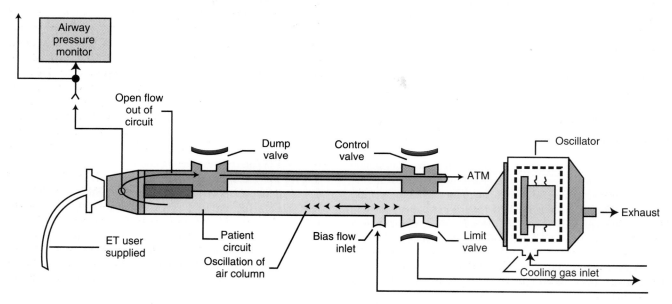

Fig. 22-29 Basic breathing circuit of the SensorMedics Model 3100A high-frequency oscillator. *ATM,* Atmosphere; *ET,* endotracheal tube. (Courtesy Viasys Respiratory Care, Inc. Yorba Linda, Calif.)

distance of the piston. The number of piston excursions determines the frequency. Two other mushroom valves function as safety releases on the circuit. See the Clinical Scenario involving HFOV below.

Clinical Scenario: Pulmonary Interstitial Emphysema (PIE)

A premature infant with severe pulmonary PIE is being ventilated on a conventional infant ventilator at a $\overline{P}_{aw}$ of 18 cm H_2O. The clinical team caring for this patient has decided to place him on HFOV. What strategy would you use, and what initial $\overline{P}_{aw}$ and fraction of inspired oxygen (F_IO_2) would you choose?

A low-volume HFOV strategy is often used for patients with an air-leak syndrome (e.g., PIE). The $\overline{P}_{aw}$ used for the conventional ventilator also should be set on the oscillator initially. The F_IO_2 should be set as high as 1.0 for the first 12 to 24 hours because the goal is to keep the arterial partial pressure of oxygen (P_aO_2) above 55 mm Hg. This strategy maintains adequate oxygenation and ventilation, while preventing extension of the air-leak syndrome. It also promotes resolution of the PIE by eliminating the potential volutrauma-producing factors. Achievement of optimal volumes (as indicated by the chest radiograph) should be avoided until the PIE has resolved. Serial chest radiographs are obtained to evaluate resolution of the condition. Once the air-leak syndrome has resolved, an optimal lung-volume strategy can be pursued (Case Study 22-7). (Chapter 23 presents information on HFOV for adults.)

Case Study 22-7

Patient Case—Acute Respiratory Distress Syndrome Managed with HFO

A 5-year-old girl with a diagnosis of ARDS secondary to sepsis and aspiration pneumonia has been on the Sensormedics 3100A oscillator for about 4 hours. The mean airway pressure is set at 28 cm H_2O, the frequency at 8 Hz, and the amplitude at 38 cm H_2O. The F_IO_2 is 0.7. Initially the ABG values and vital signs improved. However, over the past 30 minutes, the heart rate has increased and the S_pO_2 has dropped from 97% to 87%. What action should the respiratory therapist consider? *lower the MAP*

High-Frequency Jet Ventilation

Largely pioneered in the late 1970s, high-frequency jet ventilation (HFJV) remains a widely used high-frequency technique, particularly in infants. It was the first high-frequency technique to attempt delivery of a V_T smaller than dead space. HFJV originally was used to provide short-term ventilatory support during adult upper airway surgery and instrumentation, but animal studies showed that it also provided effective alveolar ventilation and gas exchange in acute lung disease.

Previously HFJV was delivered through a specially made, triple-lumen ET. Adapters are now available for converting a

conventional ET to a jet tube. A ventilator designed to deliver HFJV is the Bunnell Life Pulse (Bunnell, Salt Lake City, Utah). The principle of HFJV involves the delivery of short jet breaths, or pulsations, of an air–oxygen gas mixture under considerable pressure through an ET. The Bunnell Life Pulse can deliver frequencies in the range of 240 to 660 cycles/min.[15] Jets are delivered by electronic solenoids or fluidic valves. Most infants are well ventilated at an HFJV rate of 420 cycles/min. Small changes in the rate usually have little effect on P_aCO_2 because of patients' broad range of resonant frequency. Larger patients and those prone to gas trapping may benefit from lower HFJV rates (240 to 360 cycles/min).

Tidal volume in HFJV depends on the length of the pulsation; the amplitude, or driving pressure, of the jet; the size of the jet orifice; and the patient's R_{aw} and C_L. For infants the typical delivered V_T is 1 to 3 mL. However, a V_T that is larger or smaller than the patient's dead space volume can be delivered. Under certain conditions, gas entrainment can occur around the jet, slightly increasing V_T by a physical process called *jet mixing*, which is caused by the viscous shearing of the jet-gas layer with stagnant gas in the airway. The stagnant gas is dragged downstream in an entrainment-like effect. The volume of entrained gas varies with the patient's lung mechanics.

Often the PEEP is set much higher in HFJV than in conventional ventilation. Because jet devices deliver significantly less V_T and $\overline{P}_{aw}$ than other forms of mechanical ventilation, a higher PEEP may be used without elevating $\overline{P}_{aw}$ to potentially harmful levels.[67-69]

In most patients the conventional ventilator is operated in the CMV mode at a rate of 10 breaths/min or less. In HFJV the jet accomplishes much of the alveolar ventilation. Experience has shown that when an appropriate level of PEEP is used to achieve optimum recruitment of lung units, the jet device can effectively ventilate without the need for conventional breaths.[110] Once the patient is ready to be weaned from the ventilator, transitioning to conventional ventilation and discontinuation of the jet are relatively easy, and from that point conventional weaning can take place.

Physiology of High-Frequency Ventilation

In the high-frequency techniques in which V_T is less than dead space, the predominant means of gas transport by bulk convection is superseded by other mechanisms. However, alveoli close to the airways are still ventilated by convection, as in conventional ventilation. Many other mechanisms of gas transport in HFV are theoretical and are not completely understood. Such mechanisms include pendelluft, streaming, Taylor-type dispersion, and simple molecular diffusion (Fig. 22-30). The degree to which these mechanisms play a role depends on the HFV technique used, the characteristics of the high-frequency generator, the ventilator settings, and the patient's lung characteristics.[111]

Pendelluft, which is the exchange of gas between lung units with different time constants, is observed through photographic studies or by the measurement of different pressure values in the airways.[112,113] Although other gas transport mechanisms may bring fresh gas to the small airways, the movement of gas across lung units before it leaves the lung may enhance gas exchange between alveoli and pulmonary capillaries. Over time more gas may enter lung units with longer time constants so that these units may be recruited.

Streaming, or asymmetric velocity profiles, is thought to occur because the velocity of gas flow is higher in the center of the airway

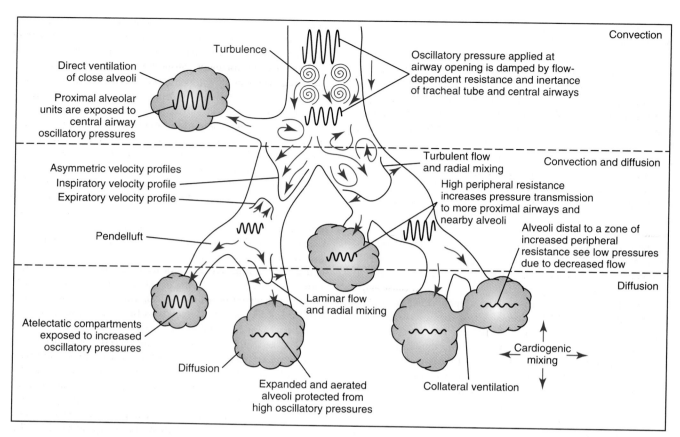

Fig. 22-30 Gas transport mechanisms and pressure damping during high-frequency oscillatory ventilation (HFOV). The major gas-transport mechanisms operating during HFOV in convection, convection-diffusion, and diffusion zones include turbulence, bulk, convection (direct ventilation of close alveoli), asymmetric inspiratory and expiratory collateral ventilation between neighboring alveoli, and molecular diffusion (see text for details). (Redrawn from Pillow JJ: High frequency oscillatory ventilation: mechanisms of gas exchange and lung mechanics, Crit Care Med. 33:S135-S141, 2005.)

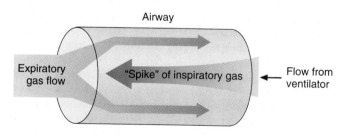

Fig. 22-31 Effect of streaming in high-frequency jet ventilation (HFJV). Pulsations from the jet push the gas forward in the center; this causes gas along the airway walls to be pushed backward.

(Fig. 22-31). Pulsations from the jet push the gas forward in the center, causing gas along the airway walls to be pushed backward. This outer layer of gas moves at a slower velocity. Because much of the gas occupying the space along the walls is dead space gas, the forward-moving alveolar gas may be used more efficiently.[114]

Taylor-type dispersion is the enhanced diffusion of gases caused by the turbulence of high gas flows reaching small airways. This is thought to be a principal mechanism of gas transport in high-frequency oscillation.[115,116] With the rapid injection of small gas volumes at high flows, the erratic formation of streams and eddies (particularly at airway bifurcations) shortens the diffusion times of gases over the distances they normally travel. With this type of enhanced gas transport, **simple molecular diffusion** likely is enhanced as well because more mixing of inspired and expired gas occurs at more distal points in the tracheobronchial tree.

The mechanism of augmented transport is further affected by the active expiration produced by the oscillator. With other ventilators, the formula for the $\dot{V}_E$ produced is $\dot{V}_E = f \times V_T$; with HFOV, the formula is $\dot{V}_E = f \times V_T^2$. Although V_T values are in the range of only 0.8 to 2 mL/kg, the interplay of gas transport mechanisms provides highly effective CO_2 elimination. $\dot{V}/\dot{Q}$ matching is improved with HFV because $\bar{P}_{aw}$ is used to achieve optimal lung volume and to maintain that volume throughout the respiratory cycle. *Reaching optimal lung volume* means that lung units that otherwise would be closed are open, providing more area for gas exchange. Moreover, the duration of gas exchange is greatly extended because no inspiration or expiration takes place.

Oxygenation is one of the factors that increases pulmonary blood flow. If a higher lung volume is achieved, pulmonary vasodilation can result because of improved oxygenation. The diameter of pulmonary vessels is yet another factor that greatly affects pulmonary blood flow. With higher lung volumes, radial traction to the walls of larger pulmonary vessels increases, enhancing blood flow.

Management Strategies for High-Frequency Ventilation

Assessment of breath sounds, heart sounds, pulmonary compliance, and other such parameters is difficult in patients receiving HFV; therefore a thorough assessment should be performed before the patient is connected to the high-frequency device. The baseline V_T should be noted if the patient initially received conventional ventilation. If possible, a chest radiograph should be taken shortly before HFV is initiated to document baseline lung inflation and to check the position of the ET.

If indicated, an initial dose of artificial surfactant is given while the patient is receiving conventional ventilation. Subsequent doses may be given after HFV has been started. Note that some clinicians prefer to keep the capability of conventional ventilation at the bedside to use during surfactant dosing; others prefer to give surfactant while manually ventilating the patient and forgo any use of conventional ventilation.

Preparations for placing a patient on HFV include repositioning the patient and completing any procedures that could cause agitation. Endotracheal suctioning is performed so that interruptions do not occur during the initial period. A pulse oximeter is put in place, and an electrocardiogram and BP are monitored continuously. Transcutaneous CO_2 monitors work well on most patients regardless of age. Monitoring of transcutaneous CO_2 is useful for noninvasively trending P_aCO_2 between blood gas draws. If a transcutaneous monitor is used, the sensor is placed on the patient and the baseline comparison to P_aCO_2 is made before HFV is initiated.

Cardiovascular assessment focuses on intravascular volume and cardiac output. A high, sustained $\overline{P}_{aw}$ can greatly reduce cardiac output if circulatory volume is not adequate. Once a patient has been placed on HFV, some practitioners prefer to administer crystalloids and colloids only if the mean arterial pressure drops. If this strategy is chosen, the patient may need to be removed from the high-frequency ventilator several times for manual ventilation until additional fluid volume can be given. Adequate sedation is provided before HFV is initiated. Some spontaneous breathing may be acceptable. However, agitation and excessive movement can interfere with high-frequency breaths and gas exchange. Paralysis is not always necessary, but some suppression of respiratory drive is desirable. Management strategies differ according to the specific type of HFV used. Generally the goal in all types is to provide effective gas exchange at the lowest possible F_IO_2 and $\overline{P}_{aw}$. Also inherent in all types of HFV is the need to escalate support frequently until a certain threshold is reached and the patient is said to be *captured* on the ventilator. Often a dramatic improvement in oxygenation or ventilation, or both, is seen when this occurs. If the patient's condition is stable, some weaning can begin almost at once.

Management of High-Frequency Oscillatory Ventilation in Infants

A recent review compared outcomes in preterm neonates using HFOV versus gentle conventional ventilation. HFOV was associated with an increase in air leaks and a reduction in surgical ligation of patent ductus arteriosus or retinopathy of prematurity. There were no differences in BPD, mortality, or neurologic insult. However, in neonates where randomization occurred earlier (1 to 4 hours), HFOV showed a significant benefit for reducing death or BPD over conventional ventilation.[117]

Unlike with the jet ventilator, which incorporates a conventional ventilator as part of its gas delivery system, the patient cannot be gradually transitioned from conventional ventilation to HFOV. Typically, manual ventilation may be the only means of optimizing alveolar recruitment and oxygenation before a patient is placed on an oscillator. Sustaining manual inflations with increasing levels of PEEP immediately before connection may enhance initial recruitment and make the transition to HFOV more successful.

Two basic treatment strategies are suggested for HFOV, depending on the patient's condition. One is the optimum lung volume strategy (Fig. 22-32). The goal of this strategy is to increase $\overline{P}_{aw}$ on the oscillator until oxygenation stabilizes. The P_aCO_2 is maintained within a range established by the management team. A chest radiograph is obtained within the first 2 hours and every 12 to 24 hours thereafter. Optimum lung inflation is indicated by radiographic findings of decreased opacification and lung expansion to the eighth or ninth posterior rib level on the right hemidiaphragm. Once this level of expansion has been established, subsequent chest radiographs should be used primarily to check for overinflation rather than to guide adjustments in $\overline{P}_{aw}$. Reducing the F_IO_2 to 0.45 to 0.5 may be possible, depending on cardiovascular status. This is followed by weaning $\overline{P}_{aw}$ (Fig. 22-33).[113] Patients with air-leak syndromes (e.g., PIE, pneumothorax, and bronchopleural fistula) are placed on HFOV using a low-volume strategy; the goals of this strategy are to prevent extension of the air-leak syndrome and to promote its resolution by eliminating factors that can potentially produce volutrauma. This strategy differs from the optimum lung volume strategy in that the lowest acceptable lung volumes are maintained using the lowest possible $\overline{P}_{aw}$. In infants with PIE, this strategy can also feature a lower frequency than is typical to allow a longer expiratory time, thus encouraging interstitial gas resorption.

The initial $\overline{P}_{aw}$ usually is set at the same level or 2 to 3 cm H_2O higher than the $\overline{P}_{aw}$ required for conventional ventilation. The amplitude and frequency are set and adjusted according to the optimum lung volume strategy algorithm (see Fig. 22-28). An F_IO_2 as high as 1 is considered acceptable during the first 12 to 24 hours.[103] The F_IO_2 usually is reduced to 0.8 before weaning the $\overline{P}_{aw}$. This is done to provide some margin in case oxygenation drops after the $\overline{P}_{aw}$ is lowered; the F_IO_2 can be increased to help restore oxygenation. The decision to wean from the $\overline{P}_{aw}$ rather than the F_IO_2 is made according to the progress seen in correcting air leaks. If they are resolving, the need to reduce $\overline{P}_{aw}$ is not as important as the need to reduce F_IO_2. Conversely, extension of air leaks may require a lower $\overline{P}_{aw}$, if possible, with a higher F_IO_2 (see Case Study 22-7). Patients with a pulmonary air leak should not be removed from the oscillator, and manual ventilation should be avoided. The ET should be suctioned with an inline suction catheter if possible. Pediatric patients with ARDS and other forms of hypoxic respiratory failure can be supported using HFOV. HFOV is typically initiated after conventional modes of ventilation have been unsuccessful. Many of the same principles that guide neonatal HFOV management can be applied to pediatric HFOV management. The major difference is that HFOV is applied using higher mean airway pressure, greater amplitude, and lower-frequency settings in pediatric patients. Compared with CV, HFOV initiated earlier in the disease process may improve gas exchange and reduce VILI in pediatric patients with ARDS.[118]

WEANING AND EXTUBATION

The length of time a patient receives mechanical ventilation is an independent risk factor for morbidity. For this reason, many

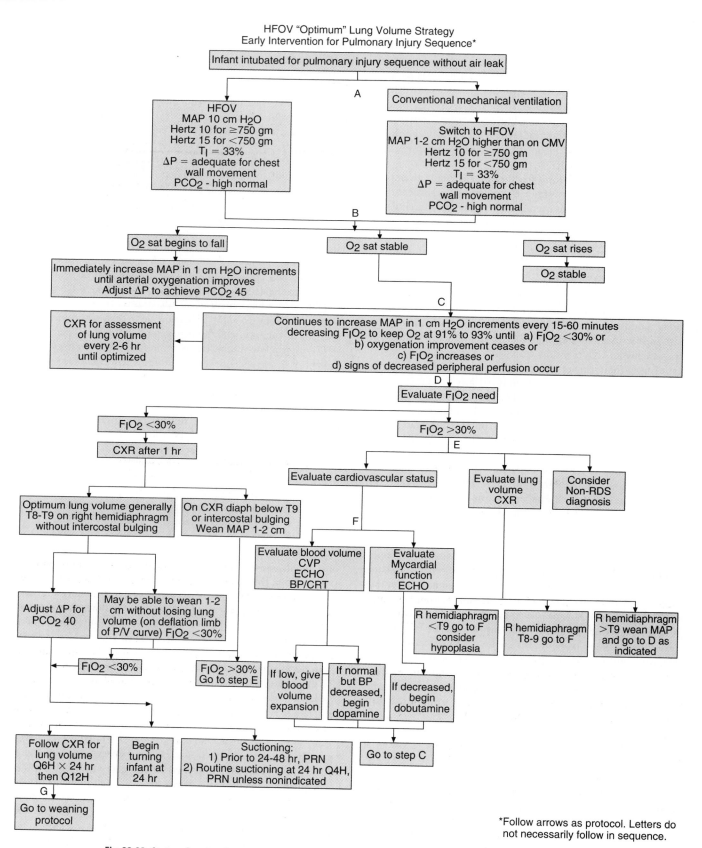

Fig. 22-32 Strategy flow chart for optimum lung volume HFOV. *CRT,* Hematocrit; *CVP,* central venous pressure; *CXR,* chest radiograph; *ECHO,* echocardiogram; *F$_i$O$_2$,* fraction of inspired oxygen; *HFOV,* high-frequency oscillatory ventilation; *MAP,* mean airway pressure; *ΔP,* pressure gradient; *PCO$_2$,* partial pressure of carbon dioxide; *P/V,* pressure/volume; *qH,* every hour; *RDS,* respiratory distress syndrome; *T8 to T9,* thoracic vertebra. (From Minton S, Gerstmann D, Stoddard R: Cardiopul Rev, PN 770118-001, Yorba Linda, Calif., 1995, SensorMedics.)

HFOV "Optimum" Lung Volume Strategy
Pulmonary Injury Sequence Without Airleak
Weaning Strategy

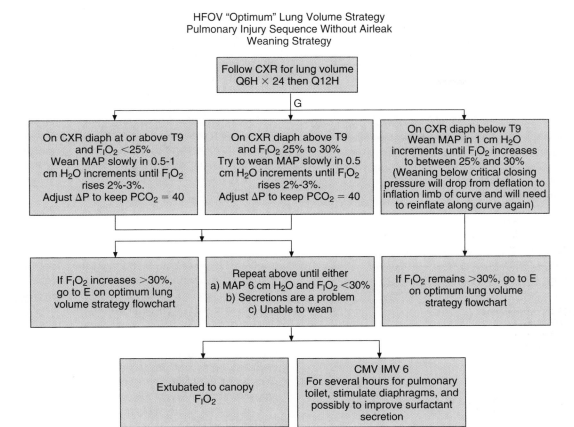

Fig. 22-33 Strategy flow chart for weaning from optimum lung volume high-frequency oscillatory ventilation. *CMV,* Continuous mandatory ventilation; *CXR,* chest radiograph; *F_iO_2,* fraction of inspired oxygen; *IMV,* intermittent mandatory ventilation; *MAP,* mean arterial pressure; *Q6H,* every 6 hours; *Q8H,* every 12 hours. (From Minton S, Gerstmann D, Stoddard R: Cardiopul Rev, PN 770118-001, Yorba Linda, Calif., 1995, SensorMedics.)

institutions have established weaning protocols in an effort to remove unnecessary obstacles to weaning and extubation. A multicenter study of the weaning of pediatric patients from the ventilator showed little difference between weaning according to clinical guidelines and weaning without following guidelines.[56] The time from start of weaning to extubation, and the rate of extubation failure, seemed to be unaffected by the use of written weaning protocols.[56] Routinely evaluating a patient for weaning readiness has been shown to be far more useful in facilitating timely ventilator discontinuation and extubation.[119] Careful attention should be paid to the balance of sedative drugs and the patient's ventilatory status because excessive sedation is the most significant factor contributing to weaning failure. Patient preparation and use of the extubation readiness test (see Box 22-8) can help achieve the earliest possible extubation.

Some institutions have established a testing procedure for determining a patient's readiness for weaning. This so-called weaning readiness test (see Box 22-8) usually is conducted in patients whose sedation score would permit extubation. The patient's enteral feedings are stopped for the test, the F_iO_2 is reduced to 0.5, and PEEP is reduced to 5 cm H_2O. If the S_pO_2 is greater than 95% on these settings or with a lower F_iO_2, the pressure support level is reduced to the minimum amount for the ET size (see Box 22-8). Once the patient has been placed on the

minimum-pressure support level for the ET size, the respiratory rate and S_pO_2 are monitored. Increases in the respiratory rate above guideline parameters, or a drop in S_pO_2, signals a failed test and suggests that additional support is needed.[56] Although the test is called an extubation readiness test, it is only one criterion in the decision on extubation. It also is a useful test for determining whether PSV might be an appropriate mode for the patient and the pressure support level that should be set on the ventilator.

Extubation failure is often attributed to glottic or subglottic injury or edema. Patients who have had airway manipulations, multiple intubations, or unplanned extubations tend to have unsuccessful extubation more often. Yet in various studies a large number of patients who had an uneventful ventilator course and planned extubation nevertheless had a failed extubation.[56,119]

An air-leak test has been recommended before extubation is scheduled, but there is controversy over whether this test can predict successful extubation or not. For this simple test, the clinician deflates the cuff of the ET, places a stethoscope directly over the larynx, and gives a manual breath; the rush of gas around the ET should be heard. The pressure at which the air leak is heard should be noted. If an air leak is present at 20 mm Hg pressure or less, the patient is unlikely to have postextubation stridor (see Chapter 20). A small number of studies support the use of dexamethasone as a prophylactic treatment to prevent postextubation

---

BOX 22-8   **Extubation Readiness Test**[120]

Procedure
1. Temporarily stop enteral feedings.
2. Reduce the fractional inspired oxygen (F_IO_2) to 0.5.
3. Reduce the positive end-expiratory pressure (PEEP) to 5 cm H_2O.
4. Evaluate the oxygen saturation by pulse oximetry (S_pO_2):
   a. If the S_pO_2 is below 95% and the F_IO_2 is less than 0.5, increase the F_IO_2 to 0.5.
   b. If the S_pO_2 is above 95%, change to pressure support ventilation (PSV) at the minimal amount for the endotracheal (ET) tube size used:
      - 3-3.5 mm: 10 cm H_2O
      - 4-4.5 mm: 8 cm H_2O
      - 5 mm or larger: 6 cm H_2O
   c. Monitor the S_pO_2, effective tidal volume (V_T), and respiratory rate (f).

Assessment
The patient is **potentially** ready for extubation if:
- The S_pO_2 is over 95%.
- The effective V_T is over 5 mL/kg.
- The respiratory rate is within the goal range for the patient's age (see chart) for up to 2 hours:

Age	Goal Range (breaths/min)
Under 6 mo	20-60
6 mo to 2 yr	15-45
2-5 yr	15-40
Over 5 yr	10-35

---

stridor. In one clinical trial the drug was given 6 to 12 hours before extubation and every 6 hours afterward, for a total of six doses.[121] This protocol is sometimes followed for patients at especially high risk for stridor and extubation failure. Steroid administration appears to be somewhat beneficial.

ADJUNCTIVE FORMS OF RESPIRATORY SUPPORT

Surfactant Replacement Therapy

Pulmonary surfactant has the remarkable ability to distribute itself in a thin layer between the alveolar surface and the alveolar gas. About 90% of human surfactant is made up of phospholipids, about 60% of which is dipalmitoylphosphatidylcholine (DPPC). DPPC, other phospholipids, and neutral lipids produce the surface-active effects in the lungs. The distribution of surfactant is thought to be caused by the low pH of the phospholipids, which makes them easily absorbed. Surfactant also contains at least three types of proteins that help distribute and regulate its life cycle and absorption. The challenge to manufacturers of artificial surfactant has been to produce a material that has the same type of surface action, can be instilled into the lung, and can immediately distribute itself to the periphery. A major problem with instilling any material into the lung is that it can obstruct gas flow and impede gas exchange.

Survanta and Infasurf (calfactant) are currently the most frequently used surfactant replacements. These preparations, which are extracted from calf-lung washings, contain some proteins plus

the major phospholipids. Both have proven highly effective at reducing mortality in very premature infants.[122]

Two strategies are suggested for surfactant replacement therapy: prophylactic therapy and rescue therapy. **Prophylactic therapy** consists of surfactant administration immediately at birth or soon after for infants who are at risk of developing RDS. **Rescue therapy** involves surfactant administration in infants who have RDS or another surfactant deficiency syndrome. Although no indications for surfactant replacement other than RDS have been established, surfactant replacement therapy is used in infants with meconium aspiration, pneumonia, and pulmonary hemorrhage. Older children and adults with ARDS also have been treated successfully with surfactant.

The procedure for administering surfactant depends on the type used and the manufacturer's recommendations. Usually the patient is placed on a conventional ventilator set at a frequency of at least 30 breaths/min and an F_IO_2 of 1.0. Each partial dose usually is followed by 30 seconds on the ventilator. Once the full dose has been given, the ventilator is adjusted back to baseline settings (or HFV can be resumed at baseline settings). Regardless of the mode of ventilation used, signs of improving pulmonary compliance are monitored. For conventional ventilation, changes in V_T and waveforms are noted and settings adjusted appropriately. If the patient is placed on an HFV, the F_IO_2 and $\bar{P}_{aw}$, S_pO_2, and ABG values are evaluated (see section on HFV previously discussed). Some clinicians prefer to obtain a chest radiograph shortly after surfactant replacement regardless of the type of ventilation used.

During and after surfactant administration, the clinician watches for signs of ET or large airway obstruction, including poor chest excursion, oxygen desaturation, and bradycardia. If the patient has preexisting obstructions, the liquid can be preferentially administered into one lung. Another problem that might be encountered during surfactant administration is reflux of the surfactant up the ET because of patient agitation and coughing. In these cases the dose may be inadvertently deposited in the pharynx because of a leak around the ET. Even without tube obstructions, hypoxemia may worsen.[123] Some patients develop prolonged periods of apnea after surfactant dosing.[124]

Other complications of surfactant replacement therapy have been reported. Pulmonary hemorrhage is a serious complication and is most often seen in very premature infants. The incidence of pulmonary hemorrhage varies inversely with birth weight.[125] Mucus plugging, especially of smaller ETs, has been reported in the hours after surfactant dosing. A long-term complication is an increase in retinopathy of prematurity in infants who have received surfactants; the cause of this is not entirely understood.[126]

Volutrauma and overdistention of the lungs have been reported in infants who have responded favorably to surfactant replacement; these conditions may be a result of failure to address increasing compliance by promptly reducing the $\bar{P}_{aw}$ delivered by the ventilator.[127] This situation underscores the importance of monitoring V_T and using VSV after the immediate postdosing period. Monitoring for changes in the shunt is crucial after surfactant replacement in patients with patent ductus arteriosus (PDA), particularly newborns with BPD.[128] Theoretically the reduced pulmonary vascular resistance produced by improved oxygenation can increase the left-to-right shunting caused by the PDA. This may prevent spontaneous closure of the ductus. A common belief is that oxygenation will worsen after the initial improvement in lung mechanics because of the effects of a PDA. The immense success of surfactant therapy in infants with RDS has prompted clinicians to use it in the treatment of ARDS in older patients. Studies have been conducted using both aerosolized administration and intratracheal instillation of surfactant.[118] The studies showed an initial improvement in the P_aO_2/F_IO_2 ratio in most subjects, but sustained improvement beyond 48 hours of treatment has not been achieved.[129] Future studies are needed to demonstrate a long-term benefit of surfactant replacement therapy in adult ARDS patients. Until that time, its use is not recommended in adults.

Prone Positioning

Pediatric patients treated for acute respiratory failure are sometimes positioned prone in an attempt to improve oxygenation. The overall beneficial effect of the prone position is to improve $\dot{V}/\dot{Q}$ matching and reduce physiological shunt (see Chapter 12). Assuming that the dorsal regions of the lung are atelectatic because the patient has been supine, repositioning into the prone position may help recruit collapsed areas. However, results from one clinical trial were unable to show any benefit in outcomes related to the use of prone positioning in pediatric patients with acute lung injury.[130]

Inhaled Nitric Oxide Therapy

Inhaled nitric oxide (INO) is a colorless, odorless gas that is also a potent pulmonary vasodilator. When given via inhalation, NO rapidly diffuses across the alveolar capillary membrane and is bound to hemoglobin and thus has little effect on the systemic circulation. The therapeutic goal of most NO regimens is to improve pulmonary blood flow and enhance arterial oxygenation. Medically its effectiveness can spare patients the need for more invasive procedures, such as **extracorporeal membrane oxygenation** (ECMO).

Several systems have been designed to administer the most common system for providing INO through circuits for spontaneously breathing patients, or through ventilator and anesthesia circuits. In one widely used system, the INOMax DS_{IR} (Ikaria, Clinton, N.J.), a pneumotachometer incorporated into an injector module is placed inline with the delivered gas. The module measures the actual flow and simultaneously injects NO to achieve the set concentration. Changes in flow or the use of a variable flow pattern do not affect the delivered NO concentration. This system also monitors the delivered NO and nitrogen dioxide (NO_2) and the F_IO_2.[131] Safe administration of INO largely depends on monitoring of the inhaled gas mixture. Two types of toxicity have been reported with INO in both animal and human subjects: pulmonary tissue toxicity and methemoglobinemia.[132] Pulmonary tissue toxicity is a well-known side effect and results when NO combines with oxygen and forms the reddish brown gas NO_2. When NO_2 is exposed to NO, dinitrogen trioxide (N_2O_3) is produced and reacts with water, forming either nitrous or nitric acid, both of which are very toxic to the alveolar epithelium.[133] The higher the concentration of oxygen, the greater the potential for the development of toxic levels of NO_2.

Many clinical situations that require administration of INO also require very high concentrations of oxygen in the gas mixture. In such cases even low-dose NO can produce toxic levels of NO_2,[134] thus underscoring the importance of NO/NO_2 monitoring in the inhalation circuit. However, when NO is administered at low doses, it usually reacts slowly with oxygen, and the formation of toxic products is small. Nonetheless, close monitoring is essential to control the therapeutic level of NO and avoid excessive levels of NO_2.

Case Study 22-8

Determining Appropriateness of Nitric Oxide Therapy

A 33-hour-old infant with respiratory distress has just been transferred to the newborn ICU. Mild cyanosis is developing, and the SpO_2 percentage is in the low 60s on supplemental oxygen. The chest radiograph is unremarkable. There is no evidence of meconium aspiration and no maternal history of infection. The peripheral pulses are weak, particularly in the lower extremities. The blood pressure is 32/12 mm Hg, and the heart rate is 190 beats/min. No murmur is noted. The respiratory rate is 80 to 100 breaths/min with moderate retractions and nasal flaring.

The patient eventually is intubated, sedated, and paralyzed. An umbilical artery catheter (UAC) is placed, and administration of dopamine and fluids is initiated. ABG values show refractory hypoxemia, a low P_aCO_2, and metabolic acidosis. The patient is placed on mechanical ventilation with 100% oxygen.

The ICU team is leaning toward a diagnosis of persistent pulmonary hypertension (PPHN), but is not ruling out congenital cyanotic heart disease. The respiratory therapist is asked her opinion about starting nitric oxide therapy. How should she respond?

Methemoglobinemia develops primarily through the oxidation of NO when it comes in contact with oxyhemoglobin. Methemoglobin occurs naturally, and its level normally is maintained partly by the enzyme methemoglobin reductase. This enzyme, which is found largely in red blood cells, converts methemoglobin to hemoglobin. The rate of methemoglobin formation rarely exceeds the ability of the reductase to convert methemoglobin to hemoglobin; therefore the methemoglobin level is usually less than 2%.

Studies of INO's effectiveness at reducing intrapulmonary shunt and improving $\dot{V}/\dot{Q}$ matching suggest that the drug is most effective when used with high-frequency ventilation.[135,136] These investigators maintain that effective recruiting of lung units enhances the effect of NO. A comprehensive review of evidence for the labeled use of INO in hypoxemic infants, devices, clinical monitoring, and management has been provided in an AARC clinical practice guideline (Case Study 22-8).[137] (See the Evolve website for this text and for additional information on NO therapy.)

SUMMARY

- Mechanical ventilation in newborn and pediatric patients involves the use of devices that recruit and maintain lung volumes, improves gas exchange and lung mechanics, assists in overcoming the resistive properties of an artificial airway, and reduces the amount of energy required to breathe.
- Neonatal and pediatric patients have smaller lungs, higher airway resistance, lower lung compliance, less surface area for gas exchange, and lower cardiovascular reserve than do adults, making them more vulnerable to rapid onset of respiratory distress.

- Neonates experiencing respiratory distress present with tachypnea, nasal flaring, and intercostal, substernal, and retrosternal retractions.
- The Silverman-Anderson respiratory scoring system is a useful clinical tool to assess the degree of respiratory distress in neonates.
- Pediatric patients experiencing respiratory distress can present with some of the same clinical manifestations as neonates. However, larger pediatric patients have ossified or stiffer chest walls and are able to sustain longer periods of WOB than neonates.
- Determining oxygenation and ventilation in neonate and pediatric patients is evaluated by ABG analysis and noninvasive techniques, such as S_pO_2 and transcutaneous CO_2 measurements. Chest radiograph evaluation is another important tool.
- The goals of mechanical ventilatory support in newborn and pediatric patients are to (1) provide adequate ventilation and oxygenation; (2) achieve adequate lung volume; (3) improve lung compliance; (4) reduce WOB; and (5) limit lung injury.
- Noninvasive respiratory support can include nasal CPAP, nasal IPPV, nasal IMV for neonates, and CPAP and BiPAP in pediatric patients.
- Used appropriately, CPAP is a less invasive and less aggressive form of therapy than other forms of ventilatory support.
- Complications of CPAP include pulmonary overdistention and can lead to ventilation/perfusion mismatching, decreased pulmonary blood flow, increased pulmonary vascular resistance, and decreased cardiac output.
- NIV, also known as *CPAP with a rate,* is an established form of ventilatory support in adults and pediatric patients wherein superimposed positive pressure inflations are combined with CPAP to re-expand atelectatic areas, improve gas exchange, reduce respiratory distress, avoid apnea, and potentially obviate invasive mechanical ventilation.
- Nasal synchronized and nasal IMV are the most commonly used breath types and pressure control is the most common mode for providing NIV in neonates.
- Nasal "sigh" positive airway pressure (SiPAP) is being used more frequently to assist spontaneously breathing infants in the NICU because it allows the neonate to breathe at a high and a low CPAP setting.
- Nasal HFV is becoming more common in clinical practice as a form of NIV as it uses smaller pressures, higher frequencies, and may be more lung protective than other NIV devices that apply higher pressure to the lungs.
- CPAP is used less often for pediatric patients than for adults; however, it is useful in children to restore FRC and reduce WOB with acute hypoxemia, neuromuscular disorders, and conditions that cause abdominal distention. It also is used to relieve the airway obstruction associated with obstructive sleep apnea or airway lesions like laryngotracheal malacia.
- Conventional mechanical ventilation or invasive mechanical ventilation involves the use of positive pressure inflations in intubated patients who are breathing spontaneously or who are heavily sedated or paralyzed, but management of such patients should always be to avoid invasive ventilation whenever possible to minimize ventilator-induced lung injury.
- Ventilator care of the newborn is often an integral part of the broader management of premature infants.

- Most newborns who require full ventilatory support are placed on infant ventilators or infant-through-adult ventilators specifically designed to respond to even the smallest of patients.
- The most frequently diagnosed cause of respiratory failure in pediatric patients under the age of 1 year was bronchiolitis; in children older than 1 year, pneumonia was most often the cause.
- Pressure-controlled ventilation is the most widely used mode of ventilation in neonates and pediatric patients. The pressure-controlled breath can be triggered by pressure or flow and is terminated based on time. It can be used during IMV and CMV breath types.
- Monitoring inspiratory pressure, PEEP, T_I, T_E, I : E ratio, V_T, frequency, mean airway pressure, and inspired oxygen concentration are all necessary with pressure-controlled ventilation.
- Older children and adults have been ventilated with volume-controlled ventilation in patients with ARDS and premature neonates with RDS.
- The most widely used form of dual-control mode used in neonates and pediatric patients is PRVC and is commonly used in patients with CMV or IMV breath types.
- VSV is well suited to infants and pediatric patients as target V_T is maintained, and self-weaning is possible.
- The goal of any lung-protective strategy is to (1) avoid repetitive opening and closing of small airways (atelectotrauma); (2) limit overinflation during inhalation (volutrauma); (3) reduce gas trapping during exhalation; and (4) alleviate pulmonary inflammation (biotrauma).
- HFV can be complicated by PIS, which includes RDS, PIE, pulmonary air-leak syndrome, oxygen toxicity, and development of BPD.
- Two potential problems are associated with HFPPV: (1) the high rate and short T_I may prevent adequate V_T delivery; and (2) because expiration is entirely passive, breath stacking can occur, causing pulmonary hyperinflation as a consequence of insufficient time for emptying of all lung units.
- HFOV has become the most widely used high-frequency technique for infants and pediatric patients because both inspiration and expiration are active, gas flow is sinusoidal rather than triangular, bulk flow rather than jet pulsations is delivered, and V_T is less than dead space.
- Assessment of breath sounds, heart sounds, pulmonary compliance, and other such parameters is difficult in patients receiving HFV; therefore a thorough assessment should be performed before the patient is connected to the high-frequency device.
- Adjunctive forms of respiratory support include surfactant replacement therapy, prone positioning, and inhaled NO_2 therapy.
- Prophylactic therapy consists of surfactant administration immediately at birth or soon after for infants who are at risk of developing RDS.
- Rescue therapy involves surfactant administration in infants who have RDS or another surfactant deficiency syndrome.
- The overall beneficial effect of the prone position is to improve $\dot{V}/\dot{Q}$ matching and reduce physiological shunt.
- The therapeutic goal of most NO (a pulmonary vasodilator) regimens is to improve pulmonary blood flow and enhance arterial oxygenation.

REVIEW QUESTIONS (See Appendix A for answers.)

1. A 6-hour-old term infant has intercostal retractions, nasal flaring, and grunting. HR is 180 beats/min, f is 70 breaths/min and regular, and S_pO_2 is 90% on room air. ABG values reveal a pH of 7.34, a P_aCO_2 of 28 mm Hg, and a P_aO_2 of 58 mm Hg. Which of the following would be most appropriate?
   A. Intubation and mechanical ventilation
   B. Intubation and CPAP
   C. Nasal CPAP
   D. No intervention necessary at this time

2. Which of the following is (are) potential complications of CPAP in newborns?
   A. Pulmonary overdistention
   B. Air-leak syndromes
   C. Increased WOB
   D. All of the above

3. A 1.4-kg neonate has been receiving nasal CPAP with the same NP tube for 2 days. The NP tube is connected to a ventilator set to deliver CPAP at 6 cm H_2O with a flow rate of 8 L/min. Over the past 2 hours, the infant's f increased from about 40 breaths/min to about 60 breaths/min. F_IO_2 had to be increased from 0.25 to 0.45 because of decreasing S_pO_2 values. Which of the following actions should be taken?
   A. Increase the flow rate
   B. Increase the CPAP level
   C. Change the NP tube
   D. Intubate the infant and begin TCPL

4. Which of the following is (are) considered essential for all infant mechanical ventilators?
   A. Pressure support capability
   B. Patient triggering
   C. Leak compensation
   D. All of the above

5. When an infant ventilator is operating in the pressure control mode, the expiratory phase of the breath cycle begins when what preset cycle is reached?
   A. Pressure
   B. Time
   C. Volume
   D. Flow

6. What is the difference between a demand flow IMV and a continuous flow IMV system in an infant ventilator delivering pressure control?
   A. A demand flow IMV system has a baseline bias flow; when the patient's inspiratory flow exceeds the bias flow, a demand valve opens to provide whatever additional flow is needed.
   B. A demand flow IMV system has a bias flow that is set by the manufacturer; it is activated only if the patient takes a spontaneous breath.
   C. A demand flow IMV system does not have a bias flow that is set by the manufacturer; patient flow triggering opens a demand valve that immediately meets the patient's inspiratory flow needs.
   D. A demand flow IMV system has a baseline flow rate that is set by the clinician; if the patient's inspiratory flow rate exceeds the set value, no additional flow is provided.

7. A previously healthy 3-year-old child is admitted to the ICU with an unconfirmed diagnosis of varicella pneumonia. The child is lethargic, the breathing is labored, and the skin is cool and mottled. The respiratory rate is 15 breaths/min, HR is 190 beats/min, temperature is 38.8° C, BP is 70/44 mm Hg, and S_pO_2 is 83% on a nonrebreathing oxygen mask. Breath sounds are distant, but coarse rales can be heard bilaterally. ABG values reveal a pH of 7.26, P_aCO_2 at 64 mm Hg, and P_aO_2 at 55 mm Hg on the nonrebreathing mask. Which of the following interventions would be appropriate based on the above information?
   A. Intubate the patient and begin CPAP
   B. Place the patient on a BiPAP system with supplemental oxygen
   C. Maintain the patient on the nonrebreathing mask, begin fluid replacement therapy to treat the low blood pressure, and obtain appropriate cultures
   D. Intubate the patient and initiate mechanical ventilation

8. For an infant about to receive mechanical ventilation, the initial PIP and T_I are best determined by:
   A. Placing the infant on the ventilator and adjusting PIP and T_I to obtain the desired V_T
   B. Manually ventilating the infant while noting the PIP and T_I that achieve the best S_pO_2 and lung aeration
   C. Placing the infant on the ventilator and adjusting PIP and T_I to obtain the desired S_pO_2
   D. Manually ventilating the infant while monitoring the waveform, noting the PIP and T_I that produce the best waveform

9. Theoretical advantages of the A/C mode on the Bird V.I.P. with both adjustable flow triggering and inspiratory flow termination for newborns are:
   A. Less potential for lung injury
   B. Reduced sedation requirements
   C. Easier weaning
   D. All of the above

10. A 3.5-kg newborn with a diagnosis of group B *Streptococcus* pneumonia is intubated with a 3-mm ID ET and is receiving mechanical ventilation with the CareFusion AVEA in the CMV mode. A monitoring device is in-line. The initial settings are as follows:
    Inspiratory Pressure = 24 cm H_2O, PEEP = 4 cm H_2O,
       F_IO_2 = 1.0, set frequency = 20 breaths/min
    Actual frequency = 50 to 55 breaths/min
    V_{Tinsp} = 45 to 50 mL, V_{Texh} = 12 to 15 mL, set T_I = 0.6 second,
       actual T_I = 0.6 second
    Flow cycle = 10%
    The infant has received little sedation and is awake and breathing but appears to be fighting the ventilator. Patient triggering seems to be occurring with every breath, but the ventilator does not flow cycle regardless of the termination sensitivity setting. Which of the following interventions would be appropriate based on the preceding information?
    A. Reintubate with a larger ET
    B. Increase the PIP
    C. Administer muscle relaxants and switch to a control mode
    D. Increase the T_I

11. A 3.1-kg term infant has just returned from the operating room after removal of a small bowel obstruction. The infant will remain paralyzed and sedated over the next 12 hours and is receiving pressure control with the following settings:

   PIP = 20 cm H_2O, PEEP = 6 cm H_2O, frequency = 22 breaths/min, T_I = 0.6 second
   F_IO_2 = 0.3, flow rate = 8 L/min
   ABG values are pH = 7.26, P_aCO_2 = 66 mm Hg,
   P_aO_2 = 78 mm Hg
   Additional data are as follows:
   V_{Texh} = 7 to 10 mL, $\dot{V}_E$ = 1.88 L/min
   S_pO_2 = 95%, BP = 68/42 mm Hg
   Based on these data, which of the following ventilator control manipulations would be most appropriate?
   A. Increase the T_I
   B. Increase the flow
   C. Increase the frequency
   D. Increase the PIP

12. A 2-year-old patient intubated with a 4-mm ID nasal ET is recovering from surgical repair of a ventricular septal defect and has been weaned from volume ventilation on SIMV to PSV (Servo-i ventilator). Since the changeover to this mode, the ventilator at times seems to trigger on and cycle off very rapidly, making the patient uncomfortable and very agitated. Which of the following should correct this problem?
   A. Reintubate the patient with a larger tube
   B. Switch to ventilator tubing with a larger diameter
   C. Check sensitivity, rise time to set pressure, and flow-cycling criteria
   D. Select a more appropriate mode

13. A newborn patient of 29 weeks' gestational age has RDS. She weighs 950 g. She is receiving conventional mechanical ventilation at a $\bar{P}_{aw}$ of 16 cm H_2O. The patient is to be changed to HFOV. Which of the following settings would you initially select?
   A. $\bar{P}_{aw}$ = 18 cm H_2O; frequency = 15 Hz
   B. $\bar{P}_{aw}$ = 16 cm H_2O; frequency = 15 Hz
   C. $\bar{P}_{aw}$ = 18 cm H_2O; frequency = 10 Hz
   D. $\bar{P}_{aw}$ = 16 cm H_2O; frequency = 10 Hz

14. An 18-month-old, 15-kg child with a diagnosis of ARDS has been mechanically ventilated for 5 days. The patient initially received volume-cycled SIMV, but now is receiving PCV at the following settings:

   PIP = 37 cm H_2O, PEEP = 8 cm H_2O, $\bar{P}_{aw}$ = 16.4 cm H_2O
   Frequency = 40 breaths/min, T_I = 0.9 second, F_IO_2 = 1
   ABG values are: pH = 7.29, P_aCO_2 = 53 mm Hg,
   P_aO_2 = 46 mm Hg, S_aO_2 = 79%
   Additional data are as follows:
   V_{Texh} = 75 to 85 mL
   $\dot{V}_E$ = 2.92 L/min
   Based on the above data, which of the following would be most appropriate?
   A. Increase the PEEP, maintain the PIP, and give sodium bicarbonate ($NaHCO_3$) to normalize the pH
   B. Change to high-frequency ventilation
   C. Maintain the present settings but give $NaHCO_3$ to normalize the pH
   D. Change to a high V_T/low f strategy

15. A patient with RDS, who developed diffuse PIE on the right side, has been on HFOV for 8 hours. Vital signs are stable, and ABG values on an F_IO_2 of 0.7 are within acceptable limits. A chest radiograph shows that the PIE is worsening and expanding to the ninth posterior rib level on the right. Which of the following ventilator management strategies should be applied to this situation?
   A. Maintain the current strategy and try to wean the F_IO_2 as soon as possible
   B. Reduce the $\bar{P}_{aw}$ even if the F_IO_2 must be increased
   C. Increase the $\bar{P}_{aw}$ and wean the F_IO_2 as much as possible
   D. Switch to conventional ventilation

16. A 640-g newborn is receiving HFOV at the following settings:
   $\bar{P}_{aw}$ = 19 cm H_2O, F_IO_2 = 0.28, frequency = 15 Hz, amplitude (P) = 34 cm H_2O
   ABG values are: pH = 7.56, P_aCO_2 = 23 mm Hg,
   P_aO_2 = 85 mm Hg
   Based on the above data, which of the following would be most appropriate?
   A. Reduce the amplitude
   B. Reduce the frequency
   C. Reduce the $\bar{P}_{aw}$
   D. Maintain the current settings

17. A full-term, 3-kg infant is on HFJV at the following settings:
   PIP = 22 cm H_2O, PEEP = 11 cm H_2O, $\bar{P}_{aw}$ = 12 cm H_2O
   Frequency = 420 cycles/min, jet T_I = 0.02 second, F_IO_2 = 0.4
   ABG values are: pH = 7.3, P_aCO_2 = 55 mm Hg,
   P_aO_2 = 90 mm Hg
   Based on the above data, which of the following control changes should be made first?
   A. Reduce the PEEP
   B. Reduce the frequency
   C. Increase the jet T_I
   D. Maintain the current settings

18. An infant is receiving pressure-controlled ventilation. Which of the following parameters most likely will need to be adjusted first after surfactant replacement therapy?
   A. T_I
   B. Frequency
   C. PIP
   D. PEEP

19. The most important advantage of nitric oxide in the treatment of pulmonary hypertension is:
   A. It does not have to be analyzed.
   B. It is selective in its effects.
   C. It is inexpensive and easy to use.
   D. It has no toxic effects.

References

1. Kumar A, Falke KJ, Geffin B, et al: Continuous positive-pressure ventilation in acute respiratory failure: effects on hemodynamics and lung function. *N Engl J Med* 283:1430–1436, 1970.
2. Gregory GA, Kitterman JA, Phibbs RH, et al: Treatment of the idiopathic respiratory-distress syndrome with continuous positive airway pressure. *N Engl J Med* 284:1333–1340, 1971.
3. Speidel BD, Dunn PM: Use of nasal continuous positive airway pressure to treat severe recurrent apnea in very preterm infants. *Lancet* 2:658–660, 1976.

4. DiBlasi RM: Nasal continuous positive airway pressure (CPAP) for the respiratory care of the newborn infant. *Respir Care* 54:1209–1235, 2009.

5. AARC Clinical Practice Guidelines: Application of continuous positive airway pressure to neonates via nasal prongs or nasopharyngeal tube or nasal mask. *Respir Care* 49:1100–1108, 2004.

6. Scopesi F, Calevo MG, Rolfe P, et al: Volume targeted ventilation (volume guarantee) in the weaning phase of premature newborn infants. *Pediatr Pulmonol* 42:864–870, 2007.

7. Van Marter LJ, Allred EN, Pagano M, et al: Do clinical markers of barotrauma and oxygen toxicity explain interhospital variation in rates of chronic lung disease? *Pediatrics* 105:1194–1201, 2000.

8. Avery ME, Tooley WH, Keller JB, et al: Is chronic lung disease in low birth weight infants preventable? A survey of eight centers. *Pediatrics* 79:26–30, 1987.

9. SUPPORT Study Group of the Eunice Kennedy Shriver NICHD Neonatal Research Network: Early CPAP versus surfactant in extremely preterm infants. *N Engl J Med* 362:1970–1979, 2010. Erratum in: *N Engl J Med* 362:2235, 2010.

10. Verder H, Bohlin K, Kamper J, et al: Nasal CPAP and surfactant for treatment of respiratory distress syndrome and prevention of bronchopulmonary dysplasia. *Acta Paediatr* 98:1400–1408, 2009.

11. Stevens TP, Harrington EW, Blennow M, et al: Early surfactant administration with brief ventilation vs. selective surfactant and continued mechanical ventilation for preterm infants with or at risk for respiratory distress syndrome. *Cochrane Database Syst Rev* (4):CD003063, 2007.

12. Davis PG, Henderson-Smart DJ: Extubation from low-rate intermittent positive airway pressure versus extubation after a trial of endotracheal continuous positive airway pressure in intubated preterm infants. *Cochrane Database Syst Rev* (4):CD001078, 2001.

13. DiBlasi RM, Richardson CP: Continuous positive airway pressure. In Walsh BK, Czervinske M, DiBlasi RM, editors: *Perinatal and pediatric respiratory care*, ed 3, St Louis, 2009, Elsevier, pp 305–318.

14. De Paoli AG, Morley CJ, Davis PG, et al: In vitro comparison of nasal continuous positive airway pressure devices for neonates. *Arch Dis Child Fetal Neonatal Ed* 87:F42–F45, 2002.

15. Johnson B, Ahlstrom H, Lindroth M, et al: CPAP: modes of action in relation to clinical application. *Pediatr Clin North Am* 27:687–699, 1980.

16. Beasley JM, Jones SEF: Continuous positive airway pressure in bronchiolitis. *BMJ* 283:1506–1508, 1981.

17. Javouhey E, Barats A, Richard N, et al: Non-invasive ventilation as primary ventilatory support for infants with severe bronchiolitis. *Intensive Care Med* 34:1608–1614, 2008.

18. Sung V, Massie J, Hochmann MA, et al: Estimating inspired oxygen concentration delivered by nasal prongs in children with bronchiolitis. *J Paediatr Child Health* 44:14–18, 2008.

19. De Paoli AG, Davis PG, Faber B, et al: Devices and pressure sources for administration of nasal continuous positive airway pressure (CPAP) in preterm neonates. *Cochrane Database Syst Rev* (23):CD002977, 2008.

20. DiBlasi RM, Salyer JW, Zignego JC, et al: The impact of imposed expiratory resistance in neonatal mechanical ventilation: Q Laboratory Evaluation. *Respir Care* 53:1450–1460, 2008.

21. Klausner JF, Lee AY, Hutchinson AA: Decreased imposed work of breathing with a new nasal continuous positive pressure device. *Pediatr Pulmonol* 22:188–194, 1996.

22. Kahn DJ, Courtney SE, Steele AM, et al: Unpredictability of delivered bubble nasal continuous positive airway pressure: role of bias flow magnitude and nares-prong air leaks. *Pediatr Res* 62:343–347, 2007.

23. Kahn DJ, Habib RH, Courtney SE: Effects of flow amplitudes on intraprong pressures during bubble versus ventilator-generated nasal continuous positive airway pressure in premature infants. *Pediatrics* 122:1009–1013, 2008.

24. Lee KY, Dunn MS, Fenwick M, et al: A comparison of underwater bubble CPAP with ventilator derived CPAP in premature neonates ready for extubation. *Biol Neonate* 73:69–75, 1998.

25. Leone TA, Rich W, Finer NN: A survey of delivery room resuscitation practices in the United States. *Pediatrics* 117:e164–e175, 2006.

26. Tanswell AK, Clubb RA, Smith BT, et al: Effects of continuous positive airway pressure on pulmonary function and blood gases of infants with respiratory distress syndrome. *Arch Dis Child* 55:33–39, 1980.

27. Speidel BD, Dunn PM: Effect of continuous positive airway pressure on breathing pattern of infants with respiratory distress syndrome. *Lancet* 1:302–304, 1975.

28. Nelson RM, Egan EA, Eitzman DV: Increased hypoxemia in neonates secondary to the use of continuous positive airway pressure. *J Pediatr* 91:87–91, 1977.

29. Czervinske M, Durbin CG, Gal TJ: Resistance to gas flow across 14 CPAP devices for newborns. *Respir Care* 31:18–21, 1986.

30. Chernick V: Lung rupture in the newborn infant. *Respir Care* 31:628–633, 1986.

31. Garland JS, Nelson DB, Rice T, et al: Increased risk of gastrointestinal perforations in neonates mechanically ventilated with either face mask or nasal prongs. *Pediatrics* 76:406–410, 1985.

32. Hayes D, Jr, Feola DJ, Murphy BS, et al: Pathogenesis of bronchopulmonary dysplasia. *Respiration* 79:425–436, 2010.

33. Aly H: Ventilation without tracheal intubation. *Pediatrics* 124:786–789, 2009.

34. Ramanathan R: Nasal respiratory support through the nares: its time has come. *J Perinatol* 30:S67–S72, 2010.

35. Bhandari V, Gavino RG, Nedrelow JH, et al: A randomized controlled trial of synchronized nasal intermittent positive pressure ventilation in RDS. *J Perinatol* 27:697–703, 2007.

36. Chang HY, Claure N, Dugard C, et al: Effects of synchronization during nasal ventilation in clinically stable preterm infant. *Pediatr Res* 1:84–89, 2011.

37. Dumpa V, Katz K, Northrup V, et al: SNIPPV vs NIPPV: does synchronization matter? *J Perinatol* 32:438–442, 2012.

38. Bhandari V, Finer NN, Ehrenkranz RA, et al: Synchronized nasal intermittent positive-pressure ventilation and neonatal outcomes. *Pediatrics* 124:517–526, 2009.

39. Davis PG, Henderson-Smart DJ: Extubation from low-rate intermittent positive airway pressure versus extubation after a trial of endotracheal continuous positive airway pressure in intubated preterm infants. *Cochrane Database Syst Rev* (4):CD001078, 2001.

40. Kugelman A, Feferkorn I, Riskin A, et al: Nasal intermittent mandatory ventilation versus nasal continuous positive airway pressure for respiratory distress syndrome: a randomized, controlled, prospective study. *J Pediatr* 150:521–526, 526.e1, 2007.

41. Kirpalani H, Millar D, Lemyre B, et al: A trial comparing noninvasive ventilation strategies in preterm infants. *N Engl J Med* 369:611–620, 2013.

42. Ancora G, Maranella E, Grandi S, et al: Role of bilevel positive airway pressure in the management of preterm newborns who have received surfactant. *Acta Paediatr* 99:1807–1811, 2010.

43. Migliori C, Motta M, Angeli A, et al: Nasal bilevel vs. continuous positive airway pressure in preterm infants. *Pediatr Pulmonol* 40:426–430, 2005.

44. Lampland AL, Plumm B, Worwa C, et al: Bi-level CPAP does not improve gas exchange when compared with conventional CPAP for the treatment of neonates recovering from respiratory distress syndrome. *Arch Dis Child Fetal Neonatal Ed* 100:F31–F34, 2015.

45. Colaizy TT, Younis UM, Bell EF, et al: Nasal high-frequency ventilation for premature infants. *Acta Paediatr* 97:1518–1522, 2008.

46. Mukerji A, Finelli M, Belik J: Nasal high-frequency oscillation for lung carbon dioxide clearance in the newborn. *Neonatology* 103:161–165, 2013.

47. Cairo JM: *Mosby's respiratory care equipment*, ed 9, St Louis, 2014, Elsevier.

48. Null DM, Alvord J, Leavitt W, et al: High-frequency nasal ventilation for 21 d maintains gas exchange with lower respiratory pressures and promotes alveolarization in preterm lambs. *Pediatr Res* 75:507–516, 2014.

49. Yañez LJ, Yunge M, Emilfork M, et al: A prospective, randomized, controlled trial of noninvasive ventilation in pediatric acute respiratory failure. *Pediatr Crit Care Med* 9:484–489, 2008.

50. Lagarde S, Semjen F, Nouette-Gaulain K, et al: Facemask pressure-controlled ventilation in children: what is the pressure limit? *Anesth Analg* 110:1676–1679, 2010.

51. Singh GK, Yu SM: Infant mortality in the United States: trends, differentials, and projections 1950 through 2010. *Am J Public Health* 85:957–964, 1995.

52. Heron M, Sutton PD, Xu J, et al: Annual summary of vital statistics: 2007. *Pediatrics* 125:4–15, 2010.

53. Cohen IL, Lambrinos J: Investigating the impact of age on outcome of mechanical ventilation using a population of 41,848 patients from a statewide database. *Chest* 107:1673–1680, 1995.

54. Angus DC, Linde-Zwirble WT, Clermont G, et al: Epidemiology of neonatal respiratory failure in the United States: projections from California and New York. *Am J Respir Crit Care Med* 164:1154–1160, 2001.

55. AARC Clinical Practice Guideline: Neonatal time-triggered, pressure-limited, time-cycled (TPTV) mechanical ventilation. *Respir Care* 39:808–816, 1994.

56. Randolph AG, Wypij D, Venkataraman ST, et al: Effect of mechanical ventilator weaning protocols on respiratory outcomes in infants and children: a randomized controlled trial. *JAMA* 288:2561–2568, 2002.

57. Randolph AG, Meert KL, O'Neal ME, et al: The feasibility of conducting clinical trials in infants and children with acute respiratory failure. *Am J Respir Crit Care Med* 167:1334–1340, 2003.

58. Betit P, Thompson JE, Benjamin PK: Mechanical ventilation. In Koff PA, Eitzman D, Neu J, editors: *Neonatal and pediatric respiratory care*, ed 2, St Louis, 1993, Mosby, pp 324–344.

59. Cools F, Offringa M: Neuromuscular paralysis for newborn infants receiving mechanical ventilation. *Cochrane Database Syst Rev* (2):CD002773, 2005.

60. Wilson BG, Cheifetz IM, Meliones JN: *Optimizing mechanical ventilation in infants and children*, Palm Springs, Calif, 1995, Bird Products.

61. Dimitriou G, Greenbough A, Cherians S: Comparison of airway pressure and airflow triggering systems using a single type of neonatal machine. *Acta Paediatr* 90:445–447, 2001.

62. Greenough A, Dimitriou G, Prendergast M, et al: Synchronized mechanical ventilation for respiratory support in newborn infants. *Cochrane Database Syst Rev* (23):CD000456, 2008.

63. Chatburn RL: Understanding mechanical ventilators. *Expert Rev Respir Med* 4:809–819, 2010.

64. Walsh BK, Czervinske MP, DiBlasi RM: *Perinatal and pediatric respiratory care*, ed 3, St Louis, 2010, Saunders.

65. Reyes ZC, Claure N, Tauscher MK, et al: Randomized controlled trial comparing synchronized intermittent mandatory ventilation and synchronized intermittent mandatory ventilation plus pressure support in preterm infants. *Pediatrics* 118:1409–1417, 2006.

66. Nicks JJ: *Graphics monitoring in the neonatal intensive care unit*, Palm Springs, Calif, 1995, Bird Products.

67. Kamlin COF, Davis PG: Long versus short inspiratory times in neonates receiving mechanical ventilation. *Cochrane Database Syst Rev* CD004503, 2003.

68. Ramsden CA, Reynolds EOR: Ventilator settings for newborn infants. *Arch Dis Child* 62:529–538, 1987.

69. Carlo WA, Chatburn RL, Martin RJ: Randomized trial of high-frequency jet ventilation versus conventional ventilation in respiratory distress syndrome. *J Pediatr* 110:275–282, 1987.

70. Claure N, Bancalari E: Methods and evidence on volume-targeted ventilation in preterm infants. *Curr Opin Pediatr* 20:125–131, 2008.

71. Heulitt MJ, Thurman TL, Holt SJ, et al: Reliability of displayed tidal volume in infants and children during dual-controlled ventilation. *Pediatr Crit Care Med* 10:661–667, 2009.

72. Klingenberg C, Wheeler KI, Davis PG, et al: A practical guide to neonatal volume guarantee ventilation. *J Perinatol* 31:575–585, 2011.

73. Dräger Medical: *Operator's Manual: Dräger Babylog 8000*, Telford, Pa., 1993, Dräger Medical.

74. Klingenberg C, Wheeler KI, Davis PG, et al: A practical guide to neonatal volume guarantee ventilation. *J Perinatol* 31:575–585, 2011.

75. Chowdhury O, Rafferty GF, Lee S, et al: Volume-targeted ventilation in infants born at or near term. *Arch Dis Child Fetal Neonatal Ed* 97:F264–F266, 2012.

76. Habashi NM: Other approaches to open lung ventilation: Airway pressure release ventilation. *Crit Care Med* 3(3 Suppl):S228–S240, 2005.

77. Kelly J: New method permits neural control of mechanical ventilation. *Pulmonary Review.com. 5 Trends in Pulmonary and Critical Care Medicine* 5(5), 2000.

78. Sinderby C, Beck J, Spahija J, et al: Inspiratory muscle unloading by neurally adjusted ventilatory assist during maximal inspiratory efforts in healthy subjects. *Chest* 131:711–717, 2007.

79. Longhini F, Ferrero F, De Luca D, et al: Neurally adjusted ventilatory assist in preterm neonates with acute respiratory failure. *Neonatology* 107:60–67, 2015.

80. Ricard JD, Dreyfuss D, Saumon G: Ventilator-induced lung injury. *Eur Respir J Suppl* 42:2s–9s, 2003.

81. Dreyfuss D, Saumon G: Barotrauma is volutrauma but which volume is the one responsible? *Intensive Care Med* 18:139–141, 1992.

82. Nilson C, Grossman G, Robertson B: Lung surfactant and the pathogenesis of neonatal bronchiolar lesions induced by artificial ventilation. *Pediatr Res* 12:249–255, 1978.

83. Hillman NH, Moss TJ, Kallapur SG, et al: Brief, large tidal volume ventilation initiates lung injury and a systemic response in fetal sheep. *Am J Crit Care Med* 176:578–581, 2007.

84. Bjorklund LJ, Ingimarsson J, Cursted T, et al: Manual ventilation with a few large breaths at birth compromises the therapeutic effect of subsequent surfactant replacement in immature lambs. *Pediatr Res* 42:348–355, 1997.

85. Muscedere JG, Mullen JBM, Gan K, et al: Tidal ventilation at low airway pressures can augment lung injury. *Am J Respir Crit Care Med* 149:1327–1334, 1994.

86. Thibeault DW, Mabry SM, Ekekezie II, et al: Collagen scaffolding during development and its deformation with chronic lung disease. *Pediatrics* 111:766–776, 2003.

87. Wheeler KI, Klingenberg C, Morley CJ, et al: Volume-targeted versus pressure-limited ventilation for preterm infants: a systematic review and meta-analysis. *Neonatology* 100:219–227, 2011.

88. Wheeler K, Klingenberg C, McCallion N, et al: Volume-targeted versus pressure-limited ventilation in the neonate. *Cochrane Database Syst Rev* (11):CD003666, 2010.

89. Abubakar K, Kezler M: Effect of volume guarantee combined with assist/control vs synchronized intermittent mandatory ventilation. *J Perinatol* 25:638–642, 2005.

90. Sunil SK, Donn SM: Volume-controlled ventilation. In Goldsmith JP, Karotkin EH, editors: *Assisted ventilation of the neonate*, ed 4, Philadelphia, 2004, W.B. Saunders, pp 171–182.

91. Lista G, Castoldi F, Fontana P, et al: Lung inflammation in preterm infants with respiratory distress syndrome: effects of ventilation with different tidal volumes. *Pediatr Pulmonol* 41:357–363, 2006.

92. Herrera CM, Gerhardt T, Claure N, et al: Effects of volume-guaranteed synchronized intermittent mandatory ventilation in preterm infants recovering from respiratory failure. *Pediatrics* 110:529–533, 2002.

93. Acute Respiratory Distress Syndrome Network: Ventilation with lower tidal volumes as compared with traditional tidal volumes for acute lung injury and the acute respiratory distress syndrome. The Multicenter Trial Group on Tidal Volume Reduction in ARDS. *N Engl J Med* 342:1301–1308, 2000.

94. Amato MB, Barbas CS, Medeiros DM, et al: Effect of preventive ventilation strategy on mortality in the acute respiratory distress syndrome. *N Engl J Med* 338:347–354, 1998.

95. Gillette MA, Hess DR: Ventilator-induced lung injury and the evolution of lung-protective strategies in acute respiratory distress syndrome. *Respir Care* 46:130–148, 2001.

96. Laffey JG, O'Croinin D, McLoughlin P, et al: Permissive hypercapnia: role in protective lung ventilatory strategies. *Intensive Care Med* 30:347–356, 2004.

97. Hickling KG: Permissive hypercapnia. *Respir Care Clin N Am* 8:155–169, 2002.

98. Sheridan RL, Kacmarek RM, McEttrick MM, et al: Permissive hypercapnia as a ventilatory strategy in burned children: effect on barotrauma, pneumonia, and mortality. *J Trauma* 39:854–859, 1995.

99. Shibata K, Cregg N, Engelberts D, et al: Hypercapnic acidosis may attenuate acute lung injury by inhibition of endogenous xanthine oxidase. *Am J Respir Crit Care Med* 158:1578–1584, 1998.

100. Laffey JG, Engelberts D, Kavanagh BP, et al: Hypercapnic acidosis worsens acute lung injury. *Am J Respir Crit Care Med* 161:141–146, 2000.

101. Emerson JM: Apparatus for vibrating portions of a patient's airway. *U.S. Patent* 2(918):917, 1959.

102. Gaylord MS, Quisell BJ, Lair ME: High frequency ventilation in the treatment of infants weighing less than 1500 grams with pulmonary interstitial emphysema: a pilot study. *Pediatrics* 79:915–921, 1987.

103. Minton SD, Gerstmann DR, Stoddard RA: Ventilator strategies to interrupt pulmonary injury sequence. *Respir Ther/J Respir Care Pract* Oct/Nov:15–31, 1992.

104. Gerstmann DR, Minton SD, Stoddard RA, et al: The Provo multicenter early high-frequency oscillatory ventilation trial: improved pulmonary and clinical outcome in respiratory distress syndrome. *Pediatrics* 98:1044–1057, 1996.

105. Sun H, Cheng R, Kang W, et al: High-frequency oscillatory ventilation versus synchronized intermittent mandatory ventilation plus pressure support in preterm infants with severe respiratory distress syndrome. *Respir Care* 59:159–169, 2014.

106. Sjöstrand U: High-frequency positive pressure ventilation (HFPPV): a review. *Crit Care Med* 8:345–364, 1980.

107. Boros SJ, Bing DR, Mammel MC, et al: Using conventional infant ventilators at unconventional rates. *Pediatrics* 74:487–492, 1984.

108. Cioffi WG, Rue LW, Graves TA, et al: Prophylactic use of high frequency percussive ventilation in patients with inhalation injury. *Ann Surg* 213:575–582, 1991.

109. Hess D, Branson R: High-frequency ventilation. *Respir Care Clin N Am* 7:577–598, 2001.

110. Smith DW, Frankel LR, Derish MT, et al: High frequency jet ventilation in children with the adult respiratory distress syndrome complicated by pulmonary barotraumas. *Pediatr Pulmonol* 15:279–286, 1993.

111. dos Santos CC, Slutsky AS: Overview of high-frequency ventilation modes, clinical rationale, and gas transport mechanisms. *Respir Care Clin N Am* 7:549–575, 2001.

112. Fredberg JJ, Keefe DH, Glass GM, et al: Alveolar pressure inhomogeneity during small amplitude high frequency oscillation. *J Appl Physiol Respir Environ Exerc Physiol* 57:788–800, 1984.

113. Lehr JL, Butler JP, Westerman PA, et al: Photographic measurement of pleural surface motion during lung oscillation. *J Appl Physiol* 59:623–633, 1985.

114. Haselton FR, Scherer PW: Bronchial bifurcations and respiratory mass transport. *Science* 208:69–71, 1980.

115. Chang HK: Mechanisms of gas transport during ventilation with high frequency oscillation. *J Appl Physiol Respir Environ Exerc Physiol* 56:553–563, 1984.

116. Baum ML, Benzer HR, Geyer AM, et al: Theoretical evaluation of gas exchange mechanisms. In Carlon CG, Howlan WS, editors: *High-frequency ventilation in intensive care and during surgery*, New York, 1985, Marcel Dekker.

117. Cools F, Askie LM, PreVILIG collaboration: Elective high-frequency oscillatory versus conventional ventilation in preterm infants: a systematic review and meta-analysis of individual patients' data. *Lancet* 375:2082–2091, 2010.

118. Pinzon A, Sica da Rocha T, Ricachinevsky C, et al: High-frequency oscillatory ventilation in children with acute respiratory distress syndrome: experience of a pediatric intensive care unit. *Rev Assoc Med Bras* 59:368–374, 2013.

119. Ely EW, Meade MO, Haponik ET, et al: Mechanical ventilator weaning protocols driven by nonphysician health care professionals: evidence-based clinical practice guidelines. *Chest* 120:454S–463S, 2001.

120. Randolph AG, Wypij D, Venkataraman ST, et al: Effect of mechanical ventilator weaning protocols on respiratory outcomes in infants and children: a randomized controlled trial. *JAMA* 288:2561–2568, 2002.

121. Anene O, Meert KL, Uy H, et al: Dexamethasone for the prevention of postextubation airway obstruction: a prospective, randomized, double-blind, placebo-controlled trial. *Crit Care Med* 24:1666–1669, 1996.

122. Hastings LK, Renfro WH, Sharma R: Comparison of beractant and calfactant in a neonatal intensive care unit. *Am J Health Syst Pharm* 61:257–260, 2004.

123. AARC Clinical Practice Guideline: Surfactant replacement therapy. *Respir Care* 39:824–829, 1994.

124. Horbar JD, Wright EC, Onstad L: Decreasing mortality associated with the introduction of surfactant therapy: an observational study of neonates weighing 601 to 1300 grams at birth. *Pediatrics* 92:191–196, 1993.

125. van Houten J, Long W, Mullett M, et al: Pulmonary hemorrhage in premature infants after treatment with synthetic surfactant: an autopsy evaluation. *J Pediatr* 120:S40–S44, 1992. (erratum in *J Pediatr* 120:762, 1992).

126. Merritt TA, Hallman M, Berry C, et al: Randomized placebo-controlled trial of human surfactant given at birth versus rescue administration in very low birth weight infants with lung immaturity. *J Pediatr* 118:581–594, 1991.

127. Goldsmith LS, Greenspan JS, Rubenstein SD, et al: Immediate improvement in lung volume after exogenous surfactant: alveolar recruitment versus increased distension. *J Pediatr* 119:424–428, 1991.

128. Heldt GP, Pesonen E, Merritt TA, et al: Closure of the ductus arteriosus and mechanics of breathing in preterm infants after surfactant replacement therapy. *Pediatr Res* 25:305–310, 1989.

129. Moller JC, Schable T, Roll C, et al: Treatment with bovine surfactant in severe acute respiratory distress syndrome in children: a randomized multicenter study. *Intensive Care Med* 29:437–446, 2003.

130. Curley MA, Hibberd PL, Fineman LD, et al: Effect of prone positioning on clinical outcomes in children with acute lung injury: a randomized controlled trial. *JAMA* 294:229–237, 2005.

131. Kirmse M, Hess D, Fujino Y, et al: Delivery of inhaled nitric oxide using the Ohmeda INOvent delivery system. *Chest* 113:1650–1657, 1998.

132. Yoshida K, Kasama K: Biotransformation of nitric oxide. *Environ Health Perspect* 73:201–205, 1987.

133. Falke KJ, Rossaint R, Keitel M, et al: Successful treatment of severe adult respiratory distress syndrome with nitric oxide: the first three patients. Second International Meeting on the Biology of Nitric Oxide, London, October, 1991.

134. Foubert L, Fleming B, Latimer R: Safety guidelines for the use of nitric oxide. *Lancet* 339:1615–1616, 1992.

135. Dobyns EL, Cornfield DN, Anas NG, et al: Multicenter randomized controlled trial of the effects of inhaled nitric oxide therapy on gas exchange in children with acute hypoxemic respiratory failure. *J Pediatr* 134:406–412, 1999.

136. Dobyns EL, Anas NG, Fortenberry JD, et al: Interactive effects of high-frequency oscillatory ventilation and inhaled nitric oxide in acute hypoxemic respiratory failure in pediatrics. *Crit Care Med* 30:2425–2429, 2000.

137. DiBlasi RM, Myers TR, Hess DR: Evidence-based clinical practice guideline: Inhaled nitric oxide for neonates with acute hypoxic respiratory failure. *Respir Care* 55:1717–1745, 2010.

Special Techniques in Ventilatory Support

SUSAN P. PILBEAM, J.M. CAIRO

OUTLINE

KEY TERMS

- Amplitude
- Electrical activity of the diaphragm (Edi)
- Heliox
- Neurally adjusted ventilatory assist (NAVA)

LEARNING OBJECTIVES *On completion of this chapter, the reader will be able to do the following:*

1. Discuss the benefits and disadvantages of airway pressure release ventilation (APRV)
2. Recommend initial settings for initiating APRV in patients with acute respiratory distress syndrome (ARDS).
3. Explain how the controls operate with the CareFusion 3100B oscillator.
4. Recommend initial ventilator settings for an adult with the 3100B unit.
5. List types of medications that may be used in transitioning from volume control continuous mandatory ventilation (VC-CMV) to high-frequency oscillatory ventilation (HFOV) for an adult.
6. Explain how the chest wiggle factor is influenced by HFOV settings.
7. Name pulmonary pathologic conditions in which heliox therapy may be beneficial.
8. Compare the difference between set tidal volume (V_T), monitored V_T, and actual V_T delivery ($V_T$del) during heliox therapy.
9. Describe how heliox used with a mechanical ventilator may affect pressures and fractional inspired oxygen concentration (F_IO_2) monitoring and delivery.
10. Explain the procedure for using heliox cylinders with a mechanical ventilator.
11. Name at least four techniques that can help to determine the correct placement of the esophageal Edi catheter.
12. Provide examples of how the Edi waveform can be of value in monitoring critically ill patients.

13. Discuss various factors that can cause a low Edi signal and a high Edi signal.
14. Describe the safety backup features and alarms available with neurally adjusted ventilator assist (NAVA).
15. Calculate an estimated pressure delivery when given the NAVA level, Edi peak, Edi minimum, and positive end-expiratory pressure (PEEP).
16. Explain what parameters (pressure, flow, volume, neural signal, time) are used to deliver a breath during NAVA ventilation.
17. Identify clinical situations in which NAVA should be used.

The ultimate goal of mechanical ventilation is to sustain life and do no harm. In an effort to achieve these outcomes, clinicians often search for alternative methods of treatment when standard procedures fail. Some of these techniques prove to be viable alternatives to standard practices and gain a foothold in clinical practice.

The inclusion of all recently explored and newly discovered techniques that can be used to ventilate and manage critically ill patients is beyond the scope of this text. We therefore present a discussion of four techniques that have received increased attention by critical care clinicians: airway pressure release ventilation, high-frequency oscillatory ventilation in the adult, heliox therapy, and monitoring the diaphragm's electrical activity and using that activity with the ventilator mode **neurally adjusted ventilatory assist (NAVA)**. Descriptions of additional techniques, such as liquid ventilation of the lung, extracorporeal membrane oxygenation, low-frequency positive pressure ventilation, extracorporeal carbon dioxide removal, intravascular oxygenation, inhaled nitric oxide, and tracheal gas insufflation are available on the Evolve website for this text.

Airway Pressure Release Ventilation

Airway pressure release ventilation (APRV) is a mode of ventilatory support designed to provide two levels of continuous positive airway pressure (CPAP) and allow spontaneous breathing at both levels when spontaneous effort is present.[1-6] APRV provides a moderately high level of pressure (P_{high}, 15 to 30 cm H_2O), which can be considered a baseline pressure. P_{high} is occasionally interrupted with a brief time at lower pressure (P_{low}, 0 to 15 cm H_2O). The brief interval at P_{low} is called release time (Fig. 23-1).

Both the high- and low-pressure levels are time triggered and time cycled when spontaneous efforts are not detected.[7] With current generation ventilators, spontaneous breathing can be accompanied by patient triggering. During APRV, if the patient is not spontaneously breathing, the pressure curve looks like pressure-controlled inverse ratio ventilation (Fig. 23-2).[8] When the patient is spontaneously breathing, the patient's breathing activity can be monitored on the ventilator's display, particularly in the flow–time and volume–time scalars during ventilation (Fig. 23-3).[9]

OTHER NAMES

In Europe, APRV is referred to as bilevel airway pressure (BiPAP).[7] It has also been called variable positive airway pressure, intermittent CPAP, CPAP with release, pressure-controlled inverse ratio ventilation with spontaneous ventilation, upside-down intermittent mandatory ventilation, and biphasic CPAP.[7,10,11] In the United States, BiPAP is often used to describe a technique in which inspiratory positive airway pressure (IPAP) and expiratory positive

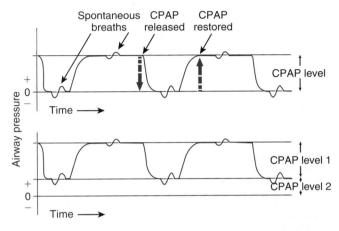

Fig. 23-1 *Top curve,* Pressure–time waveforms for airway pressure release ventilation (APRV) with a continuous positive airway pressure (CPAP) level 2 (P_{low}) of 0 cm H_2O. *Bottom curve,* Pressure–time waveform for APRV with a CPAP level 2 (P_{low}) set greater than 0 cm H_2O. Spontaneous efforts by the patient do not cycle the ventilator between low and high CPAP or high and low CPAP. A fixed time interval is set for the CPAP level 1 time and the CPAP level 2 times. (From Dupuis Y: Ventilators: theory and clinical application, ed 2, St Louis, 1992, Mosby.)

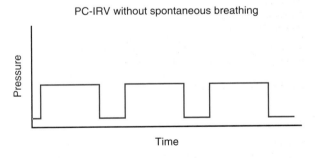

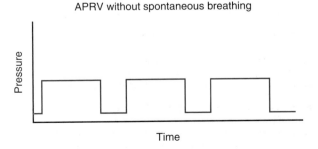

Fig. 23-2 Pressure–time curves for pressure control inverse ratio ventilation (PC-IRV) in an apneic patient *(top)* and APRV for an apneic patient *(bottom).* The waveforms appear the same.

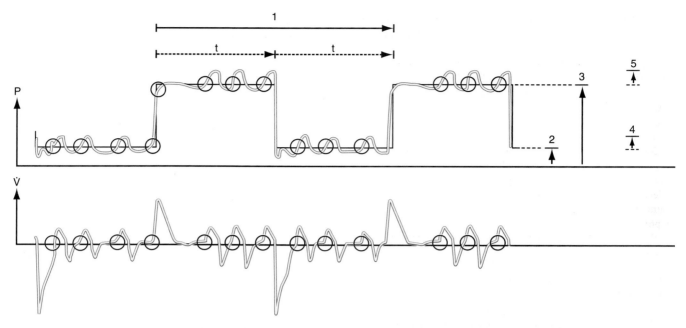

Fig. 23-3 *Top,* Pressure–time curve; *bottom,* flow–time curve during APRV, called Bi-Vent on the Servo-i ventilator. Inspiratory flows are in the upward direction and expiratory flows downward. Note the spontaneous breathing during the high pressure (P_{high}) setting and the low pressure (P_{low}) setting. (Courtesy Maquet, Inc., Bridgewater, N.J. Redrawn for this text.)

airway pressure (EPAP) levels are set for noninvasive positive pressure ventilation (NIV), where the inspiratory/expiratory (I : E) ratio is normal.[7] (See Chapter 19 for more information on BiPAP with NIV.)

The Dräger Evita was the first ventilator in the United States to provide APRV. Subsequently other intensive care unit (ICU) ventilators, such as the Hamilton G-5, the Puritan Bennett 840, the Dräger v500, the CareFusion AVEA, and the Maquet Servo-i, incorporated APRV. Interestingly, each of these manufacturers uses a different terminology for describing the APRV mode. For example, the Servo-i refers to APRV as Bi-vent; the Puritan Bennett 840 uses the term Bi-level; and the Hamilton G5 refers to APRV as Duo-PAP. The function of APRV may also be different with each ventilator. For example, the Puritan Bennett 840 Bi-level mode currently allows the setting of one pressure support level during both P_{high} and P_{low}. On the other hand, the Servo-i allows two levels of pressure support ventilation (PSV) to be set independently, one for P_{high} and a separate level for P_{low}. The benefits of pressure support with APRV have yet to be substantiated (Key Point 23-1).[7,12]

Key Point 23-1 Because the function of ventilators is frequently changed with the addition of upgraded software versions, clinicians must become familiar with these upgrades on the ventilators they plan to use with patients.

ADVANTAGES OF AIRWAY PRESSURE RELASE COMPARED WITH CONVENTIONAL VENTILATION

The original concept and the equipment for the application of APRV were first described by Stock et al in 1987.[6,13] Subsequent investigations confirmed that APRV produced lower peak pressures, better oxygenation, less circulatory interference, and better

gas exchange without compromising the patient's hemodynamic status compared with conventional ventilation for the treatment of acute respiratory distress syndrome (ARDS).[3,4,6,12,14-16] APRV requires a lower minute ventilation than VC-CMV, suggesting a reduction in physiological dead space.[9] It also provides better ventilation-perfusion matching compared with pressure support ventilation.[17] APRV improves gas exchange and lowers peak inspiratory pressure (PIP) in patients with ARDS compared with patients receiving volume-controlled inverse ratio ventilation (VC-IRV).[18] When compared with pressure-controlled inverse ratio ventilation, APRV reduces peak and mean airway pressures, increases cardiac index, decreases central venous pressure, increases urine output, increases oxygen delivery, and reduces the need for sedation and paralysis.[16,19] APRV also improves renal perfusion and function when spontaneous breathing is maintained.[20]

Because APRV can reduce airway pressure in patients with ARDS, it is also thought to be associated with a reduced risk of ventilator-induced lung injury (VILI). (Maximum alveolar pressure should be kept below 30 cm H_2O to protect the lung. See Chapter 17 for additional information on VILI.) APRV may recruit consolidated lung areas over time and prevent repeated opening and closing of alveoli.[9,12,21,22]

Patients receiving APRV have also been shown to require less sedation and analgesia when compared with patients receiving continuous mandatory ventilation. Thus APRV appears to reduce anxiety and pain, and improve patient comfort.[23,24]

Preserving Spontaneous Ventilation

Many of the advantages of APRV are likely attributable to the preservation of spontaneous breathing.[1,12,24] For example, spontaneous breathing preserves the cyclic decrease in pleural pressure, which augments venous return, thereby improving cardiac performance.[17,25] Moreover, because the patient can breathe spontaneously, the need for sedation may be reduced.[19,23,24]

Normally the mechanical delivery of air tends to ventilate areas receiving the least amount of perfusion. During a positive pressure breath in a paralyzed patient, the diaphragm is displaced toward the abdomen, with the **nondependent** regions of the lung receiving the most ventilation. At the same time, dependent areas receive the greatest perfusion.[26,27] Maintaining spontaneous ventilation tends to improve ventilation-perfusion matching by preferentially providing ventilation to dependent lung regions that receive the greatest blood flow.[23,27]

During positive pressure ventilation, atelectasis can occur near the diaphragm when activity of this muscle is absent. However, if spontaneous breathing is preserved, the formation of atelectasis is offset by the activity of the diaphragm.[28] In addition, maintaining spontaneous breathing may prevent atrophy of the diaphragm associated with the use of mechanical ventilation and paralytic agents.[28] Figure 23-4 illustrates spontaneous ventilation during APRV.

APRV and Airway Pressures During Spontaneous Breathing

In older generation ventilators, the expiratory valve closed completely during inspiration and was therefore not interactive with the patient. Current ventilators have more active expiratory values, which tend to "float open" when inspiratory pressures slightly exceed set pressures during pressure-targeted ventilation. As a result, current ventilators accommodate spontaneous breathing during APRV without pressure buildups. Because PIP during APRV does not significantly exceed the P_{high} level, complications associated with high pressures, such as overdistention of the lungs and reduced cardiac output, may be minimized (the high-pressure limit must still be set at a safe level).

DISADVANTAGES

Because APRV is a pressure-targeted mode of ventilation, volume delivery depends on lung compliance (C_L), airway resistance (R_{aw}), and the patient's spontaneous effort. The patient's volumes and gas exchange should be closely monitored. APRV does not completely support CO_2 elimination; rather, it relies on spontaneous breathing to ensure adequate CO_2 elimination.[1,7] With increased R_{aw} (increased time constants) such as occurs in patients with chronic obstructive pulmonary disease (COPD), the ability to eliminate CO_2 may be reduced because of limited emptying of the lung during the short release periods.

Another problem is not all ventilators that offer an APRV mode allow for patient triggering of breaths in the phase from P_{high} to P_{low}, and P_{low} to P_{high}.[29-31] Consequently some patient discomfort and increased work of breathing may occur during these interval changes.

Limited staff experience with this mode may make its implementation difficult in some cases. Adequate training time and offsite support services and backup from manufacturers are essential. The limited amount of clinical research data available for this method of ventilation also makes determining evidence-based application problematic.

INITIAL SETTINGS[21,32,33]

When initiating APRV, the practitioner sets two pressure levels and two time levels. Using the high pressure or P_{high} control sets the upper level of CPAP. The lower pressure, or release pressure, is set

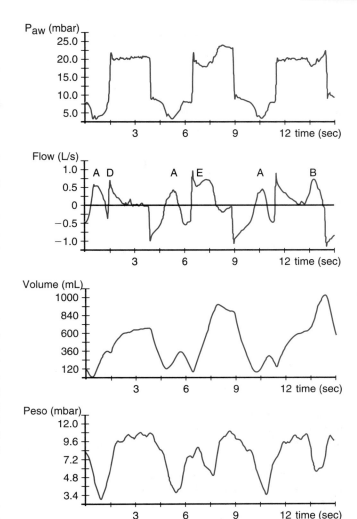

Fig. 23-4 APRV with curves for P_{aw}, flow, volume, and esophageal pressure (P_{eso}). P_{high} and P_{low} are both set at 2.5 seconds. Spontaneous breathing occurs throughout both phases. On the flow–time curve: **A,** spontaneous breaths at P_{low}; **B,** spontaneous breaths at P_{high}; **D,** a time-trigger transition from P_{low} to P_{high}; **E,** a simultaneous mandatory and spontaneous inspiration from P_{low} to P_{high}. (Redrawn from Neumann P, Golisch W, Strohmeyer A, et al: Influence of different release times on spontaneous breathing pattern during airway pressure release ventilation, Intensive Care Med 28:1742-1749, 2002.)

with a P_{low} control. A timing control commonly called T_{high} is used to set the duration of P_{high}. The P_{low} time period is set with a timer for the low time period (i.e., T_{low} control).

The respiratory frequency is based on the T_{high} and T_{low} settings. For example, if T_{low} is set at 0.5 seconds and T_{high} is 5.0 seconds, the total cycle time will be T_{low} plus T_{high}, or 5.5 seconds. The I : E ratio will be 5 : 0.5, or 10 : 1. The respiratory rate will be equal to 60 seconds divided by the total time cycle. In this example, 60 sec/5.5 sec = 11 breaths/min, or 11 cycles/min.

Tidal volume and flow delivery depend on the same factors that affect V_T and flow delivery in pressure-targeted ventilation: lung characteristics, patient effort, and pressure gradient ($\Delta P = P_{high} - P_{low}$). The higher this gradient, the more rapid the expiratory flow during release time and the higher the V_T. Minute volume ($\dot{V}_E$) depends on the patient's spontaneous effort during all time intervals plus the release interval volume change. Some clinicians suggest a target minute ventilation of 2 to 3 L/min less than the $\dot{V}_E$ on conventional ventilation.[21]

Setting High Pressure

When changing a patient from a conventional mode of ventilation to APRV, the settings for the conventional ventilator mode can serve as a guide to the APRV settings. For example, if the patient's plateau pressure ($P_{plateau}$) is 25 cm H_2O during conventional ventilation, an initial setting of 25 cm H_2O for P_{high} is appropriate. Some clinicians use the mean airway pressure ($\overline{P}_{aw}$) measured during conventional ventilation for the P_{high} setting. Generally a setting of 15 to 30 cm H_2O is used. P_{high} generally establishes a $\overline{P}_{aw}$ intended to maintain oxygenation by restoring functional residual capacity. Overdistention of the lung must be avoided, so a P_{high} of 35 cm H_2O is probably the maximum accepted level.[12,21,34] Several clinical studies have noted the use of P_{high} up to 45 cm H_2O, but this level may be damaging to the lungs unless the chest wall compliance is reduced from abdominal distention or prone positioning.[9,21]

The use of P_{high} may help in the recruitment of collapsed alveoli and the maintenance of these recruited units.[18] It can take as long as 8 hours or longer for recruitment to occur. This is reflected in a progressive improvement in oxygenation and C_L.[18]

Setting Low Pressure

Some practitioners recommend initially setting P_{low} at 0 cm H_2O. A P_{low} of 0 cm H_2O allows an unimpeded expiratory gas flow and a rapid drop in pressure.[21,32,33]

Setting High Time

T_{high} is set at a minimum of 4.0 seconds.[21,32] Values less than 4.0 seconds can affect the $\overline{P}_{aw}$ in a negative way, losing the benefits of the APRV mode. The goal is to create a nearly continuous positive pressure that recruits collapsed alveoli, maintains recruitment, and optimizes oxygenation and compliance.[21,32] T_{high} can then be progressively increased to 12 to 15 seconds in 0.5- to 2.0-second intervals until the oxygenation target is achieved.[21,32] Slow progression is better than the increase of the I : E ratio in large increments, such as 2 : 1 or 3 : 1.[5,8,21] For example, if T_{high} is 5 seconds and T_{low} is 0.5 seconds (a 10 : 1 ratio) and T_{high} is changed to 5.5 seconds, the ratio change is small (11 : 1).

Setting Low Time

During the release time, or T_{low}, the patient exhales a volume of gas. This allows ventilation and removal of CO_2 from the body. As soon as the release time period is complete, the higher level of CPAP is restored. The optimal duration of the release time and the setting of P_{low} are functions of the time constant of the respiratory system.[5] V_T depends on the C_L, R_{aw}, the duration of T_{low}, and the amount of pressure drop.[1] Complete exhalation of V_T would occur in approximately four time constants, but the actual setting of T_{low} has conflicting views.

During early trials with APRV, T_{low} settings of 1 to 1.5 seconds were suggested.[13,32] It was found that in patients with acute lung injury, after 1 second, complete emptying of the lung occurred, and after 2 seconds airway pressures remained stable with no further pressure leaving the lungs. For example, Davis et al intentionally increased T_{low} to prevent auto-PEEP.[35] They suspected that the presence of auto-PEEP was undesirable. In addition, many early trials with APRV were performed on patients with relatively normal or nearly normal pulmonary compliance, which added the variable of different pathologic conditions to the study of T_{low} settings.[4,13,34]

Several studies showed no significant deterioration in oxygenation or lung mechanics with a long release time.[30,31] In fact, a release time of 1.0 second or less, in some cases, resulted in increases in partial pressure of carbon dioxide in the arteries (P_aCO_2) and dead space ventilation, indicating that ventilation was inadequate even when spontaneous breathing was present.[2,21,29]

What seems to be essential is that T_{low} is established on the basis of the patient's pulmonary condition. For example, short T_{low} settings appear to be appropriate for patients with ARDS. Too long a release time can interfere with oxygenation and allow lung units to collapse. In the view of some practitioners, alveolar recruitment is enhanced by preventing complete exhalation in the slower compartments of the lungs, thus producing regional auto-PEEP.[21] This may help to maintain an open lung and avoid repeated collapse and re-expansion of alveoli.[36-38] Atelectasis in the injured lung can develop in seconds when airway pressure drops below a certain critical level.[21,34,39,40] In neonates with ARDS, this time may be as little as 0.2 seconds.[41]

Recently a general consensus for using APRV in patients with ARDS suggests setting T_{low} between 0.5 and 1.0 seconds, typically at 0.8 seconds.[21,32,33] The T_{low} setting should generate regional intrinsic PEEP (areas of trapped air) and enhance alveolar recruitment.[21,36] In actual practice, clinicians tend to rely on the evaluation of the expiratory gas flow waveform. When expiratory flow during a release period is approximately 50% to 75% of peak expiratory flow (T-PEFR), the airway pressure should be allowed to return to P_{high}.[21,32]

It is worth mentioning that T_{low} settings vary considerably among patients. Indeed, patients may require different settings as their lung condition changes. Establishing T_{low} is therefore not yet an exact science and should be performed with caution and careful patient monitoring.

ADJUSTING VENTILATION AND OXYGENATION[21,32,33]

Ventilation and P_aCO_2 are both determined by the release time and V_T exchange during T_{low} and by the patient's spontaneous ventilation. If the P_aCO_2 is low and the patient's spontaneous rate is low, the machine rate can be reduced by lengthening T_{high} and/or reducing T_{low}. This is done until either the spontaneous rate increases significantly, or respiratory acidosis occurs. If the patient's P_aCO_2 levels rise or tachypnea occurs, the rate can be increased.

If respiratory acidosis occurs, the patient should be evaluated for the level of sedation. It may be appropriate to reduce the level of sedation administered and allow more spontaneous ventilation. Following sedation evaluation and adjustment, if CO_2 remains high, an increase in P_{high} may be necessary. For example, suppose a patient has a pressure gradient of 20 cm H_2O (P_{high} – P_{low}; 20 – 0 cm H_2O), and this gradient produces a V_T during release of 400 mL. Imagine the patient's pulmonary edema gets worse and the patient's lungs are less compliant. For the same pressure gradient, the V_T is now 300 mL. The P_{high} level should be raised to increase the pressure gradient (P_{high} – P_{low}) and effectively increase the V_T level. In general, P_{high} should not be allowed to increase above 30 cm H_2O in order to avoid high alveolar pressures.

Another strategy for improving ventilation is shortening T_{high}. A shorter T_{high} will result in more releases per minute and increase the patient's minute ventilation. Increasing T_{high} should be done with caution since the T_{high}/P_{high} combination (higher pressure for a longer time) is what increases the mean airway pressure and the patient's oxygenation. If T_{high} is shortened so that the breath release is increased to more than 12 releases/minute, this may compromise oxygenation.[32]

Another option for improving minute ventilation is to be sure the release volume is optimized. If T-PEFR is greater than 75% and oxygenation is acceptable, consider increasing T_{low} by increments of .05 to 1.0 second increments to achieve a T-PEFR of 50%. The APRV Clinical Scenario below shows an example case of how changing T_{low} can increase V_T release. T_{low} should not be extended to the point where closure of lung units can occur (derecruitment).

Another alternative is to allow increased P_aCO_2 levels (permissive hypercapnia) and use sedation because this condition is uncomfortable for the patient. However, hypercapnia in APRV patients may not develop because these patients can achieve adequate ventilation on their own.

Oxygenation can generally be improved by increasing P_{high} or F_IO_2. P_{high} should not exceed 30 cm H_2O to avoid overdistention injury to the lung. An additional strategy is to increase T_{high}. The increase of T_{high} and P_{high} increase the mean airway pressure. The clinician should be sure that T_{low} is set optimally for the patient. Oxygenation also seems to be enhanced when spontaneous ventilation is present. Using the prone position may also provide improvement in oxygenation if maintaining an adequate P_aO_2 is difficult (e.g., requiring high pressures and high F_IO_2 values).[35,37] Once oxygenation has improved, reduction of F_IO_2 is generally recommended until an F_IO_2 of less than 0.5 is achieved. Then P_{high} can gradually be reduced.

Clinical Scenario: APRV

A 73-year-old patient with a diagnosis of severe pulmonary fibrosis is awaiting a lung transplant. He is on APRV and has a pH of 7.27 and a P_aCO_2 of 63 mm Hg. V_T during a release, with T-PEFR of 75%, ranges from 190 to 230 mL. T_{low} is set at 0.6 seconds. Oxygenation is currently acceptable. T_{low} is progressively increased to 0.8 (T-PEFR of 50%) and the V_T increases to 350 to 375 mL. The resulting ventilation change is a pH of 7.35 and a P_aCO_2 of 55 mm Hg. This is an example of how lengthening T_{low} can result in a higher V_T and improvement in ventilation in a patient with respiratory acidosis.

DISCONTINUATION

Withdrawal of APRV can begin once the patient's lung condition has improved enough so that support can be safely reduced. The technique for reducing support is to adjust P_{high} and T_{high}. P_{high} should be reduced 2 to 3 cm H_2O at a time and T_{high} lengthened in 0.5- to 2.0-second increments, depending on the patient's tolerance.[32,33] (Simultaneously T_{low} may be maintained or reduced.) P_{high} is slowly decreased until it meets P_{low}. P_{low} may be elevated slightly during the same process. During the lowering of P_{high}, some clinicians add pressure support to help compensate the spontaneous breathing efforts.[7] P_{high} and P_{low} pressures are intended to meet at the desired baseline, at which time the patient is essentially maintained at traditional CPAP or CPAP plus pressure support (PS). Before switching to CPAP, the P_{high} should be approximately 14 to 16 cm H_2O or less and the T_{high} 12 to 15 seconds (Table 23-1).[21,32]

| TABLE 23-1 | Example of Weaning APRV Settings in an Uncomplicated Case of Acute Lung Injury | | | |

P_{high} (cm H_2O)	T_{high} (s)	P_{low} (cm H_2O)	T_{low} (s)	Calculated $\bar{P}_{aw}$ (cm H_2O)
35	4.0	0	0.8	29.2
33	4.5	0	0.8	28.0
30	5.0	0	0.8	25.9
28	5.5	0	0.8	24.4
26	6.0	0	0.8	22.9
23	7.0	0	0.8	20.6
20	8.0	0	0.8	18.2
18	10.0	0	0.8	16.7
15	12.0	0	0.8	14.1

From Frawley PM, Habashi NM: Airway pressure release ventilation: theory and practice, AACN Clin Issues 12:234-246, 2001.
APRV, Airway pressure release ventilation; $\bar{P}_{aw}$, mean airway pressure.
Following the final settings, the patient was transitioned to CPAP of 12 cm of water pressure.

As the patient's condition improves, compliance will also generally improve. At P_{high} under improving conditions, the functional residual capacity is quite high and the patient tries to breathe spontaneously at this high lung volume. Therefore reducing the P_{high} allows the patient to achieve an adequate V_T at an appropriate functional residual capacity more easily. If tachypnea or respiratory acidosis occurs, or if the patient uses accessory muscles to breathe, the process should be stopped and the settings adjusted to more appropriate values.

Although APRV promises benefits such as lower PIP, better oxygenation, and reduced hazards associated with high airway pressure, there is limited evidence to support these benefits.[7] However, APRV is worth pursuing because of its potential for lung recruitment and improved ventilation/perfusion ratios, as well as its possible minimization of the compromising effects of positive pressure on cardiovascular function, particularly in patients with ARDS.

High-Frequency Oscillatory Ventilation in the Adult

High-frequency oscillatory ventilation (HFOV) has been proposed as an alternative method of respiratory support in adult patients with ARDS. Although HFOV has been used to treat neonates for some time, its use in the adult population has only recently begun to gain in popularity. The increased use of HFOV is based on the idea that it offers an alternative method of improving oxygenation in adult patients with ARDS, and at the same time, reduces the risks of VILI.

Theoretically HFOV by its design helps recruit the lung and avoid lung injury.[42-45] VT values with HFOV are quite small, with low alveolar pressures changes. Similarly maximum airway pressure (mP$_{aw}$), which is comparable to PEEP, is maintained at an adequate level to recruit the lung, at the same time avoiding repeated collapse and expansion of alveoli.[43] Overdistention of the lungs is avoided. Chapter 22 reviews the various forms of HFV, their mechanisms of action, and application in the newborn population. This section focuses on HFOV as used in the adult.

Although HFOV has been used since the late 1950s, its use in adults has only recently gained a solid footing in clinical practice.[43,44-53] The slow adoption of using HFOV in the management of adults with ARDS may be the result of several factors. First, a commercial high-frequency oscillator with sufficient power to ventilate an adult was not available until the 1990s.[54] Second, adult practitioners accustomed to using conventional ventilators were reluctant to use this technology. Indeed, in spite of its popularity among neonatal practitioners, actual outcome benefits of HFOV compared with conventional ventilation remained controversial and not well established.[39,55-57]

Two early series of case studies used high-frequency oscillation (HFO) in adult patients as a rescue technique following conventional ventilation.[57,58] In these studies patients were maintained on high levels of conventional support (high PEEP, high PIP, high $P_{plateau}$, and high F_IO_2) before being switched to HFO. Both studies showed an improvement in gas exchange when patients were switched from conventional ventilation to HFO. Mortality rate in both studies was directly related to the length of time on conventional ventilation.

In a prospective, randomized, controlled trial comparing HFOV and pressure control ventilation in adults with ARDS, HFOV was shown to be as effective and safe as pressure control ventilation. The 30-day mortality rate for patients in the HFOV group was 37%, and the mortality rate for patients receiving conventional ventilation was 52%. Although better survival appeared to occur in the HFOV group, this finding was not statistically significant.[59]

Evidence that clearly demonstrates improved survival in adults with ARDS using HFOV is not currently available. Although HFOV may improve P_aO_2 in some patients and thereby allow F_IO_2 to be lowered, this improvement may only be transitory.[60]

TECHNICAL ASPECTS

High-frequency oscillatory ventilation is a method of HFV in which gas is oscillated at high frequencies (3 to 15 Hz). The CareFusion 3100B high-frequency oscillatory ventilator (CareFusion, Viasys Corp, Yorba Linda, Calif.) is an example of an adult HFO currently available. It was approved by the Food and Drug Administration (FDA) for the United States market and introduced in 2001. Technical aspects of this specific ventilator are described elsewhere.[61]

HFOs are produced by a reciprocating piston with the 3100B. The resulting flow waveform is an approximation of a sine wave (Fig. 23-5). With HFOV, pressure is positive in the airway during the inspiratory phase (forward stroke) and negative during the expiratory phase (return stroke). Thus both inspiration and expiration are active, resulting in bulk flow rather than jet pulsations.

The diaphragm-shaped piston used in this device is magnetically driven, much like a stereo speaker. Gas is oscillated back and forth by the action of the diaphragm. The amplitude of the wave, which is set by the power control, determines the forward and backward excursion of the piston and thus helps determine V_T. A low-compliance plastic circuit provides humidified bias flow of gas to the patient (Fig. 23-6).

INITIAL CONTROL SETTINGS

Because the use of HFOV is still being researched, the following recommendations for initial settings come from available published studies.[54,55,59]

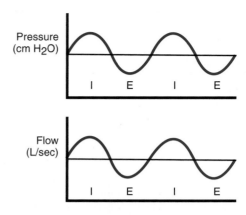

Fig. 23-5 The sinusoidal waveform generated by an oscillator. *I,* Inspiration (gas flow into the patient); *E,* expiration (active gas flow out of the patient). (From Cairo JM, Pilbeam SP: *Mosby's respiratory care equipment,* ed 8, St Louis, 2009, Mosby.)

Parameters that are set in HFOV include the following:
- mP_{aw} (analogous to $\bar{P}_{aw}$ on conventional ventilation)
- Power (the peak-to-trough pressure difference generated by the piston movement)
- Frequency (in hertz)
- Inspiratory time percentage
- Flow (bias flow)

Mean Airway Pressure

The mP_{aw} is a direct control located on the front panel of the CareFusion 3100B (Fig. 23-7). It is generated by a continuous flow of gas past the variable resistance of a mushroom valve. In the 3100B, the balloon or mushroom valve is located in the expiratory limb of the circuit (see Fig. 23-6). As the balloon is inflated, the outflow is restricted and the airway pressure increases. The mP_{aw} must be kept at the target value because it can drift. This drift can occur when other controls that affect mP_{aw} are changed.

The mP_{aw} directly affects P_aO_2 by changing lung volume. Initially, mP_{aw} is set at 3 to 5 cm H_2O above the observed $\bar{P}_{aw}$ during conventional ventilation. A starting range is typically 25 to 30 cm H_2O. As the mP_{aw} is increased, the volume in the lungs increases and the patient's diaphragm is displaced downward. For example, one goal of mP_{aw} in the neonatal population is to position the diaphragm between the eighth and ninth thoracic vertebrae on a chest radiograph. This position usually correlates with good lung expansion and an acceptable P_aO_2; it may also correlate with adequate lung expansion in the adult, that is, visualization of the ninth posterior rib above the level of the diaphragm in the midclavicular line on the chest radiograph.[59,62] The mP_{aw} should not be reduced during the first 24 hours to allow an adequate time for as many lung units as possible to be recruited. An exception to this is if mP_{aw} is initially set too high. As previously mentioned, assessment of mP_{aw} is done by observing the expansion of the thorax on a chest radiograph (Key Point 23-2). If hemodynamic monitoring is being used, further assessment of mean arterial pressure may include determining the ability of the right side of the heart to fill in the presence of the continuous high pressure in the thorax.

Key Point 23-2 Wide swings in the mP_{aw} value during ventilation may indicate leaks in the system, water in the expiratory circuit, or that the patient is making spontaneous breathing efforts.

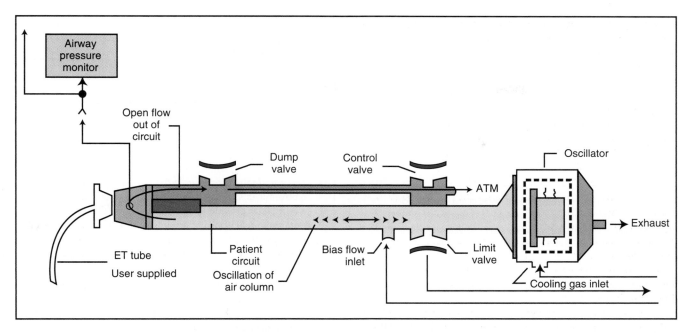

Fig. 23-6 Schematic of the CareFusion 3100B patient circuit. A dump valve located on the expiratory limb opens when the oscillator (piston) is off. The mP_{aw} control valve is located at the end of the expiratory limb. As the pressure to this valve is increased, the outflow of gas is restricted and the mP_{aw} increases. The limit valve located on the inspiratory limb is used to limit inspiratory pressure. When the set pressure limit is exceeded, this valve opens. (Courtesy CareFusion VIASYS Healthcare, San Diego, Calif.)

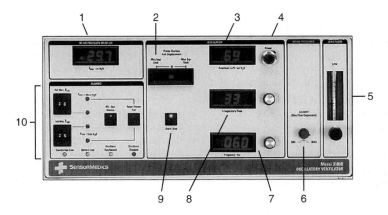

Fig. 23-7 Control panel of the CareFusion Model 3100B high-frequency oscillator. *1*, Display of mP_{aw}; *2*, indicator of piston movement; *3*, amplitude display; *4*, power control knob; *5*, bias flow display and control; *6*, adjustment for mP_{aw}; *7*, frequency control and display; *8*, $T_i\%$ control and display; *9*, on/off control for oscillating piston; *10*, alarm settings and indicators panel. (Courtesy CareFusion VIASYS Healthcare, San Diego, Calif.)

Establishing appropriate mP_{aw} during HFOV has been studied in an animal model.[63] Setting mP_{aw} at 1.5 times the lower inflection point of a static pressure–volume curve was sufficient to re-establish prelung injury P_aO_2.

Amplitude

Amplitude influences the level of ventilation (P_aCO_2) and can be adjusted by the power control, which sets the amount of piston displacement and resulting amplitude of the oscillating waveform (Fig. 23-8).[64] As amplitude is increased, the pressure gradient (ΔP) increases and V_T increases. (In HFOV, the equation dictating ventilation is not $f \times V_T$, but $f \times V_T^2$.)[62] Adjusting the power control

changes the amount of power going to the piston and the amount of piston displacement or forward-backward movement. Piston displacement affects ΔP created by a piston (oscillator) excursion (see Fig. 23-6). The settings control panel ranges from 1.0 to 10. It is adjusted by using a control located adjacent to the amplitude readout (see Fig. 23-7). A starting power setting of 6 to 7 is typical for adults. The appropriateness of the power setting is determined by observing chest wall movement or "chest-wiggle factor" (CWF). Increased amplitude is also associated with increased chest wall movement. The CWF should be visible from the level of the clavicle to the midthigh. (Assessment of chest wiggle is difficult in obese patients.) Placing a pencil or tongue depressor on the leg at the

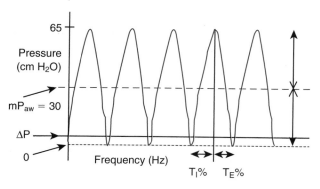

Fig. 23-8 The waveform for pressure–time produced during high-frequency oscillatory ventilation. The oscillations occur above and below the set mP_{aw} (30 cm H_2O). The amplitude of this oscillating pressure (ΔP) is approximately 70 cm H_2O, or 35 cm H_2O above and below the mP_{aw} setting. $T_E\%$, Expiratory time percent; $T_I\%$, inspiratory time percent.

midthigh level may provide a visual indicator of the wiggle at thigh level. In practice some clinicians have found that a setting that results in a ΔP of 60 to 70 cm H_2O around the mP_{aw} settings is a good starting point until arterial blood gas (ABG) results can be obtained.[64] Another recommended starting point for amplitude used by some clinicians is to determine the P_aCO_2 before HFOV and add 20 to this value. For example, if P_aCO_2 on conventional ventilation was 60 mm Hg, starting amplitude will be 80.

In addition to the actual power setting, other factors that affect the amplitude include the endotracheal tube (ET) size, R_{aw}, and C_L. Changes in R_{aw} and C_L will affect the amplitude delivery.[65] For example, at a specific power setting, a **measured** amplitude increase could be caused by an increase in R_{aw} or a decrease in C_L. The amplitude measured at the airway is significantly higher than the pressures delivered to the lung. The size of the ET, the branches of the bronchial tree, and the distance from the piston, can attenuate the pressure delivery.

Frequency

The frequency setting controls the time allowed for the piston to move forward and back. It is a secondary control for ventilation. The available range is 3 to 15 Hz (180 to 900 cycles/min). Reducing the frequency causes a greater volume displacement and thus a larger V_T and higher $\dot{V}_E$. Conversely, increasing the frequency results in a smaller volume displacement, a smaller V_T and lower $\dot{V}_E$. An initial setting for an adult is 5 to 6 Hz (300 to 360 cycles/min). One management strategy to reduce P_aCO_2 is to lower the frequency setting. (NOTE: It is not typically set lower than 3.) Generally once the frequency is established, it is usually not changed during the course of treatment. Occasionally some clinicians may change the frequency after changes in amplitude are made in an effort to alter the patient's $\dot{V}_E$ (low frequency tends to increase $\dot{V}_E$, and high frequency tends to decrease $\dot{V}_E$).

Inspiratory Time Percentage

The inspiratory time percentage ($T_I\%$) represents the portion of the respiratory cycle that the piston spends in a forward motion. An initial setting of 33% (I:E of 1:2) is usually appropriate for an adult. The $T_I\%$ control may also assist in CO_2 elimination, but to a lesser extent than amplitude and frequency. For some patients, a $T_I\%$ of 50% may improve ventilation (CO_2 removal) and lung recruitment. Once this parameter is set, it is generally not changed.

BOX 23-1 **A Recruitment Maneuver (RM) for Use During High-Frequency Oscillatory Ventilatory***

To perform a recruitment maneuver:
- Increase the F_IO_2 to 1.0.
- Stop the piston (pressure from the oscillation of the piston can be transmitted to the peripheral lung in addition to the increased setting of mP_{aw} during the maneuver).[†]
- Turn the mP_{aw} up to 40 cm H_2O for 40 to 60 seconds, or 10 cm H_2O above the mP_{aw} setting from an already established mP_{aw}, while the piston is stopped.
- Discontinue the procedure if the patient becomes hypoxemic (S_pO_2 <85%) or hemodynamically compromised (mean blood pressure <60 mm Hg, a drop of blood pressure of >20 mm Hg from baseline, an increase in heart rate to >140 beats/min, a fall in heart rate to <60 beats/min, or development of a new arrhythmia).
- After the procedure, turn the mP_{aw} to an appropriate initial setting or back to the previous setting.

*An RM should not be performed if a pneumothorax or a bubbling chest tube (active air leak) is present.
†Neonatal tubes are so small that only about 5% of the ΔP is transmitted to the distal end of the endotracheal tube (ET). However, in adults with large ETs, up to 20% of the ΔP can be transmitted to the carina level.

Bias Flow

The bias flow control is usually the first parameter set when starting HFOV. A typical range for an adult is 25 to 40 L/min (e.g., 30 L/min). Changing the bias flow affects mP_{aw}. If flow is inadequate, the set mP_{aw} cannot be reached. Low flow may result in an increase in P_aCO_2 from inadequate washout of exhaled gas. If the set bias flow is too high, dampening of active exhalation may inhibit carbon dioxide elimination. The backward motion of the piston is responsible for active exhalation (Key Point 23-3). With a high bias flow the piston may only remove air from the circuit. This may also increase the P_aCO_2 and result in auto-PEEP.

> **Key Point 23-3** In HFOV, during the expiratory phase the backward movement of the piston actively moves air out of the system.

Additional Settings

The F_IO_2 is usually set at 1.0 and decreased in increments of 0.1 (range, 0.05 to 0.10), as tolerated, to maintain the target range for P_aO_2 or oxygen saturation (S_pO_2). F_IO_2 may also be set similar to the way it is set with conventional ventilation and titrated based on S_pO_2 and ABGs. An ABG should be obtained 30 to 60 minutes after any change in mP_{aw}, amplitude, or frequency.[59]

Before transferring a patient from a conventional ventilator to the oscillator, the F_IO_2 may be increased to 1.0. After transfer, a recruitment maneuver (RM) is recommended because the patient is briefly disconnected from the ventilator (Box 23-1).[64,65] Anytime the patient becomes disconnected, the RM should be repeated. Some institutions perform an RM on a regular basis, such as every 12 hours, if an F_IO_2 of more than 0.4 is required to maintain oxygenation. This would be appropriate as long as the patient responded to an RM with an improvement in oxygenation (Key Point 23-4).[54]

A few hours after initiation of HFOV, a chest radiograph should be obtained to determine the appropriateness of the mP_{aw} setting. The chest radiograph is taken while the piston is turned on because the information desired is how well recruited the lungs are on the current setting. If more than 11 posterior ribs are showing, mP_{aw} needs to be slowly decreased in increments of 2 cm H_2O until an appropriate inflation point is reached.

Key Point 23-4 Lung recruitment may be an important aspect of HFOV, whether HFOV is being used as a rescue technique or as a primary mode to prevent VILI.

INDICATION AND EXCLUSION CRITERIA

Patients with ARDS weighing at least 35 kg and who are not responding to mechanical ventilation may be candidates for HFOV. Failure may be defined as the presence of unresponsive severe hypoxemia (F_1O_2 >0.6; PEEP 10 cm H_2O or more, with a P_aO_2 of 65 mm Hg or less) or a significant risk of VILI.[59] Indications for HFOV depend on the institutional policy. Additional indications might include the following:

- A diagnosis of H1N1 influenza infection with ARDS
- Air leaks in patients
- Early intervention to recruit the lungs
- Clinical staff comfort with using the equipment

Criteria for the use of the CareFusion 3100B HFO are listed in Box 23-2. Another exclusion criterion involves patients requiring aerosolized medications. Use of the small-volume ultrasonic-type nebulizers or a vibrating mesh nebulizer may provide a solution to the problem of aerosol delivery during HFOV.[66] Further study of this topic is certainly warranted.

MONITORING, ASSESSMENT, AND ADJUSTMENT

The oscillator should be calibrated according to the manufacturer's recommendations before use. Because patients need to be suctioned regularly (at least every 12 hours), a closed-suction catheter system should be placed in the patient circuit. The connection for a closed-suction catheter is typically placed at a right angle in the

circuit. This may affect the oscillatory pressure waveform; therefore chest excursions need to be assessed after placing the system in the circuit. A suction catheter is still required to help maintain airway patency. Some clinicians use an inline oxygen analyzer to obtain continuous monitoring of delivered F_1O_2.

The 3100B uses a standard heated humidifier with a closed feed system to maintain water level, which can provide adequate humidification. The water-feed system should be pressurized to keep water flowing into the device. Humidification can be verified when condensate appears at the distal end of the inspiratory circuit. The circuit should be kept free of water. Because of condensate, frequent checking of the circuit is required.

To transition from conventional ventilation to HFOV, sedation and analgesics may be required. The patient is sedated because vigorous spontaneous breathing efforts should be avoided during HFOV. A strong spontaneous inspiration may reduce circuit pressures below 5 cm H_2O, which can result in desaturation. A drop in pressure this low would also trigger a disconnect alarm and shut off the oscillator piston. For this reason patients are typically sedated with a combination of benzodiazepines (e.g., midazolam) and a narcotic (e.g., fentanyl).[60,64] Paralysis with such agents as pancuronium, cisatracurium, or vecuronium may also be required, particularly for the first 30 minutes or so of the procedure. (See Chapter 15 for information on these medications.) When a paralyzing agent is used, train-of-four monitoring is recommended to reduce the risk of prolonged neuromuscular blockade. Ulnar nerve placement avoids the chest, upper air area, and thigh areas—where wiggling is present—and might interfere with monitoring. (See Chapter 15 for information on train-of-four monitoring.)

Once the patient is receiving HFO, the clinician should listen for bilateral breath sounds to determine whether the intensity of breath sounds is equal over both lungs. A reduction in intensity may indicate a pneumothorax or malposition of the ET. Breath and heart sounds may be difficult to hear, so other forms of assessment should be performed (e.g., determination of C_L) once HFOV is initiated. To listen for heart sounds, the piston must be momentarily stopped while the CPAP level is maintained. Disconnecting the patient would cause derecruitment of the lungs and is therefore not recommended (Case Study 23-1).

The CWF should also be checked hourly. CWF may change with ET obstruction, right mainstem intubation, a pneumothorax, or an accidental extubation.[55]

Rotation of the patient is more difficult with HFOV than during conventional ventilation and must be performed cautiously in order not to disconnect the patient or cause an accidental extubation. A circuit disconnection with a loss of pressure will cause the oscillator to stop. For this reason, a manual resuscitator with a PEEP valve attached should be kept at the bedside. (NOTE: A circuit disconnection may occur where the expiratory valve tubing attaches to the circuit.)[64] Continuous lateral rotation also may be safely accomplished using a specialized rotating bed (e.g., RotoRest, KCI Medical, Kidlington, UK).

BOX 23-2   Indications and Precautionary Use of the CareFusion 3100B High-Frequency Oscillatory Ventilation

Indications
The 3100B is indicated for use in ventilatory support and treatment of selected patients (≥35 kg) with acute respiratory failure.

Contraindications
No contraindications exist for the use of the 3100B.

Precautionary Use
The 3100B HFO should be used with caution in the following patient conditions:
- Unstable cardiovascular status
- Acute bronchospasm
- Severe acidosis (the 3100B HFV is not designed to ventilate so much as oxygenate)
- Pregnancy
- Chronic obstructive pulmonary disease or asthma requiring the use of aerosolized bronchodilators

---

 Case Study 23-1

Patient Assessment During HFOV
A patient being ventilated by HFOV exhibits a sudden drop in S_pO_2, a reduction in CWF, tracheal deviation to the left, and a sudden drop in mP_{aw}. What is the most likely cause of these sudden changes?

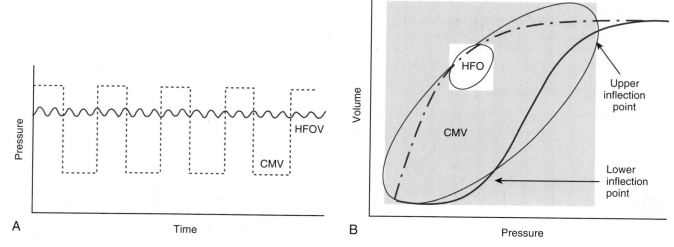

Fig. 23-9 **A,** The pressure–time curve contrasting tidal variations in pressure with conventional mechanical ventilation (CMV) *(dashed line),* and high-frequency oscillatory ventilation (HFOV) *(solid line).* **B,** Pressure–volume loop showing inflation *(solid line)* and deflation *(dashed line)* comparing the potential for overdistention and alveolar collapse during tidal breathing with CMV and HFOV *(small oval).* (From Ferguson ND, Stewart TE: The use of high-frequency oscillatory ventilation in adults with acute lung injury, Respir Care Clin N Am 7:647-661, 2001.)

ADJUSTING SETTINGS TO MAINTAIN ARTERIAL BLOOD GAS GOALS

Oxygenation during HFOV is achieved primarily by maintaining the mP_{aw} at a level sufficient to obtain optimal lung inflation.[59] At a set level of amplitude, increases in mP_{aw} result in increases in lung volume and available alveolar surface area. As long as cardiac output is not adversely affected, oxygenation generally improves (Fig. 23-9). (See Chapter 13 for lung recruitment strategies.) Conversely, decreases in mP_{aw} result in a decrease in oxygenation if lung derecruitment occurs.

An overall goal for oxygenation in patients with ARDS is a P_aO_2 of 55 to 80 mm Hg and an S_pO_2 of 88% to 95%.[67] If an F_1O_2 greater than 0.6 is required to maintain these goals, mP_{aw} can be increased by 2 to 3 cm H_2O (maximum, 45 cm H_2O) until the F_1O_2 can be decreased to less than 0.6.[59] Changes should be made slowly (every 30 minutes) to allow the opportunity for determining whether alveolar recruitment and improvement in S_pO_2 and P_aO_2 has occurred. (In neonates, alveolar recruitment may require up to 25 minutes.[59] The time required in adults is not currently known.) Before making these changes, an RM is recommended (see Box 23-1) unless a pneumothorax or an active air leak is present, and the chest drainage system to compensate for the leak is bubbling.

If severe hypoxemia persists, inhaled nitric oxide might be added or the patient may be placed in the prone position.[68]

To decrease P_aO_2, F_1O_2 is reduced in increments of 0.05 to 0.10, until an F_1O_2 of 0.6 is reached. Once F_1O_2 is 0.6 or less, reductions in F_1O_2 can be alternated with reductions in mP_{aw} (increments of 2 to 3 cm H_2O). Weaning of mP_{aw} should be done carefully and slowly until a minimum level of 20 to 24 cm H_2O is reached, and F_1O_2 is less than 0.5. These suggested changes are one approach to targeting the oxygenation goals. Some institutions may have different approaches.

The maintenance of ventilation (pH and P_aCO_2) may be more difficult with an oscillator than with a conventional ventilator. During HFOV, $\dot{V}_E$ and V_T delivery are affected by several factors, including the pressure amplitude of oscillation (ΔP), frequency, ET

size, amount of ET cuff leak, and lung characteristics (C_L and R_{aw}) (Key Point 23-5).[59]

Key Point 23-5 The ET can block part of the pressure (volume) transmission to the lower airways. The smaller the ET, the more the pressure is damped. With a large ET more pressure (volume) is transmitted to the lungs, providing better ventilation.[59]

As the piston moves, it applies cyclical pressure above and below the set mP_{aw} (see Figs. 23-8 and 23-9). As the power setting is increased and ΔP increases, V_T, and $\dot{V}_E$ increase. This improves CO_2 elimination and lowers P_aCO_2. Decreasing P_aCO_2 can generally be accomplished in most patients by changing only the amplitude to decrease the ΔP. The power setting can be increased in increments of 0.5 to 1.0 until the maximal setting is reached (10 is the maximum on the control of the 3100B). Observing changes in CWF can assess power settings.

In some cases a change in frequency may also be required to alter P_aCO_2. Decreasing the frequency (hertz) increases the time of piston movement. In addition, as frequency is reduced, the attenuation of the wave signal through the ET is diminished and a larger ΔP occurs (Key Point 23-6).[64] This increases the delivered V_T and the distal transmission of the ΔP to the lungs, thereby enhancing ventilation. Decreasing the frequency is accomplished in increments of 1 to 2 Hz until a minimum of 3 Hz is reached.[64,68] Box 23-3 provides an example of the effect of changing amplitude and frequency in HFOV.[69]

Key Point 23-6 An upward adjustment of frequency results in an increase in P_aCO_2, whereas a downward adjustment of frequency results in a decrease in P_aCO_2.[59]

Conversely, increasing the frequency reduces V_T and CO_2 elimination, and results in a higher P_aCO_2. Increasing the frequency too

BOX 23-3	Example of the Effect of Changing Amplitude and Frequency on Tidal Volume in High-Frequency Oscillatory Ventilation

Suppose the initial amplitude produces a ΔP of 50 cm H_2O, and the frequency is set at 8 Hz and the inspiratory time at 33%. If the amplitude is increased such that ΔP is increased to 60 cm H_2O, this can result in an increase in tidal volume (V_T). The same change in V_T can be accomplished by keeping the amplitude the same while decreasing the frequency from 8 Hz to 4 Hz.

BOX 23-4	Steps to Reduce P_aCO_2 During High-Frequency Oscillatory Ventilation

Increase amplitude (ΔP) incrementally.
If hypercapnia persists and amplitude (power setting) is at maximum, decrease frequency by 1 Hz to a minimum of 3 Hz.
If hypercapnia persists, increase the inspiratory time to 50%.
If hypercapnia still persists, try increasing the cuff leak.

much with HFO may actually lead to air trapping and an increase in P_aCO_2. Thus adjustments in frequency should be done cautiously. "Adequate" ventilation may be a P_aCO_2 that keeps the pH greater than 7.20 and allows permissive hypercapnia.

If high P_aCO_2 persists in spite of changes in amplitude and frequency, an increase in V_T can be accomplished by increasing T_I% from an initial setting of 33% to 50%. Notice that this may also increase mP_{aw} and the risk of air trapping.

When amplitude, frequency, and T_I% have been optimally adjusted and CO_2 remains elevated, providing a deliberate cuff leak may increase the flow of gas through and around the ET, and augment CO_2 elimination.[64] To set a cuff leak, the practitioner removes some of the air from the cuff until the mP_{aw} decreases slightly. The cuff leak is kept at this level, and the mP_{aw} is restored to its prior setting by increasing the bias flow. To confirm the cuff leak, the pilot balloon is squeezed to observe the measured mP_{aw}. Squeezing the pilot balloon should cause a rise of approximately 5 cm H_2O in mP_{aw}. ABG evaluation is performed after a cuff leak adjustment (15 to 30 minutes) to confirm that the leak was effective in lowering P_aCO_2.[59] Box 23-4 summarizes ventilator adjustments for reducing P_aCO_2 during HFOV.[59,69] To increase P_aCO_2 the previous steps can be reversed. (If the frequency [hertz] is increased, mP_{aw} may decrease.)

If a severe rise in P_aCO_2 occurs abruptly, the respiratory therapist should assess the patient immediately by manually ventilating the patient and passing a suction catheter through the ET to determine if the ET or the airway is obstructed. The ventilator circuit should also be inspected for tube crimping or obstructions (Key Point 23-7).[64]

Key Point 23-7 A significant increase in P_aCO_2 can occur as the result of a few centimeters of a suction catheter from a closed-suction system remaining in the airway. Narrowing the lumen of the ET reduces effective ventilation during HFOV.[64]

BOX 23-5	Disorders Treated with Heliox

- Postextubation stridor
- Asthma
- Tracheobronchitis
- Viral laryngitis
- Laryngotracheal bronchitis
- Bronchiolitis
- Tumors (laryngeal or mediastinal)
- Foreign body aspiration
- Vocal cord paralysis
- Dyskinesia
- Chronic obstructive pulmonary disease (COPD)

RETURNING TO CONVENTIONAL VENTILATION

Once the patient is stable with an mP_{aw} of 20 to 24 cm H_2O and a S_pO_2 of 88% or more on an F_IO_2 less than 0.5, the patient can be checked for readiness to switch back to conventional ventilation. Readiness can be evaluated by observing a resolution of initial lung injury, tolerance of suctioning (i.e., if significant desaturation does not occur), and tolerance of manual ventilation on 50% O_2 and PEEP, 10 cm H_2O or greater (S_pO_2 remains more than 90% during the procedure).[59] If the patient does well during these procedures, he or she can then be transferred to a conventional ventilator.

Some clinicians transition patients to PC-CMV with low V_T settings (6 mL/kg ideal body weight [IBW] and high PEEP levels, 10 to 15 cm H_2O).[59,64] Others favor modes such as APRV, which allows a close matching of airway pressures to the mP_{aw} on HFVO during the transition.[64]

In summary, HFOV has been available for some time for the management of infants, and now appears to be emerging as a viable option for managing adult patients with ARDS.[54,70-76] When it is used, timing is important. HFOV should be started early to avoid VILI associated with conventional ventilation. (See Chapter 17 for information on VILI.) The role of HFOV in the management of adults with ARDS needs to be verified with prospective, randomized, controlled trials.[70,77]

Heliox Therapy and Mechanical Ventilation

Helium-oxygen mixtures (**heliox**) have been used in the treatment of a number of disorders that cause airway obstruction (Box 23-5). It is approved by the FDA as a diagnostic gas; the FDA has also cleared a number of devices for the therapeutic use of heliox mixtures.[78-80]

Helium's effect is based on its low density. Box 23-6 lists some of the physical properties of helium.[81] The low density of helium reduces turbulent flow in obstructed airways and decreases respiratory muscle load and dyspnea. In cases of severe reactive airway disease (e.g., asthma), heliox delivery may reduce the work of breathing through partially obstructed airways.[81,82]

Another key property of helium regarding its medical application is the fact that it is an inert gas (Key Point 23-8).

Key Point 23-8 Because helium is an inert gas, it will not react with human tissue or with pharmaceutical agents.

BOX **23-6**	**Properties of Helium**

Except for hydrogen, helium is the most abundant element in the universe. On earth it can only be found in natural gas fields in North America (United States and Canada).[75] Helium is odorless and colorless. It has the second lowest density of any known gas, second only to hydrogen. The density of helium is 0.18 g/L. Nitrogen's density is much higher at 1.25 g/L, and oxygen is even higher at 1.43 g/L. Air is 1.29 g/L. Helium has the lowest melting point of any element and a boiling point close to absolute zero. In addition, helium has a high thermal conductivity.

BOX **23-7**	**Equations Describing Flow-Through Tubes**

The Reynold's number for a flow through a pipe is defined as:

$$Re = (2 \times \dot{V} \times \rho)/(\pi \times r \times \mu)$$

where Re is Reynold's number, $\dot{V}$ is the flow (in milliliters per second), ρ is the density of the gas (in grams per milliliter), r is the radius of the tube (in centimeters), and μ is the gas viscosity (in grams per centimeter per second).[81]

Poiseuille (laminar) flow is experimentally found to occur for a Reynold's number less than 2000. At larger Reynold's numbers ($\geq$4000) flow becomes turbulent.

In **laminar** conditions the following applies: $\Delta P = k^1$ ($\dot{V}$lam), where ΔP is the pressure difference, k^1 is the coefficient of linear resistance, (which equals $8\eta l/\pi r^4$; where η is the gas viscosity in grams per centimeter per second, l is the length of the tube in centimeters, and r is the radius of the tube in centimeters), and $\dot{V}$lam is the laminar flow (in milliliters per second). Rewritten as Poiseuille's equation for laminar flow,

$$\Delta P = (8/\eta \dot{V})/(\pi \times r^4)$$

In **turbulent** conditions, $\Delta P = k$ ($\dot{V}$ turb^2), where $\dot{V}$turb^2 is turbulent flow (in milliliters per second), and k is the coefficient of nonlinear resistance and equals $fl/4\pi^2 r^5$ (where f is the friction factor dependent on the Reynold's number and the roughness of the tubing wall). In a small tubing, $f = 0.316/Re^{1/4}$, where r is the radius (in centimeters).

GAS FLOW THROUGH THE AIRWAYS

Because heliox is effective only when turbulent flow is present, it is important to understand where and when turbulence is likely to occur. Normal airflow in the larynx and trachea is turbulent and is the predominant gas flow pattern in the larger airways of the first and second generation of bronchi (mainstem and lobar bronchi) during normal, quiet breathing. The transition to laminar flow occurs somewhere between the third and the eleventh generation of bronchi, depending on the rate of gas flow (Box 23-7).[81-83]

During laminar flow in the small airways, the driving pressure is proportional to flow and is influenced by the viscosity of the gas being breathed. Density does not affect the pressure–flow relation in laminar flow. During turbulent flow the driving pressure is proportional to the flow squared, and gas density is more important than viscosity as a determinant of flow.[81] As a low-density gas, helium provides a greater flow for a given ΔP, when flow is

turbulent. Heliox is therefore expected to be more beneficial in diseases affecting the larger airways and partially obstructed airways, where flow is turbulent. When helium reduces the Reynold's number to less than 2000, laminar flow predominates, thereby reducing R_{aw}.

HELIOX IN AVOIDING INTUBATION AND DURING MECHANICAL VENTILATION

With an acute exacerbation of asthma, central airways are narrowed from mucus plugging, mucosal edema, and smooth muscle constriction, increasing turbulent flow and R_{aw}. In the treatment of spontaneously breathing, nonintubated patients with severe asthma episodes, heliox has been shown to increase peak inspiratory flow rate. It may reduce the risk of respiratory muscle fatigue until bronchodilator and corticosteroid therapy become effective (Key Point 23-9).[81,84] Heliox has also been shown to reduce the incidence of pulsus paradoxus in patients experiencing a severe asthma exacerbation.

> **Key Point 23-9** Heliox ventilation does not cure the cause of partial airway obstruction. It should only be used as an adjunct therapy to reduce work of breathing until the obstruction can be alleviated.[81]

Early in a severe asthma exacerbation, the obstruction is located in the central airways. As time progresses (more than 96 hours), however, the peripheral airways become obstructed with secretions and edema. Thus heliox is more likely to be beneficial early in the process.[83] When heliox is required in treating asthma, it may be required for up to 12 to 24 hours and has been used in some facilities up to 5 days.[83,85] In patients with COPD or small airway disease, heliox may not be helpful in reducing R_{aw} if it occurs in the peripheral regions of the lungs.[83]

At present no guidelines exist for the indications and timing of heliox in patients with severe asthma. Some clinicians recommend using heliox when aggressive treatment with bronchodilators fails to improve the patient's condition within 30 minutes.[81] Others suggest intubation and mechanical ventilation when the patient's assessment deteriorates into acute respiratory failure and only consider heliox if the patient is then stabilized.[83] Regardless of approach, heliox does **not** replace aggressive bronchodilator and corticosteroid therapy (See Clinical Scenario on severe asthma).[81,82]

Clinical Scenario: Severe Asthma

A 24-year-old woman vacationing in Florida was admitted to a local emergency department with status asthmaticus. She was conscious on admission and indicated she had taken 80 puffs from an albuterol metered-dose inhaler (MDI) before going to the emergency department, but had no relief of her symptoms. ABGs obtained while she was breathing enriched oxygen through a nonrebreathing mask were: pH = 6.98, P_aCO_2 = 125 mm Hg, and P_aO_2 = 78 mm Hg. The patient was able to request heliox verbally. She had previously been treated with heliox successfully. Although the respiratory care department did not routinely perform this procedure, they were willing to comply.[81,82]

The patient was intubated and mechanically ventilated. She received sedation and paralyzing agents. Heliox was obtained from another local hospital and instituted within 2 hours of intubation. PIP dropped dramatically from 80 cm H_2O to 40 cm H_2O when heliox was instituted. The patient required ventilation for less than 3 days. No pneumothorax occurred during ventilation.

POSTEXTUBATION STRIDOR

In postextubation stridor, heliox can be used in addition to racemic epinephrine to reduce the work of breathing until the airway inflammation subsides. This may help avoid reintubation. In cases where stridor does not diminish after 24 to 36 hours of therapy designed to reduce upper airway inflammation, the patient may have a more serious problem, such as tracheal webbing.[83]

DEVICES FOR DELIVERING HELIOX IN SPONTANEOUSLY BREATHING PATIENTS

Heliox can be effectively delivered using a mask system, in conjunction with aerosolized bronchodilators, and with invasive and noninvasive mechanical ventilation. To achieve an optimal effect, the concentration of the helium used is generally at least 60% to 70%.[83] (Concentrations as low as 50% have been effectively used in patients with large airway obstructions.)* The most commonly used concentration of heliox is 80:20 (80% helium and 20% oxygen). This latter mixture contains the greatest amount of helium, and thus the lowest density gas, without providing subambient levels of oxygen (Key Point 23-10).

> **Key Point 23-10** It is **never** advisable to use a 100% helium cylinder in any heliox setup because of the risk that the cylinder might accidentally be used as the only gas source.

Mask Heliox

Heliox can be delivered through a mask system by two different techniques. In the first technique, two flow meters are used. One flow meter is connected to oxygen and one to a heliox cylinder. Tubing from each flow meter is connected to a T-piece that is then attached to the desired mask, usually a nonrebreather. (The one-way valve of the rebreather mask should be in place.) To set the desired F_IO_2, an oxygen analyzer is placed in line at the T-piece to determine the proper setting of each of the two flow meters. The second technique for mask delivery involves connecting the heliox directly to the nonrebreathing mask and using a nasal cannula to administer oxygen. A major drawback of this latter case is analysis of the F_IO_2 and the amount of helium delivered. Monitoring with pulse oximetry is essential in both cases.

One of the more challenging aspects of both mask systems is to determine accurately the actual flow of helium delivered. While the regulators used to connect to the heliox cylinders are specific for the cylinder, the flow meters used for delivery are usually oxygen

*Deborah Gilley, RRT-NPS, Respiratory Care, Lucile Salter Packard Children's Hospital, Palo Alto, Calif., February 2005, personal communication.

or air flow meters. Because these flow meters are calibrated to the density of oxygen and not helium, the flow displayed on the flow meter will not be accurate for indicating heliox flow. Conversion factors exist for the most common heliox mixtures that can be used to determine the actual liter flow. The factor is multiplied by the actual flow reading. The correction factor for an 80:20 heliox mixture is 1.8. A 70:30 mixture has a factor of 1.6. A 60:40 mixture has a conversion factor of 1.4. For example, if 5 L/min is displayed on the oxygen flow meter attached to an 80:20 heliox mixture, the actual flow will be 9 L/min ($5 \times 1.8 = 9$) (Case Study 23-2).

> ### Case Study 23-2
>
> **Calculating Gas Flows During Heliox Therapy**
> A patient is receiving 70:30 He : O_2 through a flow meter. The flow is set at 10 L/min. What would be a close estimate of the actual flow of gas?

In many hospitals, respiratory therapists chart the actual flow displayed on the flow meter when recording flows in the patient's chart rather than the corrected flow. The respiratory care staff should be aware of the flow delivery differences. Regardless of whether actual or corrected flow is recorded, the patient's ventilatory and oxygenation status is the most important indicator that determines if the heliox therapy is effective.[81]

Heliox should not be delivered by nasal cannula alone. Delivering heliox through the nasal cannula produces high flows that can be irritating, cold, and drying and can deliver undetected, inadvertent PEEP. Determining whether the therapy is relieving the patient's hypoxia or meeting minute ventilation needs is also difficult.

Heliox should not be used with tents or hoods. Tents and hoods leak and lose a lot of air. In addition, helium is light and will migrate to the top of the device. Because of gas layering, some situations may produce subambient oxygen concentrations (<21%) to the patient.[86,87]

Nasal CPAP for infants may be used with heliox, but the clinician must ensure the CPAP device will work effectively and safely with helium and make any necessary adaptations to the therapy. Blenders with CPAP setups that use heliox are not advised. Because of the way the blender functions, it typically has a high gas consumption.[88]

Cost and Gas Consumption During Heliox Therapy

Patients receiving heliox therapy can consume from two to six cylinders in a 24-hour period depending on the device and the heliox concentration. Therefore an adequate quantity of the cylinders should be kept in stock along with appropriate regulators and wrenches. These cylinders range in price from $55 to $155 in the United States, but can cost upwards of $275 per cylinder in Europe.[81]

Heliox and Aerosol Delivery

Aerosol delivery with heliox can easily be achieved with some simple modifications to the mask system previously described. A Y-piece can be placed between the reservoir bag and the mask, and then a nebulizer can be attached to the open limb of the Y-piece

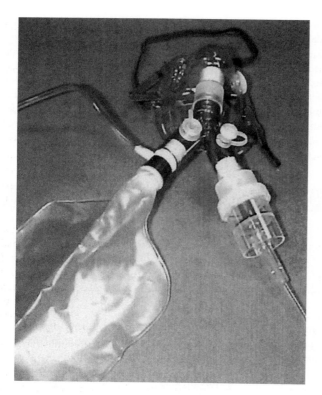

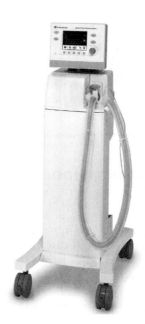

Fig. 23-11 The Aptaér Heliox Delivery System. (Courtesy Datex-Ohmeda, Inc., GE Healthcare, Madison, Wis.)

Fig. 23-10 A modified nonrebreathing mask for delivering heliox. A ventilator Y-connector allows inclusion of a standard small-volume nebulizer to provide aerosol therapy without interrupting the heliox delivery. (From Ritz R: Methods to avoid intubation, Respir Care 44:686-699, 1999.)

(Fig. 23-10). The nebulizer can be driven by either heliox or oxygen, depending on the patient's F_IO_2 requirement. A similar setup uses two flow meters hooked to one H-cylinder of heliox. One flow meter powers the reservoir bag and mask, and the other powers the nebulizer.

Heliox appears to improve the nebulizer's ability to deliver albuterol as well as aerosol deposition.[89,90] For patients receiving heliox to reduce the work of breathing associated with increased R_{aw}, the administration of aerosolized bronchodilators with an MDI may also substantially improve drug delivery.[91,92]

MANUFACTURED HELIOX DELIVERY SYSTEM

In 2004 Datex-Ohmeda, Inc., a division of General Electric Healthcare (Madison, Wis.), released the Aptaér Heliox Delivery System for sale in the United States (Fig. 23-11). This device delivers heliox to patients with severe airflow obstruction. It uses premixed heliox gases from a single gas cylinder (60:40 to 80:20 helium/oxygen mixtures). A regulator attaches directly to the cylinder. A second cylinder can be attached to the back of the unit to provide quick changeover when one is depleted.

Delivery of the gas to the patient is through a coaxial patient circuit, which consists of two tubes, one inside the other. One tube conducts inspired gas (inner tube), and the other expired gas (Fig. 23-12). The circuit is attached to the patient by a sealed face mask.

Medication delivery is provided by the Aeroneb Professional Nebulizer System (Aerogen, Mountain View, Calif.), which is incorporated into the Aptaér patient circuit (see Fig. 23-12). The

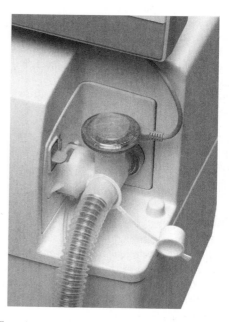

Fig. 23-12 The patient circuit demonstrating a coaxial construction with the inspiratory limb inside the expiratory limb. The Aeroneb Professional Nebulizer System from Aerogen, which is incorporated into the Aptaér Heliox Delivery System, is connected by a cable to the delivery system. (Courtesy Datex-Ohmeda, Inc., GE Healthcare, Madison, Wis.)

nebulizers system is an electronic micropump. It uses a piezoelectric element to vibrate a plate, which contains 1000 funnel-shaped openings. The vibration frequency is 100,000 cycles/sec, or approximately one tenth the frequency of ultrasonic nebulizers. Movement and vibrational frequency of the plate containing the funnel-shaped openings govern particle size. The Aeroneb consistently produces a mist with a very small particle size (2.4-μm mean mass aerodynamic diameter).

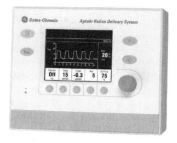

Fig. 23-13 The monitor and control screen of the Aptaér Heliox Delivery System. (Courtesy Datex-Ohmeda, Inc, GE Healthcare, Madison, Wis.)

The mode of operation of the Aptaér Heliox Delivery System is pressure support. Controls include a support pressure range of 3 to 20 cm H_2O, trigger sensitivity of −0.1 to −1.5 cm H_2O, a rise time adjustment with settings from 1 to 10 (10 being the most rapid rise to the set pressure), and the ability to adjust flow cycle from 5% to 75%. Monitored parameters include respiratory rate (0 to 122 breaths/min) and an airway pressure waveform display (pressure/time) (Fig. 23-13). Alarms are also available and include a low respiratory rate alarm (2 to 20 breaths/min), a high respiratory rate alarm (10 to 99 breaths/min), and a minimum pressure alarm (1 to 15 cm H_2O).

A dedicated system for providing heliox therapy has several advantages. The equipment needed for therapy is contained in a single cart. The Aptaér system conserves gas, and thus cylinders last longer than typical constant flow cylinder setups. The unit is equipped to provide visual displays for pressure and alarms to monitor high and low respiratory rate in addition to low pressure. It also provides gas delivery by using a pressure support mode. Additional studies are needed to determine if the Aptaér unit provides significant advantages over traditional methods of providing heliox therapy.

HELIOX AND AEROSOL DELIVERY DURING MECHANICAL VENTILATION

If a nebulizer is used for inline delivery of medications during mechanical ventilation with heliox, powering the nebulizer with oxygen and the ventilator with heliox may be advisable. The use of heliox to power the nebulizer may require a high flow and not be as effective in producing an aerosol mist.[87] The heliox in the circuit is sufficient to carry the medication to the patient. During mechanical ventilation, He : O_2 concentrations of 50 : 50 or more increase delivery of a bronchodilator (albuterol) from an MDI by more than 50%, when compared with oxygen or air.[91,92] For this reason aerosolized medications are better delivered by MDI to ventilated patients when heliox is used.

Heliox with a Mechanical Ventilator

Delivering heliox through a ventilator has been found to be effective, but presents special challenges. Because of its low density, volume and flow delivery measurements will not be accurate with most ventilators. Calculations and display of any parameter based on a flow measurement will therefore be incorrect. Ventilator values based on flow measurements are less accurate than values based on pressure measurements.[93,94] Accurate measurement of volume with heliox requires a device that is not density dependent, such as a volume displacement spirometer. However, this type of monitoring is not practical.

Delivery of heliox through mechanical ventilators can also interfere with other key functions of the ventilator, such as gas-mixing devices, inspiratory and expiratory valve function, triggering and cycling mechanisms, automatic leak compensation, monitors, and, most notably, minute volume alarms.

During volume ventilation most ventilators will show a discrepancy between the set V_T ($V_T$set) and the actual delivered V_T ($V_T$del). The magnitude of this difference, in general, is inversely related to the F_IO_2. In other words, the lower the F_IO_2 (i.e., the higher the helium percentage), the more $V_T$set exceeds $V_T$del.[94] In most ventilators a linear correlation occurs between $V_T$set and $V_T$del for any given F_IO_2. Because of this, a correction factor may be applied to the $V_T$set to obtain an actual $V_T$del for any set F_IO_2 (Box 23-8).[94-104]

Although no $V_T$set in pressure ventilation exists with heliox, discrepancy with $V_T$del as reported by the ventilator and the actual $V_T$del delivered to the patient does occur. During pressure control in most ventilators, inspired V_T reported by the ventilator ($V_T$insp) will underestimate true $V_T$del by an amount equal to that between $V_T$set and $V_T$del in volume control ventilation.[94] Because pressure ventilation is not based on flow measurements, it may be more suitable for use with mechanical ventilation with heliox. PEEP is also not dependent on flow measurements and is therefore not affected by heliox.[100]

Whatever the technical difficulties, the benefits to patients who require heliox outweigh the problems. Use of heliox reduces PIP in volume ventilation and also helps reduce P_aCO_2. To safeguard against overinflation, $P_{plateau}$ must be limited (See the Clinical Scenario on heliox).[105]

 Clinical Scenario: Heliox

....

Case 1

A 14-year-old girl with asthma is admitted to the emergency department and given continuous nebulizer therapy with albuterol (40 mg/hr), intravenous corticosteroids, intravenous terbutaline, and an aminophylline infusion to therapeutic levels. The patient is intubated, sedated, paralyzed, and placed on mechanical ventilation. With the oxygen at 70%, the ABGs on appropriate ventilator settings are as follows: pH = 7.11, P_aCO_2 = 123 mm Hg, and P_aO_2 = 68 mm Hg. End-tidal CO_2 is above the upper limit of the scale (>99 mm Hg). Heliox is started with 60% helium and 40% oxygen (60 : 40 mixture). Within minutes the P_aCO_2 drops to 63 mm Hg, P_aO_2 rises slightly to 75 mm Hg, and pH returns to the normal range.[106]

....

Case 2

One day postoperatively, a 10-year-old boy is extubated and exhibits severe stridor and respiratory distress. A nebulizer treatment with racemic epinephrine fails to relieve the stridor. The child is started on dexamethasone (Decadron), but it typically takes approximately 4 hours or more for it to become effective. Rather than reintubate the child, heliox is started (80 : 20 mixture). The stridor is immediately relieved. Five hours later, the stridor resolves apparently because of the steroid administration, and heliox is discontinued.[106]

BOX 23-8 **Ventilator Function with Heliox for Specific Models**

CareFusion AVEA *(CareFusion, Viasys Corp, San Diego, Calif.):* No significant difference in tidal volume (V_T) delivery was detected with volume control, pressure control, or pressure support ventilation, with and without heliox ratios of 80:20 and 60:40. Accuracy of volume delivery was clinically acceptable. At 80:20 V_T delivered was within manufacturer specifications of $\pm(10\% + 0.2$ mL) of actual setting. V_T delivered and measured was reasonably accurate. In pressure control mode, positive end-expiratory pressure (PEEP) and peak inspiratory pressure (PIP) were within ±1 cm H_2O of actual. Accuracy of fractional inspired oxygen concentration (F_1O_2) readings was acceptable at less than 3% variability.[94-96]

Hamilton Veolar and Hamilton Galileo *(Hamilton Medical, Bonaduz, Switzerland):* $V_T$del was consistently higher than $V_T$set. The lower the F_1O_2 (the higher the helium), the more the $V_T$del exceeded the $V_T$set. $V_T$exh underestimated actual V_T.[94,97]

Hamilton G-5: With the Heliox option, the Hamilton G-5 delivers a specific set tidal volume and displays accurate volumes for inhaled and exhaled volume delivery. It can only be used with an 80:20 mixture of helium/oxygen.

Puritan Bennett 840 *(Covidien-Nellcor Puritan Bennett, Boulder, Colo.):* Will not cycle at all (i.e., heliox cannot be used with the 840). The ventilator recognizes a low-density gas when heliox is connected to the air connect and alerts the operator. This helps protect the patient from inappropriate gases being used, but also eliminates the possibility of using this ventilator for heliox therapy.[94,97,100]

Servo-i *(Maquet, Inc., Wayne, N.J.):* Cycled consistently with all heliox mixtures tested in volume control and pressure control ventilation. O_2 analyzer was within $\pm3\%$ and blender was within $\pm1\%$. Set V_T factor (0.95) was consistent for all heliox concentrations tested. $V_T$insp was within acceptable limits. The ventilator uses ultrasonic technology to measure expiratory gas flows. Exhaled V_T display was erratic at 80:20 and 70:30 (helium/oxygen) but consistent at 60:40 and 50:50. $V_T$exp read lower than actual delivered V_T. As the helium concentration decreased, the accuracy recovered.

Correction factors can be used to determine $V_T$del by using $V_T$set. For example, $V_T$del = $V_T$set multiplied by the factor (factor for 21%, 30%, 40%, and 50% O_2 is 0.95). Correction factors can only be used to determine $V_T$del by using $V_T$exh for high F_1O_2 values (40% and 50%). For example, $V_T$del = $V_T$exh × 1.37 (for 40% O_2). At high F_1O_2 values (low helium percentage), no correction factor is available. With high helium concentrations at a set V_T of 500 mL, the low $\dot{V}_E$ alarm was breeched and could not be disabled.[98-100]

Servo-i without Heliox option: Cycled consistently with all heliox mixtures tested in volume control and pressure control ventilation. O_2 analyzer was within $\pm3\%$ and blender was within

$\pm1\%$. Set V_T factor (0.95) was consistent for all heliox concentrations tested. $V_T$insp was within acceptable limits. The ventilator uses ultrasonic technology to measure expiratory gas flows. Exhaled V_T display was erratic at 80:20 and 70:30 (helium/oxygen), but consistent at 60:40 and 50:50. $V_T$exp read lower than actual delivered V_T. As the helium concentration decreased, the accuracy recovered.

Correction factors can be used to determine $V_T$del by using $V_T$set. For example, $V_T$del = $V_T$set multiplied by the factor (factor for 21%, 30%, 40%, and 50% O_2 is 0.95). Correction factors can only be used to determine $V_T$del by using $V_T$exh for high F_1O_2 values (40% and 50%). For example, $V_T$del = $V_T$exh × 1.37 (for 40% O_2). At high F_1O_2 values (low helium percentage), no correction factor is available. With high helium concentrations at a set V_T of 500 mL, the low alarm was breeched and could not be disabled.[98-100]

Servo-i with Heliox option: With the Heliox option, the Servo-i delivers a specific set tidal volume and displays accurate volumes for inhaled and exhaled volume delivery. It can only be used with an 80:20 mixture of helium/oxygen.[103-104]

Dräger Dura-2 *(Dräger Medical, Inc. Telford, Pa.):* $V_T$del was greater than $V_T$set. $V_T$exp read higher than actual delivery. A correction factor is available to determine actual volume delivery during VC-CMV with 70:30 (helium:oxygen) and varying oxygen settings (21%, 30%, 35%). At the heliox concentration with a set F_1O_2 of 0.21, for example, the correction factor is 1.38. Divide the desired V_T by 1.38 to get the V_T value to set. The flow sensor and the oxygen analyzer must be turned off. The expiratory flow monitoring malfunction alarm is activated if it is not turned off. (Autoflow was turned off in this study.)[102] In the Dura-2 the higher the helium delivered, the lower the actual delivered F_1O_2 compared with the F_1O_2 set.

Dräger E-4 *(Dräger Medical, Inc., Telford, Pa.):* $V_T$del was higher than $V_T$set, and this difference was linear; but with $V_T$set higher than 500 mL, the relation between set and delivered was nonlinear. This problem was alleviated by inactivating the leak compensation mechanism. The ventilator gives a high-priority inoperative alarm, which cannot be silenced, but it requires inactivation of the inspiratory flow monitor. The flow sensor must be removed to accomplish ventilation with heliox. $V_T$del was consistently higher than $V_T$set so that a correction factor could be calculated from $V_T$del average. In the Evita-4, the higher the helium delivered, the lower the delivered F_1O_2 compared with the F_1O_2 set.[94,97]

eVent Medical Inspiration Mechanical Ventilator *(eVent Medical, Inc., San Clemente, Calif.):* Cycled consistently in volume control and pressure control ventilation. O_2 analyzer within $\pm1\%$ and blender was within $\pm5\%$. Conversion factors are available.[101]

Technical Considerations in Heliox Delivery

In many cases the expiratory flow sensing devices must be disconnected or disabled when heliox is used during mechanical ventilation. A clinician must always be aware of how the ventilator will function with heliox before it is used for ventilating a patient.

Delivery of heliox with mechanical ventilation is achieved by connecting the compressed air inlet hose directly to a 50-psi, 80:20 heliox gas source. In preparation for using heliox with a ventilator, two cylinders are recommended, preferably yoked together so that

when one is empty the respiratory therapist can quickly switch to the second cylinder. Cylinder trolleys, appropriate heliox regulators, and wrenches should also be on hand.[87] Early version ICU ventilators consumed approximately 4 to 6 cylinders a day. Newer ICU ventilators, such as the Servo-i and the Hamilton G-5 conserve a greater amount of gas and may use only two to three cylinders a day.[103,104] The clinician must be sure that a sufficient number of cylinders are available (Key Point 23-11). The minimum concentration of heliox recommended for use is 80:20. As previously mentioned, never use a 100% helium cylinder connected to a ventilator because of the risk of asphyxia.

Key Point 23-11 It is absolutely essential that the label on the cylinder be checked for content accuracy. It must read that the cylinder contains medical-grade (U.S.P. [United States Pharmacopeia]) helium and oxygen. The color code for heliox cylinders is typically brown and green, but do not trust the color of the cylinder.

Any heated-wire flow measuring device is likely to alarm, so a ventilator that does not have heated-wire flow monitor should be used, or the monitoring device should be disconnected. For example, the Dräger Evita XL uses a heated-wire device for measuring exhaled V_T. Failure to disconnect this device will result in continuous alarm activation. The Evita XL also has leak compensation, which should be turned off for the same reason.

As with normal ventilation, the gas should be heated and humidified. A heated-wire circuit should be used with the humidification system because of the high thermal conductivity of helium. The circuit may need to be wrapped in a plastic sleeve to help retain heat and avoid activating the temperature alarms on the humidifier.

Other potential problems must be considered. For example, an oxygen analyzer must be used to determine actual oxygen delivery during mechanical ventilation with heliox, because the setting on the front panel may not be accurate. In some ventilators that have been studied for this function, the actual delivered F_IO_2 is approximately the same as the set F_IO_2 (e.g., Hamilton Galileo, and G-5, Servo-i). The F_IO_2 delivered may also vary from the set value as the helium concentration changes in some ventilators (e.g., Dräger E-4), resulting in activation of the ventilator's internal oxygen analyzer alarm. These can be disabled or disconnected. If they are, some other form of O_2 monitoring should be provided, such as an oxygen analyzer equipped with an alarm. Activation of the oxygen alarm is often what alerts the respiratory therapist to a technical problem.

Pressure during ventilation is not a problem because pressure is not density dependent. Thus pressure ventilation is easily accomplished. In pressure control ventilation with a variety of ventilators (see Box 23-8), $V_T$del is equal to V_T measured for a range of pressures and F_IO_2 values.[94]

Heliox has a high thermal conductivity, which can affect the accuracy of the hot wire sensor. With hot wire flow monitoring, the higher the helium percentage, the greater that the flow is overestimated. The Dräger E-4 uses hot wire flow measuring, but should be used with caution (see Box 23-8).

As another example of the effect of ventilator valve function on effective ventilation with heliox, the Hamilton Galileo and G-5 ventilators use a variable orifice pneumotach. The pneumotach is located at the ventilator's Y-connector and measures both inspiratory and expiratory flows. The variable orifice pneumotach relies on turbulent flow for accuracy. Because high concentrations of helium result in laminar flow, this phenomenon lowers the resistance through the device, and reduces the ΔP across the device, causing the variable orifice pneumotach to underestimate the true flow.[94]

Because the difference between $V_T$exp and $V_T$del (see Box 23-8) is usually linear and is a function of F_IO_2, correction factors can be used to determine actual $V_T$del.[94] In some of the ventilators studied (Evita 2, Evita 4), the lower the F_IO_2 (the higher the helium percentage), the larger the discrepancy between the reported $V_T$exp on the ventilator and the actual $V_T$del. With other ventilators this relation is nonlinear and the displayed $V_T$exp is much higher than the actual $V_T$del. At these high helium concentrations, a correction factor is not available.

Only ventilators that can provide safe breath delivery should be used for heliox therapy in ventilated patients. The practitioner must keep in mind that changes can be made to ventilator function at any time by the manufacturer. These changes may affect ventilator performance differently during heliox delivery.

Heliox and NIV

Noninvasive positive pressure ventilation (NIV) with heliox has been used with both critical care and portable ventilators.[94] When heliox is used with some portable ventilators, ventilators titrated with heliox may exhibit erratic triggering and cycling, although this finding may not be clinically significant. Concentrations up to 60% helium can be delivered. Gas consumption may be high. For example, a cylinder with 4500 L of heliox being used at a flow of 18 L/min will last approximately 4 hours. With continuous therapy, this would result in the use of six cylinders in 24 hours resulting in a cost of about $500 per day.[86] This cost may be offset by a reduction in ventilator days, days in the intensive care unit, and overall hospital costs.

Despite the fact that the benefit is modest, NIV with heliox has been reported to be beneficial for patients with COPD.[107,108] Furthermore, although the benefit of heliox is seen more often in acute upper and central airway obstruction, such as in acute asthma, the ability of heliox to alleviate air trapping and unload the muscles is believed to benefit patients with COPD. This may in turn significantly reduce the length of hospital stay for this patient group. However, combining heliox and NIV is technically challenging. Importantly, the use of NIV for the treatment of acute asthma has not been well documented.[109]

Safe use of heliox during management of patients with airflow obstruction is possible if the physical properties (low density, high thermal conductivity) are kept in mind. These factors will influence work of breathing, aerosol delivery, and mechanical ventilator function. F_IO_2 and V_T delivery may be altered during heliox delivery with a mechanical ventilator. This is particularly true when hot wire technology is part of the ventilator's gas delivery or monitoring system. In most ventilators, the set V_T and delivered V_T parallel each other, and a correction factor can be used to determine the desired V_T setting. Exhaled V_T displayed may be higher or lower than the $V_T$del depending on the type of ventilator. Practitioners should study the ventilators they plan to use for heliox therapy and carefully determine equipment and cylinder requirements before using this therapy with a patient.

Monitoring the Electrical Activity of the Diaphragm and Neurally Adjusted Ventilatory Assist

For decades clinicians have used electrocardiograms to monitor the electrical activity of the heart. In fact all patients in an intensive care unit have ECG monitors with alarms in place to alert personnel of dangerous cardiac events. In contrast, clinicians have only recently gained the ability to monitor a patient's neural respiratory drive at the bedside.

A new method has been introduced to clinically monitor neural control of respiration through measurements of **electrical activity of the diaphragm (Edi)**. The principle governing this new technique is that depolarization of the diaphragm depends upon the transmission of a neural signal from the brainstem to the diaphragm. Edi measurements can therefore be used to evaluate a patient's neural control of spontaneous breathing.

REVIEW OF NEURAL CONTROL OF VENTILATION

The respiratory controller governs a person's drive to breathe. Afferent information from the peripheral and central chemoreceptors, along with neural stretch receptors and volume receptors, and information from the prefrontal cortex of the brain, are integrated and processed by the respiratory center located within the brainstem. The resulting efferent neural signal is propagated through the phrenic nerve to the diaphragm. The diaphragm then depolarizes and contracts. The greater the intensity of the neural stimulation and the greater the number of nerve fibers involved, the stronger the electrical activity measured on the muscle. In healthy individuals, the greater the neural stimulation to the diaphragm, the greater the muscle's electrical activity, the greater the diaphragm's contractile strength. This is not necessarily true in a patient with pulmonary hyperinflation, where the Edi may increase, but the strength of contraction does not increase proportionately.[110]

Previously, the only way to assess diaphragmatic activity in the clinical setting was to use an esophageal balloon to measure esophageal pressure (see Chapter 10). Although measurement of esophageal pressure (P_{es}) can provide measurements of thoracic pressure changes associated with diaphragmatic movement, its use is not without problems. For example, the accuracy of thoracic pressure measurements can be adversely affected by inappropriate positioning of the catheter balloon within the thorax, inaccurate volume filling of the catheter balloon, and patient positioning.[111,112] Consequently, a complete in vivo assessment of diaphragm function in human subjects has remained unavailable.

Without the ability to monitor the diaphragm function, it is not possible to fully address a number of the problems associated with ventilated patients. For example, does the patient demonstrate any diaphragmatic activity, or is the patient too heavily sedated or overventilated to breathe spontaneously? Is the diaphragm activated in synchrony with the triggering and cycling of the ventilator, or is patient-ventilator asynchrony present? It is believed that having the ability to monitor a patient's diaphragmatic activity at the bedside could provide clinicians with valuable information about the patient's central drive to breathe.

DIAPHRAGM ELECTRICAL ACTIVITY MONITORING

History of Diaphragm Electrical Activity Monitoring

During the past 50 years, groundbreaking research has resulted in the introduction of a technique that allowed scientists to study the function of the diaphragmatic muscle in man by means of electromyography.[110] Early laboratory studies in the 1960s showed a correlation between the activity of the phrenic nerve and the electrical activity of the diaphragm.[113] While these researchers paved the way,

| TABLE 23-2 | Edi Catheter Specifications |

EDI CATHETER GUIDE FOR SELECTING CORRECT CATHETER BASED ON PATIENT SIZE					
Patient height (cm)	<55	<55	45-85	76-160	>140
Patient weight (kg)	0.5-1.5	1.0-2.0	NA	NA	NA
French/cm	6/49	6/50	8/100	12/125	16/125 8/125

NA, Not applicable.

it would take several more decades of clinical investigation before the ability to monitor the diaphragm's electrical activity in the clinical setting was possible.[114,115]

The Edi Catheter: Its Characteristics and Placement

In 1998, Sinderby and Beck developed a catheter (Edi catheter) that allows measurements and monitoring of the diaphragm's electrical activity in the clinical setting. The catheter is basically a nasogastric tube with miniaturized electrodes near the distal tip* (See Fig. 23-14).

The Edi catheter is inserted into the esophagus through the oral route. The electrodes are positioned within the esophagus at a level that is adjacent to the diaphragm (crucial muscle of the diaphragm). This allows the electrodes to detect an Edi (or EAdi) signal. (NOTE: The distal tip itself resides in the stomach. As such, the catheter can be also be used for feeding the patient or administering medications, just as a regular nasogastric [NG] or orogastric [OG] tube.)

The Edi catheter is made of medical grade polyurethane. A barium strip is embedded along the length of the catheter for radiographic identification, although a chest radiograph is not essential for placement accuracy.[116] The Edi catheter contains a total of 10 stainless steel bipolar electrodes. The spacing between electrodes varies based on the size and length of the catheter.

A variety of catheter sizes are available for different patient sizes (premature infant to adult sizes) (see Table 23-2). The Edi catheter is inserted in a manner similar to any NG or OG tube. Once placed the catheter can be connected to the ventilator with a cable. As Fig. 23-14 illustrates, the cable connects the Edi catheter electrodes to a module located in a side slot of the Servo-i ventilator.

There are several procedures that can be used to establish that the catheter is properly positioned within the esophagus and stomach. First, the centimeter marking at the nose or mouth will coincide with a manufacturer recommended calculation used to determine the appropriate depth of insertion of the catheter. Second, the clinician can listen over the epigastric area with a stethoscope, while injecting air though the catheter feeding port. Hearing gas movement helps confirm the location of the catheter tip in the stomach. Third, there is a catheter positioning screen on

*The Edi catheter and the ability to measure the Edi is exclusively available through the Servo-i ventilator; Maquet, Inc, Wayne, N.J. Maquet uses the abbreviation Edi, rather than EAdi, which is the abbreviation that appears in the medical literature.

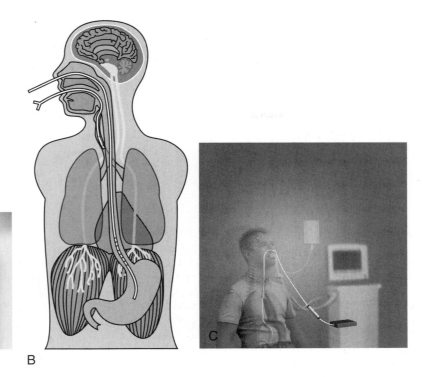

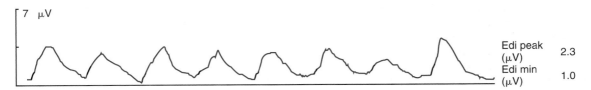

Fig. 23-14 A, Example of an Edi catheter. **B,** The catheter in the esophagus and stomach. Notice the electrodes span a certain distance so that some electrodes are located above the diaphragm and others below the diaphragm. **C,** The electrical connector from the catheter attaches to a cable connecting the catheter to the ventilator *(image on bottom).* (**A** and **C,** Courtesy Maquet, Inc, Wayne, N.J. **B,** Courtesy Dr. C Sinderby, St-Michael's Hospital, Toronto, Canada.)

7 μV

Edi peak (μV)   2.3
Edi min (μV)   1.0

Fig. 23-15 An Edi waveform. Note the Edi peak (2.3 μV) and Edi min (1.0 μV) displayed at the lower right corner of the screen. (See text for additional information.)

the ventilator that helps to establish the exact location of the electrodes within the esophagus and stomach. Fourth, the clinician can confirm the correct catheter position by performing an expiratory pause (end-expiratory occlusion) maneuver. When the patient attempts to inhale against the closed system during the pause, the Edi signal is positive (increases), while the airway pressure waveform decreases. (Additional information on these waveforms will be presented later in this section.) Fifth, a CO_2 detector can be used at the proximal end of the catheter to monitor the presence of CO_2. The presence of elevated levels of CO_2 would suggest that the catheter is in the trachea and not the stomach. Finally, a chest radiograph can be performed if hospital policy required it. Once the catheter is in place, the Edi waveform is displayed (Fig. 23-15).

The Edi waveform is basically sinusoidal in appearance. A digital display of the maximum Edi measured (Edi peak), and minimum Edi (Edi min) is provided on the right side of the screen. The values are reported in microvolts (μV).

The resting Edi peak for a healthy individual ranges from a few μV to about 10 μV. An Edi min is typically close to zero (0) μV. These values vary depending on the individual. The Edi μV

measurements are very small values when compared to the heart's electrical activity, which has an electrical amplitude 10 to 100 times that of the diaphragm.[110] The Edi will increase in normal individuals, for example, when the diaphragm is required to work harder, which occurs when an individual exercises.[117] Individuals with chronic respiratory insufficiency, such as COPD, commonly have an Edi signal 5 to 7 times stronger than a normal individual.[118-119]

Occasionally a catheter will be placed in the correct position, but there is no measurable Edi waveform or signal. An Edi signal may not be detectable on a mechanically ventilated patient for a number of reasons. For example, there may be no central respiratory drive because of sedation, hyperventilation, or brain injury. An absent Edi may also have an anatomical reason, such as a diaphragm hernia, or a severed phrenic nerve (e.g. postthoracic surgery). Even a conduction failure can result in an absent Edi, when the impulse is not conducted from the phrenic nerve to the diaphragm as a result of use of a paralytic agent, or a disease is present which blocks electrical impulse conduction.[120] Interestingly, Bordessoule and colleagues have proposed that the Edi catheter can be used to evaluate recovery from paralysis.[121]

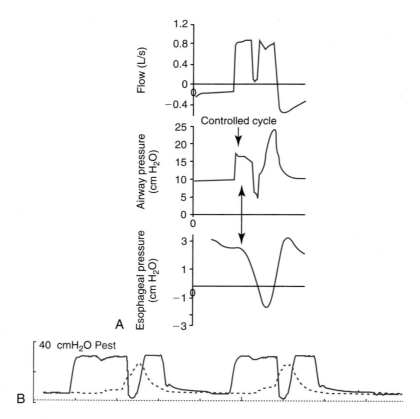

Fig. 23-16 A, The flow, pressure, and esophageal pressure curves of a patient on mechanical ventilation showing a double trigger, two consecutive breath cycles separated by a short expiratory time. Note the patient's effort indicated by the decrease in the esophageal pressure. The patient effort occurs after a mandatory breath has started and continues past the end of this breath. The pressure and flow curves decrease in apparent response to a patient effort. This seems to result in a second mandatory breath. **B,** The pressure–time curve shows double-triggered breath *(solid line)*. The Edi waveform *(dashed line demonstrates what the patient actually wants.)* The patient's neural effort starts much later than the mandatory breath provided by the ventilator. The ventilator's mandatory breath seems to end. There's a short expiratory time indicated by the pressure–time curve, but the patient's diaphragm has only begun to taper off. The ventilator has a delayed respond to the patient's effort and attempts to give another breath, while the patient is trying to exhale. (See text for additional information.) (**A,** Redrawn from Thille AW, Brochard L: Double triggering during assisted mechanical ventilation: is it a controlled, auto-triggered or patient-triggered cycle? Intensive Care Med 33:744-745, 2007. **B,** Redrawn from screen capture provided by Daniel D. Rowley, RRT-NPS, RPFT, FAARC, Pulmonary Diagnostic & Respiratory Therapy Services, University of Virginia Health System; Charlottesville, Va.)

It should be apparent from this discussion that the ability to monitor the Edi can be a valuable tool to assess ventilatory function in critical ill patients. As you will see in the following section, Edi can also be used to detect the presence of patient-ventilator asynchrony.

Detecting Patient-Ventilator Asynchrony Using the Edi Catheter

As discussed in Chapter 18, patient-ventilator asynchrony is a common problem among patients receiving mechanical ventilation. It has been estimated that 25% of mechanically ventilated patients exhibit asynchrony, which can increase the length of time that a patient requires ventilatory support.[121-124]

Patient-ventilator asynchrony can lead to a number of complications. When a patient "fights" the ventilator this can potentially result in damage to the diaphragm (ventilator-induced diaphragm dysfunction [VIDD]). This loss of diaphragmatic force-generating capacity is specifically related to the use of mechanical ventilation.[125] It is a common practice among many clinicians in the ICU to sedate the patient when asynchrony is present. However,

sedation can significantly reduce a patient's spontaneous breathing efforts, and therefore diaphragm activity. Lack of use of the diaphragm during mechanical ventilation can lead to severe diaphragm atrophy, which can occur in as short a time as 18 to 69 hours.[125,126]

Another example of asynchrony is referred to as double triggering. The etiology of double triggering was unknown, and many practitioners thought the ventilator was unable to provide the flow demand required by the patient during a breath. By using two techniques to evaluate diaphragm activity during double triggering, it is possible to determine what the patient needs versus what the ventilator is delivering (Fig. 23-16, *A* and *B*).[127,128]

The phenomenon of double trigger can occur regardless of the type of ventilator being used.[127,128] By looking at Fig. 23-16 and using either an esophageal balloon or the Edi catheter to monitor diaphragm activity, it becomes apparent that the patient is making an inspiratory effort while a mandatory breath delivery is already in progress. The ventilator is simply not coordinated with the activity of the patient's diaphragm and respiratory center. (As mentioned earlier, a common practice in these situations is to use sedation as

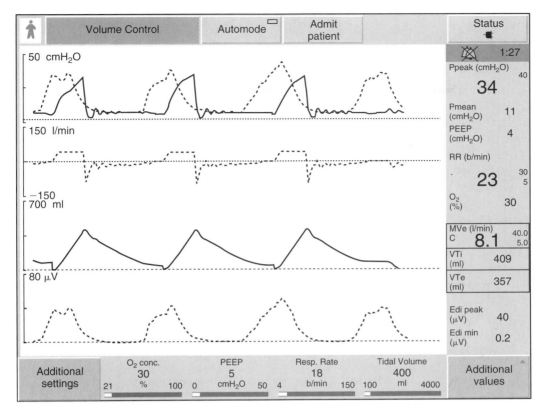

Fig. 23-17 Main screen on the Servo-i ventilator showing VC-CMV *(called "volume control")* waveforms. The top curve is the pressure–time curve *(solid line)* graph along with the Edi waveform. Note this shadow or ghost Edi waveform is identical in shape to the Edi–time waveform *(dashed line)* at the bottom of the screen. The second waveform is flow–time, the third volume–time, and the fourth the Edi waveform. Notice the lack of synchrony between what the patient wants *(Edi signal)* and what the ventilator delivers as shown in the pressure–time curve. (See text for additional information.) (Screen capture provided by Daniel D. Rowley, RRT-NPS, RPFT, FAARC, University of Virginia Health System; Charlottesville, Va.)

a means of stopping the patient from "fighting" the ventilator. However, sedation can prolong mechanical ventilation with the potential for many of its associated complications.)[129]

Using the Edi Waveform to Interpret Ventilator Synchrony

It is now possible to monitor ventilator graphics and measurements of Edi activity at the same time. This can help the clinician determine how well the set mode and parameters are in sync with the patient's drive to breathe. Figure 23-17 shows an example of the Edi compared to the pressure–time graphic during VC-CMV. The figure illustrates another example of patient-ventilator asynchrony. Notice that the ventilator breath delivery is not in synchrony with the Edi waveform. The ventilator is completely out of synchrony with the patient both in terms of when the breath starts (trigger) and when it ends (cycle).

Figure 23-18 shows an example of a patient receiving pressure support/CPAP mode on the Servo-i, which is purely a patient-triggered mode. Notice how low the Edi Peak is in this figure. One can see that the patient is triggering the breath by observing the pressure, flow, and volume curves. Remember that with PSV, all breaths are patient triggered. However, there is no Edi waveform because the diaphragm is not depolarizing and contracting. How is this possible? There are two possible explanations. First, the patient may be using accessory muscles to trigger the ventilator. A physical assessment of the patient would determine if this is true. Second,

the ventilator could be autotriggering, which the therapist could also evaluate. In this case, the patient was actually using accessory muscles to breathe, as noted by his physical examination.

Notice the ventilator settings in the example shown in Fig. 23-18 as follows: PS above PEEP is 11 cm H_2O, PEEP is 5 cm H_2O, and the F_IO_2 is set at 28%. The patient's respiratory rate is about 24 breaths/min and V_T is about 300 mL. It would appear that this patient is ready to have the level of support reduced as he is progressing toward weaning. However, when a spontaneous breathing trial was attempted, the patient failed. Under normal circumstances we might not know why he failed. However, having the Edi signal information, it is possible to determine that the diaphragm is not active. It may be necessary, in this case, to further reduce the support level in order to stimulate the patient to use his diaphragm so he can be successfully weaned.

Other types of asynchrony that may be evaluated include wasted efforts, where the patient wants to take a breath but does not receive one from the ventilator, mismatching of the neural rate with the ventilator delivery rate, and fixed levels of ventilator assist, such as a set pressure in PSV, where the level of assist does not correspond to the variable drive of the patient.

NEURALLY ADJUSTED VENTILATORY ASSIST

At this point, it would be reasonable to pose the question if you have the ability to monitor the Edi, why not use that signal to

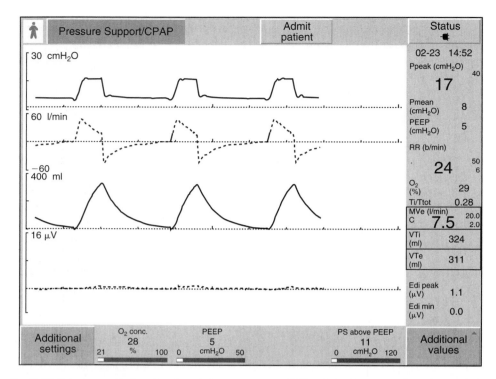

Fig. 23-18 Main screen on the Servo-i ventilator during pressure support/CPAP mode showing pressure, flow, volume, and Edi waveforms, from top to bottom. Note the Edi value is nearly zero. (See text for additional information.) (Screen capture provided by Daniel D. Rowley, RRT-NPS, RPFT, FAARC, University of Virginia Health System; Charlottesville, Va.)

control the mechanical ventilator? The high incidence of patient-ventilator asynchrony described earlier suggests that current ventilator modes and controls do not always provide the best outcomes for our patients. We currently depend on the ventilator to pneumatically measure a patient effort, using flow or pressure signals, to trigger a breath. The patient must rely on the operator's judgment to set an appropriate tidal volume, pressure, flow, and T_I.

The motivation for the development of NAVA was to allow the spontaneously breathing patient to have greater control of his or her tidal volume, T_I, and flow. In 2007 Maquet, Inc (Wayne, N.J.) received approval from the U.S. Food and Drug Administration (FDA) to include NAVA as a mode of ventilation on the Servo-i ventilator. NAVA uses the Edi, a reflection of the neural respiratory output to the diaphragm, to control triggering, breath delivery, and cycling of the ventilator.[110] A comparable mode that is available on the Puritan Bennett 840 is proportional assist ventilation (PAV), which was described in Chapter 6. Both NAVA and PAV provide breath delivery in proportion to the patient's demand.[130] The primary difference is that NAVA uses an electrical signal, the Edi, whereas PAV uses a pneumatic signal to deliver the next breath.

While the Edi catheter can be used in most ventilated patients to facilitate monitoring of the diaphragm, the NAVA mode is specifically for use in patients who are capable of spontaneous breathing, that is, patients who have an Edi signal.[110] Patients who demonstrate the following conditions would be excluded from the use of the NAVA mode:

- heavily sedated and/or paralyzed
- damaged brain center
- absence of phrenic nerve activity
- diseases that prohibit neuromuscular transmission, or
- presence of apnea (Note: some premature infants may experience periods of apnea, but because NAVA has a backup mode,

this does not necessarily exclude them from using this technique.)

Using NAVA Ventilation

The following section describes how the NAVA mode can be set up by the operator. Once the patient has an Edi catheter in place, as described earlier, it is connected to the ventilator by means of a cable that leads to a module in the side of the ventilator (Fig. 23-14). The operator then selects the NAVA mode for ventilating the patient. Triggering of a breath occurs when a 0.5-μV deflection occurs in the Edi waveform below the Edi min of the previous breath. It has been shown that complete trigger synchrony is achieved with NAVA, when compared to other modes.[131]

Delivery of pressure during inspiration is based on the strength of the Edi signal and the level of NAVA support ("NAVA level") set by the operator. The NAVA level determines the amount of pressure delivered by the ventilator in proportion to the Edi. The easiest way to think about it is that the pressure delivery is similar to pressure support. The higher the numerical value of the NAVA level (0 to 15 cm H_2O/μV), the greater the support provided by the ventilator. The pressure varies constantly during breath delivery as the Edi varies (i.e., it varies in proportion to changes in the Edi and the neural demand for a breath).[132,133] An estimated peak pressure that will be delivered during the breath is based on the following equation[134]:

$$NAVA\ P_{peak} = NAVA\ level \times (Edi\ peak - Edi\ min) + PEEP$$

For example, if the NAVA level is set at 1 cm H_2O/μV, the Edi peak is 10 μV, the Edi min is 0 μV, and the PEEP is 5 cm H_2O, then the estimated P_{peak} delivered for this particular NAVA supported breath will be equal to 1 cm H_2O/μV × (10 μV − 0 μV) + 5 cm H_2O = 15 cm H_2O. Because the Edi varies throughout inspiration, the

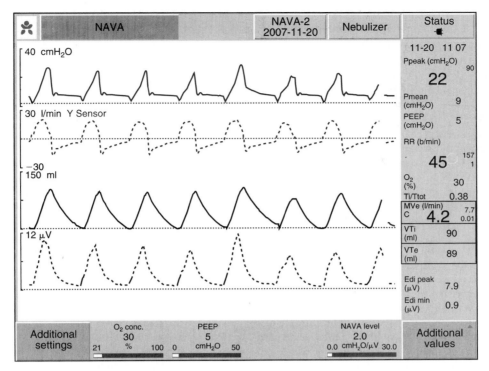

Fig. 23-19 The main screen on the Servo-i ventilator during NAVA ventilation of an infant. The waveforms, from top to bottom, are pressure, flow, volume, and time. Notice how the breath delivery is in complete synchrony with the patient's Edi signal *(drive to breathe)*. Also note that pressure, flow, and volume delivery vary breath-to-breath, a phenomenon that occurs during natural breathing. NAVA level is set at 2 cm $H_2O/\mu V$. NAVA $P_{peak\ est}$ = NAVA level × (Edi peak − Edi min) + PEEP; NAVA $P_{peak\ est}$ = 2 cm $H_2O/\mu V$ × (7.9 μV − 0.9 μV) + 5 cm H_2O; NAVA $P_{peak\ est}$ = approximately 19 cm H_2O. Displayed P_{peak} is 22 cm H_2O. This slightly higher P_{peak} represents the previous breath. (Screen capture provided by Daniel D. Rowley, RRT-NPS, RPFT, FAARC, University of Virginia Health System; Charlottesville, Va.)

amount of pressure delivered will also vary throughout inspiration. The Edi signal is measured 60 times per second so ventilator response is very rapid (Fig. 23-19).

The ventilator provides a "NAVA Preview" tool that allows the operator to estimate an appropriate NAVA level based on the patient's current mode of ventilation. For example, if the patient has acceptable blood gas results on a specific mode such as VC-CMV, the "NAVA Preview" helps the operator set a NAVA level that will be comparable to the current pressure and volume deliveries.

What if the NAVA level was accidently set at 10 cm $H_2O/\mu V$? What would be the estimated P_{peak}? Using the same values from the previous example, the Edi peak is 10 μV and the Edi min is 0 μV and the PEEP is 5 cm H_2O, the estimated P_{peak} delivered for this particular NAVA supported breath would theoretically be equal to 10 cm $H_2O/\mu V$ × (10 μV − 0 μV) + 5 cm H_2O = 105 cm H_2O! However, what happens in a case to avoid this high pressure is first the ventilator cycles and starts filling the lungs. As the lungs fill with air the stretch receptors in the lungs send signals by way of the vagus nerve to the respiratory centers of the brain. The more the receptors are stretched, the more the nerve is stimulated and the extent of the breath is inhibited (Hering-Breuer Reflex).[135] The brain then sends a signal to stop neural transmission through the phrenic nerve to the diaphragm resulting in the cessation of diaphragmatic activity. The respiratory system is therefore self-protective and the patient would not receive 105 cm H_2O. The process is extremely rapid. Additionally, there is the usual protection from the set peak pressure limit. But the pressure delivery

stops long before the upper pressure limit would be reached. It is important to note that this protective response is only for patients with intact vagal reflexes and respiratory centers. Some patients may not have an intact vagal response. For example, postlung transplant patients do not have an intact vagal reflex from the lungs. Also, in some patients that require a high CO_2 stimulation to breathe, or where the respiratory center has been impaired (injury or medications), these protective reflexes may be overridden. (In these instances, the Edi catheter may still be of benefit in monitoring the neural activity.)

Inspiration during a NAVA breath ends or cycles when the Edi decreases to 70% of the Edi peak. This represents a time when the Edi is in the process of decreasing to the Edi min (baseline), and the patient's effort is ending.

Alarms and Safety Features in NAVA

When a patient is being ventilated in the NAVA mode, there are a variety of safety features available. The clinician can set two different backup modes. The first backup mode is pressure support. In the event that the Edi signal is lost, for example if the catheter is pulled out or moved within the esophagus, or if the Edi signal and the pneumatic signal are not in sync, the ventilator will automatically switch to pressure support. An audible alarm and message will notify the operator if this is an asynchrony issue or loss of the Edi signal.

If the patient becomes apneic for some reason, for example if a large amount of sedation is administered, the backup apnea mode is pressure control. The operator can set the pressure control level above PEEP, the rate and the inspiratory time for backup pressure control mode.

The typical ventilator alarms previously discussed in Chapter 7 are also available during NAVA ventilation (i.e., upper pressure limit, high and low PEEP, high and low minute volume, high and low rate alarm, and high and low oxygen percentage).

Results of Initiating NAVA Ventilation

Several studies have reviewed changes that occur in ventilator parameters after a patient is switched to NAVA. One of this author's personal observations is that patients tend to relax and appear more comfortable after they are switched to NAVA.

When the ventilator is switching from a traditional mode of ventilation to NAVA, the mean ventilating pressures decrease, tidal volume tends to decrease and stabilizes at about 4 to 6 mL/kg IBW, and the respiratory rate tends to increase. The minute ventilation appears to remain fairly constant, unless the patient was previously hyper- or hypoventilated.[136] Once NAVA is initiated, blood gases appear to return to the patient's normal levels.[137] Oxygenation and compliance may also improve.[136,138] With NAVA the patient establishes his or her own transpulmonary pressures, volume, and respiratory rate.[110] In addition, NAVA allows a patient's respiratory center to maintain the biologically variable rhythm generation, compared to other modes such as pressure support, where the amount of support remains constant based on what the operator has selected for the patient.[139] NAVA is not affected by leaks, and in fact, is now available as noninvasive NAVA (Servo-i version 5.0 and 5.0 options).

The operator can adjust the NAVA level of support based on patient assessment. In general, if the NAVA level is increased, the support from the ventilator increases, and the Edi signal tends to decrease. This is only true if the patient does not want the assist. The patient may accept the higher pressure and keep Edi the same. Conversely, as the NAVA level is decreased, the Edi will generally increase, but again this can vary among patients.[140] These findings, of course, will vary depending on the patient's pathology. Remember it is the patient's respiratory center that is controlling ventilation during NAVA.

Weaning from NAVA

Clinicians should approach weaning from NAVA as with any mode of ventilation. The first step is to perform a weaning assessment of the patient to determine if he or she is ready to be weaned (See Chapter 20). If the criteria for weaning have been met, the level of support should then be progressively reduced. Weaning protocols in some institutions may call for a spontaneous breathing trial where all support is withdrawn. In this case the NAVA level can be set at zero and PEEP set at zero. The Edi waveform provides an excellent opportunity to evaluate the patient's response to withdrawal of support, and helps determine if the patient is ready for weaning and extubation.

The Edi catheter can remain in place following extubation by placing the ventilator in the standby mode. This allows the clinician to continue monitoring the Edi during the postextubation period. For example, the clinician can use the Edi to monitor the patient's response to the use of CPAP or a high-flow nasal cannula following extubation.[141]

Evaluating NAVA

NAVA has been shown to be a safe mode of ventilation, even in premature infants.[142] However, some clinicians argue that NAVA, unlike other modes of ventilation, requires the invasive placement of an NG tube. This is true and should be taken into account.[143] Part of the decision to use this mode should of course be based on whether or not use of an NG or OG tube is contraindicated for a patient. For example, an NG or OG tube might be contraindicated in a patient with head or facial injury. On the other hand, if the patient is likely to need an NG or OG tube, then use of the Edi catheter may be appropriate. It is also worth mentioning that the Edi catheter is more expensive than a traditional NG tube. It has been suggested, however, that the initial cost associated with purchasing these catheters may be offset by the benefits of greater patient comfort and reduced length of ventilatory support.

The use of NAVA and the Edi catheter provides a novel approach to mechanical ventilation. The idea that the operator relinquishes control of volume, pressure, flow, and rate delivery to the patient is indeed a new concept. It may be difficult for some clinicians to embrace because it is "out of the box" thinking compared to traditional ventilatory support techniques.

Early studies suggest that NAVA and the Edi catheter offer a promising alternative for the management of critically ill patients receiving mechanical ventilation.[144,145] The Edi waveform provides valuable information about a patient's respiratory center function, which in turn could ultimately improve patient-ventilator synchrony. It should be stated, however, that evidence-based practice dictates that additional studies will be required to better define the application and importance of NAVA in clinical practice.

 SUMMARY

- Airway pressure release ventilation (APRV) is a mode of ventilatory support designed to provide two levels of continuous positive airway pressure (CPAP) and allow spontaneous breathing at both levels when spontaneous effort is present.
- APRV is referred to as bilevel airway pressure, variable positive airway pressure, intermittent CPAP, CPAP with release, pressure-controlled inverse ratio ventilation with spontaneous ventilation, upside-down intermittent mandatory ventilation, and biphasic CPAP.
- APRV provides lower peak pressures, better oxygenation, less circulatory interference, and better gas exchange without compromising the patient's hemodynamic status when compared with conventional ventilation in ARDS.
- Because APRV is a pressure-targeted mode of ventilation, the patient's minute ventilation and gas exchange should be closely monitored. This is the result of the fact that volume delivery depends on lung compliance (C_L), airway resistance (R_{aw}), and the patient's spontaneous effort.
- When initiating APRV, the practitioner sets two pressure levels and two time levels. The upper level of CPAP is set with the P_{high} control and the lower CPAP level, or release pressure, is set with a P_{low} control. The duration of P_{high} is set with the T_{high} control, and the release time period is set with the T_{low} control.
- When changing from a conventional mode to APRV, the settings used with the conventional ventilator can serve as a guide to the APRV settings.
- Ventilation and P_aCO_2 are determined by the release time and V_T exchange during T_{low}, and by the patient's spontaneous ventilation. Oxygenation can generally be improved by increasing T_{high}, P_{high}, or F_IO_2.

- HFOV has been proposed as an alternative to conventional ventilation in patients with ARDS because it is believed that it offers an alternative method of improving oxygenation in adult patients, while simultaneously reducing the risks of ventilator-induced lung injury (VILI).
- With HFOV, pressure is positive in the airway during the inspiratory phase (forward stroke), and negative during the expiratory phase (return stroke). Thus both inspiration and expiration are active, resulting in bulk flow rather than jet pulsations.
- Oxygenation during HFOV is primarily achieved by maintaining the mP_{aw} at a level sufficient to obtain optimal lung inflation. $\dot{V}_E$ and V_T delivery are affected by several factors, including the pressure amplitude of oscillation, frequency, ET size, amount of ET cuff leak, and lung characteristics.
- Heliox therapy has been used in the treatment of disorders that cause airway obstruction, such as asthma and tracheobronchitis. It does not cure the cause of airway obstruction, but reduces the patient's work of breathing until the obstruction can be alleviated.
- Heliox therapy does **not** replace aggressive bronchodilator and corticosteroid therapy in the treatment of asthma.
- Heliox can be delivered using a mask system, in conjunction with aerosolized bronchodilators, and with both invasive and noninvasive mechanical ventilation. Heliox should not be delivered by nasal cannula alone. The flow through the nasal cannula is high and can be irritating, cold, and drying, and can lead to undetected, inadvertent PEEP.
- When delivering heliox through a ventilator, volume and flow delivery measurements will not be accurate with most ventilators. Heliox can also interfere with gas-mixing devices, inspiratory and expiratory valve function, triggering and cycling mechanisms, automatic leak compensation, monitors, and minute volume alarms.
- The Edi catheter allows measurement and monitoring of the diaphragm's electrical activity in the clinical setting.
- An Edi may not be detected if the patient is overly sedated, hyperventilating, or receiving neuromuscular blocking agents. The impulse may also not be detected in patients with diaphragmatic hernia, a severed phrenic nerve (e.g. postthoracic surgery), and following brain injury.
- NAVA uses the Edi measurement to control triggering, breath delivery, and cycling of the ventilator in spontaneously breathing patients. The operator can adjust the NAVA level of support based on patient assessment.
- Delivery of pressure during inspiration is based on the strength of the Edi signal and the level of NAVA support set by the operator.
- NAVA is not indicated for patients who are heavily sedated, demonstrate brainstem damage, have an absence of phrenic nerve activity, or a condition that prohibits neuromuscular transmission.
- In the event that the Edi signal is lost, or the patient becomes apneic during NAVA, the ventilator will automatically switch to pressure support, which the operator can set as the backup mode.
- Early studies suggest that NAVA may provide an effective and novel approach to mechanical ventilation of critically ill patients.

REVIEW QUESTIONS (See Appendix A for answers.)

1. Which of the following are considered a benefit of APRV compared with conventional mechanical ventilation in patients with ARDS?
   1. Less circulatory interference
   2. Better gas exchange
   3. Higher PIP
   4. Improved oxygenation
      A. 1 only
      B. 1 and 3 only
      C. 2 and 4 only
      D. 1, 2, and 4

2. The benefits of APRV compared with conventional ventilation have been primarily associated with which of the following?
   A. Preservation of spontaneous breathing
   B. Reduction in shunt fraction
   C. Less use of sedatives and analgesics
   D. Augmentation of venous return

3. Disadvantages of APRV compared with conventional ventilation include
   1. Unfamiliarity of staff with the technique
   2. Potential for patient-ventilator asynchrony if patient efforts are not matched with the ventilator
   3. Difficulty with CO_2 elimination in patients with increased R_{aw}
   4. Augmented renal perfusion when spontaneous breathing is maintained

   A. 1 only
   B. 2 only
   C. 3 and 4
   D. 1, 2, and 3

4. Which of the following represent appropriate initial settings when using APRV in patients with ARDS?
   1. P_{high} of 15 to 25 cm H_2O
   2. P_{low} of 10 to 15 cm H_2O
   3. T_{high} of 4 seconds or more
   4. T_{low} of 0.5 to 1.0 seconds
      A. 2 only
      B. 1 and 2
      C. 2 and 3
      D. 1, 3, and 4

5. The initial mP_{aw} set for HFOV in the adult is generally:
   A. 3 to 5 cm H_2O above the $\bar{P}_{aw}$ used with the conventional ventilator
   B. 10 cm H_2O above PEEP used with the conventional ventilator
   C. 15 to 25 cm H_2O
   D. 30 cm H_2O

6. Which of the following controls govern the amount of displacement of the oscillating piston during HFOV?
   1. Amplitude (power)
   2. T$_i$%
   3. Frequency
   4. mP$_{aw}$
      A. 1 only
      B. 3 only
      C. 1, 2, and 3
      D. 1, 2, and 4

7. During the transition from conventional ventilation to HFOV, the patient is often
   A. Asked to remain still
   B. Provided heavy sedation
   C. Extubated and fitted with a face mask
   D. Moved to a different unit of the hospital

8. Which of the following statements are true regarding CWF seen during HFOV?
   1. CWF should be present from the clavicles to the mid-thigh.
   2. When CWF is seen, the patient is given a paralyzing agent.
   3. Auscultation of heart sounds and breath sounds is difficult when CWF is present.
   4. When CWF is present, the patient must be disconnected from HFOV for breath sounds to be evaluated.
      A. 2 only
      B. 4 only
      C. 1 and 3
      D. 1, 2, and 4

9. Heliox therapy is most often used in which of the following pulmonary pathologies?
   A. ARDS
   B. Asthma
   C. Pulmonary embolism
   D. Pneumonia

10. Because of its density characteristics, heliox administered through a ventilator will affect which of the following?
    A. Pressure monitoring
    B. Inspiratory time
    C. Volume displays
    D. PEEP

11. Which of the following is advisable when using heliox during mechanical ventilation?
    A. Keep two large heliox cylinders in or near the patient's room.
    B. Use at least one 100% helium cylinder to save gas consumption.
    C. Use a 60:40 heliox delivery to get the most effect from gas density.
    D. Use a heated-wire volume monitoring device.

12. Heliox cannot be used in which of the following circumstances?
    A. During NIV
    B. In patients allergic to helium gas
    C. During aerosolized medication delivery
    D. When appropriate equipment is not available to deliver heliox safely

13. The Edi catheter can be used for feeding, gastric evacuation, and what other function?
    A. Monitoring the electrical activity of the diaphragm
    B. Monitoring the esophageal pressure
    C. As an optional airway
    D. As a cardiac pacemaker

14. Edi signal reflects what physiological parameter?
    A. Esophageal pressure
    B. Upper airway pressure
    C. Electrical activity of the diaphragm
    D. Neural activity of the phrenic nerve

15. The NAVA backup safety features include which of the following?
    A. Backup volume control
    B. Backup pressure control
    C. VS above PEEP
    D. IMV plus PS

16. A NAVA Level is set at 1 cm H$_2$O/μV. The Edi peak is 8 μV and the Edi min 0 μV. PEEP is set at 5 cm H$_2$O. What is an estimated pressure delivery to the patient based on these parameters?
    A. 6 cm H$_2$O
    B. 1 cm H$_2$O
    C. 13 cm H$_2$O
    D. It cannot be determined with the information given

17. A low Edi signal may be caused by which of the following?
    A. Hypoventilation
    B. Oversedation
    C. Atelectasis
    D. Increased work of breathing

18. As with pressure support, the NAVA mode can be used in which of the following situations?
    A. Paralysis
    B. Heavy sedation
    C. Injury to the respiratory brain centers
    D. Spontaneous breathing

19. Which of the following are true regarding using the Edi catheter for monitoring?
    1. The Edi can be monitored following extubation to evaluate postextubation therapy.
    2. The Edi can be used to monitor if the diaphragm is active.
    3. The Edi can be used to assess a current mode of ventilation to evaluate synchrony.
    4. The Edi can be used to stimulate the diaphragm.
       A. 1 only
       B. 2 only
       C. 3 and 4
       D. 1, 2, and 3

20. Which of the following is true regarding NAVA?
    A. Ventilator synchrony is improved.
    B. Breaths are flow-cycled.
    C. NAVA is a time-triggered mode.
    D. The amount of pressure delivered during a single breath is constant.

References

1. Branson RD, Johannigman JA: What is the evidence base for the newer ventilation modes? *Respir Care* 49:742–760, 2004.
2. Downs JB, Stock MC: Airway pressure release ventilation: a new approach in ventilatory support during acute lung injury. *Respir Care Clin N Am* 32:517–524, 1987.
3. Garner W, Downs JB, Stock MC, et al: Airway pressure release ventilation (APRV): a human trial. *Chest* 94:779–782, 1988.
4. Stock MC, Downs JB, Frolicher DA: Airway pressure release ventilation. *Crit Care Med* 15:462–466, 1987.
5. Martin LD, Wetzel RC: Optimal release time during airway pressure release ventilation in neonatal sheep. *Crit Care Med* 22:486–493, 1994.
6. Stock MC: Airway pressure release ventilation. In Perel A, Stock MC, editors: *Handbook of mechanical ventilatory support*, Baltimore, 1992, Williams & Wilkins.
7. Kallet RH: Patient-ventilator interaction during acute lung injury, and the role of spontaneous breathing: Part 2: Airway pressure release ventilation. *Respir Care* 56:190–203, 2011.
8. Stock MC: Conceptual basis for inverse ratio and airway pressure release ventilation. In Marini JJ, editor: *Seminars in respiratory medicine*, vol 14, New York, 1993, Thieme Medical, pp 270–274.
9. Varpula T, Pettila V, Nieminen H, et al: Airway pressure release ventilation and prone positioning in severe acute respiratory distress syndrome. *Acta Anaesthesiol Scand* 45:340–344, 2001.
10. Varpula T, Valta P, Niemi R, et al: Airway pressure release ventilation as a primary ventilatory mode in acute respiratory distress syndrome. *Acta Anaesthesiol Scand* 48:722–731, 2004.
11. Calzia E, Lindner KH, Witt S, et al: Pressure-time product and work of breathing during biphasic continuous positive airway pressure and assisted spontaneous breathing. *Am J Respir Crit Care Med* 150:904–910, 1994.
12. Habashi N, Andrews P: Ventilator strategies for posttraumatic acute respiratory distress syndrome: airway pressure release ventilation and the role of spontaneous breathing in critically ill patients. *Curr Opin Crit Care* 10:549–557, 2004.
13. Stock CM, Downs JB: Airway pressure release ventilation: a new approach to ventilatory support during acute lung injury. *Respir Care* 32:517–524, 1987.
14. Rasanen J, Downs JB, Stock MC: Cardiovascular effects of conventional positive pressure ventilation and airway pressure release ventilation. *Chest* 93:911–915, 1988.
15. Rasanen J, Cane RD, Downs JB, et al: Airway pressure release ventilation during acute lung injury: prospective multicenter trial. *Crit Care Med* 19:1234–1241, 1991.
16. Dart BW, IV, Maxwell RA, Richart CM, et al: Preliminary experience with airway pressure release ventilation in a trauma/surgical intensive care unit. *J Trauma* 59:71–76, 2005.
17. Putensen C, Muzt NJ, Putensen-Himmer G, et al: Spontaneous breathing during ventilator support improves ventilation-perfusion distribution in patients with respiratory distress syndrome. *Am J Respir Crit Care Med* 159:1241–1248, 1999.
18. Sydow M, Burchardi H, Ephraim E, et al: Long-term effects of two different ventilatory modes on oxygenation in acute lung injury: comparison of airway pressure release ventilation and volume-controlled inverse ratio ventilation. *Am J Respir Crit Care Med* 149:1550–1556, 1994.
19. Kaplan LJ, Bailey H, Formosa V: Airway pressure release ventilation increases cardiac performance in patients with acute lung injury/acute respiratory distress syndrome. *Crit Care* 5:221–226, 2001.
20. Hering R, Peters D, Zinserling J, et al: Effects of spontaneous breathing during airway pressure release ventilation on renal perfusion and function in patients with acute lung injury. *Intensive Care Med* 29:1426–1433, 2002.
21. Frawley PM, Habashi NM: Airway pressure release ventilation: theory and practice. *AACN Clin Issues* 12:234–246, 2001.
22. Seymour CW, Frazer M, Reilly PM, et al: Airway pressure release and biphasic intermittent positive airway pressure ventilation: Are they ready for prime time? *J Trauma* 62:1298–1308, 2007.
23. Rathgeber J, Schorn B, Falk V, et al: The influence of controlled mandatory ventilation (CMV), intermittent mandatory ventilation (IMV) and biphasic intermittent positive airway pressure (BIPAP) on duration of intubation and consumption of analgesics and sedatives: a prospective analysis in 596 patients following adult cardiac surgery. *Eur J Anaesthesiol* 14:576–582, 1997.
24. Putensen C, Zech S, Wrigge H, et al: Long-term effects of spontaneous breathing during ventilatory support in patients with acute lung injury. *Am J Respir Crit Care Med* 164:43–49, 2001.
25. Dries DJ, Marini JJ: Airway pressure release ventilation. *J Burn Care Res* 30:929–936, 2009.
26. Froese AB, Bryan AC: Effects of anesthesia and paralysis on diaphragmatic mechanics in man. *Anesthesiology* 150:242–255, 1974.
27. Neuman P, Wrigge H, Zinserling J, et al: Spontaneous breathing affects the special ventilation and perfusion distribution during mechanical ventilatory support. *Crit Care Med* 33:1090–1095, 2005.
28. Hedenstierna G, Tokics L, Linquist H, et al: Phrenic nerve stimulation during halothane anesthesia. Effects of atelectasis. *Anesthesiology* 159:1241–1248, 1994.
29. Neumann P, Golisch W, Strohmeyer A, et al: Influence of different release times on spontaneous breathing pattern during airway pressure release ventilation. *Intensive Care Med* 28:1742–1749, 2002.
30. Rouby JJ, Ben Amewr M, Jawish D, et al: Continuous positive airway pressure (CPAP) vs. intermittent mandatory pressure release ventilation (IMPRV) in patients with acute respiratory failure. *Intensive Care Med* 18:69–75, 1992.
31. Chiang AA, Steinfeld A, Gropper C, et al: Demand-flow airway pressure release ventilation as partial ventilatory support mode: comparison with synchronized intermittent mandatory ventilation and pressure support ventilation. *Crit Care Med* 22:1431–1437, 1994.
32. Habashi NM: Other approaches to open-lung ventilation: Airway pressure release ventilation. *Crit Care Med* 33(3 Suppl):S228–S240, 2005.
33. Frawley PM, Habashi NM: Airway pressure release ventilation and pediatrics: theory and practice. *Crit Care Nurs Clin North Am* 16:337–348, 2004.
34. McCunn M, Habashi NM: Airway pressure release ventilation in the acute respiratory distress syndrome following traumatic injury. *Int Anesthesiol Clin* 40:89–102, 2002.
35. Davis K, Johnson DJ, Branson RD, et al: Airway pressure release ventilation. *Arch Surg* 128:1348–1352, 1993.
36. Wrigge H, Zinserling J, Neumann P, et al: Spontaneous breathing with airway pressure release ventilation favors ventilation in dependent lung regions and counters cyclic alveolar collapse in oleic-acid-induced lung injury: a randomized controlled computed tomography trial. *Crit Care* 9:R780–R789, 2005.
37. Smith RA, Smith DB: Does airway pressure release ventilation alter lung function after acute lung injury. *Chest* 107:805–808, 1995.
38. Neumann P, Hedenstierna G: Ventilatory support by continuous positive airway pressure breathing improves gas exchange as compared with partial ventilatory support with airway pressure release ventilation. *Anesth Analg* 92:950–958, 2001.
39. Neumann P, Berglund JE, Mondejar EF, et al: Dynamics of lung collapse and recruitment during prolonged breathing in porcine lung injury. *J Appl Physiol* 85:1533–1543, 1998.
40. Neumann P, Berglund JE, Mondejar EF, et al: Effect of different pressure levels on the dynamics of lung collapse and recruitment in oleic-acid-induced lung injury. *Am J Respir Crit Care Med* 158:1636–1643, 1998.
41. Foland JA, Martin J, Novotny T, et al: Airway pressure release ventilation with a short release time in a child with acute respiratory distress syndrome. *Respir Care* 46:1019–1023, 2001.
42. Froese AB: High-frequency oscillatory ventilation for adult respiratory distress syndrome: let's get it right this time! *Crit Care Med* 25:906–908, 1997.
43. Kacmarek RM: Ventilatory adjuncts. *Respir Care* 47:319–330, 2002.
44. Mehta S, MacDonald R: Implementing and troubleshooting high-frequency oscillatory ventilation in adults in the intensive care unit. *Respir Care Clin North Am* 7:683–695, 2001.
45. Rimensberger PC, Pache JC, McKerlie C, et al: Lung recruitment and lung volume maintenance: a strategy for improving oxygenation and preventing lung injury during both conventional mechanical ventilation and high-frequency oscillation. *Intensive Care Med* 26:745–755, 2000.
46. Emerson JH: *Apparatus for vibrating portions of a patient's airway, U.S. Patent No. 2918917*, Washington, DC, 1958, U.S. Patent Office.
47. Scotter DR, Thurtell GW, Raats PAC: Dispersion resulting from sinusoidal gas flow in porous materials. *Soil Sci* 104:306–308, 1967.
48. Lunkenheimer PP, Frank I, Ising H, et al: Intrapulmonaler Gaswechsel unter simulierter Apnoe durch transtrachealen periodischen intrathorakalen druckwechsel. *Anaesthesist* 22:232–238, 1972.

49. Fukuchi Y, Roussos CS, Macklen PT, et al: Convection, diffusion and cardiogenic mixing of inspired gas in the lungs: an experimental approach. *Respir Physiol* 26:77–90, 1980.

50. Norfolk SG, Hollingsworth CL, Wolfe CR, et al: Rescue therapy in adult and pediatric patients with pH1N1 influenza infection: a tertiary center intensive care unit experience from April to October 2009. *Crit Care Med* 38:2103–2107, 2010.

51. Bohn DJ, Miyassaka K, Marchak BE, et al: Ventilation by high-frequency oscillation. *J Appl Physiol Respir, Envir Exerc Physiol* 48:710–716, 1980.

52. Butler WJ, Bohn DJ, Miyasaka K, et al: Ventilation of humans by high frequency oscillation. *Anesthesiology* 51:S368, 1979.

53. Smith RB, Sjöstrand UH, Babinsku MF: Technical considerations using high frequency positive ventilation and high frequency jet ventilation. *Int Anesth Clinics* 21(3):183–200, 1983.

54. Ferguson ND, Stewart TE: The use of high-frequency oscillatory ventilation in adults with acute lung injury. *Respir Care Clin N Am* 7:647–661, 2001.

55. Derdak S: High-frequency oscillatory ventilation for acute respiratory distress syndrome in adult patients. *Crit Care Med* 31:S317–S323, 2003.

56. Kallett RH: Evidence-based management of acute lung injury and acute respiratory distress syndrome. *Respir Care* 49:793–809, 2004.

57. Derdak S, Mehta S, Stewart T, et al: High frequency oscillatory ventilation for acute respiratory distress syndrome: a randomized controlled trial. *Am J Respir Crit Care Med* 166:801–808, 2002.

58. Fort P, Farmer C, Westerman J, et al: High-frequency oscillatory ventilation for adult respiratory distress syndrome: a pilot study. *Crit Care Med* 25:937–947, 1997.

59. Mehta S, Lapinsky SE, Hallett DC, et al: Prospective trial of high-frequency oscillation in adults with acute respiratory distress syndrome. *Crit Care Med* 29:1360–1369, 2001.

60. Fessler HE, Hess DR: Respiratory controversies in the critical care setting. Does high-frequency ventilation offer benefits over conventional ventilation in adult patients with acute respiratory distress syndrome? *Respir Care* 52:595–605, 2007.

61. Watson KF: Infant and pediatric ventilators. In Cairo JM, editor: *Mosby's respiratory care equipment*, ed 9, St Louis, 2014, Elsevier, pp 461–512.

62. Quinones A: High frequency oscillation in the adult. *AARC Times* Feb:22, 2004.

63. Luecke T, Meinhardt JP, Hermann P, et al: Setting mean airway pressure during high-frequency oscillatory ventilation according to the static pressure-volume curve in surfactant-deficient lung injury: a computed tomography study. *Anesthesiology* 99:1313–1320, 2003.

64. Van de Kieft M, Dorsey D, Derdak S: Better breathing: high-frequency oscillatory ventilation for adults with severe ARDS. *Adv Managers Respir Care* 44:47, 2004.

65. Dorsey D, Venticinque S, Derdak S: Effect of endotracheal tube size on oscillatory pressure ratio in a mechanical lung model during high-frequency oscillation. *Am J Respir Crit Care Med* 167:A179, 2003.

66. Fink JB, Barraza P, Bisgaard J: Aerosol delivery during mechanical ventilation with high-frequency oscillation: an in-vitro evaluation. *Chest* 120:277S, 2001.

67. The Acute Respiratory Distress Syndrome Network (ARDSnet): Ventilation with lower tidal volumes as compared with traditional tidal volumes for acute lung injury and the acute respiratory distress syndrome. *N Engl J Med* 342:1301–1308, 2000.

68. Mehta S, MacDonald R, Hallet DC, et al: Acute oxygenation response to inhaled nitric oxide when combined with high-frequency oscillatory ventilation in adults with acute respiratory distress syndrome. *Crit Care Med* 31:383–389, 2003.

69. Seedek KA, Tkeuchi M, Suchodulski K, et al: Determinants of tidal volume during high-frequency oscillatory ventilation. *Crit Care Med* 31:227–231, 2003.

70. Hess DR, Bigatello LM: Lung recruitment: the role of lung recruitment maneuvers. *Respir Care* 47:308–317, 2002.

71. Haas CF: Lung protective mechanical ventilation in acute respiratory distress syndrome. *Respir Care Clin North Am* 9:363–965, 2003.

72. Scotter DR, Thurtell GW, Raats PAC: Dispersion resulting from sinusoidal gas flow in porous materials. *Soil Sci* 104:306–308, 1967.

73. Lunkenheimer PP, Rafflenbeul W, Keller H, et al: Application of transtracheal pressure-oscillations as a modification of "diffusion respiration". *Br J Anaesthesiol* 44:627–628, 1972.

74. Pilbeam SP: *Mechanical ventilation: physiological and clinical applications*, ed 2, St Louis, 1992, Mosby.

75. Bohn DJ, Miyassaka K, Marchak BE, et al: Ventilation by high-frequency oscillation. *J Appl Physiol Respir Environ Exerc Physiol* 48:710–716, 1980.

76. Fukuchi Y, Roussos CS, Macklem PT, et al: Convection, diffusion and cardiogenic mixing of inspired gas in the lungs: an experimental approach. *Respir Physiol* 26:77–90, 1980.

77. Wunsch H, Mapstone J: High-frequency ventilation versus conventional ventilation for treatment of acute lung injury and acute respiratory distress syndrome. *Cochrane Database Syst Rev* CD004085, 2004.

78. Barach AL: Use of helium as a new therapeutic gas. *Proc Soc Exp Biol Med* 32:462–464, 1934.

79. Barach AL: Rare gases not essential to life. *Science* 80:593–594, 1934.

80. Barach AL: The use of helium in the treatment of asthma and obstructive lesions in the larynx and trachea. *Ann Int Med* 9:739–765, 1935.

81. Myers TR: Use of heliox in children. *Respir Care* 51:619–631, 2006.

82. Jolliet P, Tassaux D: Helium-oxygen ventilation. *Respir Care Clin North Am* 8:295–307, 2002.

83. Kallstrom TJ: Evidence-based asthma management. *Respir Care* 49:783–792, 2004.

84. Ritz R: Methods to avoid intubation. *Respir Care* 44:686–699, 1999.

85. Manthous CA, Hall JB, Caputo MA, et al: Heliox improves pulses paradoxus and peak expiratory flow in nonintubated patients with severe asthma. *Am J Respir Crit Care Med* 151:310–314, 1995.

86. Myers TR: Use of heliox in children. *Respir Care* 51:619, 2006.

87. Chatmongkolchart S, Kacmarek RM, Hess DR: Heliox delivery with noninvasive positive pressure ventilation: a laboratory study. *Respir Care* 46:248–254, 2001.

88. Fink JB: Opportunities and risk of using heliox in your clinical practice. *Respir Care* 51:651–666, 2006.

89. Fink J, Ari A: Humidity and aerosol therapy. In Cairo JM, editor: *Mosby's respiratory care equipment*, ed 9, St Louis, 2014, Elsevier, pp 158–212.

90. Hess DR, Acosta FL, Ritz RH, et al: The effect of helium on nebulizer delivery using a beta-agonist bronchodilator. *Chest* 115:184–189, 1999.

91. Kress JP, Noth I, Gehlbach BK, et al: The utility of albuterol nebulized with heliox during acute asthma exacerbation. *Am J Respir Crit Care Med* 165:1317–1321, 2002.

92. Fink J, Dhand R, Fahey P, et al: Helium:oxygen improves in vitro aerosol delivery from MDIs but reduces nebulizer efficiency. *Am J Respir Crit Care Med* 159:63–68, 1999.

93. Kita R, Cronin J, Brennan L, et al: Helium–oxygen reduces nebulizer efficiency. *Respir Care* 42:1094, 1997. (abstract).

94. McArthur C, Adams A, Suzuki S: Effects of helium/oxygen mixtures on delivered and expired tidal volume during mechanical ventilation. *Am J Respir Crit Care Med* 153:A370, 1996. (abstract).

95. Tassaux D, Jolliet P, Thouret JM, et al: Calibration of seven ICU ventilators for mechanical ventilation with helium-oxygen mixtures. *Am J Respir Crit Care Med* 160:22–32, 1999.

96. Perino CD, Hess DR: Heliox delivery using the Avea ventilator. *Respir Care* 48:1093, 2003. (abstract).

97. Rogers M, Spearman CB: Accuracy of volumes delivered and monitored by the Viasys Avea ventilator during heliox administration. *Respir Care* 48:1095, 2003.

98. Kirmse M, Hess D, Imanaka H, et al: Accurate tidal volume delivery during mechanical ventilation with helium/oxygen mixtures. *Respir Care* 41:954A, 1996.

99. Polston ST: Effects of He/O$_2$ mixtures on the performance of Siemens (now Maquet) Servo 300 and Servoi ventilators. *Respir Care* 48:1094A, 2003.

100. Brown MK: Bench test of the Siemens (now Maquet) Servoi mechanical ventilator with heliox mixtures. *Respir Care* 48:1093A, 2003.

101. Brown MK, Willms DC: A laboratory evaluation of 2 mechanical ventilators in the presence of helium-oxygen mixtures. *Respir Care* 50:354–360, 2005.

102. Brown MK: Bench test of the eVent Inspiration Mechanical Ventilator with Heliox mixtures. *Respir Care* 48:1093A, 2003.

103. Jereb D, Bauer K, Martin JE: Developing a correction factor to determine the set tidal volume when using helium through a Dräger Dura 2 ventilator. *Respir Care* 48:1093A, 2003.

104. Baxter TD, Coulliette H: A comparison of three ventilators and their oxygen consumption efficiency. *Respir Care* 2009. (abstract).

105. Donnelly D, Walsh BK: Heliox utilization by two ICU ventilators: A bench study. *Respir Care* 2009. (abstract).

106. Gluck EH: Helium-oxygen mixtures in intubated patients with status asthmaticus and respiratory acidosis. *Chest* 98:693–698, 1990.

107. Cheifetz I: Heliox in intubated patients: rationale and evidence, American Association of Respiratory Care 49th International Respir Congress, Las Vegas, December 4-7, 2003.

108. Polito A, Fessler H: Heliox in respiratory failure from obstructive lung disease. *N Engl J Med* 332:192–193, 1995. (letter).

109. Jolliet P, Tassaux D, Thouret JM, et al: Beneficial effects of helium:oxygen versus air:oxygen noninvasive pressure support in patients with decompensated chronic obstructive pulmonary disease. *Crit Care Med* 27:2422–2429, 1999.

110. Meduri GU, Cook TR, Turner RE, et al: Noninvasive positive pressure ventilation in status asthmaticus. *Chest* 110:767–774, 1996.

111. Sinderby C, Beck J: Neurally adjusted ventilatory assist (NAVA): An update and summary of experiences. *Neth J Crit Care* 11:243–252, 2007.

112. Talmor DS, Fessler HE: Are esophageal pressure measurements important in clinical decision-making in mechanically ventilated patients? *Respir Care* 55:162–172, 2010.

113. Talmor D, Sarge T, Malhotra A, et al: Mechanical ventilation guided by esophageal pressure in acute lung injury. *N Engl J Med* 359:2095–2104, 2008.

114. Lourenco RV, Cherniack NS, Malm JR, et al: Nervous output from the respiratory center during obstructed breathing. *J Appl Physiol* 21:527–533, 1966.

115. Beck J, Sinderby C, Lindstrom L, et al: Effects of lung volume on diaphragm EMG signal strength during voluntary contractions. *J Appl Physiol* 85:1123–1134, 1998.

116. Aldrich TK, Sinderby C, McKenzie DK, et al: Electrophysiological techniques for the assessment of respiratory muscle function. *Am J Respir Crit Care Med* 166:548–558, 2002.

117. Sinderby C, Spahija J, Beck J, et al: Diaphragm activation during exercise in chronic obstructive pulmonary disease. *Am J Respir Crit Care Med* 163:1637–1641, 2001.

118. Barwing J, Ambold M, Linden N, et al: Evaluation of the catheter positioning for neurally adjusted ventilatory assist. *Intensive Care Med* 35:1809–1814, 2009.

119. Sinderby C, Beck J, Spahija J, et al: Voluntary activation of the human diaphragm in health and disease. *J Appl Physiol* 85:2146–2158, 1998.

120. Beck J, Weinberg J, Hamnegard CH, et al: Diaphragmatic function in advanced Duchenne muscular dystrophy. *Neuromuscul Disord* 16:161–167, 2006.

121. Bordessoule A, Emeriaud G, Delnard N, et al: Recording diaphragm activity by an oesophageal probe: a new tool to evaluate the recovery of diaphragmatic paralysis. *Intensive Care Med* 36:1978–1979, 2010.

122. deWit M, Miller KB, Green KA, et al: Ineffective triggering predicts increased duration of mechanical ventilation. *Crit Care Med* 37:2740–2745, 2009.

123. Thille AW, Cabello B, Galia F, et al: Reduction of patient-ventilator asynchrony by reducing tidal volume during pressure-support ventilation. *Intensive Care Med* 34:1477–1486, 2008.

124. Thille AW, Rodriguez P, Cabello B, et al: Patient-ventilator asynchrony during assisted mechanical ventilation. *Intensive Care Med* 32:1515–1522, 2006.

125. Beck J, Reilly M, Grasselli G, et al: Patient-ventilator interaction during neurally adjusted assist in low birth weight infants. *Pediatr Res* 65:663–668, 2009.

126. Levin S, Nguyen T, Taylor N, et al: Rapid disuse atrophy of diaphragm fibers in mechanically ventilated humans. *N Engl J Med* 358:1327–1335, 2008.

127. Knisely AS, Leal SM, Singer DB: Abnormalities of diaphragmatic muscle in neonates with ventilated lungs. *J Pediatr* 113:1074–1077, 1988.

128. Thille AW, Brochard L: Double triggering during assisted mechanical ventilation: Is it a controlled, auto-triggered, or patient triggered cycle? Reply to Chen CW. *Intensive Care Med* 33:744–745, 2007.

129. Chiumello D, Polli F, Tallarini F, et al: Effect of different cycling-off criteria and positive end-expiratory pressure during pressure support ventilation in patients with chronic obstructive pulmonary disease. *Crit Care Med* 35:2547–2552, 2007.

130. Girard TD, Kress JP, Fuchs BD, et al: Efficacy and safety of a paired sedation and ventilator weaning protocol for mechanically ventilated patients in intensive care (awakening and breathing controlled trial); a randomized controlled trial. *Lancet* 371:126–134, 2008.

131. Sinderby C, Beck J: Proportional assist ventilation and neurally adjusted ventilatory assist—better approaches to patient ventilator synchrony? *Clin Chest Med* 29:329–342, 2008.

132. Spahija J, de Marchie M, Albert M, et al: Patient-ventilator interaction during pressure support ventilation and neurally adjusted ventilatory assist. *Crit Care Med* 38:518–526, 2010.

133. Chatburn RL, Mireles-Cabodevila E: Closed-loop control of mechanical ventilation: Description and classification of targeting schemes. *Respir Care* 56:85–102, 2011.

134. Sinderby C, Navalesi P, Beck J, et al: Neural control of mechanical ventilation. *Nat Med* 5:1433–1436, 1999.

135. Servo Education, NAVA Tutorial, Maquet Critical Care, Solna Sweden, Order No. 66 79 145, 2000.

136. Leiter JC, Manning HL: The Hering-Breuer reflex, feedback control, and mechanical ventilation: the promise of neurally adjusted ventilatory assist. *Crit Care Med* 38:1915–1916, 2010.

137. White C, Seger B, Lin L, et al: The effect of NAVA on parameters of ventilation in the pediatric intensive care unit. *Respir Care* 55:1598, A906448, 2010.

138. Howard D, Stein H: Neonates ventilated with NAVA have better blood gases than those ventilated with SIMV/PC with PS. *Respir Care* 43:2009. (abstract).

139. Coisel Y, Chanques G, Jung B, et al: Neurally adjusted ventilatory assist in critically ill postoperative patients: a crossover randomized study. *Anesthesiology* 13:925–935, 2010.

140. Demoule A, Schmidt M, Cracco C, et al: Neurally adjusted ventilatory assist increases respiratory variability and chaos in acute respiratory failure. *Am J Respir Crit Care Med* 179:a3648, 2009.

141. Brander L, Leong-Poi H, Beck J, et al: Titration and implementation of neurally adjusted ventilatory assist in critically ill patients. *Chest* 135:695–703, 2009.

142. Noblet T: Effect of bubble CPAP and high flow nasal cannula therapy on the electrical activity of the diaphragm in a premature infant. *Respir Care* 54:1537, 2009. a678892.

143. Stein H, Howard D: Neonates ventilated with NAVA do not have an increased incidence of IVH, pneumothorax or NEC/perforation compared to those ventilated with SIMV/PC with PS. *Respir Care* 43:abstract, 2009.

144. MacIntyre N: Talk to me? Toward better patient-ventilator communication. *Crit Care Med* 38:714–715, 2010. (editorial).

145. Navalesi P, Colombo D, Della Corte F: NAVA ventilation—a Review. *Minerva Anestesiol* 76:346–352, 2010.

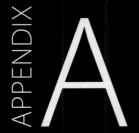

APPENDIX A

Answer Key

PART 1: REVIEW QUESTIONS ANSWER KEY

CHAPTER 1

Basic Terms and Concepts of Mechanical Ventilation

1. Figures 1-2 and 1-8 show how to draw these graphs. During spontaneous, quiet breathing, pleural pressure is always negative and ranges from approximately −5 to −10 cm H_2O. With positive pressure ventilation, pleural pressure can become positive at end inspiration but usually returns to its resting negative value (−5 cm H_2O) during exhalation.

2. $5 \times 1.36 = 6.8$ cm H_2O

3. Unit A would receive the greatest volume for the same pressure during a given inspiratory time. Unit A also has a shorter time constant. (Time constant = $R_{aw} \times C$.) Unit B fills more slowly because it has increased resistance; that is, it has a greater (longer) time constant.

4. Unit B will fill more quickly. It is less compliant than unit A, therefore its time constant ($R_{aw} \times C$) will have a smaller value. Stiff alveoli with poor compliance fill quickly, but they do not fill with the same volume for a given pressure. If pressure delivery to both units is the same, unit A will have a greater volume. Recall that $C = \Delta V/\Delta P$ and $\Delta V = C \times \Delta P$.

5. Lung units vary in filling and emptying times based on their compliance and resistance. Less compliant lung units fill faster, and those with higher R_{aw} fill more slowly.
   A. Time constant = 0.1 second
   B. Time constant = 0.025 second
   C. Time constant = 1.0 second
   D. Time constant = 0.25 second
   E. Time constant = 1.5 seconds
   F. Time constant = 0.15 second
   Units ranked in order from slowest to fastest: e, c, d, f, a, and b.
6. C
7. D
8. B
9. C
10. D
11. B
12. A
13. D
14. D
15. B
16. C
17. D

CHAPTER 2

How Ventilators Work

1. Bird Mark 7 ventilator. These devices are typically used for administering intermittent positive pressure breathing treatments.
2. Lifecare PLV-102 ventilator (Philips Respironics, Pittsburgh, Pa.).
3. Negative pressure ventilator.
4. When the ventilator begins inspiratory gas flows through the main inspiratory tube, gas also flows through the expiratory valve line to the exhalation valve, closing the valve (see Fig. 2-8, A, cutaway). During exhalation, the flow from the ventilator stops and the exhalation valve opens. The patient is able to exhale passively through the expiratory port in the exhalation valve.
5. Rotary drive piston.
6. A
7. C
8. D
9. B
10. C
11. C
12. A

CHAPTER 3

How a Breath Is Delivered

1. $P_{mus} + P_{vent} = V/C + (R_{aw} \times flow)$
2. The volume of air in the lungs depends on the elastic recoil pressure, which is the pressure resulting from alveolar tension on the volume within alveoli.
3. A

4. Pressure-targeted ventilation, pressure-controlled ventilation.
5. A
6. With pressure-controlled breaths, the pressure waveform is constant during inspiration, and volume and flow can vary with changes in lung characteristics, the set pressure, or the patient's inspiratory effort. With volume-controlled breaths, volume delivery is constant, and the volume and flow waveforms remain unchanged during inspiration. The pressure waveform can vary with changes in lung characteristics.
7. Pressure and flow.
8. C
9. B
10. A
11. Pressure rises quickly at the beginning of inspiration to a set value and tends to plateau. Flow rises quickly at the beginning of inspiration and tapers off in a descending exponential curve. Inspiration ends when flow drops to a predetermined percentage of the peak flow measured during inspiration.
12. A
13. A
14. A
15. C

CHAPTER 4

Establishing the Need for Mechanical Ventilation

1. A
2. D
3. B
4. D
5. B
6. D
7. C
8. C
9. A
10. C
11. D
12. A
13. B
14. A
15. B

CHAPTER 5

Selecting the Ventilator and the Mode

1. C
2. C
3. D
4. A
5. D
6. C
7. A pressure of 30 cm H_2O to start would provide approximately the same V_T delivery in VC-CMV and would be a safe starting point. This patient requires high pressures for delivery of V_T. P_{alv} should be kept below 30 cm H_2O.
8. Apparently the ventilator has a fixed flow and pattern during inspiration that is not adequate for the patient's needs. The therapist should increase the inspiratory flow and see if this

solves the problem. Another possible solution is to switch to another ventilator that allows additional flow on demand during VC-CMV.
9. There are several options: (1) switch the patient to PC-IMV with a lower mandatory rate; (2) switch the patient to PSV; (3) switch to VS. Although any of these options would allow for more spontaneous ventilation, it is important to monitor the S_pO_2, V_T, and V_E closely.
10. A dual control mode that limits pressure (e.g., PRVC) may be appropriate for this situation. This mode would limit pressure delivery while simultaneously allowing for a targeted volume in an effort to maintain the patient's minute ventilation.

CHAPTER 6

Initial Ventilator Settings

1. C_T = 100 mL/33 cm H_2O = 3 mL/cm H_2O
   Volume lost to circuit = 3 mL/cm H_2O × 15 cm H_2O = 45 mL
2. The V_E = 700 mL × 15 = 10.5 L/min
   Set V_T (250 mL) − Volume lost (45 mL) = About 205 mL
3. V_E = 700 mL × 15 = 10.5 L/min
   A. If the flow is set at 30 L/min using a constant flow pattern, the flow in L/sec is 30 L/60 sec = 0.5 L/sec.
   B. The TCT based on the set machine f of 12 breaths/min is 5 seconds.
   C. The TCT based on the actual machine f of 15 breaths/min is 4 seconds.
   D. The T_I based on the set f, flow, and V_T: T_I = 0.7 L/(0.5 L/sec) = 1.4 seconds.
   E. The T_E when f is 12 is 3.6 seconds.
   F. The T_E when f is 15 is 2.6 seconds.
4. C
5. The patient is actively breathing during the plateau period.
6.
   A. The patient's BSA is approximately 2.12 m^2.
   B. His ideal body weight is 160 lb, or about 73 kg.
   C. Before correction for body temperature, the $\dot{V}_E$ is 8.48 L/min. This is reduced by 18% (10% per degree Celsius). 18% of 8.48 is about 1.53 L. 8.48 − 1.53 is a final V_E of 6.95 L/min. In postoperative open heart surgery patients, the body temperature is sometimes cooler than normal. Patients warm up quickly and usually recover from the anesthesia quickly. As the patient warms up, the V_E would need to be increased. Either CMV or IMV modes would be appropriate with a safe rate and V_T setting.
   D. V_T would be targeted between 6 and 8 mL/kg IBW (i.e., 438 and 584 mL/kg). The patient weighs 210 lb; however V_T is based on IBW, not actual weight. This is a common mistake among new practitioners. (Note that the V_T would be about targeted between 570 mL and 760 mL (range of 6 to 8 mL/kg IBW) if the actual body weight of 210 lb was used). However, V_T is based on IBW, **not** actual weight; this is a common mistake among new practitioners.
   E. An appropriate rate based on a V_T of about 438 mL (0.438 = 16 breaths/min; based on a V_T of 0.584 L) would be (6.95 L/min)/0.584L = 11 breaths/min.
   F. Because the physician is concerned about pressure, a low compensating PEEP of about 3 cm H_2O would be a good starting point.

7. The patient's IBW is $105 + 5(64 - 60) = 125$ lb, or 56.8 (57) kg. However, she weighs 195 lb (about 87 kg), therefore she has a large BSA (about 1.94 m^2). Her estimated $\dot{V}_E$ (assuming normal body temperature, and so on) is 3.5×1.94, or about 6.8 L/min. If the $\dot{V}_E$ had been based on IBW, it would have underestimated her metabolic rate. However, her V_T must be based on IBW.

   Remember, when a person gains weight, his or her lungs do not get bigger.

   Using the calculated IBW, an appropriate V_T for a patient with ARDS would be in the range of 4 to 8 mL/kg. For the patient this range would be about 230 mL to 450 mL. A respiratory rate of 15 (using 8 mL/kg) to 30 (using 4 mL/kg) breaths/min would be in the target range. A higher rate may accompany a lower V_T. It might be appropriate to start in the middle of the ranges (e.g., 6 mL/kg). For example, set a V_T of 350 mL and a rate of 20 breaths/min PV would probably provide patient comfort and would be suitable for this patient, particularly based on her diagnosis. The pressure could be set to target the desired V_T.

8. Try increasing the IPAP to 11 cm H$_2$O and re-evaluate the patient. The V_T should be 420 mL to 560 mL (range, 6 to 8 mL/kg IBW), and the spontaneous rate should be below 25 breaths/min.

9. The $\dot{V}_E$ should be increased by 10%, or 5% for every degree >99° F.

10. Change to a descending waveform with volume ventilation would change the pattern of pressure delivery, resulting in a decrease in PIP. This was an actual case. After making the adjustment, the resulting PIP was 41 cm H$_2$O, and the P$_{plateau}$ was 32 cm H$_2$O without any other changes.

11. The lung characteristics are deteriorating; that is, either R$_{aw}$ is increasing or the lung compliance is decreasing, or both.

12. Volume support ventilation.

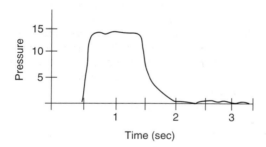

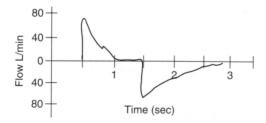

NOTE: This Figure should be read pressure–time and flow–time curves during PC-CMV.

13. About 14 cm H$_2$O.

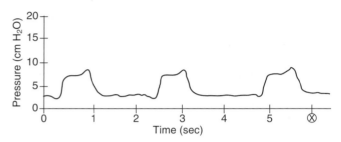

NOTE: This Figure should read pressure–time curve during PSV.

14. A

CHAPTER 7

Final Considerations in Ventilator Setup

1.
   Initial $\dot{V}_E = 4 \times 1.5 = 6$ L/min
   V_T is based on IBW
   IBW $= 106 + 6(8) = 154$ lb, or 70 kg
   V_T range of 6 to 8 mL/kg $= 280$ mL to 560 mL
   Example: At 6 mL/kg, initial $V_T = 420$ mL (0.42 L)
   Rate using selected V_T and $\dot{V}_E$: f $= \dot{V}_E/V_T = 6/0.42 = 14$;
   f $= 14$ breaths/min

2. Over a 2-hour period, the $\dot{V}_E$ increased from 6.5 L/min to 13 L/min. The patient is using accessory muscles to breathe, and the pressure–time curve indicates an inadequate flow. PIP has also increased. These findings suggest the development of air trapping, therefore evaluate for the presence of intrinsic PEEP. Increase the inspiratory gas flow and reassess the pressure–time curve. Assess the patient's ventilatory pattern to determine whether the problem persists. Another possibility is to switch to VC-IMV + PSV; however, inspiratory flow would still need to be increased and PSV would have to be set at an appropriate level. Other questions might also be asked. Can you think of any? For example, what is the S_pO_2? Have the ABG values changed? Have breath sounds changed? What does the flow–time curve look like?

3.
   (NOTE: A number of solutions are possible for this problem. The following answer is provided as one option.) Initial V_T is selected at 6 mL/kg (420 mL). Because this patient has a history of COPD, a lower V_T setting was selected to reduce the risk of lung injury. $\dot{V}_E$ is set at 8 L/min: $4 \times$ BSA $= 4 \times 1.78 = 7.12$ L/min. Increase $\dot{V}_E$ by 5% per degree Fahrenheit: T $= 102°$ F, or 15%. Increase by 1.05 L/min to a total $\dot{V}_E$ of 8.2 L/min. Rate is set at 19 breaths/min ($\dot{V}_E/V_T = f$). Flow is set at 80 L/min using the descending flow pattern. F$_I$O$_2$ is set at 0.5 initially. (NOTE: Because the patient is breathing spontaneously, a lower f and $\dot{V}_E$ could be used, depending on the clinician's preference. The F$_I$O$_2$ could be lower as well. The settings selected here would provide a minimum safe initial form of ventilation and could be adjusted based on patient assessment.)

   Resistance is estimated at P$_{ta}$/Flow, or 8 cm H$_2$O/80 L/min: 8 cm H$_2$O/(1.33 L/sec) $= 6$ cm H$_2$O/(L/sec). This answer is only an estimate because the flow is not constant. Pressure support is set at 6 cm H$_2$O. This is an example of initiating ventilatory support in a patient with COPD. Note the use of a lower V_T setting, the $\dot{V}_E$ increase because of the patient's temperature, and the use of pressure support for spontaneous breaths set high enough to overcome the resistance imposed by the airway. The patient's breathing must be evaluated to ensure comfort, patient-ventilator synchrony, and reduced WOB.

4. Postoperative patients and victims of drug overdose are examples of patients who are most likely to have normal lungs yet still require ventilation. Appropriate settings for normal lungs are as follows:

VC-CMV or PC-CMV

V_T = 6 to 8 mL/kg

f = 10 to 15 breaths/min

Descending or constant flow waveform

T_I = About 1 second initially

PEEP ≤5 cm H_2O; kept $P_{plateau}$ <30 cm H_2O

F_IO_2 ≤0.5 (titrate to patient's normal; maintain P_aO_2 >70 mm Hg and S_pO_2 ≥92%)

For this patient a V_T range of 480 to 640 mL would be appropriate. $\dot{V}_E$ would equal 4 × 1.8 = 7.2 L/min. Rate would range from 11 to 18 breaths/min. An F_IO_2 of 0.5, PEEP of 3 cm H_2O, a descending flow ramp, and VC-CMV would all be appropriate settings.

CHAPTER 8

Initial Patient Assessment

1. C. *a*, *b*, and *d* refer to times when a ventilator check is performed.
2. A
3. D
4. B. V_{Danat} is equal to about 180 mL (80 kg IBW × 2.2 lb = 176 lb). With an ET in place, the V_{Danat} is reduced by about a half to 90 mL. The HME adds about 50 mL of mechanical dead space. V_D is about 140 mL. $V_T - V_D = V_A$; V_A = 400 − 140 = 260 mL/breath.
5. B. When the flow is zero (before exhalation begins), the pressure on the pressure–time curve for the same time interval will be $P_{plateau}$.
6. A
7. C
8. D (the difference between PIP and $P_{plateau}$ is increasing).
9. An increase in R_{aw}, as might occur with bronchoconstriction or mucous plugging.
10. V_T = 0.55 mL, V_{Danat} = 150 mL, $\dot{V}_A$ = (0.55 − 0.15) × 8 = 3.2 L/min
11. A. This scenario actually describes the use of MLT. The best choice is *B*; check the cuff pressure and delivered volume. It is the safest choice without knowing whether MLT or MOV is used.
12. The cuff pressure is much too high and will result in reduced blood flow to the adjacent tracheal walls.
    The tube is too small for this patient. The best choice is *C*; change the ET to a size 8 Fr.
13. C. The change in V_T may be the result of an improvement in lung characteristics (e.g., a decrease in R_{aw} or an improvement in C_L). Listen to the breath sounds, evaluate the flow–time and volume–time curves, and check the current acid–base status. Changes in V_T may lead to respiratory alkalosis. The preset pressure may need to be reduced.
14. C. Because no air leak is heard, MOV probably has been used to inflate the ET cuff. The measurement technique is accurate if

done appropriately; that is, if the system was pressurized before the pilot balloon connection was attached to the manometer. This is a low pressure and would not interfere with tracheal blood flow.

15. Answer *A* is the most immediate fix. If the patient is to be ventilated for an extended period, it might be appropriate to change the ET (answer *B*).

CHAPTER 9

Ventilator Graphics

1. A. The arrow indicates an active exhalation by the patient.
   B. The flow cycle criterion might be increased to a higher percentage so that T_I is shorter.
   C. The expiratory flow pattern at arrow *B* indicates air trapping.
   D. Shortening the T_I might allow a longer time for exhalation and eliminate this problem. Suctioning of the patient or administration of a bronchodilator might be indicated to reduce R_{aw}. Because this is PSV, reducing the set pressure might reduce both V_T and $\dot{V}_E$, thus reducing air trapping. However, this type of adjustment would have to be monitored to ensure that the patient is still adequately ventilated.
   E. The prolonged exhalation of volume suggests airway resistance; checking a flow–volume loop might confirm this finding.
   F. It is set at a high percentage of the peak flow.
   G. The pressure–time curve does not have a concave appearance; however, the curve would not take this shape with pressure-targeted ventilation. The patient can get as much flow as needed and the pressure will be maintained. The ventilator would increase flow to achieve the set pressure if the patient were actively inhaling. As long as a rise time or slope does not reduce inspiratory flow, inadequate flow should not be a problem.

2. Answers to questions regarding the Figure featured below Question 2: Flow, pressure, and volume scalars for three different ventilation situations, *A*:
   A. The target variable is pressure. The mode could be PC-CMV, but there are not enough breaths to determine whether it is PC-CMV or PC-IMV. The breath shown is time triggered, pressure targeted, and time cycled (flow drops to zero before end inspiration).
   B. The set pressure is 20 cm H_2O.
   C. V_T is 500 mL.
   D. $P_{plateau}$ is 20 cm H_2O. Because the flow drops to zero during inspiration, there is a period of no flow before exhalation begins. The pressure at that time is the same at the ventilator and in the lungs.
   E. A leak is present; the inspired and expired volumes are not the same.

3. Answers to questions regarding the Figure featured below Question 2: Flow, pressure, and volume scalars for three different ventilation situations, *B*:
   A. The target variable is volume. The mode of ventilation is VC-CMV. You can tell it is volume targeted because it has a constant flow curve. You can tell it is CMV because you can see the beginning of a second breath and it is also a mandatory breath.
   B. The total cycle time in this example is 3.5 seconds.

C. The breath is patient-triggered.

D. Based on the pressure–time curve, the problem is inadequate flow.

4. Answers to questions regarding the Figure featured below Question 2: Flow, pressure, and volume scalars for three different ventilation situations, *C*:

A. The set flow is about 40 L/min.

B. The patient is actively inhaling during inspiration, and the ventilator is providing additional flow. This is probably a newer generation ICU ventilator with a responsive inspiratory valve.

C. Volume delivery will increase because the patient can demand more flow than the set amount.

5. Answers to question 5 regarding the Figure of P-V loop:

A. PIP is about 17.5 cm H_2O.

B. The delivered V_T is about 700 mL.

C. The pressure–volume loop begins at a pressure of zero, therefore no PEEP has been set.

D. Compliance is about 40 mL/cm H_2O.

E. P_{ta} is about 7 cm H_2O, which is slightly higher than normal.

F. The appearance of the pressure–volume loop indicates that the patient has increased R_{aw}.

6. Answers to question 6 regarding the Figure of F-V loop:

A. The target variable is volume, because the flow is constant.

B. The flow setting is 60 L/min, and the flow waveform is constant (rectangular).

C. V_T is 500 mL.

D. The artifact indicated by arrow *A* is the compressible volume from the patient circuit leaving the circuit at the beginning of exhalation.

E. Arrow *B* indicates air trapping (auto-PEEP).

F. Increased R_{aw}.

7. PIP and $P_{plateau}$ will increase, and T_I and V_T will stay the same.

8. P_{set} and T_I will remain constant, but V_T will increase.

9. Answers to question 9

A. P_{alv} is 35 cm H_2O. Compliance has nothing to do with the answer. We know the pressure because flow drops to zero during inspiration (the alveolar and preset pressures equilibrate).

B. V_T will be 0.525 L: Volume = Pressure × Compliance; Volume = 35 cm H_2O × 15 mL/cm H_2O = 525 mL (0.525 L).

C. After compliance improves to 30 mL/cm H_2O, volume delivery will increase: Volume = 35 cm H_2O × 0.03 mL/cm H_2O = 1.05 L (1050 mL). P_{ta} will be approximately the same, because the generating pressure is the same and R_{aw} is not increased. (Actually, P_{ta} will decrease slightly as the flow drops off when P_{alv} approaches the preset pressure.)

D. Reduce the preset pressure until the desired V_T is achieved. (This would be approximately half the previous setting because compliance doubled [about 17 to 18 cm H_2O].)

10. B

11. C

CHAPTER 10

Assessment of Respiratory Function

1. As Fig. 10-8 illustrates, the capnographic waveform is divided into four phases. In phase 1, the initial gas exhaled is from the conducting airways, which contain low levels of CO_2. During phase 2, alveolar gas containing CO_2 mixes with gas in the anatomical airways and the CO_2 concentration increases. In phase 3, the curve plateaus as alveolar gas is exhaled (this phase is often referred to as the *alveolar plateau*). Note that the concentration of CO_2 at the end of the alveolar phase (just before inspiration begins) is called the *end-tidal PCO_2* or $P_{ET}CO_2$. On inspiration (phase 4), the concentration falls to zero.

2. The pressure–time product, which is an assessment of transdiaphragmatic pressure during the inspiratory portion of the breathing cycle, is a way of estimating the contributions of the diaphragm during inspiration.

3. C

4. C

5. A

6. C

7. C

8. D

9. A

10. C

11. A

12. C

13. C

14. D

15. B

16. D

CHAPTER 11

Hemodynamic Monitoring

1. A

2. C

3. C

4. B

5. B

6. B

7. B

8. C

9. C

10. B

11. A

12. D

13. D

14. A

15. C

16. D

17. B

18. A

19. A

20. A

CHAPTER 12

Methods to Improve Ventilation in Patient-Ventilator Management

1.

A. Mandatory $\dot{V}_A = 8 \times (400 - 140) = 2.08$ L/min; spontaneous $\dot{V}_A = 25 \times (225 - 140) = 2.13$ L/min; total $\dot{V}_A = 2.08 + 2.13 = 4.21$ L/min

B. $C_S = 400/20 = 20$ mL/cm H_2O

C. The patient has a respiratory acidosis. In addition, his spontaneous breathing rate is high, and his spontaneous V_T is low, indicating a high WOB. His P_{set} is within safe limits. The CO_2 can be reduced by increasing the pressure to increase the V_T or by increasing the set rate. Increasing the P_{set} to 29 cm H_2O theoretically would increase the V_T to 870 mL (about 14 mL/kg) and reduce the P_aCO_2 to 40 mm Hg. This is a high V_T. On the other hand, increasing the set rate to 12 breaths/min would also reduce the CO_2 to 40 mm Hg. In addition, using PSV to overcome the work required to move air through the resistance of the ET would reduce the patient's spontaneous WOB. PSV also could be used to reduce the P_aCO_2 instead of changing the mandatory rate or volume.

2. Increase the mandatory f to 10 breaths/min to return the patient to a P_aCO_2 closer to his normal value. Add PSV of about 8 cm H_2O for spontaneous breaths to reduce spontaneous WOB.

3. IBW for this patient is 106 + 6(4) = 130 lb, or 59 kg. The set V_T is too high and has been based on actual weight, not IBW. PIP and $P_{plateau}$ are high because of the large V_T. Reduce the volume to 500 mL. The current $\dot{V}_E$ of 9 L/min results in a normal acid–base status. With $P_{plateau}$ at 35 cm H_2O for a volume of 1.00 L, C_S is about 29 mL/cm H_2O. A V_T set at 0.5 L should produce a safer $P_{plateau}$. The rate could be adjusted to 16 to 18 breaths/min, which would provide an adequate $\dot{V}_E$.

4. No change should be made at this time. If the ICP can be managed with medical intervention, the patient does not need to be hyperventilated.

5. 14 Fr (9 × 3 = 27/2 = 13.5); B. About 22 cm; C. −100 to −120 mm Hg.

6. B
7. C
8. C
9. A
10. C. Although a pMDI is more efficient, an SVN delivers more medication.
11. D
12. D
13. C
14. B
15. D
16. D
17. C
18. D

CHAPTER 13

Improving Oxygenation and Management of Acute Respiratory Distress Syndrome

1. B
2. B
3. C
4. C
5. A
6. D
7. C
8. B
9. D
10. Oxygen transport is an acceptable answer; another is C_S. More than one answer is possible. You might want to discuss your response with an instructor or mentor.
11. B
12. C
13. D

14. B. The current recommendation is to use the deflation portion of a static P-V loop to establish PEEP. Setting PEEP 2 to 4 cm H_2O above the LIP on an SPV curve is also acceptable.
15. B
16. B
17. A
18. C
19. A
20. D
21. C

CHAPTER 14

Ventilator-Associated Pneumonia

1. B
2. C
3. C
4. A
5. B
6. C
7. A
8. B
9. C
10. B

CHAPTER 15

Sedatives, Analgesics, and Paralytics

1. B
2. C
3. D
4. C
5. A
6. C
7. D
8. C
9. D
10. The TOF technique allows the clinician to assess the extent of neuromuscular blockade during pharmacologically induced paralysis. With this technique, two electrodes are placed on the skin along a nerve path, often near a hand, foot, or facial nerve. An electrical current consisting of four impulses is applied to the peripheral nerve over 2 seconds; the muscle contractions (twitches) produced provide information about the level of paralysis.

CHAPTER 16

Extrapulmonary Effects of Mechanical Ventilation

1. D
2. C
3. B
4. A
5. Decreasing P_aO_2 values in patients with respiratory failure has been shown to cause a reduction in renal function and urine flow. A P_aO_2 below 40 mm Hg (severe hypoxemia) can dramatically interfere with normal renal function.
6. A
7. B
8. The amount of blood flowing to the brain is determined by the cerebral perfusion pressure (CPP), which is calculated by

subtracting the intracranial pressure (ICP) from the mean systemic arterial blood pressure (MABP). Because PPV (with or without PEEP) can reduce cardiac output and MABP, it is reasonable to assume that CPP would also decrease during PPV in these patients.

9. C
10. A

CHAPTER 17

Effects of Positive Pressure Ventilation on the Pulmonary System

1. D
2. C
3. The RT might consider performing a recruitment maneuver that would include recruitment to open the lung, derecruitment to establish the deflation point (UIP during derecruitment) and then re-recruiting the lungs. It might be argued that a static pressure–volume curve could establish an LIP, but current research supports the use of the deflation point (see Chapter 13).
4. In patients with high chest wall and abdominal pressures, the restriction of lung movement caused by a rigid thoracic compartment may provide some protection from elevating transpulmonary pressures. The same would be true if a patient were in the prone position. In this situation the increase in $P_{plateau}$ probably is permissible and will not cause VILI. Another option might be to allow the P_aCO_2 to increase to maintain a lower $P_{plateau}$.
5. D
6. C
7. The temptation might be to sedate this patient for anxiety. Another concern might be the patient's heart, considering the ECG changes. Before any medications are administered, the patient must be assessed further. ABG analysis may reveal respiratory acidosis, because all these findings are consistent with that condition.
8. A
9. D
10. D
11. D
12. C
13. B
14. A
15. Auto-PEEP (air trapping).

CHAPTER 18

Troubleshooting and Problem Solving

1. The breath sounds and the ET marking at the teeth suggest that the tube may have migrated into the right mainstem bronchus when the patient was moved. The RT should check the original tube position from the chart. The tube must be withdrawn about 3 to 4 cm, and the breath sounds must be reevaluated. A chest radiograph may also be required.
2. D
3. C
4. D
5. D
6. Tachypnea; nasal flaring; diaphoresis; use of accessory muscles; retraction of the suprasternal, supraclavicular, and intercostal spaces; paradoxical or abnormal movement of the thorax and abdomen; abnormal findings on auscultation; tachycardia; and possibly arrhythmias and hypotension. When severe distress is confirmed (see answer to question 6), the initial step is to disconnect the patient from the ventilator and carefully begin manual ventilation. If the patient's distress immediately resolves, the problem originates with the ventilator. If the distress does not resolve, the problem originates with the patient. Continue assessment until the problem is solved.
7. Intubation apparently resulted in insertion of the tube into the right mainstem bronchus. After 4 hours of ventilation at a high oxygen percentage, the left lung has collapsed, resulting in the dull percussion of this area, the absence of breath sounds, and the tracheal shifting. The tube must be repositioned, breath sounds must be reevaluated, and a chest radiograph is necessary to confirm tube placement.
8. The most likely cause is an air leak around the tube cuff. Inflate the cuff using MLT or minimum occluding volume and measure the cuff pressure. Listen again over the tracheal area to make sure the cuff is not leaking. Another possible cause is migration of the ET upward, above the vocal cords. Check the centimeter markings at the teeth.
9. D. The drop in volume on a pressure-limited machine could be caused by leaks, a decrease in C_L, an increase in R_{aw}, or gastric distention from air swallowing from high pressures, resulting in decreased diaphragmatic excursion or a change in the patient's inspiratory effort. Perform a general visual assessment of the patient. Check around the facemask for leaks and listen to breath sounds.
10. Breath sounds suggest the presence of a pneumothorax, possibly a tension pneumothorax, in the right hemithorax. Contact a physician immediately for placement of a chest tube and continue to ventilate the patient manually with 100% oxygen.
11. The graphics demonstrate that auto-PEEP is present (flow does not return to zero before a mandatory breath begins, similar to the findings in Fig. 18-9), that the machine is not responding to patient effort, and that inspiratory flow is set too low for patient demand (concave appearance of pressuretime curve, similar to Fig. 18-3). Increase inspiratory flow to shorten T_I and lengthen T_E to try to eliminate auto-PEEP and provide the needed flow demand. If this is unsuccessful, consider using external PEEP to make triggering easier for the patient. Perhaps VC-CMV is not the best mode for this patient. Consider other alternatives, such as changing the flow waveform.
12. B. A leak exists in the system.
13. The patient will need further assessment, including vital signs, pulse oximetry, ABG values, and a chest examination. More information about the ventilator settings is needed. An immediate concern is the high cuff pressure requirements. The tube size is too small for this patient; change to a larger tube.
14. It may be appropriate to do a recruitment maneuver on this patient, because this condition is secondary, nonpulmonary ARDS. Resetting PEEP after recruitment may be indicated. Another option is to use permissive hypercapnia. Eliminate any contraindications to this treatment and assess the patient's tolerance of this ventilation technique. The patient may need sedation but may already be sedated because the I:E ratio is 1:1.
15. D. All the choices are possibly correct in this situation, depending on the circumstances.
    a. If the patient is on a facemask rather than connected with a tracheostomy or ET, heated humidity may not be necessary and in fact may be uncomfortable if used. The heated

humidifier may not have been turned, may not be set to a warm enough temperature, or may have been turned off the last time the equipment was changed.

b. The heater may not be functioning.

c. If the system had recently been changed, condensate would not have had a chance to build up in the circuit.

d. Depletion of the water supply to the humidifier reservoir could also result in lack of rain-out and inadequate humidification.

16. The patient's condition improved after treatment.

17. If a chest tube is in place, a leak may exist from the lung into the chest drainage system.

18. From the pressure graphic and the patient's description, the patient apparently is not getting sufficient inspiratory gas flow. The pressure setting seems inadequate considering the C_S and R_{aw}. The flow can be determined by rearranging the equation for calculating R_{aw}. (Note: During PSV and PCV, P_{set} may be used in place of P_{TA} to calculate the answer: $R_{aw} = P_{TA}/Flow$ [or $P_{set}/Flow$].) The maximum available flow is approximately equal to P_{set} divided by R_{aw} (Flow = P_{set}/R_{aw}). Flow = 12 cm H_2O/12 cm H_2O/L/sec = approximately 1 L/sec, or 60 L/min. This flow apparently is inadequate for the patient. The pressure needs to be increased to increase the available flow. (Note: If you got this answer correct, you're really beginning to use analytical thinking. This required the use of some advanced problem-solving skills and a modified equation that wasn't previously used. [Sometimes questions are used for teaching!])

19. The graphics show that T_I is short and flow is not returning to zero during inspiration. Increasing the T_I provides more time for Pset to reach the alveolar level and increase V_T delivery.

20. The patient's lung characteristics may have changed, and the current inspiratory pressure and/or flow are now too low, resulting in a longer T_I.

21. The machine is not set sensitive enough to the patient's inspiratory effort.

22. The patient has developed auto-PEEP since the setting change. A possible solution is to increase inspiratory gas flow to shorten T_I and increase T_E. Another possible solution is to return the ventilator to the previous settings and use a lower V_E to eliminate auto-PEEP.

23. Further information about the patient is needed before a solution can be found. Does the patient have ALI or ARDS? Is a recruitment maneuver indicated? Currently the PEEP is at zero. At the very least PEEP apparently needs to be set above the P_{FLEX} point. It would be better, depending on the patient's problem, to use the deflection point on the pressure-volume curve after a recruitment maneuver.

CHAPTER 19

Basic Concepts of Noninvasive Positive Pressure Ventilation

1. B
2. C
3. D
4. B
5. A
6. C
7. B
8. A
9. B

10. A
11. C
12. D
13. C
14. D
15. C

CHAPTER 20

Weaning and Discontinuation from Mechanical Ventilation

1. D
2. D
3. B
4. C
5. B
6. None of these techniques has proved to be unquestionably better than the others. IMV may increase weaning time compared with PSV and T-piece weaning.
7. A search for all factors that may be contributing to ventilator dependence must be undertaken with patients who require mechanical ventilation for longer than 24 hours.
8. A
9. D
10. D
11. C
12. A
13. A
14. B
15. D
16. A
17. B
18. C
19. A
20. A

CHAPTER 21

Long-Term Ventilation

1. C
2. B
3. D
4. C
5. D
6. A
7. C
8. C
9. C
10. A
11. D
12. B
13. B
14. C
15. C
16. D
17. A
18. A
19. A
20. B
21. D
22. B

23. C
24. D
25. D
26. Severity of illness, longevity of illness, multiple medications (sedatives, analgesics, psychotropics, steroids), sleep disruption, delirium, anxiety, depression.
27. Setting a long T_I and setting a PEEP level. Possibly increasing V_T if a significant leak is noted with cuff deflation.
28. Obstruct a port with the finger to direct the flow of gas through the vocal cords.
29. Deflate the cuff.
30. Comatose/unconscious patient, foam cuff in place or cuff must remain inflated, increased and/or thick secretions, severe upper airway obstruction, increased airway resistance and increased compliance that may cause air trapping (e.g., COPD), ET in place (not TT), reduced lung compliance, and laryngeal and pharyngeal dysfunction.

CHAPTER 22

Neonatal and Pediatric Mechanical Ventilation

1. C
2. D
3. C
4. B
5. B
6. A
7. D
8. B
9. D
10. A
11. D
12. C
13. C
14. B
15. B
16. A
17. A
18. C
19. B

CHAPTER 23

Special Techniques in Ventilatory Support

1. D
2. A
3. D
4. D
5. A
6. C
7. B
8. C
9. B
10. C
11. A
12. D
13. A
14. C
15. B
16. C
17. B

18. D
19. D
20. A

PART 2: CASE STUDY ANSWER KEY

CHAPTER 1: BASIC TERMS AND CONCEPTS OF MECHANICAL VENTILATION

Case Study 1-1

Determine Static Compliance (C_S) and Airway Resistance (R_{aw})

Compliance is 0.5/19, or 0.0263 L/cm H_2O (26.3 mL/cm H_2O), and R_{aw} is estimated to be 5 cm H_2O/L/s. The patient's compliance is very low, suggesting that some condition is making the lungs stiffer than normal and increasing her work of breathing. R_{aw} is low considering that the patient has an artificial airway in place.

CHAPTER 2: HOW VENTILATORS WORK

Case Study 2-1

Ventilator Selection

Because the patient's room has only piped-in oxygen, you would have to select an electrically powered ventilator with a built-in compressor. You could use an external 50 psig compressor, although some of these are very noisy. The availability of the oxygen source would allow you to provide oxygen as necessary for the patient.

CHAPTER 3: HOW A BREATH IS DELIVERED

Case Study 3-1

Patient Triggering

Problem 1: The machine is not sensitive enough to the patient's effort. The clinician should increase the ventilator sensitivity control.

Problem 2: The machine is too sensitive and is autotriggering into inspiration. The clinician should reduce the sensitivity.

Case Study 3-2

Premature Breath Cycling

The ventilator pressure-cycled when the patient coughed and increased the peak airway pressure sensed by the ventilator during the breath. With newer ICU ventilators, excess pressures are less likely to occur when a patient coughs because these devices incorporate "floating" exhalation valves.

CHAPTER 4: ESTABLISHING THE NEED FOR MECHANICAL VENTILATION

Case Study 4-1

Stroke Victim

The patient should be intubated to protect the airway and immediately evaluated for cerebral reperfusion therapy. The patient is typically admitted to the ICU after reperfusion therapy is completed for further evaluation (i.e., vital signs, S_pO_2 monitoring, ECG, breath sounds, ABG values, electrolytes, and neurologic status). Mechanical ventilation may be necessary if the patient remains unconscious and unresponsive. In cases where the patient is not receiving mechanical ventilation, aerosol therapy delivered through a Briggs T-adapter is required to prevent drying of secretions. Additional information regarding the treatment of stroke can be found at http://stroke.ahajournals.org/.

Case Study 4-2
Unexplained Acute Respiratory Failure

There are at least two possible solutions:

1. The problem may be drug related (e.g., narcotic overdose); try naloxone (Narcan).
2. Intubate and begin ventilation; assess further with vital signs, S_pO_2 monitoring, ECG, breath sounds, ABG values, electrolytes, blood alcohol levels, toxicology screening, and neurologic status evaluation.

Case Study 4-3
Ventilation in Neuromuscular Disorders

Case 1: In spite of this patient's inability to maintain a tight seal around the mouthpiece, the measured parameters are acceptable. It is prudent, however, to use a mouth seal for this patient for subsequent measurements. Continue to monitor MIP and VC for at least every 8 hours. Request an evaluation of an anticholinesterase challenge. Keep the patient NPO and provide suctioning at the bedside until swallowing ability can be evaluated. Monitor S_pO_2 and/or ABG values if symptoms become worse.

Case 2: The history and symptoms suggest Guillain-Barré syndrome. Assessment of this patient should include measurement of MIP and VC along with arterial blood gas analysis. A reduced MIP (<15 cm H_2O) and VC (<10 to 15 mL/kg) plus the presence of acute ventilatory failure would be consistent with respiratory muscle weakness associated with Guillain-Barré syndrome. Mechanical ventilation is indicated. Consider the advantages and disadvantages of using noninvasive ventilation, oral versus nasal endotracheal intubation, or consider a tracheostomy. The RT may also suggest an anticholinesterase challenge to confirm the diagnosis.

Case Study 4-4
Asthma Case

The patient's condition appears to be improving. Continue drug therapy, adjusting the medication dosages and frequency as necessary according to Expert Panel Review—3 recommendations. Continue to monitor the patient.

CHAPTER 5: SELECTING THE VENTILATOR AND THE MODE

Case Study 5-1
What Type of Breath Is It?

1. This is a patient-controlled machine breath. The V_T is delivered by the ventilator and the ventilator cycles the breath.
2. This is a spontaneous breath, and these variables describe CPAP. The patient is controlling the start time (trigger) and the V_T (cycle).

Case Study 5-2
Pressure Control (PC-CMV) or Volume Control Ventilation (VC-CMV)

1. When it is desirable to target P_aCO_2, volume control ventilation may be used because it can guarantee volume delivery and minute ventilation. With pressure control ventilation changes in lung compliance or R_{aw} will result in changes in V_T, which can ultimately affect P_aCO_2.
2. Pressure control ventilation should be used when the goal is to avoid high pressures.

CHAPTER 6: INITIAL VENTILATOR SETTINGS

Case Study 6-1
Minute Ventilation ($\dot{V}_E$) Needs

The ordered V_E is 500 mL × 12, or 6000 mL/min, or 6 L/min. The estimated $\dot{V}_E$ based on BSA (and metabolism) is 7 L/min. You might use VC-CMV with a set V_T of 500 mL and a minimum rate of 12 breaths/min. Assuming that the patient is not apneic and can also initiate spontaneous breaths, she could trigger additional breaths if needed to achieve a minute ventilation for the estimated metabolic needs.

Case Study 6-2
Minute Ventilation ($\dot{V}_E$), Tidal Volume (V_T), and Respiratory Rate

He has a BSA of 2.15 m^2. His IBW at 6 min, or 72 seconds, is 106 + 6(12) = 178 lb (81 kg). If a V_T of 7 mL/kg is used, the V_T is about 570 mL. V_E is 4 × 2.15 = 8.6 L/min, and the rate is (8.6 L/min)/(0.570 mL), or about 15 breaths/min.

Case Study 6-3
Inspiratory/Expiratory Ratio (I:E) and Flow

Her IBW is 145 lb (66 kg). (Use Fig. 6-1 and determine her BSA. Using actual weight and height BSA = 1.98 m^2.) Her V_E = BSA × 3.5 for a female. (Initial V_E = 1.98 × 3.5 = 6.93 L/min.) An initial V_T setting of 6 mL/kg IBW would be a reasonable starting point. (V_T = 6 mL/kg × 66 kg = 396 mL or approximately 400 mL.) An initial rate would be: f = V_E/V_T, f = (6.93 L/min)/400 mL = (6930 mL/min)/400 mL = 17.3 breaths/min. Setting the rate at 17 breaths/min would be appropriate. A constant flow of 30 L/min or 0.5 L/sec is set. Her T_I = V_T/flow (L/sec), T_I = 400 mL/(0.5 L/sec), T_I = 400 mL/(500 mL/sec), T_I = 0.8 sec.), her T_E = TCT − T_I; TCT = 60 sec/(17 breaths/min) = 3.5 sec; (T_E = 3.5 sec − 0.8 sec; T_E = 2.7 sec), and her I:E ratio would be 1:3.4 (T_I = 0.8 sec; T_E = 2.7 sec. I:E = (T_I/T_I)/(T_E/T_I) = (0.8 sec/0.8 sec)/(2.7 sec/0.8 sec)). This ratio would allow ample time for exhalation. In fact, the flow rate might be reduced if high peak pressures were present. (See the following section on inspiratory flow and flow patterns for more information on flow rates and peak pressures.)

Case Study 6-4
Tidal Volume (V_T) During Pressure Control Continuous Mandatory Ventilation (PC-CMV)

Assuming all other factors remain constant, the initial patient compliance (C) is 350 mL/12 cm H_2O = 29.1 mL/cm H_2O. To achieve a V_T of 550 mL, remember that C = ΔV/ΔP, and ΔP = ΔV/C; 550 mL/(29.1 mL/cm H_2O) equals a required pressure of 18.9 cm H_2O.

Case Study 6-5
Inspiratory Flow Termination in Pressure Support Ventilation (PSV)

Problem 1: The breath will end when flow drops to 12.5 L/min (i.e., 25% of peak flow).

Problem 2: The ventilator will continue to deliver flow until the maximum T_I limit is reached (usually 2 to 3 seconds, depending on the ventilator model).

Problem 3: The pressure–time graphic will show a sudden rise in the pressure at the end of the breath that is 2 to 3 cm H_2O higher than the preset pressure level. This rise in pressure will be detected by the ventilator and will pressure cycle the breath.

Case Study 6-6

Pressure-Regulated Volume Control (PRVC)

Because less pressure is required to deliver the same volume, the patient's lung characteristics may be improving. This would mean a drop in R_{aw} or an increase in C_S. The therapist may want to assess the patient to confirm this finding.

CHAPTER 7: FINAL CONSIDERATIONS IN VENTILATOR SETUP

Case Study 7-1

Auto-PEEP and Triggering

The patient must generate -8 cm H_2O to bring P_{alv} to 0, plus -1 cm H_2O to trigger the ventilator. Total effort is -9 cm H_2O.

Case Study 7-2

Key Questions for ARDS Patient

1. The initial indications for ventilation in this patient are increased WOB, impending respiratory failure, refractory hypoxemia, and inability to tolerate mask CPAP.

2. In terms of precipitating factors, he sustained a fracture of the left femur, which may cause fat emboli, and chest injuries that resulted in a pneumothorax. Bilateral fluffy infiltrates are present on a chest radiograph, and he has refractory hypoxemia (low P_aO_2 on a high F_IO_2).

3. He is 6 feet 2 inches tall and weighs 258 lb. BSA = 2.42 m²; initial $\dot{V}_E = (4 \times BSA) = 9.68$ L/min. Because this patient has experienced trauma, his metabolic rate may be elevated, which must be kept in mind when he is ventilated. IBW = 106 + 6(14) = 190 lb (86.4 kg); using values of 4 to 8 mL/kg, a V_T range of 345 mL to 690 mL is appropriate. The initial V_T of 690 mL (8 mL/kg) can be used to establish an initial f and will allow for further evaluation of the V_T setting when $P_{plateau}$ and auto-PEEP can be measured. f = $\dot{V}_E/V_T$ = 9.68/0.690 = 14 breaths/min. Flow should be set at 100 L/min to keep T_I short, and a descending ramp waveform should be used. VC-IMV + PSV or VC-CMV modes are equally acceptable. Pressure-controlled ventilation can be used instead of volume-controlled ventilation. It would be helpful to start with VC-CMV to establish the pressure needed to achieve the desired volume in pressure ventilation. PC-IMV + PSV and PC-CMV are equally acceptable. An initial PEEP of ≥5 cm H_2O and an F_IO_2 of 1 should be set.

Case Study 7-3

Troubleshooting: The Pulse Oximeter

Patients with CHF often demonstrate peripheral vasoconstriction thus limiting blood flow to their extremities. The pulse oximeter cannot register a value unless it detects a pulse (see Chapter 10). The respiratory therapist could try warming the patient's hand or using another site, such as the other hand or a toe. Testing the function of the pulse oximeter to see whether it is working properly is also a good idea.

CHAPTER 8: INITIAL PATIENT ASSESSMENT

Case Study 8-1

The Importance of Documentation

The legal inference is that if treatment is not documented, it is not done. The therapist must prove that he provided care despite a lack of documentation. He argued that he did not want to repeat the same information over and over and that he had "charted by exception." Fearing that a jury might not believe the therapist, the hospital settled the case out of court.

Case Study 8-2

Circuit Disconnect

The low-pressure alarm did not activate for several reasons. First, it may have been set too low and was not sensitive enough to the drop in pressure. Second, the bedding may have been occluding the Y-connector, thus keeping the pressure in the circuit above the low-pressure alarm level. The low-pressure alarm and the low V_T alarm must be set appropriately to avoid these types of situations. With a low volume returning to the exhalation side of the ventilator, the drop in V_T would have been detected and the low V_T alarm would have been activated. This would have alerted the respiratory therapist to a problem before the patient's monitor indicated tachycardia.

Case Study 8-3

Cuff Inflation Techniques

The MLT was used to set the cuff pressure so that a small leak existed at 13:00. This can be noted by the difference of 20 mL between the set volume (520 mL) and the measure exhaled volume (500 mL). Several hours later (the set volume is the same), the patient's condition improves such that less pressure is required to deliver the same volume. With a lower ventilating pressure, a leak no longer exists around the cuff. Note that the cuff pressure (20 mm Hg) is equal to about 27 cm H_2O. This is enough cuff pressure to prevent a leak when the ventilating pressure is only 23 cm H_2O. The MLT could be repeated if maintaining a leak is desirable for this patient.

Case Study 8-4

Patient Assessment Cases

Problem 1: Findings suggest that the patient has a respiratory infection. A chest radiograph and laboratory studies, including a white blood cell count, might confirm this diagnosis. The low-pitched rattles heard on auscultation (rhonchi) indicate secretions in the large airways. The patient may need to be suctioned. Also, a culture and sensitivity test of a sputum sample may be in order. Antibiotics may be indicated.

Problem 2: Pneumothorax on the left side.

Problem 3: Right mainstem intubation.

Case Study 8-5

Evaluating C_S and R_{aw} During Mechanical Ventilation

Problem 1: The increase in PIP and P_{TA} while $P_{plateau}$ remains constant indicates a change in R_{aw}. Listen to the breath sounds and try to determine the cause of the change (e.g., secretions, kink in the ET tube, or bronchospasm).

Problem 2: The decrease in V_T indicates a change in lung characteristics. Listen to the breath sounds and try to determine whether R_{aw} may have increased (i.e., presence of low-pitched rattling breath sounds [rhonchi] or wheezing) or whether the tube has become progressively occluded or is obstructed in some way. Crackles or changes in the percussion note may indicate a change in lung parenchyma that might reduce compliance (e.g., the development of pneumonia) or a completely obstructed airway that is causing the distal portion of the lung to collapse. Try to determine the cause of the change and correct it. Increase the set pressure to maintain ventilation if necessary.

CHAPTER 9: VENTILATOR GRAPHICS

Case Study 9-1

The two different breath types can be easily distinguishable by analyzing the pressure and flow scalars (see Fig. 9-11).

CHAPTER 10: ASSESSMENT OF RESPIRATORY FUNCTION

Case Study 10-1

Causes of Cyanosis

The patient had an adverse reaction to the benzocaine and developed methemoglobinemia, which could be verified by performing CO-oximetry. CO-oximetry would allow you to directly measure methemoglobin levels in the patient's blood. The treatment of acute methemoglobinemia is intravenous administration of methylene blue.

Case Study 10-2

Capnography During Intubation

Capnography is often used to assess the ET placement. In this case the ET was placed in the esophagus thus preventing the detection of any exhaled CO_2. Listening to breath sounds and reviewing the patient's chest radiographs can confirm this finding.

Case Study 10-3

Dead Space Ventilation

The application of +10 cm H_2O of PEEP may have caused a reduction in pulmonary perfusion resulting in an increase in dead space ventilation, which is evidenced by the shifting of the $SBCO_2$ curve to the right and the reduction in PCO_2. The reduction in S_pO_2 is consistent with an altered V/Q ratio, which would be associated with compression of the pulmonary capillaries by an excessive amount of $PEEP_E$ being administered.

CHAPTER 11: HEMODYNAMIC MONITORING

Case Study 11-1

Evaluation of Pressure Tracing

1. The catheter is located in a pulmonary artery.
2. Systolic and diastolic pressures are approximately 40/25 mm Hg. These values are measured during exhalation.

Case Study 11-2

Cardiac Index and Stroke Index

C.I. = $\dot{Q}$/BSA = (3 L/min)/(1.7 m²) = 1.76 L/min/m²

S.I. = SV/BSA; SV = $\dot{Q}$/HR = 3 L/min/110 beats/min = 0.027 L/beat or 27 mL/beat. S.I. = SV/BSA = 27 mL/beat/1.76 m² = 15.34 mL/beat/m². Cardiac index and stroke index are both lower than normal.

Case Study 11-3

Application of the Fick Principle

At 13:00 $\dot{Q}$ = (350/[20 – 14] × 10) = 4.7 L/min. At 15:00 $\dot{Q}$ is (350/[20 – 12] × 10) = 4.4 L/min. The decrease in $C\overline{V}O_2$ is associated with a decrease in cardiac output.

Case Study 11-4

Stroke Work

Left ventricular stroke work (LSW) = MAP × SV × 0.00136. And,

LSWI = LSW/BSA.

Before the medication LSW = 80 × 60 × 0.00136 = 6.53 kg-m. LSWI = 6.53 kg-m/1.5 m² = 4.35 kg-m/m². After the medication LSW = 100 × 70 × 0.00136 = 9.52 kg-m. LSWI = 9.52 kg-m/1.5 m² = 6.35 kg-m/m².

Case Study 11-5

Hemodynamic Monitoring: After Open-Heart Surgery

Calculate $C(a-\overline{v})O_2$ for before and after treatment: (ignore the dissolved portion).

Before: C_aO_2 = 0.90 × 13 × 1.34 = 15.7 vol%; $C\overline{v}O_2$ = 0.75 × 13 × 1.34 = 13.1 vol%; $C(a-\overline{v})O_2$ = 2.6 vol%. Calculate cardiac output before: $\dot{Q}$ = ($\dot{V}O_2$/$C(a-\overline{v})O_2$) × 100 = (250/2.6) × 100 = 9620 mL/min or 9.62 L/min.

After: C_aO_2 = 0.98 × 13 × 1.34 = 17.1 vol%; $C\overline{v}_2$ = 0.65 × 13 × 1.34 = 11.3 vol%; $C(a-\overline{v})O_2$ = 5.8 vol%.

Calculate cardiac output after: $\dot{Q}$ = ($\dot{V}O_2$/$C(a-\overline{v})O_2$) × 100 = (230/5.8) × 100 = 3956 mL/min or 3.96 L/min.

Cardiac output has dropped and the $C(a-\overline{v})O_2$ has increased as a result.

Case Study 11-6

Hemodynamic Monitoring: Chest Injury

It was determined that the pulmonary artery was torn during surgery and the patient's liver had been injured by a retractor. The low Hb is one indication of internal bleeding. The patient's hemodynamic status appears to be good. The only value that was significantly out of the normal range was the pulmonary artery pressure (PAP), which was probably elevated because of the medications that the patient was receiving.

Case Study 11-7

ICU and Hemodynamic Assessment

This case describes a patient with a pulmonary embolism, which is suggested by the refractory hypoxemia present. The fact that the PAP pressures are elevated with a normal PAOP is representative of a pulmonary condition as opposed to left heart failure. The CVP is within normal limits, indicating that the condition is acute because the right side of the heart has not yet been affected by the elevated pulmonary artery pressures.

CHAPTER 12: METHODS TO IMPROVE VENTILATION IN PATIENT-VENTILATOR MANAGEMENT

Case Study 12-1

Hyperventilation

The flow–time scalar shows that flow does not return to zero during exhalation before another mandatory breath occurs. Auto-PEEP (air trapping) is present. It is important to check ventilating pressures and keep $P_{plateau}$ below 30 cm H_2O to prevent lung injury. The physician should be notified that, in an effort to normalize the pH, the high $\dot{V}_E$ is causing auto-PEEP.

Case Study 12-2

Assessment During Suctioning

A sudden tachycardia is a possible complication of suctioning. The respiratory therapist should immediately stop the procedure, provide oxygen (100%), and ensure that the patient is receiving adequate ventilation, preferably using the ventilator to do so.

Case Study 12-3

Evaluation of Bronchodilator Therapy

Yes, the PIP decreased, the P_{TA} decreased by nearly 50%, and the PEFR increased by more than 50%.

Case Study 12-4

Evaluating Fluid Status

The most likely problem is low fluid volume. Fluid replacement is recommended.

CHAPTER 13: IMPROVING OXYGENATION AND MANAGEMENT OF ACUTE RESPIRATORY DISTRESS SYNDROME

Case Study 13-1

Myasthenia Gravis

The patient has respiratory acidosis. The P_aO_2 indicates moderate hypoxemia. A common reaction by clinicians in this situation is to increase the F_IO_2. However, the cause of the hypoxemia is the elevated CO_2. An increase in P_aCO_2 of 1 mm Hg will reduce the P_aO_2 by 1.25 mm Hg (see Chapter 1). The P_aCO_2 is about 40 mm Hg above normal, therefore the P_aO_2 will be about 50 mm Hg below its actual value. The most appropriate way to increase the P_aO_2 is to increase ventilation.

Case Study 13-2

Changing F_IO_2

Desired $F_IO_2 = (60 \times 0.75)/40 = 1.13$

No, this is not possible. You cannot give more than 100% oxygen. Along with increasing the F_IO_2 to 1, another method of improving oxygenation is to use PEEP.

Case Study 13-3

Problem Solving: Infant CPAP

This is a common problem encountered when using CPAP in the treatment of infants. The flow from the CPAP device is leaking out of the infant's mouth because the infant is crying. The CPAP levels cannot be maintained. Once the infant stops crying, the problem will correct itself.

Case Study 13-4

Selecting Optimum PEEP

P_aO_2 progressively increases as expected with an increase in PEEP and FRC. $P\bar{v}O_2$ is low initially (about 50% saturation, assuming that pH is close to normal), progressively improves to 38 mm Hg, and then declines. At the same setting (20 cm H_2O PEEP), BP falls. $P\bar{v}O_2$ declines because of a drop in cardiac output (assuming that $\dot{V}O_2$ is constant). The optimum PEEP level for the patient at this time is 15 cm H_2O. The next step is to reduce the F_IO_2.

Case Study 13-5

Changing Patient Position

The most likely cause is a ventilation/perfusion mismatch caused by rotation of the affected lung in the dependent position. With unilateral lung disease, it is best to position the good lung down, in the dependent position.

Another possible problem is thromboembolism; repositioning of patients sometimes causes clots to move.

A third possible problem is a compromised airway; the airway would need to be checked for proper function.

CHAPTER 14: VENTILATOR-ASSOCIATED PNEUMONIA

Case Study 14-1

Patient Case—VAP

His CPIS is 7 and his condition does warrant initiation of a broad range antibiotic.

Case Study 14-2

Patient Case—Methicillin-Resistant S. aureus

An appropriate antibiotic regimen would include Linezolid (600 mg every 12 hours) or vancomycin (15 mg/kg every 12 hours).

CHAPTER 15: SEDATIVES, ANALGESICS, AND PARALYTICS

Case Study 15-1

Patient Case—Discontinuing Lorazepam

Long-term use (longer than just a few months) of lorazepam can lead to physical dependence. The most common side effects that can occur when this patient suddenly stops taking his medication include nausea, vomiting, agitation, and insomnia. Other possible side effects include tremors, muscle cramping and spasms, and seizures.

Case Study 15-2

Patient Case—Agitated Patient

Fentanyl, which is a synthetic opioid, would be an effective choice for treating this patient. Fentanyl possesses analgesic and sedative properties. Morphine would not normally be used with this type of patient due to her unstable hemodynamic status.

Case Study 15-3

Patient Case—Asynchrony

Asynchrony cannot be corrected through ventilator adjustment, therefore it is appropriate to use a sedative and, if necessary, a paralyzing agent to reduce patient-ventilator asynchrony.

Case Study 15-4

Patient Case—Neuromuscular Blocking Agent

The NMBA that would be appropriate for this patient would be a depolarizing agent such as succinylcholine. It is indicated in patients who are hemodynamically stable. It can cause increases in intracranial pressure and should not be used in patients with cerebral edema and head trauma. Succinylcholine has been widely used for cases of emergency intubation because of its relatively low cost, rapid onset of action, and short duration of action.

CHAPTER 16: EXTRAPULMONARY EFFECTS OF MECHANICAL VENTILATION

Case Study 16-1

The Effects of Ventilator Changes on Blood Pressure

The increases in V_T and respiratory rate have resulted in a substantial increase in the mean airway pressure, which in turn has caused the patient's BP to drop. With this large a V_T and this high an RR, auto-PEEP may also be contributing to the rising peak and mean airway pressures. The RT should determine whether the V_T setting is appropriate for this patient (maximum ~8 mL/kg IBW). The RT also might recommend the use of VC-IMV or PC-IMV, rather than VC-CMV, and reduce the mandatory rate. PSV might be added to support spontaneous breaths.

CHAPTER 17: EFFECTS OF POSITIVE PRESSURE VENTILATION ON THE PULMONARY SYSTEM

Case Study 17-1

Peak Pressure Alarm Activating

Physical findings indicate the presence of a right-sided pneumothorax. A physician should be contacted immediately for an order for a chest radiograph and to begin treatment. The respiratory therapist should stay with the patient and make sure the pneumothorax does not become a tension pneumothorax. Appropriate emergency equipment (e.g., an emergency resuscitation cart) should be kept close at hand. Depending on the circumstances, the respiratory therapist may need to ventilate the patient manually until treatment can be administered.

Case Study 17-2

Patient Case—Acute Pancreatitis

The crackles in the basilar and posterior areas may indicate atelectasis and the opening and closing of alveoli in dependent areas. An increase in PEEP is indicated, and a recruitment maneuver might also be considered (see Chapter 13).

Case Study 17-3

Appropriate Ventilator Changes

The ABG values after 7 days of PPV are normal. However, this patient's baseline ABG values suggest chronic CO_2 retention. The patient has been hyperventilated with the ventilator, and the kidneys have reduced the bicarbonate level to normal. When the mandatory rate is reduced for weaning, the patient's P_aCO_2 rises, stimulating spontaneous ventilation. Unfortunately, the patient cannot maintain a normal P_aCO_2 and pH, as suggested by the high spontaneous rate. To correct the problem, the patient's mandatory rate must be reduced gradually until normal baseline ABG values are restored (i.e., pH = 7.38, P_aCO_2 = 51 mm Hg, P_aO_2 = 58 mm Hg, HCO_3^- = 29 mEq/L). Appropriate PSV for spontaneous breaths should also be provided.

Case Study 17-4

Difficulty Triggering in a Patient with COPD

The new V_E is 11.7 L/min. The increase in V_E resulted in auto-PEEP, which caused the rise in PIP and the transient drop in exhaled V_T that occurred after the change. Also, the patient is unable to trigger the ventilator, another possible indication of air trapping.

CHAPTER 18: TROUBLESHOOTING AND PROBLEM SOLVING

Case Study 18-1

Evaluating Severe Respiratory Distress in a Ventilated Patient

The patency of the airway can be used to rule out upper airway obstruction; auscultation of the patient's breath sounds can be used to rule out any sudden change in the patient's lung condition, such as the presence of secretions or the occurrence of a pneumothorax. The sudden oxygen desaturation that occurs simultaneously with a drop in end-tidal CO_2 suggests the possibility of a pulmonary embolus. This cannot be confirmed easily and requires further radiographic evaluation.

In this case a pulmonary embolism was later confirmed. Aside from attempts to increase oxygenation, little can be done for this problem through ventilator management and immediate medical intervention is required.

Case Study 18-2

Evaluating Peak Inspiratory Pressure (PIP) and Plateau Pressure ($P_{plateau}$) in Volume-Controlled (VC) Ventilation

Based on the pressure findings, C_L is progressively decreasing. PIP and $P_{plateau}$ are increasing while the difference between them (P_{ta}) remains relatively constant, which suggests that R_{aw} has not changed. ARDS is a possible diagnosis based on the physical findings, the chest radiograph, and the patient's history.

Case Study 18-3

Evaluating PIP and Volume in Pressure Control Ventilation

This patient, with a history of asthma, may be experiencing increased bronchial constriction and increased secretions. The drop in volume may be associated with increased R_{aw}. The flow–volume loop indicates increased R_{aw}, and the wheezing supports this finding. Activation of the alarms resulted from two different causes. The high pressure alarm was activated by the patient's coughing and forceful exhalations; the low volume alarm was activated by the reduction in volume delivery associated with increased R_{aw} during pressure ventilation. The patient most likely needs bronchodilator therapy and possibly IV corticosteroids and suctioning.

Case Study 18-4

Problem Solving Using Ventilator Graphics

The flow–time and volume–time curves in Fig. 18-7 show a greater inspired volume than exhaled volume, which indicates a leak in the system.

Case Study 18-5

Evaluating a Ventilator Problem

In this situation the exhalation valve was malfunctioning. A gas leak apparently occurred through the valve, causing the baseline pressure to begin dropping. The ventilator increased gas flow delivery to try to compensate for the drop in PEEP. This moved air through the exhalation valve, which was measured by the flow transducer, resulting in an upward swing of the volume curve at the end of exhalation. The problem was corrected when the expiratory valve was changed. Perhaps you can think of another possible cause of this situation.

CHAPTER 19: BASIC CONCEPTS OF NONINVASIVE POSITIVE PRESSURE VENTILATION

Case Study 19-1

Patient Selection for NIV

Oxygenation and respiratory status appear to be acceptable, but close assessment reveals several risk factors that may compromise the patient's safety. The patient's ability to cough and swallow have deteriorated, reflecting her inability to protect the airway adequately. This places her at a very high risk for aspiration. The patient also has become more agitated and confused in the past hour, which could indicate worsening hypercarbia. The correct action at this time would be to intubate the patient and initiate invasive ventilation. Delaying this process would cause further clinical deterioration and increase morbidity and mortality.

Case Study 19-2

Monitoring and Adjusting NIV

The symptoms of dyspnea, agitation, and increased respiratory rate reveal inadequate clinical improvement from NIV. Two things need to be considered at this time. Currently, the patient's average exhaled V_T is only 3 to 4 mL/kg of the patient's body weight; this contributes to his rapid respiratory rate and may promote auto-PEEP. The practitioner should attempt to increase the patient's exhaled V_T to 6 to 8 mL/kg by increasing IPAP. The use of a full-face mask may increase the potential for CO_2 rebreathing, especially if EPAP levels are not set adequately. Increasing EPAP levels will increase the flow of gas to the mask during exhalation and reduce the potential for rebreathing of CO_2. Increasing EPAP also may reduce WOB. However, if EPAP is increased without increasing IPAP, the gradient between IPAP and EPAP (or the pressure support level) will decrease, resulting in a lower delivered V_T. Therefore, if EPAP is increased, IPAP also must be increased to ensure adequate pressure support for greater V_T delivery to the patient. (NOTE: If auto-PEEP is present, elevating EPAP may also make it easier for the patient to trigger a breath [see Chapter 7].)

Case Study 19-3

Common Complications of NIV

Improvement in gas exchange and other symptoms related to chronic hypoventilation may take several weeks to occur for those who use NIV only intermittently. Patients who can tolerate NIV for at least 4 to 6 hours in each 24-hour period are most likely to show improvement in symptoms. This patient's lack of compliance and intolerance of NIV is most likely responsible for his poor physiological improvement. Nasal dryness and congestion is a common complication of NIV, and every effort should be made to minimize its occurrence. A room-temperature humidifier attached to the CPAP machine adds moisture and often is helpful for patients with nasal drying or congestion. Cold, dry air coming directly from the CPAP mask may increase nasal resistance by means of increased nasal congestion. Heated humidification is more expensive but may be attempted in particularly difficult cases. Nasal irritation and congestion may be treated with nasal sprays containing steroids, ipratropium, or antihistamines. Patients with persistent difficulties may benefit from referral to an ear, nose, and throat specialist.

Treatment with decongestants, inhaled (nasal) steroids, or cromolyn sodium; humidification; and in some cases nasal surgery can control nasal symptoms in most patients. However, a few will continue to find nasal CPAP uncomfortable because of high nasal resistance.

CHAPTER 20: WEANING AND DISCONTINUATION FROM MECHANICAL VENTILATION

Case Study 20-1

Evaluation of Weaning Attempt

The patient's spontaneous rate has risen progressively as the spontaneous V_T has decreased. Without any further information, these two findings strongly suggest that the patient's WOB has dramatically increased as the mandatory IMV rate has decreased. To assist the patient, return the IMV rate to a higher level (e.g., 4 breaths/min or more) and add PSV to support the patient's spontaneous breathing efforts. The use of low levels of PEEP/CPAP (3 to 5 cm H_2O) is also appropriate. Furthermore, evening is approaching. The patient probably needs to rest for the night, which means a return to full ventilatory support.

Case Study 20-2

Calculation of Rapid Shallow Breathing Index (RSBI)

Patient 1: The index is 10/0.4, or 25, which indicates readiness to wean from mechanical ventilation.

Patient 2: The index is 30/0.25, or 120; therefore weaning is not recommended.

Case Study 20-3

Failed Weaning Attempt

One possible cause relates to cardiac function. Based on the patient's history of a myocardial infarction, he may be experiencing increased left ventricular preload and a shift in blood volume to the central veins, which may lead to cardiogenic pulmonary edema, as demonstrated by the rise in wedge pressure, albeit no dysrhythmias are present. One solution to this problem might be the administration of diuretics in an effort to reduce the fluid volume and treat the cardiac problem.

CHAPTER 21: LONG-TERM VENTILATION

Case Study 21-1

Patient Case—Difficulty Weaning

It would be appropriate to assess the patient further to determine why he is having difficulty weaning from the ventilator and whether he meets the criteria for discharge. It may be related to his chronic condition (ALS) or his previous MIs left him unable to support ventilation. In either case, he may require slower weaning attempts. If his condition is medically stable and meets the criteria for discharge, transfer to an intermediate or long-term care facility probably would be the best course.

Case Study 21-2

Patient Case—Communication Difficulty

The respiratory therapist might consider a speaking valve. This might help the patient phonate without requiring a change of the tracheostomy tube. Careful evaluation of the patient's ability to use the valve would be required to ensure that the apparatus is beneficial considering the level of ventilatory support.

CHAPTER 22: NEONATAL AND PEDIATRIC MECHANICAL VENTILATION

Case Study 22-1

Assessment and Treatment of a Newborn

Clinical assessment of this patient should include prompt measurement of vital signs and S_pO_2. Clinical signs call for nasal CPAP or surfactant administration. The patient should be attached to an electrocardiograph–respiratory rate monitor, and a chest radiograph should be taken immediately. The typical approach for a patient this size is to first start with nasal CPAP and if the infant shows ongoing signs of respiratory distress and increasing oxygenation, then a blood gas should be obtained. Additionally, he may benefit from a dose of surfactant with immediate extubation to CPAP. ABG analysis should be considered. Based on the history and clinical presentation, respiratory distress syndrome is the most likely diagnosis and should be ruled out first.

Case Study 22-2

Adjustments to Home Therapy

The RT primarily faces the challenge of helping to clear and manage this patient's secretions. The patient may have developed pneumonia.

However, the chest radiograph showed extensive atelectasis in the right middle and lower lobes. Atelectasis was also seen on the left at the lingular area. Many patients with neuromuscular disorders can be ventilated quite effectively with noninvasive devices. However, secretions, which can obstruct and cause plugging of the airways, persistently affect some patients.

The RT immediately recruited the parents to help develop a home care plan that would provide cough assist and chest physical therapy. On the RT's recommendation, the patient was admitted to the hospital's intermediate care unit. The clinical staff, along with the parents, introduced the patient to the cough-assist device, which had never been used with this patient. The parents were taught to perform chest physical therapy. Although some nasotracheal suctioning was necessary on the first day of admission, this was soon replaced with frequent use of the cough-assist device, followed by suctioning of the hypopharynx with a Yankauer suction tube. The RT also evaluated the patient on a BiPAP ventilator and determined that both IPAP and EPAP should be increased.

Case Study 22-3
Patient Case—Acute Status Asthmaticus

Despite the helium/oxygen mixture, R_{aw} for this patient probably is quite high. The RT should evaluate pressure and flow scalar waveforms. It may be that with the T_I of 0.9 second, the set inspiratory pressure cannot be reached before the time limit. Flow, which normally tapers to zero in pressure control breaths, may be terminated prematurely. Some clinicians call this situation *flow chop*. The RT should recommend an increase in the T_I and adjustment of the inspiratory time, which would probably achieve a higher V_T. Also, the RT should monitor the patient's flow during the expiratory phase of each breath. It might be necessary to reduce the ventilator rate, providing additional expiratory time to allow expiratory flow to return to baseline.

Case Study 22-4
Recommending Changes in Ventilator Settings

Although many patients treated for pneumonia respond very well to the Pressure Control/CMV, some develop areas of atelectasis. This may be a result of secretions and airway plugging, or it may be associated with a progressive loss of pulmonary compliance secondary to the acute pneumonitis. An early sign of progressive lung collapse is tachypnea with deteriorating V_T on this mode of ventilation. Although the patient's $\dot{V}_E$ has not dropped, oxygenation has been affected. Some might consider keeping the patient on this mode and increasing the inspiratory pressure and PEEP settings. Because the clinical condition is worsening, the patient should be switched from a pressure control mode to a volume control mode. The change to a volume control mode of ventilation will restore lung volumes, particularly FRC and V_T. It is becoming increasingly more common to use volume control or dual-control modes of ventilation in patients to prevent lung collapse that may not be able to be maintained during pressure control.

Case Study 22-5
Evaluation of PRVC Dual-Control Mode

In this example the patient is not tolerating PRVC due to a leaky ET. In some cases, dual-control modes should not be advocated with leaky ETs. In this particular case, the ventilator servo-controls or adjusts pressure based on a measured inspiratory tidal volume. However, because there is a large leak present, the ventilator is initially sensing a tidal volume that is greater than the preset volume, improved compliance, and the ventilator weans the inspiratory pressure. A larger ET leak during PRVC can result in erroneous weaning

of the inspiratory pressure, placing the patient at greater risk for hypoventilation and lung collapse. Conversely, dual-control modes that regulate pressure based on exhaled tidal volume may over-expand lung units. Patients that have large ET leaks may be better supported using pressure control modes that will hold a constant pressure in the lungs without the risk of inappropriate weaning of the inspiratory pressure.

Case Study 22-6
Interpretation and Response to Monitored Data

The physician and RCP should continue to monitor the $\dot{V}CO_2$. With an increase in PEEP, additional lung units probably have been recruited, leading to an increase in CO_2 elimination at the airway. In this situation the $\dot{V}CO_2$ usually rises to a plateau and then drops slightly. If an inappropriate amount of PEEP had been added, the $\dot{V}CO_2$ most likely would have decreased because of an increase in dead space.

Case Study 22-7
Patient Case—Acute Respiratory Distress Syndrome Managed with HFO

The RT should suggest lowering the mean airway pressure setting. Significant recruitment of lung units may have taken place over the short time the patient has been on the oscillator. The mean airway pressure may be so high at this point that overdistention could be contributing to dead space ventilation. In this situation, reducing the mean airway pressure for a short time often is a good idea to see whether oxygenation improves.

Case Study 22-8
Determining Appropriateness of Nitric Oxide Therapy

RTs often are called upon to administer nitric oxide to patients whose condition is refractory to oxygen therapy. It is essential that the underlying cause of the hypoxemia be identified before iNO is given. In some cases administration of iNO could worsen the patient's condition. Almost all infants and children who are candidates for iNO should undergo echocardiography (ECHO). In this infant's case, the RT asked whether ECHO had been done to confirm a diagnosis of PPHN. ECHO was ordered, and a critical coarctation of the aorta was identified. It was also determined that the aortic arch was moderately hypoplastic. Although the infant's condition was serious, he was relatively hemodynamically stable because of right-to-left shunting, presumably through the PDA and patent foramen ovale (PFO). If nitric oxide had been given, pulmonary vasodilation would have occurred, reducing the shunting of blood from the pulmonary to the systemic circulation. The result most likely would have been profound systemic hypotension.

CHAPTER 23: SPECIAL TECHNIQUES IN VENTILATORY SUPPORT

Case Study 23-1
Patient Assessment During HFOV

The most likely cause is a pneumothorax. Given the tracheal shift, it may be a tension pneumothorax.

Case Study 23-2
Calculating Gas Flows During Heliox Therapy

The correction factor for 70:30 is 1.6. At a flow of 10 L/min, the actual flow will be 1.6×10, or 16 L/min.

PART 3: CRITICAL CARE CONCEPTS ANSWER KEY

CHAPTER 1: BASIC TERMS AND CONCEPTS OF MECHANICAL VENTILATION

Critical Care Concept 1-1

Calculate Pressure

Remember that if $C = \Delta V / \Delta P$, then ΔP is $\Delta V / C$. With a volume of 0.5 L and a compliance of 0.1 L/cm H_2O, Pressure = 5 L/0.1 cm H_2O, or 5 cm H_2O. A P_{alv} change of 5 cm H_2O would be required to achieve a 0.5 L V_T in a person with normal C_L.

CHAPTER 2: HOW VENTILATORS WORK

Critical Care Concept 2-1

Open Loop or Closed Loop

This is a closed-loop system. The ventilator is providing a specific F_IO_2 and monitors S_pO_2. The ventilator can detect changes in S_pO_2 and change the F_IO_2 setting. Whether this is a good idea is a matter of opinion. It can be argued that this would provide a safeguard for patients who suddenly become hypoxemic. It could also be argued that oxygen saturation monitors are not reliable enough and could give erroneous readings, resulting in an inappropriate ventilator response.

CHAPTER 5: SELECTING THE VENTILATOR AND THE MODE

Critical Care Concept 5-1

Volume-Controlled Breaths with Changing Lung Characteristics

1. About 1 second and it does not change between *A*, *B*, or *C*.
2. This is a constant flow waveform, also called a *rectangular* or *square* waveform.
3. The V_T is about 500 mL.
4. PIP at *A* is about 14 cm H_2O, at *B* it is about 25 cm H_2O, and at *C* it is about 12 cm H_2O.
5. Lung compliance decreases with pneumonia, ARDS, pulmonary fibrosis, or pulmonary scarring, such as can occur with lung cancer. Compliance also decreases with pneumothorax and pleural effusions. Changes in the abdominal wall, such as occur with ascites, can elevate the diaphragm and reduce compliance. Placing a patient in the prone position reduces thoracic compliance. Burns and surgical incisions in the chest wall reduce thoracic compliance.
6. If compliance remains the same but airway resistance increases, more pressure will be required to deliver gas flow. PIP will increase.

Critical Care Concept 5-2

Pressure-Controlled Breaths with Changing Lung Characteristics

1. The pressure curve is constant.
2. The waveform during inspiration is basically a descending (decelerating) ramp. It might also be called an *exponential descending flow waveform*.

3. The flow–time curve in *A* drops to zero just at the end of inspiration. The flow curve in *C* drops to zero before the end of inspiration.
4. The volume curve in *C* has a short plateau at the top that begins when flow drops to zero during inspiration and ends when exhalation starts. It is flat because the volume is not changing. Because the flow is zero during this time interval, no more volume is going into the lungs.
5. The volume delivery at *B* is higher than at *A* because the lungs in *B* are more compliant than the lungs in *A*.

CHAPTER 6: INITIAL VENTILATOR SETTINGS

Critical Care Concept 6-1

Tidal Volume (V_T) and Ideal Body Weight (IBW)

The lowest V_T would be 390 mL (6 mL/kg × 65 kg = 390 mL) and the highest V_T would be 520 mL (8 mL/kg × 65 kg = 520 mL). A woman of the same height (5 feet 6 inches) would have an IBW of 61 kg. The female's lowest V_T would be 366 mL (6 mL/kg × 61 kg = 366 mL) and the highest V_T would be 732 mL (8 mL/kg × 61 kg = 488 mL).

Critical Care Concept 6-2

Inspiratory Flow in a Time-Cycled Ventilator

TCT = 5 seconds (60 sec/12 breaths = 5 seconds for each breath); I : E ratio = 1 : 4; T_I = 5 sec/5 = 1 second; T_E = 4 seconds. Inspiration must be delivered in 1 second. Flow = Volume/Time = 0.5 L/1 sec. Convert time to a minute; flow = (0.5 L)/sec = (0.5 L × 60 sec)/(1 sec × 1 min) = 30 L/min.

CHAPTER 11: HEMODYNAMIC MONITORING

Critical Care Concept 11-1

Fick Principle

Q = VO_2 / ($C_aO_2 - C_vO_2$)

   Q = 300 mL/min / (180 mL/L of whole blood – 130 mL/L of whole blood)

   Q = 6 L/min

CHAPTER 16: EXTRAPULMONARY EFFECTS OF MECHANICAL VENTILATION

Critical Care Concept 16-1

Calculating Cardiac Transmural Pressure

Problem 1: First, convert to similar units: 1 mm Hg = 1.36 cm H_2O; therefore 150 mm Hg = 204 cm H_2O. $P_{TM} = P_{inside} - P_{outside} = $ (204 cm H_2) – (+10 cm H_2O) = 194 cm H_2O

Problem 2: P_{TM} = (204 cm H_2) – (–10 cm H_2O) = 214 cm H_2O

The higher P_{TM} value during spontaneous breathing increased the LV afterload compared with PPV.

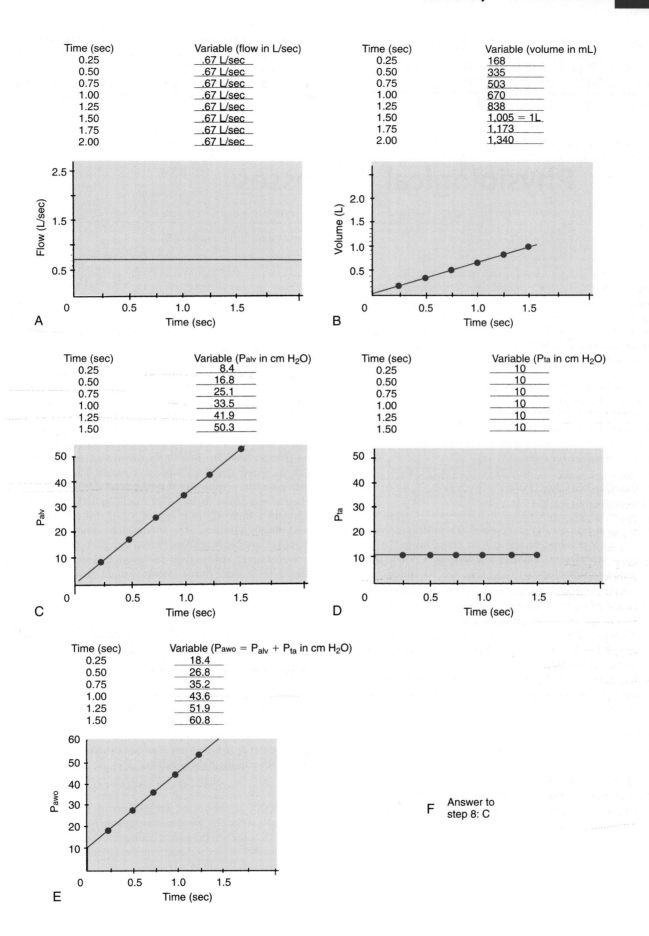

Time (sec)	Variable (flow in L/sec)
0.25	.67 L/sec
0.50	.67 L/sec
0.75	.67 L/sec
1.00	.67 L/sec
1.25	.67 L/sec
1.50	.67 L/sec
1.75	.67 L/sec
2.00	.67 L/sec

A

Time (sec)	Variable (volume in mL)
0.25	168
0.50	335
0.75	503
1.00	670
1.25	838
1.50	1,005 = 1L
1.75	1,173
2.00	1,340

B

Time (sec)	Variable (P_{alv} in cm H_2O)
0.25	8.4
0.50	16.8
0.75	25.1
1.00	33.5
1.25	41.9
1.50	50.3

C

Time (sec)	Variable (P_{ta} in cm H_2O)
0.25	10
0.50	10
0.75	10
1.00	10
1.25	10
1.50	10

D

Time (sec)	Variable ($P_{awo} = P_{alv} + P_{ta}$ in cm H_2O)
0.25	18.4
0.50	26.8
0.75	35.2
1.00	43.6
1.25	51.9
1.50	60.8

E

F Answer to
step 8: C

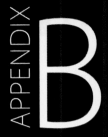

Review of Abnormal Physiological Processes

MISMATCHING OF PULMONARY PERFUSION AND VENTILATION

Pathologic pulmonary conditions can result in loss of perfusion and/or loss of ventilation to various areas of the lung. These abnormal conditions include dead space, intrapulmonary shunt, ventilation/perfusion abnormalities (also called $\dot{V}/\dot{Q}$ mismatching), and diffusion defects. Figure B-1 illustrates an extreme case of uneven ventilation and uneven blood flow. Each of these various conditions will be reviewed.

PHYSIOLOGICAL DEAD SPACE AND ITS CLINICAL MONITORING

Physiological dead space (V_D) is defined as ventilation of lung areas, which are not perfused, resulting in no gas exchange (i.e., ventilation without perfusion). Physiological dead space (V_{Dphys}) is divided into anatomical dead space (V_{Danat}) (Fig. B-2, *A*), which comprises the conductive airways down to the level of the respiratory bronchioles where gas exchange begins, and alveolar dead space (V_{Dalv}), where alveoli are ventilated but unperfused or underperfused, respectively. Physiological dead space is therefore the sum of the anatomical and alveolar dead space: $V_{Dphys} = V_{Danat} + V_{Dalv}$.[1]

V_{Danat} is about 1 mL/lb of ideal body weight (IBW) or about 2 mL/kg of IBW. In an average-sized, 150-pound adult, the anatomical dead space is about 150 mL per breath. In normal healthy individuals, physiological dead space and anatomical dead space are approximately equal, and V_{Dalv} is not significant. Anatomical dead space seldom changes in clinical situations. V_{Danat} can be lower than normal when an endotracheal tube or a tracheostomy tube is in place, bypassing the upper airway. V_D can be artificially increased by adding mechanical dead space (V_{Dmech}). (This will be discussed in more detail later.)

Increased V_{Dalv} can occur with such conditions as pulmonary thromboemboli, pulmonary vascular injury, pulmonary vascular disorders, chronic obstructive pulmonary disease (COPD), and regional hypotension. Increases in V_{Dalv} cause $\dot{V}/\dot{Q}$ mismatching. V_{Dalv} can produce hypoxemia and hypercarbia. Patients with increased V_{Dalv} often have the following characteristic findings: normal lung volumes; normal lung mechanics; increased ventilation (hypoxemic response); normal distribution of ventilation in most cases; uneven distribution of capillary blood flow in the lungs; decreased diffusing capacity; hypoxemia; and normal or increased partial pressure of arterial carbon dioxide (P_aCO_2). Pulmonary embolism is an example of a classic dead space disorder. Pulmonary embolism reduces pulmonary perfusion without necessarily altering ventilation (Fig. B-2, *B*).

Patients receiving mechanical ventilation can have increased V_{Dalv} if high ventilating pressures cause overexpansion of the alveoli, which in turn exerts pressure on adjacent capillaries, reducing effective flow (Fig. B-2, *C*). Increased V_{Dalv} can also be present with increased shunting. Suppose a patient had left lower lobe atelectasis. The perfusion to that area would likely be near normal, whereas ventilation to that area would be reduced. This would represent a shunt ($\dot{Q}$ in excess of $\dot{V}$). If this patient was being mechanically ventilated, the affected lobe might not be as well ventilated as other lung areas. Pressurized gas would favor uncompromised areas, reduce their perfusion, and cause a dead space effect to those areas. Thus, a combined shunt and dead space condition would exist, as illustrated by the extreme case in Figure B-1.

If a patient with COPD were given therapeutic oxygen, the oxygen might decrease the pulmonary artery pressure by opening up pulmonary capillaries that were previously constricted because of alveolar hypoxemia. However, these newly opened capillaries would allow blood to flow past unventilated alveoli and thus divert pulmonary blood flow away from areas of better ventilation. The result might cause an increased V_{Dalv}.

For these various reasons, it is beneficial to monitor V_D in critically ill patients and monitor for changes in V_{Dphys}. One way is to measure the dead space to tidal volume ratio (V_D/V_T). Normal V_D/V_T is about 0.25 to 0.40. V_D/V_T can be calculated from the Enghoff modification of the Bohr equation:

$$V_D/V_T = (P_aCO_2 - P_ECO_2)/P_aCO_2$$

where P_ECO_2 is the mixed expired partial pressure of carbon dioxide, V_D is the physiological dead space, V_T is the tidal volume, and P_aCO_2 is the arterial partial pressure for carbon dioxide.

Figure B-3 shows a classic representation of a procedure for determining V_D/V_T. In this example:

$$P_aCO_2 = 40 \text{ mm Hg}, P_ECO_2 = 20 \text{ mm Hg},$$
$$V_T = 500, \text{ and } V_D/V_T = (40-20)/40 = 0.50$$

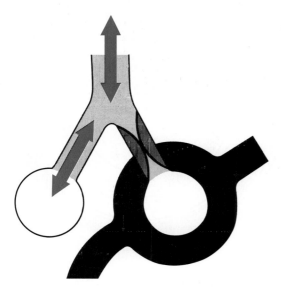

Fig. B-1 Extreme cases of uneven ventilation and uneven pulmonary perfusion. *Circles* represent groups of alveoli with their pulmonary capillary blood flow. *Gray areas* represent the conductive airways (anatomical dead space), and *arrows* represent the distribution of ventilation. The alveolus on the left receives all the ventilation but no perfusion, representing an extreme case of alveolar dead space. The alveolus on the right receives all of the blood flow but is not ventilated because of an obstructed airway. This represents an extreme case of intrapulmonary shunt. (From Comroe JH, Forster RE, DuBois AB, et al: The lung: clinical physiology and pulmonary function tests, ed 2, Chicago, 1973, Year Book Med Publishers.)

The amount of ventilation that is not involved in gas exchange (unperfused alveoli) is 50%. Because the V_T is 500 mL, the V_D will be 0.50×500 mL, or 250 mL.

Use of end-tidal CO_2 monitoring can also be useful in tracking changes in dead space. For example, when a pulmonary embolism occurs, there may be a significant decrease in the end-tidal PCO_2 and an increase in the arterial-to-end-tidal PCO_2 gradient (see Chapter 10). However, this finding by itself is not conclusive evidence of increased V_{Dalv} because end-tidal PCO_2 decreases with increased alveolar ventilation ($\dot{V}_A$) and an improvement in $\dot{V}/\dot{Q}$ matching. Another technique for determining physiological dead space is to use volumetric capnography, as described in Chapter 10.

CALCULATION OF MECHANICAL DEAD SPACE VOLUME NEEDED TO INCREASE P_aCO_2

On very rare occasions it may be beneficial to increase a patient's P_aCO_2 when hypocapnia is associated with an increase in minute ventilation that cannot be controlled for some reason (see Chapter 6, Mechanical Dead Space Considerations). When adding V_{Dmech} is desirable, the amount needed can be calculated using the equation in Box B-1. The dead space is added between the endotracheal tube and the patient Y-connector on the ventilator circuit.

SOME CAUSES OF HYPOXEMIA

Changes in the lung that compromise the ability of oxygen to transfer from the alveolus to the pulmonary capillary result in hypoxemia. This hypoxemia results in lower than normal partial pressure of arterial oxygen (P_aO_2) and a higher than normal

Types of respiratory dead space

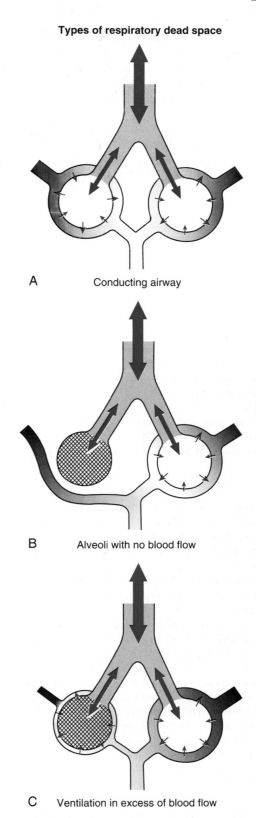

A   Conducting airway

B   Alveoli with no blood flow

C   Ventilation in excess of blood flow

Fig. B-2 Three types of dead space. **A,** Anatomic dead space represented by the conductive airways. **B,** Alveolar dead space because of alveoli with no blood flow. **C,** Alveolar dead space because of ventilation in excess of perfusion (alveolus on the left). See text for further explanation. (From Comroe JH, Forster RE, DuBois AB, et al: The lung: clinical physiology and pulmonary function tests, ed 2, Chicago, 1973, Year Book Med Publishers.)

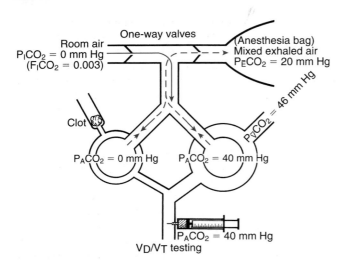

Fig. B-3 Schematic representation of the procedure for measuring P_ICO_2 (inspired partial pressure of CO_2), F_ICO_2 (fraction of inspired CO_2), P_ACO_2 (partial pressure of CO_2 in the alveolus), $P\overline{V}CO_2$ (partial pressure of mixed venous CO_2), P_ECO_2 (mixed expired CO_2), and P_aCO_2 (arterial PCO_2) for the calculation of the dead space to tidal volume ratio (V_D/V_T). See text for further explanation.

BOX **B-1**	**Calculation of Mechanical Dead Space Volume Needed to Increase P_aCO_2**

$$V_{Dmech} = \frac{PaCO_2' - PaCO_2}{PaCO_2' - (PaCO_2 - P_ACO_2)} \times (V_T - V_{Danat})$$

where V_{Dmech} = mechanical dead space to add
P_aCO_2 = actual P_aCO_2
$P_aCO_2{}^I$ = desired P_aCO_2
P_ACO_2 = alveolar CO_2

1. Assume that $\dot{V}/\dot{Q}$ is normal, then $P_aCO_2 - P_ACO_2$ is <10 mm Hg. Use $P_aCO_2 - P_ACO_2$ = 5 mm Hg
   Example: P_aCO_2 = 40 mm Hg
   P_ACO_2 = 30 mm Hg
   V_T = 900 mL
   V_{Danat} = 200 mL

$$V_{Dmech} = \frac{40 - 30}{40 - 5} \times (900 - 200) = 200 \text{ mL}$$

2. Add 200 mL V_{Dmech} to achieve a P_aCO_2 = 40 mm Hg
3. To determine the volume of a length of large-bore corrugated tubing:
   a. Fill the tubing with water and pour it into a graduated cylinder
   b. Add the V_{Dmech} between the endotracheal tube and the patient circuit Y-connector
   c. Increase the patient's O_2 percentage slightly to correct for the decreased F_IO_2 brought on by using V_{Dmech}

$P_{(A-a)}O_2$ owing to one of three general causes: shunt, ventilation/perfusion abnormalities ($\dot{V}/\dot{Q}$ mismatching), and diffusion defects. Each of these will be described.

Shunt

Shunt is defined as that portion of blood from cardiac output that does not participate in gas exchange with alveolar air, i.e., perfusion without ventilation. There are three different types of

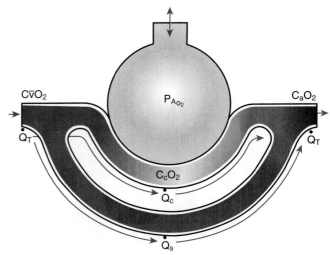

Fig. B-4 Normal alveolar gas exchange is presented by the exchange of gas between alveolar air (presented by the balloon-shaped alveolus) and the normal alveolar capillary (vessel adjacent to the alveolus). Shunted blood is represented by the blood vessel that is not in contact with the alveolus. Mixed venous oxygen content ($C\overline{v}O_2$), alveolar capillary content (C_cO_2), arterial oxygen content (C_aO_2), cardiac output ($\dot{Q}_T$), and the shunted portion of cardiac output ($\dot{Q}_S$). See text for further explanation. (From Shapiro BA: Clinical application of blood gases, Chicago, 1973, Year Book Med Publishers.)

shunts: anatomic shunt, capillary shunt, and perfusion in excess of ventilation.[2]

Normal anatomic shunts are present in everyone. These shunts are called *right-to-left shunts* because blood that would ideally return to the right side of the heart (deoxygenated blood) drains into vessels served by the left side of the heart (oxygenated blood). The normal anatomic shunt includes deoxygenated blood from bronchial veins, pleural veins, and thebesian veins, which all drain directly into the left heart (i.e., arterial blood). Normal anatomic shunt represents about 2% to 3% of normal cardiac output. Abnormal anatomic shunts can occur with vascular tumors in the lung or ventricular septal wall defects. In this latter case blood flows from the right to the left side of the heart bypassing the pulmonary circulation. Any condition in which blood from the systemic circulation flows from the right heart to the left heart without entering the pulmonary circulation is therefore considered an anatomic shunt.

A capillary shunt is the result of blood flowing into the left heart from the pulmonary circulation without passing through ventilated regions of the lung. This intrapulmonary shunting causes hypoxemia that does not respond to oxygen therapy. In other words, there is no significant improvement in P_aO_2 with increases in fractional inspired oxygen (F_IO_2) (refractory hypoxemia). Figure B-4 illustrates an example of a capillary shunt. Even if the partial pressure of alveolar oxygen (P_AO_2) is increased with administration of oxygen, the increased P_AO_2 never comes in contact with the shunted blood. Thus, shunted blood mixing with normal arterial content results in a lower than normal P_aO_2 and arterial oxygen content (C_aO_2).

Intrapulmonary shunts are associated with atelectasis, pulmonary edema, pneumonia, pneumothorax, complete airway obstruction, consolidation of the lung, acute respiratory distress syndrome, and, on rare occasions, arterial-to-venous fistulas. *True shunt* is the sum of anatomic and intrapulmonary capillary shunts.

Perfusion in excess of ventilation causes a *shunt effect,* which is also referred to as *venous admixture.* A shunt-like effect can occur in either poorly ventilated alveolar units that are well perfused or in alveolar-capillary units, in which oxygen diffusion is impaired. Blood leaving these poorly ventilated areas is low in oxygen. Thus, a shunt-like effect occurs because of a $\dot{V}/\dot{Q}$ inequality. $\dot{V}/\dot{Q}$ abnormalities can also cause dead space effects and are complex and variable. (See section on Ventilation/Perfusion Abnormalities for further explanation.)

Calculation of Shunt

Because cardiopulmonary disorders can cause either dead space or shunt abnormalities, it is important to be able to evaluate each of these characteristic disorders. Dead space has been described previously. Calculation of a pulmonary shunt relies on the Fick equation:

$$\dot{V}O_2 = \dot{Q}_T \times (C_aO_2 - C\bar{v}O_2),$$

which states that the total oxygen consumption ($\dot{V}O_2$) expressed in milliliters per minute is equal to the cardiac output ($\dot{Q}_T$) expressed in 100 mL per min, multiplied by the arterial-to-venous oxygen content difference ($C_aO_2 - C\bar{v}O_2$) expressed in milliliters of oxygen divided by 100 mL of blood (vol%).

Figure B-4 illustrates how the total cardiac output is composed of that portion of cardiac output that participates in gas exchange with alveolar air ($\dot{Q}_C$), and the shunted portion of the cardiac output that does not exchange with alveolar air ($\dot{Q}_S$).[2,3] Calculation of the pulmonary shunt can be determined by the following classic shunt equation (the derivation of the shunt equation is not included in this discussion):

$$\dot{Q}_S/\dot{Q}_T = (C_cO_2 - C_aO_2)/(C_cO_2 - C\bar{v}O_2)$$

where $\dot{Q}_S$ is the shunted portion of the cardiac output, $\dot{Q}_T$ is total cardiac output, C_cO_2 is the content of oxygen of the pulmonary end-capillary after oxygenation of the blood, C_aO_2 is the arterial O_2 content, and $C\bar{v}O_2$ is the mixed venous oxygen content (i.e., pulmonary capillary blood before oxygenation). C_cO_2 is calculated based on the assumption that pulmonary end-capillary PO_2 is the same as P_AO_2. Mixed venous blood can be obtained using a right heart balloon flotation catheter inserted into the pulmonary artery (see Chapter 11).

In many cases, clinicians often use a *clinical shunt equation* to estimate cardiac output and shunt. This equation, which is derived from the classic shunt equation, uses oxygen pressures rather than using oxygen content values. The clinical shunt equation is

$$\dot{Q}_S/\dot{Q}_T = \frac{[(P_AO_2 - P_aO_2) \times 0.003]}{[3.5 + (P_AO_2 - P_aO_2) \times 0.003]}$$

Alveolar P_AO_2 is determined by the following equation:

$$P_AO_2 = [(F_1O_2) \times (P_B - PH_2O)] - \{P_aCO_2 \times [F_1O_2 + (1 - F_1O_2)/R]\}$$

where P_AO_2 is the alveolar partial pressure of oxygen, F_1O_2 is the fraction of inspired oxygen, P_B is the barometric pressure, PH_2O is water vapor pressure (at $37°$ C $= 47$ mm Hg), and R is the respiratory quotient (R $= \dot{V}CO_2/\dot{V}O_2$). An R value of 0.8 is commonly substituted in the equation and represents a normal value.

The clinical shunt equation estimates oxygen content by first assuming that the hemoglobin is the same in arterial, capillary, and mixed venous blood. It also assumes that if the P_aO_2 is >150 mm Hg, both the pulmonary and arterial hemoglobin is fully saturated (SO_2

$= 100\%$). The PO_2 of capillary, arterial, and mixed venous oxygen is then multiplied by 0.003, which is the solubility coefficient of oxygen. The equation also assumes that arterial and alveolar oxygen tensions are equal. Because central venous blood samples are not commonly available, the previous equation makes another assumption. It assumes that the $a - \bar{v}$ oxygen content difference is normal, if the clinician establishes that the following circumstances are true[1]:

1. The patient's cardiovascular status is basically normal (i.e., blood pressure, heart rate, pulse pressure, etc.)
2. The metabolic rate is basically normal (i.e., no fever is present and the patient is resting)
3. The perfusion is basically normal (i.e., the skin is warm and dry, capillary refill is good, urine output is normal, etc.)

Patients meeting these three criteria will typically have an arterial-to-mixed venous difference of about 3.5%. Thus, an average arterial-to-mixed venous oxygen difference of 3.5 is substituted into the equation.

Practitioners have often used the *clinical shunt equation,* assuming it provides useful information for ventilated patients. However, it has been shown that the equation will be inaccurate at any F_1O_2 because of all the assumptions made in its derivation. In addition, at F_1O_2 values >0.6, the equation will be as much as 10% to 12% inaccurate when compared with the classic shunt equation.[4] Clinicians are advised to not make the assumptions used in the clinical shunt equation but to try and determine as much information as possible and accurately apply the classic shunt equation. Other resources are also available for more accurately estimating pulmonary shunt.[5]

Ventilation/Perfusion Abnormalities

Ideally, ventilation should be perfectly matched with pulmonary perfusion and $\dot{V}/\dot{Q}$ should be equal to 1.0. However, because of many factors, $\dot{V}/\dot{Q}$ varies throughout the lung even in normal individuals. Distribution of gas volume (ventilation) varies based on regional differences in resting lung volumes and transpulmonary pressure (i.e., the difference between alveolar and pleural pressures). Ventilation increases (in relation to overall ventilation) from the apex to the base of the lung in the upright individual. Distribution of pulmonary blood is affected primarily by gravity. Pulmonary blood flow also increases (relative to total pulmonary perfusion) from apex to base, and changes in perfusion are more dramatic than changes in ventilation as blood flow progresses toward the bases. $\dot{V}/\dot{Q}$ is much higher at the top of the lung (i.e., it is about 3.3). Ventilation and perfusion are nearly equal in the middle of the lung (i.e., $\dot{V}/\dot{Q}$ is about 1). In the bases of the lungs both ventilation and perfusion are better than at the apex of the lung. In addition, the lung bases are better perfused than ventilated so the $\dot{V}/\dot{Q}$ is considerably lower in the bases and equals about 0.66.[6]

A ventilation/perfusion abnormality ($\dot{V}/\dot{Q}$ mismatching) is defined as an abnormal mismatching of gas exchange and pulmonary perfusion. A high $\dot{V}/\dot{Q}$ indicates that ventilation is greater than normal, and perfusion is less than normal, or both. In cases in which a high $\dot{V}/\dot{Q}$ ratio exists, the PO_2 is higher and the PCO_2 lower than normal. With a low $\dot{V}/\dot{Q}$ ratio, ventilation is less than normal and perfusion is greater than normal, or both. With a low $\dot{V}/\dot{Q}$ ratio, the alveolar PO_2 is lower and the alveolar PCO_2 is higher than normal.[1,6] The hypoxemia associated with a low $\dot{V}/\dot{Q}$ ratio (shunt effect) does not respond well to oxygen therapy.

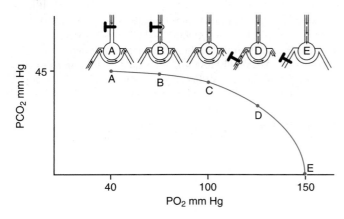

Fig. B-5 The relationship between PO_2 (mm Hg) and PCO_2 (mm Hg) with changes in the ratio of ventilation and perfusion. See text for further explanation. (Redrawn from Deshpande VM, Pilbeam SP, Dixon RJ: *A comprehensive review in respiratory care*, Norwalk, Conn., 1988, Appleton & Lange.)

Figure B-5 graphically illustrates the effect of regional lung changes of the $\dot{V}/\dot{Q}$ relationship on PO_2 and PCO_2 in the lung.[6] At *A* of the graph, perfusion is present without ventilation, resulting in PO_2 and PCO_2 similar to venous blood (PCO_2 is about 46 mm Hg and PO_2 is about 40 mm Hg). This represents a pulmonary shunt, and $\dot{V}/\dot{Q}$ will be zero. At *B*, perfusion is in excess of ventilation, representing a *shunt effect*. PO_2 in this region of the lung is low. $\dot{V}/\dot{Q}$ ratio will equal about 0.4 to 0.5. Many conditions can produce this effect, including hypoventilation, partial airway obstruction (e.g., COPD), and pulmonary interstitial disease. Pulmonary disorders with this type of $\dot{V}/\dot{Q}$ mismatching are more likely to respond to oxygen therapy. Point *C* represents a normal $\dot{V}/\dot{Q}$ relationship of 0.8, resulting in normal PO_2 and PCO_2. Point *D* illustrates ventilation in excess of perfusion. In this case the excess ventilation does not completely take part in gas exchange, producing a dead space effect. Pulmonary capillary blood from these areas is well oxygenated and may have a CO_2 lower than normal (regional hyperventilation). $\dot{V}/\dot{Q}$ values will be in excess of 1.0. Conditions that might cause this type of $\dot{V}/\dot{Q}$ mismatching are positive pressure ventilation and a decreased cardiac output. Point *E* illustrates ventilation without perfusion and is known as V_{Dalv}. A classic example of this type of $\dot{V}/\dot{Q}$ mismatch is pulmonary embolism, which was described earlier in the section on dead space. With no perfusion, alveolar PO_2 (P_AO_2) for a person breathing room air will be about 150 mm Hg and alveolar PCO_2 (P_ACO_2) will be zero in affected areas. Resulting exhaled gases will contain lower than normal PCO_2 values. $\dot{V}/\dot{Q}$ will approach infinity (i.e., one divided by zero).

In summary, the adequacy of gas exchange is a sum of the $\dot{V}/\dot{Q}$ distribution of gas throughout the lung. In general, inadequate ventilation relative to a normal perfusion (low $\dot{V}/\dot{Q}$ and shunt) has the greatest effect on oxygen uptake by the lung and results in hypoxemia. On the other hand, an excessive amount of ventilation relative to perfusion affects CO_2 elimination and can result in hypercapnia in severe cases.[6]

Diffusion Defects

A diffusion defect is a pathologic condition resulting from impaired gas exchange across the alveolar-capillary membrane resulting in hypoxemia that is generally responsive to oxygen therapy. Diffusion defects occur through three possible mechanisms: a reduction of alveolar surface area, a thickened alveolar-capillary membrane, or a lower than normal oxygen pressure gradient.

A reduced surface area can occur after surgery in which, for example, a pulmonary lobe is removed (lobectomy). It can also occur in diseases that destroy alveolar tissue, such as emphysema. These structural changes to the lungs are not reversible.

Diffusion defects can also occur as a result of an increase in the thickness of the alveolar-capillary membrane, which can occur with pneumonia, pulmonary or interstitial edema, pulmonary fibrosis, or any condition that thickens one or all of the components of the alveolar-capillary membrane.

A lower than normal alveolar-to-arterial oxygen tension gradient usually results from a lower than normal P_AO_2. It is rare that PO_2 is lower than normal with the exception of individuals residing at high altitudes (e.g. living at 10,000 feet above sea level). With a low P_AO_2, the pressure gradient between the alveolus and the pulmonary capillary will be lower than normal, thus reducing the rate of gas transfer across the alveolar-capillary membrane.[1,6]

References

1. Levitzky MG: *Pulmonary physiology*, ed 8, New York, 2013, McGraw-Hill Medical, pp 58–90.
2. Shapiro BA: *Clinical application of blood gases*, Chicago, 1973, Year Book Med Publishers.
3. Comroe JH, Forster RE, DuBois AB, et al: *The lung: clinical physiology and pulmonary function tests*, ed 2, Chicago, 1973, Year Book Med Publishers.
4. Warner MA, Divertie MB, Offord KP, et al: Clinical implications of variation in total venoarterial shunt fraction calculated by different methods during severe acute respiratory failure. *Mayo Clin Proc* 58:654–659, 1983.
5. Cairo JM: *Mosby's respiratory care equipment*, ed 9, St. Louis, 2014, Elsevier, p 314.
6. West JB: *Pulmonary pathophysiology—the essentials*, Baltimore, 1992, Williams & Wilkins.

Graphics Exercises

GRAPHING VENTILATOR WAVEFORMS

This exercise is designed to help the reader understand graphic waveforms produced by a microprocessor-controlled ventilator. By performing these graphing exercises and calculations, the reader also will gain a better understanding of the interrelationship of flow, volume, pressure, and time waveforms generated during mechanical ventilation.

Problem 1

Assume that you have a patient who is being ventilated using volume-controlled continuous mandatory ventilation (VC-CMV) set to deliver a constant flow of gas during inspiration until it reaches the volume ordered by the physician. You are given the following information about the patient's lung characteristics and the ventilator parameters:

- Compliance (C) is 0.2 L/cm H_2O
- Airway resistance (R_{aw}) is 15 cm H_2O/L/sec
- Flow rate is constant at 40 L/min
- Ordered tidal volume (V_T) is 1 L (1000 mL)
- End-expiratory pressure is zero (no positive end-expiratory pressure [PEEP])

Perform the following steps using the preceding information:

- Calculate the flow rate in L/sec.
- Record under variable (Fig. C-1, *A*) the flow at each quarter second of time that will be present during inspiration. Graph the flow at quarter-second intervals (Fig. C-1, *A*).
- Calculate and graph the volume delivered at each quarter-second interval during inspiration: Volume (V) = Time (T) × Flow (Fig. C-1, *B*).

    Note that the ordered V_T of 1 L (1000 mL) was delivered in about 1.5 seconds. A volume-cycled ventilator would stop the inspiratory phase at this point. For all graphs from this point on, calculations need to be made only for times up to 1.5 seconds.

- Using the volume, calculate and graph the alveolar pressure. Recall that C = $\Delta V/\Delta P$; $\Delta P = P_{alv} - EEP$ and EEP = 0; $P_{alv} = \Delta V/C$. The volume is taken from the calculations of volume in step 3 for each quarter-second interval (Fig. C-1, *C*).
- Calculate and graph the transairway pressure (P_{TA}). Recall that $R_{aw} = P_{TA}/Flow$. Therefore $P_{TA} = R_{aw} \times Flow$, $P_{TA} = 15 \times 0.67 = 10$ cm H_2O. Both R_{aw} and flow have constant values. P_{TA} will have the same value for each quarter-second interval (Fig. C-1, *D*).

- Add the values of P_{alv} and P_{TA} to determine the airway opening pressure (P_{awo}) at each quarter-second interval. Graph these values. Note that at the zero point on the *x* and *y* axes, the P_{awo} will not go to zero. The pressure rises rapidly as the flow begins to go to the patient because the gas flow encounters the resistance of the circuit, the endotracheal tube (ET), and the patient's airways. The P_{awo} value just near zero on the *x* axis is approximately equal to the P_{TA} just to the right of the *y* axis (Fig. C-1, *E*).
- Compare the curves produced in the preceding exercise; the graph for flow has the same waveform as the graph for:
    - P_{alv}
    - PIP
    - P_{TA}

CHANGES IN WAVEFORMS WITH CHANGES IN LUNG CHARACTERISTICS

Ventilator Working Pressure

A ventilator that can generate pressures that greatly exceed those reached at the upper airway can deliver any waveform pattern for flow, volume, or pressure. These waveforms do not change regardless of changes in lung characteristics. Some ventilators deliver pressures of 400 to 700 cm H_2O, far greater than what is needed to ventilate the human lung (10 to 35 cm H_2O).

The following sections discuss how pressure waveforms change during volume ventilation (constant flow) and how volume and flow waveforms change during pressure ventilation (constant pressure) with changes in lung characteristics.

Constant Flow Volume Ventilation with High Working Pressure

During volume ventilation (constant flow), the volume waveform increases linearly and volume delivery is constant. Inspiration usually is time cycled or volume cycled (Fig. C-2). As a patient's lungs become less compliant or R_{aw} increases, the pressure waveforms are affected; however, the volume and flow curves remain the same. Clinically, a decrease in compliance increases peak inspiratory pressure (PIP) and $P_{plateau}$ (Fig. C-3). An increase in R_{aw} also increases PIP, whereas alveolar pressure ($P_{plateau}$) remains fairly constant. The difference between the two (P_{TA}) increases (Fig. C-4). The ventilator provides a constant volume, even with changes in

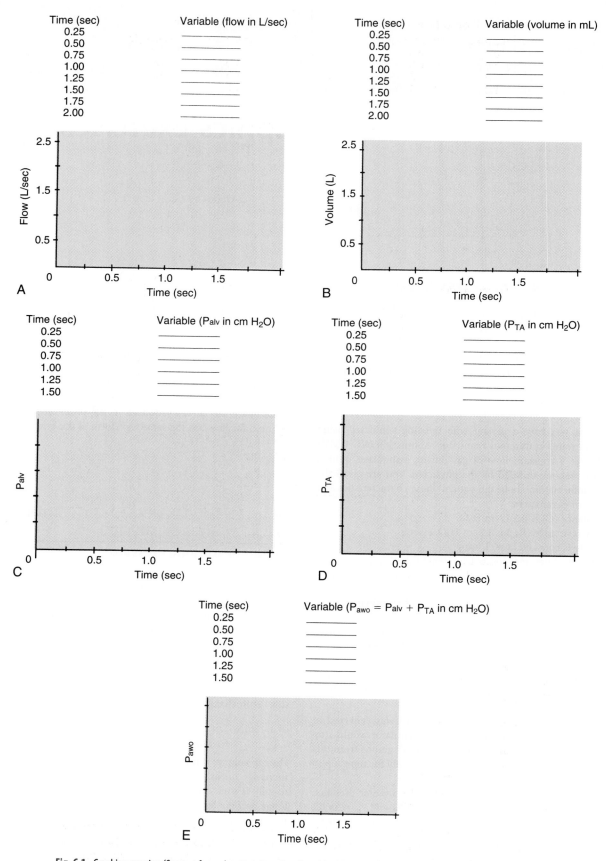

Time (sec)	Variable (flow in L/sec)
0.25	_____
0.50	_____
0.75	_____
1.00	_____
1.25	_____
1.50	_____
1.75	_____
2.00	_____

Time (sec)	Variable (volume in mL)
0.25	_____
0.50	_____
0.75	_____
1.00	_____
1.25	_____
1.50	_____
1.75	_____
2.00	_____

Time (sec)	Variable (P_{alv} in cm H_2O)
0.25	_____
0.50	_____
0.75	_____
1.00	_____
1.25	_____
1.50	_____

Time (sec)	Variable (P_{TA} in cm H_2O)
0.25	_____
0.50	_____
0.75	_____
1.00	_____
1.25	_____
1.50	_____

Time (sec)	Variable ($P_{awo} = P_{alv} + P_{TA}$ in cm H_2O)
0.25	_____
0.50	_____
0.75	_____
1.00	_____
1.25	_____
1.50	_____

Fig. C-1 Graphing exercise. (See text for explanation. Note that the tables of Time/Variable appear directly above each graph.) (Answers to this problem can be found in Appendix A.)

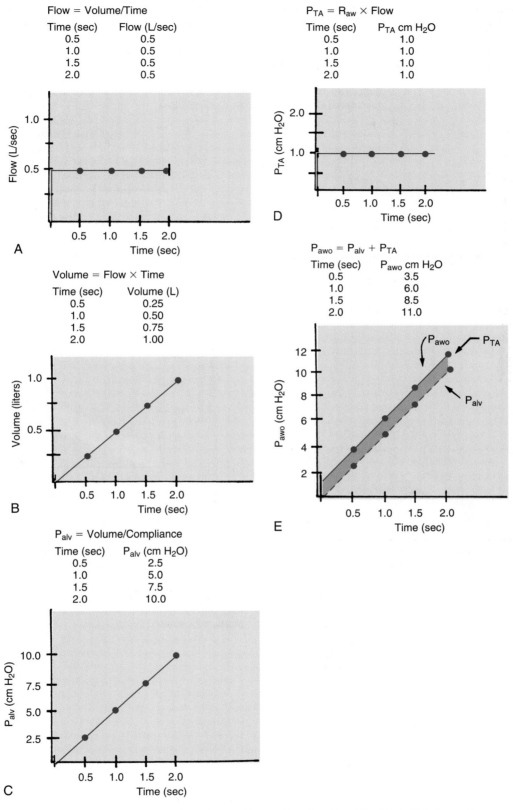

Flow = Volume/Time

Time (sec)	Flow (L/sec)
0.5	0.5
1.0	0.5
1.5	0.5
2.0	0.5

$P_{TA} = R_{aw} \times$ Flow

Time (sec)	P_{TA} cm H_2O
0.5	1.0
1.0	1.0
1.5	1.0
2.0	1.0

Volume = Flow × Time

Time (sec)	Volume (L)
0.5	0.25
1.0	0.50
1.5	0.75
2.0	1.00

$P_{awo} = P_{alv} + P_{TA}$

Time (sec)	P_{awo} cm H_2O
0.5	3.5
1.0	6.0
1.5	8.5
2.0	11.0

P_{alv} = Volume/Compliance

Time (sec)	P_{alv} (cm H_2O)
0.5	2.5
1.0	5.0
1.5	7.5
2.0	10.0

Fig. C-2 Curves for constant (rectangular) flow under normal lung conditions (compliance [C] = 0.1 L/cm H_2O; airway resistance [R_{aw}] = 2 cm H_2O/L/sec); inspiratory time [T_I] = 2 seconds. **A,** Flow is constant at 0.5 L/sec. **B,** Volume increases at a constant rate during inspiration, achieving a tidal volume (V_T) of 1 L. **C,** P_{alv} increases at a constant rate, as does volume, to a maximum of 10 cm H_2O. **D,** Because flow is constant, P_{TA} is constant; this assumes that resistance and flow do not change. **E,** P_{TA} is 1 cm H_2O/L/sec. P_{TA} = Flow × R_{aw}. P_{alv}, Alveolar pressure; P_{awo}, upper airway pressure; P_{TA}, pressure lost to airways.

Time (sec)	P_{alv} (cm H_2O)
0.5	5
1.0	10
1.5	15
2.0	20

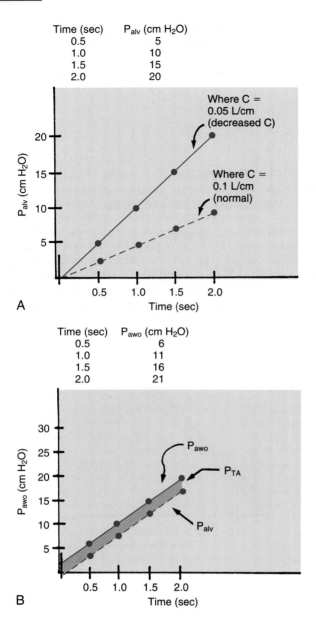

A

Time (sec)	P_{awo} (cm H_2O)
0.5	6
1.0	11
1.5	16
2.0	21

B

Fig. C-3 **A,** Flow is constant at 0.5 L/sec. $T_I = 2$ seconds. The volume coming from the ventilator remains the same at 1 L even though compliance (C) is reduced. P_{alv} has doubled (20 cm H_2O) in this situation because compliance is half its previous value. The *dashed line* represents the curve for normal compliance (C = 0.1 L/cm H_2O), and the *solid line* represents the curve for reduced compliance (C = 0.05 L/cm H_2O). **B,** Because flow and airway resistance (R_{aw}) are constant, the pressure lost to the airways is constant ($P_{TA} = 1$ cm H_2O). P_{TA} is the *shaded area*. The upper airway pressure is much higher than normal because compliance is reduced. P_{alv}, Alveolar pressure; P_{awo}, upper airway pressure; P_{TA}, pressure lost to airways.

Time (sec)	P_{TA} (cm H_2O)
0.5	2.0
1.0	2.0
1.5	2.0
2.0	2.0

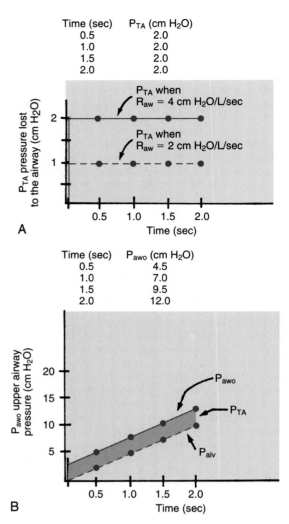

A

Time (sec)	P_{awo} (cm H_2O)
0.5	4.5
1.0	7.0
1.5	9.5
2.0	12.0

B

Fig. C-4 Constant flow ventilator. The following inspiratory curves are produced when airway resistance (R_{aw}) is increased to 4 cm H_2O/L/sec and compliance is normal (C = 0.1 L/cm H_2O). **A,** Pressure lost to the airways (P_{TA}) is the product of flow and airway resistance (Flow × R_{aw}). With an increase in R_{aw}, P_{TA} increases to 2 cm H_2O *(solid line)* compared with normal at 1 cm H_2O *(dashed line)*. **B,** Upper airway pressure (P_{awo}), the sum of alveolar pressure (P_{alv}) and P_{TA}, increases to a maximum of 12 cm H_2O because P_{TA} is increased *(shaded area)*. The difference between the peak and the plateau, or P_{alv}, increases.

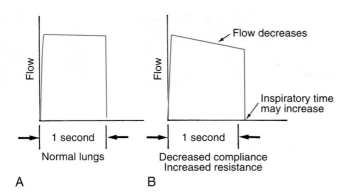

Fig. C-5 Inspiratory curves represent the changes in flow that can occur using constant flow in a ventilator with moderate to low pressure-generating capabilities. **A,** Under normal conditions, flow is constant. **B,** As compliance decreases and resistance increases significantly, flow decreases slightly. If the ventilator is volume cycled, volume is delivered from the ventilator, but inspiratory time (T_I) may increase. This affects the inspiratory-to-expiratory ratio (I : E). These changes in lung characteristics increase P_{alv} and P_{awo} as long as the ventilator is not pressure cycled out of inspiration by reaching the pre-set pressure limit.

lung characteristics, as long as the ventilator is time cycled or volume cycled. If it prematurely pressure cycles as a result of reaching the set pressure limit, volume decreases.

Using other types of flow waveforms produces changes similar to those seen for $P_{plateau}$, P_{TA}, and P_{awo}. Reduced compliance increases PIP and $P_{plateau}$. Increased R_{aw} increases P_{TA}.

Constant Flow Volume Ventilation with Low Working Pressure

Under normal lung conditions, a constant flow ventilator with low to moderate working pressure (40 to 120 cm H_2O) creates a constant flow waveform similar to that shown in Figure C-5, *A*.

When compliance is significantly reduced and resistance is increased, PIP rises and flow decreases during inspiration because of the decrease in the pressure gradient between the ventilator and the alveoli. When the driving mechanism no longer generates an adequate working pressure, the ventilator no longer provides a constant flow. This is not necessarily a disadvantage. The resulting modified descending ramp waveform may actually be more desirable for improving gas distribution in the lungs, but it can alter inspiratory time (T_I) (see Fig. C-5, *B*).

Glossary

A

absorption atelectasis Atelectasis (lung collapse) resulting from the absorption of oxygen from obstructed or partially obstructed alveoli.

acinus The smallest division of a gland; a subdivision of the lung consisting of the tissue distal to a terminal bronchiole including respiratory bronchioles, alveolar ducts, alveoli, and all other structures within.

acute cardiogenic pulmonary edema Defined as fluid accumulation in the air spaces and parenchyma of the lungs due to increased capillary hydrostatic pressure secondary to elevated pulmonary venous pressure.

Acute Physiology and Chronic Health Evaluation (APACHE) A method of classifying the severity of illnesses in patients; a scoring system used to predict outcome.

acute respiratory failure (ARF) Any condition in which respiratory activity is completely absent or is inadequate to maintain oxygen uptake and carbon dioxide clearance.

acute severe asthma Also known as status asthmaticus. Severe asthma episode unresponsive to repeated courses of beta2-agonist therapy. Emergency that requires immediate recognition and treatment.

adaptive support ventilation A patient-centered method of closed-loop mechanical ventilation that increases or decreases ventilatory support based on monitored patient parameters.

afterload The impedance that the ventricles must overcome to eject blood into the great vessels.

airway opening pressure (P_{awo}) Pressure at the upper airway (nose and mouth); also called mouth pressure (P_M), airway pressure (P_{aw}), upper airway pressure, mask pressure, or proximal airway pressure.

airway pressure (P_{aw}) Pressure in the upper airway; also called mouth pressure (P_M), airway pressure (P_{aw}), upper airway pressure, mask pressure, or proximal airway pressure.

alveolar distending pressure The pressure difference between the inside of the lung and the outside of the lung, which is responsible for maintaining alveolar inflation; also called transpulmonary pressure.

amplitude The maximum value of a periodic curve or wave measured along the vertical axis.

analgesic An agent that reduces pain without causing a loss of consciousness.

anesthetic A drug or agent that is used to abolish the sensation of pain.

anterograde amnesia Condition in which the acquisition and encoding of new information that can potentially lead to memories of unpleasant experiences is prevented.

ascites An abnormal accumulation of fluid in the peritoneal space.

assisted breaths When all or part of the breath is generated by the ventilator and the ventilator is providing part of the work of breathing for the patient.

assist-control (A/C) ventilation See *continuous mandatory ventilation*.

asynchrony (dyssynchrony) See *patient-ventilator asynchrony*.

automatic tube compensation A feature available in some ventilators that provides adjustable compensation for the work of breathing through an artificial airway.

auto-PEEP Inadvertent PEEP that is not set by the operator but results in a build up of positive pressure in the lungs at the end of exhalation; commonly caused by high minute ventilation settings, particularly in the presence of airway obstruction, which result in incomplete exhalation of an inspired volume.

B

back pressure Pressure that builds in a tube or circuit and increases and extends backward through the tube if the normal point of exit (egress) is blocked and not restored.

balloon-tipped, flow-directed catheter The balloon-tipped, flow-directed catheter (also referred to as the Swan-Ganz catheter or pulmonary artery catheter) is a multiple-lumen catheter constructed of radiopaque polyvinylchloride.

barotraumas Injury to the lung parenchyma caused by excessive pressures in the lungs.

baseline pressure The pressure from which inspiration begins and at which expiration ends during mechanical ventilation; also known as *expiratory pressure*. Normal baseline pressure is atmospheric. Positive pressures can be applied to increase the baseline above atmospheric.

biofilm A thin, mucous film of bacteria that attaches to a surface.

Biot respirations Periods of apnea (10 to 30 seconds) followed by periods of breathing at a uniform depth; associated with central nervous system disorders (e.g., meningitis) and increased intracranial pressure.

bradycardia Heart rates in the adult less than 60 beats/min.

bronchial alveolar lavage (BAL) Medical procedure in which a bronchoscope is passed through the mouth or nose into the lungs and fluid is instilled into a small part of the lung and then recollected for examination.

bronchomalacia Weak cartilage in the walls of the bronchial tubes, occurring in children under 6 months, presenting with noisy breathing and/or wheezing. There is collapse of a main stem bronchus, on expiration.

bronchopleural fistula A hole or opening between the lung and pleural space producing an air communication between the two.

bronchopulmonary dysplasia (BPD) A chronic respiratory disorder that often occurs in infants exposed to long-term ventilation. Lung tissue is scarred and pulmonary arterial walls thickened. Mismatching of ventilation and pulmonary perfusion exists.

C

capnography Graphic display of exhaled carbon dioxide concentration using a capnograph.

cardiac index Cardiac output divided by body surface area.

cardiac tamponade Compression of the heart caused by fluid or air in the pericardial sac; also caused by positive pressure in the lungs around the outside of the heart.

cardiac transmural pressure The pressure difference between the inside of the heart and the intrathoracic pressure.

cardiac work An estimate of the amount of work the heart must perform to eject the stroke volume.

cardiogenic pulmonary edema (CPE) Accumulation of fluid (plasma) in the pulmonary interstitial and alveolar spaces as a result of increased pulmonary capillary pressure typically associated with left heart failure.

central venous lines Catheters placed near or in the right atrium to measure central venous pressure.

chest-abdominal paradox When the chest wall and abdomen move the opposite of normal during breathing. The chest wall goes inward on inspiration while the abdomen is moving outward, and vice versa. See also *respiratory alternans*.

chest cuirass The shell-like device that fits over the thorax for the delivery of a negative pressure ventilation.

Cheyne-Stokes respiration A pattern of breathing with apneas lasting 10 to 30 seconds followed by gradual increase in the depth and rate of breaths; associated with cerebral disorders, congestive heart failure, and alterations in acid–base status such as in metabolic problems.

choanal atresia A congenital abnormality in which a bony or membranous obstruction blocks the passage between the nose and pharynx; can result in serious respiratory problems in the neonate.

cleft palate A congenital defect in which a fissure occurs in the midline of the palate; often associated with a cleft in the upper lip.

Clinical Pulmonary Infection Score (CPIS) An approach to clinical diagnosis that includes six clinical assessments with each item given a score of 0 to 2 points. The assessment criteria include fever, leukocyte count, quantity and purulence of tracheal secretions, oxygenation status, the type of radiographic abnormality, and results of a tracheal aspirate culture and Gram stain.

closed-loop system A feedback control scheme in which the actual output is measured and compared with the desired input set on the control panel (user interface). An error signal is sent to the controller if a specified difference is found between the input value and the measured output.

community-acquired pneumonia (CAP) A common infectious respiratory disease characterized by inflammation of lung tissue, acquired outside the hospital setting by inhalation or aspiration of pathogenic organisms into a lung segment or lobe. A pneumonia contracted from the environment as opposed to being acquired within a medical facility (e.g., hospital-acquired pneumonia), CAP is usually more sensitive to antibiotics.

compliance (C) The relative ease with which the structure distends; the opposite, or inverse, of elastance (e). C = 1/e or e = 1/C.

compressible volume The volume of gas in the patient (ventilator) circuit that stays in the circuit during inspiration; also referred to as the compressible volume or the volume lost as a result of tubing compliance (C_T).

continuous mandatory ventilation (CMV) Term used most often to describe a mode that is time or patient triggered, volume or pressure targeted, and volume or time cycled. Every breath is mandatory. Also known as *controlled mechanical ventilation* and *continuous mechanical ventilation*.

continuous positive airway pressure (CPAP) Positive pressure applied to the spontaneously breathing patient during both inspiration and expiration; used for the treatment of obstructive sleep apnea and to increase mean airway pressure in critically ill patients who are able to do some spontaneous breathing.

contractility Cardiac contractility is related to the force that the ventricle generates during each cardiac cycle. The value can be estimated by using the ejection fraction.

control system The internal components of a ventilator that interpret what the operator sets on the control panel (user interface).

control variable The primary variable the ventilator control circuit adjusts to cause inspiration.

control ventilation Time triggering of all breaths, with breath rate established by the ventilator.

cor pulmonale Enlargement (hypertrophy) or failure of the right heart and pulmonary hypertension caused by certain pulmonary parenchymal or pulmonary vascular disorders.

critical opening pressure The pressure required to open a collapsed lung unit.

Cushing response A normal response to acute increases in intracranial pressure, which results in hypertension with bradycardia.

cycle variable The phase variable that ends inspiration.

cycling mechanism The variable by which the ventilator marks the end of inspiration.

cytokines A group of low-molecular weight proteins secreted by specific cells; involved in cell-to-cell communication and a variety of immune responses.

D

decannulation Removal of a tracheostomy tube.

deep sulcus sign (chest radiograph) A radiographic sign indicative of the presence of a pneumothorax.

de-escalation An important method that can be used to reduce the incidence of MDR (multidrug-resistant organisms) pathogens because it reduces unnecessary use of antibiotics.

deflation point The upper inflection point on the deflation portion of the curve (UIPd) also called deflection point or deflation point. Point at which lungs begin to collapse.

deflection point Part of the information obtained during a lung recruitment maneuver. Following a full inspiration to total lung capacity, a deflation is performed and graphs are established for pressure–volume points similar to the inflation curve. A deflection point occurs where a large number of lung units collapse very quickly. The deflection point is the upper inflection point during deflation.

delay time control A comfort feature incorporated in many noninvasive pressure-targeted ventilators that allows the user to set a period of time that must elapse before inspiratory and expiratory pressures achieve prescribed levels. A very low pressure and continuous flow of gas will continue through the circuit during this interval of time. It is most often used in conjunction with the ramp feature. See *ramp*.

depolarizing agent An agent that causes skeletal muscle paralysis by causing a reversal of the resting membrane potential in excitable cell membranes.

diastole The period of cardiac relaxation and filling during the cardiac cycle.

double-circuit ventilator A ventilator in which the primary power source generates a gas flow that compresses another mechanism such as a bag or bellows.

dP/dT Change in pressure relative to time.

drive mechanism The mechanical device that causes gas flow to the patient.

dyssynchrony (asynchrony) See *patient-ventilator asynchrony*.

E

early-onset pneumonia VAP (ventilator-associated pneumonia) that develops between 48 and 72 hours following tracheal intubation.

ejection fraction Calculated as the ratio of the stroke volume to the ventricular end-diastolic volume.

elastance (e) The tendency of a structure to return to its original form after being stretched or acted on by an outside force. Elastance (e) is the inverse of compliance (C); e = 1/C.

electrical activity of the diaphragm (Edi) A minimally invasive bedside technique used in conjunction with neurally adjusted ventilator assist (NAVA) that gives information on the patient's diaphragm activity.

endogenous Growing inside the body; originating from inside the body or produced from internal causes. Compare *exogenous*.

erosive esophagitis Inflammation of the mucosal lining of the esophagus in which erosion occurs to the tissues. Causes include infection and irritation from a nasogastric tube or from backflow of gastric fluids from the stomach into the esophagus.

esophageal pressure Pressure measured from a balloon placed in the esophagus; used to estimate pressures and pressure changes in the pleural space.

exogenous Located or originating from outside the body, e.g., a foreign bacteria causing an infection.

expiratory positive airway pressure (EPAP) The application of positive pressure to the airway during exhalation. Compare *inspiratory positive airway pressure.*

external circuit See *patient circuit.*

external respiration The movement of O_2 and CO_2 across the alveolar capillary membrane.

extracorporeal membrane oxygenation A procedure in which venous blood is pumped out of the body to a heart–lung machine, where it is oxygenated and returned to the body.

extrinsic PEEP Positive end-expiratory pressure applied by the operator.

exudative Related to the oozing of fluid and other substances from cells and tissues; usually a result of infection or injury.

F

fiberoptic bronchoscopy Technique to examine breathing passages (airways) of the lungs using a thin flexible or rigid tube called a bronchoscope that is placed in the nose or mouth. The tip contains a very small camera that projects onto a video screen.

fibrosing alveolitis A form of alveolar inflammation accompanied by dyspnea and hypoxia. Chest radiographs show diffuse infiltrates and thickening of the alveolar septa. It occurs with advanced rheumatoid arthritis and other immune disorders.

Fick principle A method for determining perfusion through an organ; based on the oxygen consumption and arterial-to-venous O_2 content difference.

flow cycling When the cycle variable is flow. Inspiration ends when a specific flow is measured during inspiration by the ventilator. For example, pressure support ventilation is flow cycled.

flow limited A ventilator is considered flow limited if the flow during ventilation reaches a maximum value before the end of inspiration but does not exceed that value.

flow resistor A device with an orifice of fixed size placed in the expiratory limb of a breathing circuit; used to achieve positive expiratory pressure by creating a resistance to exhaled gas flow. As the diameter of the orifice increases in size, the provided pressure level decreases, and vice versa. Changes in the rate of gas flow also change the pressure. The higher the expired gas flow, the higher the expiratory pressure generated.

flow triggering Inspiratory flow from the ventilator begins when a set drop of flow through the patient circuit is detected during exhalation.

fractional hemoglobin saturation Calculated by dividing the amount of oxyhemoglobin measured by the amount of all four types of hemoglobin present, or fractional $O_2Hb = O_2Hb/(HHb + O_2Hb + COHb + MetHb)$.

French size A unit of measure. The French size divided by π (3.1416) equals the external diameter of a catheter in millimeters.

full ventilatory support (FVS) When the ventilator provides all the energy necessary to maintain effective alveolar ventilation.

functional hemoglobin saturation Calculated by dividing the oxyhemoglobin concentration by the concentration of hemoglobin capable of carrying oxygen, or functional $O_2Hb = O_2Hb/(HHb + O_2Hb)$.

functional residual capacity The volume of gas remaining in the lungs at the end of a normal exhalation.

G

gastroprotective agents Agents such as antacids that reduce the risk of gastrointestinal bleeding.

gastrostomy or jejunostomy tube A tube used to introduce nutrients into the stomach or to remove fluids, gas, or poisons; also called a *stomach tube.*

glabella The smooth area on the frontal bone between the superciliary arches.

H

health care–associated pneumonia (HCAP) Afflicts patients who have resided in a long-term care facility or received acute care in an acute care hospital for a specified time before developing pneumonia (i.e., 2 or more days within 90 days of the infection).

heliox A mixture of helium and oxygen, usually in concentrations of 80% helium and 20% oxygen or 70% helium and 30% oxygen; used to reduce the work of breathing by lowering the density of the gas mixture.

hematogenous Originating in the blood or transported in the blood.

hertz (Hz) Unit of measure equivalent to 60 cycles (oscillations) per minute.

heterogeneous Composed of different parts or elements.

high-frequency jet ventilation Ventilation that uses rates between about 100 and 600 breaths/min; operates by using a nozzle or an injector, which creates a high-velocity jet of air directed into the lungs. Exhalation is passive.

high-frequency oscillatory ventilation (HFOV) Uses rates into the thousands, up to about 4000 cycles/min. HFOV ventilators use either a small piston or a device similar to a stereo speaker, both of which deliver gas in a "to-and-fro" motion, pushing gas in during inspiration and drawing gas out during exhalation.

high-frequency positive pressure ventilation High-frequency ventilation that employs a conventional positive pressure set at high respiratory rates (60-100 breaths/min) with lower than normal tidal volumes.

homeostasis A consistency or balance in the internal environment of the body, maintained normally by adaptive responses that promote survival and well-being.

homogeneous Comprising similar parts or elements.

hospital-acquired pneumonia (HAP) Pneumonia that occurs 48 hours or longer after admission to the hospital and results from an infection that was not incubating at the time of admission.

humidity deficit The difference between what is provided by the humidifier and the amount of humidity required by the patient.

hyperinflation See *overinflation.*

hyperosmolar A substance or condition with increased osmolarity.

hyperthyroidism A condition that results from increased activity of the thyroid gland. An increase in metabolic activity occurs that is characterized by nervousness, tremors, hunger, weight loss, fatigue, palpitations, and related symptoms.

hypoventilation A respiratory condition resulting in elevated blood carbon dioxide and generalized reduction in respiratory function.

hypoxemia Lower than normal oxygen pressure in the arterial blood.

hypoxia Lower than normal oxygen pressure in the alveolus or at the tissue level resulting in an inadequate amount of oxygen available to the body cells to meet their metabolic needs.

hysteresis Can be thought of as a lagging of one of two associated phenomena; that is, two associated phenomena fail to coincide or occur simultaneously. An example of hysteresis is the difference between the inspiratory and expiratory curves in a pressure–volume loop for the lungs.

I

iatrogenic Caused by a medical procedure or treatment.

ileus An obstruction of the intestinal tract associated with immobility of the bowel or a mechanical blockage of the bowel.

incisura A small negative deflection on the pressure–time tracing present in the aortic and pulmonary artery pressure tracings; caused by the transient reversal of blood flow toward the heart during the last part of systole that pushes against the respective semilunar valve.

independent lung ventilation A form of mechanical ventilation.

indirect calorimetry Estimate of the caloric expenditure of the body by measurement of exhaled gas volumes and fractional concentrations of oxygen and carbon dioxide rather than direct heat production from the body.

inflammatory mediators Chemical substances produced by the body that are involved in the inflammatory response.

inflection point Occurs during deflation (also sometimes called the *deflection point*) and represents collapse of a significant number of lung units following full inflation (recruitment) of the lungs.

inspiratory positive airway pressure (IPAP) The application of positive pressure to the airway during inspiration. Compare *expiratory positive airway pressure*.

inspissated secretions Airway secretions that are thickened or hardened through the loss or evaporation of the liquid portion.

intermittent abdominal pressure ventilator (IAPV) A motorized inflatable bladder that fits over the abdomen and assists spontaneous breathing. The motor inflates the bladder, which in turn pushes the diaphragm upwards to facilitate exhalation. When the bladder deflates, the diaphragm returns to its resting position allowing for passive inhalation. See *pneumobelt*.

intermittent positive pressure breathing (IPPB) The application of positive pressure breaths to the upper airway on a periodic basis; used to provide short-term or intermittent mechanical ventilation for the purpose of augmenting lung expansion, delivering aerosol medication, or assisting ventilation.

intermittent positive pressure ventilation (IPPV) A general term for mechanical ventilation provided by positive pressure. The acronym *IPPV* can also be used to mean *invasive positive pressure ventilation* in which the patient has an endotracheal or tracheostomy tube in place to connect to the ventilator.

internal pneumatic circuit A series of gas-conducting tubes on the inside of a ventilator that direct the gas flow within the ventilator to the outside of the ventilator for delivery to the patient.

internal respiration The movement of O_2 and CO_2 between the cells and the blood.

international normalized ratio (PT/INR) Calculation made to standardize prothrombin time. INR depends on the ratio of the patient's prothrombin time and the normal mean prothrombin time. Prothrombin time shows how fast the blood clots in patients receiving oral anticoagulant medication.

intrinsic PEEP (PEEP$_I$) See *auto-PEEP*.

iron lung A negative pressure ventilator. Also called a *tank ventilator*, *artificial lung*, or *Drinker respirator*.

ischemia A reduction in the flow or supply of oxygenated blood to a body organ or area; may be accompanied by severe pain and organ dysfunction, e.g., cardiac ischemia when an adequate oxygenated blood flow to the heart is lacking.

isothermic saturation boundary The point in the airway where inspired air is warmed and humidified to 100% relative humidity at 37° C and contains 44 mg/L of water (absolute humidity). This point is approximately at the level of the fourth to fifth generation of subsegmental bronchi and varies with rate of gas flow, minute ventilation, and ambient air conditions.

K

ketoacidosis Acidosis accompanied by an increase in ketones; occurs primarily as a complication of diabetes mellitus.

kinetic therapy The use of automated rotating beds to reduce the incidence of ventilator-associated pneumonia (VAP), particularly in surgical patients or patients with neurologic problems.

L

late-onset pneumonia Pneumonia that develops later than 72 hours after exposure to a hospital or clinic setting.

limit variable The phase variable whose size is set at some predetermined maximum that cannot be exceeded during inspiration.

lower inflection point A point of significant change in the slope of a static pressure–volume curve at the beginning of lung inflation; indicate the pressure at which large numbers of alveoli are beginning to be recruited; sometimes called P_{FLEX}.

M

mandatory breaths Breaths for which the ventilator determines the start time (time triggered based on the set rate) or the volume (volume targeted) or pressure (pressure targeted) or both the start time **and** the tidal volume or pressure delivered.

mandatory minute ventilation (MMV) A closed-loop system in which the ventilator monitors set parameters and makes adjustments based on those parameters and the patient's spontaneous breathing efforts. The operator sets a minute ventilation ($\dot{V}_E$) lower than the patient's spontaneous $\dot{V}_E$. If monitored $\dot{V}_E$ falls below the minimum set $\dot{V}_E$, the ventilator increases support to the patient, and vice versa. Also called *minimum* $\dot{V}_E$.

mask pressure Term often used to describe the airway opening pressure.

mechanical dead space The amount of rebreathed volume in a ventilator circuit.

meconium aspiration syndrome The inhalation of meconium by the fetus or newborn, resulting in blockage of the airways, failure of the lungs to expand, potential pneumonia, and possible respiratory failure.

minute ventilation The volume of gas per minute inhaled or exhaled from a person's lungs. The calculation of minute ventilation is the product of rate and tidal volume.

miosis The constriction of the pupil of the eye to 2 mm or less.

mouth pressure (P_M) Pressure at the upper airway (mouth); also called airway opening pressure (P_{awo}), airway pressure (P_{aw}), upper airway pressure, mask pressure, or proximal airway pressure.

multidrug-resistant (MDR) microorganism A bacteria that resists distinct drugs or chemicals of a wide variety of structure and function targeted at eradicating the organism.

multiorgan failure Modified organ function in an acutely ill patient requiring medical treatment to achieve homeostasis.

multisystem organ failure (multiple organ dysfunction syndrome [MODS]) Severe pathologic failure occurring all at once of many organ systems, such as the lungs, gastrointestinal tract, liver, and heart; may accompany acute lung injury or acute respiratory distress syndrome.

N

negative end-expiratory pressure (NEEP) Negative pressure applied to the airway at the end of exhalation during mechanical ventilation.

neonate A newborn less than 4 weeks of age.

neural adjusted ventilator assist (NAVA) A mode of mechanical ventilation that provides respiratory assistance for the patient in comparison to and in synchrony with the patient's respiratory efforts.

nocturnal hypoventilation An elevated P_aCO_2 and accompanying fall in oxygen saturation that occurs in response to a progressive fall in minute ventilation occurring during sleep, most often in the REM stage.

nondepolarizing agent An agent that causes skeletal muscle paralysis by causing competitive inhibition of acetylcholine at the muscle receptor site.

noninvasive positive pressure ventilation (NIV) The delivery of positive pressure mechanical ventilation to the lungs without the use of an artificial airway.

nosocomial infection Infections in hospitals and other health care facilities.

O

obstructive sleep apnea (OSA) A condition characterized by episodes of breathing cessation during sleep. Relaxation of the muscles of the upper part of the throat during sleep causes the upper airway to close, blocking the upper airway (oropharynx) and preventing air from entering the lungs. This results in failure of air movement through the obstructed passage while breathing efforts persist. At least five episodes of apnea (lack of air movement) lasting 10 or more seconds are characteristic of OSA.

oliguria A diminished output of urine relative to fluid intake.

open-loop system A control scheme in which a variable is set and the operating system makes no comparisons between output and input signals and no changes to the designated variable; an "unintelligent" system; the opposite of a closed-loop system.

operational verification procedure (OVP) A checklist used to verify that the ventilator systems are fully functional and safe before use with a patient; sometimes a part of the respiratory therapy department's policy and procedure manual. The self-test performed by the ventilator may be part of the OVP.

overdistension See *overinflation* and *hyperinflation*.

overinflation When excessive pressure or volume delivery during mechanical ventilation causes too much stretching of lung parenchyma; overdistension or hyperinflation.

P

paralytic agent Drug used to facilitate invasive procedures (e.g., surgery, endotracheal intubation) and to prevent movement and ensure the stability of artificial airways. Paralysis may also be used to decrease mean airway pressure (P_{aw}) during uncoordinated or uncontrolled mechanical ventilation.

partial ventilatory support (PVS) Any amount of mechanical ventilation with ventilator rates that are less than those used with continuous mandatory ventilation (CMV), in which the patient is participating in the work of breathing to help maintain effective alveolar ventilation.

patent ductus arteriosus (PDA) An abnormal opening between the pulmonary artery and the aorta resulting when the ductus arteriosus does not close at birth.

patient circuit A series of gas-conducting tubes that conduct gas from the ventilator output connector to the patient and from the patient to the ventilator exhalation valve; also called the ventilator circuit.

patient triggering When inspiration begins due to the ventilator's sensing a change in pressure, flow, or volume due to a patient effort.

patient-ventilator asynchrony A situation in which the patient breathing pattern and ventilator breathing pattern are not harmonious.

patient-ventilator system check See *ventilator flow sheet*.

peak airway pressure The highest pressure achieved during inspiration on positive pressure ventilation; also called *peak pressure* and *peak inspiratory pressure*.

peak inspiratory pressure See *peak airway pressure*.

peak pressure See *peak airway pressure*.

pediatric An infant, child, and adolescent from birth to 21 years of age.

perivascular Pertaining to an area around a blood vessel.

permissive hypercapnia Higher than normal P_aCO_2 values resulting from ventilator strategies used to protect the lung from injury associated with the ventilator.

phase variable A signal that is measured and used by the ventilator to begin some part (phase) of the breathing cycle.

physiological shunt The total shunt fraction.

plateau pressure A pressure measurement taken during positive pressure ventilation after a breath has been delivered to the patient and before exhalation has begun. A condition of no flow exists, reflecting the pressure in the lungs and patient circuit.

pneumobelt A belt containing a bladder that inflates during exhalation to move the diaphragm upwards (cephalad) to assist exhalation. Inhalation is passive.

polymicrobial Infection by multiple pathogenic microorganisms.

polyneuritis Inflammation of many nerves at once or disseminated neuritis.

positive end-expiratory pressure (PEEP) Pressure above atmospheric, applied to the airway during exhalation, that increases the functional residual capacity.

preload The filling pressure of the ventricle at the end of ventricular diastole.

pressure control A mode of ventilation that is normally patient or time triggered, pressure targeted, and time cycled.

pressure cycling Inspiration ends when the ventilator measures a set pressure during inspiration.

pressure gradient A pressure difference between two points, one pressure being higher than the other.

pressure limit A set maximum pressure that cannot be exceeded.

pressure support A mode of ventilation that is normally patient triggered, pressure targeted, and flow cycled.

pressure-targeted ventilators Ventilators that provide multiple modes for presetting the maximum inflation pressure rather than a fixed tidal volume.

pressure triggering When a change in pressure starts gas flow from the ventilator to deliver inspiration.

problem An unwelcome or harmful matter requiring immediate attention that must be dealt with and overcome.

prone positioning Placing the body with the chest (ventral side) down and back (dorsal side) up.

prophylactic therapy Therapy aimed at defending against or preventing disease.

protected specimen brush (PBS) An invasive microbiologic procedure to culture lower respiratory secretions often necessary to ensure effective treatment of patients with ventilator-associated pneumonia (VAP).

proximal airway pressure Term used to indicate an estimate of the alveolar distending pressure.

pruritus Itching leading to the desire to scratch.

pulmonary angiogram A radiologic image of the pulmonary vasculature bed obtained by injecting an opaque contrast medium into the pulmonary circulation.

pulmonary artery catheter (PAC) A long, thin flow-directed tube with a balloon tip on the end (also known as Swan-Ganz) that allows it to flow into the right chamber of the heart.

pulmonary vascular resistance The afterload the right ventricle must overcome to eject blood into the pulmonary circulation.

pulse oximetry A technique that uses a sensor placed on a digit, an earlobe, the forehead, or the bridge of the nose to determine oxygen saturation and pulse rate. Pulse oximetry actually combines two physical techniques: (1) the spectrophotometric technique, which is used to determine a patient's percent arterial oxyhemoglobin, and (2) optical plethysmography, which is used to estimate the pulse rate.

pulse pressure The difference between the systolic and diastolic pressure.

pulsus paradoxus A systolic blood pressure that is more than 10 mm Hg lower during inspiration than during expiration.

Q

qualitative Measures the quality of something rather than its quantity.

quantitative Measures the quantity of something rather than its quality.

R

ramp A comfort feature incorporated in many noninvasive pressure-targeted ventilators that allows an incremental rise in set pressures over a set period of time; most often used in conjunction with the *delay time control*.

Ramsay "sedation" scale A graduated single-category scale that is used to assess the level of sedation in an individual receiving sedation.

recruitment maneuver Denotes activating an intentional transient increase in transpulmonary pressure to open unstable airless alveoli.

relative humidity The actual or absolute amount of humidity in a gas compared with its maximum carrying capacity at that temperature, calculated as a percent. Relative humidity (absolute)/ (maximum capacity) × 100.

rescue therapy A life-threatening event requiring nonsurgical treatment.

residual volume The volume of air in the lungs following a maximum exhalation.

resistance Frictional forces associated with ventilation due to the anatomical structure of the conductive airways and the resistance to gas flow through the airways, and the tissue viscous resistance of the lungs and adjacent tissues and organs as the lungs expand and contract.

respiration The movement of gas molecules across a membrane.

respiratory alternans Alternation between using the diaphragm to breath and the accessory muscles of respiration; an indication of end-stage respiratory muscle fatigue.

respirometer A device used to measure breathing variables such as tidal volume and vital capacity.

respite care Allowing caregivers of a ventilator-assisted individual to have an opportunity to rest and relax by providing another caregiver to care for the patient.

retrograde To direct or turn backward.

rocking bed A motorized bed that moves continuously in a longitudinal plane. Expiration is assisted when the head is in the down position and the abdominal contents and diaphragm are moved by gravity toward the thorax (cephalad).

S

scalar A way to specify the waveforms for pressure, flow, and volume that are graphed against time (e.g., pressure, flow, and volume scalars). The resulting waveform is referred to as a *scalar*.

sedative Used to reduce anxiety and agitation and to promote sleep and anterograde amnesia.

simethicone agents A nonprescription agent that reduces the surface tension of gas bubbles in stomach.

single-circuit ventilator A ventilator in which the internal pneumatic circuit allows the gas to go directly from its power source into the patient.

spontaneous breaths A breath or inspiratory gas flow that is started by the patient (patient triggered) and tidal volume delivery is determined by the patient (patient cycled). With spontaneous breaths, the amount of volume and/or pressure delivered is based on patient demand and not by a preselected amount set on a ventilator.

static compliance/static effective compliance Compliance measurement obtained during conditions of no gas flow. Compliance is equal to a volume change divided by a pressure change.

status asthmaticus A severe and prolonged asthma episode that is poorly responsive to adrenergic agents; associated with decreased airway diameter due to bronchospasm, increased mucous plugging, and inflammation of the airway. Signs and symptoms of potential respiratory failure may be present.

stroke index Stroke volume divided by body surface area.

stroke work Cardiac work; calculated by using mean blood pressure multiplied by the stroke volume multiplied by a correction factor.

superinfection An infection that develops during drug treatment for another infection, caused by a different microorganism that is resistant to the treatment used for the first infection.

Swan-Ganz catheter A multilumen, balloon-tipped, pulmonary artery catheter originally designed by Swan, Ganz, and colleagues.

systemic vascular resistance The afterload the left ventricle must overcome to eject blood into the aorta and systemic circulation.

T

tachycardia Heart rates in the adult greater than 100 beats/min.

threshold resistor A device that provides a constant pressure throughout expiration regardless of the rate of gas flow; used in the exhalation line of a ventilator. The exhaled air proceeds unimpeded through the resistor until pressure falls to a preset value (PEEP). At that time, the exhaled gas flow stops and the system pressure is maintained.

thrombolytic therapy Drug therapy directed at dissolving a clot, e.g., administration of streptokinase or urokinase to dissolve an arterial clot in a patient with an acute myocardial infarction resulting from clots in the coronary vessels.

thrombotic mediators Chemical substances produced by the body that cause an abnormal vascular condition, resulting in a clot developing inside a blood vessel in the body.

time constant The product of compliance (C) and resistance (R).

time cycling When the ventilator ends inspiration after measuring a specific time that has elapsed during the inspiratory phase.

time triggering The beginning of inspiration initiated by a ventilator when it detects that a certain period of time has elapsed. Time is commonly based on a rate or frequency control setting.

tracheoesophageal fistula A congenital malformation resulting in a tube-like opening between the trachea and esophagus.

tracheomalacia Erosion of the tracheal wall, often associated with excessive pressure from an endotracheal or tracheostomy tube cuff, which reduces effective blood flow through the tracheal wall resulting in injury to the tissue.

train-of-four monitoring An electrophysiological technique used to assess the effectiveness of neuromuscular blocking agents. An electrical current consisting of four impulses is applied to the peripheral nerve over 2 seconds, and the muscle contractions (twitches) produced provide information about the level of muscle paralysis.

transairway pressure The difference between airway pressure and alveolar pressure.

transcutaneous monitoring A noninvasive method of indirectly assessing ABGs. Unlike pulse oximetry and capnography, which rely on spectrophotometric analysis, transcutaneous monitoring uses modified blood gas electrodes to measure the oxygen and carbon dioxide tensions at the skin surface.

transpulmonary pressure The difference between alveolar pressure and pleural pressure.

transpyloric Across the pyloric region of the stomach.

transrespiratory pressure The difference between airway opening pressure and body surface pressure ($P_{TR} = P_{awo} - P_{bs}$).

transthoracic pressure The difference between alveolar pressure and body surface pressure; also called *trans-chest wall pressure*.

trigger variable The phase variable that begins inspiration.

tubing compliance (C_T) System compressibility; reflects the amount (in mL) of gas compressed in the ventilator circuit for every centimeter of water pressure generated by the ventilator during the inspiratory phase. (C_T = change in volume divided by change in pressure [$\Delta V/\Delta P$] in mL/cm H_2O).

U

upper airway pressure Term used to describe airway opening pressure.

upper inflection point A point of significant change in the upper slope of a static pressure–volume curve at the end of lung inflation near total lung capacity (TLC). The change indicates a point at which large numbers of alveoli are being overinflated.

user interface The dials, knobs, controls, and touch screen devices used by the ventilator operator to determine how the ventilator will function.

V

ventilation The movement of air into and out of the lungs.

ventilator-associated pneumonia (VAP) Pneumonia that develops 48 hours after a patient has been placed on mechanical ventilation.

ventilator flow sheet A regularly performed check of the patient-ventilator system, usually done by the respiratory therapy staff;

includes patient assessment data and monitored information, as well as ventilator parameters or parameter changes. Can be handwritten or computer based and is usually performed every 2 to 4 hours, unless an unusual event requires earlier checking.

vital capacity (VC) The total amount of air that can be exhaled after a maximum inspiration. The sum of the inspiratory reserve volume, the tidal volume (V_T), and the expiratory reserve volume.

volume cycled Inspiration ends when a preset volume is delivered to the patient.

volume limit A maximum volume that is set by the clinician that is set and cannot be exceeded.

volume triggering When the ventilator detects a small drop in volume in the patient circuit during the later part of exhalation and begins inspiration.

volutrauma A form of lung injury associated with excessive volume delivery by a ventilator resulting in tissue injury at the alveolar level.

W

weaning The process of discontinuing ventilation and liberating the patient from the ventilator.

Z

zero end-expiratory pressure (ZEEP) A baseline pressure of zero during the expiratory phase of mechanical ventilation.

Index

Page numbers followed by "*f*" indicate figures, "*t*" indicate tables, and "*b*" indicate boxes.